P9-DTG-230

Wound Care

A Collaborative Practice Manual for Health Professionals

FOURTH EDITION

Edited by

Carrie Sussman, PT, DPT

Owner and Operator

Sussman Physical Therapy, Inc.

Wound Care Management Services

Torrance, California

Barbara M. Bates-Jensen, PhD, RN, FAAN

Associate Professor

School of Nursing & David Geffen School of Medicine, Division of Geriatrics

University of California, Los Angeles

Los Angeles, California

Veterans Administration Greater Los Angeles Healthcare System

Geriatric Research Education Clinical Center

Los Angeles, California

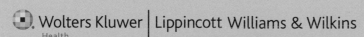
. Wolters Kluwer | Lippincott Williams & Wilkins
Health

Philadelphia • Baltimore • New York • London
Buenos Aires • Hong Kong • Sydney • Tokyo

Acquisitions Editor: Emily Lupash
Product Manager: Paula C. Williams
Marketing Manager: Allison Powell
Designer: Terry Mallon
Compositor: SPi Global

Fourth Edition

Copyright © 2012 Lippincott Williams & Wilkins, a Wolters Kluwer business

351 West Camden Street   Two Commerce Square
Baltimore, MD 21201   2001 Market Street
                        Philadelphia, PA 19103

Printed in China

All rights reserved. This book is protected by copyright. No part of this book may be reproduced or transmitted in any form or by any means, including as photocopies or scanned-in or other electronic copies, or utilized by any information storage and retrieval system without written permission from the copyright owner, except for brief quotations embodied in critical articles and reviews. Materials appearing in this book prepared by individuals as part of their official duties as U.S. government employees are not covered by the above-mentioned copyright. To request permission, please contact Lippincott Williams & Wilkins at Two Commerce Square, 2001 Market Street, Philadelphia, PA 19103, via email at permissions@lww.com, or via website at lww.com (products and services).

Library of Congress Cataloging-in-Publication Data
Wound care : a collaborative practice manual for health professionals / [edited by] Carrie Sussman, Barbara Bates-Jensen. — 4th ed.
    p. ; cm.
  Includes bibliographical references and index.
  ISBN 978-1-60831-715-8
  1. Wounds and injuries—Treatment. 2. Physical therapy. 3. Nursing. I. Sussman, Carrie. II. Bates-Jensen, Barbara M.
  [DNLM: 1. Wounds and Injuries—rehabilitation. 2. Physical Therapy Modalities. 3. Wounds and Injuries—diagnosis. 4. Wounds and Injuries—nursing. WO 700]
  RD93.W683 2011
  617.1—dc23

                                          2011027050

DISCLAIMER

Care has been taken to confirm the accuracy of the information present and to describe generally accepted practices. However, the authors, editors, and publisher are not responsible for errors or omissions or for any consequences from application of the information in this book and make no warranty, expressed or implied, with respect to the currency, completeness, or accuracy of the contents of the publication. Application of this information in a particular situation remains the professional responsibility of the practitioner; the clinical treatments described and recommended may not be considered absolute and universal recommendations.

The authors, editors, and publisher have exerted every effort to ensure that drug selection and dosage set forth in this text are in accordance with the current recommendations and practice at the time of publication. However, in view of ongoing research, changes in government regulations, and the constant flow of information relating to drug therapy and drug reactions, the reader is urged to check the package insert for each drug for any change in indications and dosage and for added warnings and precautions. This is particularly important when the recommended agent is a new or infrequently employed drug.

Some drugs and medical devices presented in this publication have Food and Drug Administration (FDA) clearance for limited use in restricted research settings. It is the responsibility of the health care provider to ascertain the FDA status of each drug or device planned for use in their clinical practice.

To purchase additional copies of this book, call our customer service department at (800) 638-3030 or fax orders to (301) 223-2320. International customers should call (301) 223-2300.

Visit Lippincott Williams & Wilkins on the Internet: http://www.lww.com. Lippincott Williams & Wilkins customer service representatives are available from 8:30 am to 6:00 pm, EST.

9 8 7 6 5 4 3 2 1

CCS0811

To the Global Community of
Health Professionals and Patients
who have shared their knowledge
with us and made this book possible.

FOREWORD

Clinicians around the world continue to strive to provide uncompromised excellence in the delivery of evidenced-based wound care. With the explosion of knowledge and multiple media sources (internet, etc.), clinicians struggle to decipher "real" information from simple sham. There remain few references that provide current information that can guide the clinician in providing appropriate evidenced-based wound care. Lucky for us, the 4th edition of *Wound Care: A Collaborative Practice Manual for Health Professionals* fills this very important gap.

The 4th edition has been expanded to 30 chapters. These chapters are logically divided into four sections: Introduction to Wound Care Diagnosis; Management of Wound Etiology; Management of Wound Characteristics; and Management of Wound Healing with Biophysical Agents. As the sections note, it forces both novice and experienced clinicians to not only consider the wound type, but more importantly it guides the clinicians to consider the multidimensionality of providing relevant wound care. This physiological-environmental-societal approach allows the clinician to not only manage the wound, but to consider the wound in the context of the whole patient and their caregivers. Simply said, the clinician can't manage a wound successfully without the context of managing all aspects of the patient's environment. What also makes this edition a keepsake is the addition of two new chapters on burns and the wise use of hyperbaric oxygen.

The book chapter authors are all global leaders in wound management. This is a unique strength of the 4th edition. Given the multiple disciplines, contributing their expertise to numerous book chapters clearly underscores the multidisciplinary as well as interdisciplinary nature of providing relevant wound care in the 21st century. All book chapters have been significantly updated with a brand new format. Moreover, each book chapter provides ample case studies and examples to translate the didactic content to practice. This translational approach is critical to ensure that the clinicians after reading each book chapter actually "get it". Another major strength of the 4th edition is the wise use of tables that can be readily used as practice tools in the practice arena.

As new knowledge in the management of wound care is developed, this will remain the "go to" textbook to synthesize and codify that knowledge so it is relevant to clinicians. I am confident that there are few wound care textbooks that can provide such relevant evidenced-based information to the novice as well as the expert wound care clinician. In this regard, the 4th edition remains in the vanguard.

Respectfully,
Courtney H. Lyder, ND, GNP, FAAN
Dean and Assistant Director, UCLA Health System
Professor of Nursing, Medicine and Public Health
Executive Director, Patient Safety Institute
University of California, Los Angeles School of Nursing

PREFACE

When the first edition of *Wound Care: A Collaborative Practice Manual for Physical Therapists and Nurses* was published in 1998, you told us about the importance that this work has for you. That has fueled our efforts to keep the book current. The book has grown from 20 chapters and 481 pages to its current size with 30 chapters. New chapters have been added to each edition and former chapters updated as you have asked for more information and topics. Our readership now includes a multidisciplinary global audience so our name changed with the third edition to *Wound Care: A Collaborative Practice Manual for Health Professionals*. We are grateful for your loyalty and to the loyalty of our valued contributors, most of whom have remained aboard for each new edition. Along the way, new contributors have joined the team to share their expertise and knowledge with us. In this, the fourth edition, we have made many changes that are highlighted below.

A NEW LOOK FOR THE FOURTH EDITION

The fourth edition of *Wound Care: A Collaborative Practice Manual for Health Professionals* is really a new book with a new look. In response to requests by many of our readers, we are now four color throughout. The hierarchy of information is color coded for ease in determining levels of information presented. See Exhibit P.1 for a key to the hierarchy of information levels and associated box color coding. You may notice a theme. All special information color bars begin with gold, something to put into the bank. We would like to thank the talented art team at Lippincott Williams & Wilkins for their user-friendly design, use of color, and execution. We look forward to hearing your reactions.

Photographs sometimes appear in more than one chapter as teaching tools for different subjects. One of our learning objectives is to teach the observer to look at many aspects of a wound for different purposes, and flipping back and forth between chapters to look at a photograph breaks up the learning experience at inopportune times. Color photographs of wounds are utilized as much as possible to bring reality to the learning situation.

Like in previous editions, cross-referencing of materials is done. When information occurs in detail in another chapter, the reader is referred to the appropriate chapter to find that information. Our intention is to avoid redundancy and to integrate the information between chapters wherever and whenever possible.

NEW FEATURES OF THE FOURTH EDITION

In response to requests from our audience of readers and educators, we implemented a number of changes. Two new chapters have been added to the fourth edition: Chapter 15 Management of Burns and Chapter 30 Hyperbaric Oxygen. The vascular ulcer and pressure ulcer chapters are entirely new. All chapters have been reviewed, edited, and updated to reflect current information and evidence about medical science and wound management practice since the third edition. Information organization has been revised into a more logical sequence to meet another objective, which is to facilitate the learning process by being concise and cohesive in presentation.

We have omitted the appendix of wound dressing products because they represent a market in constant flux and other sources are better ways to locate sources and products. Chapter 20, Management of the Wound Environment with Dressings and Topical Agents, provides information and guidelines about product classes to guide you in your clinical decision making about dressing and topical agent products.

ASSEMBLING A WORLD-CLASS INTERDISCIPLINARY TEAM

From the beginning of the development of the Wound Care textbook we, the editors, have recognized the value of an interdisciplinary, collaborative message. We have chosen contributors whose expertise reflects that of the real world of wound caring. Five world-class experts in wound management have joined our list of returning outstanding contributors. We are honored to have all of them aboard.

Collaboration and use of interdisciplinary talent is evident throughout the book with multiple coauthored chapters. A further objective of Wound Care is to encourage collaborative, interdisciplinary practice across all borders and continents. We recognize our expanding global impact and and the important contribution of our multinational contributors and sources such as those found in our resource and reference materials.

ORGANIZATION OF THE FOURTH EDITION

The sections of the fourth edition have been reorganized and rearranged for more logical flow. As in prior editions, we have retained the same four divisions or parts but have rearranged them so that wound etiology comes before wound characteristics for more logical exposition.

EXHIBIT P.1

Hierarchy of Chapter Information Levels with Key to Color Coding in Text

Level of Information	Color Code
Main Section	Fuchsia
First Level Subsection	Blue
Second Level Subsection	Green
Third Level Subsection	Orange
Tables	Orange and Burgundy
Review Questions	Green and Blue
Clinical Wisdoms	Gold/Green
Research Wisdoms	Gold/Purple
Case Studies	Gold/Orange
Exhibits	Gold/Fuchsia

Part I Introduction to Wound Care Diagnosis

Part I, Introduction to Wound Care Diagnosis, Chapters 1 to 7, presents information on assessment, evaluation, diagnosis, and prognosis skills. Together these chapters provide a foundation for clinicians caring for the patient with a wound. Wound photographs, procedures, flow diagrams, assessment and screening forms, case studies, and referral criteria are provided to enable clinicians easy access to necessary tools for practice. Chapter 1 begins with The Wound Care Process followed by Chapter 2, Skin and Soft Tissue Anatomy and Wound Healing Physiology. Chapter 3 focuses on Assessment of the Patient, Skin, and Wound. In Chapter 5, several tools for evaluating and predicting wound healing are presented. This chapter includes the assessment tools in appendices. Chapters about vascular assessment and assessment and management of nutritional status complete Part I.

Part II Management by Wound Etiology

Part II, Management by Wound Etiology, Chapters 8 to 16, provides chapters on the physiology and pathophysiology associated with different wound etiologies. This section begins with Chapter 8 on management of the acute surgical wounds. The newly revised Chapter 9 presents information on the pathophysiology, detection, and prevention of pressure ulcers and is followed by Chapter 10 on Management and prevention of pressure ulcers with therapeutic positioning. Chapter 11 is our entirely new chapter on diagnosis and management of vascular ulcers. We follow with diagnosis and management of the neuropathic foot and other common foot problems in Chapters 12 and 13. The final three chapters in this section deal with difficult wound situations: malignant wounds and fistulas, a new chapter devoted to burns, and scar management. Each chapter includes photographs and case studies that illustrate issues related to wounds specific to that etiology.

Part III Management by Wound Characteristics

Part III, Management by Wound Characteristics, Chapters 17 to 22, consists of chapters that outline the steps required to prepare the wound for healing. These chapters include specific details and photographs showing signs and symptoms of each characteristic along with narrative text explaining the significance of each characteristics. Chapters include step-by-step procedures for specific tests, treatments, and interventions. Case studies, self-care teaching guidelines, and referral criteria facilitate management of specific wound characteristics for clinicians. Chapter 17 begins the section with discussion on Management of Necrotic Tissue, followed by Chapter 18 Management of Exudate and Infection, and Chapter 19 Management of Edema. The next two chapters in this section provide information on topical treatment of wounds and include Chapter 20 Management of the Wound Environment with Dressings and Topical Agents followed by Chapter 21 Management of the Wound with Advanced Therapies. The final chapter in Part III is Management of Wound Pain including the neuroanatomy, physiology, pathogenesis of pain and current pharmocologic and non pharmocologic interventions.

Part IV Management of Wound Healing with Biophysical Agents

Part IV, Management of Wound Healing with Biophysical Agents, Chapters 23 to 30, looks at eight exogenous and endogenous biophysical energy sources, their applied physiology, and efficacy on aspects of as well as complete wound healing. The introduction, longer than that of other sections, is there to help you understand the relationships between the energies, how to choose between them, and how to value their addition to wound therapy. All chapters have been updated. Updated evidence tables are a special feature found in most of the chapters for quick review. The first three chapters concern energies derived from the electromagnetic spectrum. The beginning chapter is electrical stimulation, followed by pulsed radio frequency and pulsed electromagnetic fields, variants of electrotherapy, and phototherapy (ultraviolet and laser). The rest of the chapters presents use of other physical properties like mechanical energy to promote biophysical cellular and tissue responses. These chapters include ultrasound (high and low frequency, therapeutic and diagnostic), hydrotherapy (and heat), pulsed lavage with suction (negative pressure), and negative wound pressure therapy. We end our final section with a new chapter on hyperbaric oxygen therapy.

OUR AUDIENCE

Our audience has identified themselves as both seasoned and novice wound clinicians from many health-care disciplines in addition to researchers, industry representatives, and academicians who select our textbook for their students in various health-care fields to teach wound management skills. Over the four editions, our audience has grown and expanded globally, reaching more people in countries around the world. We are gratified by your acceptance of our work and that of our collaborators. We appreciate the opportunities you have given us to help you and your patients heal.

MAKING A DIFFERENCE: A VISION

As we work with you to improve wound care for patients and clinicians globally, we want you to know that a portion of all proceeds from the Wound Care book will be donated to the UCLA Bates-Jensen Wound REACH Foundation (http://www.ouchrace.com or http://nursing.ulca.edu/ouchrace) whose vision is "Raising Money for Wound REACH, Research, Education, And Clinical Health: Improving Wound Care Globally". The UCLA Bates-Jensen Wound REACH Foundation raises funds to improve Wound Research Education And Clinical Health here in the United States and around the world by conducting charity race events, the OUCH! Races. Proceeds from the events go to support local improvement in wound care through education and research and to support development of sustainable wound clinics in resource-poor countries through education and clinical care. We think the vision of the foundation is closely aligned to our vision for this 4th edition of *Wound Care: A Collaborative Practice Manual for Health Professionals,* and we hope you agree.

ADDITIONAL RESOURCES

Wound Care: A Collaborative Practice Manual for Health Professionals includes additional resources for both instructors and students that are available on the book's companion Web site at http://thePoint.lww.com/Sussman4e

Instructor Resources

Approved adopting instructors will be given access to the following additional resources:

- Case Studies
- Image Bank
- Test Bank
- Answers to Chapter Review Questions

Student Resources

Students who have purchased *Wound Care: A Collaborative Practice Manual for Health Professionals* have access to the following additional resources:

- Case Studies

In addition, purchasers of the text can access the searchable full text on-line by going to the *Wound Care: A Collaborative Practice Manual for Health Professionals* Web site at http://thePoint.lww.com/Sussman4e

See the inside front cover of this text for more details, including the passcode you will need to gain access to the Web site.

Thank you.

Carrie Sussman
Barbara M. Bates-Jensen

CONTRIBUTORS

Karen Wientjes Albaugh, PT, DPT, MPH, CWS
Assistant Professor
Neumann University
Aston, Pennsylvania
Clinical Specialist
Optimum Physical Therapy Assoc.
West Chester, Pennsylvania

Barbara M. Bates-Jensen PhD, RN, FAAN
Associate Professor
School of Nursing and David Geffen School of Medicine,
Division of Geriatrics
University of California, Los Angeles
Associate Director
UCLA/Jewish Home for Aging Borun Center for Gerontological
Research
Los Angeles, California
National Associate Director
Research and Implementation for Pressure Ulcers
Veterans Administration Spinal Cord Injury QUERI
Chicago, Illinois
Veterans Administration Greater Los Angeles Healthcare System
Geriatric Research Education Clinical Center
Los Angeles, California

Autumn Bell, PT, CWS, CLT
Adjunct Professor
Winston-Salem State University
Waxhaw, North Carolina

Martin Borhani, MD
Chief, Division of Vascular Surgery
Associate Professor, Clinical Surgery
University of Illinois at Chicago
University of Illinois Medical Center at Chicago
Chicago, Illinois

Joan Conlan, CPed
Owner (Thera-ped)
Siskiyou Medical Group
Mt. Shasta, California

Teresa Conner-Kerr, PT, PhD, CWS, CLT
Chair and Professor
Physical Therapy, School of Health Sciences
Winston-Salem State University
Winston-Salem, North Carolina

Mary Dyson, PhD, LDH (Hon), FAIUM (Hon), FSCP (Hon), CBiol, MIBiol
Centre for Cardiovascular Biology and Medicine
Guy's Hospital Campus, Kings College
University of London
England, United Kingdom

Nancy Elftman, CO, CPed
Owner
Hands on Foot
La Verne, California

William J. Ennis, DO, MBA
Professor of Clinical Surgery
Wound Healing Tissue Repair
University of Illinois at Chicago
Chief Section Wound Healing
Wound Healing Tissue Repair
University of Illinois at Chicago Medical Center
Chicago, Illinois

Evonne Fowler, RN, CNS, CWON
Wound/Ostomy/Skin Care Specialist
San Gorgonio Medical Center
Banning, California

Allen Gabriel
Assistant Professor
Plastic Surgery
Loma Linda, California
Chief of Plastic Surgery
Southwest Washington Medical Center
Vancouver, Washington

Mark S. Granick, MD
Professor & Chief of Plastic Surgery
New Jersey Medical School
The University Hospital
Newark, New Jersey

Subhas C. Gupta, MD, PhD, FRCS (C)
Chairman, Department of Plastic Surgery
Loma Linda University Medical Center
Loma Linda, California

Teresa Kelechi, PhD, GCNS-BC, CWCN
College of Nursing
Medical University of South Carolina
Charleston, South Carolina

Harriett B. Loehne, PT, DPT, CWS, FACCWS
Clinical Educator
Department of Wound Management & Hyperbaric Medicine
Archbold Medical Center
Thomasville, Georgia

Courtney H. Lyder, ND, GNP, FAAN
Dean and Assistant Director
UCLA Health System
Professor of Nursing, Medicine and Public Health
Executive Director, Patient Safety Institute,
University of California, Los Angeles School of Nursing
Los Angeles, California

Patricio Meneses, PhD
Research Director
Wound Care Program
St. James Hospital
Olympia Fields, Illinois

Jeffrey A. Niezgoda, MD, FACHM, MAPWCA
Medical Director
The Center for Comprehensive Wound Care & Hyperbaric
Oxygen Therapy
St. Luke's Medical Center/Aurora Health Care
Milwaukee, Wisconsin

Liza Ovington, PhD, CWS
Medical Director
Ethicon Inc. (Johnson & Johnson)
Allentown, Pennsylvania

Craig Pastor, MD
Resident
Plastic Surgery
New Jersey Medical School
Newark, New Jersey

Gregory K. Patterson, MD
South Georgia Surgical Associates
Thomasville, Georgia

Mary Ellen Posthauer, RD, CD, LD
President
M.E.P. Healthcare Dietary Services, Inc.
Evansville, Indiana

Laurie M. Rappl, PT, DPT, CWS
Clinical Development Liason
Cytomedix, Inc.
Simpsonville, South Carolina

Gregory Scott Schultz, PhD
UF Research Foundation Professor
Department of Obstetrics & Gynecology
University of Florida
Gainesville, Florida

Susie Seaman, CFNP, MSN, CWOCN
Nurse Practitioner
Wound Clinic
Sharp Rees-Stealy Medical Group
San Diego, California

Thomas E. Serena, MD, FACS, MAPWCA, FACHM
The Serena Group
Warren, Pennsylvania

Geoffrey Sussman, OAM FPS, FAIPM, FACP, FAWA
Associate Professor
Monash University Australia,
Victoria, Australia
Auckland University, New Zealand
Visiting Consultant
Austin Hospital
Melbourne, Australia

Nancy Tomaselli, RN, MSN, CS, CRNP, CWOCN, LNC
President & CEO
Premier Health Solutions, LLC
Cherry Hill, New Jersey

Terry Treadwell, MD, FACS
Medical Director
Institute for Advanced Wound Care
Baptist Medical Center South
Montgomery, Alabama

Matthew J. Trovato, MD
Plastic Surgery Resident
Division of Plastic Surgery
Department of Surgery
University of Medicine and Dentistry of New Jersey
New Jersey Medical School
Newark, New Jersey

R. Scott Ward, PT, PhD
Professor and Chair
Department of Physical Therapy
University of Utah
Staff
University of Utah Burn Center
Salt Lake City, Utah

John E. T. Williams, RN, MSN
Staff Nurse
Department of Oncology
New York-Presbyterian/Weill Cornell Medical Center
New York, New York

REVIEWERS

Simone Bollaerts, BN, IWCC
Professor of Nursing
Mohawk College of Applied Arts and Technology
Hamilton, Ontario, Canada

Gail Bursch, MSEd—PT
Director of Clinical Education
Belmont University
Nashville, Tennessee

Michael Chiacchiero, DPT
Assistant Professor, Physical Therapy
College of Staten Island
Staten Island, New York

Mary Dockter, PhD, Med
Head of Physical Therapy Program
University of Mary
Bismark, North Dakota

Martha Henao Bloyer, MSPT
Director of Clinical Education
Florida International University
Miami, Florida

Susan Lowe, BSPT, MS Exercise Physiology, DPT, GCS
Associate Clinical Professor
Northeastern University
Boston, Massachusetts

Janelle K. O'Connell, PhD, PT, DPT
Professor and Department Head
Hardin-Simmons University
Abilene, Texas

Rose Ortega, BSPT, MS in Health Science Education, Post-Professional DPT
Physical Therapy, Clinical Assistant Professor
Stony Brook University
Stony Brook, New York

Clare E. Safran-Norton, PhD, MS, OCS, BSPT
Assistant Professor
Simmons College
Boston, Massachusetts

Mary Walden, MSN, CWOCN
Instructor
Itawamba Community College
Fulton, Mississippi

APPRECIATIONS AND ACKNOWLEDGMENTS

No book is ever written without the support, cooperation, and empathy of others. *Wound Care: A Collaborative Practice Manual for Health Professionals* is no exception. Each edition of Wound Care has grown up upon the structure of prior editions. Therefore, we would like to acknowledge our appreciation to the many individuals who share in the achievements of Wound Care since the first edition, published in 1998. We are very grateful to each one of you who has sustained and built relationships with us and the book including

Paula Williams, Laura M. Bonazzoli, Jennifer Clements, Emily Lupash, and Chitra Subramaniam, and those whose names are unknown at Lippincott Williams & Wilkins/Wolters Kluwer of the United States and India who have contributed their professional publishing skills toward making our writing, the art, illustrations, and the color design into a superb fourth edition.

Our phenomenal, extraordinary contributors, ranging from world experts to graduate students, who have given unstintingly of their time, knowledge, research, photos, tables, and illustrations and above all their commitment to sharing and teaching to make this book into a global success.

Generous authors, publishers, companies, and colleagues who have allowed us to publish their information, photographs, and tables to illustrate the text.

The University of California, Los Angeles, Biomedical library resources and the reference staff of Western University of Health Science Pomerantz Library who have been quick to respond to requests for journal articles delivering them promptly via e-mail for the last two editions, thus making it possible to incorporate new information as required.

We have been blessed with phenomenal support persons for each edition. For this edition, a good friend, physical therapist associate and wound care specialist, Anne Myers, PT, DPT, GCW, CWS, joined the team to help put this book together. She has reviewed chapters and labored for these many months with the many not so small details associated with preparation of the manuscript and the publication. Kyelynn Chiong and Deborah Johnsen were helpful and diligent with organization and final details.

This review of appreciation would not be complete without recognizing the contribution of our families and friends who have been there the whole time encouraging, making allowances for tight schedules and temperaments and often making meals. To our husbands and children, who have offered every support possible: Robert Sussman, of blessed memory, Cliff Sussman and Audrey Sussman Cloven, and Ron Jensen, and Holly and Thomas Jensen, who have grown up along with the book, thank you for helping us sweat the big and small stuff for so long and without whom this fourth edition would not have become a reality.

Carrie Sussman
Barbara M. Bates-Jensen

CONTENTS

PART FOUR:
Management of Wound Healing with Biophysical Agent Technologies   **573**

Introduction to Wound Care

Carrie Sussman

A diagnostic process is used to direct and guide treatment of wounds and allows health professionals to apply their skills and knowledge to the appropriate treatment of client situations that they can and should treat legally and independently. Recognizing its value, health professionals, besides physicians, have developed expertise in the role of diagnostician and have been integrating diagnosis into their practice for many years. But because the incorporation of diagnosis into the allied health care professions is still in its infancy, many find the role of diagnostician unfamiliar. These clinicians may lack both understanding of and practical experience in the process of diagnosis. For these clinicians, a number of questions need to be answered:

- What does a diagnosis really mean?
- What kind of information needs to be collected to yield a diagnosis?
- How are diagnoses differentiated from one another?
- How is a diagnosis tailored to a patient's functional problem or human response to health or illness?
- How does diagnosis relate to prognosis and outcomes?
- How does the wound diagnosis direct interventions?
- Advanced clinicians who are familiar with classification systems and diagnostic methods will have additional questions:
- Can and should the medical diagnosis be part of the clinical functional diagnostic statement?
- What kind of functional diagnostic statement should be written for a person at risk for wounds?
- What is the difference between diagnosis and classification?

Part I begins with an introduction to the diagnostic process and provides an overview of the whole wound care process. It seeks to answer these questions and provide specific information about wound diagnosis. Guidelines for writing functional diagnoses that are meaningful and related to the prognosis and treatment interventions are included and apply across health-care disciplines.

Whereas physicians and podiatrists focus on etiology-based diagnosis, nurses and physical therapists use similar taxonomy. The nursing process includes a standardized language or taxonomy. Nurses have taxonomy for impaired tissue integrity, impaired skin integrity, and ineffective peripheral tissue perfusion. Further, nursing's role includes the promotion of health as well as activities to contribute to adjustment to or recovery from illness. Thus, nurses can focus on prevention and health promotion activities. The nursing process is used as a problem solving approach to provide nursing care to individuals, communities, and populations.[1] Physical therapists use disablement terminology, including the terms *impairment*, *disability*, and *handicap* in their management model.[2]

In addition, both nurses and physical therapists incorporate functional impairment and disability into the diagnostic process. For example, a nurse determines the client's response to health or illness as positive functioning, altered functioning, or at risk for altered functioning.[1] Notice that nurses can use a diagnosis that incorporates risk, which could work equally well for a physical therapist. Moreover, nursing diagnoses specifically identify collaborative problems that the health-care clinical team needs for joint management. The most appropriate joint manager for wounds may be the dietitian, the nurse, the physician, the physical therapist, or the podiatrist. Functional diagnosis requires an understanding of functional impairment, which differs from the pathogenesis or etiology of the problem. Instead, a *functional impairment* is a system or organ impairment that prevents normal functioning.[3] It describes a functional change as physiologic, anatomic, structural, or functional at the tissue, organ, or body system level.[4] In impaired wound healing, a functional impairment occurs at one of these three levels in the body.

Chapter 2 describes skin and deep tissue anatomy, acute wound healing physiology, and chronic wound healing factors. Chapter 3 considers the whole patient which incorporates intrinsic, extrinsic, and iatrogenic factors that can influence wound healing. Next, Chapter 3 along with Chapters 4 to 7 teaches assessment, examinations, tests, and measurements that are an integral part of establishing a diagnosis. The same chapters describe methods and procedures for collecting information and interpreting the findings.

By the time they finish Part I, clinicians will understand skin and soft tissue anatomy, acute and chronic wound healing physiology, patient health- and care-related factors that affect wound healing. They will be able to perform the required tests and measurements necessary to determine a functional wound diagnosis, develop a prognosis, select appropriate interventions, and document the diagnostic process and findings with a functional outcomes report. In Parts II, III, and IV, clinicians will learn the management skills and appropriate interventions required for different wound-related problems.

References

1. Doenges ME, Moorhouse MF, Murr AC. *Nursing Diagnosis Manual: Planning, Individualizing, and Documenting Client Care*. Philadelphia, PA: F.A. Davis Company; 2005.
2. American Physical Therapy Association. A guide to physical therapy practice, I: a description of patient management. *Phys Ther*. 1995;75:707–764.
3. Jette AM. Physical disablement concepts for physical therapy research and practice. *Phys Ther*. 1994;74:380–386.
4. World Health Organization. *International Classification of Functioning, Disability and Health*. Geneva, Switzerland: World Health Organization; 2001.

1

The Wound Care Process

Carrie Sussman and Barbara M. Bates-Jensen

CHAPTER OBJECTIVES

At the completion of this chapter, the reader will be able to:

1. Describe each step in the wound care process.
2. Identify key data to collect during assessment.
3. Differentiate between behavioral and functional outcomes.
4. Explain the importance of determining prognosis.
5. Describe the process of evaluation using outcomes.

This chapter describes the process used for management of patients with acute and chronic wounds. Although their descriptive terminology may differ slightly, health-care practitioners employ essentially the same decision-making process in managing patient problems: assessment, diagnosis, goals, interventions, and evaluation. To simplify terminology and guide health-care practitioners, this textbook presents the wound care process in four steps, each with two or three parts:

a. Assessment—includes review of the reason for referral, collection of patient history, systems review/physical assessment, and wound assessment
b. Diagnosis—includes examination strategy, evaluation, and diagnosis
c. Goals—includes prognosis, establishment of goals and outcomes, and evaluation of progress
d. Intervention—described in subsequent chapters

Examinations and specific measurements, as well as special test procedures, are found in Chapters 3 and 7, as well as in other chapters. We present the wound care process as appropriate for all health-care practitioners who manage patients with wounds; however, throughout this chapter, we also present information that is specific to nursing and physical therapy.

STEP 1: ASSESSMENT

The assessment process assists in clinical decision making by preventing undirected care and inappropriate treatment. Clinicians perform a thorough assessment for all patients before determining the need for special examinations and interventions. This process begins when the patient is admitted to the agency or when referred for services.

Assessment involves gathering data from the patient history and physical examination. The patient history determines which relevant system reviews should be included in the physical examination. The history and systems review determine whether the patient is a candidate for services and the direction of the treatment plan. For nurses, the assessment process provides the framework for planning comprehensive wound care and for making referrals for physical therapy or other services. For all providers, proper *utilization management* is mandatory in today's health-care environment. Utilization management, which is part of the process of prospective management, is designed to ensure that only medically necessary, reasonable, and appropriate services are provided.[1] The interdisciplinary nature inherent in caring for a patient with a wound requires clinicians to carefully determine candidacy for services before initiating referral or treatment. For example, many practitioners believe that a referral to physical therapy automatically confers candidacy for wound care; however, not all patients are appropriately referred. The physical therapist needs to review the case, make the appropriate assessments, and determine candidacy and then advise the referring provider of recommendations. Many patients with a wound have comorbidities and coimpairments. For such patients, collaborative interdisciplinary management is critical to prevent iatrogenic effects caused by inappropriate selection of interventions or handling of a wound and to reduce extrinsic and intrinsic complications (see Chapter 3).

Standardized forms are the best tools for collecting assessment data quickly and efficiently, thus ensuring that important information is not lost. When both the clinician and the patient complete assessment forms, data from the interview is more likely to be maintained. In addition, engaging the patient in his or her own care from the beginning promotes mutually satisfactory outcomes. Although clinicians will find important information in the patient's medical record, the patient (or a significant other or caregiver) can often provide additional insights and information not otherwise available. A self-administered patient history form helps the clinician focus on the interview and saves time. Samples of a self-administered patient history form and a focused assessment form for physical therapists and nurses are presented in Appendices 1A and 1B.

Review of Admission/Referral

The referral is the first step in documenting the patient history. But what is the referral process? The initial referral for wound care management is usually made to a nurse; if the nurse determines the need for physical therapy or other services, these health-care practitioners are brought into the team. In order to refer appropriately, nurses need to understand the expectations of and projected outcomes from physical therapy and other health professionals. In some health-care settings, a wound care team decides which services are necessary for wound management and makes the appropriate referrals.

It is essential for a physical therapist or other health-care professional to know the reason a patient was referred. Typically, patients referred to a physical therapist for wound healing have not shown signs of normal wound repair. Most often, other treatment interventions are in use or have been attempted with limited or no success. Patients may be referred to occupational therapy for environmental adjustments related to their wound or to an orthotist for management of off-loading and positioning. Clinicians often make a referral to other health-care practitioners in an attempt to optimize wound repair. However, referrals can be made for reasons beyond improved wound healing. For example, a patient may be referred for help in cleaning and debriding a necrotic wound, for enhancement of the inflammatory process, to reinitiate wound repair, to decrease bacterial burden or palliative care. For the patient who presents with factors that impair wound healing, the reason for referral is to achieve a clean, stable wound that can be managed effectively by the nurse or caregiver at home. In other cases, pain management can be the reason for referral, and physical agents and/or electrotherapeutic modalities prescribed.

In addition to understanding the reason for the referral, health-care practitioners should understand the expected outcome. Wound closure may not be the highest priority. Of course, the selected intervention must match the expected outcomes to meet the referral objectives. For example, a patient with a foot ulcer secondary to pressure and insensitivity is fearful of amputation and loss of ability to walk. The patient's main concern is limb salvage, and expectations are high. In contrast, the family of a debilitated long-term care patient may desire only comfort for their family member, with no expectations of wound closure. Note that family and caregiver perceptions of various interventions may differ from the clinician's view. For example, a family member may perceive physical therapy as a heroic and painful measure, whereas a clinician may consider it a normal procedure. The nurse or physician must address these issues before making referrals.

Patient History

Patient history information is commonly collected in three ways:

- By interviewing the patient, family, significant others, and/or caregivers
- By consulting with other health-care practitioners
- By reviewing the medical record

CLINICAL WISDOM

Patient History Data Needed to Determine Care Direction

- Reason for admission or referral
- Expectations and perceptions about wound healing
- Psychosocial-cultural-economic history
- Present medical comorbidities
- Current wound status

Ideally, in the continuum of care, the patient's historical information is transmitted via the patient's paper or electronic medical record, but this is not always the case. You may need to piece together the history from the other sources named above. If only a limited amount of medical and social information is collected, then you will need to choose diagnostic options based on that limited data. Obviously, it is more effective to plan appropriate care with a complete history.

Remember that one of the primary goals of the patient interview is to begin to develop a therapeutic relationship with the patient and family. History taking allows you to assess and diagnose patient problems and to place the problems within the context of the individual patient's life. Important skills you will use during the patient history include listening, observing, and asking questions. Here, we discuss the five components of a thorough patient history: the chief complaint and health history, the sociologic history, the psychological history, the cultural history, and the nutritional history.

Chief Complaint and Health History

The chief complaint and health history includes a full description of the patient's chief complaint, including symptoms; a review of the patient's past history; current health information; and data about the health of family members.

Chief Complaint

Begin the patient history by determining the patient's chief complaint or major reason for seeking care, as well as the duration of the problem. Why is the patient seeking help at this time? The reason may be as simple as convenience or as complicated as a wound problem that has worsened. Investigate motivations the patient may have beyond the obvious problem by asking a question such as, "How did you hope that I could help you today?"

Explore the meaning of the wound to the patient. Questions such as, "What do you think caused your wound?" "Why do you think it started when it did?" and "How long do you think the wound will last?" can reveal the patient's level of understanding of the health problem. Based on their answers, you can develop a plan of care that is sensitive to the patient's needs and level of understanding.

Seek a complete understanding of the patient's symptoms, that is, the subjective feelings of the patient, during the interview. Prompt the patient to include seven criteria in describing his or her symptoms:

1. Location
2. Character

CLINICAL WISDOM

Questions to Elicit Extent of Wound Symptoms

1. *Location:* Where do you feel the wound? Do you feel it anywhere else? Show me where it hurts.
2. *Character:* What does it feel like?
3. *Pain Severity:* On a scale of 0 to 10, with 10 being the worst pain you could imagine, how would you rate the discomfort you have now? How does the wound interfere with your usual activities? How bad is it?
4. *Emotional Feelings:* On a scale of 0 to 10 with 10 being agonizing, how distressed do you feel about having this wound? Has it changed how you feel about yourself and your interpersonal relations?
5. *Timing/Duration:* When did you first notice the wound? How often have you had wounds?
6. *Setting:* Does the wound occur in a certain place or under certain circumstances? Is it associated with any specific activity?
7. *Antecedents and Consequences:* What makes it better? What makes it worse?
8. *Other Associated Symptoms:* Have you noticed any other changes?

Answers to these questions should provide a thorough understanding of the patient's wound symptoms.

3. Severity
4. Timing
5. Setting in which the symptom occurs
6. Antecedents and consequences of the symptom
7. Other associated symptoms

Review the patient's present health and present illness status to learn additional information about his or her reasons for seeking care. Describe the patient's usual health and then focus on the present problem, investigating the chief complaint thoroughly, as described above. For interpretation and analysis of the patient's problem, it is helpful to document the chief complaint data in chronologic order.

Past Health History

Next, review the patient's past health history. Information about how the patient responded to past problems may provide an indication of the patient's potential response to treatment of the current problem. Much of this information may be available in the patient's medical record. If not, make sure to obtain the following information:

- Past general health
- Childhood illnesses, accidents, or injuries with any associated disabilities
- Hospitalizations
- Surgeries
- Major acute or chronic illnesses
- Immunizations
- Medications and transfusions
- Allergies

Current Health Information

Current health information includes allergies, health habits, medications, exercise patterns, and sleep habits.

Allergic reactions usually affect the gastrointestinal tract, respiratory tract, and skin. Thus, specific allergies may influence your choice of interventions for the patient's wound care regimen. Make sure to investigate environmental, animal, food, product, and medication allergies. Some products used for wound care can contribute to an allergic reaction. An example is latex, which is found in dressings, gloves, and plastic tubing. Tape is also often associated with skin allergies. Sulfonamide is a common drug allergen that is contained in silver sulfadiazine (Silvadene), a topical therapy widely used for wound care.

Evaluate current and past lifestyle habits relevant to the health of the patient, including use of alcohol, tobacco, illicit substances, and caffeine. Alcohol, tobacco, and illicit substance use, in particular, present significant problems for tissue perfusion and nutrition for wound healing.

Complete a full medication profile, including prescription and over-the-counter medications, names, dosages, frequency, intended effect, and compliance with the regimen. Many medications interfere with wound healing or may interact with wound therapy.

Evaluate the patient's usual routine to determine patterns of physical and sedentary activities. Ask the patient to describe a typical day's activities. Exercise patterns influence healing of several wound types, such as venous disease ulcers.

Finally, investigate the patient's sleep pattern and whether he or she perceives the sleep to be adequate and satisfactory. Ask the patient where he or she usually sleeps. Patients with severe arterial insufficiency may sleep sitting up in recliner chairs because of the pain associated with the disease. Likewise, patients with chronic obstructive pulmonary disease (COPD) may sleep sitting up because of difficulty breathing in the supine position.

Family Health History

The family health history provides information about the general health of the patient's relatives. Family health information is helpful in the identification of genetic, familial, and environmental illnesses. Specific areas to target are diabetes mellitus, heart disease, and stroke, as these diseases can impair wound healing and are risk factors for further wounding. If the patient has a family history of any of these diseases, he or she may have early signs of the disease as yet undiagnosed and is at higher risk of eventual disease development.

Social History

Diagnosis and management of a patient's wound is best accomplished within the context of the whole person, so it is important to gather information about the patient's social, psychological, and nutritional status. Social data fall into seven areas, each of which is discussed briefly below:

1. Relationships with family and significant others
2. Environment
3. Occupational history
4. Economic status and resources
5. Educational level
6. Daily life
7. Patterns of healthcare

Information about relationships with family and significant others includes the patient's position and role in the family, the persons living with the patient, the persons to whom the patient relates, and any recent family changes or crises. This information is important, because the role of the patient within the family can dictate treatment decisions. For example, a grandmother with venous disease ulcers may be the primary caregiver of young grandchildren; thus, it would be unrealistic to expect her to comply with a therapeutic regimen that includes frequent, lengthy periods of elevating her lower extremities. The family support system is another critical factor when determining wound care management programs, and answers to questions such as, "Who will change the wound dressing and perform procedures?" "Who prepares meals?" and "Who will transport the patient to the clinic?" can influence treatment options.

Aspects of the patient's environment can play a significant role in the patient's health and illness. Ask questions about the home, community, and work environments. Home-care patients can present challenging environments for wound repair. For example, an elderly woman living alone with four cats in a two-room trailer with minimal bathroom facilities will require management strategies that differ from those used with a middle-aged man living with a spouse and children in a three-bedroom house in the suburbs. In addition, the community environment may provide additional resources for the patient, such as senior citizen centers, health fairs, or a neighborhood grocery store that delivers to the home. The work environment, along with the occupational history, can identify job-related health risks and provide information on the ability of a patient to eliminate certain risk factors for impaired healing. For example, a grocery clerk with a venous disease ulcer will need support in transferring to a job that does not require standing for long periods of time.

Information about the patient's economic status and resources is important to determine adequacy for therapy compliance. It is not necessary to know a patient's exact income, but ask whether the patient feels the income is adequate and elicit the source of the income. It is important to identify patients with inadequate resources and to make appropriate referrals for financial assistance. Assess the patient's health insurance resources, including the source of insurance coverage and resources available to obtain necessary dressing supplies. If prolonged wound healing is expected, a discussion of financial reserves may be desirable. Some patients have insurance coverage that pays for all dressing supplies, whereas other patients have insurance coverage that pays for only certain types of supplies (e.g., gauze, but not tape). Still other patients have no coverage for supplies at all. Also determine whether the patient has adequate resources available to pay for a caregiver if one is needed to help with dressing changes or other aspects of care.

In order to plan for patient teaching, you'll need to know the patient's level of education. These data are also important when planning methods of patient self-care.

Ask the patient to describe a typical day and to identify any differences on the weekend. Answers to questions about their typical daily routine, as well as social and recreational activities, should provide you with valuable insights into the patient's lifestyle and possible health risks. These answers should also help you make sound clinical judgments about the patient's past health promotion and prevention activities, and use of healthcare, including determining whether there has been continuity of care.

Psychological History
The psychological history includes an assessment of the patient's

- Cognitive abilities (including learning style, memory, and comprehension)
- Responses to illness (coping patterns and reaction to illness)
- Responses to care (compliance)

At this point in the history taking, you will usually have some idea of the patient's comprehension, memory, and overall cognitive status. If mental function is still unclear, administer an examination such as the mini-mental status exam. Previous coping patterns and reactions to illness provide insight into possible reactions to the current situation. Has the patient had difficulties with wound healing in the past? Is there a history of chronic wounds? How has the patient responded to previous chronic wounds? Information about the patient's response to previous care and compliance with other therapy regimens can identify potential difficulties with adhering to the current treatment plan.

Cultural History
In today's culturally diverse world, patients often have culturally determined values, beliefs, and behaviors that differ significantly from those of the clinician. These differences often arise in the areas of health and wellness, healthcare, and self-care. Thus, you should assume nothing and routinely assess the patient's and caregiver's culture prior to determining goals of care and the overall treatment plan. Be particularly sensitive when performing this assessment.

Nutritional History
Nutrition plays a major role in wound healing (see Chapter 7). During the patient history, determine the patient's usual daily food intake, risk for malnutrition, and specific nutritional deficiencies. Evaluate the patient's weight in comparison with his or her usual weight. Ask the patient to recall all foods eaten in the past 24 hours and determine whether this is a normal eating pattern for the patient. Involvement of the dietician or nutritionist is recommended if the nutrition history reflects nutritional needs.

Systems Review and Physical Assessment
Together, the systems review portion of the patient history and the physical assessment of each system provide information on comorbidities that can impair wound healing. The individual's capacity to heal can be limited by the effects of specific diseases on tissue integrity and perfusion, patient mobility, compliance, nutrition, and risk for wound infection. Throughout the patient history, systems review, and physical assessment, consider these host factors that may affect wound healing as part of your systems review and physical assessment. Chapter 3 details systems to be reviewed that include

- Respiratory system
- Cardiovascular system
- Gastrointestinal system
- Genitourinary system
- Peripheral vascular system
- Neurologic
- Musculotskeletal system
- Hematologic system
- Endocrine system

Although the review of systems with physical assessment guidelines presented in Chapter 3 is not inclusive, it identifies the areas of greatest concern when managing patients with wounds. A complete history and physical examination provides the context for the wound itself; after completing it, you can begin to plan interventions. If the information you are able to glean from the history and physical assessment is very limited, you will need to base your clinical decision about the appropriateness of the referral on the reason for referral, expected outcomes, and your personal observations of the patient.

Most clinicians can complete the general history, systems review, and physical assessment in about 30 to 40 minutes for a single wound. An experienced clinician can perform a basic physical assessment in 10 to 15 minutes. Typically, not all information is gathered at one time; portions of the history and physical assessment can be gathered over a period of several days after multiple clinic or home visits.

Wound Assessment

Wound assessment involves evaluation of a composite of wound characteristics, including location, shape, size, depth, edges, undermining or pocketing and tunneling, necrotic tissue characteristics, characteristics of drainage or **exudate**, drainage that contains dead cells and debris, surrounding skin color, peripheral tissue edema and induration, and the presence of granulation tissue and epithelialization (also see Chapter 3 on wound assessment, Chapter 4 on tools, and Chapter 5 on wound measurement).

Wound History

Following are key questions to elicit information about the history of the wound:

- "How long has the wound been present?"
- "Is there a history of previous wounds?"
- "What interventions have been used, and have they been successful?"
- "What types of health-care providers have been involved in the management of the wound?"

If the patient has been seen by providers from several disciplines and has undergone multiple interventions without successful progress toward healing, the patient's candidacy for more aggressive intervention is questionable. Examine carefully the patient's previous therapy and response to therapy in order to avoid repeating unsuccessful interventions. Some patients do not heal. However, careful evaluation of past interventions with attention to appropriateness of topical wound care, prevention strategies, risk factor and comorbidity management, and use of adjunct therapy, such as a whirlpool or electrical stimulation, can reveal inconsistencies in treatment approach.

Patient Candidacy for Specialized Services

As noted earlier, during the assessment process, the clinician focuses on how the medical history and systems review affect the candidacy of the patient. For instance, although physical therapists may determine the candidacy of the patient for services, this is not an option in nursing; the nurse typically has no role in determining whether to provide nursing services to the patient. However, the nurse may assist in determination of appropriate therapy for patients when other disciplines are involved.

Sometimes, the medical history and systems review findings suggest that the patient's problem requires consultation, that is, it is outside the scope of your knowledge, experience, or expertise. In other cases, you may determine that the intervention originally suggested would be inappropriate. In physical therapy, you would then identify the patient as a noncandidate for the referred service. It would then become the responsibility of the clinician to refer the patient to another practitioner who is skilled and knowledgeable in a different area or better equipped to manage the identified problem or recommend an alternative strategy. Following are examples of criteria that would trigger a referral:

- Vascular testing should be considered if hair loss, skin pallor or cyanosis, or cold temperature of the feet is found on assessment.
- Callus and hemorrhagic spots on the callus indicate deeper tissue damage and warrant further assessment for high pressure.
- Toenail abnormalities should be referred if this is not an area of expertise for the examiner.
- An abscess in a tunnel or sinus tract requires immediate referral for surgical management.
- Undermining or tunneling (i.e., a black hole without a bottom) should be immediately referred for surgical management.
- Signs of granulation tissue infection (e.g., superficial bridging, friable tissue, bleeding on contact, pain in the wound, and regression of healing) require medical intervention.

STEP 2: DIAGNOSIS

At this point in the diagnostic process, you will have identified the risk factors for impaired healing, based on data you collected during the history and systems review. The specific information you gather about a patient determines your examination strategy; thus, not all patients will receive the same examination. The examination strategy is typically more focused and specific than the general assessment.

Examination Strategy

There are two parts to the examination: Part 1 includes testing for factors related to the patient's comorbidities and Part 2 looks at key features of the wound assessment.

Examination: Part 1

The first part of the examination involves testing for factors related to the physiologic or anatomic status of the comorbidities that impair healing, such as vascular or sensory impairment. These tests carry significant weight in the prediction of healing and development of the prognosis. For example, a low ankle-brachial index score indicates severe occlusive disease and is a predictor of failure to heal without reperfusion. Loss of protective sensation in the feet indicates a high risk for ulceration from pressure or trauma and an intervention strategy is warranted.

A patient with a low ankle-brachial index would not be considered a candidate for physical therapy services or aggressive wound healing interventions because of the severity of vascular system impairment. In this case, a nurse would manage the patient's wound and refer the patient to a vascular surgeon.

A patient with an insensitive foot due to neuropathy would be a candidate for physical therapy because this condition would constitute a medical necessity, requiring the skills of a physical therapist. The physical therapist would predict a functional outcome of risk reduction following interventions of pressure elimination and stimulation, leading to healing.

In both cases, the ulcerations are related to underlying medical pathology. In the former case, the ulcer would not be expected to respond unless the underlying pathology were addressed. In the latter case, ulcer management would be appropriate, along with risk reduction management. As you can see, the interpretation of the data from the history and physical examination sets the stage for functional diagnosis and allows for triage of cases that should be referred or managed conservatively.

Examination: Part 2

This part of the examination strategy looks at four key features of the wound assessment:

- Evaluation of the surrounding skin
- Assessment of the wound tissue
- Observation of wound drainage
- Size measurements

The sequence of the examination depends on visual observation and palpation of the impaired tissues. Be sure to choose tests and measures that are specific to the wound situation. For example, temperature testing may be the best way to distinguish the presence of inflammatory processes in pressure ulcers in patients with darkly pigmented skin. A wound tracing may be the best method to measure the irregular shape of a venous ulcer.

After completing the examination portion of the diagnostic process, your task is to interpret the physiologic and anatomic systems information and wound assessment data, bringing all of the information together like the pieces of a puzzle to develop a functional diagnosis.[2]

Evaluation and Diagnosis

The **evaluation** aspect of the wound care process involves analysis of the findings you have collected. The purpose of evaluation is to draw conclusions about a patient's specific problems and needs so that you can implement effective interventions. In short, evaluation leads to clinical judgments.

"Diagnosis" refers to the process itself, as well as the conclusion reached after the evaluation data have been organized.[3]

Diagnosis involves forming a clinical judgment by identifying a problem—that is, a disease/condition or human response—through the scientific evaluation of signs and symptoms, history, and diagnostic studies. Problem identification is a process of diagnostic reasoning in which judgments, decisions, and conclusions are made about the data collected to determine whether intervention is needed.[4] Thus, in many respects, a diagnosis is analogous to a research hypothesis: A research hypothesis directs the research study, and a diagnosis directs the patient's care plan. Both a research hypothesis and diagnosis are chosen based on available data and information, and both can be proven correct or incorrect as the study or care plan progresses.

Both nurses and physical therapists base diagnoses on the symptoms or the sequelae of the injurious process, such as impaired wound healing. *Nursing diagnoses* identify specific human responses to existing or potential health problems. These problems may be physical, sociologic, or psychological. In contrast, physical therapists establish diagnoses for the specific conditions requiring attention. A *physical therapy diagnosis* is defined as "a label encompassing a cluster of signs, symptoms, syndromes, or categories."[3] The purpose of a diagnosis is to guide the clinician in determining the most appropriate intervention strategy for the individual. When assessment does not provide adequate information to formulate a diagnosis, the interventions may need to be limited to alleviation of symptoms and remediation of deficits.

Distinguishing Between Impairments and Disabilities

Physical therapists evaluate the functional implications of impairments and disabilities. *Impairment* is defined as a loss or abnormality of psychological, physiologic, or anatomic structure or function.[5] It may thus involve the loss of function of a body system or organ due to illness or injury.[6] An example is the loss of function of skin and underlying soft tissue due to wounding or underlying pathology. An underlying pathology can create the susceptibility to loss of function; for example, "undue susceptibility to pressure ulcers" and "undue insensitivity to pain."[8]

The definition of *disability* is any restriction or lack of ability to perform an activity in the manner or within the range considered normal for a human being. Disability can result from impairment or from the person's response to the impairment. It can be reversible or irreversible. Disability reflects a deviation in performance or behavior within a task or activity.[6] Examples are an individual who has musculoskeletal disablement that leads to difficulty walking or moving, and an individual with integumentary disablement related to the inability of the body to progress from the inflammatory phase of healing to the proliferative phase.

Functional Diagnosis

Physical therapists use *functional diagnosis* to describe the consequences of disease and to justify the medical necessity of management by a physical therapist. In wound care, functional diagnosis is an assessment of the related impairments and associated disabilities that affect the status of a wound and its ability to heal. Examples of functional diagnoses include the following:

- Impaired sensation (inability to detect pressure or light touch)
- Impaired circulation (ankle-brachial index below 0.8) of lower extremities
- Impaired lower extremity strength and joint range of motion (including manual muscle testing and range of motion), resulting in persistent pressure to buttocks
- Impaired healing associated with chronic inflammation phase

STEP 3: PROGNOSIS AND GOALS

Once the diagnosis is established, the clinician predicts, or prognoses, the expected outcome and selects an intervention. **Prognosis** is defined as a prediction of the maximal improvement expected from an intervention and how long it will take. It is thus a useful tool for goal setting. Prognosis may also include prediction of *improvement* at different intervals during treatment.[5]

Some clinicians are intimidated by the idea of predicting outcomes; however, they are in the best position to do so if they are knowledgeable about the effects of the interventions prescribed and administered. Patients would not expose themselves to interventions with unpredictable results, and payers would not reimburse providers for services with unexpected benefits and indefinite costs. In the current health-care environment, a sound understanding of prognosis and outcomes is important for all health-care practitioners.

Wound Prognosis Options

The prognosis options for wounds are limited. One system for evaluating wound healing defines healing as *minimally, acceptably*, or *ideally* healed. An ideally healed wound results in return of the fully restored dermis and epidermis with intact barrier function. An acceptably healed wound has a resurfaced epithelium capable of sustained functional integrity during activities of daily living. A minimally healed wound is characterized by closure but without a sustained functional result and may recur. In all these definitions, complete closure of the wound is expected.[7]

For some individuals and some wounds, closure is not an option. Rather, the best prognosis is a change in the wound healing phase from an impaired or early phase of repair to a more advanced phase of repair. A change in wound healing phase is a functional outcome prediction. This method monitors a real change in the organ function of the skin and soft tissues, which is a measure of reduced functional impairment.

The prognosis that a wound is not expected to improve should lead to referral for other management. Nurses may be expected to care for the wound, but the patient may need services including palliative care that can be provided by a physical therapy, dietary, or orthotic intervention.

Goals

A **goal** is precisely defined as the desired or expected result of an intervention. Goal setting differs somewhat for different clinical disciplines involved in wound care. Here we are limiting the discussion of goal setting to the disciplines of nursing and physical therapy. Other disciplines would have similar goals that apply to their area of expertise.

Nursing Goals

Nurses must set priorities, establish goals, and identify desired outcomes for patients. Goals are important because they assist in determining outcomes of care and measuring the effectiveness of interventions. Goals must be measurable, objective, and based on the prioritized needs of the patient.

Short-term goals are typically actions that must be taken before a patient is discharged or moved to another level of care. Long-term goals may require continued attention by a patient and/or caregiver long after discharge. Short-term goals should move a patient toward the long-term goal.

Physical Therapy Goals

Physical therapists are also required to establish short-term and long-term goals. These goals should be measurable, objective, functional, and very specific. Traditionally, a short-term goal was one that would be achieved in 30 days or less and usually corresponded to the end of the billing period or length of stay.

Long-term goals were those predicted to be met by the time of discharge. There has also been a shift in terminology away from using the term *goal* and replacing it with *expected outcome*. In contrast, an *outcome* is the actual result or status after the intervention.

Completing the wound care process with recommendations is one outcome of physical therapy services. Physical therapists target specific, measurable outcomes for specific interventions. To make them functional outcomes, they must meet the criteria described below. *Target outcomes* are short-term, specific expectations of a change in impairment status. Since a prognosis is the expected outcome after a course of care, it represents the long-term goal.

Examples of wound healing prognoses include the following:

1. Ideally healed closure
2. Acceptably healed closure
3. Minimally healed closure
4. Clean and stable open wound
5. Wound ready for surgical closure
6. Not expected to improve

Evaluation of Progress and Outcomes

As just noted, an **outcome** is the result of what is done, that is, the change resulting from an intervention. Outcomes are measured using *performance indicators*, objective measurements used to monitor change resulting from an intervention. Providers, payers, regulators, and clinicians all work toward establishing reliable performance indicators to report clinical outcomes. Exhibit 1.1 lists examples of wound-related performance indicators, with outcomes and functional outcomes for each.

Two types of outcomes are behavioral and functional. Payer groups have an interest in both types.[8] Thus, we'll discuss each in detail shortly.

Reporting Outcomes

The reporting of outcomes is not to be confused with *process*; that is, an intervention or activity performed to achieve a result. Outcomes must be specific, realistic, time oriented, objective, patient centered, and measurable. Once established, outcomes serve as an evaluation tool.

Terms Frequently Misused When Reporting Outcomes

This section discusses some terms that are commonly misused when reporting outcomes, and the appropriate way to report an outcome.

Reduced risk of infection is a topic of confusion, and clinicians must understand that it is not an outcome. Freedom from infection or reduction in exudate, odor, or culture results are measurable outcomes. For any of these outcomes to be functional outcomes, they must change the way the body system functions. Freedom from infection can be an outcome of wound cleansing, but it becomes a functional outcome when wound healing progresses to the next phase of repair. The functional outcome would be correctly written as, "The wound is infection-free, and the wound healing has progressed from the inflammatory phase to the proliferative phase."

A troublesome word in healthcare is *maintained*, which implies no change. *Controlled* should not be mistaken for *maintained*. For example, if edema has fluctuated from treatment

EXHIBIT 1.1

Examples of Performance Indicators with Wound Outcomes and Functional Wound Outcomes

Performance Indicators	Wound Outcomes	Functional Wound Outcomes
1. Change in wound and surrounding skin attributes	Progression through the phases of wound healing (inflammation, proliferation, and epithelialization)	1. Clean, stable wound ready for surgical closure
2. Reduced severity of wound in depth or size		2. Dressing changes needed biweekly instead of daily
3. Change in wound exudate characteristics or undermining		3. Exudate managed; patient returns to work
4. Closure		4. Return to work/leisure activities
1. Temperature comparison	Oxygenation or perfusion of tissue	1. Progress to next wound healing phase
2. Transcutaneous partial pressure of oxygen level		2. Pain level no longer interferes with ADL
3. Laser Doppler		
1. Girth measurements	Edema reduced or controlled	1. Patient able to *don compression hose*
2. Volume meter measurements		2. Leg ulcers are smaller, require less frequent dressing changes
3. Palpation grading system		
1. Wound exudate characteristics	Infection controlled	1. Wound exudate odor controlled, able to return to community
2. Wound and surrounding skin attributes		2. Pain alleviated, patient resumes walking
3. Culture		
1. Free of necrosis	Clean, stable wound	1. Frequency of visits reduced
2. Proliferation phase tissue attributes		2. Physical therapy intervention no longer required
3. Change in depth or size		3. Patient can now manage wound dressings changes
1. Braden Scale score	Reduced risk of pressure ulceration	1. Repositions self in bed
2. Functional activities performance		2. Patient performs self-care activities while in wheelchair
3. Comprehension testing		3. Patient demonstrates use of hand mirror to monitor skin
1. Wound closure	Acceptable healed scar	1. Patient identifies risk factors for reulceration
2. Functional activities performed related to use of scar tissue		2. Patient uses protective equipment correctly under scar tissue to perform functional activities in wheelchair

to treatment, and then stabilizes as a result of intervention, the outcome is that edema is controlled. A functional outcome for controlled edema would be stated as, "The edema in the tissues surrounding the wound is controlled." The functional outcome of control of the edema is that the wound progresses to the next phase of healing.

Maximized and *minimized* are similarly confused with outcomes. For example, "maximized participation in activities of daily living" does not reflect the functional outcome of an intervention with an orthotic device. A functional outcome reports the result of the intervention, such as, "The patient performs activities of daily living wearing/using orthotic equipment, and has returned to work and/or resumed leisure activities." An example of misuse of *minimized* as an outcome is "minimized stresses precipitating or perpetuating injury." Correct use is, "Functional outcome—patient/caregiver identified stress-reduction methods to minimize risk of injury."

Improved is defined as "to make better or enhance in value." This is a subjective measure, not a measurable outcome. An outcome reports the objective result of improvement. For example, increased vital capacity measured in liters (performance indicator) is a measurable change in the pulmonary system, with a result of increased oxygenation of tissues for wound healing. The functional outcome is "wound progresses to next phase of healing."

Provided is sometimes confused with an outcome, although it is an action by the clinician, not an outcome of the intervention. An example of improper use is "provided electrical stimulation to enhance circulation." This describes the rationale for the intervention, not the outcome.

Promoted is another inappropriately used term. For example, "promoted angiogenesis" is a process. Angiogenesis is an expected outcome of treatment and represents an attribute of wound healing. The performance indicators of angiogenesis are change in wound attributes, phase, or size. The outcome is wound progression through the proliferative phase.

Behavioral Outcomes

Behavioral outcomes include behaviors that can be observed or monitored to determine whether an acceptable or positive outcome is achieved within the desired time frame. Like all outcomes, behavioral outcomes must be specific, realistic, time oriented, objective, patient centered, and measurable.

Use measurable action verbs to describe behavioral outcomes. For example, the verb *understand* is not measurable; we cannot measure a person's understanding. The same is true for the verbs *feel, learn, know,* and *accept.* But *identify* is measurable; the patient can be tested to determine whether he or she can identify. Other appropriate action verbs include *list, record, name, state, describe, explain, demonstrate, use, schedule, differentiate, compare, relate, design, prepare, formulate, select, choose, increase, decrease, stand, walk,* and *participate.*

Examples of behavioral outcomes for a patient with a wound include: "The patient will describe the signs of wound infection and identify correct action within 24 hours" and "The patient will demonstrate wound dressing application within 2 days." Correct documentation that the target outcome was met would include: "Patient is able to describe the signs of infection and list the steps for corrective action. Patient is able to demonstrate correct wound dressing application."

Functional Outcomes

A *functional outcome* helps to communicate a change in function to the patient, caregiver, and payer. Physical therapists usually work with patients who have experienced loss of functional abilities, and they use functional tests that measure physical attributes to predict the function that the patient is expected to achieve after a course of treatment. *Function* in this context refers to activities and actions that are meaningful to the patient or caregiver. You should make a determination about meaningful function while completing the "reason for referral" portion of the assessment.

To constitute a functional outcome, the results must meet three criteria[9]:

1. The result is meaningful.
2. The result is practical.
3. The result can be sustained over time outside the treatment setting.

Meaningful is defined as being of value to the patient, caregiver, or both. *Practical* means that the outcome is applicable to the patient's life situation. *Sustainable over time* refers to functional abilities achieved through an intervention that are maintained by the patient or caregiver outside the clinical setting (e.g., a patient demonstrates the ability to apply a dressing and stocking during two follow-up visits).[10]

Standardized tests and measurement tools are useful to monitor and track change over time. The Bates-Jensen Wound Assessment Toll (BWAT), formerly called the Pressure Sore Status Tool (PSST), the Sussman Wound Healing Tool (SWHT), and the Pressure Ulcer Scale for Healing (PUSH), described in Chapter 4, can be used to document the outcomes of changes in wound attributes by changes in test scores, and can then be applied to function. For example, using the BWAT to monitor exudate amounts, a change in score on that test item from 4 (moderate exudate) to 2 (scant exudate) would indicate reduced drainage. This outcome is measurable and objective, and meets the criteria for a valid outcome. However, this information alone does not constitute a functional outcome. To interpret this score as a functional outcome, a statement must connect the findings with meaning to the patient, practical effect, and sustainable result. A correct statement of functional outcomes would be, "Wound exudate BWAT has reduced from 4 (moderate) to 2 (scant) exudate, patient demonstrates ability to monitor for signs of infection and action to take, and patient is now able to return to work and will be seen for intermittent follow-up."

Functional outcomes should be documented throughout the course of care, not just at discharge. Factors you can use to demonstrate intermittent functional change include change in patient lifestyle, change in patient safety, and adaptation to impairment or disability. These statements should be patient centered and measurable (Exhibit 1.2).

EXHIBIT 1.2

Example of Functional Outcomes Documented Throughout Course of Care

Initial Statement: Patient is unable to sit in wheelchair without trauma to integument.

Initial Target Outcome: Patient is sitting for 2 hours in adaptive seating system in 2 weeks.

Interim Outcome After 1 Week: Patient sits for 1 hour in adaptive seating system.

Discharge Statement: Patient sits in adaptive seating system for 2 hours without disruption of integumentary integrity.

EXHIBIT **1.3**

How to Write Outcome Statements and Functional Outcomes

When reporting outcomes, use the following guidelines:
1. An outcome expresses the *result* of an intervention—not the intervention or the process—to reach an outcome (e.g., wound resurfacing/closure).
2. A behavioral outcome can be learned information (e.g., demonstrates application of wound dressing). This outcome would follow an intervention of instruction.
3. Coordination of treatment including: interdisciplinary, communication, and documentation of care outcomes used to ensure proper utilization management include.

Functional outcomes are written to describe results of treatment on function and include three parts:
1. Description of a meaningful functional change to a body system (e.g., progression through the phases of healing)
2. Description of a practical result of a change in a body system (e.g., wound is minimally exudative)
3. Description of the sustainable result or change in the impairment status or disability resulting from the intervention (e.g., pressure elimination allows the patient to sit up in wheelchair 2 hours twice a day)

A change in wound tissue attributes and size can also be used as a functional outcome; for example, "Free of necrosis, reduced risk of infection, and size reduced 50%, wound is clean and stable, decreased frequency of visits required" (Exhibit 1.3).

REEVALUATION

Reevaluation is an ongoing, dynamic process that follows regular reexamination of the effects of treatment. Clinicians use performance indicators to measure a patient's progress toward the outcome within the desired time frame. For example, if the target outcome is "Patient's wound will demonstrate 25% reduction in size within 2 weeks," the clinician would monitor wound size throughout the 2-week period of time, and then determine whether the wound had reduced in surface area by 25% at the end of week 2. If the wound decreased in size more than 25%, the outcome was exceeded. If the wound decreased in size by 25%, the outcome was acceptably met. If the wound failed to decrease in size by 25%, the outcome was not met, and the goals must be adjusted and interventions reviewed.

What happens if an outcome is not met? Failure to achieve goals can be related to a change in the patient's overall condition, ineffective therapy, or inadequate adherence to the treatment regimen. When this occurs, you may decide to adjust goals and outcomes, develop new goals, and modify interventions. That

said, because utilization management attempts to influence the clinical path from the beginning, in order to reduce deviation from an expected course and produce optimal outcomes, your adjustment of goals and expected outcomes should be minimal. Multiple approximations to reach the target outcome are not tolerated by patients or third-party payers.

The *APTA Guide to PT Practice*[11] lists wound management guidelines regarding range of visits and length of episodic care by physical therapists for patients with wounds. This range represents the lower and upper limits of services that an anticipated 80% of patients/clients with such wounds will need to receive to reach the predicted goals and outcomes (prognosis). Multiple factors can modify the duration of the episode of care, frequency, and number of visits.

CONCLUSION

The wound care process described in this chapter is intended as a framework for clinicians working with patients with wounds; it will be especially helpful to clinicians who are new to wound care. Even for experienced clinicians, review of this key material will likely be helpful. Use of clinical judgment with diagnostic reasoning is one of the essential practice tools that nurses, physical therapists, and other health-care practitioners use with the patients they serve.

REVIEW QUESTIONS

1. Steps of the wound care process include
   A. assessment, diagnosis, prognosis/ goals
   B. assessment, history, reason for referral
   C. examination, prognosis, candidacy
   D. wound assessment, history, prognosis

2. Wound healing prognosis options include
   A. mimimally, acceptably, ideally healed
   B. closure, remodeling, hypergranulation
   C. change in wound characteristics
   D. none of the above

3. A functional outcome must be
   A. meaningful to the patient's function
   B. communicate change in function including progression of healing
   C. meaningful, practical, sustained outside the treatment setting
   D. all of the above

4. 3 terms often misused when reporting outcomes are
   A. debridement, dressing change, cleansing
   B. promote, provided, risk reduction
   C. healed, closure, infection free
   D. treatment provided as before, minimal exudate, closure

5. Performance indicators for wounds include
   A. change in wound attributes
   B. change in girth measurements
   C. change in wound exudate
   D. all of the above

REFERENCES

1. Clifton DW. Utilization management: whose job is it? *Rehab Manage.* 1996;38:44.
2. Swanson G. *The Guide to Physical Therapist Practice.* Vol 1. Presented at California chapter, APTA, October 1995; San Diego, CA.
3. American Physical Therapy Association. Guide to Physical Therapy Practice. *Phys Ther.* 2001;81(1):S695.
4. Doenges MD, Moorhouse MF, Burley JT. *Application of Nursing Process and Nursing Diagnosis.* 2nd ed. Philadelphia, PA: FA Davis; 1995.
5. Jette AM. Physical disablement concepts for physical therapy research and practice. *Phys Ther.* 1994;74:380–386.
6. Swanson G. *The IDH Guidebook for Physical Therapy.* Long Beach, CA: Swanson and Company; 1995.
7. Lazarus GS, Cooper DM, Knighton DR, et al. Definitions and guidelines for assessment of wounds and evaluation of healing. *Arch Dermatol.* 1994;130:489–493.
8. Swanson G. What is an outcome? And what does it mean to you? *Ultra/sounds.* (California Private Practice Special Interest Group—California APTA). 1995;94(51):7.
9. Swanson G. Functional outcome report: the next generation in physical therapy reporting in documenting physical therapy outcomes. In: Stuart D, Ablen S, eds. *Documenting Physical Therapy Outcomes.* Chicago, IL: CV Mosby, 1993:101–134.
10. Staley M, Richard R, et al. Functional outcomes for the patient with burn injuries. *J Burn Care Rehabil.* 1996;17(4):362–367.
11. Guide to physical therapist practice. *Phys Ther.* 1997;77:1593–1605.

APPENDIX
1A

Patient History Form

Medical Record # _____   Name _____
Street Address _____
City, State, Zip _____
Telephone Number (_____) _____
Sex: M/F _____   Height: _____   Weight: _____
Religious Preference: _____
What is your primary reason for seeking wound care today? _____
_____
How long has your wound existed? _____
_____
Who referred you here? _____
Who has been treating you before today? _____
Can you describe what you have been using on your wound? _____
_____
Who has been helping you with your wound care? _____
How have you been paying for your supplies? _____
Have you ever had surgery? _____   Type: _____
Do you have any allergies? Medications (Sulfa, Penicillin) _____   Other? _____
Do you smoke? _____   Packs per day: _____   # of years: _____
Do you use recreational or illicit drugs? If so, how often? _____
Do you drink alcohol? If so, how often? _____
Do you have any pain? _____
On a scale of 0–10 (0 = No Pain, 10 = Severe Pain), what is your pain level now?   0 – 1 – 2 – 3 – 4 – 5 – 6 – 7 – 8 – 9 – 10
What over-the-counter medications do you take (Tylenol, aspirin, antacids, vitamins, etc.)? _____
_____
What prescription medications do you take? Please include drug, dose, and frequency: _____
_____

Have you ever been told you had or do you currently have any of the following:

	Past	Present		Past	Present
Stroke:			Hypertension:		
Gangrene:			Cancer:		
Problems with circulation:			Chemotherapy:		
Arterial:			Radiation therapy:		
Venous:			Alternative treatments:		
Diabetes:			Swollen glands:		
Parkinson's:			Muscle spasms:		
Alzheimer's:			Polio or post-polio syndrome:		
Congestive heart failure:			Quadriplegia/paraplegia:		
Problems sleeping:			Myelomeningocele:		
Emphysema:			Decreased sensation:		
Bronchitis:			Arthritis:		
Chronic obstructive pulmonary disease:			Decreased activity:		
Problems controlling urine:			HIV or AIDS:		
Problems controlling bowels:			Hepatitis B:		
Atherosclerosis/arteriosclerosis:			Decreased appetite:		
Malnutrition:			Problems with mobility:		
Dehydration:			Changes in weight greater than 10 pounds:		
Thyroid disorder:			Pacemaker:		

Source: Copyright © Dean P. Kane, MD, FACS, PA.

Focused Assessment for Wounds

Medical Record # _____ Name _____

Attending Physician: _____

Referral Source: _____ MD _____ Nurse _____ Other

Site: __ Office __ Acute Hospital __ Subacute Center __ Nursing Home __ Assisted Living __ Home __ Other

    Facility Name / Address / Pt. bed #: _____

Physical Exam: _____ year-old M F acquired non-healing wound(s) on   / / .

Prior wound management includes: _____

    _____

Past Medical History is positive for the following:

Allergies _____	Alcoholism _____
CVA _____	NIDDM _____
Gangrene _____	Complications of DM _____
PVD _____	Weakness _____
Arterial insufficiency _____	Paraplegia/quadriplegia _____
CAD _____	Immobility/contractures _____
IDDM _____	Parkinson's _____

Vitals: T/P/R _____ BP: L/R _____ (sit/stand/lying)

Braden Scale:

Sensory/MS	1. totally limited	2. very limited	3. slightly limited	4. no impairment
Moisture	1. constantly moist	2. very moist	3. occasionally moist	4. dry
Activity	1. bedfast	2. chairfast	3. walks w/assist	4. walks frequently
Mobility	1. 100% immobile	2. very limited	3. slightly limited	4. full mobility
Nutrition	1. very poor	2. <1/2 daily portion	3. most of portion	4. eats everything
Friction/Shear	1. frequent sliding	2. feeble corrections	3. independent correction	

                Braden Scale Total: _____

Mental Status: <u>Alert & Oriented X3:</u> Other: _____

Skin: (moist, dry, flaky, scaly, condition of nails): _____ Turgor: <u>good / med / poor</u>

   <u>Rubor, cyanosis, atrophy, dermatitis, hair loss, rash, erythema.</u>

EENT (Eyes sunken, swollen lymph nodes): _____ Mucous Membranes Moist: _____

Neuro (Cranial nerves, sensation): _____

Endocrine (Blood sugar/other): _____

Respiratory: <u>Lungs Clear:</u> <u>Other:</u> _____

Cardiac: <u>Regular Rate & Rhythm:</u> Other: _____

Abdomen: <u>G-Tube: Soft/Supple/Without Masses or Tenderness:</u> Other: _____

Perineal: Skin intact _____ Other: _____

Lower Extremities: Ankle-Brachial Index: L: _____ R: _____

  Pulses Palpable: Dorsalis Pedis _____ Posterior Tibial _____ Popliteal _____

  Pulse Quality: Bounding _____ Strong _____ Weak _____ Barely Palpable _____

  Doppler: L+ _____ : R+ _____

  Edema _____ Circumference: (L) _____ : (R) _____

Functional Assessment: ADLs: Independent _____ Minimal Assist _____ Mod Assist _____ Total Assist _____

Labs/Nutrition: Hct: _____ % TP: _____ Alb: _____ Prealbumin: _____ Other: _____

             WBC: _____ % O2 Sat: _____ Lytes: _____

Suggested Tests/Examinations: _____

Adapted with permission from Dean P. Kane, MD, FACS, PA.

APPENDIX
1C

Sample Case Report Using HCFA-700

DEPARTMENT OF HEALTH AND HUMAN SERVICES
HEALTH CARE FINANCING ADMINISTRATION

FORM APPROVED
OMB NO. 0938-0227

PLAN OF TREATMENT FOR OUTPATIENT REHABILITATION *(COMPLETE FOR INITIAL CLAIMS ONLY)*

1. PATIENT'S LAST NAME	FIRST NAME	M.I.	2. PROVIDER NO.	3. HICN
Luck	George			

4. PROVIDER NAME	5. MEDICAL RECORD NO *(Optional)*	6. ONSET DATE	7. SOC. DATE
		10/09/01	11/27/01

8. TYPE:	9. PRIMARY DIAGNOSIS *(Pertinent Medical D.X.)*	10. TREATMENT DIAGNOSIS	11. VISITS FROM SOC.
☐ PT ☐ OT ☐ SLP ☐ CR	CHF, COPD, multiple decubitus,	2 wounds with impaired wound healing secondary to eschar and chronic	15
☐ RT ☐ PS ☐ SN ☐ SW	weakness, debility	inflammatory phase. Impaired mobility, transfers, gait (707, 707.7)	

12 PLAN OF TREATMENT FUNCTIONAL GOALS

GOALS *(Short Term)*   Tissue Attribute changes expected:
Necrosis-free and wound healing progression to proliferative phase
  Wounds #1 & 2   21 days
Reduce risk of pressure ulcers (Reduce Braden score to 19/22) 15 days
Transfers and Gait with FWW to bathroom SBA   15 days

OUTCOME *(Long Term)*:

Target Performance Status:
Patient has improvement potential: Wounds will heal following intervention.
Functional independent bed mobility, transfer and gait with assist device will
be restored to enable patient to return to prior living situation in 6 weeks.

PLAN
1. Wound not improving with routine dressing changes, pressure relief & enzymatic debridement
2. Wounds #1 & 2 require a) sharp debride b) HVPC (electrical stimulation) to stimulate cells of repair and circulation for healing
3. Ther ex., balance, gait training to reduce risk of pressure ulcers and enhance circulation for healing current ulcers

13. SIGNATURE *(professional establishing POC including prof. designation)*	14. FREQ/DURATION *(e.g., 3/Wk × 4 Wk)*
	6x/wk daily x 6 wks (36 days)

I CERTIFY THE NEED FOR THESE SERVICES FURNISHED UNDER THIS PLAN OF TREATMENT AND WHILE UNDER MY CARE ☒ N/A	17. CERTIFICATION
15. PHYSICIAN SIGNATURE	16 DATE	FROM THROUGH ☒ N/A

18. ON FILE *(Print/type physician's name)* ☒

20. INITIAL ASSESSMENT *(History, medical complications, level of function at start of care. Reason for referral)*	19. PRIOR HOSPITALIZATION
	FROM 10/08/01 TO 11/26/06 ☐ N/A

<u>Reason for Referral</u>: Loss of mobility (e.g., unable to reposition in bed or ambulate); necrotic pressure ulcers R upper back and coccyx. Wants to regain prior level of indep. Gait with cane. Heal pressure ulcers for return to retirement home.

Hx: Mild dementia, indep. in gait w/cane; fell in shower and was unable to move; sustained pressure ulcers R upper back and coccyx, CHF, COPD.

<u>Systems Review</u>: 1) Cardiopulmonary system disabilities affect oxygen transport to tissues for repair. 2) Musculoskeletal impairments due to weakness (MMS BLE 3-/5 limit bed mobility, inability to transfer or ambulate without assist of 2 w/4ww ? few feet. Diminished balance. 3) Neuromuscular impairment due to reduced cerebral oxygen causes mild functional loss of mentation, impaired mobility, and awareness of need to reposition. Risk of pressure ulcers is moderate (Braden Risk score 17/23).

<u>Results of test and measures</u>: Wound Severity Dx (stage) delayed until both wounds are debrided.

<u>Wound healing tissue assessment</u>: 1) R upper Back: presence of tissue attributes "good for healing"; adherence of wound edges; and "not good for healing": necrosis and depth of 0.2cm; 2) coccyx: presence of attributes "not for healing": erythema, necrosis, absence of attributes "good for healing."

<u>Wound Size</u>: R Up Back: 17.7cm² Coccyx: 4.3cm². depth >0.2

21. FUNCTIONAL LEVEL *(End of billing period)*   PROGRESS REPORT   ☐ CONTINUE SERVICES OR ☐ DC SERVICES

1) Change in Wound Status: a) R upper back: progressed to proliferative phase of healing. Wound is erythema-free, necrosis-free and has factors "good for healing": Contraction sustained ? 2 weeks, edges are adhered. Wound is reduced in size from 17.5cm² to 12.3cm² (decreased 25%). b) Coccyx: increased size and extent from 34.4cm² to 37.41cm² after debriding. Severity Dx: Stage IV pressure ulcer. Tissue attributes present: "not good for healing" include: Undermining at 9:00 position, necrosis and erythema; good for healing attributes include: granulation-significant reduction in depth from 2.0 cm to 1.5 cm, appearance of contraction and sustained wound contraction for 2 weeks (reduced size). Wound is at end of acute inflammatory phase and progressing to proliferative phase. 2) Change in Mobility Status: a) Braden risk score 19/23; b) Performs transfers and gait with min-assist using FWW for 15 feet; c) Change in balance improved from fair to fair+ with functional change. Reduced risk of falling and pressure ulcers.

22. SERVICE DATES
FROM 11/27/01   THROUGH 11/30/01

FORM HCFA-700 (11-91)
STF CCR0224F

Source: Reprinted from Department of Health and Human Services, Health Care Financing Administration.

Skin and Soft Tissue Anatomy and Wound Healing Physiology

Carrie Sussman and Barbara M. Bates-Jensen

CHAPTER OBJECTIVES

At the completion of this chapter, the reader will be able to:

1. Identify structures that are part of skin and soft tissue anatomy.
2. Determine wound severity based on depth of tissue loss.
3. List three acute wound healing models.
4. Identify and list the benchmarks of each of the four phases of wound healing.
5. List the benchmarks of wound phase changes for acute and chronic wound healing.
6. Describe the role of basic scientific research in understanding pathophysiology and developing wound treatments.
7. Apply knowledge of the wound microenvironment to identification of factors that can affect the healing process.

Skin and soft tissue anatomy set the stage for understanding the significance and relationship between the depth of loss of the tissue integrity that occurs with wounding and the role of the anatomical structures in regeneration and repair. Skin and soft tissue anatomy are also the basis for classification systems that have been developed to diagnose wound severity. Classification systems for wounds are presented in Chapter 3. Scientific study of the physiology of wound healing has progressed greatly in the past few decades. From an initial understanding of acute wound healing and the development of an acute wound healing model, research progressed to identify the cellular physiology and microenvironment of acute wounds. Current research is also focused on comparing acute wound healing mechanisms and the microenvironment with factors affecting wound chronicity.[1,2] Still, all of these areas of research are works in progress, continuing to provide new information for both acute and chronic wound classifications.

As a clinician, you need to understand the basic anatomy of the skin and soft tissues and the science of wound healing and stay abreast of new research discoveries related to both acute and chronic wounds. Only by doing so will you be able to approach clinical decision making with confidence. At the same time, scientists, engineers, and manufacturers are also applying the growing scientific knowledge about wound healing to the development of products that promote positive outcomes and mitigate the negative factors in healing wounds. Ideally, all of these research findings and resources will be transferred to the clinical setting as best practices in wound management.

The basic science presented in this chapter is not comprehensive. Yet, it should enable you to understand the anatomy and fundamental physiological processes of wound healing and how they may affect outcomes of clinical care. The chapter covers skin and soft tissue anatomy, wound classification systems related to skin integrity and basic acute wound healing models, chronic wound healing, fetal wound healing, the physiology of acute and chronic wound healing by phase, factors that interrupt acute wound healing processes and can lead to chronicity, and factors that can affect the healing process. Chapter 3 connects the concepts of basic wound healing science to the clinical assessment.

ANATOMY AND PHYSIOLOGY OF THE SKIN AND SOFT TISSUES

In this section, we briefly review the anatomy and physiology of young and aged skin and subcutaneous soft tissues to help you appreciate how aging and the depth of loss of skin and soft tissue affect how wounds heal as well as the role of the different structures in tissue regeneration or repair. Figure 2.1 is a diagram of skin and soft tissues, which is included here to help you visualize the anatomic arrangement of the structures.

As we will see shortly, wounds are defined according to the level of skin and soft tissue structure lost.

Young Skin

The skin or integument is the largest organ in the body and consists of two primary layers. The outermost layer, the *epidermis*,

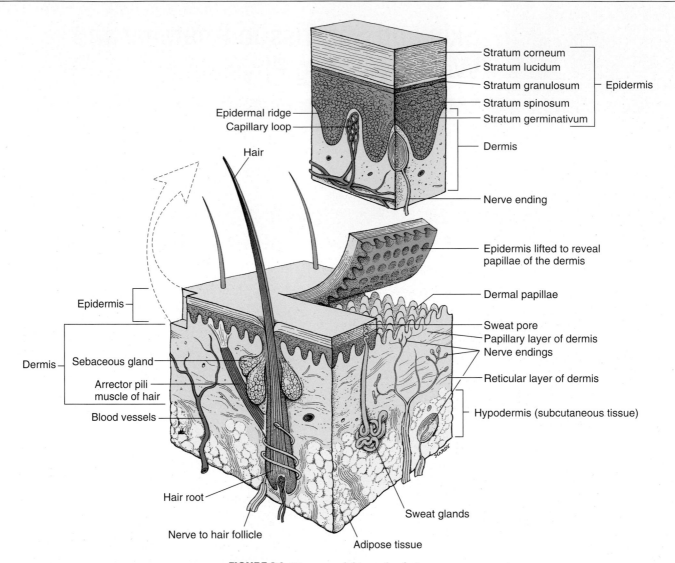

FIGURE 2.1 Diagram of skin and soft tissues.

is itself composed of several layers of epithelium. The first epidermal layer is the stratum corneum, also known as the horny layer, which is composed of keratinocytes. The innermost skin layer is the *dermis*, a connective tissue layer that contains neurons and blood vessels.

The primary function of the skin is protection—from bacteria and other microbes, from mechanical trauma, harmful chemicals, and excessive heat, cold, moisture, dryness, and ultraviolet radiation. Thus, when the skin is injured, the body is subject to invasion by outside agents, loss of body fluids, and other problems. In addition to its barrier function, skin is important for thermal regulation, vitamin D metabolism, and immune defense. Also, skin health is a mirror of general health, and skin failure often accompanies other system failures within the body.

Epidermis

The **epidermis** consists almost entirely of *keratinocytes*, cells that produce keratin, a fibrous protein. The epidermal keratinocytes are arranged into five layers as shown in Figure 2.2. The most superficial is the stratum corneum. Deeper layers of the epidermis include the stratum lucidum, stratum granulosum, stratum

spinosum, and stratum basale (also called the stratum germinativum). Keratinocytes arise from the stratum basale and, as they mature, they migrate upward toward the stratum corneum, increasing their keratin load. Keratinocytes reproduce continuously and produce a protein called keratin, which is insoluble in water and prevents water loss and entrance of irritants into the body. They live for only a few weeks and, by the time they reach the skin surface, have died. In fact, the stratum corneum consists entirely of dead keratinocytes. Deposits of dry keratin on the skin surface are called *scale*. Hyperkeratosis (thickened layers of keratin) is often found on the heels and can indicate loss of sebaceous glands and sweat gland functions.

In addition to keratinocytes, the epidermis contains other functional cells. For instance, *Langerhans cells*, which are immune cells that help fight infection, and *melanocytes*, which produce the pigment protein melanin as well as have an immune function.[3] An important function of the epidermis in wound healing is to close the wound quickly and efficiently. As we'll discuss in detail later in this chapter, epidermal wounds heal primarily by cell migration called *epithelialization*. Clusters of keratinocytes migrate into the area of damage and cover the defect. These lead cells are phagocytic and clear the surface

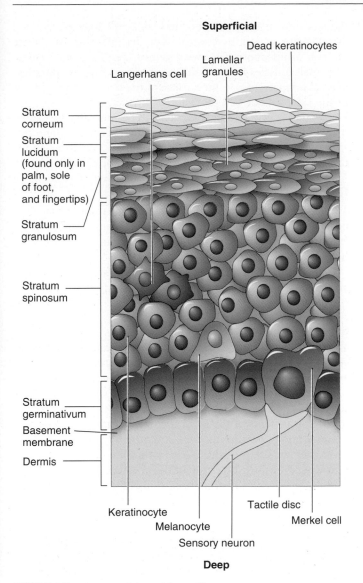

Superficial

Langerhans cell
Lamellar granules
Dead keratinocytes

Stratum corneum

Stratum lucidum (found only in palm, sole of foot, and fingertips)

Stratum granulosum

Stratum spinosum

Stratum germinativum

Basement membrane

Dermis

Keratinocyte

Melanocyte

Sensory neuron

Tactile disc

Merkel cell

Deep

FIGURE 2.2 Diagram of the epidermal layers.

of debris and plasma clots. Repair cells originate from local sources, primarily the dermal appendages and from adjacent intact skin areas. Healing occurs rapidly, and the skin is *regenerated* and is left unscarred.

pH of the Stratum Corneum

The normal pH of the stratum corneum is between 4 and 6.5. This low pH forms an *acid mantle* that enhances the skin's barrier function. Recent studies have demonstrated that enzymatic activity is involved in the formation of this acid mantle. Together, the acid mantle and stratum corneum make the skin less permeable to water and other polar compounds and indirectly protect the skin from invasion by microorganisms.

Damage to the stratum corneum increases the skin pH and, thus, the susceptibility of the skin to bacterial skin infections.[4] For example, hand washing three times a day with cleansing agents alters the acid mantle for several hours, and multiple washings alter the barrier functions, including the skin pH, for up to 14 hours. Increased alkalinity can also be caused by perspiration or urine and stool from incontinence. Systemic diseases, such as diabetes, chronic renal failure, and cerebrovascular

disease, can also cause increased skin pH. Wound dressings and diapers have also been known to raise skin pH.[4]

If the pH of the skin shifts toward alkaline, it can become prone to secondary bacterial and fungal infections. These thrive, for example, in the perineal skin. Other problems associated with increased skin surface pH include eczema, contact dermatitis, atopic dermatitis, perineal dermatitis, and dry skin.

An association between wound surface pH and wound healing has been made. The pH of open wounds tends to be alkaline or neutral (range 6.5–8.5). As new epithelium is formed at the wound edges, the pH on the surface is restored.[5]

Maintenance of the Stratum Corneum

Hydration and lubrication of the stratum corneum are important in keeping the skin intact. Extremes of either dryness or hydration are equally damaging, as is mechanical trauma. Indeed, any disruption in the stratum corneum allows increased transepidermal water loss, impairing the barrier function.[6] Barrier disruption causes a localized inflammatory cascade, which can prompt inflammatory skin diseases such as eczema. For example, removal of wound dressing adhesives can strip the stratum corneum and cause noticeable transepidermal water loss.[7] This in turn triggers an inflammatory wound healing response, proportional to the amount of damage to the skin.

Following such insults, normal adult skin has the capacity to recover its barrier function within 6 hours. Recovery of the barrier is slower in aged skin. During recovery, there is an increase in lipid production within the stratum corneum. Application of effective moisturizer products containing the appropriate mix of lipids can reduce the epidermal water loss during the recovery period. In particular, petrolatum and lanolin-based skin care products have been shown to enhance barrier recovery by reducing water loss and inhibiting the inflammatory reaction of the cells.[6,8]

Skin cleansers and moisturizers that have low or neutral pH are recommended for maintaining the acid mantle of the skin. Soaps are more alkaline than most synthetic detergents and nonionic surfactants (which are slightly acidic or neutral) and should not be used to clean open wounds.[4]

Melanin and Skin Color

Melanin pigmentation accounts for the variation in skin color among humans from very dark to very light. Although the number of melanocytes present in dark and light skin is similar, the size and activity of the melanocytes are greater in dark skin than in light skin. In people with dark skin, the melanin pigmentation is concentrated in a layer of the stratum corneum that can be wiped off when washing. Of course, this does not mean that

RESEARCH WISDOM

Effect of Hand washing on Skin Health of Health-Care Professionals

Health-care professionals wash their hands between each patient, typically more than three times per day, and often develop eczema, contact dermatitis, atopic dermatitis, and dry skin.

CLINICAL WISDOM

Care of Darkly Pigmented Skin

Care of darkly pigmented skin requires keeping the skin lubricated. Petrolatum, lanolin-based lotions, and sparing use of soaps are recommended.[9]

all the color is removed, just the superficial layer. In addition, although the thickness of the stratum corneum in both dark and light skin is the same, the cells in dark skin are more compact and have more cell layers. For this reason, dark skin is more resistant to external irritants. Healthy dark skin is usually smooth and dry, whereas dry dark skin can have an ashen appearance.[9]

Basement Membrane and Dermal-Epidermal Junction

The *basement membrane* is a thin layer of protein that both separates and connects the epidermis and dermis at the dermal epidermal junction.

Dermal Appendages

Dermal appendages, which include hair follicles, sebaceous and sweat glands, fingernails, and toenails, originate in the epidermis and migrate into the dermis.[10] Hair follicles and sebaceous and sweat glands contribute epithelial cells for rapid closure of wounds that do not penetrate through the dermis. The sebaceous glands are responsible for secretions that lubricate the skin, keeping it soft and flexible. They are most numerous in

the face and in the palms of the hands and soles of the feet. Sweat gland secretions control skin pH and thereby reduce the risk of infection. The sweat glands, dermal blood vessels, and small muscles in the skin (responsible for goose pimples) control temperature on the surface of the body. Nerve endings in the skin include receptors for pain, touch, heat, and cold. Loss of these nerve endings, as occurs in peripheral neuropathy, increases the risk for skin breakdown by decreasing the tolerance of the tissues to external forces. Figure 2.3 shows an annotated sonogram of the skin and the dermal appendages.

Dermis

The **dermis**, or the true skin, is a vascular structure that supports and nourishes the epidermis.[10] In addition, sensory nerve endings in the dermis transmit signals regarding pain, pressure, heat, and cold.

The dermis is divided into two layers: the superficial dermis and deep dermis. Figures 2.4 and 2.5 show superficial and deep dermis structures.

Superficial (Papillary) Dermis

The superficial dermis is connective tissue. It consists of an extracellular matrix (ECM) (collagen, elastin, and ground substances) and fibroblasts, which produce the collagen and elastin components that give the skin its turgor and toughness. Fibroblasts also secrete fibronectin and hyaluronic acid (HA) or hyaluronan, major components of the ECM that are primarily proteins and can be found in skin, joints, eyes, and most other organs and tissues. They are also thought to have important biological roles in skin wound healing, by virtue of the presence in high amounts in skin. The hyalurnan content in skin is further elevated transiently in granulation tissue during the wound healing process.[11]

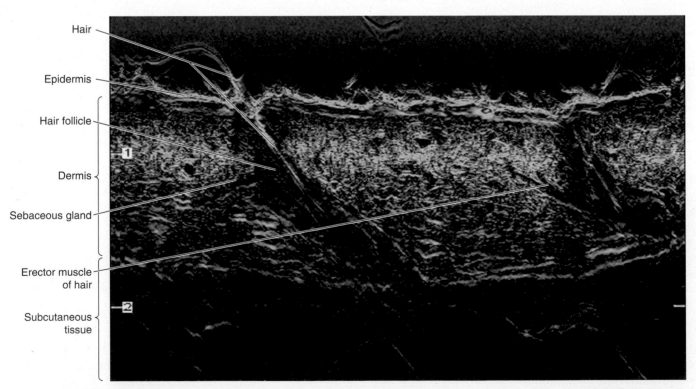

FIGURE 2.3 Sonogram of the skin shows the dermal appendages and layers of the skin. (Copyright © Paul Wilson, Longport Inc.)

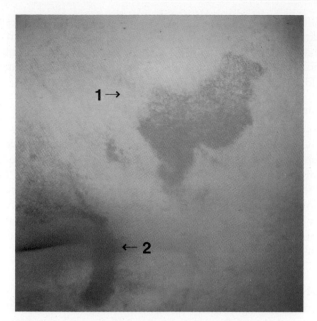

FIGURE 2.4 Superficial Dermis (1) and (2) macerated dermis.

The superficial dermis also contains blood vessels, lymphatics, epithelial cells, small muscles, and neurons. The dermal vascular supply is responsible for nourishing the epidermis, regulating body temperature and skin color. One mechanism of thermoregulation is via blood flow. In this skin layer, there are capillary loops, which are the source of nutrition for the tissues and which also function for thermal regulation through skin surface heat exchange.[12] Younger people have the ability for the dermal vessels to vasodilate as blood flow increases and permit heat to be dissipated from the skin.

Deep (Reticular) Dermis

The deep dermis is located over the subcutaneous fat; it contains larger networks of blood vessels and collagen fibers to provide tensile strength.[10] The well-vascularized dermis will withstand pressure for longer periods of time than will subcutaneous tissue or muscle.

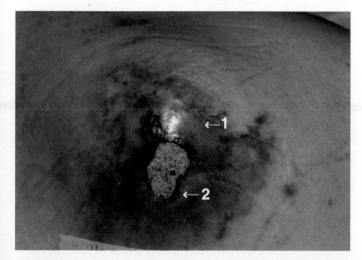

FIGURE 2.5 Acute inflammatory phase, partial-thickness stage II pressure ulcer located over bony prominence. Note: (1) Erythema and edema. (2) Reticular layer of dermis. (Copyright © B.M. Bates-Jensen.)

CLINICAL WISDOM

Because of the highly vascularized anatomy of the dermis, dermal wounds can exude serum, blood, or pus, that lead to formation of clots or crusts; however, they typically heal rapidly.

It also consists of fibroelastic connective tissue, which is yellow and composed mainly of collagen. Fibroblasts are also present in this tissue layer. Wounds that breach this level of tissue are considered to be partial-thickness wounds. They will heal by regeneration as described in the upcoming section about the healing cascade.

Aged Skin

The skin aging process is continuous, and by the fourth decade, morphological changes are seen histologically that affect the function and appearance of the skin including change in skin topography (e.g., lines, wrinkles, and texture) and microcirculation.[12] Since many patients who have poor or nonhealing wounds are elderly, age related changes to the skin are very relevant to wound healing but are not often given adequate consideration due to a lack of awareness and/or knowledge. Therefore, the following materials are included to help you understand the underlying anatomic and physiologic changes that occur in the skin during aging, which affect the speed and healing of wounds in otherwise healthy elders.

Epidermis

During aging, several changes occur in the epidermis that alter function and appearance of the skin structures. These include

- Epidermal changes
- Thickening of the stratum corneum
- Appearance of redness
- Decrease in both Langerhans cells and melanocytes
- Keratinocytes and senescence
- Atrophy of the basal membrane and flattening of the dermal epidermal junction

Epidermal Changes

Age-associated epidermal changes include the atrophy of the epidermis. It becomes thinner and more transparent, and there is increased visibility of the vascular structure in the dermis giving the appearance of redness.[12] There is a thinning of the stratum spinosum and thickening of the stratum corneum. The later thickening is not directly age related but is the body reaction over time to protect the skin from sunlight.[3]

Langerhans Cells

Langerhans cells are the most important antigen-presenting cell population in the skin. Melanocytes are abundant in the hair follicles and also have immune function. In elderly skin, both cell types are decreased in number and Langerhans cells have reduced antigen-trapping capacity, which may explain the diminished cutaneous immune function in the elderly.[3,13]

Keratinocytes

Keratinocyte proliferative activity decreases and the cells become senescent or approach senescence. Senescent cells survive a long time but are unable to divide or die by the process of apoptosis. Cells accumulate with DNA mutations and protein damage until transformation to an "immortal cell" occurs, thus producing a dysfunctional skin repair process due to ineffective DNA repair mechanism resulting in genetic instability and mutations.[3] When the cells stop reproducing or do so slowly, the ability to reepithelialize a wound is impaired. More about this is explained ahead under chronic epithelialization.

Basement Membrane and Dermal-Epidermal Junction

As skin ages, the basement membrane atrophies, and there is a flattening of the dermal-epidermal junction, reduced dermal-epidermal adhesion, and a decrease in epidermal thickness.[3] A consequence of these, and other soon to be explained changes, is limitation of heat transfer to the deeper tissues allowing heat to accumulate at the surface and creating the risk of hyperthermia related skin damage.[14] Another major consequence related to the flattening of the epidermal-dermal junction is the increased fragility of aged skin to shear stress and the readiness of the skin to form blisters.[3]

Dermis

Age-related changes also occur in the dermis including

- Damage to the elastic and collagen fibers
- Increasing skin stiffness
- Papillary capillary loop decrease
- Diminished skin blood flow and risk of hyperthermia
- Sympathetic nervous system (SNS) impairment
- Loss of endothelial vascular activity

Elastic and Collagen

Aging skin suffers superficial dermis changes including damage to elastic and collagen fiber organization with the result that the tensile or breaking strength of the collagen is impaired and the skin is more easily broken or torn.[3]

Capillary Loops

As we learned, the dermis is nourished by the blood flow in capillary loops; as aging progresses, the number of loops decreases and the distance between loops increases and over time they disappear. Perhaps this is why persons over 80 do not have increased skin blood flow in response to thermal stimulation.[15] However, elders exhibit increased blood flow in remaining microvessels, but this may be due to SNS impairment as explained next.[12]

Sympathetic Nervous System

SNS impairment occurs with aging and that affects the dermal vasculature. Since blood flow is dependent on peripheral vascular resistance, which is under SNS control, and blood flow controls thermoregulation, impaired SNS function markedly impairs thermoregulatory control.[16] The reserve capability of the vascular system to vasodilate in response to increased blood flow is reduced and plateaus at a certain point in elderly skin, putting the skin at risk for hyperthermia and burns from inability to dissipate heat quickly enough from the skin.[17]

Diabetes causes early aging of the body and that includes the skin. What has been said about elders can be applied to the diabetic population as well. In this population, the skin blood flow response is profoundly more diminished than in the elderly or even absent.[18]

Impairment of Vascular Endothelial Cells

As part of the aging process, there is damage of the vascular endothelial cells of blood vessels in the skin as well as elsewhere, which causes reduced nitric oxide (NO) and other vasodilator production. NO function is described more fully on page 21. Thus, due to another age related change, the microcirculation capacity needed for heat dissipation of the skin is severely impaired, which allows the skin to heat up more quickly at the same temperature than for younger subjects and to become vulnerable to damage.

Other Soft Tissue Types and the Skeleton

It is critically important for you to be knowledgeable about the anatomy of the structures beneath the skin as well as the skin itself. Once the skin, epidermis, and dermis are breached, other tissues are exposed including superficial fascia, deep fascia, subcutaneous fat, skeletal muscle, tendon, ligament, nerve, bursa, and skeleton. Breach of the tissues beneath the dermis is considered a **full-thickness wound** meaning that it penetrates through the full thickness of the skin layers. Wounds with this loss of tissue integrity will heal by *repair* and **scar formation**, which is described below.

Figure 2.6 is a cadaver dissection of a lower leg that shows the anatomy of the soft tissues located beneath the skin and can be used as a guide through this section.

Different anatomical locations have different depths and types of soft tissue covering the skeleton. For example, over the sacrum, anterior tibial, ankle, and scapula, there is minimal soft tissue. Over the buttocks and calf, there are muscle masses and other soft tissues. All of these anatomical structures are seen in open full-thickness and deeper wounds during wound assessment. Appropriate evaluation of the type and depth of tissue loss is critical for developing a wound severity diagnosis, to appropriately use wound classification systems described in Chapter 3, as well as to spare critical structures during wound debridement and cleansing procedures and to develop a plan of care.

Superficial Fascia

Superficial fascia is located directly beneath the dermis and when healthy looks like a fine mesh network and functions to let the skin move freely. Fascia then wraps around the subcutaneous fat.

Deep Fascia

Deep fascia is a dense fibrous connective tissue that envelopes and separates muscles, tendons, ligaments, blood vessels, nerves, and bones. Healthy deep fascia has a gleaming appearance. In some areas, it attaches muscles to bones such as the iliotibial band that connects the gluteus maximus to the femur. The space between muscle bundles is called the fascial plane. Fascial planes are seen in wounds that have been surgically or sharp debrided where the integrity of the tissue

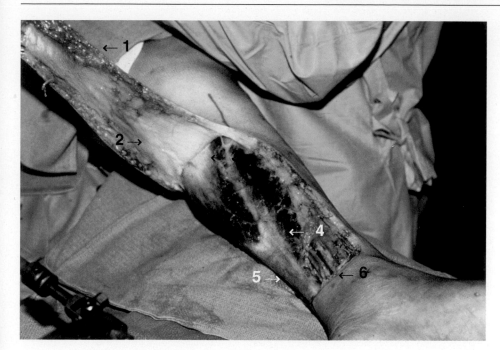

FIGURE 2.6 Full-thickness skin resected from calf. Note: (1) Vascularized dermis. (2) Yellow, healthy fat tissue. (3) White fibrous fascia. (4) Dark red muscle tissue. (5) Tendon covered with peritenon. (6) Blood vessel. (Copyright © J. Wethe.)

is lost. This tissue is composed of collagen and elastin fibers. Although it is an avascular tissue, it is richly innervated by pain nociceptors. Fascia is fragile and can be readily torn by finger pressure. When the fascia is torn along a fascial plane, a separation occurs between the layers and is commonly called a tunnel. Tunnels are areas where infection can travel and an abscess may form.

Subcutaneous Fat

Subcutaneous fat is located directly beneath the dermis. Function of the subcutaneous fat is thermal regulation. Heat transfer to the deeper tissues is impaired by thick subcutaneous fat layers and this contributes to warmer skin temperature when heat is added to the body (e.g., warm room and warm water).[15] Aging also reduces the thickness of the subcutaneous fat layer.[18] The healthy appearance of subcutaneous fat is pale yellow, waxy, globular, and oily and glistens like shown in Figure 2.7.

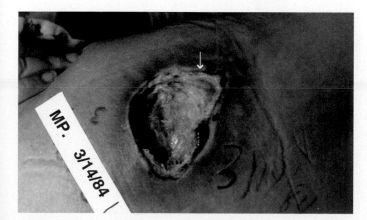

FIGURE 2.7 Subcutaneous fat in full-thickness wound. Eschar after debridement. Necrotic fat and fascia often called slough. Restart of inflammatory phase. Absence of proliferative phase. (Copyright © C. Sussman.)

When exposed to air and drying, the appearance changes as the fat congeals and turns to a tan or yellow-brown color. When fat is observed in a wound, like shown in Figure 2.7, it is classified as a full-thickness wound.[19] Classification systems for wounds are discussed in detail in Chapter 3.

Skeletal Muscle

Skeletal muscle is striated, looks like that shown in Figure 2.8, and will jump or spring back when pinched. Healthy muscle is well vascularized and deep red in color. Because of its high levels of vascularity, it is extremely sensitive to hypoxic and ischemic states caused by pressure. Poorly vascularized or ischemic muscle will be pink, pale, and/or cyanotic (bluish).

Tendon

Tendon is an extension of muscle whose function is to connect muscles to bones. It consists of a tough band of inelastic connective tissue covered with a fascial sheath called peritenon. Peritenon is essential for tissue healing. As a part of the muscle, tendon has muscle characteristics of jumping when touched or pinched. Tendons have few blood vessels but are innervated with sensory nerve fibers near the musculotendinous junction. Exposed tendons will dry and the peritenon sheath may die. Tendons are often observed in full-thickness foot and hand wounds. Figure 2.9 is a drawing of a foot with tendons, ligaments, and associated blood vessels.

Ligaments

Ligaments are strong fibrous bands of connective tissue that connect bones together. They are more flexible than extensible and some limit motion. Ligaments contain nerve endings that are important in reflex mechanisms and in the perception of movement and position. The appearance of ligaments is pearly white, and they are flatter and more loosely woven than tendons and have a shiny fascia covering. In the ankle, ligaments are very superficial and may be seen if skin is removed.[20]

FIGURE 2.8 Skeletal muscle. Surgical dissection demonstrating the extent of the tunneling process, forming a sinus tract. (Copyright © J. Wethe.)

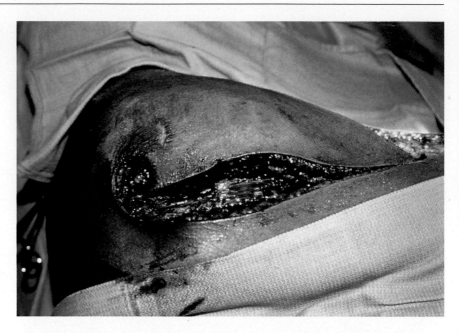

Nerves

Nerves likely to be seen in wounds are long strands of yellow/gray tissue. Major peripheral nerves that can be seen are usually 2 to 3 mm in diameter. Avoid handling the nerve as they are easily damaged. Smaller nerves will not be visible to the naked eye but their presence needs to be understood.

Bursa (Plural, Bursae)

Bursae are synovial fluid-filled sacs composed of fibrous connective tissue that is lined with synovial membrane. The function of the bursa is to provide shock absorption between bones, tendons, and muscles. They are found around joints including the elbow, the trochanter, ischium, and the knee. Leaking synovial fluid can be identified by its sticky, mucous-like fluid.

Bones

Bones are the hard skeletal frame of the body. The appearance of bone is white, shiny, and hard and covered with a sheath of connective tissue called periosteum. Healthy periosteum feels smooth and looks shiny. In the absence of periosteum, the bone may feel rough and repair compromised.

FIGURE 2.9 Drawing of foot with tendons and ligaments and blood supply.

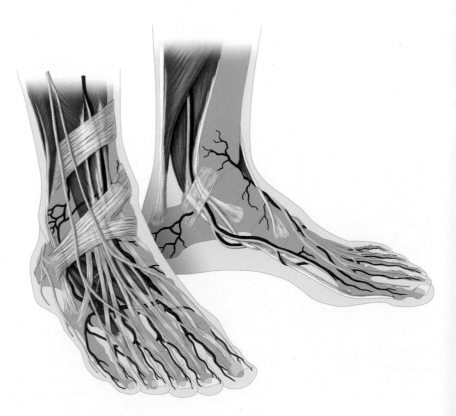

WOUND HEALING PHYSIOLOGY: AN OVERVIEW

Anatomic depth of tissue loss due to wounding is predictive of healing.[21,22] Superficial wounds involve the epidermis as shown in Figure 2.4. They are resolved by subcutaneous inflammatory processes, with the exception of wounds with intact skin that also have deep tissue injury and can manifest later as deep wounds such as shown in Figure 2.10 and 2.11. Partial-thickness wounds, which do not extend beneath the dermis, heal by epithelialization or regeneration and heal faster than subcutaneous and full-thickness wounds that heal by secondary intention or repair. **Epithelialization** is the resurfacing of a wound by new epithelial cells, which are mostly keratinocytes derived from the wound edges and dermal appendages. In partial-thickness wounds, the skin is **regenerated** and has the properties of the original skin. Full-thickness and subcutaneous wounds heal by secondary intention, which concludes with scar formation, and scar tissue lacks the properties of the original tissues. **Secondary intention** refers to a process in which the wound is **repaired** by the generation of granulation tissue, whose appearance is like a bunch of granules piled upon each other that fills the wound space and enables closure. Granulation tissue is the manifestation of the process of **fibroplasia**, laying down of the **extracellular matrix**, an intricate system of glycosaminoglycans (GAGs) and proteins that provides the framework to support **angiogenesis**, growth of new blood vessels, and to fill the wound space. **Contraction** is the drawing together of the wound edges like the stings of a purse and speeds closure. Granulation tissue is eventually reabsorbed and replaced by **scar tissue**, collagen fibers that are deposited in the granulation tissue. Figure 2.12 shows a diagrammatic representation of first and secondary intention healing.

Five basic wound healing models are discussed in this book.

1. **Superficial wound healing.** A wound involving only the epidermis.

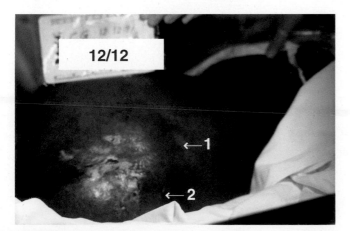

FIGURE 2.10 Suspected deep tissue pressure ulcer. Ulceration with multiple, small, stage II open areas. Wound is in acute inflammatory phase. Note onset date 12/12. Note: (1) Clear line of demarcation between healthy tissues and inflamed tissues. (2) Evidence of discoloration, edema, and induration, suggesting underlying tissue death. Assess tissue temperature and pain. (Copyright © C. Sussman.)

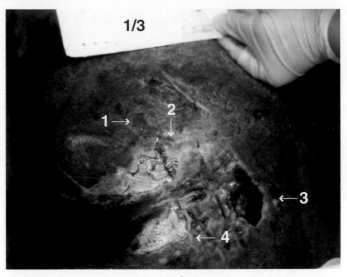

FIGURE 2.11 Same pressure ulcer as Figure 2.10. Three weeks later, the skin shows evidence of the severe tissue destruction that occurred at the time of trauma. Note delayed manifestation of injury at the skin level. The date was 1/3. Note: (1) Continued demarcation of inflamed tissue. (2) Irregular, diffuse wound edges. (3) Black and adherent eschar. (4) Partial-thickness skin loss; there is enlargement of stage II ulcers compared with those in Figure 2.10. The correct staging for this sacrococcygeal pressure ulcer is at minimum a stage III. Once eschar is removed, the true depth of tissue loss can be determined. Documentation should reflect a combined area of wounding, including all three visible ulcers and the area of inflammation; this is the overall size estimate for the pressure ulcer. Inflammation is now chronic. (Copyright © C. Sussman.)

2. **Partial-thickness, wound healing.** A wound involving the epidermis and the uppermost layers of the dermis.
3. **Full-thickness/second intention wound healing.** Any wound extending through all layers of the epidermis, dermis, into subcutaneous tissues and deeper structures that heals by secondary intention.
4. **Primary or first intention wound healing.** A wound healing process in which a wound is cleaned, the edges approximated by a surgeon, and then held in place with sutures or another method.
5. **Delayed primary intention wound healing.** A dirty wound is left open to allow cleansing and then closed by the surgeon.

There are similarities among all five models. This section briefly discusses the superficial, partial-thickness, and full-thickness/secondary intention wound healing models. An overview of chronic wound healing is then presented, followed by fetal wound healing. Chapter 8 covers the primary intention and delayed primary intention healing models that occur in surgical wounds.

Superficial Wound Healing

Alterations in the superficial skin, such as those caused by pressure (e.g., in stage I pressure ulcers), first-degree burns, and contusions, activate an inflammatory repair process that is comparable to that of open wounds.[23] Superficial skin involvement can also indicate deeper soft tissue trauma, which warrants investigation for changes in skin color, temperature (e.g., warmth, followed by coolness, indicating

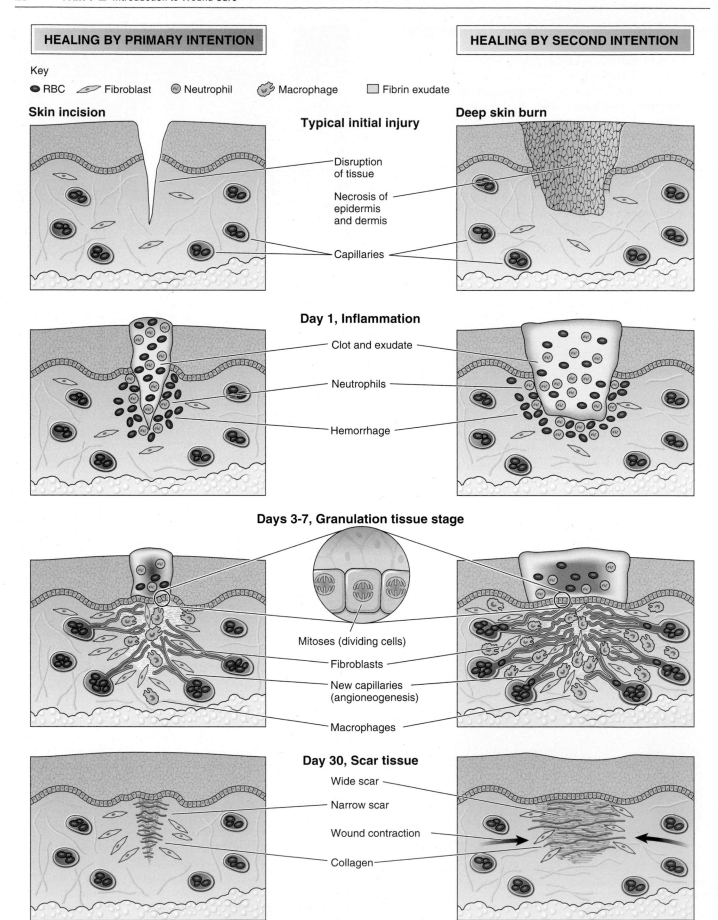

FIGURE 2.12 Healing by first and secondary intention.

tissue death [devitalization]), tissue tension or swelling (indicating tissue congestion), and sensation.

If deep tissue death occurs, the tissues can rupture and become a deep cavity. This often occurs in stage I pressure ulcers and is referred to as the *erupting volcano* effect. This effect is now attributed to deep tissue injury, and is manifested under the skin as a purple discoloration, leading to the name "purple ulcers." Figure 2.10 shows what initially appeared to be superficial and partial-thickness (stages I and II) pressure ulcers, but there are also signs of purple deep discoloration in the surrounding tissues suggestive of deep tissue injury. The true degree of involvement manifested itself 3 weeks after they are first diagnosed (Fig. 2.11). It is significant that the manifestation doesn't occur immediately because the staging of the ulcer will not be possible until that happens. (Chapter 3 discusses assessment of suspected deep tissue injury and staging.)

In superficial wound healing, the soft tissues usually heal by themselves over time, but intervention at this stage can hasten return to functional activities, such as work and homemaking. For example, athletes are often assessed and treated immediately for superficial soft tissue injuries, with reduced loss of playing time, less pain, and less tissue swelling from congestion in the tissues. Tissue swelling can limit functional activities, resulting in diminished mobility and placing the individual at risk for further wounding.

Partial-Thickness Wound Healing

Wounds with partial-thickness loss of the dermis heal principally by epithelialization, see Figure 2.5. Epithelialization is the body's attempt to protect itself from invasion or debris by beginning to close the wound; this process begins immediately following injury.

Epithelial cells at the wound edges, as well as from the dermal appendages—sebaceous glands, sweat glands, and hair follicles—provide a supply of intact epithelial cells to assist in resurfacing the wound by lateral migration.[24,25] If dermal appendages are

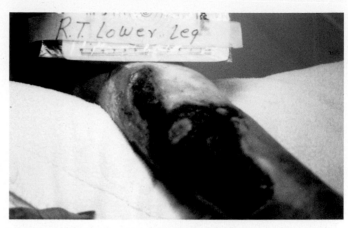

FIGURE 2.13 Note islands of epidermal tissue which indicate probable presence of dermal appendages. (Copyright © C. Sussman.)

present, islands of epidermis can appear throughout the wound surface and speed the resurfacing process. The resulting epithelium is often indistinguishable from the surrounding skin, and the normal function of the skin is restored. Figures 2.13 and 2.14 show a wound resurfacing from islands of epidermis. Examples of partial-thickness wounds are abrasions, skin tears, stage II pressure ulcers, and second-degree burns.

Full-Thickness or Secondary Intention Healing

Secondary intention healing is the most effective method of healing full-thickness wounds. It is necessary because, when a large amount of tissue is removed or destroyed, a gap occurs, and either the wound edges cannot be approximated or nonviable wound margins are present or both (Figure 2.15). Wounds with a high microorganism count, debris, or skin necrosis are also left to close by secondary intention (Figure 2.16).

Full-thickness secondary intention healing principally occurs by *contraction*, a reduction of the wound surface area by the drawing together of the wound edges

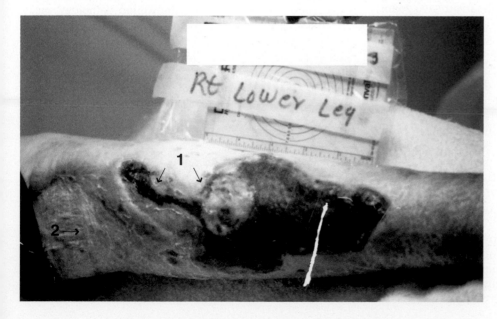

FIGURE 2.14 Same wound as Figure 2.13. Note: (1) Epidermal migration from wound edges, island, and wound shape changes. (2) Progression to the acute epithelialization phase. (3) Hyperkeratotic skin changes due to old burn wounds and poor circulation. (Copyright © C. Sussman.)

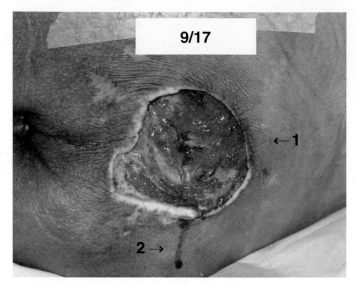

FIGURE 2.15 Full thickness Wound Healing by Secondary Intention. (Copyright © B.M. Bates-Jensen.)

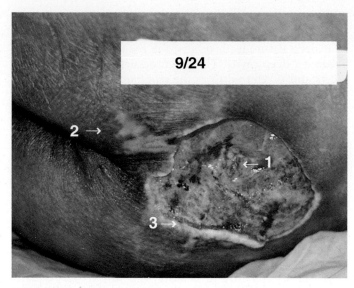

FIGURE 2.16 Same ulcer as Figure 2.15 with attributes of infection. Note change in color of granulation tissue from red to dusky pink. (Copyright © B.M. Bates-Jensen.)

(Figures 2.17– 2.19). This results in scar tissue formation. In this process, the anatomic structure of the scar tissue does not replicate that of the tissue being replaced (e.g., muscles, tendons, or nerves); thus, original tissue function is lost. In addition, the surface tissue will not be equal in elasticity or tensile strength to the original.[24] Sometimes, defects are too large or will result in suboptimal reconstruction of the skin defect if surgically closed by primary intention. Then healing by secondary intention is preferred.

If a wound is located in an area where contraction will produce disfiguring or nonfunctional deformities, the process of healing by secondary intention can be allowed initially, in order to develop a strong, healthy wound bed. Then it is interrupted, and a skin graft is placed on the granulating wound bed. **Autologous** skin transplants are taken from the person's own body and grafted to the wound surface. Donor sites are chosen from appropriate body surfaces. Skin grafts are divided into two main categories: full-thickness skin grafts (FTSGs) and split thickness skin grafts (STSGs). STSGs are thin (0.008–0.018 mm). FTSGs are thicker (0.018–0.030 mm). Both include the epidermis and FTSGs include the dermis as well. STSGs include only part of the dermis. The donor site then becomes a secondary wound, which will need to heal. FTSGs are used to correct defects when cosmesis is a primary concern and the defect to be corrected is not too large. STSGs are used if cosmesis is not a concern or if FTSG is precluded. Skin grafting is used for nonhealing cutaneous ulcers, to replace tissue in full-thickness burns and for reconstruction of skin after removal of malignancies.[26] Chapter 8 covers surgical wounds and grafts and Chapter 15 grafts and burns.

Healing of full-thickness wounds by secondary intention involves a process that is divided into four overlapping phases of repair: inflammation, epithelialization, proliferation, and remodeling. Each of these phases will be discussed in detail later in this chapter.

Chronic Wound Healing

Secondary intention is the healing model associated with chronic wounds.[27] A **chronic wound** Exhibit 2.1 is defined as one that has "failed to proceed through an orderly and timely process to produce anatomic and functional integrity, or proceeded through the repair process without establishing a sustained anatomic and functional result."[27]

Orderly refers to the progression of the wound through the biological sequences that comprise the phases of repair of acute wounds described shortly. Orderliness can be interrupted during any of the phases of healing, but only recently have the causative factors for these interruptions been identified. Causative factors that affect the orderly progression of the healing process are presented in this chapter for each phase of wound healing.

Timeliness relates to the progression of the phases of repair in a manner that will heal the wound expeditiously. Timeliness is determined by the nature of the wound pathology, medical status of the patient, and environmental factors.[27] Those wounds that *do not* repair themselves in an orderly and timely manner are classified as chronic wounds; those that do are classified as acute wounds.

EXHIBIT	**2.1**

Examples of Chronic Wounds

- Ischemic arterial ulcers
- Diabetic vascular and neuropathic ulcers
- Venous ulcers
- Vasculitic ulcers
- Rheumatoid ulcers
- Pressure ulcers

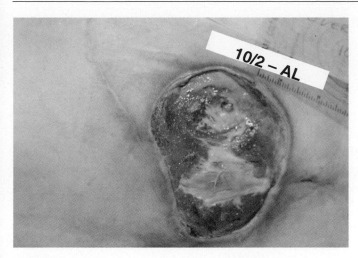

FIGURE 2.17 Epidermal ridge formation with rolled edges. (Copyright © C. Sussman.)

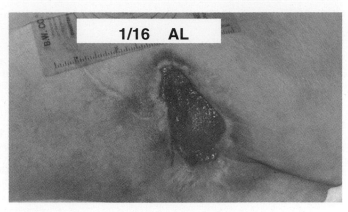

FIGURE 2.19 Same wound as in Figures 2.17 and 2.18. Note sustained wound contraction and progression of epithelialization and proliferative phase. (Copyright © C. Sussman.)

Fetal Wound Healing

Researchers are studying what can be learned from fetal wound healing that will be useful in promoting improved wound healing. It has been known for some time that fetuses who undergo surgery in utero do not form scars.[28–30] Fetal wounds are continually bathed in amniotic fluid, which has a rich content of HA and fibronectin, as well as growth factors crucial to fetal development. HA is a key structural and functional component of the ECM, which fosters an environment that promotes cell proliferation and tissue regeneration and repair.[25,31] HA is laid down in the matrix of both fetal and adult wounds, but its sustained deposition is unique to fetal wounds. Many questions remain to be answered regarding fetal wound healing. There are many differences between fetal development and adult repair and regeneration. For example, the transplacental circulation provides a partial pressure of oxygen of 20 mm Hg, which is markedly lower than that in adults, signifying that the fetus lives in a hypoxic environment.[32] This is in marked contrast to the adult environment, where oxygen is a critical factor in prevention of infection and in the repair process. There are also differences in the fetal and adult immune systems, the histology of fetal skin during development, the function of adult versus fetal fibroblasts in collagen synthesis, the absence of myofibroblasts, and the absence of an inflammatory phase.[33,34]

An example of the effects of HA and amniotic fluid on healing of surgical wounds was reported by Byl et al. in two studies.[35,36] Amniotic fluid, HA, and normal saline were applied to controlled incisional wounds. The surgeons were blinded to the fluids applied. Incisions treated with HA and amniotic fluid both healed faster than the saline-treated wounds; in fact, they appeared to close within minutes of application. The healing was quicker, and the quality of the scar was better in the HA and amniotic fluid incisions than in the saline-treated incisions. The tensile strengths of the wounds treated with amniotic fluid and HA were slightly weaker than those of the saline-treated group at the end of 1 week; however, after 2 weeks, all groups had equal tensile strength.

Four Phases of Wound Healing

The physiological process of acute wound healing includes four phases: inflammation, epithelialization, proliferation, and remodeling. Rather than a series of distinct steps, these phases have been described as a cascade of overlapping events that occurs in a reasonably predictable fashion. A diagram by Hunt and Van Winkle[1] (Figure 2.20) features inflammation the central activity of wound healing—in its center. On either side are proliferation and epithelialization—the concurrent events that occur as a consequence of injury. The lower portion of the diagram represents the coming together of the phases, leading to the remodeling phase of wound healing. The interpretation of this diagram is that the four phases occur in an orderly,

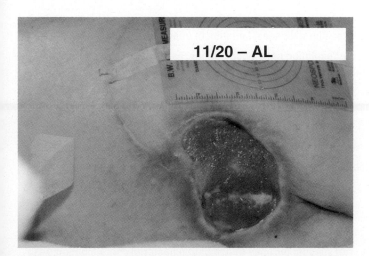

FIGURE 2.18 This is the same wound as Figure 2.17 that is progressing through the proliferative phase. It is contracting and changing size and shape. (Copyright © C. Sussman.)

RESEARCH WISDOM

HA is a gel that is degraded in vivo and breaks down rapidly when applied to wounds. A wound dressing called Hyaff (ConvaTec, a Bristol Myers Squibb company, Princeton, NJ) has recently been produced from HA. When applied to the wound, this dressing creates an HA-rich tissue interface and moist wound environment conducive to granulation and healing (see Chapter 20).[37]

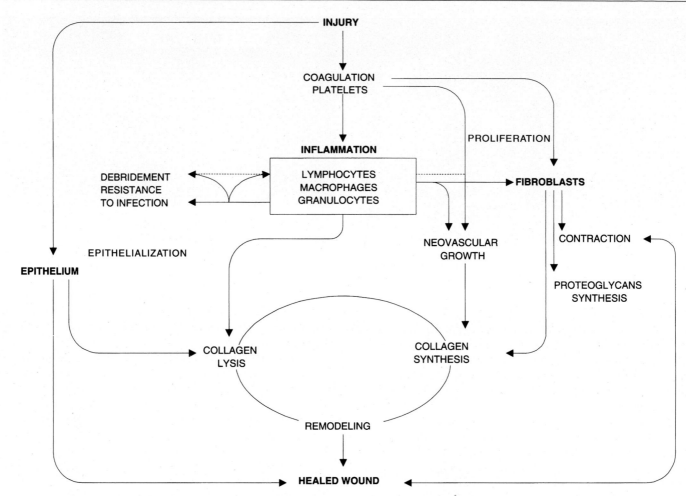

FIGURE 2.20 Diagram of wound repair. (Reprinted with permission from Hunt TK, Van Winkle W. Fundamentals of Wound Management in Surgery, Wound Healing: Normal Repair. South Plainfield, NJ: Chirurgecom, Inc, 1976.)

TABLE 2.1	**Terminology Associated with Wound Healing Physiology**

Term	Definition (Reference)
Angiogenesis	Development of new blood vessels in injured tissues. Function of endothelial cells.
Apoptosis	A mechanism for cell deletion in the regulation of cell populations, as of B and T lymphocytes following cytokine depletion. Often used synonymously with *programmed cell death.*
Basement membrane	Thin layer of extracellular material found between the layers of the epithelia or between the epithelia and connective tissue. Also called *basal lamina*.[39]
Chemoattractants	Cause cell migration.
Chemotaxis	Attraction of a cell in response to a chemical signal.
Chronic wound	Wound that has "failed to proceed through an orderly and timely process to produce anatomic and functional integrity, or proceeded through the repair process without establishing a sustained anatomic and functional result."[27]
Collagenases	Enzymes that cleave (break) the bonds of the polypeptide chains in collagen at specific sites, aiding in its resorption during periods of connective tissue growth or repair.[39]
Complement system	Eleven proteins found in plasma with specific purpose of combating bacterial contamination. Also chemotactic for phagocytes; substances most responsible for acute inflammation.[24]
ECM	Intricate system of GAGs and proteins secreted by cells; provides the framework for tissues.[39]

TABLE 2.1	Terminology Associated with Wound Healing Physiology (*continued*)
Term	**Definition (Reference)**
Free radicals	Highly reactive molecular species that have at least one unpaired electron in the outer shell. Attempt to react with other molecules to achieve an electrically more stable state in which the electron is paired with another. Important for normal cell functions, including metabolism and defense against infection.[74]
Galvanotaxis	Attraction of a cell in response to an electrical signal.
GAGs	Polysaccharides that contain amino acids, sugars, and glycoprotein. Termed *proteoglycans*.[97]
Growth factors (GFs)	Extracellular polypeptides—proteins able to affect cell reproduction, movement, and function. Term encompasses items c, d, and e, below. Regulators of the wound healing cascade. May be deficient in chronic wounds.[39]
a. Autocrine stimulation	GF produced by a cell acting on itself.
b. Paracrine stimulation	GF produced by one cell type acting on another in the local area.
c. Endocrine stimulation	GF produced by one cell type acting on distant cells.
d. Cytokines	Refers to diverse group of polypeptides and glycoproteins that are important mediators of inflammation. Anti-inflammatory cytokines inhibit production of proinflammatory cytokines, counter their action or both
e. Interleukins (ILs)	A group of proinflammatory cytokines
f. Colony-stimulating factor	Term for GF used by hematologists.[120]
Hemostasis	Coagulation to stop bleeding and initiate the wound healing process.
Hydroxyproline (HoPro)	A polypeptide chain of insoluble collagen.
Integrins	Regulate a wide range of cellular functions during growth, development, differentiation, and the immune response. Serve a critical function in cell adhesion and signaling during wound healing, where they are fundamental to reepithelialization and granulation tissue formation.[94]
Ligand	A molecule that binds to another molecule, used especially to refer to a small molecule that binds specifically to a larger molecule.[121]
MMPs	Proteolytic enzymes that degrade proteins and ECM macromolecules. MMPs have the ability to degrade a variety of ECM components, which is of benefit in the developmental and remodeling processes in healthy tissues.[94] Synthesized and secreted by multiple cell types involved in wound healing in response to biochemical signals.
Mitogens	Cause cell growth.
Mitogenic	Causing mitosis or cellular proliferation.
Neovascularization	Development of new blood vessels; another term for angiogenesis.
Phagocytosis	Ingestion, destruction, and digestion of cellular particulate matter.[39]
Proteases	Proteolytic enzymes that degrade proteins.[39]
Substrates	Substances acted upon by an enzyme, such as substances necessary for new tissue growth: protein, vitamin C, zinc.
Tensile strength	The most longitudinal stress that a substance can withstand without tearing apart.
TIMPs	Secreted proteins that are widely distributed in tissues and fluids and serve as specific inhibitors for the MMPs. Synthesized and secreted by same multiple cell types as MMPs.[52]

overlapping fashion. Incidentally, the literature identifies either three or four phases of repair, depending on whether epithelialization is included as part of proliferation or as a separate phase. The wound healing model used in this text is based on four phases.

The biologic repair process is the same for all acute wounds, open or closed, regardless of etiology. However, the sequence of repair is completed more quickly in primary healing and when involvement is limited to superficial and partial-thickness skin. Slower healing occurs when there is full-thickness skin loss extending into and through the subcutaneous tissue.[38] Table 2.1 defines key terminology associated with wound healing physiology to facilitate understanding.

Attributes that distinguish the healing of chronic wounds from that of acute wounds are continually being studied. Thus, after we explain the process of normal wound healing in a particular phase in each of the sections that follow, we go on to discuss the attributes and processes that may be responsible for chronic wound healing in that phase. Table 2.2 summarizes factors and their effects on chronic wound healing during each phase of repair.

TABLE 2.2   Summary of Factors and Effects during Each Phase of Wound Healing in Chronic Wounds

Chronic Inflammatory Phase	Chronic Epithelialization Phase	Chronic Proliferative Phase	Chronic Remodeling Phase
Different stimulus of repair	Diminished keratinocyte migration due to	Different composition of fibronectin:	Imbalance of collagen synthesis and degradation:
a. From within	a. Lack of moist environment	a. Partially degraded into fragments	a. Impaired scar tensile strength
b. Gradual	b. Lack of oxygen	b. Fragments may perpetuate activity of matrix proteases	b. Overproduction of collagen: hypertrophic scarring
c. Slowed	c. Lack of nutritious tissue base	c. Inhibit healing	c. Imbalance of fibrotic and antifibrotic cytokines: hypergranulation
	d. Lack of stimulation by appropriate cytokine		
Inadequate perfusion and oxygenation:	Keratinocyte migration obstructed by wound edges that are	Excess activity of proteases causes:	Hyperoxygenation:
a. Muted phase process	a. Rolled	a. Accelerated rate of connective tissue breakdown	a. Hypertrophy of granulation tissue
b. Ischemic tissue barrier to angiogenesis	b. Thickened	b. Destruction of polypeptide-signaling molecules	b. Impediment to epidermal cell migration
	c. Nonproductive	c. Production of metalloproteinases that do not lyse collagen	
Free radicals and oxygen reperfusion injury:	Keratinocyte migration slowed due to	Chronic wound fluid inhibition of:	Impairment of scar tensile strength:
a. Large production of free radicals	a. Large gap	a. Cellular proliferation: endothelial cells, keratinocytes, fibroblasts	a. Wound breakdown
b. Disruption in normal defense against free radicals	b. Slow filling of "dead space"	b. Cell adhesion	b. Dehiscence
c. Capillary plugging by neutrophils		Repeated trauma and infection:	
		a. Increases the presence of proinflammatory cytokines	
		b. Increases the presence of tissue inhibitors (metalloproteinases)	
		c. Lowers the level of growth factors	
		Impediments to wound healing:	
		a. Elevated levels of MMPs	
		b. Imbalance between levels of MMPs and their inhibitors (TIMPs)	
		Large tissue defect:	
		a. Prolongs proliferation of tissue to fill the space	

TABLE 2.2	Summary of Factors and Effects during Each Phase of Wound Healing in Chronic Wounds (*continued*)		
Chronic Inflammatory Phase	**Chronic Epithelialization Phase**	**Chronic Proliferative Phase**	**Chronic Remodeling Phase**
		Substrates relationship to stalling or plateauing:	
		a. Inadequate substrates	
		b. Bacterial competition for substrates necessary for tissue repair	
		c. Continued lysis of new growth faster than synthesis of new material	
		Long-term wound hypoxia effects:	
		a. Negative effect on collagen production	
		b. Decreased fibroblast proliferation	
		c. Decreased tissue growth	
		Impaired wound contraction:	
		a. Wound remains large	
		b. Delayed reepithelialization	

Adapted from Bates-Jensen B. A Quantitative Analysis of Wound Characteristics as Early Predictors of Healing in Pressure Sores. Dissertation Abstracts International, Volume 59, Number 11, University of California, Los Angeles; 1999, with permission.

INFLAMMATORY PHASE

Inflammation is a normal reaction of the body's immune system to tissue injury. The classic observable signs and symptoms of inflammation are also the benchmarks of the inflammatory phase and include changes in

- Color in the surrounding skin (red, blue, purple)
- Temperature (heat)
- Turgor (swelling)
- Sensation (pain)
- Function (reduced function)

These benchmarks, some of which can be seen in the wounds in Figure 2.4 are only minimally manifested with normal healing; thus, when severe as in Figure 2.21, they should be regarded as clinical signs of excessive inflammation that are characteristic of impending infection.[39] The inflammation response is sometimes referred to as a "flare" because the suddenness of the response, color, and associated temperature changes are reminiscent of the flaring up of a fire. The descriptions of the physiologic events that are presented in the following sections will explain the scientific basis for the classic signs and symptoms of inflammation: reddening of the surrounding tissues (or, in individuals with darkly pigmented skin, a purple or violaceous discoloration), pain, heat, and edema.

Inflammation is essential for orderly, timely healing. The physiology of inflammation is well regulated in the normally healing acute wound and typically lasts 3 to 7 days. Acute inflammation begins soon after the injury, setting into motion a biologic cascade of events. The major goals of the inflammatory phase of healing are to provide for **hemostasis** (controlled bleeding) and the breakdown and removal of cellular, extracellular, and pathogen debris; this produces a clean wound site for tissue restoration and initiation of the repair process. **Growth factors** (cytokines) are signaling biochemical substances that are expressed at the time of injury within the wound,

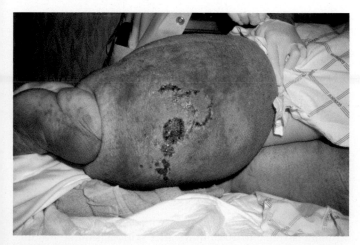

FIGURE 2.21 Clinical signs of excessive inflammation, the "flare" or erythema, turgor, and reduced ankle function are present. (Courtesy of A. Myer.)

FIGURE 2.22 The phases of acute wound healing.

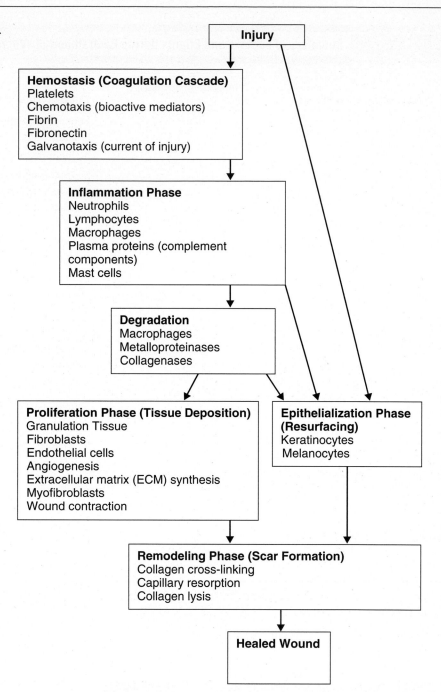

communicate with and attract responder cells and regulate the repair process. Growth factors are explained more fully on page 20.

Figure 2.22 shows an algorithm of healing through a distinct but overlapping series of processes, leading to scar formation and normal wound healing. The following is a description of the key processes of the acute inflammatory phase, including

- Coagulation cascade to achieve platelet activation and hemostasis
- Hypoxia and regulation via the oxygen-tension gradient
- Oxygen and antibacterial effects
- Nitric oxide and cellular signaling
- Vasodilation
- Hypothermia

- Complement system activation to control infection
- Neutrophil, mast, macrophage, and fibroblast cell functions
- Growth factors and other regulatory proteins
- "Current of injury" stimulus for the repair process

As noted earlier, after describing normal inflammation, we will discuss the attributes and processes that may be responsible for chronic wound healing during the inflammatory phase.

Platelets, Hemostasis, and the Coagulation Cascade

The coagulation cascade begins with clotting and vasoconstriction lasting 5 to 10 minutes after skin incision, to produce hemostasis at the site of wounding immediately after injury to control hemorrhaging and reduce blood loss (Figure 2.23).

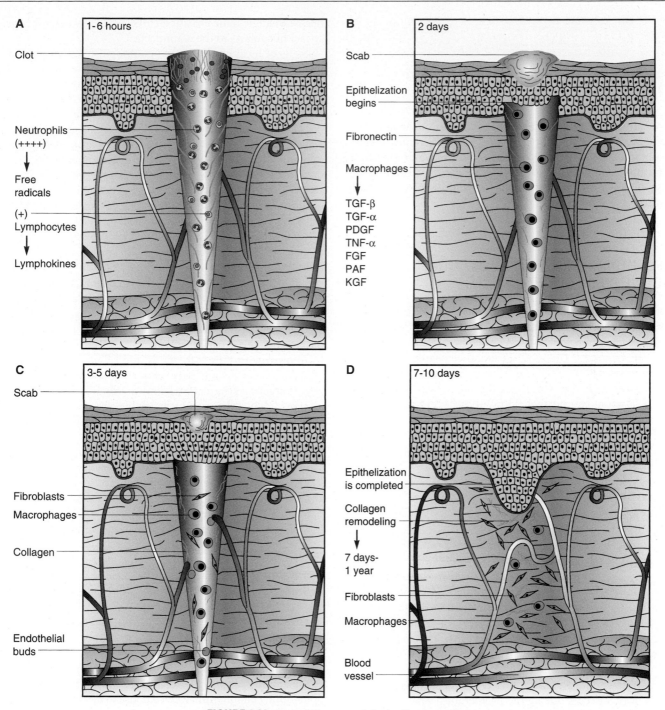

FIGURE 2.23 Growth factors and the healing cascade.

Hemostasis is initiated as the first major function of the platelets. **Platelets**, white blood cells that are normally present in the intravascular space, are activated by collagen or microfibrils from the subendothelial layers that are exposed when injury occurs resulting in *platelet aggregation* (*clotting*) and *degranulation*. This process known as *platelet activation* induces changes in platelet structure and function necessary for coagulation to occur, including thrombin, fibrinous clot production, and, ultimately, hemostasis.[39] The fibrin clot becomes the primary foundation for collagen deposition, which will be necessary for tissue repair, and the pathway for the influx of monocytes and fibroblasts to the wound site.[40] The second, equally important function of the platelet is the secretion of cytokines and growth factors with multiple functions, including recruitment of leukocytes, and fibroblasts to the injury site.[41] Growth factors and other regulatory peptides like cytokines are discussed on page 20. Fibrin clots also seal off the lymphatic flow to prevent spreading of infection. However, immediately after the formation of the fibrinous clot, the process of **fibrinolysis** to lyse the clot begins.[42] Unplugging of the capillaries and vasodilation follows and permits entrance of fluid into the wound space, which activates the complement system that is explained on page 22. Coagulation and the ensuing events described above are known as the coagulation cascade.

RESEARCH WISDOM

Evaluating Postoperative Healing by Monitoring Temperature

In postoperative patients, you can determine the temperature pattern of healing by taking daily measurements of local skin temperatures following surgery. The measurements can be obtained using liquid crystal strips (see Chapter 3). If the zone of warmth does not decrease in width by the fourth postoperative day, the possibility of wound infection and disturbed healing exists.[46]

HYPOTHERMIA, PLATELET ACTIVATION, AND THE COAGULATION CASCADE

Hypothermia, often associated with surgery, inhibits platelet activation and increases bleeding time. Even a 0.2°C lowering of core body temperature will trigger peripheral vasoconstriction and tissue hypoxia.[43] Unless corrected, the coagulation cascade may not proceed normally, and there is increased risk of blood loss and infection. Rewarming of the blood will restore both platelet function and normal clotting time.[44,45] Hypothermia is often undetected.

Fibronectin secretion is an adhesive glycoprotein secreted during the inflammatory phase as part of the process of ECM formation.

Wound Space Hypoxia and Regulation via the Oxygen-Tension Gradient

Vasoconstriction, coagulation, and lack of blood flow quickly deplete oxygen delivery to the wound space, producing an environmental change to the state of hypoxia. Soon after wounding, an oxygen-tension gradient develops between the surrounding tissues and the wound space. This gradient is a key factor in initiating the healing cascade and stimulating tissue repair. If the normal gradient of oxygen is eliminated, a macrophage-free tissue space may be created causing the process of **angiogenesis**, new blood vessel growth by the endothelial cells, to be temporarily or permanently inhibited. Hypoxia itself acts as a signal that recruits endothelial responder cells and stimulates angiogenesis, which occurs during the proliferation phase. Hypoxia, however, puts the tissues at risk for infection by impairing the function of neutrophils, lymphocytes, macrophages, and fibroblasts. Local hypoxia also causes a shift to anaerobic glycolysis with increased lactate production, which is involved in activation of both angiogenesis and collagen synthesis (see page 27), activities essential for later tissue repair. Unrelated trauma, like a surgical procedure, to a site remote from an existing wound also can retard the rate of healing, alter the tensions of respiratory gases, and cause increased susceptibility to wound infection in the existing wound, probably due to decreased nutritive blood flow.[47]

Lactate accumulation from white blood cells at the site contributes to a hyperlactic and acidotic wound space.[38,48,49] In conjunction with the lactate produced through anaerobic metabolism and from white blood cells, hypoxia stimulates the release of angiogenic growth factors (AGFs) by macrophages to attract fibroblasts to the wound site.[50,51]

Signs of local hypoxia often go undetected. One example is the case of perioperative hypothermia-induced vasoconstriction and tissue hypoxia, which have been shown to triple the incidence of perioperative surgical wound infection.[43]

Thus, it should not be surprising that research on the activities of GFs shows that they provide the key biochemistry for the wound healing process. Platelets, macrophages, and epidermal cells are the primary cells that produce and release GFs. As such, they are the critical components initiating the wound healing cascade. These include *platelet-derived growth factor* (PDGF), epidermal growth factor (EGF), *transforming growth factor-ß* (TGF-ß), *heparin-binding epidermal growth factor* (HB-EGF), and *insulin-like growth factor-1* (IGF-1), all of which facilitate cell migration of neutrophils and macrophages to the area of injury.[39,41] PDGF is multifunctional, playing multiple roles in wound healing, including release of endothelial growth factor (VEGF) and basic fibroblast growth factor (bFGF) early in the inflammatory phase. For example, TGF-ß and PDGF are specific chemoattractants for macrophages during the inflammatory phase continuing into the proliferative phase (discussed on page 23)[39] (see Figure 2.23).

A key role of GFs is to act as intercellular communicators. GFs can act on distant cells (endocrine stimulation), adjacent cells (paracrine stimulation), and themselves (autocrine stimulation).[39] They deliver messages that are released to nonimmune cells and result in cell proliferation, such as the synthesis of granulation tissue.

Cells have the ability to increase (upregulate) or decrease (down regulate) their receptors in response to environmental signals. Cell receptors are not stationary on the cell surface, and their numbers can vary from time to time. They also can bind with one or more kinds of messages.[52] Cell surface receptors on the target cell receive the message, bind to the cell, and produce a biological response in the receiving cell. Some GFs deliver messages related to cell proliferation like cell reproduction by mitosis (mitogenesis), others cause cell migration (via chemotaxis) or cell synthesis, and still others perform regulatory functions.

Cytokines are signaling molecules—peptides, proteins, or glycoproteins—that are essential in cellular communication throughout the body that play two critical roles in inflammation: Proinflammatory cytokines communicate with immune system cells and attract those cells to the area of injury for the purpose of mounting an inflammatory response to destroy foreign organisms and debris. In acute wounds, the level of proinflammatory cytokines peaks in a few days and remains low in the absence of infection.[53] Anti-inflammatory cytokines have powerful inhibitory actions on the inflammatory cells. Table 2.3 is a key to growth factor acronyms used for representation of the inflammatory phase, indicating the release of multiple cytokines, the cytokines, and an identification of their cellular sources and functions.

A third group of regulatory proteins is collectively known as *chemokines*. Chemokines have two primary functions: they regulate the trafficking of leukocyte populations during normal health and development, and direct the recruitment and activation of neutrophils, lymphocytes, macrophages, eosinophils, and basophils during inflammation.[53] Together GFs, cytokines, and chemokines are the key molecular regulators of wound healing. These multiple cell types associated with wound healing

TABLE 2.3	Key to Acronyms Used	
Cellular Sources	Cytokines	Function
Platelets	PDGF	Chemotactic for neutrophils
	TGF-β	Directs collagen matrix expression in late phase of wound repair
Macrophages	PDGF	
	TNF-α	Induces MMP transcription; Proinflammatory; Stimulates synthesis of Nitric oxide
	IL-1	Proinflammatory; Stimulates synthesis of Nitric oxide (NO)
		Amplifies inflammatory response through increased synthesis of IL-1 and IL-6
	IL-6	Proinflammatory
	G-CSF—Granulocyte colony-stimulating factor	Proinflammatory
	GM-CSF—Granulocyte-macrophage colony-stimulating factor	Necrotic ECM degradation
Keratinocytes	IL-6	Stimulate Keratinocytes
		Induce Keratinocyte proliferation
	VEGF—Vascular endothelial growth factor	Potent stimulus for angiogenesis
Fibroblasts	KGF-2—Keratinocyte growth factor	Enable cellular migration the ECM; directs epithelialization
	IL-1	Proinflammatory; amplifies inflammatory response through increased synthesis of IL-1 and IL-6
	TGF-β	Directs collagen matrix expression; upregulated TIMPs
Endothelial cells	VEGF	Potent stimulus for angiogenesis; upregulated in presence of NO

plus other cell types (e.g., epithelial, endothelial, and fibroblasts) receive specific chemical communication from proinflammatory cytokines (e.g., tumor necrosis factor α [TNF-α], interleukin-1 [IL-1], interleukin-6 [IL-6]), which trigger synthesis of a family of 20 proteolytic enzymes, called *matrix metalloproteinases* (*MMPs*). MMPs have been identified as critical in achieving tissue degradation. MMPs require calcium ions for structural conformation and zinc ions in their active site for function.

Balancing the activities of MMPs are endogenous enzyme inhibitors called *tissue inhibitors of metalloproteinase* (TIMPs). Four different TIMPs have been identified, and they are synthesized by the same cells that produce MMPs. If the balance of MMPs and TIMPs is disrupted, a shift to high levels of MMPs can occur, resulting in excessive tissue degradation or destruction of other protein components in the ECM, including growth factors, cell surface receptors, and even the TIMPs.[52] This imbalance affects wound chronicity and chronic wound healing. There is considerable overlap in target cell specificity and actions among the groups. Transmission of these regulatory messages, whether between cells of the same or different types, requires a fluid medium in which to disperse the message; thus, a moist environment is essential. On the other end, there must be a receptor to receive the message.

Immediately after injury, the body employs several built-in check-and-balance systems to ensure that over proliferation does not occur. For example, extended exposure to some growth factors (at least 4 hours) is required before cell division can occur.[39]

Another check-and-balance system involves endothelial growth factor (VEGF), which is a potent stimulus for *neovascularization* also known as *angiogenesis*, (growth of new blood vessels)

and endostatin, a potent inhibitor of angiogenesis; both are products of the platelets, which initiate the healing cascade. The function of these two antagonists is to regulate programmed cell death (apoptosis) and speed removal of damaged cells, while endothelial cells work to restore the vascular system and wound space to homeostatic state of the tissues as expeditiously as possible.[55]

Oxygen and Antibacterial Effects

Oxygen is essential for wound healing, both in preventing infection and meeting the metabolic demands of the tissues. Although neutrophils and macrophages are attracted to a hypoxic environment, once they arrive at the wound site, they require oxygen to kill bacteria. They do not function efficiently in a hypoxic environment, where microorganisms can proliferate at a faster rate than the neutrophils can phagocytise them, leading to infection.[56] Oxygen also has been demonstrated to function equivalently to an "antibiotic" for prevention of wound infections.[57–60] In addition, fibroblasts are aerobic cells that require oxygen for cell function, including division and

---

RESEARCH WISDOM

1. One reason that moisture-retentive dressings are a vital part of wound healing is because they provide the moist environment necessary for cellular communications.[52]
2. Although a moist wound environment is desirable for acute wound healing, chronic wound fluid has been shown to have an inhibitory effect on fibroblasts.[53,54]

collagen synthesis.[61] Finally, oxygen is needed for the hydroxylation of proline necessary for useful collagen production in the remodeled wound. Oxygen is available in the blood in two forms: bound to hemoglobin and dissolved in plasma. The oxygen dissolved in plasma can be adequate for wound healing if tissue perfusion is satisfactory.[53]

Nitric Oxide and Cellular Signaling

NO is a small, bioactive gaseous free radical that is formed from the amino acid L-arginine by three distinct isoforms of nitric oxide synthase (iNOS). All three isoforms are proteins. L-arginine is a semiessential amino acid that is in short supply after injury, but it is the critical substrate for NO synthesis.[63] Chapter 7 details how arginine nutritional supplementation is used to support NO synthesis. NO has been described as a "driver of skin repair" because as a key cellular signaling agent it is responsible for vasodilation and thrombolysis of the fibrinous clot following hemostasis while also playing two significant roles in angiogenesis: as an "actor" of and as a "director of"angiogenesis.[64] One of its attributes that appears to allow it to play different roles is the ability to cross cell membranes without mediation of channels or receptors.

Many cells participate in NO synthesis during all phases of wound healing beginning in the early inflammatory phase with expression by the macrophages, and keratinocytes and then during the proliferative phase by the fibroblasts.[65]

NO synthesis occurs for 10 to 14 days following wounding, after which time it gradually decreases as the wound progresses toward healing.[66] This regulatory process is very important since low concentrations of NO stimulate angiogenesis as the wound progresses to the proliferative phase, but higher concentration, typical of inflammatory responses, is inhibitory of angiogenesis.[67] Dysregulation of NO may be a causative factor in tissue ischemia, necrosis, and chronic inflammation.[67] The critical role of NO in fibroblast collagen synthesis is supported by the finding that in vivo NO inhibition results in reduced wound collagen formation and accumulation, cell proliferation, and wound contraction in distinct ways in human and animal models of wound healing.[68] Although iNOS gene deletion delays healing, and arginine and NO administration improves healing, the exact mechanisms of action of NO on wound healing parameters are still unknown [66,68,69] In addition to skin reparative effects, NO has been shown to kill *Staphylococcus aureus*, prevent replication of DNA viruses within cells, and serve as an immune regulator.[2] Chapter 27 has information about how warmth increases blood flow that stresses the lining of the blood vessels, which enhances endothelial cell NO production.

RESEARCH WISDOM

Evidence-based Ways to Facilitate Oxygen Delivery

Facilitate delivery of oxygen to wound tissues by keeping the patient warm and well-hydrated.[61,62] Improve tissue oxygen levels by administering oxygen by nasal cannula at 5 L/min.[57] Precaution: CO_2 retainers.

VASODILATION

As already mentioned, vasoconstriction at the wound site is followed within several minutes by vasodilation. In addition to NO, other humoral and neurogenic factors, such as bradykinin, histamine, and prostaglandins are responsible for causing vasodilation of the tissues surrounding the wound. Vasodilation prompts the following changes:

- *Increased perfusion.* Increased perfusion brings needed nutrients to meet the increased metabolic demands of the tissues.
- *Increased vessel permeability.* Vasodilation is accompanied by increased capillary pressure and permeability of small blood and lymphatic vessels. This permits the plasma protein molecules to migrate into the surrounding tissues. This results in edema, erythema (redness or purplish color in darkly pigmented skin), and stimulation of the pain afferents. Vasodilation also aids in movement of inflammatory cells from the vasculature into the site of injury.

Increased temperature. Increased perfusion increases local tissue temperature, a response known as *hyperemia.* Hyperemia is not an inflammatory reaction. Pain, as a consequence of the trauma to the tissues, irritates nerve endings and produces reflex hyperemia.[46] In addition, increased metabolic activities and higher vascularity result in higher tissue temperatures. The rise in tissue temperature provides an environment favorable for cell mitosis and enhanced cellular activities.[70,71]

The Complement System

A noncellular (i.e., humoral) group of substances precedes the arrival of neutrophils to the wound space. This system, called the *complement system*, consists of approximately 11 proteins that normally reside in the plasma. Components of the complement system are responsible for acute inflammation through their ability to cause both humoral (i.e., protein) and cellular (i.e., phagocytic) defense mechanisms to move from the intravascular to the extravascular space, where bacteria accumulate. The primary function of the complement system is to facilitate bacterial destruction.

Complement activation can be prompted by any of several specific substances, most often bacteria. The complement system acts either through the classical pathway of *lysing* bacterial cell walls, thereby destroying the infecting organism, or the alternate pathway of *opsonizing* the invader (i.e., coating the antigen with antibody), which makes the invader more appealing and recognizable to the phagocytic cells. In addition, complement acts as a chemotactic agent for attracting phagocytic cells, neutrophils, and macrophages to the site of infection, and enhances their mechanism for oxidative killing.[24]

Two antibodies, IgG and IgM, directly activate the classical pathway of the complement system. These antibodies are produced by the lymphocytes located in the spleen, lymph nodes, and submucosa of the gastrointestinal, respiratory, and genital tracts. They produce specific antibodies in response to specific antigens. These antibodies can neutralize viruses and lyse gram-negative bacteria; as such, they are potent inhibitors of antigens.[24]

Neutrophils

Neutrophils (polymorphonuclear neutrophilic leukocytes) migrate into the wound space, usually within the first

24 hours after wounding, and remain from 6 hours to several days.[24] Neutrophils are granulocytic leukocytes that function as phagocytic cells to clean the site of debris and bacteria. Initially, neutrophils are the most prevalent type of white blood cell at the injury site. They use a special enzyme system to produce and employ free radicals to attack invading bacteria.[72] Neutrophils proliferate in hypoxic, acidotic environments and produce superoxide to fight bacteria and enhance the effectiveness of antibiotics. When the bacterial count is low or declines, the neutrophils stay at the site for only a minimal period of time. High bacterial counts prolong neutrophil activation and inflammation.[73]

The neutrophil is considered to be a primary cell responsible for cleansing wounds of microorganisms; therefore, inadequate numbers of neutrophils will retard healing in infected wounds. When bacterial counts in the wound exceed 10^5 organisms per gram of tissue or mL of fluid, infection becomes apparent in the wound site.[25] The wound produces pus, which is the accumulation of dead neutrophils that have phagocytized debris in the wound. Neutrophils have a short life span because they cannot regenerate the stores of lysosomal enzymes and other enzymes they used to destroy foreign substances. In addition to prompting pus formation, neutrophils produce numerous toxic by-products that, if there is excessive neutrophil activity due to high bacterial counts, negatively affect the wound tissue and even healthy tissue.[24]

When the wound is predominantly clean, neutrophil accumulation resolves. Whether it resolves or is prolonged (as may be the case in chronic wound healing), the monocyte becomes the primary white blood cell in the wounded tissues.[50] Once in the wounded area, monocytes mature into macrophages.

Mast Cells

Mast cells are specialized secretory cells. In the resting state, mast cells contain granules, which serve as histamine-binding sites. Histamine, a vasoactive amine, is initially released from the mast cells after injury. It plays an important role in vascular dilation and permeability, inducing temporary mild edema. In low doses, histamine can stimulate collagen formation and healing.[54]

Clotting factor II, or **prothrombin**, is a vitamin K–dependent proenzyme that functions in the blood coagulation cascade. Once the body has produced enough platelet and prothrombin reaction, the mast cell produces heparin. Heparin then stimulates the migration of endothelial cells which figure in the process of angiogenesis. It also accelerates the activity of the leukocytes (neutrophils and eosinophils) in the thrombolysis of the hematoma, clotted blood that occurs in the wound following damage to the blood vessels at the time of wounding.[74] This is essential for the progression of the inflammatory phase. Other substances derived from the mast cells, eosinophil and neutrophil chemotactic factors, attract leukocytic cells. These cells act as chemical signals for the recruitment of macrophages, which lead to a modulation of the inflammatory phase. Macrophages also promote later phases in the repair process through recruitment of fibroblasts.[75,76] Mast cells themselves promote fibroblast proliferation through the release of tumor necrosis factor β (TNF-β), which is a weak mitogen for fibroblasts. **Mitogens** cause cell mitosis and cellular proliferation.[39]

RESEARCH WISDOM

Physical Agents Affect Mast Cell Function

Electrical stimulation, pulsed radiofrequency stimulation, and ultrasound have been shown to affect mast cell function and promote thrombolysis and absorption of hematoma (see Chapters 23, 24, and 26).

Macrophages

Macrophages are key players in both the inflammatory and proliferative phases of wound healing and arrive in the wound space approximately 2 to 3 days post injury. The life span of the macrophage is estimated to be months to years; it is a component of wound fluid for a long period of time, transcending all phases of healing.[24]

Macrophages perform several important functions during the inflammatory phase, including the following:

1. Macrophages secrete collagenases and elastases, enzymes, which break down injured tissue and release cytokines. Macrophage released cytokines, amplify the inflammatory response by **chemotaxis** (biochemical attraction of cells), inducing fibroblasts and endothelial cells to synthesize and secrete more proinflammatory cytokines (IL-1 and IL-6) and colony stimulating factors (G-CSF and GM-CSF).[2]
2. Macrophages phagocytize debris by ingesting microorganisms. They also control infection by excreting ascorbic acid, hydrogen peroxide, and lactic acid. The body interprets the buildup of these excreted byproducts as a signal to send more macrophages. The result of the increased macrophage population is a prolonged, more intense inflammatory response.
3. Macrophages initiate autolytic debridement through synthesis and secretion of collagenases in preparation for the laying down of the new collagen matrix.[39]
4. Macrophages initiate angiogenesis as well as the formation of granulation tissue in preparation for the proliferative phase that follows. Macrophage-derived growth factors play a pivotal role in new tissue formation, as evidenced by the fact that new tissue formation in macrophage-depleted animal wounds demonstrates defective repair. Reestablishment of the blood supply is essential for delivering nutrients to the newly forming tissue.
5. Macrophages also release NO, which, as just mentioned, kills pathogens.

Macrophages are the essential cells for transition from the inflammatory to the proliferative phase of healing because of these activities.[51]

Fibroblasts

Fibroblasts respond to the chemotactic signals from growth factors released by platelets, macrophages, granulocytes, and keratinocytes during the inflammatory phase. These growth factors stimulate fibroblast proliferation. Alignment of the fibroblast cells within the wound site during the inflammatory phase is an early indication of the strength that will eventually be imparted to the wound. Alignment of the fibroblasts along the wound axis and

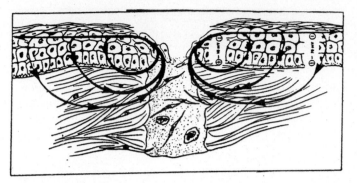

FIGURE 2.24 Current path in wounded section of the skin. Disruption in the epidermis has provided a return path for current driven by transepithelial potential. (Reprinted with permission from Jaffe LF, Vanable JW. Electric fields and wound healing. *Clin Dermatol.* 1984(3):233–234, with permission from Elsevier Science.)

creation of cell-to-cell linkages aid in the contraction of the wound and the strength of the final scar tissue.[24] During the inflammatory phase, the fibroblasts differentiate into a specialized cell called the *myofibroblast.* Myofibroblast functions are explained on page 28.

Current of Injury

Endogenous biologic electrical currents are another component of healing. All body cells, including bone, skin, muscle, and nerve cells, possess injury currents. In the 1960s, Becker demonstrated the existence of a direct-current electrical system that controls tissue healing, which he named the *current of injury.*[77]

Polarity is a key component of the current of injury. Multiple experiments have demonstrated that a negative charge exists on the surface of the skin with respect to the deeper skin layers. This results in weak electrical potentials across the skin, creating a "skin battery" effect. The human body has an average charge on the skin surface of -23 mV.[78] The battery is driven by a sodium ion (NA^+) pump, initiated by the sodium ions passing through the cells of the epithelium via specific channels in the outer membrane. Once in the cell, they diffuse to other cells of the epithelium. Then, they are actively transported from these cells via electrogenic "pumps" located in all of the plasma membranes of the epithelium except the outer membrane. The result is the transport of NA^+ from the fluid bathing the epithelium to the internal body fluids, as well as generation of a potential of 50 mV across the epithelium.[79]

A break in the integrity of the skin causes a net flow of ionic current through the low-resistance pathway of the injured cells and drainage that line the wound; if the wound space becomes dry, the voltage gradient will stop.[59,60] Figure 2.24 represents the flow of the ionic current between the skin surface and wound space. During the repair process, there is a distinct pattern of current flow and polarity switching; cells of repair are attracted to either the positive or the negative poles, a phenomenon called *galvanotaxis.* Macrophages and neutrophils are attracted to the positive pole.[80,81] When the wound is inflamed or infected, neutrophils are attracted to the negative pole.[82] The negative pole also attracts fibroblasts,[83] which stimulate protein and DNA synthesis, and increases CA^{2+} uptake, fibroblast proliferation, and collagen synthesis.[84] Negative polarity facilitates migration of epidermal cells and is also associated with suppression of bacterial growth.[85–89] When healing is complete, the current ceases. Clearly, there are significant research data to support the concept that electrical current plays an important role in the cell physiology of wound healing. Exogenous application of electrical stimulation, as a treatment intervention, to mimic the current of injury and accelerate wound healing has important clinical value. Clinical application and validity are discussed in Chapter 23.

INFLAMMATORY PHASE IN CHRONIC WOUNDS

Defining the critical attributes and benchmarks of the inflammatory phase of chronic wound healing is difficult because researchers have only recently begun to distinguish the differences between the normal acute wound healing process and that observed in chronic wound healing. Several factors that have been identified as causing an interruption in the inflammatory phase of repair include the stimulus for repair, inadequate perfusion and ischemia, free radicals and oxygen reperfusion injury, the balance of inflammatory cytokines and proteases, and the levels of growth factors present.[85]

Stimulus for Repair

One of the primary differences between acute and chronic wound healing is the stimulus for repair. In acute wounds, there is vascular disruption from the outside of the body to the inside of the body, initiating the hemostasis process and, thus, the wound healing cascade. In chronic wounds, the injury or stimulus for repair may come from within and can be gradual in onset.

Inadequate Perfusion and Ischemia

Acute tissue trauma to normally healthy tissues changes the vascular perfusion to the wounded tissues resulting in *tissue ischemia* or inadequate tissue perfusion. In some cases, the ischemic tissue slows or stops the healing cascade and then itself becomes an obstacle to healing because it is a barrier to angiogenesis.[48] Small thromboses in the tissues produce multiple sites of hemostasis, autonomic nervous system is activated producing physiological stress that results in vasoconstriction, and free radicals that cause oxygen reperfusion injury (described in page 25) leaving the tissues ischemic resulting in a slow and laborious course of healing.[48,86] Underlying pathologic vascular conditions like insufficiency, venous and/or arterial, is known to interfere with the process of hemostasis and the coagulation cascade. Because hemostasis is the stimulus for the wound healing cascade, the process is muted and the wound ends in a chronic or absent phases of inflammation. Angiogenic stimulation by GF and chemokines is suppressed and the angiogenic process retreats from the wound edge causing the wounds to heal slowly, as the angiogenic stimuli become increasingly

---

CLINICAL WISDOM

Moist Wound Healing and the Current of Injury

Acute wounds benefit from contact with acute wound fluid, which provides a moist environment for cell migration and galvanotaxis.[90]

more removed from the initial wound edge. New blood vessels coalesce or drop out, resulting in a predominantly ischemic wound site.[48,86]

Tissue ischemia triggers a series of events that includes the production of inflammatory mediators, mechanical capillary plugging by leukocytes, and oxygen metabolite formation, which leads to further tissue damage.[72,87] The wound healing process can begin with the entry of white blood cells into the damaged tissues from blood vessel disruption. However, in ischemic tissues, even this process may be slowed. Once the injury is present, the leukocytes attempt to initiate the inflammatory stage of healing; however, many are unable to enter the wound tissue by passing through the capillary walls, because of increased rigidity of vessels and capillary plugging.[72] The leukocytes that do enter the wound tissue have difficulty performing bactericidal activities, because underlying ischemia decreases oxygen content in the wound bed.[56,87]

Inadequate perfusion often affects the healing of lower extremity wounds. Arterial ulcers are associated with macrovascular and microvascular disease that leads to tissue ischemia. Pressure ulcers are the consequence of compression of the base tissues and closure of the capillaries, also leading to ischemia. Infection also contributes to ischemia when neutrophils are deposited in the walls and lumen of the small vessels.[53] Smoking, psychophysiological stress, and pain can all increase the sympathetic tone of the vascular system and decrease tissue perfusion. Smoking also decreases microcirculation. Calcium deposits in microvasculature, such as occurs in diabetics, reduce blood flow and contribute to ischemia and can progress to anoxia and necrosis often seen as a secondary complication of diabetes.

Free Radicals

The mechanisms for capillary plugging by neutrophils and delayed entry into the wounded tissues are related to formation of oxygen-free radicals and reperfusion injury.

Reactive oxygen species (ROS) is a collective term for oxygen-free radicals. Oxygen-free radicals take part in many metabolic processes, acting as part of the defense mechanism against infection. Free-radical species are generated during the process of oxidative phosphorylation and the electron transfer chain within the mitochondria. Normally, the free-radical species generated during these processes are used in a well-controlled manner; they serve useful functions in the cell metabolic processes, and do not escape to a significant degree from the mitochondria to other parts of the cell. Free radicals are chemically very reactive and, if they do escape, can cause severe damage to many chemical compounds that are part of the cell, especially the lipids that make up the cell membrane. Fortunately, enzymes within the cells usually catalyze the safe breakdown of oxygen-free radicals, thus protecting the cell from these compounds. In addition, tocopherol (a vitamin E component) in the lipid membrane and ascorbic acid (vitamin C) act as free-radical scavengers that can safely break down free radicals.[72] Free radicals are also implicated in the development of leg ulcers, in which the protective mechanisms become deranged during ischemia and overwhelmed after reperfusion by the extent of free-radical production.[72]

Oxygen Reperfusion Injury

When blood flow is reestablished to the ischemic tissue, further damage to the tissues occurs from the disruption of the normal mechanisms of defense against injury from oxygen-free radicals. This is referred to as *reperfusion injury*. When blood flow resumes to an ischemic site, the new availability of oxygen causes the conversion of an enzyme called xanthine dehydrogenase, which the body uses in normal metabolism, to xanthine oxidase. This chemical reaction releases large numbers of free radicals.[72] This overwhelms the normal free-radical defense mechanisms and leads to extensive injury of the endothelium by lipid peroxidation, with ultimate destruction of the microcirculation. The consequence of these events is cell death.

In addition, an already difficult situation can be complicated by the escape of free radicals from the mitochondria.[72] Additional free radicals are released by neutrophils in response to activation of compounds released by endothelial cells during reperfusion. Both neutrophil activation and the availability of xanthine oxidase increase free radicals at the wound site, which results in increased endothelial damage.[54] When activated to produce free radicals, neutrophils lose their ability to deform to enter capillaries and adhere more easily to the endothelium, occluding capillaries.[72] Capillary occlusion and the neutrophils' inability to deform may explain the decreased levels of functioning neutrophils and macrophages present in chronic wounds.[72] Current research is focused on prevention of the most damaging features of ischemia and the resulting reperfusion injury. Clinicians need to be aware of the implications of new treatments that may be developed as a consequence of this research.

EPITHELIALIZATION PHASE

Epithelialization, a second phase of wound healing, involves resurfacing or *reepithelialization* of the wound and changes in the wound edges. Reepithelialization, which means restoring the denuded wound surface, protects the body from invasion by outside organisms, commences immediately after trauma, and occurs concurrently with the other phases of wound healing (Figure 2.14).[2]

Role of Keratinocytes

The process of reepithelialization is the function of the keratinocytes, which make up the layers of the dermis and epidermis as well as the linings of various body organs and dermal appendages (e.g., sebaceous glands, sweat glands, and hair follicles). Derived from epidermal stem cells that are located in the bulge area of the hair follicle, keratinocytes migrate from there into the basal layers of the epidermis and are capable of proliferating and differentiating to produce the epidermis. That is, the epidermis is replenished by epidermal stem cells and progenitors arising from the keratinocytes. Keratinocytes synthesize insoluble proteins that cross-link to form a protective, cornified layer, the stratum corneum, which functions to keep pathogens out and water in.[88] Keratinocytes respond to signals from the macrophages, neutrophils, and the current of injury within hours after injury. As soon as the skin barrier is broken by a wound, the proinflammatory cytokine IL-1, which is stored in skin cells, is released. Within hours, keratinocytes respond to signals from the macrophages, neutrophils, and the current of injury by entering an activation cycle.[88] Keratinocyte activation is transmitted to other neighboring cells (primarily fibroblasts), which in turn release multiple growth factors and initiate the wound healing cascade.[88]

Keratinocytes respond to signals from released growth factors by advancing in a sheet to resurface the open space. The leading edges of the advancing keratinocytes become phagocytic; they clean the debris, including clotted material, from their path. Cell sheets continue to migrate until the wound is covered and a new basement membrane is generated. Multilayered epithelial cells appear to migrate either as a moving sheet or in a complex "leapfrog" manner (epiboly). The wound environment speeds the migration of keratinocytes toward one another from the edges of the wound and the dermal appendages.

Full-thickness wounds involve loss of the dermal appendages, which are an important source of new keratinocytes. As a consequence, epithelial cells can migrate only from the wound edges. The advancing front of epidermal cells cannot cover a cavity, so they dive down and curl under at the edges. For example, full-thickness pressure wounds develop a buildup of epithelial cells at the wound edges, forming an epidermal ridge that curls under the edges and slows closure. The situation is as though the epithelial cells get tired of waiting for granulation tissue to fill in the wound defect, so they prematurely proliferate and migrate over the edge, as shown in Figure 2.17 and form and epidermal ridge. The migration of epithelial cells is also oxygen-dependent; when there are low levels of oxygen, epithelial migration cannot debride the wound.

In surgical wounds that are sutured, epidermal migration begins within the first 24 hours. In healthy adults, it is usually complete within 48 to 72 hours postoperatively. In other wounds, skin trauma results in tissue degeneration, with broad, indistinct areas and edges that are difficult to see. This forms a shallow lesion, with more distinct, thin, separate edges. As tissue trauma progresses, the reaction intensifies, with a thickening and rolling inward of the epidermis. The edge is well-defined, sharply outlining the ulcer, with little or no evidence of new tissue growth. Repeated trauma and attempts to repair the wound edges result in fibrosis and scarring. The edges of the wound become indurated and firm,[89] a condition that can impair the migratory ability of the keratinocytes.[91]

Once the wound has been resurfaced by epithelial cells, the cells begin the process of differentiating and maturing forming scar tissue. Tissue properties of elasticity and tensile strength of the replaced epidermal layers affect the function of the skin as it overrides bony prominences and moving muscles or tendons because it is less elastic and more *friable*, easily torn, than the original. The *tensile strength*, breaking strength of the fibers, of the remodeled skin will not exceed 70% to 80% of the original. The quality of the scar tissue is an indication of the final outcome.

The fact that closure has been achieved by reepithelialization does not mean that the wound is fully healed. At this time, the new skin has a tensile strength of approximately 15% of normal compared to the 70% to 80% of the original that it will possess when it is remodeled and mature. It must be treated carefully to avoid trauma, which can cause edema and infection, and can lead to reinflammation. Chronic inflammation compounds the problems of impaired scar quality since it causes a thickening of the skin and less elastic remodeled tissue.[92]

EPITHELIALIZATION PHASE IN CHRONIC WOUNDS

As is true for interruption of the inflammatory phase, if the reepithelialization process is interrupted or arrested, the result is a chronic wound. Any factor that diminishes keratinocyte migration may arrest the reepithelialization process. Such factors are discussed below.[85]

Histological analysis of biopsies from chronic ulcers reveals a different appearance of the epidermis. It is mitotically active and hyperproliferative; however, keratinocytes are unable to migrate. It seems that those keratinocytes at the chronic wound edge are only partially activated. The differentiation process is also incomplete and incapable of proceeding. One consequence is that cells grown from the nonhealing wound edge fail to respond to GFs and cytokines.[88]

Delayed reepithelialization due to diminished keratinocyte migration can also occur because of lack of a moist, oxygen-rich, nutritious tissue base. This is the case, for example, with debris-filled chronic wounds.[51] Decreased keratinocyte migration can also be due to a lack of stimulation, caused by failure of the appropriate cytokine to be released during the initial processes of the inflammatory phase of healing.[51,93]

Keratinocyte migration can be difficult in chronic wounds because of the rolled, thickened, nonproductive wound edge. Additionally, reepithelialization or wound resurfacing may be delayed until the wound has filled sufficiently with granulation tissue to provide a moist environment for keratinocyte migration. In wounds with significant tissue loss, reepithelialization is slowed by virtue of the larger area requiring resurfacing. If wound contraction is impaired and the wound remains large, reepithelialization is also affected.

Research related to chronic wound healing in the epithelialization phase provides new insight into the process of reepithelialization of the skin surface and identifies the weak links. Tissue engineers are taking advantage of the new science and developing products in the form of human skin equivalents that can be grown and combined with a patient's own keratinocytes to reconstruct skin.

PROLIFERATIVE PHASE

The **proliferative phase** (Figure 2.25) of wound healing overlaps with and succeeds the inflammatory phase, beginning 3 to 5 days postinjury and continuing for 3 weeks in acute wounds that heal by primary intention[50] (see Figure 2.12). The goals of this healing phase are to fill in the wound defect with new tissue and restore the integrity of the skin. New tissue formation is the benchmark for the start of this phase. The processes involved in the proliferative phase are *angiogenesis* (growth of new blood vessels), *collagen synthesis* (ECM formation), and wound *contraction* (the drawing together of the wound edges as shown in Figures 2.17 to 2.19.[2]

Oxygen and nutrition demands remain very high to support the cells of repair (i.e., fibroblasts, myofibroblasts, endothelial cells, and epidermal cells), which reproduce at a rapid rate to create the collagen matrix. Nutrients, including zinc, iron, copper, vitamin C, and oxygen, are essential for fibroblast synthesis of the collagen matrix. The macrophages and neutrophils work to control infection as long as the wound remains open. The combination of these activities raises tissue temperatures. The

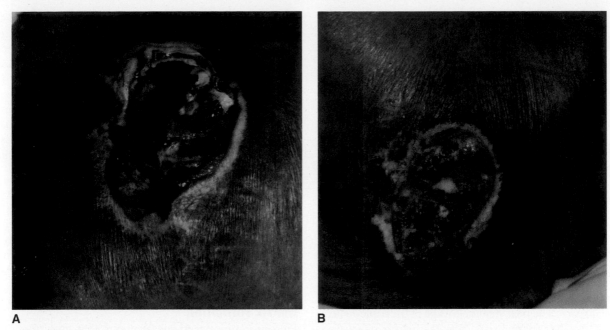

FIGURE 2.25 A. Acute proliferative phase. Note the attached wound edges from the 12:00 to 6:00 positions and how well vascularized granulation tissue fills up one side of the ulcer. A new pink border of epithelium surrounds the granulation tissue. **B:** Same wound as in (**A**). All of the wound edges are now attached to the wound base. Note the presence of fibrin (*yellow*) within the granulation tissue. Ready for epithelialization phase. (Copyright © B.M. Bates-Jensen.)

wound needs warmth at this time to promote cellular division and manage infection.

Integrins

In unwounded tissues, cells that are involved in repair are stationary; however, after wounding, they change into migrating cells. Migrating cells express specialized receptors called *integrins*.[52] Integrins serve a critical function in cell adhesion and signaling during wound healing. They are critical for a duality of events: reepithelialization and formation of granulation tissue because of their ability to recognize and respond to various components during formation of the ECM.[94]

Growth Factors—Proliferative Phase

As wound healing progresses from the inflammatory to proliferative phase, the keratinocytes, fibroblasts, and endothelial cells synthesize growth factors. As we will see, GFs function to promote cell migration, proliferation, angiogenesis, and synthesis of the ECM components.[53] AGFs, TGF-β, TNF-α, IL-1, and bFGF are the GFs involved.[39]

Angiogenesis

Restoration of vascular integrity begins in the inflammatory phase but becomes a major activity during the proliferative phase. During this phase, angiogenesis, growth of new blood vessels by the endothelial cells (also known as *neovascularization*), takes place. Angiogenesis occurs as new capillary buds, arising from intact vessels adjacent to the wound, extend into the wound bed. As endothelial cells proliferate, grow into the wound space, and create capillaries, they connect to form a new network of vessels to fill the tissue defect. In the early stages of vessel growth, the vessels have loose junctions and gaps in the endothelial lining.[51] As a result, the initial capillaries are fragile

and permeable, allowing passage of fluids from the intravascular to the extravascular space; thus, new tissue is often edematous in appearance.[51] The thick capillary bed, which fills the matrix, supplies the nutrients and oxygen necessary for the wound to heal. To the naked eye, the capillary loops look like small granules, explaining the name *granulation* tissue.[27] Granulation tissue first appears as pale pink buds; as it fills with new blood vessels, it becomes bright, "beefy," and red, as shown in Figure 2.25. In Figure 2.25A,B, the granulation begins at one side of the wound and "marches" across the wound bed.

At this time, the granulation tissue is very fragile and unable to withstand any trauma. Trauma to the new tissue will cause bleeding that can reinitiate the inflammatory process and cause the laying down of excessive collagen; this results in poor elasticity and a less desirable scar. Protection of the new granulation tissue is very important.

Even when mature, granulation tissue will remain structurally and functionally different from the tissues it replaces. It will not differentiate into nerves, muscles, tendons, or other tissue.[24]

Fibroblasts

Fibroblasts mainly participate in the biosynthesis of collagen to form the ECM, which acts as a mold, precursor, plastic material, and cementing substance in the wound healing process. Fibroblasts secrete collagen until the wound is filled; then, collagen production ceases as the fibroblast is downregulated. This process of fibrous tissue formation is called *fibroplasia*. Wound healing by fibroplasia requires that the wound be shaped like a boat or bowl to ensure that granulation tissue fills the base before the epithelial edges of the wound meet. Wounds that are not of this shape are at risk for premature surface healing, leaving a cavity under the skin that will subsequently break

CLINICAL WISDOM

Granulation Tissue Complications

A change from healthy red granulation tissue to dark red or a dusky pink color is a sign that warrants further investigation and possible intervention (Figs. 2.15 and 2.16). Wound fluid can also change in color and/or quantity. Pain may increase; this is often a sign of infection.

down.[2,95] The optimal wound conditions for supporting fibroblast production of collagen and ground substances includes an acidic, low-oxygen wound bed.

Fibroblasts synthesize three polypeptide chains that coil to form a right-handed triple helix.[92] Now called *procollagen*, these spiraled chains are extruded from the fibroblast into the extracellular space. The next step is cleavage of the triple-helical molecule at specific terminal sites. Now the helix is referred to as a *tropocollagen molecule*. Tropocollagen, thus transformed, amassed and convolving with other tropcollagen molecules, form a collagen fibril, then combine with ground substance to form the ECM or scaffolding of repair that will support blood vessel growth by the endothelial cells.[24,96] The endothelial cells migrate and proliferate along the scaffolding, building new capillaries that are capable of providing oxygen and nourishment to the new collagen.[51,66]

Tropocollagen, a precursor to collagen, is a soluble substance that is transformed into hydroxyproline (HoPro), insoluble collagen, by a process called *hydroxylation of praline*. Ferrous iron, a reducing agent (e.g., ascorbic acid), *alpha ketoglutarate* (a collagen boosting agent), and oxygen are required to achieve this transformation. In research, the measurement of HoPro is used to assess collagen deposition, with collagen estimated as seven times the value of HoPro.[97] In vitro and in vivo studies show that collagen hydroxylation, cross-linking, and deposition are proportional to the arterial partial pressure of oxygen. Hydroxyproline deposition is proportional to wound tensile strength in rats.[61] Another reason is that the oxygen gradient is critical to the wound healing process.

Collagen Types

Tropocollagen polymerizes (joins with many small particles to create a large molecule) to form various types of collagen.[23] Types I and III collagen are important to our discussion, because they are found in the dermis and are involved with wound healing. New tissue growth in the wound follows a characteristic pattern:[51,66]

- *Production of type III collagen*. Type III collagen is the predominant type of collagen synthesized in the wound.[66]
- Type III collagen is poorly cross-linked and not aligned in the same manner as type I collagen; as such, it provides minimal tensile strength to the new tissue.[51] Type III collagen fibrils are small (40–60 nm), but elastic. They help the tissue withstand a load over time, a quality referred to as *creep resistance*. The proportion of small to large fibrils changes over the life span, with type III gradually replaced by type I.

- *Production of type I collagen*. Early immature type III collagen is gradually replaced with the normal adult type I collagen throughout the proliferation phase of healing and continuing through the remodeling phase of healing. Type I collagen fibrils have a larger diameter (100–500 mm) than type III, and are less elastic. These fibers are organized and arranged in parallel lines along mechanical stress points, giving tissue strength.[51] Approximately 80% of dermal collagen is type I, and these fibers provide the tensile strength to the tissue. The proportion of large-diameter to small-diameter fibrils determines the overall dermal tensile strength.[96]

At this point, about 3 weeks after wounding, the greatest mass of collagen assembled by the tensile strength is roughly only 15% of normal. This new scar will not tolerate mobilization or rough handling, both of which will ultimately lead to creation of a new wound and further scarring.[92] Wound *dehiscence* (separation of all the layers of an incision or wound) occur most frequently during this phase.[23]

Matrix Formation

Fibrous connective tissue elements that give strength to the ECM include collagen, elastin, **fibronectin** (an adhesive glycoprotein secreted during the inflammatory phase as part of the process of ECM formation) and *reticulin* (young collagen fibers).[98] Elastin derives its name from its elastic properties. It is found in skin, lungs, blood vessels, and the bladder, and functions to maintain tissue shape.[23] Matrix proteins, including collagen, form the basal lamina over which the keratinocytes migrate. Laminin is a component of the basement membrane that functions to inhibit keratinocyte migration.[53]

Cross-Linking of Collagen

Once the collagen fibrils are formed, they are very disorganized. This disorganization is why early scar tissue is weak with poor tensile strength. Cross-linkage is necessary for wound tensile strength. As the proliferative phase gives way to the remodeling phase of wound healing, the collagen is remodeled into ordered, structured formations, which increase the tensile strength of the scar tissue. The number of collagen filaments does not give the collagen matrix durability or tensile strength; rather, tensile strength depends on the microscopic welding, or bonding, of one filament to another. The sites at which these bonds occur are called *cross-links*. Intermolecular bonds are the major force holding the collagen molecules together. The greater the number of these bonds, the greater the strength of the collagen filament. In an anoxic wound, cross-linking is inhibited.

Ground Substance

Ground substance is primarily water, salts, and GAGs. GAGs are polysaccharides that contain amino acids, sugars, and glycoprotein (called *proteoglycans*).[96] GAGs are hydrophilic substances, so they attract large amounts of water and sodium. The *turgor* (feeling of fullness) normally associated with connective tissue is a manifestation of the accumulation of fluid by the GAGs. Ground substance has semiliquid gel properties[24] Turgor will be discussed as part of wound assessment in Chapter 3.

Myofibroblasts and Contraction

Wound contraction pulls the wound edges together for the purpose of closing the wound. In effect, this reduces the open area and, if successful, results in a smaller wound, with less need for repair by scar formation.

Myofibroblasts are important in wound contraction. They contain an actin and myosin contractile system similar to that found in smooth muscle cells,[61] which allows them to contract and extend. The myofibroblast connects itself to the wound skin margins and pulls the epidermal layer inward. The myofibroblast ring forms what has been described as a "picture frame" beneath the skin of the contracting wound. The contracting forces start out equal in all wounds, but the shape of the "picture frame" predicts the resultant speed of contraction. Linear wounds contract rapidly, square and rectangular wounds contract at a moderate pace, and circular wounds contract slowly. One characteristic of pressure ulcers is that they take on a circular shape, which is an indicator that they will contract slowly (see Figure 2.17).[92] Wound contraction is manifested by a change in wound shape and reduction in the open area of the wound. This occurs at the final stage of wound repair (see Figure 2.19).

Partial-thickness wounds heal with very little wound contraction. However, in full-thickness wounds, contraction can account for up to a 40% decrease in wound size.[51,93] For successful healing, contraction needs to be balanced. A diminished level of contraction leads to delayed healing, with possible excess bleeding and infection. Conversely, excess contraction can lead to loss of function from tissue contractures.[51]

Wound contraction can be extremely beneficial in the closure of wounds in areas such as the buttocks and trochanter, but it can be harmful in areas such as the hand and around the neck and face, where it can cause disfigurement and excessive scarring. Rapid, uncontrolled wound contraction in these areas must be avoided. Tissue that draws together too tightly can cause deformity of the repaired scar and impairment of tissue function. Skin grafting is used to reduce contraction in undesirable locations. The thickness of the skin graft influences the degree of contraction suppression. Pressure garments are another method of controlling wound contraction (see Chapter 16).

PROLIFERATIVE PHASE IN CHRONIC WOUNDS

Several differences exist for the chronic wound in the proliferative phase.[85] These processes and differences are described here.

Fibroblast Senescence

Vande Berg et al. studied fibroblast senescence in pressure ulcers.[99] For this purpose, the study hypothesis defined cell populations as senescent when they failed to undergo 0.5 doubling after a 1-week period.[99] Findings from the research included[99]

1. Fibroblast populations grown from normal, unulcerated skin undergo more doublings than those from the ulcer margin or wound bed before becoming senescent.
2. Small fibroblasts have more doubling compared with large fibroblasts.
3. Fibroblasts from patients of all ages become senescent after fewer population doublings than fibroblasts from adjacent normal skin.
4. As fibroblast cell populations age, the number of senescent cells appear to increase, while cells in the proliferating pool decrease.

RESEARCH WISDOM

Best Time to Apply Skin Grafts

Text Split-thickness skin grafts suppress contraction by 31%, and full-thickness skin grafts diminish contraction by 55%. The best time for application of skin grafts is during the inflammatory phase, before contraction begins.[92]

5. Myofibroblasts appear to attempt wound contraction, but their efforts may be compromised by cellular senescence and/or necrosis.

The literature review associated with this study pointed out that diabetic patients show premature fibroblast senescence and decreased fibroblast division; moreover, senescent fibroblasts lose their ability to bind to collagen.[99]

Fibronectin Composition

Fibronectin is a matrix protein critical in the laying down of collagen. Wysocki demonstrated differences in the composition of fibronectin in chronic wounds, as compared with acute wounds.[100] The fibronectin in chronic wounds was partially degraded, whereas it remained intact in acute wounds. The small fibronectin fragments found in chronic wounds may perpetuate the activity of matrix proteases and inhibit healing.[101] Indeed, the excess activity of proteases, which breaks down connective tissue faster than it is formed and destroys important polypeptide-signaling molecules that coordinate healing, may play a role in persistent nonhealing wounds.[102]

Parks[103] has shown that chronic wounds exhibit production of stromelysins (metalloproteinases that do not lyse collagen), which may represent the unregulated production of proteinase that contributes to the inability of some chronic wounds to heal.

Chronic Wound Fluid

The desire to learn more about the wound microenvironment has led researchers to look at wound fluid as a reflection of the microenvironment from which it was collected. Human studies of wound fluids are complicated by the inability to carefully control the variables related to the wound, the patient, and the way wound fluids are collected, leading to varied results. However, considerable efforts have been made by investigators to study fluid from both acute and chronic wounds.

It is fairly well-accepted that fluid from acute wounds is mitogenic for wound-associated cells, and fluid collected from chronic wounds is inhibitory to these cells of regeneration.[104,105] Analysis and study of wound fluid is providing an important insight into the healing of chronic wounds. It has been suggested that chronic wound fluid analysis could be used to identify potential biomarkers of wound chronicity, leading to new treatment strategies and possibly customized treatment based on the identified biomarkers. This concept has already been applied to secreted biofluids of other chronic inflammatory conditions such as osteoarthritis and periodontal disease to determine disease and metabolic activity.[54]

Chronic wound fluid has been shown to inhibit proliferation of endothelial cells, keratinocytes, fibroblasts, and cell adhesion.[106,107] In nonhealing wounds, proinflammatory cytokines and proteases are present at high levels compared to the relatively low levels and narrower range of GFs present in healing wounds. When there is an increase in proinflammatory cytokines, there is an accompanying elevation of proteases production. This may be due to the presence of bacteria and their endotoxins, as well as the presence of platelet degranulation products.[52]

Recently, the focus of chronic wound fluid research has been on the proinflammatory cytokines and proteases, but there is also interest in the potential of ECM components in wound fluid as biomarkers of wound healing pathology.[54] It is no longer recommended to allow wounds to bathe in chronic wound fluid such as occurs under an occlusive dressing, because of the potential for defective remodeling, as will be described in a following chapter section.

Protracted Inflammatory and Proliferative Responses

Repeated trauma and infection of chronic wounds changes chronic wound fluid mediator concentrations by increasing the presence of proinflammatory cytokines and tissue inhibitors or metalloproteinases, and lowering the level of growth factors compared with acute wounds and creates imbalances that appear to impede proliferative responses necessary for pressure ulcer healing.[108-111] This is of clinical significance because healing has been associated with reduced levels of MMPs and an increase in TIMP activities.[54] Another, clinically significant, outcome of research on wound fluid is temperature change effects on chronic wound fluid mediators. Inhibitory effects are abolished by heating the wound fluid to100°C, and heating it to 38°C has a significant effect.[105] Clinically, this has importance in the selection of interventions that affect tissue temperature and is discussed in several chapters.

Dead Space or Large Tissue Gap

Full-thickness ulcers often present with a "dead space" or "tissue gap," which prolongs proliferation because of the larger tissue defect that needs to be filled with new connective tissue and blood vessels.[56] Prolongation of the proliferative phase of healing can be observed in many chronic wounds. In these cases, the wound progresses to a certain point of new tissue growth and then "stalls" or "plateaus," with no further evidence of proliferation. The cessation of proliferation may be related to inadequate substrates necessary for new tissue growth, such as protein, vitamin C, and zinc.[48] Inadequate substrate availability may be due to increased levels of bacteria in the wound environment or continued lysis of new growth faster than new material can be synthesized. The increased bacteria levels may compete with healthy cells for the substrates necessary for healing and thus prevent further tissue growth.[56]

Siddiqui and colleagues[112] suggested an alternate cause of decreased tissue proliferation. Using an in vitro system, their study demonstrated decreased collagen production and fibroblast proliferation in a chronically hypoxic wound environment, suggesting that long-term wound hypoxia exerts a negative influence on tissue proliferation.

REMODELING PHASE

The final phase of wound healing is the **remodeling phase**, which begins as granulation tissue forms in the wound site during the proliferative phase and continues for 1 to 2 years postinjury until the tissue reaches maturation.[51,113] During the remodeling phase, scar tissue is rebuilt, and tensile strength increases from the 15% to 20% strength associated with the initial scar tissue, to as much as 80% of the preinjury tissues by the end of the remodeling phase.[93,94]

The remodeling phase shows most clearly the overlapping of all of the phases of wound healing. Typically, it is described as the end of the proliferative phase, which is about 3 weeks postacute injury. Actually, collagen matrix formation and remodeling begin concurrently with the formation of granulation tissue.[23]

As we will see shortly, remodeling requires maintenance of a delicate equilibrium between collagen synthesis and lysis. Regulation of the remodeling process is the function of growth factors, primarily TGF-β, PDGF, and FGF, which are stimulated during tissue injury and repair by specific MMPs called *collagenases*.[39]

Matrix Remodeling

ECM and collagen deposition continuously and gradually changes from the time it is initially produced in the wound bed, and this process continues even after tissue continuity is restored.[51] Type III collagen, originally produced by the fibroblasts, is gradually lysed by lysosomal proteases and tissue collagenases, and type I collagen is produced to replace the lost tissues. The lysis of old collagen and production of new collagen lead to a change in the orientation of the scar tissue: as noted earlier, type I collagen fibrils are laid down parallel to the lines of tension in the wound in an organized fashion, with strong cross-linking and bundle construction.[51] Proteoglycans are deposited with the new type I collagen, increasing the wound's resilience to deformation.[51] Also during this phase, the highly vascular and cellular granulation scar tissue is gradually replaced with less vascular and less cellular tissues.[56]

Matrix Metalloproteinases and Collagen Lysis or Degradation

Numerous proteases have been implicated in the proteolytic degradation of the ECM, most prominent among which are members of the MMP family. MMPs have been divided into collagenases, gelatinases, stromelysins, and matrilysins.[114]

Recall that collagenase and other proteolytic enzymes are produced during the inflammatory phase and throughout the proliferative phase as regulators of fibroplasia. Collagenase can cleave, or break, the cross-linkage of the tropocollagen molecules, aiding in its reabsorption during periods of connective tissue growth or repair.[28] In a healthy wound, collagenase regulates the balance between synthesis and lysis of collagen. It is this ability to break down collagen that makes collagenase useful as a debriding agent. Breaking of the cross-linkage makes the tropocollagen molecule soluble so that it can be excreted from the body. The balance between collagen synthesis and collagen lysis is delicate, with a goal that one process should not exceed the other. However, as the wound matures during remodeling, collagen lysis increases. The organization of collagen fibers as they are laid down by the fibroblasts is part of this regulatory process; better organization produces a better functional outcome of more elastic, smoother, and stronger fibers for the repaired scar tissues.

Scar Formation

As mentioned, collagen synthesis and lyses are well regulated process leading to **scar formation** and wound remodeling. In uncomplicated healing, TGFβ-1 is expressed early during the inflammatory phase. TGFβ-1 levels drop and TGFβ-3 levels rise during the late proliferative phase. These receptors, along with the corresponding TGF-β isoforms, decrease in density during granulation tissue remodeling when healing is well-regulated. In addition to GFs, their corresponding receptors are also expressed.[33,34]

Clinical manifestations of the remodeling phase of healing include changes in the appearance of scar tissue. **Normotrophic** or normal scaring results in a visible scar that is not raised above the surface of the surrounding tissue. As collagen synthesis and degradation (lysis) proceed, the vascularity and cellularity of the scar tissue diminish, with loss in scar tissue mass and obvious changes in the visual appearance of the wound site. The scar changes from bright red or pink to a silvery gray or white, and the site becomes less bulky, flattening over time until a normotrophic scar is achieved.[56,113] Additionally, the scar tissue becomes more flexible as it matures.[56] As long as the scar exhibits a rosier appearance than normal, remodeling or maturation of the immature scar is underway[92] An example is a surgical scar on the incision line. Initially, it is bright red; then, over time, it blanches and conforms to the body contours. The entire

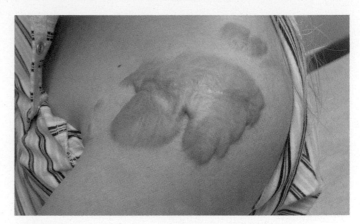

FIGURE 2.26 Hypertrophic scarring.

process of wound remodeling until maturation takes from 3 weeks to 2 years postinjury.[92] Chapter 16 explains normal scar formation processes, complications, and methods of managing scar formation for the most cosmetic and functional outcomes.

REMODELING PHASE IN CHRONIC WOUNDS

The remodeling phase in chronic wounds is altered if there is dysregulation of the remodeling process. The ratio of this activity is an important determinant of the progress of wound healing and formation of hypertrophic scarring and hypergranulation tissue. Figure 2.26 shows hypertrophic scaring and Figure 2.27 shows hypergranulation tissue.

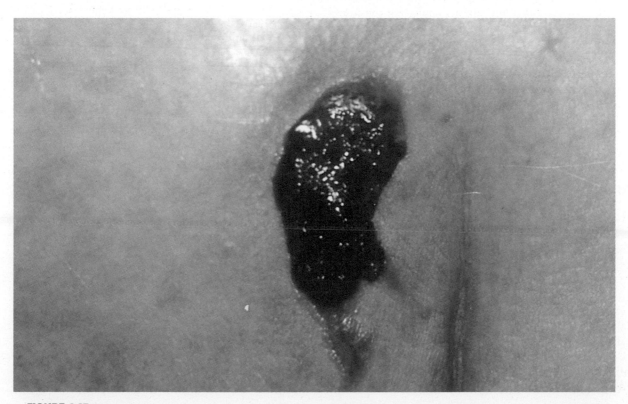

FIGURE 2.27 Wound is in chronic proliferative phase. Note hypergranulation tissue and absence of epithelialization phase. (Copyright © B.M. Bates-Jensen.)

EXHIBIT 2.2

Twelve Possible Wound Healing Phase Diagnoses

1. Acute Inflammation
2. Chronic inflammation
3. Absence of inflammation
4. Proliferation
5. Chronic proliferation
6. Absence of proliferation
7. Epithelialization
8. Chronic epithelialization
9. Absence of epithelialization
10. Remodeling
11. Chronic remodeling
12. Absence of remodeling

When both collagen synthesis and lysis are out of balance, they never seem to reach equilibrium; the result is proliferative scarring or excessive healing. Thus, the repair process continues without an apparent "turn-off switch."[85] There appears to be several reasons for this. Collagen synthesis is oxygen-dependent, but collagen lysis is not. One result of dysregulation, excess oxygen delivery to tissue, is thought to produce *hypergranulation*. Hypergranulation refers to over production of granulation tissue in excess of the surface of the surrounding tissue. Other terms used to describe *hypergranulation* include *exuberant granulation, hyperplasia or "proud flesh,"* and they are synonymous. Hypergranulation inhibits epidermal cell movements because they must now move against gravity, which they are now unable to do and thus cannot cover and resurface the wound.

Excessive scarring is associated with dysregulation and the failure to eliminate TGF-β receptors, which are expressed by overactive fibroblasts during the remodeling phase. The result is persistent overproduction of matrix proteins and fibrosis.[33,34]

SUMMARY

Acute wound healing has been studied extensively, and information learned over time has been extrapolated and applied to chronic wound healing based on the assumption that chronic wound healing is "abnormal." Research has identified chronic wound healing as a different process in many ways, as described in this chapter. The current thinking is that imbalances exist in the molecular environment of healing and nonhealing wounds. When the scales are tipped toward low levels of inflammatory cytokines and proteases, and mitotically competent cells are present, the balance will produce high mitogenic activity and healing. When high levels of inflammatory cytokines and proteases are present along with

RESEARCH WISDOM

Hypergranulation in Horses

In the veterinary community, there has been significant interest in hypergranulation because it is a frequent complication of wound healing on the legs of horses. Predisposing factors for hypergranulation in horses include tissue hypoperfusion, infection, trauma, and bandaging of wounds.[115–118] In horses, the initial inflammatory reaction tends to be protracted, and this leads to the perseverance of TGFβ-1 well into the proliferative phase; this is suggested as the predisposing factor that leads to production of excessive granulation tissue. One study of horses reported findings that TGFβ-1 and TGFβ-3 expression in normal and exuberant wound healing are different. The latter tend to have higher concentrations of fibrogenic TGFβ-1 and lower concentrations of antifibrotic, antiscarring TGFβ-3. However, the differences were not statistically significant. Based on the study results, the authors suggest that production of exuberant granulation is related to bandaging (dressing) of the wound, which is associated with higher concentration of fibrogenic TGFβ-1 and decreased expression of antifibrotic TGFβ-3. Healing appeared normal in wounds in which the TGFβ-3 concentrations were higher.[117]

Different dressing types appear to be related to hypergranulation formation.[119] Silicone gel dressings were found to prevent hypergranulation and improve tissue quality. Possible rationale includes

1) Microvessel occlusion, which occurs significantly more often in wounds that were dressed with silicone
2) Gradual decrease in oxygen tension in the tissue until the point of anoxia, when fibroblasts no longer function adequately and undergo apoptosis, and the ratio of collagen synthesis to degradation is altered in favor of degradation minimizing fibrosis
3) Diminished expression of mutant p53, an indirect inhibitor of apoptosis also found in these wounds. Exuberant granulation typically does not go on to wound closure.[48]

CLINICAL WISDOM

Wound dressings appear to play a significant role in exuberant granulation tissue formation and hypertrophic scarring, in humans, related to prolonged contact of the wound tissue with wound fluid. Dressings are described in Chapter 20.

senescent cells, there is low mitogenic activity, and the result is a chronic wound.[53] Understanding the differences between acute and chronic wound healing is a work in progress; as scientists demonstrate new findings, this information is being used to customize treatment interventions. Other chapters in this book are devoted to those interventions.

REVIEW QUESTIONS

1. The erupting volcano effect is attributed to which type of pressure ulcer?
   A. Deep Tissue Injury
   B. Stage II
   C. Stage III
   D. Stage IV

2. Experts agree that fetal tissue is different from adult tissue. Which of the following statements is true regarding fetal tissue and healing?
   A. Contraction is a usual event along with minimal scarring.
   B. Low levels of adrenal steroids and an immature immune system affects cellular activity.
   C. Amniotic fluid surrounding the fetus has no effect on the healing response of the fetus.
   D. When amniotic fluid is removed there is an abrupt transition to adult like healing.

3. The shape of the myofibroblast "picture frame" beneath the skin can be predictive of the speed of wound contraction. Which statement is true?
   A. Linear wounds contract moderately.
   B. Circular wounds contract slowly.
   C. Rectangular wounds contract rapidly.
   D. Square wounds contract slowly.

4. Chronic wound fluid has been shown to:
   A. Inhibit proliferation of endothelial cells.
   B. Promote proliferation of keratinocytes.
   C. Inhibit proliferation of proinflammatory cytokines.
   D. Promote proliferation of fifibroblasts.

5. High levels of matrix metalloproteinases (MMPs) can result in:
   A. Excessive tissue degradation.
   B. Maintenance of growth factor levels.
   C. Promotion of cell surface receptors.
   D. Promotion of tissue inhibitors of metalloproteinase (TIMPS)

REFERENCES

1. Hunt TK, Van Winkle W. *Fundamentals of Wound Management in Surgery, Wound Healing: Normal Repair.* South Plainfield, NJ: Chirurgecom; 1976.
2. Goldman R. Growth factors and chronic wound healing: past, present and future. *Adv Skin Wound Care.* 2004;17(1):24–35.
3. Wulf HC, Sandby-Møller J, Kobayasi T, et al. Skin aging and natural photoprotection. *Micron.* 2004;35(3):185–191.
4. Yosipovitch G, Hu J. The importance of skin pH. *Skin Aging.* 2003;11:88–93.
5. Schultz GS, Mozingo D, Romanelli M, et al. Wound Healing and TIME; new concepts and scientific applications. *Wound Repair Regen.* 2005;13(4):S1–S11.
6. Halkier-Sorenson L. Understanding skin barrier dysfunction in dry skin patients. *Skin and Wound Care.* 1999;7:60–64.
7. Dykes P, Heggie R, Hill S. Effects of adhesive dressings on the stratum corneum of the skin. *J Wound Care.* 2001;10(2):7–10.
8. Langemo D, Hunter S, Anderson J, et al. Incorporating a body wash and skin protectant into skin care protocols reduces skin breakdown in two nursing homes. *Extended Care Products News.* 2003:36–37.
9. Maklebust J, Sieggreen M. Glossary. In: Maklebust J, Sieggreen M, ed. *Pressure Ulcers: Guidelines for Prevention and Nursing Management.* West Dundee, IL: S.N. Publications; 1996:8–9.
10. Sibbald RG, Cameron J, Alavi A. Dermatological aspects of wound care. In: Krasner DL, Rodehaver GT, Sibbald RG, eds. *Chronic Wound Care: A clinical Source Book for Healthcare Professionals.* 3rd ed. Wayne, PA: HMP Communications; 2001:273–285.
11. Chen John WY, Abatangelo G. Functions of hyaluronan in wound repair. *Wound Repair Regen.* 1999;7(2):79–89.2.

12. Li L, Mac-Mary S, Marsaut D, et al. Age related changes in skin topography and microcirculation. *Arch Dermatol Res.* 2006;297:412–416.
13. Gilhar A, Ullmann Y, Karry R, et al. Aging of human epidermis: the role or apoptosis, FAS and telomerase. *Br J Dermatol.* 2004;150:56–63.
14. Petrofsky JS, Lohann III E, Suh HJ, et al. The effect of Aging on conductive heat exhange in the skin at two environmental temperatures. *Med Sci Monit.* 2006;12(10):CR400–CR408.
15. Petrofsky J, Bains G, Prowse M, et al. Dry heat, moist heat and body fat: are heating modalities really effective in people who are overweight? *J Med Eng Technol.* 2009;33(5):361–369.
16. Grassi G, Seravalle G, Turri C, et al. Impairment of thermoregulatory control of skin sympathetic nerve traffic in the elderly. *Circulation.* 2003;108(6):729–735.
17. McLellan K, Petrofshy JS, Zimmerman G, et al. Multiple stressors and the response of vascular endothelial cells: the effect of aging and diabetes. *Diabetes Technol Ther.* 2009;11(2):73–77.
18. Petrofsky J, McLellan K, Bains G, et al. Skin heat dissipation: the influence of diabetes, skin thickness and subcutaneous fat thickness. *Diabetes Technol Ther.* 2008;10(6):487–493.
19. Black J, Baharestani M, Black S, et al. An overview of tissue types in pressure ulcers: a consensus panel recommendation. *Ostomy Wound Manage.* 2010;56(4):28–44.
20. Kendall FP, McCreary EK, Provance PG, et al. Muscle testing and function with posture and pain. 5th Edition, Lippincott Williams and Wilkins, Baltimore, MD: 2005;9.
21. Van Rijswijk L. Frequence of reassessment of pressure ulcer, NPUAP Proceedings. *Adv Wound Care.* 1995;8(suppl 4):19–24.
22. Ferrell BA, Osterweil D, Christenson P. A randomized trial of low-air-loss beds for treatment of pressure ulcers. *JAMA.* 1993;269:494–497.

23. Hunt TK, Hussain M. Can wound healing be a paradigm for tissue repair? *Med Sci Sports Exerc*. 1994;26:755–758.

24. Cooper DM. The physiology of wound healing: an overview. In: Krasner D, ed. *Chronic Wound Care: A Clinical Source Book for Healthcare Professionals*. Vol. 1. King of Prussia, PA: Health Management Publications; 1990:1–10.

25. Winter GD. Formation of the scab and the rate of epithelization of superficial wounds in the skin of the young domestic pig. *Nature*. 1962;193:293–294.

26. Grande DJ, Mezebish DS. Skin grafting. *Emedicine* [online]. October 1, 2008. Accessed May 4, 2010.

27. Lazarus GS, Cooper DM, Knighton DM, et al. Definitions and guidelines for assessment of wounds and evaluation of healing. *Arch Dermatol*. 1994;130:489–493.

28. Adzick NS, Harrison MR, Glick PI, et al. Comparison of fetal, newborn and adult wound healing by histologic, enzyme-histochemical and hydroxyproline determination. *J Pediatr Surg*. 1985;20:315.

29. Harrison MR, Langer JC, Adzick N, et al. Correction of congenital diaphragmatic hernia in utero. V: initial clinical experience. *J Pediatr Surg*. 1990;25:47.

30. Harrison MR, Adzick NS, Longaker MT, et al. Successful repair in utero of a fetal diaphragmatic hernia after removal of herniated viscera from the left thorax. *N Engl J Med*. 1990;322:1582.

31. Mast B. The skin. In: Cohen I, Diegelmann RF, Lindblad WJ, ed. *Wound Healing Biochemical and Clinical Aspects*. Philadelphia, PA: WB Saunders; 1992:344–355.

32. Hock RJ. The physiology of high altitude. *Aci Amer*. 1987;22:52.

33. Schmid P, Itin P, Cherry G, et al. Enhanced expression of transforming growth factor-beta type I and type II receptors in wound granulation tissue and hypertrophic scar. *Am J Pathol*. 1998;152(2): 485–493.

34. Robson MC. Proliferative scarring. *Surg Clin North Am*. 2003;83:557–569.

35. Byl N, McKenzie A, Stern R, et al. Amniotic fluid modulates wound healing. *Eur J Rehab Med*. 1993;2:184–190.

36. Byl N, McKenzie A, West J, et al. Pulsed micro amperage stimulation: a controlled study of healing of surgically induced wounds in Yucatan pigs. *Phys Ther*. 1994;74:201–218.

37. Edmonds M. Hyaluronic Acid in Recalcitrant Ulcers. Paper presented at: Evidence Based Outcomes in Wound Management; March 31, Dallas, TX; 2000.

38. Hunt TK, Heppenstall RB, Pines E, et al. *Soft and Hard Tissue Repair: Biological and Clinical Aspects*. New York, NY: Praegar Publishers; 1984.

39. Kerstein MD, Bensing KA, Brill LR, et al. *The Physiology of Wound Healing*. Philadelphia, PA: The Oxford Institute for Continuing Education and Allegheny University of Health Sciences; 1998.

40. Grinnell F, Billingham RE, Burgess L. Distribution of fibronectin during wound healing in vivo. *J Invest Dermatol*. 1981;76(3): 181–189.

41. Doherty D, Haslett C, Tonnesen M, et al. Human monocyte adherence: a primary effect of chemotactic factors on the monocyte to stimulate adherence to human endothelium. *J Immunol*. 1987;138(6):1762–1771.

42. Steed D. The role of growth factors in wound healing. *Surg Clin North Am*. 1997:575–586.

43. Sessler DI. Mild perioperative hypothermia. *N Engl J Med*. 1997;336(24):1730–1736.

44. Michaelson AD, MacGregor H, Barnard MR, et al. Reversible inhibition of human platelet activation by hypothermia in vivo and in vitro. *Thromb Haemost*. 1994;71(5):633–640.

45. Valeri CR, Khabbaz K, Khuri SF, et al. Effect of skin temperature on platelet function in patients undergoing extracorporeal bypass. *J Thorac Cardiovasc Surg*. 1992;104(1):108–116.

46. Horzic M, Bunoza D, Maric K. Contact thermography in a study of primary healing of surgical wounds. *Ostomy Wound Manage*. 1996;42(1):36–42.

47. Conolly WB, Hunt T, Sonne M, et al. Influence of distant trauma on local wound infection. *Surg Gynecol Obstet*. 1969;128(4): 713–717.

48. Hunt T, Hopf H. Wound healing and wound infection: What surgeons and anesthesiologists can do. *Surg Clin North Am*. 1997;77(3): 587–606.

49. Knighton DR, Silver IA, Hunt TK. Regulation of wound-angiogenesis: effect of oxygen gradients and inspired oxygen concentration. *Surgery*. 1981;90:262.

50. Clark R. Wound repair: overview and general considerations. In: Clark R, ed. *The Molecular and Cellular Biology of Wound Repair*. New York, NY: Plenum Press; 1996:3–50.

51. Calvin M. Cutaneous wound repair. *Wounds: A Compendium of Clinical Research and Practice*. 1998;10(1):12–32.

52. Ovington Lisa G, Cullen B. Matrix metalloprotease modulation and growth factor protection. *Wounds: A Compendium of Clinical Research and Practice*. 2002;14:1–13.

53. Schultz GS, Sibbald GR, Falanga V, et al. Wound bed preparation: a systematic approach to wound management. *Wound Repair Regen*. 2003;11(1):S1–S28.

54. Moseley R, Stewart JE, Stephens P, et al. Extracellular matrix metabolites as potential biomarkers of disease activity in wound fluid: lession learned from other inflammatory diseases? *Br J Dermatol*. 2004;150:401–413.

55. Sanchez-Fidalgo S, Martin-Lacave I, Illanes M, et al. Angiogenesis, cell proliferation and apoptosis in gastric ulcer healing. Effect of a selective cox-2 inhibitor. *Eur J Pharmacol*. 2004;505(1–3): 187–194.

56 Suh D, Hunt T. Time line of wound healing. *ClinPodiatr Med Surg*. 1998;15(1):1–9.

57. Knighton DR, Halliday B, Hunt TK, et al. Oxygen as an antibiotic: the effect of inspired oxygen on infection. *Arch Surg*. 1984;119: 199–204.

58. Hohn DC, et al. Effect of O_2 tension on microbicidal function of leukocytes in wounds and in vitro. *Surg Forum*. 1976;27:18–20.

59. Goodson WH, Andrews WS, Thakral KK, et al. Wound oxygen tension of large vs. small wounds in man. *Surg Forum*. 1979;30: 92–95.

60. Phillips T, Machado F, Trout R, et al. Prognostic indicators in venous ulcers. *J Am Acad Dermatol*. 2000;43(4):627–630.

61. Byl N. Electrical stimulation for tissue repair: basic information. In: Nelson R, Hayes KW, Currier DP, eds. *Clinical Electrotherapy*. 3rd ed. Samford, CT: Appleton & Lange; 1999.

62. Jonsson K, Jensen JA, Goodson WH III, et al. Tissue oxygenation, anemia, and perfusion in relation to wound healing in surgical patients. *Ann Surg*. 1991;214(5):605–613.

63. Boykin JV. The nitric oxide connection: hyperbaric oxygen therapy, becaplermin, and diabetic ulcer management. *Adv in Skin and Wound Care*. 2000;13(4):169–174.

64. Debats BJG, Wolfs TGAM, Gotoh T, et al. Role of arginine in superficial wound healing in man. *Nitric oxide*. 2009;21:175–183.

65. Frank S, Kampfer H, Wetzler C, et al. Nitric oxide drives skin repair: novel functions of an established mediator. *Kidney Int*. 2002;61(3)882–888.

66. Witte M, Barbul A. General principles of wound healing. *Surg Clin N Am*. 1997;77(3):509–528.

67. Izenberg JS, Frazier WA, Roberts DD. Thrombospoondin-1 is a central regulator of nitric oxide signaling in vascular physiology. *Cell Mol Life Sci*. 2008;65(5):728–742.

68. Schaeffer MR, Tantry U, Gross SS, et al. Nitric oxide regulates wound healing. *J Surg Res*. 1996;63:237–240.

69. Schaffer MR, Tantry U, Efron PA, et al. Diabetes impaired healing and reduced nitric oxide synthesis: a possible pathophysiologic correlation. *Surgery*. 1997;121(5):513–519.

70. Lock PM. The effect of temperature on mitotic activity at the edge of experimental wounds. Paper presented at: Symposium on Wound Healing: Plastic, Surgical and Dermatologic Aspects, 1979; Molndal, Sweden.

71. Myers JA. Wound healing and use of modern surgical dressing. *Pharm J*. 1982;229:103–104.

72. Coleridge-Smith PD. Oxygen, oxygen free radicals and reperfusion injury. In: Krasner D, Kane D, eds. *Chronic Wound Care: A Clinical Source Book for Healthcare Professionals*. Vol 1. Wayne, PA: Health Management Publications, Inc.; 1997:348–353.

73. Knighton DR. HTIene. The defenses of the wound. In: Howard RJ SR, ed. *Surgical Infectious Diseases*. 2nd ed. Stamford, CT: Appleton & Lange; 1988:188–193.

74. Ross J. Utilization of pulsed high peak power electromagnetic energy (diapulse therapy) to accelerate healing processes. Paper presented at: Digest International Symposium, Antennas and Propagation Society; June 20–22, 1977; Stanford, CA.

75. Dyson M, Luke D. Induction of mast cell degranulation in skin by ultrasound. *IEEE Trans Ultrason Ferroelectr Freq Control*. 1986;33: 194–201.

76. Dexter TM, Stoddart RW, Quazzaz STA. What are mast cells for? *Nature*. 1981;291:110–111.

77. Becker RO. The significance of bioelectric potentials. *Med Times*. 1967;95:657–659.

78. Foulds IS, Barker AT. Human skin battery potentials and their possible role in wound healing. *Br J Dermatol*. 1983;109:515–522.

79. Vanable J Jr. Natural and applied voltages in vertebrate regeneration and healing. In: Liss AR, ed. *Integumentary Potentials and Wound Healing*. New York, NY: 1989.

80. Orinda N, Feldman JD. Directional protrusive pseudopodial activity and motility in macrophages induced by extracellular electric fields. *Cell Motil*. 1982;2:243–255.

81. Fukishima K, Senda N, Inui H, et al. Study of galvanotaxis of leukocytes. *Med J Osaka Univ*. 1953;4:195–208.

82. Kloth LC. Electrical stimulation in tissue repair. In: McColloch JM KL, Feeder JA, ed. *Wound Healing Alternatives in Management*. 2nd ed. Philadelphia, PA: F.A. Davis; 1995:292.

83. Erickson CA, Nuccitelli R. Embryonic fibroblast motility and orientation can be influenced by physiological electric fields. *Cell Biol*. 1981;98:296–307.

84. Bourguignon GJ, Bourguignon LYW. Electric stimulation of protein and DNA synthesis in human fibroblasts. *FASEB J*. 1987;1:398.

85. Bates-Jensen B. *A Quantitative Analysis of Wound Characteristics as Early Predictors of Healing in Pressure Sores. Dissertation Abstracts International, Volume 59, Number 11* University of California, Los Angeles; 1999.

86. Eaglstein W, Falanga V. Chronic wounds. *Surg Clin North Am*. 1997;77(3):689–700.

87. Wipke-Tevis D, Stotts N. Leukocytes, ischemia, and wound healing: s critical interaction. *Wounds*. 1991;3(6):227–238.

88. Tomic-Canic M. Keratinocyte cross-talks in wounds. *Suppl Wounds*. 2005:3–9.

89. Shea JD. Pressure sore: classification and management. *Clin Orthop*. 1975;112:89–100.

90. Jaffe LP, Vanable JW. Electric field and wound healing. *Clin Dermatol*. 1984(3):233–234.

91. Seiler WD, Stahelin HB. Implications for research. *Wounds*. 1994;6:101–106.

92. Hardy MA. The biology of scar formation. *Phys Ther*. 1989;69(12):1014–1023.

93. Kirsner R, Eaglstein W. The wound healing process. *Dermatol Clin*. 1993;11:629–640.

94. Steffensen B, Hakkinen L, Larjava H. Proteolytic events of wound-healing—coordinated interactions among matrix metalloproteinases (MMPs), integrins, and extracellular matrix molecules. *Crit Rev Oral Biol Med*. 2001;12(5):373–398.

95. Harding KG, Bale S. Wound care: putting theory into practice in the United Kingdom. In: Krasner D, Kane D, eds. *Chronic Wound Care: A Clinical Source Book for Healthcare Professionals*. Vol 1. 2nd ed. Wayne, PA: Health Management Publications; 1997: 115–123.

96. Weiss EL. Connective tissue in wound healing. In: McCulloch J KL, Feedar J, ed. *Wound Healing Alternatives in Management*. 2nd ed. Philadelphia, PA: F.A. Davis; 1995:26–28.

97. Byl N, McKenzie AL, West JM, et al. Low-dose ultrasound effects on wound healing: a controlled study with Yucatan pigs. *Arch Phys Med Rehabil*. 1992;73:656–663.

98. Bertone M, Dini V, Romanelli P, et al. Objective analysis of heterologous collagen efficacy in hard to heal venous leg ulcers *Wounds*. 2008;20(9):245–249.

99. Vande Berg JS, Rudolph R, Hollan C, et al. Fibroblast senescence in pressure ulcers. *Wound Repair Regen*. 1998;6(1):38–49.

100. Wysocki A. Fibronectin in acute and chronic wounds. *J ET Nurs*. 1992;19(5):166–170.

101. Hynes R. Molecular biology of fibronectin. *Ann Rev Cell Biol*. 1985;1:67–90.

102. Grinnell F, Zhu M. Identification of neutrophil elastase as the proteinase in burn wound fluid responsible for degradation of fibronectin. *J Invest Dermatol*. 1994;103(2):155–161.

103. Parks W. The production, role, and regulation of matrix metalloproteinases in the healing epidermis. *Wounds*. 1995;7(5 suppl A): 23A–37A.

104. Staiano-Coico L, Higgins PJ, Schwartz SB, et al. Wound fluids: a reflection of the state of healing. *Ostomy Wound Manage*. 2000;46(1A):85S–93S.

105. Park H-Y, Shon K, Phillips T. The effect of heat on inhibitory effects of chronic wound fluid on fibroblasts in vitro. *Wounds: A Compendium of Clinical Research and Practice*. 1998;10(6):189–192.

106. Bucalo B, Eaglstein W, Falanga V. Inhibition of cell proliferation by chronic wound fluid. *Wound Repair Regen*. 1989;1(3):181–186.

107. Grinnell F, Ho C, Wysocki A. Degradation of fibronectin and vitronectin in chronic wound fluid: Analysis by cell blotting, immunoblotting, and cell adhesion assays. *J Invest Dermatol*. 1992;98(4):410–416.

108. Bennett N, Schultz GS. Growth factors and wound healing: Part II. Role in normal and chronic wound healing. *Am J Surg*. 1993;166(1):74–81.

109. Cooper D, Yu EZ, Hennessey P, et al. Determination of endogenous cytokines in chronic wounds. *Ann Surg*. 1994;219(6):688–691.

110. Pierce G, Tarpley J, Tseng J, et al. Detection of platelet-derived growth factor (PDGF)-AA in actively healing human wounds treated with recombinant PDGF-BB and absence of PDGF in chronic non-healing wounds. *J Clin Invest*. 1995;96(3):1336–1350.

111. Yager D, Zhang L, Liang H, et al. Wound fluids in human pressure ulcers contain elevated matrix metaloproteinase levels and activity compared to surgical wound fluids. *J Invest Dermatol*. 1996;107(5):743–748.

112. Siddiqui A, Galiano RD, Connors D, et al. Differential effects of oxygen on human dermal fibroblasts: acute versus chronic hypoxia. *Wound Repair Regen*. 1996;4(2):211–218.

113. Gogia P. Physiology of wound healing. In: Gogia P, ed. *Clinical Wound Manage*. Thorofare, NJ: Slack; 1995:1–12.

114. Stamenkovic I. Extracellular matrix remodelling: the role of matrix metalloproteinases. *J Pathol*. 2003;200(4):448–464.

115. Engelen M, Besche B, Lefay MP, et al. Effects of ketanserin on hypergranulation tissue formation, infection, and healing of equine lower limb wounds. *Can Vet J*. 2004;45(2):44–49.

116. Berry DB II, Sullins KE. Effects of topical application of antimicrobials and bandaging on healing and granulation tissue formation in wounds of the distal aspect of the limbs in horses. *Am J Vet Res.* 2003;64.(1):88–92.

117. Theoret CL, Barber SM, Moyana TN, et al. Preliminary observations on expression of transforming growth factors beta 1 and beta 3 in equine rull-thickness skin wounds healing normally or with exuberant granulation tissue. *Vet Surg.* 2002;31(3):266–273.

118. De martin I, Theoret CL. Spatial and Temporal Expression of Types I and II Receptors for Transforming Growth Factor TGF-β; in Normal Equine Skin and Dermal Wounds. *Vet Surg.* 2004;33(1):70–76.

119. Ducharme-Desjarlais M, Celeste CJ, Lepault E, et al. Effect of a silicone-containing dressing on exuberant granulation tissue formation and wound repair in horses. *Am J Vet Res.* 2005;66(7):1133–1139.

120. Fylling CP. Growth factors: a new era in wound healing. In: Diane K, Kane D, eds. *Chronic Wound Car: A Sourcebook for Healthcare Professionals.* 2nd ed. Wayne, PA: Health Management Publications, Inc.; 1997:344–346.

121. Thomas ST. *Management and Dressings.* The Pharmaceutical Press; 1990.

CHAPTER 3

Assessment of the Patient, Skin, and Wound

Carrie Sussman

CHAPTER OBJECTIVES

At the completion of this chapter, the reader will be able to:

1. Identify patient-related factors that effect wound healing.
2. Perform tests and assess adjacent tissues and periwound status.
3. Perform tests and evaluate wound status.
4. Apply classification systems to diagnose wound severity.
5. Explain and apply the concept of wound phase diagnosis, based on the status of the phase of wound healing.

Holistic patient care requires looking at the whole patient including pertinent internal and environmental factors as well as inappropriate management factors that have the potential to interfere with wound healing. Thus, the first portion of Chapter 3 begins by considering these factors. Next is instruction about assessment and evaluation of attributes of the skin and wound. In the following sections, you will learn how the data gleaned from these assessments lead to wound classification and to two wound diagnoses pertaining to the wound healing status.

FACTORS AFFECTING WOUND HEALING

Wound healing processes are complex and sensitive to internal and external environmental forces. In this section, we review internal (host) and external (environmental) factors as well as inappropriate management (iatrogenic) factors that need to be identified and assessed that may interfere with wound healing. We begin this section by looking at the patient and three groups of factors that influence whether a wound will go on to heal or become chronic or refractory:

- Underlying pathology (intrinsic factors)
- Environmental influences (extrinsic factors)
- Inappropriate management (iatrogenic factors)

These factors that affect wound healing are summarized in Table 3.1.

The Patient's Health Status

We begin with the patient's health status including his or her internal and external environment, to identify factors such as comorbidities that will aid in predicting the healing response.

Chronic wounds affect millions of people and are a particular problem of the elderly who are most likely to have comorbidities assumed to impair healing. Few studies have identified specific comorbidities that can be attributed to effecting healing and nonhealing. Two retrospective reviews showed that patients with comorbid conditions of cerebral vascular accident (CVA), neuropathy, and dementia were statistically never likely to heal ($p < .0001$).[1,2] Other important comorbidities identified associated with the never healing included malnutrition, infection,[1] diabetes mellitus (DM), depression, dementia, and degenerative arthritis.[2] Other statistically significant factors identified here as predictive of nonhealing were a high number of chronic ulcers and lower hemoglobin counts.[2] Hypertension, cardiovascular/respiratory diseases, senile dementia, and neurologic disease are conditions identified as associated with development of pressure ulcers.[3] The effects of chronic and comorbid illness on predicting wound healing must be considered as part of the holistic patient evaluation. From what we know, it is reasonable to say that early identification of factors that predict wound healing response will help you triage cases, reduce variability in cost and care, and improve the prognosis and outcome for planned interventions.

Underlying Pathology (Intrinsic Factors)

Underlying pathology includes the intrinsic factors related to the patient's health status that can affect skin integrity and/or healing. Intrinsic factors affecting health and wound healing considered here include age, body systems and associated chronic diseases, perfusion and oxygenation, immunosuppression, neurologically impaired skin, confusion and mental status wound extent and duration, and skin changes at the end of life.

TABLE 3.1	Factors Affecting Wound Healing	
Intrinsic Related to Medical Status	**Extrinsic Related to Environment**	**Iatrogenic Related to Wound Management**
Age	Medications	Local ischemia
Chronic Disease	Nutrition	Inappropriate wound care
Perfusion and oxygenation	Irradiation and chemotherapy	Trauma
Immunosuppression	Psychophysiologic stress	Wound extent and duration
Neurologically impaired skin	Wound bioburden and infection	

Age

Inflammation, cell migration, proliferation, and maturation responses slow with aging.[4,5] A major skin change that occurs with aging is thinning of the epidermis, which increases the risk of injury from shearing and friction, resulting in skin tears and ulceration. The skin also loses its impenetrability to substances in the environment, so irritants and certain drugs are more readily absorbed. The reproductive function of epidermal and fibroblast cells diminishes with age, and replacement is slowed. Elastin fibers are lost, and the skin becomes less elastic. There is diminished vascularity of the dermis, and the dermis atrophies, which slows wound contraction and increases the risk of wound dehiscence.[6] Wound dehiscence is two to three times higher in patients over age 60, yet, as Eaglstein[5] notes, the causative factors may be infection, inadequate protein intake, and other medical complications—not solely age.

Aging and chronic disease states often go together, and both delay repair processes; this is due to delayed cellular response to the injury stimulus, delayed collagen deposition, and decreased tensile strength in the remodeled tissue. The regeneration process can be diminished as a result of impaired circulatory function. Because chronic disease is more common in older adults, age is at least a marker for conditions that predispose to chronic wounds, and it is typically identified as a cofactor in impaired healing.[7] Despite these factors, aging alone is not a major factor in chronic wound healing. Research now demonstrates that healing is only slightly retarded in healthy elderly individuals without chronic disease states, compared with that of a young population.[1,2,8] Patient age does not significantly affect the healing time for leg ulcers associated with venous insufficiency[9] or for neuropathic foot ulcers using total contact casting.[10] However, age appears to affect the risk for skin breakdown in individuals who are older than 85 years; this group demonstrated a 30% risk of developing pressure ulcers.[11]

Chronic Diseases

Cardiopulmonary morbidities. Chronic diseases of all kinds affect the cardiopulmonary system and oxygen-transport pathway that delivers oxygen from the lungs to the tissues and removes carbon dioxide. Oxygenation and oxygen balance in the tissues are key requirements for healing. The cardiopulmonary system is affected by hematologic, neuromuscular, musculoskeletal, endocrine, and immunologic conditions.[12] For example, in patients with chronic obstructive pulmonary disease, breathing functions are compromised. This reduces efficient respiratory function, which affects lung volumes, flow rates, and the delivery of oxygen to and removal of carbon dioxide from the tissues that are required for healing. Impaired cardiopulmonary function affects mobility that is considered a risk factor for skin ulceration.

Diabetes mellitus. Patients with *DM* are at risk for poor wound healing, due to the effects of high blood glucose levels on leukocyte function, predisposing them to increased risk of infection.[13] The microvascular and neuropathic components of diabetes also place these patients at increased susceptibility to impaired healing.[14] The rest of this section and Chapter 12 discuss in more detail how DM influences multiple body systems associated with wound healing.

Immune suppression. In cases of immune suppression, such as is common in patients who have diabetes, cancer, human immunodeficiency virus (HIV) infection, and acquired immune deficiency syndrome, or those who are undergoing immunosuppressive therapy, the body lacks the ability to produce an inflammation phase that initiates the cascade of repair. Absence or impairment of inflammation at the onset of trauma will impair the healing cascade through all phases of healing.[15]

Perfusion and Oxygenation

All phases of wound healing require adequate perfusion to bring nutrients and oxygen to the tissues, thus the lack of perfusion is a significant barrier to healing. Several factors influence perfusion including

Peripheral vascular impairment. Wound healing is dependent on a well-vascularized wound bed to sustain the growth of new tissue and immunological response of the tissues to counter infection, which means that adequate perfusion is required. Impaired peripheral vascular function such as chronic arterial hypertension secondary to peripheral arterial atheroma (hardening of the arteries) restricts blood flow and tissue perfusion because the blood vessels do not dilate but instead create blood flow resistance. A low flow state occurs that is usually located in the lower extremities, and the result is risk for arterial ulceration from severe tissue ischemia and the mechanisms of ischemic reperfusion injury, which were described in Chapter 2. Diabetes also leads to increased susceptibility to peripheral arterial atheroma, which can progress to stenosis and occlusion, ischemia, and ulceration.[16] Oxygen-free-radical activity, also described in Chapter 2, is elevated in individuals with DM and has been implicated in the etiology of vascular complications that may be related to ulceration and poor healing.[16] Chronic venous hypertension leads to leukocyte accumulation in the skin and other tissues of the leg, which initiate the damage that eventually leads to skin ulceration.[16] In addition to generating oxygen-free radicals, these cells replace proteolytic enzymes and inflammatory cytokines that lead to skin ulceration.[16] Thus, when reviewing the medical history, it is important to consider vascular changes such as these as intrinsic factors that will predict the development and healing of vascular ulcers. Perfusion assessment methods are described in Chapter 7. Chapter 11 covers the diagnosis and management of vascular ulcers.

Blood volume. Hypovolemia, the lack of adequate intravascular blood volume, has been shown to impair healing because there is insufficient volume to transport oxygen and nutrients to the tissues and remove waste products.[17] Prolonged hypovolemia impairs collagen production and diminishes leukocyte activities.[8] There are no external signs of mild hypovolemia; its diagnosis is made by measuring the transcutaneous partial pressure of oxygen in the blood (Chapter 6). Hypovolemia should be considered in situations that are common to the chronic wound population, such as the use of diuretics, renal dialysis, and blood loss.

Fluid administration can correct hypovolemia.[8] Hartmann et al.[18] reported that, according to measurements of subcutaneous oxygen tension, fluid replacement improved tissue perfusion[19] and improved accumulation of collagen in healing wounds by day 7 in 29 patients after major abdominal surgery ($p < .05$).[18] Fluid replacement thus can be used to improve tissue perfusion.[19] When replacing fluids, care must be taken to maximize intravascular volume without causing fluid overload, as over hydration can lead to difficulties related to edema. Thus, fluid balance is the key principle to follow to promote wound healing. For example, in anemia, there is reduced hemoglobin and thus reduced oxygen-carrying capacity of the blood. However, research data suggest that anemia does not impair wound healing when there is adequate *perfusion* and *blood volume*.[17]

Immunosuppression

Wound healing is also delayed in patients with HIV or cancer, in those undergoing immunosuppressive therapy, and in severely malnourished individuals.[20] Immunosuppression retards or prevents the inflammatory response and affects all phases of wound healing.[15]

Neurologically Impaired Skin

Neurologically impaired skin is related to several different pathologies. Two such conditions that are often associated with wounds are peripheral neuropathy (PN) and spinal cord injury (SCI).

Peripheral neuropathy is a complication associated with such conditions as chronic diabetes, alcoholism, and chemotherapy and involves the loss of neuronal signaling and transmission. PN usually occurs first in the feet and is progressive in the case of diabetes and other progressive conditions and with repeated series of chemotherapy and ongoing alcoholism. Chemotherapy-induced sensory peripheral neuropathy (CIPN) is a relatively common side effect reported in 30% to 50% of patients who are treated with these agents. CIPN is underestimated and underdiagnosed but is becoming more prevalent as survival rates and lifespan of cancer survivors increase.[21] Therefore, the incidence of skin trauma due to insensitivity can also be expected to rise. Three types of PN can occur: sensory,

motor, and autonomic. Sensory neuropathy is the loss of the ability to recognize and react to sensations of touch, pain, pressure, and kinesthesia (position). It also frequently includes symptoms of burning and paresthesias. Other signs of PN are reports of gait and balance dysfunction. Motor neuropathy is the loss of the motor control of the muscles, and the results are the development of muscle atrophy and imbalance that contributes to structural changes and deformities. Neuropathy of the autonomic nervous system (ANS) impairs the function of the sweat and sebaceous glands located in the skin. When ANS function is impaired in the feet, the skin becomes dry and cracked, providing a portal of entry for infection. The skin acidity also changes, resulting in impairment of the ability to control surface bacteria. Because of an impaired immune system, another complication of diabetes, when infection occurs, these individuals are unable to generate an inflammatory phase of repair and overcome the infection. Chapter 12 describes the examinations for testing for neuropathy, including photos of the consequences of polyneuropathy.

Spinal cord injury results in alteration of the functions of the same three nervous system components: sensory, motor, and autonomic and all may be affected at the same time depending on the extent and location of cord injury. In progressive conditions like PN, neuronal changes occur slowly and progressively over time. If the SCI lesion is above the 6th thoracic level, ANS function is impaired in the early stages postinjury, and the individual is often unable to maintain a constant body temperature. This is due to loss of the ability to dissipate and retain heat from the interior of the body to the periphery via vasomotor responses to heating. Reflex sweating is also lost with injury at these levels, which places the individual with an SCI at risk for overheating.[22] Another complication of SCI is loss of vasomotor tone; this leads to dilation of the veins of the lower extremity, with resultant peripheral edema and frequent deep vein thrombosis.[23]

Neurologically impaired skin in persons with SCI undergoes metabolic changes that can take 3 to 5 years to stabilize following the SCI.[22] These changes include the following:

- The rate of collagen catabolism increases immediately, and significantly, and there is a rapid increase in the rate of collagen catabolism.
- Decreased enzyme activity related to defective collagen biosynthesis in the skin below the level of injury decreases; the increased rate of catabolism of collagen, coupled with defective collagen biosynthesis, produces fragile skin that is more subject to skin breakdown.
- Decrease in the proportion of type I collagen, allowing type III collagen greater prominence in the skin below the level of injury. Recall that properties of type III collagen include thinner, weaker, and has more widely spaced fibrils that contribute to the fragility of the neurologically impaired skin.
- Decrease in the density of adrenergic receptors in the skin below the level of injury could be the cause of abnormal vascular reactions.
- Large increase in the level of glycoaminoglycans (GAGs) excreted in the urine increases, robbing the skin of the elasticity necessary to adapt to mechanical insults.

Motor function loss, paralysis, produces muscle atrophy, which reduces muscle bulk over bony prominences and exposes the skin covering them to mechanical forces. It also limits ability to reposition and to be mobile. Sensory loss causes skin insensitivity and loss of signaling of impending damage. The combination of these changes increases the vulnerability of the skin to ulceration as well as negatively affecting ulcer healing.[22]

Mental Status Changes (Dementia)

Changes in mental status often accompany aging. When there is obvious dementia, it is readily recognized; however, when there is mild cognitive impairment (MCI), it may be unobserved. When a patient with MCI has a wound, he or she may not be able to adhere to a wound management care plan. When you interview a patient, look for symptoms of MCI such as forgetfulness of recent events, inability to understand words, and difficulty focusing on the interview or tasks. Ask a caregiver about personality changes.

Delirium, an acute confusional state, is characterized by reduced attention, changes in cognition, or perceptual disturbances.[24] Delirium and depression may often coexist. Development of delirium is often associated with the use of multiple medications to treat a variety of medical conditions and risk of infection. Delirium can have devastating consequences and in many cases is both preventable and treatable. Suspicion of delirium requires an urgent referral to geriatric medicine or geriatric psychiatry.[24]

Depression is a common finding among elders. Elderly possess several factors that predispose them to depression. Depression is correlated with a sedentary lifestyle, female gender, cigarette smoking, and alcohol consumption. The later behaviors increase as the depression increases. This population is dependent on others and has the presence of multiple disease conditions and associated disabilities, which may include a wound. The occurrence of depression in community-dwelling older adults is reported to be as high as 20% to 37%. Patients who reside in nursing homes have a 15% to 25% prevalence of depression. Older adults also are embarrassed by these changes and often talk about somatic symptoms like aches and pains, and gastric problems diverting attention from the problems of depression. Subclinical depression often goes undetected and untreated due to the common misconception that depression is a part of normal aging or because of social taboos associated with depression or psychiatric care. Depression is characterized by diminished appetite and significant weight loss; loss of interest in activities of daily living; lack of sleep and lethargy; restlessness; decreased capacity to concentrate, act, think, and do problem solving activities; feelings of worthlessness; loss of self-esteem; feelings of guilt; and suicidal or thoughts of death. Major depression is characterized by five or more of these symptoms.[25] All of these factors are associated with impaired ability of wounds to heal.

Undernutrition (Malnutrition) and Dehydration

Undernutrition, formerly referred to as malnutrition, is defined as a state in which there is a nutritional deficiency or an excess or imbalance of energy protein and other nutrients essential for support of bodily functions including healing.[26] Undernutrition affects the hosts' resistance to infection.[27] The causal relationship between undernutrition and skin breakdown is at this point unclear, but it is clear that providing and consuming sufficient kilocalories are necessary for tissue repair.[26] In addition, the patient must be able to chew, swallow, and consume enough nutrients to support tissue growth. Adequate hydration

was mentioned earlier as a requirement for adequate blood volume to perfuse tissues and deliver nutrients and oxygen to tissues as well as other important bodily activities. Chapter 7 discusses nutritional assessment and treatment in detail.

Wound Extent and Duration

Research supports that the extent of wound surface area, multiple wounds, and wound depth are factors in time to healing[1,2] since they impair the hosts' ability to combat infection and to repair.[6,8,28–31] Patients with venous ulcers that are initially large in size or who have moderate arterial insufficiency (ankle-brachial index [ABI] of 0.5–0.8, see Chapter 6) have associated delayed healing times.[9] Injuries with large surface areas and multiple wounds, which increase the total body surface area to be repaired, increase the need for oxygen, nutrients, and adaptive resources for healing because there is more damaged tissue to repair and therefore take longer to heal.

In addition to wound size, duration of ulceration is an important factor influencing wound healing. Researchers looking at factors that can be used to predict wound healing have identified duration and size as two factors that are predictive of healing outcomes. Percentage of healing of ulcerated area at week 3 was a good predictor of 100% healing. Shorter duration of ulceration and smaller size were predictive of reduced time to heal.[32] Ulcers that are large, long-standing, and slow to heal after 3 weeks of optimal therapy are unlikely to change their course.[33] It is now possible to identify and diagnose correctly those ulcers that are unlikely to respond to standard care, and consideration should be given to introduce alternative therapies.[33] Chapter 4 presents information about healing percentage and size change predictors of healing.

Skin Changes at the Life's End (SCALE)

In this section, we have reviewed systems and conditions that are predictive of problems with wound healing or nonhealing. One system deserving special consideration is the skin. The skin is the largest organ in the body and it is subject to failure as are other organs. Kennedy observed that patients at the end of life may experience a skin failure phenomena that is a subset of pressure ulcers that she identified as having the following characteristics: sudden onset; may be pear, butterfly, or horseshoe shape; often located on the sacrum or coccyx but can appear in other areas, with irregular borders, showing colors of red, yellow, and black; and usually precedes death by a short period of time. This is now referred to as a Kennedy Terminal Ulcer (KTU)[34,35] (Fig. 3.1).

Case studies have appeared in the literature that also document this phenomena.[36] The pathogenesis of these ulcers has been attributed to hypoperfusion that occurs in conjunction with multiorgan system dysfunction or failures.[37,38] However, at this time, this is only a suspicion. Research regarding the etiology and pathogenesis of this phenomena is under study.

Since KTU are considered a type of pressure ulcer, a persistent question in health care is whether all pressure ulcers are avoidable. To address this question, a panel of experts convened to consider this problem and the result is 10 consensus statements about skin changes at the end of life. The panel recognized that at the end of life skin, the largest organ in the body, like any other organ undergoes "Physiological changes that occur as a result of the dying process (days or weeks) (that) may affect the skin and soft tissues and may manifest as observable

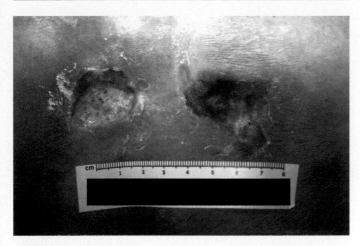

FIGURE 3.1 Photo of KTU (Photograph used with permission of Karen Lou Kennedy.)

(objective) changes in skin color, turgor, or integrity, or as subjective symptoms such as localized pain. These changes can be unavoidable and may occur with the application of appropriate interventions that meet or exceed the standard of care."[38] This is the first consensus statement by the SCALE expert panel recognizing that current knowledge of skin changes at life's end are limited and that skin changes are insidious and difficult to prospectively determine. The panel came up with nine additional statements to address this problem. All statements from the panel along with a glossary of terms and references are available online at www.gaymar.com. The patient's circle of care (members of the family, significant others, caregivers, and health-care professionals) needs to be educated regarding identifying and managing SCALE. Therefore, the topic is raised here as we proceed to learn about wound assessment attributes. For detailed information about pressure ulcers, see Chapter 9.

Extrinsic (Environmental) Factors

Extrinsic factors come from sources in the environment that affect the body or wound, such as medications, nutrition, irradiation and chemotherapy, wound bioburden and infection, and psychophysiologic stress.

Medications

Anticoagulation and anti-inflammatory agents. Many patients with chronic wounds have multiple comorbidities requiring medications that interfere with platelet activation. These include anticoagulation agents (e.g., warfarin or heparin), antiplatelet aggregation medications (e.g., clopidogrel, aspirin, or other salicylates), and/or nonaspirin nonsteroidal anti-inflammatory drugs (NSAIDS) (e.g., ibuprofen or cyclooxygenase [COX-2] inhibitors) medications. All of these drugs interfere with platelet activation.[39] Even a baby aspirin, 81 mg, can cause maximum inhibition of platelet function and primary hemostasis.[39] The effects of NSAIDs and aspirin on platelets is reversible, and the degree of intensity and duration of inhibition of platelet function by NSAIDs is dose-dependent. Many individuals are on a prophylactic regime of baby aspirin, so this should be checked as part of the medical history. Platelet function returns to normal within 12 hours of administration of these drugs.[39]

Nonaspirin NSAIDs can have both negative and beneficial effects on the coagulation cascade. Early in the inflammatory phase, these drugs can blunt the coagulation response, setting the stage for delayed wound healing as well as having negative effects on progression to the proliferative phase when angiogenesis is occurring, because they alter the balance of antiangiogenic and proangiogenic factors.[40] However, they may be beneficial in controlling inflammation during the resolution of the inflammatory phase but should be discontinued, if possible, during the proliferative phase, because in the proliferative phase, they inhibit angiogenesis by altering the balance of antiangiogenic and proangiogenic factors and have a direct effect on endothelial cells. Subsequently, there may be deleterious effects on mitogenic activity of fibroblast growth factor (FGF) that can reduce proliferation of fibroblasts. Consequently, the ratio of proliferation by the fibroblasts to apoptosis is diminished with both NSAIDs and COX-2.[41] This results in decreased collagen production in the proliferative/angiogenic phase.[42]

Another consequence of using these medications on a regular basis is that people who use them bruise easily, an effect that may increase the risk of pressure ulceration. Finally, NSAIDs have other adverse effects, including gastrointestinal bleeding and delayed healing of colonic anastomoses.[40] Your clinical judgment is required to evaluate the risks and benefits of these medications for patients with wounds.

Steroids. Steroids are another class of medication of concern in wound healing. Steroids are prescribed for a diverse group of disorders, ranging from asthma to polymyalgia rheumatica. Steroids delay all phases of wound repair. They inhibit macrophage levels, reduce immune-competent lymphocytes, decrease antibody production, and diminish antigen processing.[7,43] Applications of topical vitamin A and systemic vitamin A supplementation are effective in counteracting the effects of steroid medication.[44]

Other common medications. Some other common medications that can alter wound healing include antiprostaglandins and antineoplastics. Specific agents implicated in CIPN include the platinum agents (e.g., cisplatin), taxanes (e.g., paclitaxel and docetaxel), vinca alkaloids, and thalidomide, which is also an antiangiogenesis agent.[21] Phenylbutazone and vitamin E also disrupt normal healing.[7] Data suggest that local anesthetics also cause some cellular impairment of healing, but pain relief can be achieved with no clinically significant impairment in the rate of healing.[7] Prolonged use of antibiotics appears to suppress rate of wound healing.[1]

Nutrition

Protein and calories. Protein energy malnutrition (*PEM*) and insufficient calories are comorbidities related to impaired wound healing. Multiple studies cite this and other forms of malnutrition as a risk factor for wound healing.[45–47] A nutritional assessment should be considered for all patients with wounds who have comorbidities, and it is required for individuals who are unable to take food by mouth or who experience weight loss.

Chapter 7 presents the requirements and methods to do nutritional assessment, the effects of nutrition on wound healing, and nutrition interventions to prevent skin breakdown and promote healing.

Irradiation and Chemotherapy

Radiation therapy is given for the purpose of disrupting cell mitosis, and has ongoing effects for the remainder of the individual's life.[7] The extent, dosage, frequency, and location of irradiation in relation to the wound site will determine its effects on wound healing. Injuries to the cells of repair (fibroblasts and endothelial cells) and the vasculature of the area put tissues that have been irradiated at risk for breakdown and poor healing. The damage may not be visible on the skin surface and may be suppressed or have a latent appearance. Thus, an individual who experienced radiation therapy may show signs of poor wound healing months or years after completion of the radiation therapy treatments. Injuries to the cells of repair (fibroblasts and endothelial cells) and the vasculature of the area put tissues that have been irradiated at risk for breakdown and poor healing. The extent, dosage, frequency, and location of irradiation in relation to the wound site will determine its effect on wound healing. These effects of irradiation on tissue are not easily reversed.[6] Recovery depends on the dose of radiation and the half-life of the various cells.[7]

Chemotherapy is accomplished with anticancer drugs that damage DNA or prevent DNA repair; thus, these drugs can interfere with tissue repair. The primary effects of chemotherapy occur during the treatment period and immediately after it.[7] However, some drugs, such as methotrexate, are used for other medical reasons on a long-term basis and can interfere with tissue repair. Another consequence of chemotherapy as mentioned earlier is induced PN with loss of protective sensation; this puts tissues, particularly those of the feet, at risk for breakdown similar to other peripheral neuropathies. As chemotherapeutic agents become more common, and individuals receive repeat episodes of care, the incidence of impaired wound healing and induced PN is likely to rise.

Bioburden and Infection

Excessive bioburden from necrotic tissue and infection has been identified as a barrier to preparing the wound bed for healing and the development of a chronic wound. For example, epidermal cells normally march forward as a sheet and lyse the necrotic debris from the wound edges; however, they are impaired in this process of phagocytosis if obstructed by a large quantity of devitalized material. Devitalized tissue and foreign matter debris contribute to the proliferation of bacteria in the wound, which, in turn, overwhelms the body with infection and can lead to sepsis. In such situations, the body cannot cleanse the wound without intervention.

It is imperative to clean the wound down to healthy bleeding tissue to restart the inflammatory phase and the biologic cascade of healing. Bleeding creates a new acute inflammatory phase and serves as a signal source for the responder cells. However, if there is inadequate circulation, the response may fail to occur or be inadequate to initiate a new inflammation response. Frequent sharp and mechanical debridement over the first 3 months of care also appears to retard healing.[1] Chapter 16 has detailed information about management of necrotic tissue.

Psychoneuroimmunology and Psychophysiologic Stress

Psychoneuroimmunology (PNI) is a multidisciplinary field of study research that has the central premise that studies interrelationships between the behavioral, nervous, endocrine, and immune systems. Thirty years ago, Ader proposed that these are components of an integrated system of body defenses.[48] Chapter 22 has more information about how these protective systems work together. The PNI premise accounts for many of the current theories about the impact of stress on health outcomes. The effects of PNI interactions—especially those involving stress—on wound healing are the subject of a significant amount of research and the mechanisms of action are only just beginning to be understood. The following is a brief description of how some of the identified mechanisms may affect healing outcomes, and discuss as well PNI interventions used to reduce the effects of stress.

Anatomically, there is a close interaction between the nervous, endocrine, and immune systems and studies demonstrate the existence of physical and chemical links between them at the cellular level.[49] Close communication between the mind and these body systems occurs in both health and disease states.[50] For example, the brain can start, influence, and stop biologic skin events, and negative emotions have the ability to change the functions of the skin by producing signs such as pallor, sweat, horripilation, itching, and/or redness.[51] This is demonstrated by ways in which the skin acts as part of the "diffuse brain" in its ability to modify the quality of perceptions and feelings.

As noted above, one of the most studied aspects of PNI is the interrelationship between stress and the nervous, endocrine, and immune systems. Stress can be positive or negative. Positive stress allows us to perform all of our daily functions, whereas negative stress may weaken the immune system. An example of positive stress is exercise. Emery found that although cortisol levels in healthy elderly adults rose with exercise, this group demonstrated more rapid healing than a comparison group of sedentary healthy elderly, possibly because the exercise activity increased blood flow to the area and improved tissue oxygen levels while enhancing neuroendocrine function.[52] In contrast, it is estimated that negative stress contributes to 50% to 80% of illnesses. Stress is recognized as a risk factor in addictions, obesity, high blood pressure, peptic ulcers, colitis, asthma, insomnia, migraine headaches, and lower back pain. Close communication between the body and mind occurs in both health and disease states.[50]

Cortisol and wound healing. Stress and depression induce the release of pituitary and adrenal hormones, adrenalin, noradrenalin, and cortisol by the endocrine system, and this in turn influences effects of immune function and wound healing. Cortisol is a key regulatory substance. For example, cortisol can up or down regulate proinflammatory cytokine production that appears to be a self-maintaining phenomena associated with both chronic infection and delayed wound healing. Increased cortisol levels suppress migration of neutrophils and inhibit synthesis of proinflammatory mediators like Interleukin-1 (IL 1), Interlukin-6, and impair activation of metal metalloprotease enzymes like MMP-9. This can lead to decreased macrophage function and subsequent suppression of fibroblast proliferation, as well as matrix degradation that affects the duration and strength of the wound.[53] Thus, it is not surprising that high preoperative stress levels are predictive of postsurgical reduction in levels of IL-1 and MMP-9, resulting in more painful, poorer, and slower healing.[53] In another study, paraplegic college students were found to have more skin breakdown during final examination periods than at other times of the school year.[54] Also, caregivers of Alzheimer's patients who experienced wounds were found to take longer to heal than individuals who did not live in such stressful situations.[55] In contrast, the use of guided imagery for relaxation and wound healing of surgical patients has been found to reduce cortisol levels and inflammation. This work parallels the subsequent findings by Braden that individuals with lower cortisol levels did not develop pressure sores.[56] In another study, satisfaction with life activities was inversely related to the incidence of pressure sore development.[57]

Sleep and Wound Healing

Growth hormone, which is essential for tissue repair, is released during the deepest stage of sleep. Thus, interrupted sleep or sleep of short duration can interfere with wound healing, whereas adequate, restful sleep may promote the physiological processes involved with wound healing.[58] The interaction between stress and the growth hormone–somatomedin system is not entirely understood. Lee and Stotts reviewed the effect of the growth hormone–insulin-like growth factors (IGFs), formerly called somatomedin, system on healing, as well as the negative effects of sleep changes and stress on the system. They described the importance of the anabolic function of growth hormone on tissue repair and recommended interventions targeted at healthy functioning of the growth hormone–IGF system. Suggested PNI interventions include promoting adequate time for uninterrupted sleep and encouraging exercise as a mild stressor to promote secretion of growth hormone.[59] North reviewed the effect of sleep on wound healing, concluding that sleep and relaxation may affect the physiological processes involved with wound healing.[58] The exploratory studies and reviews described here have focused on acute wound healing, but studies on the effect of stress as a causative factor in the development of chronic wound healing by interruption of the healing cascade would be useful.

Satisfaction with life activities has been inversely related to the incidence of pressure ulcer development.[57]

Stress-Induced Vascular Changes and Wound Healing

West also examined the role of stress, but looked at the effect of perioperative stress on the repair process, concluding that perioperative stress appears to decreases tissue and wound oxygen tension via vasoconstriction related to high levels of circulating catecholamines.[57] In contrast, biofeedback relaxation training for patients with chronic leg ulcers increased tissue perfusion in the experimental group, which had 87.5% healing compared to 44% healing for the control group.[60]

Noise and Wound Healing

Noise as a stressor has also been explored in relation to wound healing. McCarthy and colleagues reviewed the potential impact of noise on wound healing.[61] Using an animal model, this group of researchers demonstrated impairment in leukocyte function in rats exposed to noise stress, compared with rats not exposed to noise stress. Wysocki in another study demonstrated decreased healing in rats when they were exposed to intermittent noise.[62]

Learned Elements in Wound Healing

The nervous system changes as new information is learned by a process called neuroplasticity. Negative learning such as "learned pain" leads to degradation of nervous system representation that adversely affects the cells of repair, maintenance of inflammation, adequate protein synthesis, and circulation. Chapter 22 has more information about learned pain and neuroplastic changes that effect wound healing.

Reversal of Psychophysiologic Stress

The patient may be able to reverse the adverse effects of stress through PNI interventions including hypnosis, progressive muscle relaxation, exercise, classical conditioning, self-disclosure, visual imagery, visualizing the process of healing (e.g., increasing blood flow to the affected area by imagining the phagocytic cells gobbling up bacteria and debris), and positive self-talk about healing.[51,52,60]

Iatrogenic Factors in Chronic Wound Healing

Iatrogenic factors are related to the specific way that a wound is managed. These include a failure to prevent local ischemia, inappropriate wound care, and additional trauma.

Local Ischemia

Local ischemia can occur in many different ways. For example, failure to prevent chronic ischemia from pressure over a bony prominence, or inappropriate application of compression to a limb with mixed venous and arterial disease. Individuals who smoke experience nicotine-induced vasoconstriction and tissue ischemia. Persons with a history of tobacco use are 76% more likely to develop a pressure ulcer than are nonsmokers[63]

Inappropriate Wound Care

Inappropriate wound care has been implicated as a factor in development of a chronic wound.[6,8] It includes the misuse of topical agents (e.g., antiseptics) or poor technique in the application of dressings and tape that results in tears and blisters on surrounding skin or the wound bed. Inappropriate wound care has been implicated as a factor in development of a chronic wound.[6,8] Wound desiccation from lack of dressing or inappropriate dressing choice is not uncommon. Drying out of the wound interferes with the "current of injury" function (described in Chapter 2) (Fig. 3.2),[64] as well as with the mitotic and migratory function of cells. Dressing changes and wound cleansing disrupt the wound environment, causing chilling of the wound and surrounding tissues. Lock found that it takes up to 40 minutes for the tissues to regain

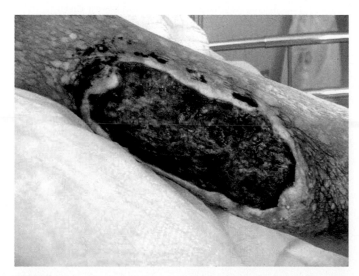

FIGURE 3.2 Desiccated leg ulcer that shows absence of proliferative and epitheliazation phase. When treated properly went on to heal (Copyright © A. Myer.)

their usual temperature, and chilling impairs cell mitosis for up to 3 hours.[65] Chilling also severely disrupts leukocytic activity and oxyhemoglobin dissociation.[66] Persistent use of antimicrobial dressings and frequent dressing changes appears to be associated with higher likelihood of nonhealing.[1]

Containment of wound fluid on the wound with moisture-retentive dressings to maintain a moist wound environment for cell migration and communication has been part of wound management for many years. Although this may be useful for acute wounds, it has since been learned that bathing the wound in chronic wound fluid has a negative effect on the wound healing microenvironment, as described above.[27] For more information about wound care products, (see Chapter 19.)

Additional Trauma

Additional trauma even at a distance from a wound retards the rate of healing due to alteration of the tensions of respiratory gases in previous wounds and causes increased susceptibility to wound infection, probably due to decreased nutritive blood flow.[67] Additional trauma direct to the wound can be attributed to many different causes, including

- High-pressure irrigation, such as in a whirlpool or with a Water Pik™
- Sharp or mechanical debridement
- Improper pressure to new granulation tissue, traumatizing the fragile tissue and initiating a new inflammatory response, which retards healing and causes abnormal scarring
- Improper handling during removal of dressings, compression wraps, or stockings, causing trauma to venous ulcers whose surrounding skin is often extremely fragile

To address the problem of wound trauma, specialized dressings and adhesives have been developed (see Chapter 20).

THE WOUND ASSESSMENT PROCESS

For many years, it was assumed that the healing processes for acute and chronic wounds were equivalent, and that findings from one could be directly applied to the other. However, that opinion has shifted as more is understood about disruption in wound healing physiology and barriers to orderly healing. In this context, the search for the best method of wound assessment is ongoing.

Groups of experts meet and publish reports on best practices for clinicians, such as the wound bed preparation approach to wound management, MEASURE, a proposed wound assessment framework.[27,68] There is consensus by these experts that global assessment is needed when wounds are not healing as expected in order to analyze the probable underlying causes. In these cases, a plan for management of the whole patient, not just the wound, needs to be prepared. What follows adheres to these principles.

Certain familiar terms are used somewhat differently when discussing wound care:

- *Tests* are the instruments or means by which wound events are assessed or measured.
- *Examination* is the process of determining the values of the tests.
- *Assessment* is the systematic process of assigning numbers or grades to wound events during the examination.
- *Evaluation* is the process of making clinical judgments based on the data gathered from the examination. Skills of *evaluation* are necessary for interpreting the appropriateness, significance, reliability, and validity of the tests and measurements.

Both assessment and evaluation require an understanding of the condition, the ability to recognize the importance and value of the information, and the skills to collect this information appropriately and methodically.[69] One thing that differentiates assessment from evaluation is the scope of practice and skill set of the examiner. For example, performing tests and examinations and monitoring tissue attributes are within the scope of practice of physical therapist (PT) assistants and licensed practical/vocational nurses. Evaluation of the data is a skill that is in the purview of licensed PTs, registered nurses, nurse specialists, physician assistants, nurse practitioners, and podiatrists who have advanced skills and knowledge of wound management.

Purpose and Frequency

Wound assessment data are collected for five purposes:

1. Examine the severity (stage) of the lesion
2. Determine the status of wound healing
3. Establish a baseline for the wound
4. Prepare a plan of care
5. Report observed changes in the wound over time

Assessment data enable clinicians to communicate clearly about a patient's wound, provide for continuity in the plan of care, and allow for evaluation of treatment modalities.

Baseline assessment, monitoring, and reassessment are the keys to establishing a plan of care and evaluating the achievement of target outcomes and progress toward goals. For a successful assessment process, start by selecting valid, significant tests and measurements. Continue to use the same tests throughout the course of care to evaluate progress and revise the treatment plan as required.

After the initial or baseline examination, reassess wound attributes at regular intervals in order to measure any change in the status of the ulcer or in risk factors.[70] How frequent should these regular intervals be? One study of category/stage III and category/stage IV pressure ulcers found that the percentage of reduction in the ulcer area after 2 weeks of treatment was predictive of healing time.[70] Thus, reassessment at 2-week intervals is commonly advised. If, after 2 to 4 weeks of appropriate treatment, reassessment indicates that the wound has deteriorated or has failed to improve, the plan of care should be modified, and adjunctive treatment should be considered.[71]

Between full reassessments, wounds must be continually monitored. Monitoring is a means of checking the wound briefly but frequently such as during dressing changes and other treatment applications or signs and symptoms that should trigger a

---

CLINICAL WISDOM

Avoiding Adverse Treatment Effects

Careful evaluation of each treatment and technique, based on wound assessment, can avoid adverse treatment effects and change the course of the wound.

CLINICAL WISDOM

Monitoring Wound Progress

Teach family members and other caregivers to monitor the wound at each dressing change. Help them to identify signs of wound infection, such as large amounts of purulent exudate (pus red or purplish color of nearby skin, warmth, increased tenderness or pain at the site, and elevated temperature). Caregivers should also be aware of healing characteristics, such as bright red color, new skin, and small amounts of clear drainage.

full reassessment, such as increased wound exudate or bruising of the adjacent (i.e., tissues extending away from the periwound) or periwound skin. The periwound skin refers to the tissues immediately surrounding the wound. Monitoring includes gross evaluation for signs and symptoms of wound complications, such as erythema (redness) of nearby skin, and presence of a yellowish drainage, commonly called pus, which is indicative of infection. It should also include progress toward wound healing, such as granulation tissue growth (indicated by red color of newly vascularized tissues) and reepithelialization (new skin observed as pale pink color even in darkly pigmented surrounding skin). Monitoring, unlike assessment, may be performed by unskilled caregivers, such as the patient, the patient's family, or a nurse attendant.

Different care settings have different requirements that designate specific individuals to perform the assessment and monitoring functions. For example, in the home setting, a nonprofessional caregiver may monitor the wound attributes, but a nurse or PT assesses the findings. The caregiver may gather data at dressing changes and predetermined intervals and report changes to the nurse or PT, who evaluates the results of the treatment plan. The professional wound case manager may see the patient's wound only intermittently for a complete reassessment. In a skilled nursing facility, requirements by federal licensing agencies typically prescribe intervals for reassessment. If the patient is in an acute or subacute setting where there are very short lengths of stay, there may be only a single assessment.

Data Collection and Documentation: Forms and Procedures

Data is better organized and more consistent when it is collected on a form, whether on paper or an electronic template. Although many forms exist, the most common is the skin care flow sheet used by nurses. Methods of recording assessment data should allow for the tracking of each assessment item over time, in objective and measurable terms that show changes in wound status. The Sussman Wound Healing Tool (SWHT) and Bates-Jensen Wound Assessment Tool (BWAT), and Pressure Ulcer Scale for Healing (PUSH) tool, mentioned earlier, can be used to record findings and measure each attribute objectively. Both forms, with instructions, are described in Chapter 5.

Useful forms for tissue assessment usually include the following items:

- Periwound skin attributes
- Wound tissue attributes
- Wound exudate characteristics

Regardless of which instrument is used to collect findings, all attributes on the form should be considered. If the attribute is not applicable, the notation "N/A" should be made to fill the blank. If an attribute is absent, record a zero. If present, a grade or check is required. Leaving a blank space on the form implies that the attribute was not considered or assessed.

If the patient's medical diagnosis suggests possible related medical impairments associated with the wound and periwound skin (e.g., neuropathy or vascular disease), multiple forms may be required to report all the necessary elements relating to the patient's condition. Later chapters include forms specific to recording data related to specific problems.

Documentation requirements for wound assessment should be part of a facility's policies and procedures. Documentation should be accurate and clearly reflect the patient's condition, examinations performed, findings, care rendered, and proper notification of the physician of significant findings. Documentation of similar findings by practitioners in the same department or facility should be consistent and reflect facility policies.[72] Remember, medical records can be subpoenaed into court, sometimes several years after the assessment. "Documentation can be either your shield against a potential malpractice lawsuit or the sword that strikes you down."[72]

ASSESSMENT OF SKIN AND WOUND ATTRIBUTES

In this section, we discuss procedures that require you to use your senses to assess the physical characteristics of the skin and wound, that is, the *skin and wound attributes*. For instance, you will use your vision to observe surrounding tissues and the wound; smell to identify healthy from unhealthy tissues; touch to palpate skin and soft tissue contours, temperature, and

CASE STUDY

Dangers of Differing Clinical Procedures and Facility Policies

A PT debrided a toenail on a patient with a medical history of neuropathy associated with diabetes. The toe became infected, leading to below-the-knee amputation of the leg. The PT's action was called into question in a malpractice lawsuit. The debridement procedure followed by the PT was acceptable and documented, but it was the facility's policy to have a patient with diabetic neuropathy evaluated in the vascular laboratory for transcutaneous oxygen levels before debridement. The PT did not document an evaluation of the patient for circulatory status prior to performing the debridement procedure. As a consequence, the PT's action was called into question, and he became the defendant in a malpractice lawsuit.

nervous system responses such as pain and guarding; and hearing to evaluate blood flow with a Doppler ultrasound and to listen to the patient's responses to tests and questions. Note that your assessment findings should reflect a composite of wound attributes. A single attribute cannot provide the data necessary to determine the treatment plan, nor will it allow for the monitoring of progress or degradation of the wound. The attributes for wound assessment include all of the following:

- Location
- Age of wound
- Size of the wound
- Stage or depth of tissue involvement
- Presence of undermining or tunneling
- Presence or absence of tissue attributes that prevent healing (e.g., necrotic tissue in the wound and erythema of the periwound tissue)
- Presence or absence of tissue attributes that aid healing (e.g., condition of the wound edges, granulation tissue, and epithelialization)
- Exudate characteristics
- Pain status

There are two schools of thought regarding tissue assessment: The first looks only at the wound tissue, whereas the second examines adjacent soft tissue structures, periwound skin, and the wound tissue. Because the adjacent and periwound skin are intimately involved in the circulatory response to wounds, and the risk for infection, it is prudent to evaluate all areas. The examination of the wound and periwound skin provides data related to the wound healing phase diagnosis discussed in a later section. Exhibit 3.1 lists the common indexes for wound assessment.

Assessment of the wound is separate from assessment of the etiology of the wound, although the examinations chosen for the assessment can relate to or provide clues to the etiology. For example, wounds caused by venous insufficiency typically appear on the lower leg above the ankle; a brawny color is often seen in the adjacent tissues, edema is likely to be present, and the periwound skin may be fragile. A patient diagnosed with a diabetic ulcer and insensitivity will often have an ulcer on the plantar surface of the foot. There may be areas of callus over bony prominence, bony deformities, and hyperkeratosis of the heel, which are related to polyneuropathy. Therefore, soft tissues adjacent to the area of wounding should be assessed for the attributes of location, sensation, circulation, texture, and color. These findings will be used to establish a treatment plan, and predict wound outcomes.

Observation and Palpation Techniques

Observation and palpation are classic components of physical assessment of skin and wound attributes. They are used to determine alteration in soft tissue characteristics, including the skin, subcutaneous fascia, and muscles leading to a soft tissue or structural diagnosis.[73] Proper lighting and positioning of the patient and tissue to be assessed will improve observation.

Effective palpation technique requires you to use light pressure and slow movements. Pressing too hard and trying to examine the area too quickly can send confusing messages to your hands' sensory receptors. It's also helpful to reduce other sensory inputs in the environment (noise, traffic, conversation). This will help you to concentrate and focus on the palpation examination.

Finally, you need a common language of easily understood terms with which to communicate your findings. Paired descriptors, such as *superficial-deep, moist-dry, warm-cold, painful-nonpainful, rough-smooth, hard-soft*, and *thick-thin*, are useful to accurately describe findings. The state of tissue changes can be reported as acute, subacute, chronic (persistent), or absent.

EXHIBIT **3.1**

Indexes for Wound Assessment

- Anatomic location
- Size: length, width
- Volume: depth (also stage if initial assessment; note if unable to stage)
- Undermining/tunneling
- Age of wound in weeks or months
- Attributes preventing healing: necrotic tissue (including eschar[140], hemorrhage (purple deep tissue injury), periwound erythema and edema, edges undermined (not connected)
- Attributes characteristic of healing: granulation tissue, new epithelium, attached wound edges
- Wound exudate: color, amount, odor, consistency
- Pain: to touch, pressure, tissue tension, all of the time or only during treatment
- Temperature: excess warmth, coolness, normal body temperature for the area

---

CLINICAL WISDOM

Assessment Toolbox

A penlight, small mirror with a long handle, infrared and/or liquid crystal thermometer, and tuning fork are handy items to keep in the assessment toolbox.

Begin the tissue examination by evaluating for symmetry with the contralateral limb and adjacent structures, using both observation and palpation. Look for symmetry of tissue color, texture, contour, hardness/softness, and temperature. When compared with an area of normal skin and soft tissue, any differences in the skin, subcutaneous tissue, fascia, and muscle should be noted.

In palpation, the hands are important, sensitive diagnostic instruments. Your hands should be clean, and your fingernails short. It is important to develop a palpatory sense using different parts of your hands for different tests:

- The palms of the hands are best used to detect changes in soft tissue contours (induration, edema).
- The thumbs are useful in applying pressure to check for hardness or softness at different tissue depths.
- The finger pads are more sensitive to texture (fibrotic tissues) and fine discrimination.
- The back of the hands can get a sense of temperature, warmth or coolness. Follow-up with appropriate testing.

CLINICAL WISDOM

Requirements for a Successful Palpatory Examination

1. Light pressure
2. Slow movement
3. Concentration
4. Standardized language to communicate findings

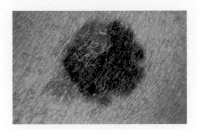

FIGURE 3.3 Photo of melanoma.

They can also be graded on a scale of 0 to 3+; for example, pitting edema, discussed shortly, uses this grading scale. The use of a grading scale is also helpful in reporting response to treatment intervention.

Assessment of Adjacent and Periwound Tissues

The tissues adjacent to and immediately surrounding a closed or open wound provide many clues to the patient's overall health status, the health of the integumentary system, the body's ability to respond to the wound, and the precise phase of wound healing. The attributes of the adjacent tissues and periwound skin that you should assess, which are described in the following sections, include the following:

- Skin texture (e.g., dryness, thickness, turgor)
- Scar tissue
- Callus
- Maceration
- Edema
- Color
- Depth of tissue injury
- Temperature
- Hair distribution
- Toenails
- Blisters
- Sensation (pain, protective sensation, thermal sensation, and vibratory perception threshold [VPT])

Skin Texture

Smooth, flexible skin has a feeling of fullness and resistance to tissue deformation that is called *turgor*. Turgor is a sign of skin health. In aging skin, atrophy and thinning of both the epithelial and the fatty layers commonly result in a loss of turgor. The areas most affected by loss of subcutaneous fat are the upper

RESEARCH WISDOM

ABCD Rule

While checking the skin, observe for ABCD signs of early melanoma:

A: asymmetry—uneven edges, lopsided in shape
B: borders—irregular (scalloped, poorly defined)
C: color—black or shades of brown, red, white, occasionally blue
D: diameter—greater than 5 mm (larger than a pencil eraser)

and lower extremities. This causes more prominent bony protuberances on the hips, knees, ankles, and bony areas of the feet, which results in a higher risk of pressure ulcer formation.

Other changes of aging skin include loss of elasticity because of shrinkage of both collagen and elastin. There is a weakening of the juncture between the epidermis and dermis causing the skin layers to "slide" across each other and placing the person at risk for skin tears. Sebaceous glands and their secretions are diminished, which results in skin that is dry, often itchy, and easily torn.[74] Impaired circulation also contributes to changes in the skin; it is usually associated with aging, but can be due to a disease process, such as neuropathy associated with diabetes. This disease impairs the secretion of sweat and sebaceous glands, which in turn contributes to the slow resurfacing of partial-thickness dermal ulcers. Loss of sweat changes the pH of the skin, making it more susceptible to infection and bacterial penetration.

To assess skin texture, use observation and palpation. Look for evidence of dryness, such as flaking or scaling. To check skin turgor, gently pinch the tissues with thumb and forefinger, and observe how they respond. For example, in older patients, loss of elasticity can be exhibited by the tissues' slow return to normal after pinching. Tenting of the skin when pinched can be an early indicator of dehydration. In older patients, it is best to check for general skin turgor on the forehead or sternal area. Palpate by gently rubbing your fingers across the patient's skin and feeling for sliding of the epidermis away from the dermis.

Skin inspection is an opportunity to spot suspicious signs of early melanoma. If a suspicious skin lesion is noted, ask the patient how long the area of skin has been discolored, whether it has changed shape or size in the past 6 weeks to 6 months, and whether it has been examined by a physician. The ABCD rule with a 90% positive value is a valid screening tool for early melanoma (Fig. 3.3).[75]

Scar Tissue

Inspection of the adjacent skin should include checking for scar tissue. If present, scar tissue should be assessed for smoothness, flexibility, thickness, and toughness. Scar tissue that is mature has greater density and toughness and is less resilient than surrounding skin. New scar tissue is thinner and more flexible than mature scar tissue and is less resilient to stress. Wounding in an area of scarring will have less tensile strength when healed than will a new wound and will be more likely to break down (Fig. 3.4A).

New scar tissue is bright pink in appearance. As the scar tissue matures, it becomes nearly the same color as the periwound skin, except in individuals with darkly pigmented skin. Hypopigmentation frequently follows injuries to dark skin. Loss of skin color can create more anxiety for individuals than the wound itself. If the wounding disruption is less than full-thickness loss of the epidermis, repigmentation will usually

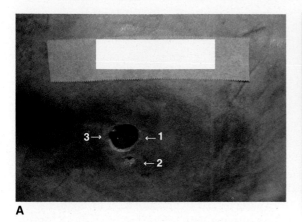
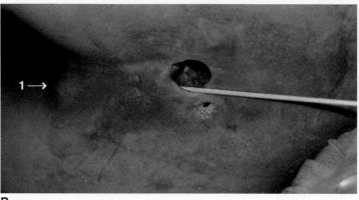

A   **B**

FIGURE 3.4 A: Wound with tunneling before insertion of a cotton-tipped applicator. Note: (1) Ulcer reoccurrence at site of old scar tissue, (2) Skin bridge between two open ulcers, (3) Surrounding skin has unblanchable erythema; wound edges rolled under demonstrate chronic inflammatory phase, (4) Absence of proliferative phase. **B:** Same wound as in (A). The wound's overall size is much larger than the surface open area. Tunneling is present. Note the bulge from the end of the cotton-tipped applicator. (Copyright © B.M. Bates-Jensen.)

occur over time. However, new skin covering deeper lesions and new lesions will appear pink.[76] The scar area can even turn white. Hypopigmented areas are more susceptible to sunburn than are normally pigmented areas. For some individuals, burns and physical trauma can be followed by localized areas of hyperpigmentation. Like hypopigmentation, hyperpigmentation causes anxiety in many individuals.

Observe for abnormal scarring characteristics. Hypertrophic scarring results from excessive collagen deposition, causing a very thick scar mass that remains within the area of the original wound. These scars are unattractive and disfiguring, and can cause itching or pain that interferes with functional mobility (Fig. 3.5).

Hypertropic scars are differentiated from **keloids**, which are also thickened but extend beyond the boundaries of the original wound (Fig. 3.6).[77] Although keloids are found in people of all races, scarring is of special concern to African American individuals and some Asians because of the frequency of keloid formation in these populations. Frequency of occurrence is equal among men and women.

Keloids are similar to benign tumor growths in that they continue to grow long after the wound is closed and can reach a large size. Any attempt to cut or use dermabrasion to buff away a keloid will result in even more scarring.[76] In keloids, the mechanism of collagen deposition is totally out of control. Areas with keloids can be itchy, tender, or painful.[78] New therapies are being used to control this phenomenon, but if a patient reports a previous keloid or a familial tendency to form keloids, special attention should be made to address this problem at the time of initial assessment.

Hyperkeratotic scarring involves hypertrophy of the horny layer of the epidermis. It is commonly seen in diabetic patients and can be located in adjacent and periwound tissue (Fig. 3.7) (see Chapter 16).

Callus

Callus formation is a protective function of the skin to shearing forces of a prominent bone against an unyielding surface—most often, a shoe. The most commonly encountered calluses are located on the plantar surface of the foot, along the medial

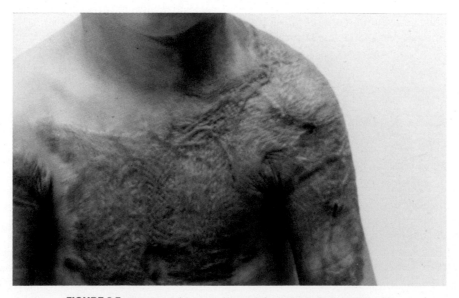

FIGURE 3.5 Hypertrophic scar. (Copyright © 2001, R. Scott Ward.)

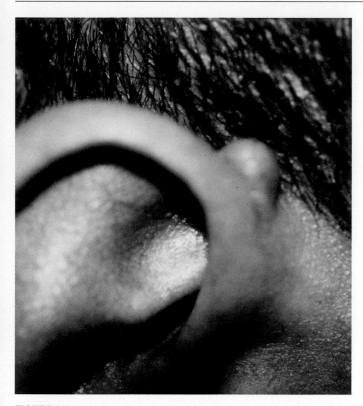

FIGURE 3.6 Keloid scar. (Copyright © 2001, R. Scott Ward.)

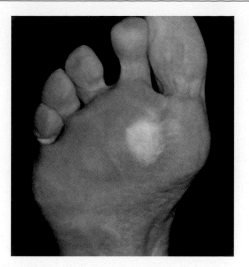

FIGURE 3.8 Callus on plantar surface of foot.

Maceration of Skin and Moisture Balance

Maceration is defined as "the softening of a tissue by soaking until the connective tissue fibers are so dissolved that the tissue components can be teased apart."[74] Where it occurs, the stratum corneum takes on a soft, white, spongy texture (Fig. 3.9). Softened tissue is easily traumatized by pressure and contributes to the development of pressure ulcers.[74]

Determine the cause of the maceration. The source of moisture can be perspiration, soaking in a tub, wound exudate, or incontinence (urine or feces), as well as wound dressing products.

Macerated skin is thinner than adjacent skin. Palpate very gently to avoid trauma. Exposure to friction and shear should

side of the great toe, over the metatarsal heads, and around the heel margin (Fig. 3.8).

Untreated, callus buildup will continue, creating additional shear forces between the bony prominence and soft tissues, and resulting in breakdown of the interposing soft tissues. Hemorrhage on a callus indicates probable trauma and perhaps ulceration beneath.

The location of the callus is a due to the underlying pathologic condition.[79] For example, neuropathy often leads to muscle imbalance and subsequent uneven weight distribution and high pressure and shear along the metatarsal heads, which results in callus formation in those areas. The presence of a callus indicates the need for further assessment of the foot. Chapter 12 contains illustrations and more information about callus management.

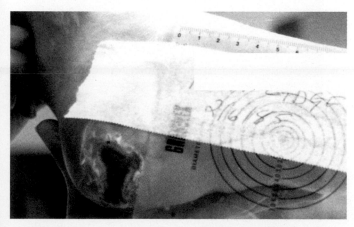

FIGURE 3.7 There is an absence of the epithelialization phase. Hyperkeratosis on heel ulcer of a 100-year-old woman. (Copyright © C. Sussman.)

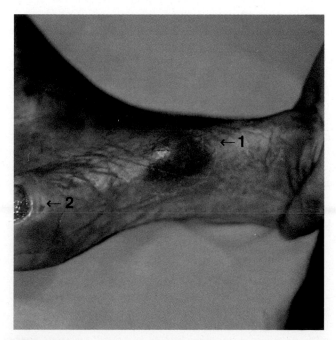

FIGURE 3.9 Intact skin with subcutaneous microvascular bleeding (unblanchable erythema), suggesting deeper trauma located over a bony surface. This wound would be classified as a stage I pressure ulcer. (2) Note maceration of the periwound skin. (Copyright © B.M. Bates-Jensen.)

CLINICAL WISDOM

Observation and Palpation of Calluses

Calluses often appear as thickened areas on the sole of the foot and are usually lighter in color (often yellow) than the adjacent areas. When palpated, the callus area will feel firm or hard to touch. There may also be some scaling or flaking, roughness, or cracking of the callus. A cracked callus is a portal for infection. Buildup of callus around a wound signals an area of high pressure, and further examination is required.

be avoided. Skin moisture barrier products can be used to reduce the impact of moisture on the skin, but they need to be evaluated based on the needs of the patient.

Excessive sweating can be related to medication, infection, or the environment, and may not be controllable.[81] Excessive sweating is a problem in skin folds, such as under the breasts. Obese individuals have many skin folds that need to be examined because they are a common site of yeast infection. Absorbent products to control the moisture need to be evaluated to meet the requirements of the individual. Moisture control should include use of support surfaces and chair cushion coverings, because moisture and temperature affect tissue load tolerance. Moist skin has a higher coefficient of friction than dry skin; in that state, it has reduced tissue integrity. Cotton or air exchange covers for seat cushions are recommended because they can better dissipate moisture and heat on the surface, and promote better skin moisture balance.

As described, too much moisture can affect skin integrity. Likewise, a dry or desiccated wound is out of balance and slows keratinocyte migration. A dry state can be beneficial if the wound is located on the heel, has a dry eschar, and shows no signs of edema, erythema, or drainage; however, even these wounds should be monitored daily.[41]

Edema

Edema is "the presence of abnormally large amounts of fluid in the intercellular tissue spaces of the body, usually referring to demonstrable amounts in the subcutaneous tissues. It may be localized, due to venous or lymphatic obstruction or increased vascular permeability, or systemic, due to heart failure or renal disease."[82] Edema is another example of moisture imbalance.

CLINICAL WISDOM

Good moisture balance of the skin can be achieved by choosing a dressing product that manages wound exudate and does not macerate the skin. Protect the periwound skin by applying petrolatum or a zinc oxide paste combined with petrolatum to make it less stiff and easier to apply with a tongue depressor. The zinc oxide does not need to be removed during dressing changes. To ease removal of zinc oxide from the skin, apply petrolatum or oil.[80]

The presence of edema can be associated with the inflammatory phase, the result of dependence of a limb, or an indication of circulatory impairment or congestive heart failure. One consequence of trauma is increased extracellular fluid in the tissues that both blocks the lymphatic system and causes increased capillary permeability. The function of edema following injury is to block the spread of infection. The result is a swelling that is hard; the application of pressure to the swollen area does not distort the tissues. The term *brawny edema* refers to this type of swelling and is associated with the inflammatory phase. Traumatic edema is usually accompanied by pain, whereas swelling resulting from lymphedema or systemic causes is usually painless.[83]

There are two types of edema: nonpitting and pitting. Nonpitting edema is identified by skin that is stretched and shiny, with hardness of the underlying tissues. Pitting edema is identified by firmly pressing a finger down into the tissues and waiting 5 seconds. If the tissues fail to resume the previous position after pressure is released, and an indentation remains, pitting edema is present. Pitting edema is often observed with dependence of a limb and with tissue congestion associated with congestive heart failure, venous insufficiency, and lymphedema. It is measured on a severity scale of 0–3+, where 0 = not present, 1+ = minimal, 2+ = moderate, and 3+ = severe (Fig. 3.10).

When examining for edema, look for body symmetry and review the patient's medical history. Bilateral edema of the lower extremities can be a sign of a systemic problem, such as congestive heart failure, cirrhosis, malnutrition, or obesity. It may also be caused by dependence on or use of certain drugs. Drug-induced edema is often pitting edema and can be caused by hormonal drugs, including corticosteroids, estrogens, progesterones, and testosterone. Other drugs to consider include nonsteroidal anti-inflammatory and antihypertensive drugs. Symptoms usually resolve if the drug is withdrawn.[83]

Systemic edema can extend from the lower extremities into the abdomen, which is termed *ascites*. Unilateral edema of the lower extremity of sudden onset can be due to acute deep vein thrombophlebitis and is a medical red flag that requires immediate referral to a physician. Other causes of unilateral edema include chronic venous insufficiency, lymphedema, cellulitis, abscess, osteomyelitis, Charcot joint, popliteal aneurysm,

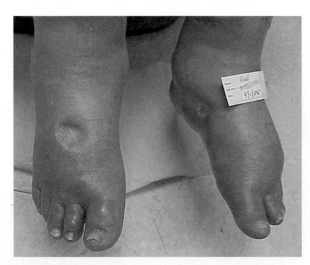

FIGURE 3.10 Pitting edema. (Copyright © Evonne Fowler, RN, CNS, CWOCN.)

dependence, and revascularization. Deep vein thrombophlebitis, chronic venous insufficiency, and lymphedema are the three most common causes.[83]

If the etiology of the edema is uncertain, consult with a physician before planning further testing or an intervention. If edema remains in the tissue, the large protein molecules can clog the lymphatic channels and cause fibrosis. Management of edema is another way to clinically manage moisture balance. Chapter 10 describes the management of edema.

Measurement of edema. Tissue volume increases when edema is present, stretching and expanding the tissue with a change in circumference or girth. Accurate assessment of edema is essential for early intervention and to evaluate the outcomes of treatment interventions. Edema is often evaluated and diagnosed by visual inspection, palpation for change in contour of the tissues, and by photographs. However, visual diagnosis is not as accurate as measurement.[84] Two methods used for measurement of the extent of edema formation are girth and volume.

After visual inspection, girth measurement of the limb is the most common method used in clinical practice because it is simple to perform. Research findings validate the sensitivity of girth measurements as a way to evaluate changes in edema over time.[84] Measurements should be taken at one or more reproducible reference points on the limb. (Fig. 3.11). Clinical variation in edema status is considered improved if the edema is diagnosed by girth measurement at the initial visit and then reduced at the follow-up visit, unchanged if girth is the same at both visits, and worsened if the measurement increases between the first and second assessments. A change of 1.5 cm between two measurements is reported as a valid, reliable estimate of improvement or worsening of edema. Smaller changes between assessments were evaluated but were less accurate.[84] A simple form, such as that shown in Exhibit 3.2 either handwritten or preprinted, that lists the measurements of both limbs side by side is a useful guide for consistency and completeness of the measurements. It is also useful for comparing baseline with retest measurements quickly and easily. Change in edema measurements is one way to assess treatment outcomes.

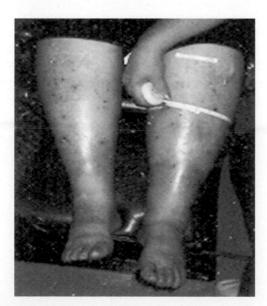

FIGURE 3.11 Correct measurement of an edematous leg. (Copyright © Evonne Fowler, RN, CNS, CWOCN.)

EXHIBIT 3.2

Lower Extremity Girth Measurement Form

Date						
	Right	Left	Right	Left	Right	Left
Locations:						
Metatarsal heads						
Both malleoli						
3 cm ↑ lateral malleolus						
12 cm ↑ lateral malleolus						
18 cm ↑ lateral malleolus						
Lower edge of patella						

The procedure for girth measurements is as follows:

1. Mark and record the bony landmarks on the limb to guide the measurements, including the metatarsal heads, both malleoli, 3 cm above the lateral malleolus, 12 cm above the lateral malleolus, 18 cm above the lateral malleolus, and the lower edge of the patella.
2. Use a flexible tape measure to measure the circumference around these landmarks.
3. Measure both limbs.
4. Record measurements (for both limbs) side by side. Repeat at next assessment. Compare.

Volumetric measurement is made by using water displacement and is considered the gold standard. Volume meters are made of a heavy Lucite and come in different sizes for immersion of a foot and ankle, leg above the knee, or hand (Fig. 3.12). These meters are strong and durable. The water displacement method presents several problems, including the time to set up; transport of the apparatus, which may contain 1000 mL of water; inability to immerse the entire extremity in the tank; and unsuitable patient conditions, such as immersion of a limb that has an open wound.

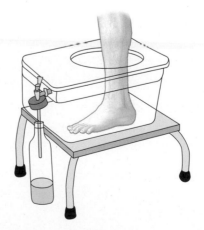

FIGURE 3.12 Volumetric edema measurement.

The procedure for volume displacement measurement is as follows:

1. Fill volume meter with tepid water (~95°F or 37°C).
2. Immerse the affected extremity in water.
3. Catch overflow in a graduated cylinder to measure volume displaced.
4. Repeat with both limbs.
5. Record volume displacements to both limbs side by side on a form.

Reassessment of edema. When reassessment of edema is preformed, the target outcomes to track are that the edema will be absent, reduced, or controlled. Baseline girth or volume measurements that were larger for the affected limb or area at baseline will be equal to or closer to the measurements of the unaffected limbs.

If both limbs are affected, it is not possible to do an opposite limb comparison, and measurements will be compared with the same limb or area. Palpation and observation, as well as decreased measurements, are used for evaluating changes in edema. Change in severity of pitting is another measurement with which to report changes in edema. Controlled edema means that, following an initial reduction, the edema has not returned to the prior level and remains in the tissues.

Color

Assessment of adjacent skin color provides clues to skin health and general health, including circulation, and is used clinically to check for ischemia. For example, cyanosis would suggest hypoxia and the need for further testing. It's important to distinguish between *transient erythema*, a component of reactive hyperemia, and *persistent erythema*. Transient erythema can be detected in lightly pigmented skin by applying pressure to the skin. The pressure closes capillaries and induces a blanching of the skin color that returns to normal when pressure is released. (Make sure you remove pressure from the area and expose it to ambient room temperature for 5–10 minutes before examining). If the color does not return to that of the adjacent skin within 20 to 30 minutes after removal of pressure, it is considered *unblanchable erythema*, or *persistent erythema*.[85] Histology of unblanchable erythema shows erythrostasis in the capillaries and venules, followed by hemorrhage (Figs. 3.9 and 3.13).[86] Unblanchable erythema is one of the hallmarks of stage I pressure ulcers. The same indexes cannot be used in *darkly pigmented skin*. Exhibit 3.3 has tips for assessing unblanchable erythema.

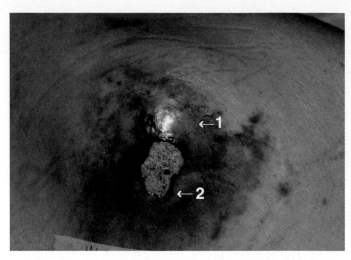

FIGURE 3.13 Acute inflammatory phase, partial-thickness stage II pressure ulcer located over bony prominence. Note: (1) Erythema and edema, (2) Reticular layer of dermis. (Copyright © B.M. Bates-Jensen.)

Color Assessment for Darkly Pigmented Skin

Identification of stage I pressure ulcers has historically relied heavily on color changes in the skin; however, color changes may be difficult to observe in darkly pigmented skin.[76] Darkly pigmented skin is defined as skin tones that "remain unchanged (do not blanch) when pressure is applied over a bony prominence, irrespective of the patient's race or ethnicity."[87] Darkly pigmented skin is usually found in African Americans, Africans, Caribbean individuals, Hispanics, Asians, Pacific Islanders, Middle Easterners, Native Americans, and Eskimos

When assessing patients with darkly pigmented skin who are at high risk for pressure ulcers, careful attention should be paid to color changes at sites located over bony prominences. Look for color changes that differ from the patient's usual skin color (as described by the patient or those who are familiar with the patient's usual skin color, or as observed in an area of healthy tissue).[87] Consider conditions that can cause changes in skin color, such as vasoconstriction (pallor) caused by lying on a cold surface or hyperemia (redness or deepening of skin tones) from lying on a bony prominence. As with light-colored skin, remove pressure and allow the area to be exposed to ambient room temperature for 5 to 10 minutes before examining. When darkly pigmented skin is inflamed, the site of inflammation is darker and appears bluish or purplish (eggplant-like color)

EXHIBIT 3.3

Tips for Evaluating Blanchable Erythema[122]

- Blanchable Erythema "If the reddened area blanches when gentle pressure is applied, the microcirculation is intact."[122]

- Too little pressure: blanching may not occur
- Too much pressure: further tissue damage is possible
- Hard to determine blanching and nonblanching erythema if vascular refill time is short
- Use of a transparent pressure disc makes it easier to observe whether the reddened area blanches when pressure is exerted. Use of the disc can standardize the amount of pressure.

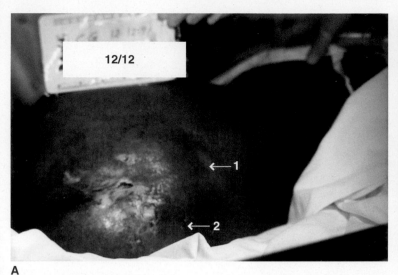

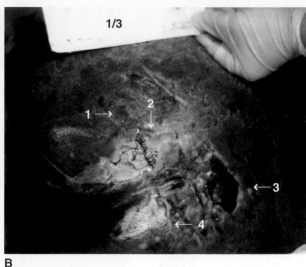

FIGURE 3.14 **A:** Pressure ulceration with multiple, small, stage II open areas. Wound is in acute inflammatory phase onset date 12/12. Note: (1) Clear line of demarcation between healthy tissues and inflamed tissues; (2) Evidence of discoloration, edema, and induration, suggesting underlying tissue death. Assess tissue temperature and pain. **B:** Same pressure ulceration as in (A). Three weeks later, the skin shows evidence of the severe tissue destruction that occurred at the time of trauma. Note delayed manifestation of injury at the skin level. The date was 1/3. Note: (1) Continued demarcation of inflamed tissue; (2) Irregular, diffuse wound edges; (3) Black and adherent eschar; (4) Partial-thickness skin loss; there is enlargement of stage II ulcers compared with those in (A). The correct staging for this sacrococcygeal pressure ulcer is at unstageable. Once eschar is removed, the true depth of tissue loss can be determined. Documentation should reflect a combined area of wounding, including all three visible ulcers and the area of inflammation; this is the overall size estimate for the pressure ulcer. Inflammation is now chronic. (Copyright © C. Sussman.)

(Figs. 3.14A and 3.15). This is comparable to the erythema or redness seen in persons with lighter skin tones.[87] Changes in color can indicate hemorrhage of the microvasculature in the skin or deep tissue trauma that will later rupture and form a

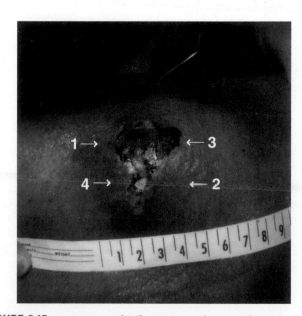

FIGURE 3.15 Assessment of inflammatory phase attributes in darkly pigmented skin. Note: (1) Erythema gives skin a reddish-brown glow, (2) Hemorrhage of microvasculature gives skin a purplish gray hue, (3) Eschar-note tissue texture change to hard black, (4) The color of adjacent skin is used as reference for normal skin tones. (Copyright © B.M. Bates-Jensen.)

crater. When there is an extremely high melanin content, the color of the skin can be so dark that it is difficult to assess any changes in color.[74]

Another complicating factor in identifying erythema in darkly pigmented skin is differentiating inflammation from the darkening of the skin caused by hemosiderin staining, which is a sign of wound chronicity or repeated injury. Hemosiderin staining usually occurs close to the wound edges, whereas injury-related color changes usually extend out a considerable distance and are accompanied by the other signs of inflammation. Figure 3.16 shows hemosiderin staining at the margins of a wound in a dark-skinned person. The mechanism of hemosiderin staining is described later in this chapter. Color changes are apparent around acute (inflamed—red or violet) and chronic open wounds (pigmentation—dark brown). If color is not a reliable indicator, use other clinical indicators, such as sensation (pain), temperature (heat or coolness), and tissue tension (edema or induration and hardness) to confirm the diagnosis of inflammation in darkly pigmented skin.

Assessment of tissue circulatory status by use of color is also difficult in darkly pigmented skin. Consider the effects of gravity on vasomotor changes in the tissues of the extremities in elevated and dependent positions. Color changes will appear more subtle than those in light skin. Assess the patient from a neutral position and then with the area elevated approximately 15° and dependent for about 5 minutes, and compare.[88] Assessment of capillary refill time for individuals with darkly pigmented skin should be attempted at the tips of the second or third fingers.[89] Also consider examining the nail beds. If they are not pigmented, apply pressure to the second or third fingers; if the skin

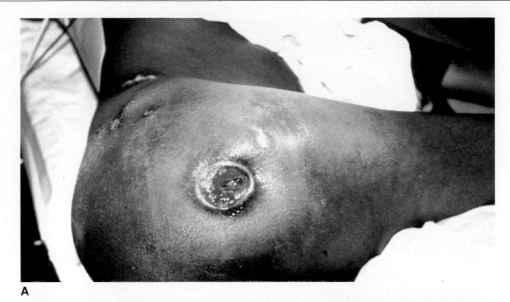

A

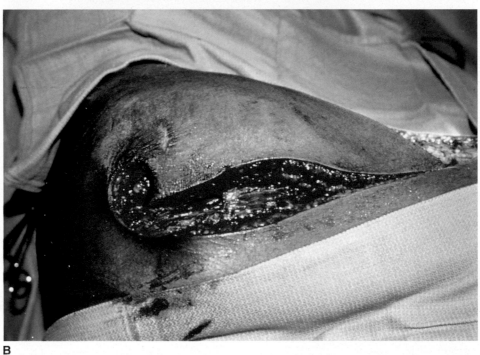

B

FIGURE 3.16 A: Hemosiderin staining (hemosiderosis) in darkly pigmented skin. **B:** Same wound as in (A) with surgical dissection demonstrating the extent of the tunneling process, forming a sinus tract. (Copyright © J. Wethe.)

under the nail blanches, it will provide a color comparison for assessing pallor or cyanosis. The speed of color return following the slow release of pressure is an indicator of the quality of vasomotor function. The slower the return of color, the more diminished is the vasomotor function. Compare the speed of return with that in your own nail bed or that of another person with normal vascularity.[88]

Importance of Lighting in Color Assessment

Proper lighting is important for accurate assessment of all skin tones. Avoid fluorescent light, which casts a blue color to the skin. Use natural or halogen lighting to assess skin tones. Flash photographs are recommended, because the flash makes the

demarcation between normal skin tones and those that are traumatized easier to see, and the picture provides a visual record of the patient's skin status.[87] Notice the demarcation between normal skin tones and the traumatized area in Figure 3.14A. The patient or a family member who is familiar with the patient's natural skin tones should be the primary person to provide information about skin color changes.

Deep Tissue Injury

Trauma to the skin and subcutaneous tissue causes rupture of the blood vessels and subcutaneous bleeding or hemorrhage, called **ecchymosis** (bruising); this is a sign of deep tissue injury. Ecchymosis appears as a purple discoloration in white skin and

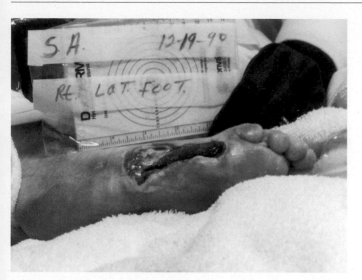

FIGURE 3.17 Soft, soggy necrosis and ecchymosis often referred to as "purple" ulcer. Foot shows signs of cellulitis and edema. Chronic inflammatory phase. (Copyright © C. Sussman.)

a deepening to a purple color in darkly pigmented skin. In the literature, these areas have been described as "purple ulcers."[90] With purple ulcers, the skin over the hemorrhagic area can be taut, shiny, and edematous (Figs. 3.17 and Fig. 3.14A). It can be intact or, in some cases, it can be rubbed off.[90] Purple ulcers typically develop as a consequence of an acute injury, such as trauma from pressure, bumping, or shearing, as well as trauma to new granulation tissue and venous leakage from venous insufficiency (Fig. 3.18). They can also develop as an adverse effect of oral anticoagulant therapy.[91,92] In fact, use of these medications predisposes tissues to subcutaneous hemorrhage with minimal amounts of pressure, friction, and shear. Proper labeling for this class of pressure ulcers is important because they are dangerous lesions with the potential for rapid deterioration. Labeling provides the means for appropriate diagnosis

and the development of efficacious interventions to address the problem. Figure 3.14B is the same wound as shown in Figure 3.14A that showed suspected deep tissue injury (sDTI) and has manifested as a large deep pressure ulcer. However, at this point, it is still unstageable. Staging is used to describe the depth of tissue injury and will be explained in the next chapter section. The term *unstageable* is often used to diagnose eschar-covered lesions, and it has come to be interpreted as wounds that will be staged once they are debrided. However, deep tissue injury lesions should *not* be debrided. As such, labeling a deep tissue "purple ulcer" as unstageable can have the unintended consequence of a care plan that does not include offloading.[93]

An analysis of wound attribute relationships to healing, using the SWHT (see Chapter 5), ranked the presence of hemorrhage as the most significant predictor of poor prognosis for healing.[94] Why do purple ulcers slow or complicate healing? First, hemorrhage occurs followed by clotting (thrombosis) that cuts off oxygen to the tissues, with subsequent hypoxia and ischemia. Rapid deterioration of the tissues following injury can be a combination of direct ischemic injury and reperfusion injury from oxygen-free radicals, cytokines, and neutrophilic adhesion to microvascular endothelium.[95] When hypoxia is prolonged, the initial damage can be due to ischemia. However, a short period of ischemia followed by reperfusion can result in damage that is more severe than the injury itself. If the blood clot is not lysed (thrombolysis) and reabsorbed into the tissues in a timely fashion, tissue necrosis will occur. It is not known exactly how long clotted blood can remain in the tissues before necrosis occurs.

Purple ulcers are now classified according to the current National Pressure Ulcer Advisory Panel (NPUAP) staging system as suspected deep tissue injury (sDTI). However, the significance of these ulcers is seldom recognized. NPUAP has attempted to raise awareness of this unstageable type of ulcer through a consensus conference of the pressure ulcer community,[96] a white paper,[95] and a literature review identifying limitations in the current staging systems' attempts to categorize

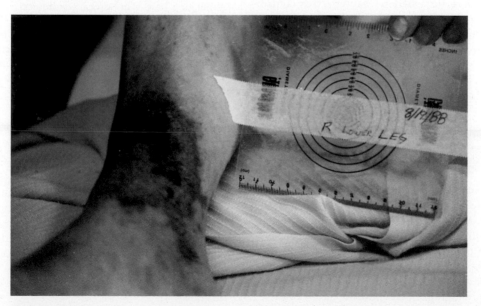

FIGURE 3.18 Wound is in acute inflammatory phase and shows subcutaneous hemorrhage (ecchymosis) associated with venous disease. (Copyright © C. Sussman.)

CLINICAL WISDOM

Education of Clinicians about Deep Tissue Injury

Health-care providers need to be educated about the phenomenon of deep tissue injury and how to identify, describe, and document purple ulcers during the skin assessment.

these lesions.[97] Action subsequently taken includes revising the NPUAP pressure ulcer classification system to include sDTI pressure ulcer. NPUAP pressure ulcer classification system is fully described in a following section. Further research is needed to fully understand and reliably diagnose and predict the natural history of these lesions, the extent of tissue damage under the intact skin, and the viability of injured tissue, and to identify the most efficacious treatments for deep tissue injury.[95]

Another type of hemorrhagic condition for assessment is rupture of the vessels around a wound and seepage from venous hypertension that cause deposition of blood in the subcutaneous tissues. The blood stains the tissues by deposition of hemosiderin from lysed red blood cells, turning the skin a rust-brown color that is called *hemosiderosis*. Hemosiderosis is seen as a ring around pressure ulcers (Fig. 3.16A) or a brown discoloration of the skin of the lower leg in patients with venous disease (Fig. 3.19). The discoloration can be permanent or gradually disappear.

Hair Distribution

Body hair is distributed over all four extremities, extending down to the digits. Over time, body hair diminishes and is eventually lost. The diminished presence of hair is seen in aging skin and in individuals with impaired circulation. As circulation in a leg decreases, hair is lost distally. Hair distribution can be used as an indicator of the level of vascular impairment and the need for vascular testing. Hair follicles are important to wound healing because, as discussed in Chapter 2, they contribute epidermal cells for resurfacing partial-thickness wounds. As such, the absence of hair is a factor in the prognosis of wound healing if there is a partial-thickness wound in an area where hair is usually found, such as the lower leg.

RESEARCH WISDOM

Electrical stimulation, pulsed radiofrequency stimulation, and ultrasound facilitate thrombolysis, when started soon after injury (e.g., within 48–72 hours). However, in one reported case, therapeutic ultrasound was not started to treat a large rectus sheath hematoma until 9 days after the diagnosis, and hematoma was completely resolved following 20 sessions (five times per week for 4 weeks).[91] Efficacy studies reported in the literature and photographs that show the effects of these interventions are described in Chapters 23–25.

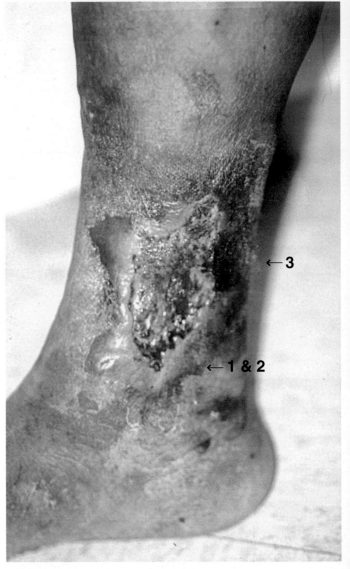

FIGURE 3.19 Shallow and irregularly shaped lesion with a good granulating base. The associated physical signs of chronic venous insufficiency, such as hyperpigmentation, chronic scarring, and skin contraction in the ankle region, are readily identified. Note the classic characteristics of venous disease: (1) Irregular edges, (2) Shallow ulcer, (3) Evidence of hyperpigmentation (hemosiderosis), (4) Location above the medial malleolus. (Copyright © C. Donayre.)

Toenails

Part of a comprehensive examination of the feet includes the toenails. Assess the color, thickness, and shape, and note any irregularities. Hypertrophic, thick nails are a commonly seen toenail pathology. Some toenails are shaped like a ram's horn. Ingrown toenails and fungal and pseudomonas infections, which give the toenail a green color, can also be observed. Findings of toenail abnormalities are considered referral criteria unless the clinician has knowledge and training in foot and nail care.[98] Chapters 12 and 13 include specific information that guides the assessment and care of feet.

Blisters

Trauma to the epidermis gives rise to blisters. Blisters can contain clear fluid or, if the trauma is deeper than the epidermis

CLINICAL WISDOM

Assessment of Hair Distribution as an Indicator of Peripheral Circulation

1. An easy checkpoint for adequate tissue perfusion to the lower extremities is examination of the great toes for hair growth. Hair growth on the great toes implies adequate circulation to support the hair follicles. When working with female patients, remember to ask if they shave the hair on their great toes.
2. Move up the leg proximally from the ankle and assess the most distal point at which hair distribution stops. Next, palpate for skin temperature and pulses, and observe skin color in any areas denuded of hair for circulatory changes.

and ruptures blood vessels, the fluid can be bloody or brown (Fig. 3.20A). The blister roof is nature's best dressing, but it can hide deep tissue damage (Fig. 3.20B). Removal of the blister roof is controversial. If the blister fluid is clear, tissue damage may not extend into the dermis or deeper; the wound will likely heal under the blister roof, and the epidermis will eventually fall off. The blister roof should not be disturbed and, in fact, may require protection. However, if the fluid is bloody, brown, or cloudy as in Figure 3.20A, deep tissue damage may be present, and unroofing the blister can be the only way to determine the extent of trauma (Fig. 3.20B). Ultrasound technology to identify depth of tissue edema and trauma, such as under a blister, is being tested with good outcomes (see Chapter 26).

Assessment of the tissue under the blister without breaking the blister is helpful in evaluating when the blister needs to be unroofed. The validity of using digital palpation to determine tissue resilience (i.e., less resilient or less stiff compared with

A

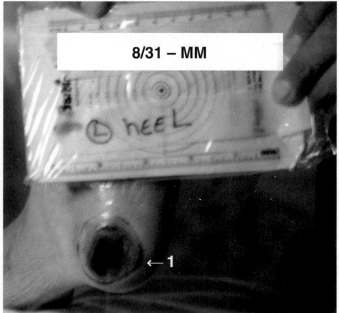

B

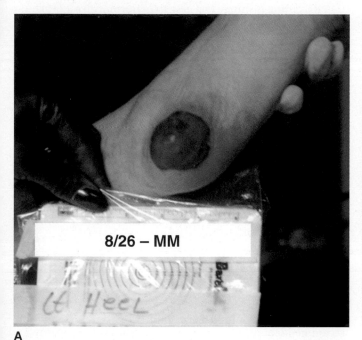

C

FIGURE 3.20 A: Unstageable bloody filled blister. Legend should change to leave off day of identification. **B:** Same wound as in (A). Note apparent necrosis without blister roof. Note area of sDTI. **C:** Same wound as in Figure 3.20a with the blister opened and it is now stageable. Category/Stage III pressure ulcer. Note area of sDTI. (Copyright © C. Sussman.)

adjacent tissue) has been demonstrated. Gently press down with a fingertip on the tissue beneath the blister roof and compress it. Release and feel for the resiliency of the subcutaneous tissues. If there is good resilience (i.e., it bounces back when the pressure is removed), the deep tissues may be mildly congested. However, if the tissue feels soft, spongy, or boggy, there is high probability of tissue congestion and probable necrosis.[85] The common term for this characteristic is "mushy" or "boggy." Practice and careful concentration are needed to perform this palpation examination. One tip is to try pressing the skin down on the contralateral location (e.g., on the heel) to compare the resiliency.

Sensation

Sensory testing procedures and expected outcomes are described in this section. They include pain, protective sensation, thermal sensation, and VPT.

Pain

Accreditation standards for health-care facilities in the United States require each patient's pain to be measured regularly and proper relief supplied.[99] Severe pain or tenderness, either within or around the wound, can indicate the presence of infection, deep tissue destruction, or ischemia. In recognition of the significant effect of pain on wound healing and wound management, Chapter 22 is devoted entirely to that topic, addressing the issues of wound pain and wound healing, including pain physiology, pain issues, pain assessment, and treatment strategies.

Protective Sensation

Testing for protective sensation, defined as loss of the ability to feel or perceive a minimal amount of touch/pressure using Semmes-Weinstein monofilaments, is indicated if sensory loss is suspected. Neuropathy from many causes, including diabetes, Guillain-Barré syndrome, alcoholism, chemotherapy, and Charcot-Marie-Tooth disease, results in the loss of protective sensation. A minimal protective sensation threshold is the key to protecting the neuropathic foot from ulceration.

A safe, accurate method for testing protective sensation has been developed using Semmes-Weinstein monofilaments.[100] The monofilaments come in different force levels. Levels 4.17, 5.07, and 6.10 are used to check for protective sensation. Force levels increase as the numbers increase. The object of the test is to determine if the patient can detect pressure when the monofilament is placed against the skin and the force applied is sufficient to buckle the monofilament. Testing is usually performed on the sole of the foot. The inability to sense the 5.07 monofilament is the threshold for loss of protective sensation and indicates a limited ability to use protective sensations. If the patient can distinguish this level of sensation at several points on the feet, the sensation is considered to be adequate to avoid trauma.[101] Many individuals with PN do not feel the largest monofilament (6.10), which indicates a loss of protective sensation of 75 g. This finding should trigger the prompt referral to a specialist for appropriate protective footwear and should be followed closely (see Chapter 12).

Thermal Sensation

The test for thermal sensation is performed using test tubes or small narrow bottles filled with warm water. Be sure to test in a normal area before applying to possible insensate areas to avoid burns. Research reports that the lateral aspect of the foot is the area most sensitive to thermal sensation.[102] If a patient is unable to sense warmth, he or she is at high risk of burns if heat is applied to the skin. Testing for cold can be performed by applying a cold tuning fork. If a patient is unable to sense cold, he or she is at risk for injury from exposure to cold; the feet should be protected from frostbite if the patient is going to be exposed to very cold temperatures. Thermal allodynia can also be detected in hypersensitive areas.

Vibratory Perception Threshold

VPT is a measure of progressive PN for aging adults and individuals with immune-mediated polyneuropathies including diabetes. In all groups, VPT is better perceived in the upper extremities compared with the lower. There is a significant age-related decline in VPT at all locations. VPT is recommended as a part of routine neurologic examination, as well as for patients with diabetes and other risk factors for skin ulceration.[103,104]

VPT testing is simple and easy to perform with a 128 Hz tuning fork.[103–105] The simplest method is the on/off method, which is reliable for testing VPT at the foot.[105] The test procedure is as follows:

1. Before testing the VPT at the foot, give the patient a preliminary test by placing the vibrating tuning fork on the sternum, so that the vibratory sensation can be readily recognized.
2. Ask the patient to shut the eyes and keep them closed.
3. Ask the patient to report the start of the vibration sensation and the cessation of vibration (on-off).
4. Strike the tuning fork and place it on the bony prominence on the dorsum of the great toe proximal to the nail bed.
5. Repeat the test eight times at the same location, recording the on/off report.
6. VPT is defined as "the total number of times the application of the vibrating tuning fork and the dampening of vibration was NOT felt. Scores can range from 0–8."[105]

Note that VPT is a screening test used to predict risk for ulceration, rather than a wound assessment technique. Screening is recommended annually for patients without neuropathy and every 6 months for individuals who have neuropathy but do not have deformity or vascular disease. Patients who have neuropathy with deformity or vascular disease diagnoses should be evaluated every 3 months. If ulceration is part of the patient history, evaluation should be performed every 1 to 3 months.[106] Any patient identified as having abnormal values at screening should be referred for further medical workup and special education, such as foot care education programs, as described in other chapters. VPT results are a trigger to evaluate candidates for this intervention, as well as to validate the outcome of the intervention.

Skin Temperature

Baseline skin temperature is one objective measurement of circulation that can be used to evaluate inflammation, and diagnose infection and monitor circulatory response to treatment. Local body temperature can be tested by palpation, with a thermistor, liquid crystal skin thermometer, or with an infrared thermometer.

Palpation

Palpation using the assessors hands is a subjective measurement of skin temperature, which has limited reliability detecting subtle differences in skin temperature.[107,108]

Thermistor

Temperature can also be measured using a thermistor, which is a probe placed against the skin that takes a reading. These devices are difficult to attach to the body surface resulting in poor surface contact, which limits the accuracy of the readings and take significant time to equilibrate.[108] Therefore, these devices are not recommended for assessment purposes.

Liquid Crystal Skin Thermography

A liquid crystal skin thermometer is a thermosensitive strip that changes color in a few seconds after contact with the skin to indicate skin temperature. It is a semiquantitative method that relies on color to measure periwound and adjacent skin temperature.

Liquid crystal strips are available with different temperature ranges. Use of an inexpensive liquid crystal skin fever thermometer strip that changes color with temperature change is a simple, accurate, and useful way to assess the temperature of periwound skin. These devices are reliable and have been clinically tested for evaluation of primary wound healing status of surgical wounds. The method is quick, simple, reliable, and inexpensive.[109] Strips are available with a range of 80°F to 100°F (26°C–38°C).

A higher temperature of both periwound and adjacent skin measured on the liquid crystal compared with contralateral area is an indication of increased circulatory perfusion. This is the heat described as a classic sign of inflammation, which includes hyperemia associated with increased blood flow but can also be an indicator of infection.[108] Assessment and judgment of an experienced clinician are needed to make an appropriate diagnosis. Cooler periwound skin temperature compared with adjacent and contralateral skin should be considered an indicator of wound chronicity.

The procedure for measuring skin temperature with a liquid crystal strip is as follows:

1. Ensure that the area of skin to be tested has been pressure-free and exposed to ambient air temperature for at least 5 to 10 minutes before testing. (A sheet can cover the patient for privacy and to avoid chilling.)
2. Dry the skin of sweat before each measurement, because moisture on the skin considerably modifies the image.[109]
3. Place a single layer of plastic against the skin as a hygienic barrier (this does not interfere with temperature accuracy). This step and the following can be eliminated if the strip is disposable. Strips can be reused for a single patient if the barrier is used.
4. Lay the temperature strip flat on the plastic barrier.
5. Hold the strip in place at both ends lightly, to avoid compressing capillaries. Wait for the color of the strip to change, allowing at least 1 full minute for the change to occur. In very inflamed tissues, color change can occur immediately, but it may change more as it is held for the full minute.
6. Read the temperature while the strip is still against the skin.

7. For large wounds, measure at the wound edge at the 12:00 and 6:00 positions and near the expected outer margin of the periwound erythema/discoloration. Repeat at the 3:00 and 9:00 positions.
8. For small wounds, measure by placing the liquid crystal strip across the wound diameter.
9. Record temperature at each point.

Infrared Thermometer

A radiometer or infrared scan determines temperature by measurement of surface reflection of infrared radiation. These devices can reliably be used in the clinic with minimal training. In addition, personal infrared thermometers may prove to be an effective means of reducing risk of ulceration in high-risk patients by providing an easy-to-use tool that encourages vigilant monitoring, provides immediate feedback about a pending problem, and empowers the patient to take action when change is measured. Chapter 12 has explicit directions for use of the infrared scanner.

Utility of Skin Temperature Assessment

Skin temperature is a useful measure for assessing many types of wounds and tissue status including the following situations:

Surgical wounds. Changes in wound temperature are readily apparent during the first 8 postoperative days. During the first 3 postoperative days, the temperatures of the wound and adjacent tissues are typically the same. However, by postoperative day 4, there should be a discernible change, with the temperatures of the wound and surrounding tissues decreasing gradually. Zones of warmth around the wound become narrower, with significantly greater warmth over the incision than in the surrounding tissues. The heat measured in adjacent skin areas is not an inflammatory reaction; rather, it is reactive hyperemia. Hyperemia is the consequence of humoral substances released from cellular damage at the time of wounding—chiefly histamine—and pain that triggers neurogenic reactions, including vasodilation.[109] Only a narrow zone adjacent to the wound is due to inflammation. During the early postoperative period, the two areas are indistinguishable from one another. As the wound heals, the area of warmth narrows, decreases in temperature, and represents the area of true inflammation.

Wound temperature depends on the degree of vascularity of the tissues: a higher grade of vascularity will result in a higher tissue temperature.[109] If the expected outcomes (i.e., that the wound and adjacent skin temperatures decrease by the fourth postoperative day) are not met, this indicates that the wound is not healing as expected and secondary intention healing (see Chapter 2) is imminent because of tissue necrosis or bacterial contamination.[109]

Inflammation. An increase in skin temperature of 4°F compared with the contralateral side[110] can indicate inflammation that has not manifested on the surface, such as a pressure ulcer over a bony prominence or the presence of infection (e.g., an abscess) or Charcot arthropathy (see Chapter 12). It is a very useful tool for assessing inflammation and wounding in darkly pigmented individuals in whom the margins of erythema are difficult to see. Skin temperature can be measured at locations on the margins of discoloration and at the center over the bony prominence. The clock method (i.e., measuring the temperature at the 12:00, 3:00, 6:00, and 9:00 positions around the wounded tissue) is useful for recording this measurement in large wounds. Expect periwound temperature to decrease as the wound heals.[110]

Infection. Infrared thermometry is a reliable instrument for detecting increased periwound skin temperature. Evaluation of venous leg ulcers demonstrates a statistically significant relationship between periwound skin temperature and the presence of wound infection.[108]

Increased blood flow. To measure the effects of an intervention, take a baseline temperature measurement before treatment and repeat the measurement after treatment. Skin temperature should rise after treatment with increased blood flow. If the target outcome of the intervention is to initiate the acute inflammatory phase, with resultant hyperemia and mild inflammation, measurement of tissue temperatures will help to verify the outcome.

Ischemia. Ischemia may be detected by measurement of skin temperature. Like warmth, coolness without trauma can be an indicator of circulatory status. Sometimes, there is an initial increase in skin temperature that is followed by coolness after trauma. Some areas of the body naturally have less warmth, such as the feet, toes, and fingers. The areas of the trunk or over well-perfused muscle tissues have greater warmth. If there is coolness in the digits or feet, or other signs and symptoms, such as lack of hair, altered skin color, pulse, or texture, the area should be evaluated for circulation. If those signs are also suggestive of circulatory impairment, further circulatory examination is warranted. Coolness can also be an indicator of impaired tissue viability or tissue death following ischemia.

A quantitative measure of tissue temperature as part of the assessment of wounds is not yet a standard of clinical practice. Journal articles describe temperature measurement as a useful method of assessment for inflammatory processes.[108,109,111–114] All of the procedures described in this chapter are simple, noninvasive, and quick. Most importantly, they have validity and clinical significance, and they are more reliable than clinical observation or manual palpation.[108,109]

RESEARCH WISDOM

A patient can have unapparent, mild core hypothermia that will affect wound healing and resistance to infection. The tympanic membrane temperature is an accurate measure of core body temperature.[109]

WOUND CLASSIFICATION SYSTEMS

Differential Diagnosis of Wound Etiology

In Part II of this book, you will learn in detail about the management of wounds of different etiology. This is just a brief introduction to the differential diagnosis of wound etiology of five types of ulcers discussed in this chapter and is adapted from Woundpedia (www.woundpedia.com).

Surgical wounds usually go on to heal without complications and do not need specialized wound care. Local surgical factors such as infection, edema, seroma and hematoma formation, wound tension, wound trauma, wound drainage, the presence of drainage devices, muscle spasticity, and wound dressings all affect postoperative wound healing.[115]

Pressure ulcers also known as decubitus, pressure sores or bedsores are lesions caused by factors such as constant pressure, friction, or shear, usually occurring over bony prominences.[115]

Vascular pathology is associated with the majority of leg ulcers. Almost 70% of leg ulcers have a venous etiology; approximately 20% to 25% are due to arterial insufficiency; and some of these have a mixed vascular etiology. The remaining leg ulcers have a variety of less common causes, including infection, malignancy, vasculitis and other conditions and most are not discussed in this text.

Venous leg ulcers result from venous hypertension due to valve dysfunction, venous obstruction, and/or failure of calf

---

TABLE 3.2	Wound Classification Systems and Wound Types				
Wound Classification Systems	Pressure Ulcers	Venous Ulcers	Arterial and Ischemic Ulcers	Diabetic Ulcers (Neuropathic)	Other Wounds
Pressure ulcer staging	X		X (Those with a pressure component)	X (Those with a pressure component)	Stage II classification is appropriate for skin tears and tape damage
Wagner Ulcer dysvascular Classification System			X	X	
University of Texas Diabetic Classification				X	
Depth of tissue injury	X (full-thickness wounds require examination of deep tissue involvement)	X (full-thickness wounds require examination of deep tissue involvement)	X (full-thickness wounds require examination of deep tissue involvement)	X (full-thickness wounds require examination of deep tissue involvement)	Useful for skin tears, burns, and other skin wounds surgical secondary intention healing
Red, yellow, and black	X	X	X	X	

muscle pump function. They usually occur on the medial side of the lower leg and are accompanied by edema that may be weeping. Skin changes including hemosiderosis and hyperkeratosis are signs that often accompany this condition. They often take a prolonged time to heal, frequently months to more than a year, and they commonly recur. Venous reflux testing (Chapter 6) confirms this diagnosis.

Arterial ulcers result from inadequate perfusion of skin and subcutaneous tissue, and they are primarily a complication of peripheral arterial disease (PAD). A punched-out appearance, with a pale, dry poorly perfused base is characteristic of arterial ulcers. The foot and leg may be cold, pale or bluish, with shiny, taut skin and dependent rubor, and possibly gangrenous toes. Pain is common, especially after exertion or leg elevation. A decreased ABI confirms the diagnosis (see Chapter 6). Arterial insufficiency may be slowly or rapidly progressive, and early diagnosis is critical to prevent further tissue death.[115]

Diabetic foot ulcers are a major complication, occurring in approximately 15% of people with DM, and are a preceding factor in approximately 85% of lower limb amputations. Poor diabetes control may result in PN and vascular disease. PN raises the likelihood of both trauma to the foot and inability to detect abnormal pressures that may predispose patients to develop foot ulcers. Sensory testing and vascular testing provide a differential diagnosis for neuropathic ulcers.

Wound Classification Systems

A *wound classification system* is a hierarchical system that classifies or categorizes wounds by severity according to different characteristics, such as level of tissue involvement, color of wound, and so forth. Documenting assessment findings and diagnosing wounds following a standardized classification system allows you to communicate effectively with other health-care providers. Note that each wound classification system was researched and designed for use with one specific wound type; thus, it is inappropriate to use the same classification system for all wounds you encounter. Since each system measures only one characteristic of the wound (e.g., the depth of tissue loss), it should not be viewed as a complete assessment independent of other indicators. A complete wound assessment and written description is still required.

Avoid using any wound classification system "in reverse" as a method of measuring wound healing. Biologically, wounds do not heal in the manner suggested by reversing a staging system, and classification systems were not developed for use in assessing healing. This inappropriate use can actually hinder tracking of progress.

The five wound classification systems presented in this chapter are[116–118]

1. Classification by depth of tissue injury
2. NPUAP pressure ulcer staging criteria
3. Wagner staging system for grading severity of dysvascular ulcers
4. University of Texas Treatment-Based Diabetic Foot Classification System
5. Marion Laboratories red/yellow/black color system. Table 3.2 presents the four wound classification system discussed in this section and identifies the types of wounds most appropriate for use with each system.

Classification by Depth of Tissue Injury

In Chapter 2, we identified four types of wounds, distinguished by depth of tissue injury: superficial, partial-thickness, full-thickness, and subcutaneous (see Table 3.3). This "generic" classification system identifies specific anatomic levels of the tissues involved, but does not report their condition or color. It is commonly used for wounds that are not categorized as pressure ulcers or neuropathic ulcers, such as skin tears, donor sites, vascular ulcers (venous ulcers in particular), surgical wounds, and burns. However, in some cases, these classifications do have parallels in other systems. For example, superficial wounds are equivalent to NPUAP stage I pressure ulcer or, on the Wagner scale, a grade 0 dysvascular ulcer.

Anatomic depth of tissue loss is predictive of healing.[29,69] Superficial wounds are often resolved by subcutaneous inflammatory processes, with the exception of wounds with intact skin that also have deep tissue injury and can manifest later as deep wounds. Partial-thickness wounds, which heal by epithelialization, heal faster than full-thickness and subcutaneous wounds. Full-thickness and subcutaneous wounds heal by secondary

TABLE 3.3	Classification by Depth of Tissue Loss	
Thickness of Skin Loss	**Definition**	**Clinical Examples/Healing Process**
Superficial wounds	Effects only the epidermis	Sunburn, stage I pressure ulcer, stage 0 diabetic ulcer; heal by inflammation
Partial-thickness skin loss	Extends through the epidermis, into, but not through, the dermis	Skin tears, abrasions, tape damage, blisters, perineal dermatitis from incontinence; heal by epidermal resurfacing or epithelialization
Full-thickness skin loss	Extends through the epidermis and dermis into subcutaneous fat and deeper structures	Donor sites, venous ulcers, surgical wounds; heal by granulation tissue formation and contraction
Subcutaneous tissue wounds	Additional classification level for full-thickness wounds that extend into, or beyond, the subcutaneous tissue	Surgical wounds, arterial/ischemic wounds; heal by granulation tissue formation and contraction

EXHIBIT **3.4**

Examples of Chronic Wounds

- Ischemic arterial ulcers
- Diabetic vascular and neuropathic ulcers
- Venous ulcers
- Vasculitic ulcers
- Rheumatoid ulcers
- Pressure ulcers

intention, a combination of fibroplasia or granulation tissue formation and contraction.

At the beginning of Chapter 2, we defined a chronic wound as "one that deviates from the expected sequence of repair in terms of time, appearance, and response to aggressive and appropriate treatment".[119] When the response to wounding does not conform to the described acute phased model of wound recovery after a period of 2 to 4 weeks, the wound may have become "stuck" and unable to progress through the phases of healing without intervention. This wound would then be classified as a chronic wound.

The typical medical model for diagnosing chronic wounds is to use the pathophysiology associated with ulcers. For example, there are ischemic arterial ulcers, diabetic ulcers (both vascular and neuropathic), pressure ulcers, vasculitic ulcers, venous ulcers, and rheumatoid ulcers. All of the ulcers listed in Exhibit 3.4 are considered chronic wounds.

National Pressure Ulcer Advisor Panel Pressure Ulcer Staging System

The NPUAP pressure ulcer staging system is probably one of the most widely known wound classification systems. It was developed by the NPUAP and used by the Agency for Health Care Research and Quality (AHRQ) based upon an earlier pressure

ulcer staging system proposed by Shea.[120] The earlier four-stage systems described pressure ulcers using depth of anatomic tissue loss and the involvement of soft tissue layers and was redefined in 2007 by adding two stages on deep tissue injury and unstageable pressure ulcers with descriptions of each. It is a diagnosis of severity of tissue insult *before healing starts*. The NPUAP system is most often applied to pressure ulcers, but it is also used (sometimes inappropriately) to classify other types of wounds. It is best used for wounds with a pressure or tissue perfusion etiologic factor, such as with arterial/ischemic wounds and diabetic neuropathic ulcers.

The NPUAP staging system is widely accepted and commonly used to describe wound severity, organize treatment protocols, and select and reimburse treatment products for pressure ulcers. For example, the AHRQ adopted the NPUAP staging system for use in two sets of clinical practice guidelines.[71,121] The new definitions are included in the 2009, International Prevention and Treatment of Pressure Ulcer Clinical Practice Guideline with the addition of the term category/stage. Figures 3.9, 3.13, 3.17, and 3.22–3.28 present diagrams and photos illustrating the NPUAP and European Pressure Ulcer Advisory Panel (EPUAP) 2009 Pressure Ulcer Classification system.[26]

The pressure ulcer staging system has many problems. For example, the definition of a category/stage I pressure ulcer does not account for the severity of soft tissue trauma beneath the unbroken skin, such as that seen with purple ulcers. Thus, NPUAP proposes that this trauma should be referred to as "suspected pressure-related deep tissue injury under intact skin" or "suspected deep tissue injury (sDTI)."[97]

Furthermore, category/ stage I lesions vary in presentation and pose validity concerns. For example, some stage I lesions indicate deep tissue damage that is just beginning to manifest on the skin, whereas others indicate only superficial insult in which damage may be reversible and may not be indicative of underlying tissue death. There are also problems reliably assessing stage I ulcers in dark-skinned patients. Identification and interpretation of skin color changes in darkly pigmented skin require special assessment strategies described later in this chapter. An ultrasound scanner image that can detect tissue damage and provide early identification of stage I pressure ulcers is demonstrated in Figure 3.29A–C. Chapter 26 discusses has information to interpret with

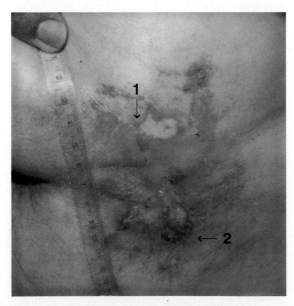

FIGURE 3.21 Perineal dermatitis with partial-thickness skin loss that is not a pressure ulcer. (Copyright © B.M Bates-Jensen.)

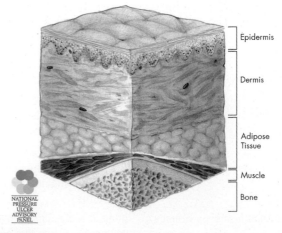

FIGURE 3.22 Diagram Normal Skin © National Pressure Ulcer Advisory Panel. 2007.

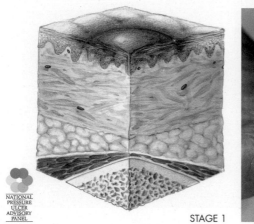

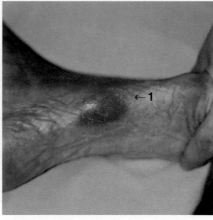

STAGE 1

FIGURE 3.23 Diagram **Stage I:** Intact skin with nonblanchable redness of a localized area usually over a bony prominence. Darkly pigmented skin may not have visible blanching; its color may differ from the surrounding area. **Further description:** The area may be painful, firm, soft, warmer, or cooler as compared to adjacent tissue. Stage I may be difficult to detect in individuals with dark skin tones. May indicate "at risk" persons (a heralding sign of risk). (Copyright © National Pressure Ulcer Advisory Panel. 2007.)

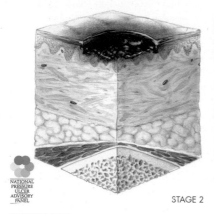

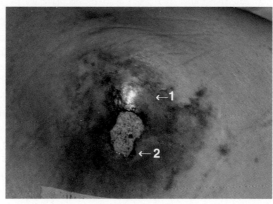

STAGE 2

FIGURE 3.24 Diagram **Stage II:** Partial-thickness loss of dermis presenting as a shallow open ulcer with a red pink wound bed, without slough. May also present as an intact or open/ruptured serum-filled blister. **Further description:** Presents as a shiny or dry shallow ulcer without slough or bruising. This stage should not be used to describe skin tears, tape burns, perineal dermatitis, maceration, or excoriation. Bruising indicates sDTI. (Copyright © National Pressure Ulcer Advisory Panel. 2007.)

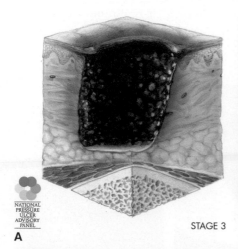

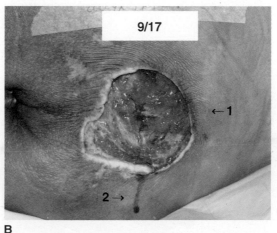

STAGE 3

A   **B**

FIGURE 3.25 **A:** Diagram **Stage III:** Full-thickness tissue loss. Subcutaneous fat may be visible but bone, tendon, and muscle are not exposed. Slough may be present but does not obscure the depth of tissue loss. May include undermining and tunneling. **Further description:** The depth of a stage III pressure ulcer varies by anatomical location. The bridge of the nose, ear, occiput, and malleolus do not have subcutaneous tissue and stage III ulcers can be shallow. In contrast, areas of significant adiposity can develop extremely deep stage III pressure ulcers. Bone/tendon is not visible or directly palpable. (Copyright © National Pressure Ulcer Advisory Panel. 2007.) **B:** Photo of category/stage III pressure ulcer. (Copyright © B.M. Bates-Jensen.)

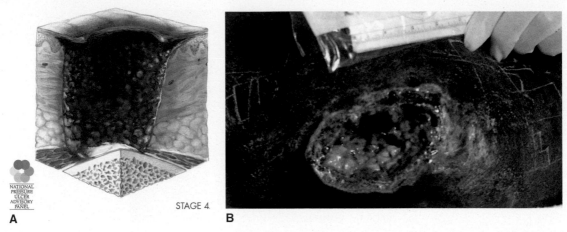

FIGURE 3.26 A: Diagram **Stage IV:** Full-thickness tissue loss with exposed bone, tendon, or muscle. Slough or eschar may be present on some parts of the wound bed. Often include undermining and tunneling. **Further description:** The depth of a stage IV pressure ulcer varies by anatomical location. The bridge of the nose, ear, occiput, and malleolus do not have subcutaneous tissue and these ulcers can be shallow. Stage IV ulcers can extend into muscle and/or supporting structures (e.g., fascia, tendon, or joint capsule) making osteomyelitis possible. Exposed bone/tendon is visible or directly palpable. Copyright © (National Pressure Ulcer Advisory Panel. 2007.) **B:** Photo of category/stage IV pressure ulcer. Necrotic fatty tissue. (Copyright © C. Sussman.)

the information shown on the scan. Category/Stage II pressure ulcers are lesions that exhibit partial-thickness skin loss or a blister, which leads to superficial and partial-thickness damage to the epidermis and dermis[26] (Fig. 3.12). Pressure ulcers will present with a shallow open red/pink wound bed, without slough or maybe an open/ruptured serum-filled blister. Theoretically, pressure ulcer trauma starts at the bony tissue interface and works outward, eventually manifesting as damage on the skin. Conversely, stage II lesions start at the epidermis or skin and can progress to deeper layers. Figure 3.20A shows a bloody fluid-filled blister but it cannot be staged because the tissue under blister is not visible. Figure 3.20C shows the same wound as Figure 3.20A with the blister opened and it is now stageable.

EPUAP defines incontinence ulcers as "skin lesions not caused by pressure or shear."[122] This information is introduced here as a clarification to reduce confusion and misdiagnosis of lesions in this category. Distinguishing features of lesions caused by incontinence include location (not necessarily over bony prominences), edema, wet skin, incontinence of urine or feces, and color (more purple)[122] (Fig. 3.21).

Pressure ulcers with necrotic tissue filling the wound bed are full-thickness wounds, category/stage III or category/stage IV (Fig. 3.26B). Staging of pressure ulcers covered by eschar and necrotic tissue cannot be accomplished until removal of necrotic tissue allows for determination of the extent of depth of tissue involvement and are designated as "unstageable—depth unknown" (Fig. 3.28C). They remain unstageable until viable tissue is observed at the base of the wound. Then they are staged based on the anatomical structures exposed. Likewise, with deep tissue injuries, associated with pressure, the level of tissue insult cannot be categorized/staged until the full impact of the lesion manifests. It is also difficult to define stages in

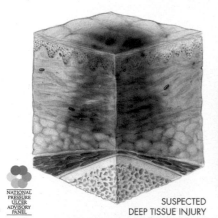

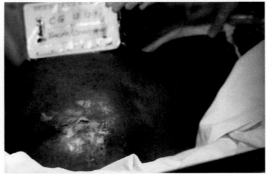

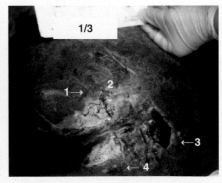

FIGURE 3.27 Diagram **Suspected Deep Tissue Injury:** Purple or maroon localized area of discolored intact skin or blood-filled blister due to damage of underlying soft tissue from pressure and/or shear. The area may be preceded by tissue that is painful, firm, mushy, boggy, warmer, or cooler as compared to adjacent tissue. **Further description:** Deep tissue injury may be difficult to detect in individuals with dark skin tones. Evolution may include a thin blister over a dark wound bed. The wound may further evolve and become covered by thin eschar. Evolution may be rapid exposing additional layers of tissue even with optimal treatment. (Copyright © National Pressure Ulcer Advisory Panel. 2007.)

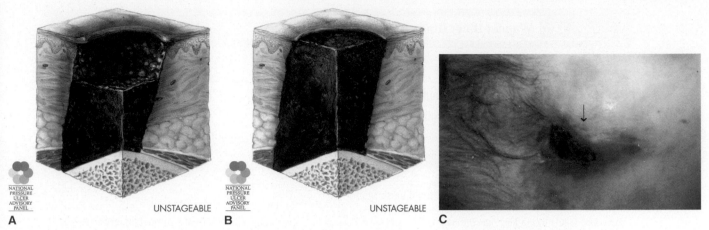

A   B   C

FIGURE 3.28 **A:** Diagram **Unstageable:** Full-thickness tissue loss in which the base of the ulcer is covered by slough (yellow, tan, gray, green, or brown) and/or eschar (tan, brown, or black) in the wound bed. **Further description:** Until enough slough and/or eschar is removed to expose the base of the wound, the true depth, and therefore stage, cannot be determined. Stable (dry, adherent, intact without erythema or fluctuance) eschar on the heels serves as "the body's natural (biological) cover" and should not be removed. (Copyright © National Pressure Ulcer Advisory Panel. 2007.) **B:** Diagram of unstageable pressure ulcer. (Copyright © National Pressure Ulcer Advisory Panel 2007.) **C:** Photo of Unstageable pressure ulcer. (Copyright © B.M. Bates-Jensen.)

patients with supportive devices because of the difficulty in accurately assessing the wound without removal of the devices. Finally, accurate, meaningful communication is difficult, because clinicians may not have the experience necessary to recognize the various tissue layers that identify the category, stage, or grade. In addition, clinicians may define stages differently. Staging requires practice and skill that develops with

time spent examining wounds. The NPUAP has a teaching aide for staging pressure ulcers available on its Web site www.npuap.org.

We noted earlier that classification systems are misapplied when used to monitor healing. This is as true for the NPUAP system as it is for other classification systems. For example, a category/stage IV pressure ulcer cannot "heal" and become a

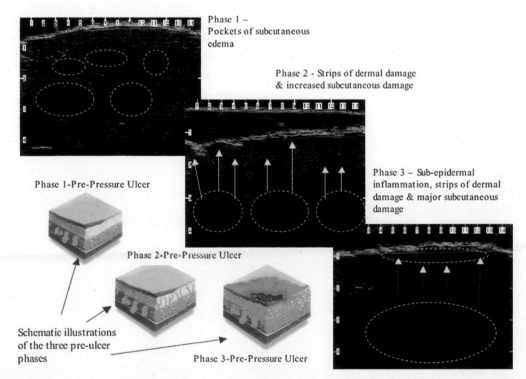

Phase 1 –
Pockets of subcutaneous edema

Phase 2 - Strips of dermal damage & increased subcutaneous damage

Phase 3 – Sub-epidermal inflammation, strips of dermal damage & major subcutaneous damage

Phase 1-Pre-Pressure Ulcer

Phase 2-Pre-Pressure Ulcer

Schematic illustrations of the three pre-ulcer phases

Phase 3-Pre-Pressure Ulcer

FIGURE 3.29 Using the EPISCAN, pressure ulcers have been found to develop in the subcutaneous tissue over a hard prominence, typically a bone, and then spread out through the dermis to the epidermis, where at some point, an open wound often develops. Studies have shown that the early phases of pressure ulcer development can be used to initiate earlier and more targeted intervention, and that this can significantly and cost-effectively reduce the occurrence of open pressure ulcers. (Copyright P. Wilson.)

TABLE 3.4	Wagner Ulcer Grade Classification

Grade	Characteristics
0	Preulcerative lesions; healed ulcers; presence of bony deformity
1	Superficial ulcer without subcutaneous tissue involvement
2	Penetration through the subcutaneous tissue; may expose bone, tendon, ligament, or joint capsule
3	Osteitis, abscess, or osteomyelitis
4	Gangrene of digit
5	Gangrene of the foot requiring disarticulation

Copyright © 2011 by the American Orthopardic Foot and Ankle Society, Inc., originally published in Food & Ankle. 1981;(2):64–122 and reproduced here with permission.

CLINICAL WISDOM

Reverse Staging or Back Staging of Pressure Ulcers

Reverse staging or back staging of pressure ulcers is an inappropriate way to define a healing wound. Once the ulcer is staged, the stage and wound severity diagnosis do not change; rather, correct terminology is *healing stage II* (or *III* or *IV*).

category/stage II pressure ulcer. The purpose of staging pressure ulcers is to document the maximum anatomic depth of tissue involved (after all necrotic tissue is removed) and to determine the extent of tissue damage only. Staging can also aid examination of the wound *severity*, but not wound *healing*.

The SWHT, PUSH, and the BWAT are tools for monitoring wound healing attributes described in Chapter 6.

Wagner Ulcer Grade Classification

The Wagner Ulcer Grade Classification system is used to establish the presence of depth and infection in a wound. This system was developed for the diagnosis and treatment of the dysvascular foot.[118] It is commonly used as an assessment instrument in the evaluation of diabetic foot ulcers, but is limited in its ability to identify and describe vascular disease and infection as independent risk factors.[123] The system includes six grades, progressing from 0 to 5 in the order of severity of breakdown in the diabetic, neuropathic foot (Table 3.4). The 0 classification evaluates for predisposing factors leading to breakdown; along with grades 1–3, it is used for risk management. Photos of the grades appear in Chapter 12.

The University of Texas Treatment-Based Diabetic Foot Classification System

The University of Texas Treatment-Based Diabetic Foot Classification System is a matrix of grades used for situations in which neuropathy is present and information is needed about infection, circulation (PVD), and the combination of infection and ischemia in order to assign risk and predict outcome (Table 3.5).[117] Each ulcer is given both a numeric grade (0–III) and an alphabetic stage (A–D). Letter "A" denotes wound depth. Other letters denote ischemia and infection categories. However, this system lacks consideration of biomechanics and neuropathy. Analysis of this system reveals that it is a better predictor of group outcome than of individual patient outcome.[117]

TABLE 3.5	University of Texas, San Antonio Classification			
	Grade 0	I	II	III
S				
T A	Preulcerative or postulcerative lesion; completely epithelialized	Superficial wound (not involving tendon, capsule or bone)	Wound penetrating to tendon or capsule	Wound penetrating to bone or joint
A B	Infection	Infection	Infection	Infection
G C	Ischemia	Ischemia	Ischemia	Ischemia
E D	Infection and Ischemia	Infection and Ischemia	Infection and Ischemia	Infection and Ischemia

Reprinted with permission from Armstrong DG, Lavery L, Harkless LB. Validation of a diabetic wound classification system: the contribution of depth, infection, and ischemia to risk of amputation. *Diabetes Car PMID: 9589255 [PubMed - indexed for MEDLINE].* May 1998;21(5):855–859.

Therefore, this is the favored classification system for neuropathic ulcers.[123]

Marion Laboratories Red, Yellow, Black Classification System

The Marion Laboratories system of classification by color is popular because of its simplicity and ease of use. Three colors—red, yellow, and black—are used to describe the wound's surface color, with each color corresponding to specific therapy needs:[89]

- The red wound is clean, healing, and granulating.
- Yellow signals possible infection, the need for cleaning or debridement, or the presence of necrotic tissue.
- The black wound is necrotic and needs cleaning and debridement.

Red is considered the most desired characteristic, yellow is less desirable, and black is least desirable. If all three types are present, select the least desirable as the basis for treatment. Table 3.6 shows the red, yellow, and black classification system with clinical manifestations. Examples of wounds that would be classified as red, yellow or black are shown accompanying the NPUAP staging diagrams.

WOUND SEVERITY DIAGNOSIS

The more tissue layers that a wound penetrates, the more severe the wound is considered. This *wound severity diagnosis* influences further wound assessment strategies and treatment decisions. It can also be used to predict healing time and risk for nonhealing and complications, which in turn influences prediction of length of stay and reimbursement. For example, a category/stage IV pressure ulcer requires more care and a longer length of stay than does a category/stage II pressure ulcer, and the risk of complications is greater.

Wound severity diagnosis statements for all wound care clinicians are similar, in that all use diagnoses that reflect impairments of the involved tissues. In medicine, wound diagnoses are made based on identified pathological conditions such as venous ulcer or diabetic ulcer.

Nurses use nursing diagnoses to classify skin and tissue impairments, and to assist with developing care plans for wound care patients. Nursing diagnoses are expressed as specific diagnostic statements that include the diagnostic category and the "related to" stem statement. For example, *impaired tissue integrity* is a broad diagnosis that would be correctly applied to category/ stage III and category/stage IV pressure ulcers. *Impaired skin integrity* is a subcategory that correctly applies to partial-thickness or full-thickness loss of skin. *Impaired skin integrity* should not be used as a diagnosis for surgical incisions or deep tissue wounds. The diagnosis of *risk for infection related to surgical incision* is more appropriate, because of the disruption of the skin during surgery, making it more vulnerable to infection.

The "related to" stem statements aid in communicating with other health-care professionals and planning care by targeting the defining characteristics for the diagnostic statement. For example, the diagnosis statement *impaired skin integrity* would be followed by a statement such as *impaired skin integrity related to friction and moisture from urinary incontinence*. For nurses, the "related to" stem statement usually reflects etiologic factors in wound development and directs the plan of care and specific interventions.[124]

PTs also use wound severity diagnoses that relate to depth of wound penetration. Wound diagnosis statements include a stem statement that indicates depth of skin involvement, such as *superficial skin involvement* or *partial-thickness skin involvement and scar formation, full-thickness skin involvement and scar formation*, or *involvement extending into fascia, muscle*, or *bone*. An example of a complete statement is *impaired integumentary integrity secondary to partial-thickness skin involvement and scar formation*.[125] The statement refers to the functional impairment of the skin and different tissues, which has implications for disability.

The concept that the depth of tissue involvement or wound stage is a measure of wound severity is regularly accepted by all health-care disciplines, and this concept is used to select examinations, plan treatment, and predict functional outcomes.

EVALUATION OF WOUND HEALING STATUS

This section explains how to evaluate the status of wound healing. Chapter 2 presents acute and chronic wound healing physiology; therefore, you may wish to review pertinent sections for explanation of the mechanisms that may underlie your assessment findings. After the assessment, you will be able to determine a *wound healing phase diagnosis*; that is, a diagnosis of the functional status of healing based on the phase of the wound at the time of the assessment.[126] The wound healing phase diagnosis is useful to demonstrate medical necessity for advanced interventions, which are described shortly. (See Table 3.7).

Wound healing begins with the inflammatory phase, progresses to the proliferative phase and epithelialization phase,

TABLE 3.6	Marion laboratories Red, Yellow, and Black Wound Classification System	

Color	Indication
Red	Clean; healing; granulation
Yellow	Possible infection; needs cleaning; necrotic
Black	Needs cleaning; necrotic

Data from Cuzzell JZ. The new RYB color code. *American Journal of Nursing.* 1988;88(10):1342-1346 And Stotts NA. Seeing red & yellow & black: the three color concept of wound care. *Nursing.* 1990;2:59–61.

TABLE 3.7	Wound Healing "Phase Diagnosis" and Prognosis		
Wound Healing Phase	**Acute Wound Healing "Phase Diagnosis"**	**Chronic Wound Healing "Phase Diagnosis"**	**Absence of Wound Healing "Phase Diagnosis"**
Inflammatory	Acute inflammatory	Chronic inflammatory	Absence of inflammatory
Proliferative	Acute proliferative	Chronic proliferative	Absence of proliferative
Epithelialization	Acute epithelialization	Chronic epithelialization	Absence of epithelialization
Prognosis	Orderly, timely progression through phases of healing	Reinitiate acute phase, then progress through phases of healing. Progress to a clean, stable wound.	Initiate healing phase, if able, and progress through phases. Or progress to a clean, stable wound. If unable to initiate healing phase, refer.
Outcome	Healed wound	Healed wound clean stable wound	

and then enters the remodeling phase. Careful assessment of the wound and periwound tissue establishes the present, *predominant* wound healing phase, which is the primary "phase diagnosis" for the wound at that time.

Identifying the Aspect of the Wound Healing Phase

In order to determine the phase of wound healing, you need to be able to recognize the signs and symptoms of the three potential aspects of each phase: acute (progressing), chronic ("stuck" or plateaued), and absent (not apparent). Each aspect of each phase has benchmarks that are indicators of the phase status. There are also benchmarks that signify transition to the next phase(s) or absence of the subsequent phases(s). Tables 3.7 through 3.10 list the wound healing phase diagnoses and related wound healing phase benchmarks, which are also discussed in more detail below.

Acute Aspect

As normal acute wounds heal, there is an orderly, timely overlapping progression through the wound healing phases: inflammatory to proliferative/epithelialization, to remodeling.

Chronic Aspect

Failure of the orderly, timely progression of healing through the successive phases results in a chronic wound. Chronic wounds can fail to initiate or stall in any phase of wound healing. When a wound stalls, plateaus, or simply gets stuck in one wound healing phase, the wound becomes chronic with respect to that phase. For example, wounds that experience repeated trauma from dressing changes or debridement often become stuck in the inflammatory phase of wound healing. This phase diagnosis would be *chronic inflammatory phase*. Another example is the wound that fills with granulation tissue but does not stop proliferating, instead going on to form hypergranulation tissue (Fig. 3.42). At this point, the wound appears stuck building the collagen matrix and is unable to progress to remodeling. This wound is in the *chronic proliferative phase*. A final example is the wound with chronic scar formation, such as with hypertrophy or keloid scars (Figs. 3.5 and 3.6) that do not stop laying down collagen and progress to remodeling. This is *chronic epithelialization*.

Absent Aspect

The wound that fails to pass through a wound healing phase lacks attributes of that phase and is referred to as being in the *absence of inflammatory phase*, *absence of proliferative phase*, or *absence of epithelialization phase* (see Fig. 3.2). Wounds that fail to progress through a wound healing phase differ from those that get stuck or exhibit characteristics of chronicity in a phase. Wounds that lack an inflammatory response, for example, do not demonstrate signs of inflammation, whereas wounds with chronic inflammation show signs of a continued inflammatory response. Absence of the wound healing phase indicates that the wound has not initiated the phase, for whatever reasons (e.g., lack of circulation). Absence of the wound healing phase signifies either the inability to heal or the need for help from an intervention to initiate the acute phase, leading to progression through phases (e.g., reperfusion through surgical intervention, debridement of senescent cells, or enhanced blood flow from a physical agent).

Identifying the Wound Healing Phase Diagnosis

Since phases overlap, benchmarks for multiple wound healing phases can be apparent at the same time. But as noted earlier, if the wound is transitioning from one phase to the next, the wound healing phase diagnosis is defined by the *predominant* phase appearance.

Inflammatory is the wound healing phase diagnosis if the identified attributes of acute or chronic inflammation are at least 50% to 75% of what would be expected (Figs. 3.13, 3.17, 3.18 and 3.34). Although a wound in the chronic inflammatory phase is also in absence of the proliferative phase and absence of the epithelialization phase, the chronic inflammatory phase would be the *primary* wound healing phase diagnosis.

When the wound attributes of the acute inflammatory phase are less than 50% of what are expected and there is significant proliferation of granulation tissue in the wound bed, the primary wound phase diagnosis changes to the proliferative phase (Fig. 3.31B). A wound healing phase diagnosis of *acute proliferative phase* means that most (50% or greater) of the wound surface appearance attributes (granulation tissue and contraction) are observed.

A diagnosis for a wound "halfway" between the inflammatory and proliferative phases exists: If less than 50% of the proliferative phase attributes are identified, the wound is primarily in an inflammatory phase and has not yet reached the proliferative phase for diagnostic purposes. The diagnosis would be written *inflammatory phase/proliferative phase*. Some clinicians call this *late inflammatory* or *early proliferative phase*.

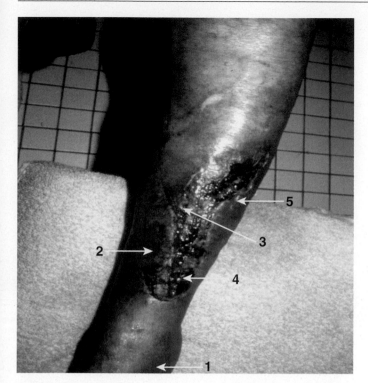

FIGURE 3.30 Traumatic wound in acute inflammatory phase. Note: (1) Adjacent tissue erythema, (2) Periwound erythema, (3) Hemorrhagic tissue, (4) Sanguinous drainage, (5) Location over anterior tibia, (6) Classification: full thickness. (Copyright © A. Myer.)

A wound phase diagnosis of *epithelialization phase* is based on findings that the wound is resurfacing. Partial-thickness wounds that are resurfacing from the middle or edges are in the *epithelialization phase*. Wounds that are greater than 50% attached at the edges and do not have steep walls that are epithelializing also are diagnosed as being in the *epithelialization phase* (Fig. 3.31C). Wounds in the acute epithelialization phase have an excellent prognosis for healing, whereas wounds in the chronic epithelialization phase need an intervention to restart the healing process. The prognosis then would be that the wound will heal with intervention. Wounds that have absence of the epithelialization phase of healing are at high risk for nonhealing unless contributing conditions can be altered, e.g., by reperfusion, application of moisture-retentive dressings, or stimulation with biophysical agents, as described in Part IV of this text.

ASSESSING WOUNDS IN THE INFLAMMATORY PHASE

Assessment of the periwound and wound tissues during the inflammatory phase includes four categories of wound attributes:

- Adjacent and periwound tissue appearance
- Wound bed tissue appearance (color and texture)
- Wound edges
- Exudate characteristics (odor, type, and quantity)

In this section, the attributes of the wound and the periwound tissues that serve as benchmarks of the phase are described during acute inflammation, chronic inflammation, and absence of inflammation. Figures 3.30 and 3.41A,B show a wound that went from the chronic inflammatory phase to the

acute inflammatory phase and subsequently progressed to the proliferative and then to epithelialization and remodeling phase.

Acute Inflammation

Signs of acute inflammation (e.g., erythema, pain, edema, heat, loss of function) often extend well beyond the immediate wound and periwound tissues into adjacent tissues. Initially, they indicate a healthy response and are a prerequisite to normal healing. Use the characteristics observed during acute inflammation as a reference point for the evaluation of impaired responses.

Adjacent and Periwound Tissue Assessment

The major attributes of adjacent and periwound tissues that are observed and palpated in the inflammatory phase are color, firmness/texture, temperature, and pain.

Skin Color

Erythema is one of the classic characteristics of the acute inflammatory phase. Initially, the adjacent skin can be erythematous due to reactive hyperemia. Erythema may not be evident in individuals with darkly pigmented skin (see previous discussion on skin color attributes). Reddened skin with streaks leading away from the area can indicate cellulitis, a skin infection. If observed, check the patient's history for fever, chills, history of recurrent cellulitis, or medications being used to treat the condition. If no treatment has been initiated, these findings should be reported immediately to a physician.

Edema and Induration

The edema of the acute inflammatory phase is localized and brawny. It feels firm and distorts the swollen tissues, causing the skin to become taut, shiny, and raised from the contours of the surrounding tissues. This edema results from trauma (e.g., pressure ulcers, burns, and surgical debridement) and is related to the release of histamines. Histamines cause vasodilation and increase vascular permeability, resulting in the movement of fluid in the interstitial spaces. Edema is usually accompanied by pain.

Induration is abnormal hardening of the tissue at the wound margin from consolidation of edema in the tissues. To test for induration, attempt to pinch the tissues gently; if induration is present, the tissues cannot be pinched. Induration follows reflex hyperemia or chronic venous congestion.[74]

Skin Temperature

Skin temperature should be tested as previously described. During acute inflammation, expect the temperature of the wound and adjacent tissues to be the same. As healing progresses, the temperature of the adjacent wound tissue will gradually decline, and the area of increased temperature will narrow.[109]

Pain

Chapter 22 is devoted to wound pain with specific assessment guidelines. Therefore, this discussion is very limited. Assess spontaneous or induced pain in the adjacent tissues by palpation or patient/family report, or both. Quantify using an accepted pain scale like the visual analog scale. Pain can indicate infection or subcutaneous tissue damage that is not visible, such as in pressure ulcers or vascular disease. Report of the sudden onset of pain accompanied by edema in a leg is a common

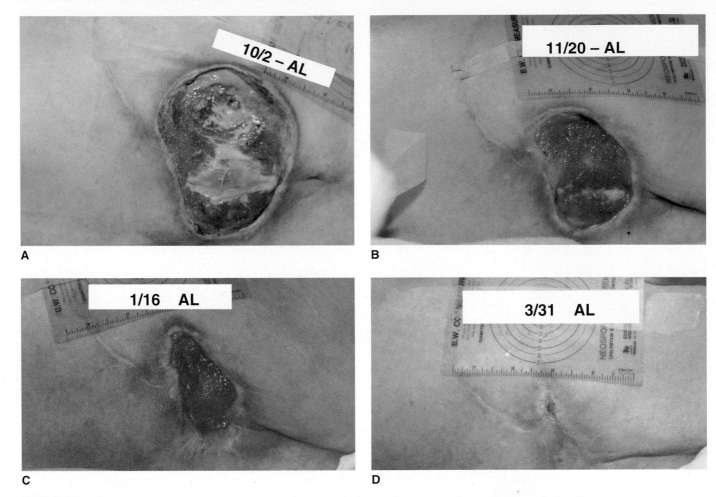

FIGURE 3.31 A: Chronic wound: converted to acute inflammatory phase. This is a sacral wound with stringy, yellow slough evident. Note example of epidermal ridge formation of wound edges. Predominant wound healing phase diagnosis: acute inflammatory/proliferative phase. Wound severity diagnosis: impaired integumentary integrity secondary to skin involvement extending into fascia, muscle, and bone (Stage IV pressure ulcer). **B:** Same wound as in (A), progressing through the proliferative phase. The wound is contracting and proliferating. Note changes in size, shape, and depth, as well as new healthy granulation tissue compared with (A). **C:** Note sustained wound contraction. Note epithelialization and proliferative phases. **D:** The wound is completely resurfaced and is in the remodeling phase. (Copyright © C. Sussman.)

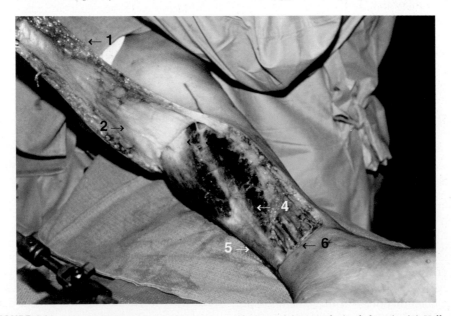

FIGURE 3.32 Full-thickness skin resected from calf. Note: (1) Vascularized dermis; (2) Yellow, healthy fat tissue; (3) White fibrous fascia; (4) Dark red muscle tissue; (5) Tendon covered with peritenon; (6) Blood vessel. (Copyright © J. Wethe.)

CLINICAL WISDOM

Excessive Inflammatory Signs and Infection

Excessive signs of acute inflammation should be considered a signal of impending wound infection.[127]

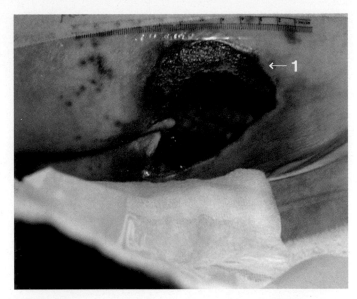

FIGURE 3.33 Cave, or undermining, of the wound edges. Note the shelf. (Copyright © C. Sussman.)

indicator of deep vein thrombosis and wound infection. Pain in the calf or during palpation over a vein accompanied by unilateral edema is an indicator of thrombophlebitis, and immediate referral is required. The absence of pain in an obviously infected or inflamed wound should be investigated as an indication of neuropathy and the need for further assessment of sensation.

Wound Bed Tissue Assessment

Assess the wound bed for depth, undermining and tunneling, and exposure of subcutaneous and deeper tissues.

Depth

A partial-thickness skin loss creates a shallow crater that looks red or pink, or shows the yellow reticular layer—a thin, yellow, mesh-like covering that constitutes the deep layer of the dermis (Fig. 3.12). If the crater is bright and shiny, it is healthy and viable and should be left intact. Refer back to Chapter 2 and Figure 3.38 to view the anatomy of the tissues deep to the skin. If the wound penetrates through the dermis into the subcutaneous tissue, it will appear as though it contains yellow fat (such as chicken fat) or white connective tissue, called *fascia*. Fascia covers and wraps around all muscles, tendons, blood vessels, and nerves. Wounds that extend through the subcutaneous tissue into the muscle can have a pink or dark red appearance with a shiny layer of fascia on top.

Undermining and Tunneling

Excavation of the subcutaneous tissues during debridement creates a "cave," or undermining, of the wound edges. Undermining can lead to separation of fascial planes (Figs. 3.4A,B and 3.33). Muscles lie together in bundles that are held together by fascia; when the fascia is cut, the muscle bundles separate. Separation of the fascial layers opens tunnels along the fascial planes between the muscles under the skin. Tunnels can join together and form sinus tracts (Fig. 3.16B). Infection can travel through these tunnels, leading to abscess.

Exposure of Subcutaneous and Deeper Tissues

When debriding or treating deep or undermined wounds, it is likely that muscle tissue or tendons will be exposed. Muscle tissue can be identified by appearance (striated) and by activity (it jumps or twitches when palpated). Muscles are connected to bones by tendons. These are rope-like structures covered with a sheath of white fascia called *peritenon*. Sparing the peritenon during wound care procedures facilitates the growth of new granulation tissue over the intact peritenon.

Penetration of a wound into a joint can expose several anatomic structures, including ligaments, which are white and striated; joint capsule, which is white and shiny; and cartilage, which is white, hard, and smooth, and is located on the ends of bones. Bone is white and hard, and covered with a clear or white membrane called *periosteum*. Loss of peritenon or periosteum will compromise a skin graft. Wounds that can be probed to bone are considered to have osteomyelitis, and immediate referral is warranted.

Assessment of Wound Edges

Palpate wound edges for firmness and texture. Observe the margins for curling. During acute inflammation, the wound edges are often indistinct or diffuse as in Fig. 3.30, and they change shape as wound contraction and epithelialization begins to cover the wound surface. Wound edges can be attached to the wound base or separated from it, forming walls with the base of the wound at a depth from the skin surface as in Fig. 3.33. This is considered a key factor in wound resurfacing. When undermining occurs, the wound edge is not attached, and epithelialization cannot advance, because the keratinocytes are unable to advance across the gap. Repetitive injury to the wound edges can cause them to become firm, fibrotic, and indurated; this in turn can affect the ability of epithelialization to progress.[68] Figure 3.35A–D shows examples of wound edges. Chapter 5 has detailed descriptions of different types of wound edges.

Assessment of Wound Drainage

Wound drainage during the acute inflammatory phase is an indication of the status of the clotting mechanisms and infection. During assessment, record the presence or absence, color, odor, quantity, and quality of the wound drainage.

Wound drainage that contains proteins, dead cells, and debris is called *exudate* and is typically brown or grey, although it may be viscous and look like pus (Fig. 3.36A,F). Bloody exudate is called *sanguineous drainage*. Sanguineous wounds may have impaired clotting due to anticoagulant or antiplatelet pharmaceutical products (e.g., aspirin or Plavix) or disease processes such as hemophilia. A medical history, including a pharmacologic history, and systems review are indicated to determine the causes of the sanguineous drainage (Fig. 3.36F).

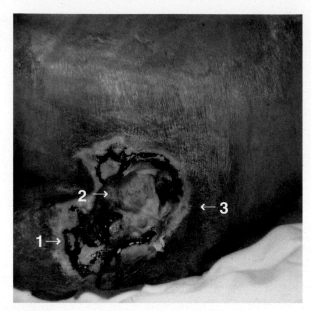

FIGURE 3.34 Chronic inflammatory phase. Note the following wound characteristics: (1) Sanguineous drainage, (2) Muscle exposure, (3) Hemosiderin staining surrounding the wound. (Copyright © B.M. Bates-Jensen.)

Copious or persistent sanguineous drainage should be reported to a physician immediately, as it may be a sign of internal bleeding.

In contrast, clear fluid drainage is called *transudate*. The presence of transudate indicates diffusion of plasma fluid from the blood into the surrounding tissues. Serous transudate is a clear yellow fluid that exudes from the wound. It is usually odorless, and is present in varying amounts during the inflammatory phase (Fig. 3.36B,E).

Chronic Inflammation

Inflammation that persists for weeks or months is referred to as chronic (or persistent). Chronic inflammation occurs when the macrophages and neutrophils fail to phagocytose necrotic matter, ingest foreign debris, and fight infection.[128] Therefore, necrotic matter and foreign debris is typically found in the wound bed. Chronic inflammation is also related to the release of histamine from the mast cells and reflex hyperemia associated with vasodilation of the surrounding vasculature. Repeated trauma to a wound can also develop into chronic inflammation.

Adjacent and Periwound Tissue Assessment

Chronic inflammation in the periwound area appears as a halo of erythema in lightly pigmented skin and a dark halo in darkly pigmented skin. The latter may be easily mistaken because of its similar appearance to hemosiderin staining. Arterial ulcers over the malleolus and pressure ulcers are frequently seen with a halo of erythema, but they lack the blood flow to progress the wound (Fig. 3.37).

There is minimal temperature change or cooling, compared with adjacent uninjured tissues. Edema may prompt some minimal firmness in the periwound tissues. Usually, the pain response is minimal. Intense pain may be associated with arterial vascular disease or infection.

Wound Bed Tissue Assessment

In wounds in the chronic inflammatory phase, necrotic tissue usually covers all or part of the wound surface. Necrotic tissue varies in color and may be black, yellow, tan, brown, or gray. Soft necrotic tissue, such as fibrin or slough, can be present in the wound bed. Fibrin forms on the wound surface of venous ulcers. *Slough* is necrotic fat and fascia adhering to the layer beneath it. See Figures 3.17, 3.26B, 3.28C, 3.38, and 3.39 for different appearances of necrotic tissue.

During assessment, record the presence and color of necrotic tissue. Wounds that are in the chronic inflammatory phase of healing often have a combination of several attributes. For example, a wound can have black and yellow necrotic tissue, as well as pink granulation tissue or healthy muscle tissue (Fig. 3.34) and sanguinous drainage.

In wounds that are chronically inflamed, a portion of the wound surface is often in the proliferative phase with granulation tissue present, but the proliferation fails to progress possibly due to infection. Not all pink tissue is granulation tissue: muscle tissue that lies beneath newly removed necrotic tissue is pink or dark red.

Signs of acute inflammation may be absent. If, however, cellulitis or other infection is present, streaks of redness will often be seen in the periwound and adjacent skin extending away from the wound, and pain can become intense (Fig. 3.37). Signs and symptoms of systemic infection that can lead to sepsis include fever of 101°F (39.4°C) or higher; chills; manifestation of shock, including restlessness, lethargy, and confusion; and decreased systolic blood pressure.[89] These are red flags that require immediate medical follow-up.

Chronic Wound Drainage

Prolonged, chronic inflammation is the result of a bacteria-filled wound.[128] When there is a high bacterial count ($>10^5$), signs of active infection are seen. Wound drainage characteristics, including color, odor, and volume, are often used as indicators of active wound infection. During assessment, record the presence or absence, color, odor, and quantity of exudate. The BWAT includes a nominal Likert scale to rate each one of these aspects. (See Chapter 5).

Exudate Color

Exudate color can suggest the type of infection. Normally, wound exudate is serous—a clear or light-yellow fluid. Exudate from an infected wound can be yellow, tan, brown, or green. Wound drainage that has a yellow/gray or green color, has a foul odor, and/or is viscous, is commonly referred to as *pus*. Pus is a result of the demise of neutrophils after they have phagocytosed debris and excessive bacterial loads. Green exudates are usually associated with an anaerobic infection. The wound dressing should be examined after removal for evidence of the attributes of the wound exudate (Fig. 3.36A–F).

Exudate Odor

Not all malodorous exudate signifies infection. The odor can result from solubilization of necrotic tissue by enzymatic debriding agents or autolysis. In assessing exudate odor, begin by cleansing exudate from the wound to determine whether the

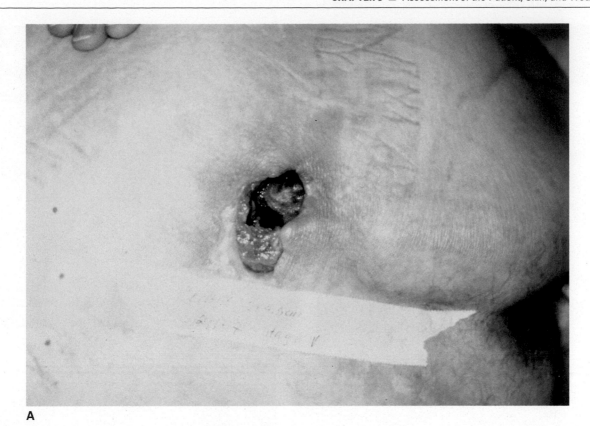

A

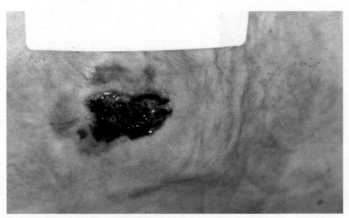

B

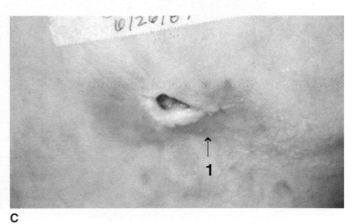

C

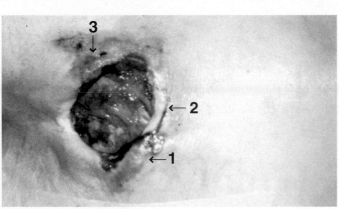

D

FIGURE 3.35 Wound edges. **A:** Absence of proliferative phase. Wound with no epithelialization present. The wound is clean, but nonproliferating. **B:** Same wound as in Figure 3.41A. Wound is in acute proliferative phase with evidence of new epithelial migration. indicating wound improvement. **C:** There is an absence of the epithelialization phase due to chronic fibrosis and scarring at the wound edge. Edges achieve a unique, grayish hue in both dark and lightly pigmented skin. Note rolled and thickened attributes. Chronic proliferative phase. **D:** Example of knowledge gained from careful examination of the wound edge. This is a chronic, deep ulcer that does not bleed easily. Wound is in chronic proliferative phase. Note: (1) New pressure-induced damage (hemorrhage), (2) Maceration from wound fluid, (3) Friction injury with signs of inflammation. (Copyright © B.M. Bates-Jensen.)

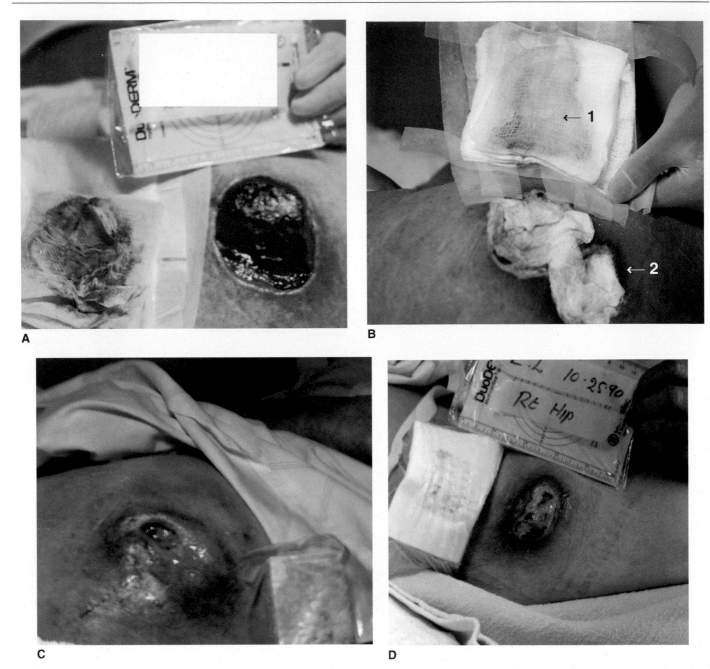

FIGURE 3.36 Assesment of wound Drainage. **A:** Wound appears "clean," but it is in the chronic proliferative phase. The quantity of exudate is determined by the amount of dressing saturated by the drainage. Note: (1) Moderate to large amount of sanguineous exudate, (2) Moderate to large amount of purulent exudate. Evaluate for infection. **B:** Wound with packing still present. Note: (1) Moderate amount of serous exudate on dressing, (2) Green color of exudate suggests possible infection. **C:** Wound with composite dressing shows scant amount of serous exudate. Wound is in chronic inflammatory phase. There is an absence of proliferative phase. Wound is stage III pressure ulcer. **D:** Wound with composite dressing. Dressing shows scant amount of serosanguineous exudate. The wound bed shows a gelatinous mass that may be gelatinous edema. Bright pink skin is scar tissue. Evaluate for trauma. (Copyright © C. Sussman.)

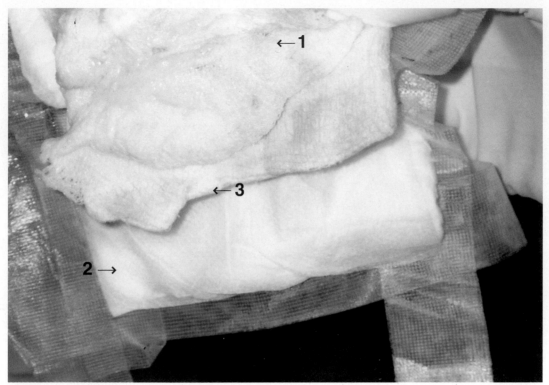

E

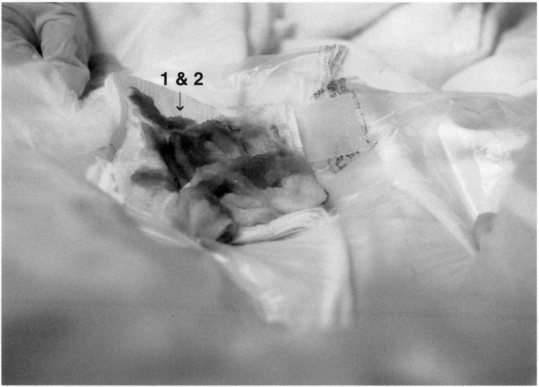

F

FIGURE 3.36 (*continued*) **E:** Large amount of serous drainage. Note: (1) Drainage flows into secondary dressing; (2) Green tinge to edges of dressing, suggesting anaerobic infection (e.g., pseudomonas). Monitor for a degenerative change in exudate type from present serous to purulent (e.g., greener, thicker, and more opaque). **F:** Large amount of purulent exudate. Note: (1) Thick, opaque, cloudy appearance; (2) Green and red color. Assess for odor. (Copyright © C. Sussman.)

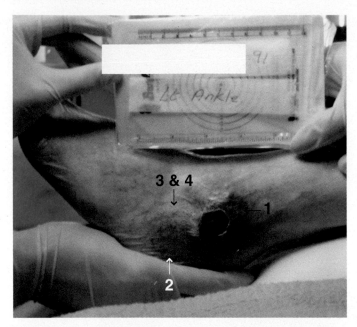

FIGURE 3.37 Classic ischemic ulcer. Note: (1) Chronic inflammation with cellulitis; (2) Punched-out, ulcer edges; (3) covering of dry, black eschar; (4) Location over lateral malleolus. (Copyright © C. Sussman.)

RESEARCH WISDOM

Wounds with early signs of infection are treated with a regimen of oral antibiotics for 2 to 4 weeks, and those that have late healing signs of infection are treated with topical antibiotics.[129] The prognosis is that the wound will resume progression through the phases of healing following intervention with antibiotics.

All chronic wounds are colonized with bacteria; however, at times the bacteria overwhelm the host and become critically colonized and progress to infection. During assessment, the clinician will identify certain attributes that may be indicators of infection. Cutting and Harding did an extensive literature review to determine criteria suggesting wound infection in granulating wounds.[130] These include

- Delayed or stalled healing compared with the norm for the site or condition
- Discoloration of the granulation tissue
- Friable granulation tissue that bleeds easily
- Unexpected pain or tenderness
- Pocketing at the base of the wound
- Bridging of the soft tissue
- Abnormal smell
- Wound breakdown

Sibbald et al. developed a mnemonic guide that parallels the same indicators of chronic bacterial damage identified by Cutting and Harding and called this system NERDS (non-healing, exudate, red friable granulation tissue, necrotic debris and/or smell). Three or more of these attributes are considered positive indicators of infection in chronic wounds.[131] However, symptoms of deep infection more closely reflect classic signs and symptoms of infection. Chapter 18 is devoted to management of wound excudate and infection.

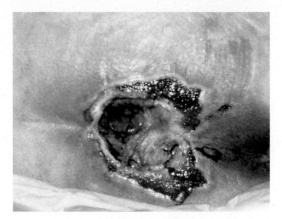

FIGURE 3.38 Soft, soggy, black eschar in the absence of an inflammatory phase. Typical location and butterfly shape associated with a Kennedy Terminal Ulcer. (Copyright © B.M. Bates-Jensen.)

odor is transient or internal. If enzymatic or autolytic methods of debridement are used, the odor and debris should be removed by cleansing. If odor remains, or the exudate that is expressed from the wound or adjacent tissues has color or odor, consider infection. Check for other symptoms of infection, such as heat, fever, and lethargy (Refer to chapter 18.)

Exudate Volume

Exudate volume is considered an indicator of wound outcome.[70] Estimate the amount of wound exudate as scant/minimal, small, moderate, or large/copious from examining the wound dressing or by expressing it from the wound. The absence of exudate or dryness of the wound bed can indicate desiccation and the need for adding moisture (Fig. 3.36D).

Gelatinous Edema

Following a secondary trauma to the wound bed, such as sharp or enzymatic debridement, leaking plasma proteins from the damaged or irritated capillaries can allow moisture to accumulate and form an opaque, gelatinous mass visible in the base of the wound. The edematous mass contains many substances, all of which contribute to sustaining the chronic inflammatory response. This gelatinous edema is considered a benchmark

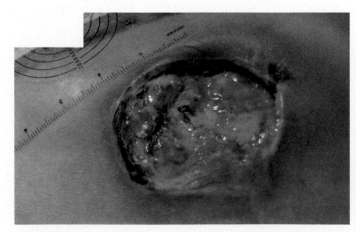

FIGURE 3.39 Chronic wound with yellow, mucinous slough. (chronic wound exudate) (Copyright © C. Sussman.)

CLINICAL WISDOM

Distinguishing Granulation Tissue from Muscle

To distinguish granulation tissue from healthy muscle, palpate the tissue with a gloved finger. Granulation tissue feels soft and spongy. It will not "jump" if pinched, but it may bleed. Muscle tissue is firm and resilient to pressure. It will jump or twitch if pinched or probed.

of the chronic inflammatory phase, and should be recorded if present (Fig. 3.36C).[132]

Absence of Inflammation

Absence of the inflammatory phase, or the inability of the body to present an immune response to wounding, can be due to many causes, including an immune-suppression state (e.g., HIV infection/AIDS, cancer, diabetes, drug or radiation therapy, overuse of antiseptics, and severe ischemia). The absence of an inflammatory response prevents the wound from progressing through the biologic cascade of repair. It is different from chronic inflammation, with distinct signs and symptoms.

Lack of tissue perfusion is a common cause for an absent inflammatory phase. For example, a patient with an ulcer on an ischemic foot with an eschar over a wound on the heel has an absence of inflammation. Lack of perfusion is a barrier to healing. Unless reperfusion is an option, it may not be possible or appropriate in such a case to remove the eschar. In this case, the eschar is nature's best protection from the entry of infection. Protection of the eschar and the limb from trauma to

prevent opening of the body to infection and new wounding is the preferred treatment strategy (Fig. 3.40).[71] In order for the wound to heal, interventions are necessary to restart the inflammatory response. However, because of the comorbidity related to the problem, palliative care would be the best option.

Adjacent and Periwound Tissue Assessment

The absence of an inflammatory phase is recognized by the absence of a vascular response to wounding, including the absence of color changes in the periwound skin and the absence of tension or hardness. However, there may be a boggy feeling and minimal temperature difference or coolness compared with adjacent tissue. Minimal pulses are palpable. Such findings should trigger further investigation of the vascular status of the patient.

Wound Bed Tissue and Drainage Assessment

Wound bed tissue can be covered with hard, dry eschar to seal off debris and infection from the wound (Fig. 3.40).

Wound drainage can be scant, or the tissues can be dry. Dryness can be due to hemostasis sealing off the blood supply to the tissues without adequate perfusion to progress the healing, ischemia reperfusion injury, or improper treatment. Table 3.8 summarizes the findings during the inflammatory phase.

ASSESSING WOUNDS IN THE PROLIFERATIVE PHASE

Like the inflammatory phase, the proliferative phase can be described with three aspects: acute, chronic, or absent.

- The acute proliferative phase is the active biologic process of proliferation, including extracellular matrix (ECM) synthesis, granulation tissue formation and degradation, and wound contraction.

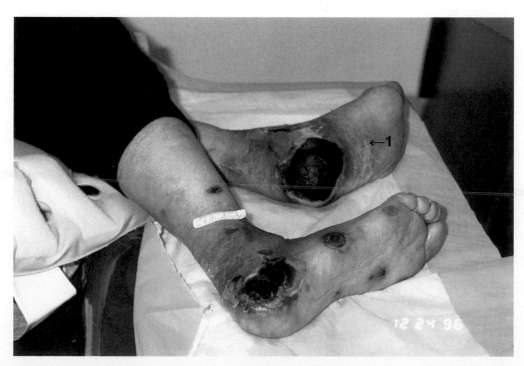

FIGURE 3.40 Severe arterial ischemic disease with multiple ischemic ulcers below the ankle bilaterally. There is an absence of the inflammatory phase with hard, dry, black eschar covering. Note trophic changes on foot, evidence of scaling. Do not debride. (Copyright © E. Fowler.)

| TABLE 3.8 | **Wound Healing Phase Diagnosis: Aspects of Inflammatory Phase** | | |

Periwound Skin and Wound Tissue Characteristics	Acute Inflammatory Phase	Chronic Inflammatory Phase	Absence of Inflammatory Phase
Periwound skin color	• Unblanchable erythema in light-skinned patients • Discoloration or deepening of normal color in darkly pigmented patients • Ecchymosis (purplish bruising)	• Halo of erythema or darkening • Hemosiderin (rust-brown) staining • Hemosiderin staining • Ecchymosis	• Pale or ashen skin color • Absence of erythema or darkening • Hemosiderin staining • Ecchymosis
Edema and induration	• Firmness • Taut, shiny skin • Localized swelling • Consolidation (hardness) between adjacent tissues • Gelatinous edema may be seen on wound tissue	• Minimal firmness • Absent • May feel boggy	
Tissue temperature	• Elevated initially, decreases as inflammation progresses	• Minimal change or coolness	• Minimal change or coolness
Pain	• Present; wound is tender and painful unless neuropathy is present	• Minimal pain unless arterial etiology or infection, then can have intense pain	• Minimal or no pain unless arterial etiology, then can have intense pain
Wound tissue	• Blister with clear or bloody fluid • Shallow or deep crater with red to pink color • Red muscle • White, shiny fascia • Yellow reticular layer of dermis with granulation buds	• Necrotic; varies in color from yellow to brown to black • Necrotic tissue covering full or partial surface area • Soft or hard necrotic tissue • Yellow fibrin or slough • Portion of wound can have granulation tissue • Can also appear as clean, pale pink	• Covered with hard, dry eschar • Necrotic; varies in color from yellow to brown to black • Scab
Undermining/tunneling	• Can be present in deep wounds • Has potential for infection and abscess	• Can be present in deep wounds • Has potential for infection and abscess	• Can be present in deep wounds • Has potential for infection and abscess
Wound edges	• Diffuse, indistinct; can still be demarcating from healthy tissues	• Distinct; edges can be rolled or thickened • Is not continuous with wound bed if deep wound cavity	• Has distinct, well-defined wound edges • Can be attached to necrotic tissue
Wound drainage	• Serous or serosanguineous	• Infection • Viscous • Malodor • Pus (yellow, tan, gray, or green) • Moderate to large amount	• Scant or dry

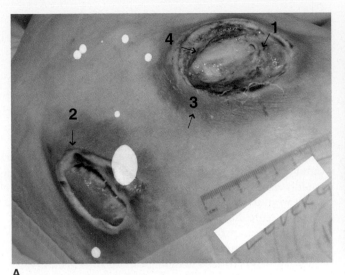
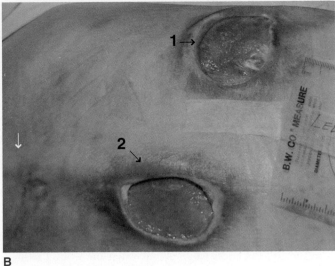

A   **B**

FIGURE 3.41 **A:** Chronic inflammatory phase. Note: (1) Yellow, stringy slough; (2) Edema; (3) Skin color changes (red), erythema; (4) Rib bone noted in superior ulcer. Wound severity diagnosis: Impaired integumentary integrity secondary to skin involvement extending into fascia, muscle, and bone (Stage IV pressure ulcer). **B:** Same wound as in Figure 3.35A. Note: (1) Softening of the rolled epidermal ridge edge around granulation base, (2) Brown hemosiderin staining (hemosiderosis). Wound healing phase: acute proliferative phase. (Copyright © C. Sussman.)

- The chronic proliferative phase is characterized by a wound that is stuck in the proliferative phase, hyperproliferating, or not progressing to the next phase of epithelialization and remodeling.
- Absence of the proliferative phase is characterized by a wound bed that lacks signs of ECM development or is not contracting (see Fig. 3.35A).

Assessment of each of these three aspects of the proliferative phase is described next, using the same four categories of wound attributes discussed for the inflammatory phase: adjacent and periwound tissue, wound bed tissue, wound edges, and wound drainage.

Acute Proliferative Phase

Signs of acute proliferation indicate a healthy response and normal healing. They are also benchmarks against which to evaluate impaired responses.

Adjacent and Periwound Tissue Assessment

During the acute proliferative phase, periwound skin regains color and contour symmetry with that of adjacent skin (i.e., edema is resolved). With recovering chronic wounds, however, you will likely see hemosiderin staining (pigmentation) around the wound margins (Fig. 3.41B). Ecchymosis should be resolved. Skin turgor is normal and is not stretched or taut because the edema and induration are resolved (absent). Firmness is absent or minimal.

Periwound skin temperature, when palpated or measured with an LCD skin thermometer, is the same as the adjacent skin or slightly elevated, due to the enhanced perfusion of tissues and higher metabolic activities associated with healing. A temperature gradient of 4°F or greater indicates inflammation and possible infection, and further evaluation is needed.

Minimal pain is experienced during this phase. Pain may be entirely absent in patients with neuropathy. Sudden onset of pain suggests possible infection.

As previously described, wound undermining and tunneling occurs following debridement of the skin and subcutaneous tissue (Fig. 3.33). The extent of undermining or tunneling is a measure of the total soft tissue involved in the wound. Tunneling may be unobservable from the surface and yet have a great extent, as shown in Figure 3.16A,B of the same wound. In the proliferative phase, undermining and tunneling close as the tissues reestablish continuity during the laying down of the collagen matrix and granulation tissue (Fig. 3.41A,B). Reduction of the extent of undermining/tunneling is a measure of the progression of proliferation and reduced overall wound size. Record findings of undermining and tunneling as part of the tissue assessment. If the tunneling extends beyond approximately 15 cm, notify the physician. Chapter 4 describes how to measure undermining/tunneling and calculate the extent of the overall wound.

Wound Bed Assessment

Granulation tissue develops during this phase. Granulation buds are clearly seen in Figure 3.41B. Wounds that have a bowl-shaped cavity will fill with ECM and granulation tissue during the acute proliferative phase to create a surface across which epidermal cells can migrate. Notice in these photos how the cavity is filling to create a level surface with the adjacent skin.

The acute proliferative phase, which overlaps with the late inflammatory phase, starts when the wound bed tissue begins to show red or pink granulation buds. The collagen matrix is laid down and is infiltrated by and supports the growing capillary bed, giving it a red color. Reduced depth in a full-thickness wound is a measure of proliferation activity. The collagen matrix does not replace the structures or functions of the tissues that occupied the cavity prior to injury; rather, this is scar tissue. The prevailing opinion is that this deep red color indicates a healthy, healing wound. Figure 3.36B is such a wound. A contrary opinion is presented shortly.

Another feature that has been reported to appear during the acute proliferative phase of healing in a number of patients is the development of a yellow, fibrinous membrane on the surface of the granulation tissue. When removal of this membrane has been attempted, it has recurred within a few days. Wounds that develop this yellow membrane appear to be less susceptible to infection and heal in a normal fashion. It is important to recognize this membrane during examination and avoid unnecessarily disrupting it.[129]

Assessment of Wound Edges

The wound edges are soft to firm and flexible to touch. Edges will roll in full-thickness wounds, but when the wound tissue fills the cavity to a point even with the edge of the wound, the edges will flatten, and epithelialization and contraction will continue together (Fig 3.31B,C and 3.41B). At this point, the wound acquires a distinctive wound shape or "picture frame." The cells that control the movement of the picture frame, the myofibroblasts, are located beneath the wound edge. The cells are contractile and will move forward, drawing the wound together, as in the drawing together of purse strings, shrinking the size of the open area measurably. The shape that the wound now assumes predicts the resulting speed of contraction. Linear wounds contract rapidly. Square or rectangular wounds contract at a moderate pace. Circular wounds contract slowly.

Wound contraction is a major activity of the acute proliferative phase of healing. Contraction reduces the areas that need to close by epithelialization. Contraction in areas such as the gluteals and abdomen is typically uncomplicated, but contracture is troublesome in areas such as the head, neck, and hand. Drawing together too tightly in those areas will cause a defect or contracture that can impair function and cosmesis. Wounds that would have a poor outcome if allowed to close by contraction warrant surgical intervention at the start of the proliferative phase.[133]

Assessment of Wound Drainage

During the acute proliferative phase, the wound drainage is serosanguineous and of moderate to minimal quantity and odor.

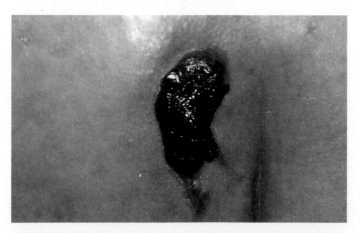

FIGURE 3.42 Hypergranulation tissue; *chronic proliferative phase.* (Copyright © B.M. Bates-Jensen.)

Chronic Proliferative Phase

Chronic proliferation develops when tissue integrity is not reestablished in a timely fashion.

Adjacent and Periwound Tissue Assessment

In the chronic proliferative phase, the color of the skin at the wound edges can blanch or begin to draw together very tightly (Fig. 3.35D). Gelatinous edema can be present, signifying an episode of trauma.

Compared with the temperature of the adjacent skin, periwound skin during the chronic proliferative phase can be cool or mildly elevated. There may be signs of intense pain, indicating that the wound has been traumatized and is undergoing another episode of acute inflammation, or infection may be present.

Tunneling can extend a long distance, presenting an opportunity for infection to travel up the fascial plane. Tissues in the tunnel can be necrotic. Tunneling can become a sinus tract, a cavity, or channel underlying a wound that involves an area larger than the visible surface of the wound (Fig. 3.16A,B). An abscess can form in the tunnel or sinus tract.[70] When undermining/tunneling persists in a proliferating wound and the assessment findings include a black hole that has no reachable bottom, the wound requires urgent medical management.

Wound Bed Tissue Assessment

Wound bed tissue in the chronic proliferative phase is commonly caused by infection. The presence of infection may be indicated by a livid red surface color (Fig. 3.36A) or represent a change from healthy red to pale pink. An example is Figure 3.25B, which was progressing through the proliferative phase. Seven days later, it had attributes of infection, proliferation had ceased, and the wound was in the chronic proliferative phase and the change was attributed to infection (Fig. 3.43). Other features of infection that can be observed in granulating wounds include superficial bridging, friable tissue, bleeding on contact, pain in the wound, and a delay in healing. There are two stages in the proliferative phase when the granulation tissue can show these characteristics of infection: approximately 10 days postoperatively and at the end stage of healing, when the wound has progressed satisfactorily, but then becomes indolent.[129]

Other factors that can contribute to chronic proliferation include poor vascular supply, desiccation, hemorrhage, and hypergranulation (Fig. 3.34). Poor vascular supply is indicated by pale pink, blanched to dull, and dusky red granulation tissue. Desiccated granulation tissue is dark, dull, and garnet red as seen in Figure 3.3. Hemorrhage can result from trauma to the fragile tissues, such as from pressure. Hemorrhaging of the granulation tissue vessels causes acute inflammation in the area and promotes scarring. The surface on the granulation tissue looks like a purple bruise. In Figure 3.44, note the small hemorrhagic area at the center of the wound, indicating rupture of blood vessels.

An imbalance of collagen synthesis and degradation can allow the collagen to proliferate unchecked, creating a hump of granulation tissue called "hypergranulation." When hypergranulation tissue overflows the wound bed, the epithelial cells cannot "climb the hill" of granulation tissue against gravity; the result is that the epithelialization process is halted. It is as if the proliferative "switch" is stuck and won't turn off, leaving the wound in a chronic proliferative phase. In this state, the tissue is predisposed to infection (Fig. 3.42).

Assessment of Wound Edges

One sign that a wound is in the chronic proliferative phase is when wound edges roll in and become hard and fibrotic, inhibiting further wound contraction. Figure 3.35C is an example of rolled fibrotic edges. Wounds of different pathogeneses develop this problem, including pressure ulcers and venous ulcers. This is apparently due to imbalances in the wound biochemistry that controls tissue deposition and degradation during the proliferative phase. Another area of research suggests that impaired senescent cells are present in specific cellular patterns in the edges of nonhealing wound that are different from those of healing wounds and the true "healing edge" of the wound lies further away from the wound edge than traditionally thought. The true "healing edge" is the wound margin where cells capable of migration and wound healing are found. Scientists are developing tools, like bar coding scanners, that can be used to identify the healing wound margins and thus guide wound debridement and improve healing outcomes.[137]

Assessment of Wound Drainage

Chronic proliferative exudate can be a yellow, gelatinous, viscous material on the wound granulation base, which indicates the wound has been traumatized. This appearance should not be confused with residue from wound dressings, such as amorphous hydrogels, or hydrocolloids or treatments, such as antimicrobial ointments.

An infected wound in chronic proliferation can have a malodorous, viscous, reddish-brown, green, or gray exudate. Figure 3.36A shows an apparently clean wound; however, the wound dressing shows signs of moderate to large amounts of sanguineous and purulent, reddish-brown exudate. This is a benchmark of the chronic proliferative phase and the wound needs treatment to recover.

Absence of Proliferative Phase

The absence of proliferation may be caused by interference in the healing cascade due to one or more of the following factors.

CLINICAL WISDOM

Management of Hypergranulation

Because hypergranulation inhibits the reepithelialization of the wound surface, it must be prevented or controlled. Methods for preventing and controlling hypergranulation include the following:

1. Cauterization, by applying silver nitrate sticks to the surface, will necrose the superficial granulation tissue, which can then be wiped off.
2. Excess hypergranulation tissue can be trimmed by rubbing with a gauze sponge or snipping with scissors. This can trigger a new inflammatory cascade.
3. The application of hypertonic saline is a nontoxic method of reducing hypergranulation (see Chapter 20).
4. The application or avoidance of certain wound dressings: silicone gel dressings have preventative potential,[134] and polyurethane foam-type dressings reduce hypergranulation.[135] Occlusive moisture-retentive dressings appear to enhance the development of hypergranulation[136] (see Chapter 20).

Adjacent and Periwound Tissue Assessment

The presence of hemosiderin staining or a halo of erythema surrounding the wound signifies a wound that is also in the chronic inflammatory phase. The skin can show signs of ecchymosis. Edema and pain are minimal or absent. Temperature is the same as adjacent skin, or coolness is present signifying poor perfusion.

Wound Bed Tissue Assessment

A wound in the absence of proliferative phase is either not producing granulation tissue or not contracting (Fig. 3.35A). The wound bed tissue can appear dry, dull red, and desiccated, like

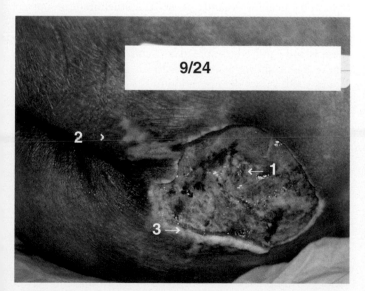

FIGURE 3.43 Chronic proliferative phase with attributes of infection. Note: (1) Hemorrhagic area of trauma; (2) Hypopigmentation; (3) Dull, pink granulation tissue. (Copyright © B.M. Bates-Jensen.)

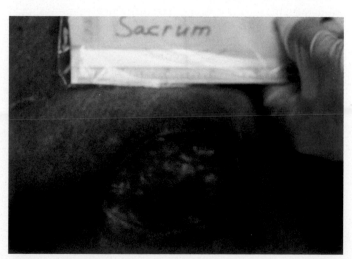

FIGURE 3.44 Wound is in chronic proliferative phase. Note: (1) Trauma to granulation tissue caused hemorrhagic spot that may go on to necrose, (2) Hemosiderin staining from prior bleeding surrounds ulcer. (Copyright © C. Sussman.)

CLINICAL WISDOM

Describing a Wound in the Proliferative Phase

The following is an example of a narrative note describing a wound in the acute proliferative phase:

Evaluation: The wound on the right hip has red granulation tissue. The wound edges are firm and soft. Wound is contracting into a rectangular shape.
Wound healing phase diagnosis: The wound healing phase diagnosis is acute proliferative phase.

dried raw meat, or it can contain pale pink granulation tissue (see Figure 3.2). There is no change in wound depth in a 2- to 4-week time frame. Wounds that are simultaneously in the chronic inflammatory phase or absence of inflammatory phase often have a surface appearance of necrotic tissue and/or hemorrhage/ecchymosis. Any signs of ecchymosis signify a restart of the inflammatory process within the wound. The chronic inflammatory phase and absence of the proliferative phase can both be used as wound healing diagnoses for the same wound. The prognosis would be for the wound to progress to the acute proliferative phase. The medical history and systems review should guide you to investigate the reasons behind the impairments to the proliferation process.

Assessment of Wound Edges

Wound edges can be rolled or jagged, and the wound shape is irregular. The wound does not change shape, signifying lack of wound contraction. Deep wounds can lack continuity of wound bed and edges. The wound does not reduce in size.

Assessment of Wound Drainage

Wounds lack exudate or have scant serous exudate. The wound in Figure 3.36D is in the chronic inflammatory phase and has absence of a proliferative phase. Note the scant amount of serous exudate on the wound dressing. Treatment interventions should be reviewed to determine why the wound lacks moisture. Table 3.9 summarizes the findings during the proliferative phase.

ASSESSING WOUNDS IN THE EPITHELIALIZATION PHASE

Acute Epithelialization Phase
Adjacent and Periwound Tissue Assessment

Because acute epithelialization begins at the time of wounding concurrently with the inflammatory phase and overlapping with the other phases, expect the signs of acute inflammation in the periwound skin. As the acute inflammatory process subsides, the periwound skin should return to the usual color for ethnicity, and to the temperature of adjacent tissues. It should be firm, but not hard, edematous, or fibrotic. Maceration of the periwound skin and new epidermis can occur from leakage of wound exudate or the use of products that moisten the skin and saturate the cells. Maceration is especially damaging to new epithelium. Macerated skin appears pale and wrinkled, and feels

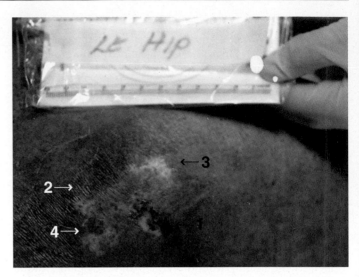

FIGURE 3.45 A,B. Assessment of epithelialization and remodeling attributes in darkly pigmented skin. Note: (1) New epithelial tissue is light red, (2) New scar tissue lacks melanin and is bright pink, (3) Old scar tissue lacks melanin and is silvery white, (4) Residual hemosiderin staining. (Copyright © C. Sussman.)

soft and thin to touch, making it very susceptible to trauma, such as from pressure.

Assessment of Wound Bed Tissue and Wound Edges

Within hours of wounding, epithelial cells start migrating toward the center from the wound edges to cover the defect with new skin. The wound edges must be adhered to the wound base for epithelial cell migration to cover the wound. Gradually, the epithelium spreads across the wound bed, as shown in Figure 3.31A–D. The migrating tissue is connected to the adjacent skin and pulls it along to cover the opening.[133]

The new skin will be bright pink, regardless of normal pigmentation, and may never regain the melanin factors that color skin (Fig. 3.45). New skin is formed as a very thin sheet, and it takes several weeks for it to thicken. If the wound is less than full-thickness, islands of pink epithelium can appear in the wound bed from migrating cells donated by the dermal appendages, hair follicles, and sweat glands. Cells from these islands and edges spread out and cover the open area. Figure 3.48A shows a wound with an island of epithelium. Figure 3.48B shows the migration of the epithelium across the wound from the edges and island. Notice how the edges of the new epithelium are jagged.

Full-thickness wounds lose these island contributors, and they never regenerate.[138] Full-thickness wounds begin to epithelialize when the edges are attached and even with the wound so that there are no sides or walls, and the epithelial cells can migrate from the edge across the wound surface. Edges are soft to firm and flexible to touch, as shown in Figure 3.47. This wound went on to heal by epithelialization from the wound edges.

Wounds can bypass this phase of repair if it is necessary to place a skin graft or muscle flap to close the wound. Large wounds and wounds in areas where contraction will be harmful or will simply take too long to cover the wound can benefit from surgical repair. The wound shown in Figure 3.51B was closed at that time by a split-thickness skin graft to speed the repair process.

TABLE 3.9	Wound Healing Phase Diagnosis: Aspects of Proliferative Phase		
Periwound Skin and Wound Tissue Characteristics	**Acute Proliferative Phase**	**Chronic Proliferative Phase**	**Absence of Proliferative Phase**
Periwound skin color	• Continuity with adjacent skin • Hemosiderin staining if recovering chronic wound	• Continuity with adjacent skin • Paler than adjacent skin • Hemosiderin staining	• Hemosiderin staining if chronic wound • Halo of erythema if in chronic inflammatory phase • Ecchymosis
Edema and induration	• Absent	• Gelatinous edema can be present, signifying trauma	• Minimal edema present
Tissue temperature	• Temperature can be minimally elevated if wound is well-perfused	• Minimal change	• Minimal change or coolness
Pain	• Pain-free or minimal pain • Inappropriate indicator in presence of neuropathy	• Painful, can indicate local inflammation; if intense, consider infection	• Minimal or absent • Intense if infection present
Wound tissue	• Shiny, bright red to pink granulation • Sustained reduction in wound depth • Sustained wound contraction • Reduced size • Covering of yellow fibrinous membrane on granulation tissue • Livid red	• Hypergranulation • Desiccation (dark red color) • Poor vascularization (pale pink) • Ecchymosis on granulation	• Necrotic tissue—stuck in chronic inflammatory phase • Ecchymosis on granulation inflammation restarting • Dull red—desiccated granulation • Pale pink granulation • Lacking change in wound depth • Unsustained contraction—no reduction in size of surface area
Undermining/ tunneling	• Can be present in deep wounds • Closes as proliferation progresses	• Can be present in deep wounds • Fails to close or can extend • Has potential for infection and abscess	• Can be present in deep wounds • Fails to close or can extend • Has potential for infection and abscess
Wound edges	• Soft to firm • Flexible to touch • Rolled if full-thickness • Change in wound shape from irregular to regular • Reduction in size of surface area • Drawing together • Adherence of wound edges by end of phase	• Tight drawing together to reduce size—contracture • Absence of continuity of wound bed and edges • Fibrotic • Fibrotic • Ecchymosis on wound edge	• Unchanged size • Rolled or jagged, irregular edges • No change of shape—not drawing together • Absence of continuity of wound bed and edges
Wound drainage	• Serosanguineous or serous in moderate to minimal amount for wound size	• Yellow gelatinous following trauma • Infection: viscous malodorous, red/brown, green, purulent • Large amount	• Serous drainage, scant to minimal amounts • Desiccated and dry

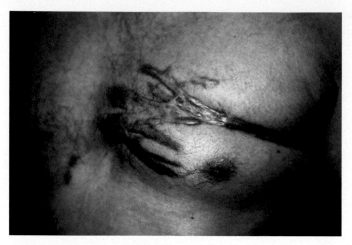

FIGURE 3.46 Immature keloid scar; *chronic epithalialigation stage.* (Copyright © 2001, R. Scott Ward.)

Assessment of Wound Drainage

A scant or small amount of serous or serosanguineous wound exudate is expected. The wound must be kept moist during this phase of healing, because desiccation will destroy the epithelial cells.

CLINICAL WISDOM

Maintaining a Moist Wound Bed for Epithelialization

Amorphous hydrogel dressings are useful wound moisturizers. Along with moisture-permeable films and sheet hydrogels, they provide the warm, moist, homeostatic environment that is critical for epithelialization. Avoid hydrocolloids or other strong adhesives on new or fragile skin.

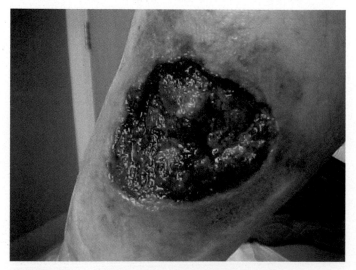

FIGURE 3.47 Full-thickness skin loss in the acute proliferative phase. The wound is a full thickness venous leg ulcer. Wound edges are soft and flexible to touch.

CLINICAL WISDOM

Protection of Skin from Maceration

Skin barriers are products that can be used over the periwound skin and new scar tissue to protect them from maceration.

Chronic Epithelialization Phase

If the edge of the wound is separated from the wound base creating a gap such as shown in Figure 3.35C, the keratinocytes will still initially attempt to epithelialize the wound by migrating to the periwound edge and then curling over, creating a rolled edge. Repeated cellular attempts to cross the gap result in thickening of this edge. Eventually, the cells seem to run out of reproductive capacity and become senescent as described earlier. Presence of thickened fibrotic wound edges is characteristic of wounds of long duration. When palpated they will feel hard, rigid, and indurated, and the wound is now in chronic epithelialization phase.

Adjacent and Periwound Tissue Assessment

The characteristics of the skin can be the same as those seen in the chronic inflammatory and absence of inflammatory phases. The periwound skin can show signs of ischemia, such as a pale or ashen color in the elevated position that deepens to dark purple with dependence (rubor). Pain can be constant and throbbing, or intermittent claudication during walking, if it is associated with arterial occlusive disease. The appearance of the adjacent skin is usually dry, shiny, taut, and/or hairless. These characteristics indicate the loss of hair follicles and sweat and/or sebaceous glands, which benchmark the phase.

The wound shown in Figure 3.49 is in both the chronic epithelialization and chronic inflammatory phases. In the same wound, the appearance of adjacent and periwound skin changed as chronicity was altered and the acute epithelialization and proliferative phases were initiated.

Assessment of Wound Bed Tissue

Wound bed tissue that is hypergranulating can develop a chronic epithelialization phase because the epithelial cells cannot migrate over the hump of granulation tissue against gravity (Fig. 3.42). In this case, the granulation tissue must be trimmed back to a level even with the periwound skin for epithelialization to resume.

Assessment of Wound Edges

Epithelialization of deep wounds occurs only at the edges and can involve thickening and rolling under of the edges. When the cells cannot continue to migrate across the wound, they build up an epithelial ridge along the edge of the wound, as seen in Figures 3.31A and 3.36A. Pressure ulcers typically develop a round shape when this occurs. In wounds in chronic epithelialization, the cells pile up on each other until the rolled, thickened edges become fibrotic. The wound edges need to be modified and the wound bed filled before wound epithelialization can be reinitiated. With full-thickness and deeper wounds,

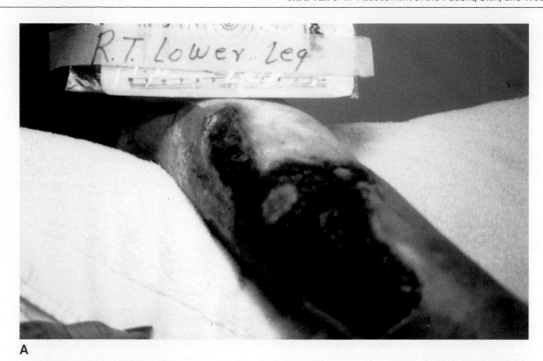

A

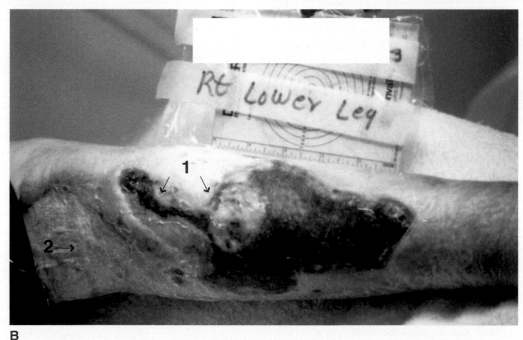

B

FIGURE 3.48 A: Note beefy, red granulation tissue and island of epidermal tissue in full-thickness wound. The wound was in the acute proliferative phase on 12/28. **B:** Same wound as in Figure 3.47A. Note: (1) Epidermal migration from wound edges, island, and wound shape changes; (2) Progression to the acute epithelialization phase by 2/17; (3) Hyperkeratotic skin changes due to old burn wounds and poor circulation. (Copyright © C. Sussman.)

the process of healing by epithelialization at the wound edges will be arrested if (1) a large amount of wound debris interferes with epithelialization, or (2) the wound edges fall off into a deep wound bed with steep walls or do not adhere to the wound bed.

Hyperkeratosis (overgrowth of the horny layer of the skin) is another abnormality of the epithelialization phase. Figure 3.7 shows a wound with hyperkeratosis and the irregular shape of a heel ulcer in a 100-year-old woman. Additional photos of

hyperkeratosis and the management of the problem are shown in Chapter 12. Chronic epithelialization affects scar formation as shown in Figure 3.46. Hypertrophic and keloid scars are aberrations of the epithelialization phase. Chapter 16 discusses scars.

Assessment of Wound Drainage
The wound can be dry with no wound drainage. Epithelial cells migrate best in a warm, moist environment; thus, if no exudates or only scant exudate is assessed, additional moisture

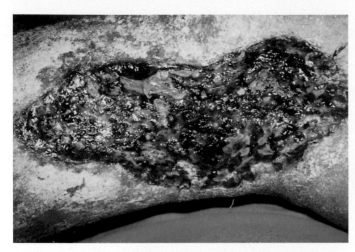

FIGURE 3.49 Pyoderma gangrenosum ulcer in both chronic inflammatory and chronic epithelialization phases. (Copyright © H. Loehne.)

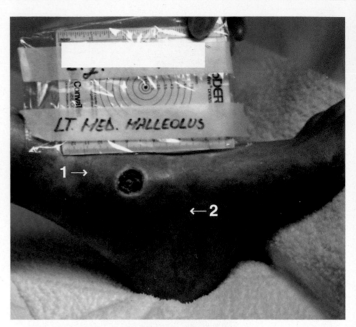

FIGURE 3.50 Ischemic ulcer in chronic proliferative phase and absence of epithelialization phase. Note: (1) Punched-out ulcer appearance with rolled wound edges, (2) Dependent rubor. (Copyright © C. Sussman.)

may be needed to facilitate epithelialization. Wound dryness can be due to improper dressing selection, loss of dressing, dehydration of the wound or patient, or other iatrogenic conditions.

On the other hand, there may be heavy exudate from a partial-thickness ulcer that should be epithelializing, but the exudate washes out the epidermal cells faster than they can migrate and attach to the wound surface. Excessive moisture associated with certain wound products can also cause this to occur and needs to be managed.

Absence of Epithelialization Phase

Absence of the epithelialization phase can be due to many factors, such as failure of the wound to fill with the ECM, desiccation of the tissues, scar tissue from a prior wound that is not donating epithelial cells, or repetitive trauma to the wound edges. Figure 3-46 is an example of a wound in this phase.

Adjacent and Periwound Tissue Assessment

The color of the adjacent and periwound skin offers clues to the etiology of absence of the epithelialization phase. Absence of this phase can be related to a condition such as arterial obstructive disease (AOD). AOD limits blood supply and oxygen to the tissues and impairs the ability of the skin to repair itself. Examination of adjacent skin will reveal absence of hair, dependent rubor, and pallor on elevation. The wound will have a punched-out appearance and a very limited ring of epidermal tissue around it that does not migrate across the wound, as shown in Figure 3.50. If no prior vascular testing has been reported, further assessment of the vascular system is warranted.

Periwound skin that is dry, flaky, macerated, or has an irregular texture provides limited epidermal cells to resurface the wound. This wound will lack epithelialization activity.

Skin temperature is a reflection of blood supply. Skin temperature cooler than 92°F–96°F on the torso and lower in the extremities (75°F–80°F) indicates that blood supply to the skin may be limited; warmer skin can be due to infection.

Chronic edema, which can be caused by tissue congestion, such as lymphedema, congestive heart failure, or venous insufficiency, stretches the skin and fills the interstitial spaces with excess fluid, including large protein molecules. When the capacity of the tissue to hold fluid is exceeded, the fluid leaks through the skin. As a result of this disease process, changes occur in the vascularity of the tissues, leading to the loss of dermal appendages and dry stasis eczema. These changes are known as *lipodermatosclerosis*.[139] Skin changes associated with this disease process are shown in Figure 3.51A,B. Patients with lipodermatosclerosis can show absence of epithelialization phase. More information on lipodermatosclerosis is presented in Chapter 12.

Assessment of Wound Bed Tissue

As noted previously, throughout the wound healing process, the inflammatory, proliferative, and epithelialization phases overlap. This overlapping can be seen when assessing hypogranulation of wound bed tissue in the absence of epithelialization phase: Hypogranulation occurs because of the absence of the proliferative phase. This failure to fill the wound bed means there will be no surface for the epidermal cells to migrate across to cover the wound.

Assessment of Wound Edges

Another intrinsic factor that causes absence of epithelialization is decreased epidermal proliferation due to cellular senescence and delayed cellular migration, which are attributed to aging. In this case, there is slow or absent new skin growth from the edges or islands. Absence of epithelialization attributes includes dry, flaky, hyperkeratotic skin at the wound edges. The dryness can be associated with a dry wound environment.

Assessment of Wound Drainage

Table 3.10 summarizes the findings during the epithelialization phase.

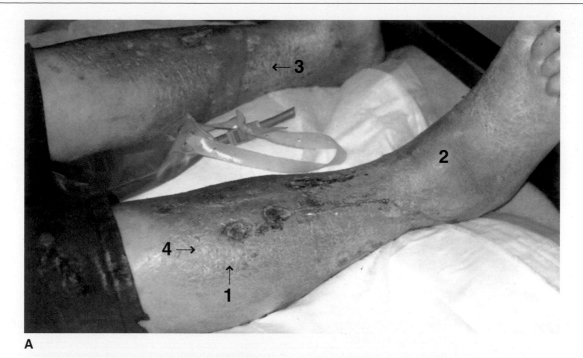

A

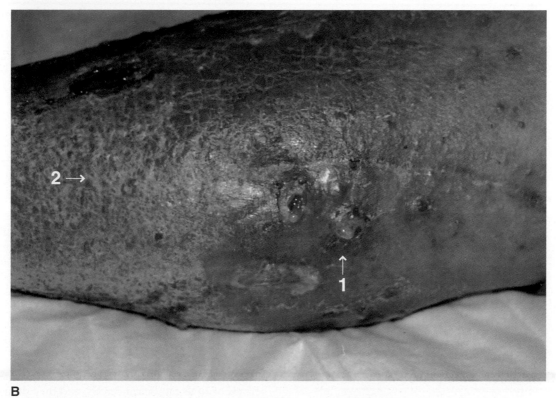

B

FIGURE 3.51 A: Stasis dermatitis. There is an absence of the epithelialization phase. Note evidence of: (1) Brawny edema, (2) Trophic skin changes, (3) Hemosiderin staining (hyperpigmentation), (4) Multiple shallow ulcers. **B:** Close-up view of same leg as in Figure 3.54A. Note evidence of (1) Edema leakage through wounds, (2) Scaling and crusting (trophic changes) due to lipodermatosclerosis. (Copyright © B.M Bates-Jensen.)

| TABLE **3.10** | **Wound Healing Phase Diagnosis: Aspects of Epithelialization Phase** | | |

Periwound Skin and Wound Tissue Characteristics	Acute Epithelialization Phase	Chronic Epithelialization Phase	Absence of Epithelialization Phase
Periwound skin	• Early phase has same characteristics as acute inflammatory phase • Returns to normal color for ethnicity as inflammation subsides • Hemosiderin staining if chronic wound	• Can be same as chronic or absence of inflammatory phase • Can be ischemic (pale) or ashen • Can be purplish with dependency • Dry, flaky (hyperkeratotic—can be due to desiccation or aging skin) • Maceration: pale, wrinkled, soft, thin • Hemosiderin staining	• Scar tissue • Same as chronic or absence of inflammatory phase • Dry with hyperkeratosis or lipodermatosclerosis
Wound tissue	• Even with wound edges • Pink/red granulation • Reduction in wound surface area	• Not connected with wound edge • Hypergranulation	• Absence of resurfacing from edges or dermal appendages • Hypogranulation • Presence of scab or necrotic tissue
Undermining/tunneling	• Steep walls limit migration	• Steep walls limit migration	• Steep walls limit migration
Wound edges	• New skin moves out from wound edge and dermal appendages in irregular pattern • Bright pink color, regardless of usual skin pigmentation • Texture is soft to firm and flexible to touch, thin	• Epithelial ridge • Rolled under or thickened • Dry, flaky skin • Rounding off of wound shape	• Fibrotic wound edge • Rounding off of wound shape and edges • Macerated • Dry, flaky skin
Wound drainage	• Minimal to scant serous or serosanguineous	• Absent, dry; if hypergranulation, minimal/moderate	• Absent, dry
Scar tissue	• Thin layers of scar tissue • Thickens over time • Deep pink color initially; changes to bright pink color, regardless of normal skin pigmentation	• Hypertrophic scarring • Keloid scarring • Hyperkeratotic scarring	• Weak, friable epithelial tissue • Breaks or washes out

REFERRAL CRITERIA

A patient's problems must be identified and if indicated referred early to the medical provider who is most appropriate, according to the patient's wound severity or wound healing phase diagnosis. Make a referral when your findings require the attention of another practitioner more skilled or more knowledgeable in management of the identified problem.

Referral depends on location, available resources, and other significant factors. For example, skin lesions such as scales, papules (e.g., warts and tumors), vesicles (e.g., chickenpox), shingles, and skin cancers are examples of skin conditions that can be seen on the adjacent skin and should be referred to a

dermatologist. Wounds with a history of nonhealing for long periods of time can be cancerous, and they should be referred to a dermatologist for biopsy evaluation. Deep wounds that can be probed to the bone should be considered positive for osteomyelitis and require immediate referral to an orthopedic surgeon. Wounds that are in the chronic inflammatory phase often need enhanced perfusion to heal. Vascular assessment would be a primary consideration, and a vascular surgeon may be the most qualified professional to evaluate and treat. A wound with deep tunneling should be referred to a plastic surgeon. PTs are skilled in exercise, use of physical agents, and electrotherapeutic modalities, all of which enhance perfusion to tissues. Exhibit 3.5 lists possible referral sources, and Exhibit 3.6 lists red flags for referral.

EXHIBIT 3.5

Referral Sources

Physicians	Nurses	Allied Health Professionals
Dermatologist	Dermatology Nurse	Physical Therapist
Orthopedic Surgeon	Wound Ostomy Continence Nurse (WOCN)	Podiatrist
Plastic Surgeon	Geriatric Nurse Practitioner	Vascular Technician
Vascular Surgeon	Vascular Nurse	

SELF-CARE TEACHING GUIDELINES

Patients and caregivers should be brought into the wound team at the time of assessment. In many cases, the patient or a family member or other caregiver will be required to monitor the skin and wound. A simple, 10-point observation tool , such as the one provided in Figure 3.52 can be used to educate them about self assessment of their skin and wounds.

CONCLUSION

Assessment begins with looking at the whole patient and determining comorbidities and other factors that will predict the healing response. Wound classification systems are used to identify wound severity by the depth of tissue impairment, leading to an impairment finding of *impaired skin integrity* (if the dermis is not penetrated) or *impaired tissue integrity* (if the wound extends through the dermis and deeper). Wound healing assessment by physiologic wound healing phase includes

EXHIBIT 3.6

Red Flags for Referral

- Unilateral edema of the lower extremity of sudden onset; may be due to acute deep vein thrombophlebitis
- Findings of gross toenail abnormalities needing foot care
- Loss of protective sensation; requires prompt referral to a specialist for appropriate protective footwear and should be followed closely.
- Inability to initiate and progress through the phases of healing; prognosis for the wound is nonhealing
- Wounds that can be probed to bone; patient is considered to have osteomyelitis, and emergent referral is needed.
- Excessive signs of acute inflammation; should be considered as a signal of impending wound infection

CLINICAL WISDOM

Describing a Wound in the Epithelialization Phase

The following is an example of a narrative note describing a wound in the epithelialization phase:

Evaluation: A wound on the left medial ankle is adhered at 75% of the edges, and epithelialization is progressing over 50% of the open area.
Wound healing phase diagnosis: The wound is in the acute epithelialization phase.

three aspects for each physiologic phase: acute, chronic, and absent. Each phase includes attributes and benchmarks for the acute, chronic, or absent state of the phase by signs found in the adjacent, periwound, and wound tissues.

At the baseline assessment, you need to determine where the wound is within the trajectory of healing. This knowledge will help you to plan treatment, make a diagnosis and prognosis of healing, select interventions, predict outcomes, and triage patients. Trajectories of healing are presented in Chapter 4. Collection tools to measure, grade, record, and monitor findings are described in Chapters 4 and 5.

Documentation requirements for wound assessment should be part of a facility's policies and procedures. Documentation should be accurate, clearly reflect the patient's condition, and consistent with documentation by other professionals in the same department or facility. If it is not documented, it did not happen.

10 Point Observation Tool

1. Changes in how the skin looks.

2. Changes in the color of the skin over bony areas (learn to identify the color of skin that is normal for you).

3. Changes in the color of the wound tissue (more red, more yellow, more black).

4. Reddened areas where you have worn shoes or braces.

5. Skin irritations, sores, or foreign bodies (check the soles of your feet with a mirror to see if there are any foreign items lodged there or areas of redness or tenderness).

6. Signs of excess moisture, redness, or cracking under skin folds (breast, stomach, around rectum, genitals).

7. Swelling of the feet and ankles.

8. New blisters, scrapes, cuts, or bruises.

9. Foul wound odor after wound is cleansed .

10. Any pain in the wound or surrounding skin.

Report any changes in the skin or wound to your health-care provider. Research shows that contacting your health-care provider at the first sign of a problem can prevent bad things from happening.

FIGURE 3.52 10 Point Observation Tool.

REVIEW QUESTIONS

1. Intrinsic factors that can affect wound healing include all of the following except
   A. age
   B. immunosuppression
   C. confusion

2. Which of the medications following characteristics of peripheral neuropathy is correct?
   A. Sensory neuropathy involves symptoms of paresthesia and coolness.
   B. Motor neuropathy involves muscle imbalance and deformities.
   C. Autonomic neuropathy involves improved function of sebaceous glands.
   D. None of the above.

3. When assessing darkly pigmented skin consider

   A. color changes over bony prominences
   B. the type of lighting
   C. conditions that may cause color changes
   D. all of the above

4. The NPUAP staging system is commonly used to
   A. assess all wound types
   B. describe wound severity
   C. guarantee reimbursement
   D. describe pressure ulcer severity

5. Poor vascular supply, desiccation, hemorrhage, and hypergranulation are factors that can contribute to
   A. chronic proliferation
   B. chronic inflammation
   C. infection
   D. all of the above

REFERENCES

1. Jones KR, Fennie K, Lenihan A. Chronic wounds: Factors Influencing healing within 3 months and nonhealing after 5–6 months of care. *Wounds: A Compendium of Clinical Research and Practice.* 2007;19(3):51–63.

2. Takahashi PY, Kiemele LJ, Chandra A, et al. A retrospective cohort study of factors that affect healing in long-term care residents with chronic wounds. *Ostom Wound Manage.* 2009;55(1):32–37.

3. Chacon JMF, Nagaoka C, Blanes L, et al. Pressure ulcer risk factors among the elderly living in long-term institutions. *Wound: A Compendium of Clinical Research and Practice.* 2010;22(4):106–113.

4. Jones PL, Millman A. Wound healing and the aged patient. *Nurs Clin N Am.* 1990;25(1):263–277.

5. Eaglstein W. Wound healing and aging. *Clin Geriatr Med.* 1989;5(1):183–188.

6. Mulder G, Brazinsky BA, Seeley J. Factors complicating wound repair. In: McCulloch JM, Kloth LC, Feeder JA, eds. *Wound Healing Alternatives in Management.* 2nd ed. Philadelphia, PA: F.A. Davis; 1995:47–59.

7. Stotts N, Wipke-Tevis D. Co-factors in Impaired Wound Healing. In: Krasner D, Kane D, eds. *Chronic Wound Care: A Clinical Sourcebook for Health Care Professionals.* 2nd ed. Wayne, PA: Health Management Publications; 1997:64–71.

8. Stotts NA, Wipke-Tevis D. Co-factors in impaired wound healing. *Ostom Wound Manage.* 1996;42:44–56.

9. Marston W, Carlin R, Passman M, et al. Healing rates and cost efficacy of outpatient compression treatment for leg ulcers associated with venous insufficiency. *J Vasc Surg.* 1999;30(3):491–498.

10. Sinacore DR, Muller MJ. Pedal ulcers in older adults with diabetes mellitus. *Topics Geriatr Rehabil.* 2000;16(2):11–23.

11. Voss AC, Bender S, Cook AS, et al. Pressure Ulcer Prevention in LTC: Implementation of the National Pressure Ulcer Long-term Care Study (NPULS) Prevention Program. Paper presented at: Symposium for Advanced Wound Care; April 2000; Dallas, TX.

12. Dean E. Oxygen transport deficits in systemic disease and implications for physical therapy. *Phys Ther.* 1997;77:187–202.

13. Yue D, McLennan S, Marsh M, et al. Effects of experimental diabetes, uremia, and malnutrition on wound healing. *Diabetes.* 1987;36(3):295–299.

14. Rosenberg C. Wound healing in the patient with diabetes mellitus. *Nurs Clin N Am.* 1990;25(1):247–261.

15. Norris S, Provo B, Stotts NA. Physiology of wound healing and risk factors that impede the healing process. *AACN.* 1990;1:545–552.

16. Coleridge-Smith PD. Oxygen, oxygen free radicals and reperfusion injury. In: Krasner D, Kane D, eds. *Chronic Wound Care: A Clinical Source Book for Healthcare Professionals.* Vol. 1. Wayne, PA: Health Management Publications, Inc.; 1997:348–353.

17. Hunt Tk, Rabkin J, Von Smitten K. Effects of edema and anemia on wound healing and infection. *Curr Stud Hematol Blood Transf.* 1986;53:101–111.

18. Hartmann M, Jonsson K, Zederfeldt B. Effect of tissue perfusion and oxygenation on accumulation of collagen in healing wounds. Randomized study in patients after major abdominal operations. *Eur J Surg.* 1992;158(10):521–526.

19. Jonsson K, Jensen J, Goodson WD, et al. Assessment of perfusion inpostoperative patients using tissue oxygen measurements. *Br J Surg.* 1987;74(4):263–267.

20. Mosiello G, Tufaro A, Kerstein M. Wound healing and complications in the immunosuppressed patient. *Wounds.* 1994;6(3):883–887.

21. Pignataro RM, Swisher AK. Chemotherapy induced peripheral neuropathy: Risk factors, pathophysiology, assessment and potential physical therapy interventions. *Rehab Oncol.* 2010; 28(2):10–18.

22. Garber SL, Biddle AK, Click CN, et al. *Pressure Ulcer Prevention and Treatment Following Spinal Cord Injury: A Clinical Practice Guideline for Health-care Professionals.* Jackson Heights, NY: Paralyzed Veterans of America; 2000.

23. Twist D. Acrocyanosis in a spinal cord injured patient—effect of computer-controlled neuromuscular electrical stimulation: a case report. *Phys Ther.* 1990;70:45–49.

24. Reddy M, Holroyd.-Leduc J., Cheung C, et al., eds. Geriatric principles in the practice of chronic wound care. *Chronic Wound Care: A Clinical Source book for Healthcare Professionals.* Malvern, PA: HMP Communications; 2007.

25. Ozarde P, Bottomley J. Depression and the elderly. *Gerinotes.* 2010;17(5):12–16.

26. National Pressure Ulcer Advisory Panel and European Pressure Ulcer Advisory Panel. Prevention and treatment of pressure ulcers. *Clinical Practice Guideline.* Washington, DC: National Pressure Ulcer Advisory Panel; 2009.

27. Schultz GS, Sibbald GR, Falanga V, et al. Wound bed preparation: A systematic approach to wound management. *Wound Repair Regen.* 2003;11(1):S1–S28.

28. Gorse G, Messner R. Improved pressure sore healing with hydrocolloid dressings. *Archives Dermatol.* 1987;123:766–771.

29. Ferrell B, Osterweil D, Christenson P. A randomized trial of low-air-loss beds for treatment of pressure ulcers. *JAMA.* 1993;269:494–497.

30. Gentzkow G, Pollack S, Kloth L, et al. Improved healing of pressure ulcers using dermapulse, a new electrical stimulation device. *Wounds.* 1991;3(5):158–169.

31. van Rijswijk L. Full-thickness pressure ulcers: patient and wound healing characteristics. *Decubitus.* 1993;6(1):16–21.

32. Skene AL, Smith J, Dore CJ, et al. Venous leg ulcers: a prognostic index to predict time to healing. *BMJ.* 1992;305(6862):1119–1121.

33. Phillips T, Machado F, Trout R, et al. Prognostic indicators in venous ulcers. *J Am Acad Dermatol.* 2000;43(4):627–630.

34. Kennedy KL. The prevalence of pressure ulcer in an intermediate care facility. *Decubitus.* 1989;2(2):44–45.

35. Kennedy-Evans KL. Understanding the Kennedy Terminal Ulcer. *Ostom Wound Manage.* 55(9):6.

36. Schank JE. Kennedy Terminal Ulcer: The "Ah-Ha!" moment. *Ostom Wound Manage.* 2009;55(9):40–44.

37. Langemo DK, Brown G. Skin fails too: acute,chronic, and end-stage skin failure. *Adv Skin Wound Care.* 2006;19(4):206–211.

38. Sibbald RG, et al. Skin changes at life's end (SCALE): Final consensus statement. *Adv Skin Wound Care.* 2010;23(5):237–238.

39. Schafer AI. Effects of nonsteroidal antiinflammatory drugs on platelet function and systemic hemostasis. *J Clin Pharmacol.* 1995;35(3):209–219.

40. Salcido R. Do Antiinflammatories Have a Role in Wound Healing. Paper presented at: Clinical Symposium on Advances in Skin and Wound Care; October 23–26, 2005; Las Vegas, NV.

41. Sanchez-Fidalgo S, Martin-Lacave I, Illanes M, et al. Angiogenesis, cell proliferation and apoptosis in gastric ulcer healing. Effect of a selective cox-2 inhibitor. *Eur J Pharmacol.* 2004;505(1–3):187–194.

42. Jones KG, et al. Inhibition of angiogenesis by nonsteroidal antiinflammatory drugs: insight into mechanisms and implicaitons for cancer growth and ulcer healing. *Nat Med.* 1999;5(5):1418–1423.

43. Leiebowitch SJ, Ross R. The role of the macrophage in wound repair. *Am J Pathol.* 1975;78:71–91.

44. Hunt TK, Rabkin J, von Smitten K. Vitamin A and wound healing. *J Am Acad Dermatol.* 1986;15:817.

45. Allman RM, Laprade CA, Noel LB, et al. Pressure sores among hospitalized patients. *Ann Intern Med.* 1987;105:337–342.

46. Bergstrom N, Braden B. A prospective study of pressure sore risk among institutionalized elderly. *J Am Geriat Soc.* 1992;40:747–758.

47. Breslow RA, Hallfrisch J, Goldberg AP. Malnutrition in tube fed nursing home patients with pressure sores. *J Parenter Enteral Nutr.* 1991;15:663–668.

48. Ader R. On the development of psychoneuroimmunology. *Eur J Pharmacol.* 2000;405:167–176.

49. Eller LS. Effects of cognitive-behavioral interventions on quality of life in persons with HIV. *Int J Nurs Stud.* 1999;36:223–233.

50. Masek K, Petrovicky P, Zi'dek Z, et al. Past, present and future of psychoneuoimmunology. *Toxicology.* 2000;142:179–188.

51. Urpe M, Buggiani G, Lotti T. Stress and psychoneuroimmunologic factors in dermatology. *Dermatol Clin.* 2005;23(4):609–617.

52. Emery CF, Kiecolt-Glaser JK, Glaser R, et al. Exercise accelerates wound healing among healthy older adults: A preliminary investigation. *J Gerontol Sci Med Sci Med Sci.* 2005;60A(11):1432–1436.

53. Broadbent E, Petrie KJ, Alley PG, et al. Psychological stress impairs early wound repair following surgery. *Psychosom Med.* 2003;65:865–869.

54. Crenshaw R, Vistnes L. A decade of pressure sore research *J Rehab Res Dev.* 1989;26:63–74.

55. Kiecolt-Glase JK, Marucha PT, Malarkey WB, et al. Slowing of wound healing by psychological stress. *Lancet.* 1995;346,1194–1196.

56. Braden B. The relationship between stress and pressure sore formation. *Ostom Wound Manage.* 1998;44(3A 1Suppl):26S–36S.

57. West J. Wound healing in the surgical patient: Influence of the perioperative stress response on perfusion. *AACN Clin Issues.* 1990;1(3):595–601.

58. North A. The effect of sleep on wound healing. *Ostom Wound Manage.* 1990;27:56–58.

59. Lee KA, Stotts N. Support of the growth hormone-somatomedin system to facilitate heaing. *Heart Lung J Crit Care.* 1990;19(2):157–164.

60. Rice B, Kalker A, Schindler J, et al. Effect of biofeedback-assisted relaxation training on foot ulcer healing. *J Am Podiatr Med Assoc.* 2001;91(3):132–141.

61. McCarthy D, Ouimet M, Daun J. Shades of Florence Nightingale: Potential impact of noise stress on wound healing. *Holist Nurs Pract.* 1991;5(4):39–48.

62. Wysocki A. The effect of intermittent nise exposure on wound healing. *Adv Wound Care.* 1996;9(1):35–39.

63. Ross Products Division. *Executive Summary—Phase I Prevention Results: The National Pressure Ulcer Long-term Care Study.* Columbus, OH, Ross Products Division; September 14, 1999.

64. Illingsworth C, Barker A. Measurement of electrical currents emerging during the regeneration of amputated finger tips in children. *Clin Phys Physiol Meas.* 1980;1:87.

65. Lock P. The effect of temperature on mitosis at the edge of experimental wounds. In: Lundgren A, Sover A, eds. *Symposia on Wound Healing: Plastic, Surgical and Dermatologic Aspects.* 1980; Molndal, Sweden.

66. Thomas S. *Wound Management and Dressings.* London: The Pharmaceutical Press; 1990.

67. Conolly WB, Hunt T, Sonne M, et al. Influence of distant trauma on local wound infection. *Surg Gynecol Obstet.* 1969;128(4):713–717.

68. Keast DH, Bowering C, Keith EA, et al. MEASURE: A proposed assessment framework for developing best practice recommendations for wound assessment. *Wound Repair Regen.* 2004;12:1–17.

69. van Rijswijk L. Frequence of reassessmnet of pressure ulcers, NPUAP Proceedings. *Adv Wound Care.* 1995;8(Suppl 4):19–24.

70. van Rijswijk L, Polansky M. Predictors of time to healing deep pressure ulcers. *Ostom Wound Manage.* 1994;40(8):40–42, 44, 46–48.

71. Bergstrom N, Allman Richard M, Alvarez OM, et al. *Clinical Practice Guideline: Treatment of Pressure Ulcers.* Rockville MD: US Department of Health and Human Services Public Health Service Agency for Health Care Policy and Research; 1994:15.

72. Abeln S. Reporting risk check-up. *PT Magazine.* Vol 5; 1997:38.

73. Greenman PE. Principles of structured diagnosis. *Principles of Manual Medicine.* 2nd ed. Baltimore, MD: Williams & Wilkins; 1996:13–20.

74. Maklebust J, Sieggreen M. Etiology and pathophysiology of pressure ulcers. In: *Maklebust J, Sieggreen M.* 1st ed. West Dundee, IL: S.N. Publications; 1991:19–27.

75. Nachbar F, Stolz W, Merkle T, et al. The ABCD rule of dermatoscopy. High prospective value in the diagnosis of doubtful melanocytic skin lesions. *J Am Acad Dermatol.* 1994;30(4):551–559.

76. Throne N. The problem of the black skin. *Nurs Times;* 1969:999–1001.

77. Weiss EL. Connective tissue in wound healing. In: McCulloch JM, Kloth LC, Feedar J, eds. *Wound Healing Alternatives in Management.* 2nd ed. Philadelphia, PA: F.A. Davis; 1995:26–28.

78. Maklebust J, Sieggreen M. Glossary. In: Maklebust J SM, ed. *Pressure Ulcers: Guidelines for Prevention and Nursing Management.* West Dundee, IL: S.N. Publications; 1996:8–9.

79. Harkless LB, Dennis K. Role of the podiatrist. In: Levin ME, O'Neal L, Bowker JH, eds. *The Diabetic Foot.* 5th ed. St. Louis, MO: Mosby-Year Book; 1993:516–517.

80. Sibbald RG, Cameron J. Dermatological aspects of wound care. In: Krasner D, Rodeheaver G, Sibblad RG, eds. *Chronic Wound Care: A*

Clinical Source Book for Healthcare Professionals. 3rd ed. Wayne, PA: HMP Communications; 2001:273–285.

81. Sibbald RG, Williamson D, Orsted H. Preparing the wound bed—debridement, bacterial balance, and moisture balance. *Ostom Wound Manage.* 2000;46(11):14–35.

82. Dorland. Dorland's Illustrated Medical Dictionary. *W.B. Saunders (Harcourt Health Services)* [electronic]. Available at: http://www.mercksource.com/pp/us/cns/cns_hl_dorlands. Accessed September 19, 2005.

83. Ruschhaupt WF III. Vascular disease of diverse origin. In: Young JR Graor R.A., Olin J.W. and Bartholomew J.R., eds. *Peripheral Vascular Diseases.* St. Louis, MO: Mosby-Year Book; 1991:639–650.

84. Berard Anick KX, Zuccarelli F, Abenhaim L. Validity of the Leg-o-meter, an instrument to measure leg circumference. *Angiology.* 2002;53(1):21–28.

85. Sprigle S, Linden M, Riordan B. Analysis of localized erythema using clinical indicators and spectroscopy. *Ostom Wound Manage.* 2003;49(3):42–52.

86. Parish CP, Witkowski JA. Decubitus ulcers: How to intervene effectively. *Drug Ther;* 1983:not numbered.

87. Bennett M. Report of the task force on the implications for darkly pigmented intact skin in the prediction and prevention of pressure ulcers. *Adv Wound Care.* 1995;8:34–35.

88. Roach LB. Assessment: Color changes in dark skin. *Nursing.* 1977:48–51.

89. Cuzzell JZ. The new RYB color code. *Am J Nurs.* 1988;88(10):1342–1346.

90. Dailey C. "Purple" ulcers. *J ET Nurs.* 1992;19:106.

91. Berna-Serna JD, Sanchez-Garre J, Madrigal M, et al. Ultrasound therapy in rectus sheath hematoma. *Phys Ther.* 2005;85(4):352–357.

92. Liefeldt L, Destanis P, Rupp K, et al. The hazards of whirlpooling. *Lancet.* 2003;361(9356):534.

93. Yosipovitch G, Hu J. The importance of skin pH. *Skin & Aging.* Vol. 11; 2003:88–93.

94. Sussman C, Swanson G. The utility of Sussman wound healing tool in predicting wound healing outcomes in physical therapy. *Adv Wound Care.* 1997;10(5):74–77.

95. Panel NPUA. *Deep tissue injury – White paper.* Washington, DC, National Pressure Ulcer Advisory Panel; 2005.

96. Panel NPUA. Deep Tissue Injury. Paper presented at: Merging Missions Consensus Conference; February 25–26, 2005; Tampa, FL.

97. Ankrom MA, Bennet RG, Sprigle S, et al. National Pressure Ulcer Advisory Panel. Pressure-related deep tissue injury under intact skin and the current pressure ulcer staging systems. *Adv Skin Wound Care.* 2005;18(1):35–42.

98. Fishman T. Foot and Nail Care. Paper presented at: First Annual Wound Conference; October, 1995; Boca Raton, FL.

99. (JCAHO) JCoAoHO. Pain Management Standards (Standard RI 2.8 and PE 1.4). In: JCAHO, ed. *Comprehensive Accreditation Manual for Hospitals;* 2001.

100. Birke J. Management of the insensate foot. In: Kloth LC, McCulloch JM, eds. *Wound Healing: Alt Manage.* 3rd ed. Philadelphia, PA: FA Davis; 2001:385–408.

101. Cavanagh PR, Ulbricht JS. Biomechanics of the foot in diabetes mellitus. In: Levin ME, O'Neal LW, Bowker JH, eds. *The Diabetic Foot.* 5th ed. St. Louis, MO: Mosby-Year Book; 1993:225.

102. Levin ME. Pathogenesis and management of diabetic foot lesions. In: Levin ME, O'Neal LW, Bowker JH, eds. *The Diabetic Foot.* 5th ed. St. Louis, MO: Mosby-Year Book; 1993:43.

103. Martina ISJ, van Koningsweld R, Schmitz PIM, et al. for the European Inflammatory Neuropathy Cause and Treatment (INCAT) group. Measuring vibration threshold with a graduated tuning fork in normal aging and in patients with polyneuropathy. *J Neurol Neurosurg Psychiatr.* 1998;65:743–747.

104. Merkiesa ISJ, Schmitz P, van der Mechéa FGA, et al. for the Inflammatory Neuropathy Cause and Treatment (INCAT) Group. Reliability and responsiveness of a graduated tuning fork in immune mediated polyneuropathies. *J Neurol Neurosurg Psychiatr.* 2000;68:669–671.

105. Perkins BA, Olaleye D, Zinman B, et al. Simple Screening Tests for Peripheral Neuropathy in the Diabetes Clinic. *Diabetes Care.* 2001;24(2):250–256.

106. Peters EJG, Lavery LA. Effectiveness of the diabetic foot risk classification system of the international working group on the diabetic foot. *Diabetes Care.* 2001;24:1442–1447.

107. Murff RT, et al. How effective is manual palpation in detecting subtle temperature differences? *Clin Podiatr Med Surg.* 1998; 15(1):151–154.

108. Fierheller M, Sibbald RG. A clinical investigation into the relationship between increased periwound skin temperature and local wound infection in patients with chronic leg ulcers. *Adv Skin Wound Care.* 2010;23(8):369–379.

109. Horzic M, Bunoza D, Maric K. Contact thermography in a study of primary healing of surgical wounds. *Ostomy Wound Manage.* 1996;42(1):36–42.

110. Armstrong DG, Lavery LA, Liswood PJ, et al. Infrared dermal thermometry for the high-risk diabetic foot. *Phys Ther.* 1997;77(2):169–177.

111. Pernet A, Villano JB. Thermography as a preoperative and followup method for surgery of the hand. *Int Surg.* 1984;69(2):171–173.

112. Chan AW, MacFarlane IA, Bowsher DR. Contact thermography of painful diabetic neuropathic foot. *Diabetes Care.* 1991;10:918–922.

113. Benbow SJ, Chan AW, Bowsher DR, et al. The prediction of diabetic neuropathic plantar foot ulceration by liquid-crystal contact thermography. *Diabetes Care.* 1994;17(8):835–839.

114. Kohler A, Hoffmann R, Platz A, et al. Diagnostic value of duplex ultrasound and liquid crystal contact thermography in preclinical detection of deep vein thrombosis after proximal femur fractures. *Arch Orthop Trauma Surg.* 1998;117(1–2):39–42.

115. Woundpedia

116. Panel NPUA. Pressure ulcer and risk assessment: consensus development conference statement. *Decubitus.* 1989;(2):23–28.

117. Armstrong DG, Lavery LA, Harkless LB. Validation of a diabetic wound classification system. The contribution of depth, infection, and ischemia to risk of amputation. *Diabetes Care.* 1998;21(5):855–859.

118. Wagner FEW. The dysvascular foot: A system for diagnosis and treatment. *Foot Ankle.* 1981;(2):64–122.

119. Mulder GD, Jeter KF, Fairchild PA, eds. *Clinician's Pocket Guide to Chronic Wound Repair.* Spartanburg, SC: Wound Healing Publications; 1991.

120. Shea JD. Pressure sore: Classification and management. *Clin Orthop.* 1975;112:89–100.

121. Bergstrom N, Allman RM, Carlson CE, et al. *Pressure Ulcers in Adults: Prediction and Preventions.* Rockville, MD: US Dept of Health and Human Services; 1992. 3.

122. European Pressure Ulcer Advisory Panel (EPUAP). *Pressure Ulcer Classification.* 2004.

123. Snyder RJ, Kirsner R, Warriner III RA, et al. Consensus recommendations on advancing the standard of care for treating neuropathic foot ulcers in patients with diabetes. *Ostom Wound Manage.* 2010;56(Suppl 4):S1–S24.

124. Carpenito LJ. *Nursing Diagnosis, Application to Clinical Practice.* 6th ed. Philadelphia, PA: JB Lippincott; 1995.

125. Metzger-Donovan D, Biggs K, Sussman C, et al. Guide to physical therapist practice, II. *Phys Ther.* 1997;77:1163–1650.

126. Sussman C. Case Presentation: Patient with a Pressure Ulcer. Paper presented at: American Physical Therapy Association Scientific Meeting, 1996; Minneapolis, MN.

127. Kerstein MD, Bensing KA, Brill LR, et al. *The Physiology of Wound Healing.* Philadelphia, PA: The Oxford Institute for Continuing Education and Allegheny University of Health Sciences; March 1998.

128. Cooper DM. The physiology of wound healing: An overview. In: Krasner D, ed. *Chronic Wound Care: A Clinical Source Book for Healthcare Professionals.* Vol 1. King of Prussia, PA: Health Management Publications; 1990:1–10.

129. Harding KG, Bale S. Wound Care: putting theory into practice in the United Kingdom. In: Krasner D, Kane D, eds. *Chronic Wound Care: A Clinical Source Book for Healthcare Professionals* Vol 1. 1st ed. Wayne, PA: Health Management Publications; 1990:115–123.

130. Cutting KF, Harding KG. Criteria to idenify wound infection. *J Wound Care.* 1994;3(4):198–201.

131. Sibbald RG, Woo K., Ayello EA. Increased bacterial burden and infection: the storey of NERDS and STONEES. *Adv Skin Wound Care* 2006;19:347–61.

132. Feedar JA. Clinical management of chronic wounds. In: McCulloch JM, Kloth LC, Feedar J, ed. *Wound Healing Alternatives in Management.* 2nd ed. Philadelphia, PA: F.A. Davis; 1995:140.

133. Hardy MA. The Biology of Scar Formation. *Phys Ther.* 1989;69(12):1014–1023.

134. Ducharme-Desjarlais M, Celeste CJ, Lepault E, et al. Effect of a silicone-containing dressing on exuberant granulation tissue formation and wound repair in horses. *Am J Vet Res.* 2005;66(7):1133–1139.

135. Harris A, Rolstad BS. Hypergranulation tissue: A nontraumatic method of management. *Ostom Wound Manage.* 1994;40(5):20–22, 24, 26–30.

136. Berry DB 2nd, Sullins KE. Effects of topical application of antimicrobials and bandaging on healing and granulation tissue ormation in wounds of the distal aspect of the limbs in horses. *Am J Vet Res.* 2003;64(1):88–92.

137. Tomic-Canic M, Brem H. Using gene transcription patterns (bar coding scans) to guide wound debridement and healing. Tomic when looking at the edge of a chronic wound most clinicians would. *Adv Skin Wound Care* 2008;21(10):487–92.

138. Knighton D, Fiegel VD, Doucette MM. Wound repair: The growth factor revolution. In: D Knighton, ed. *Chronic Wound Care: A Clinical Source Book for Health Care Professionals.* Wayne, PA: Health Management Publications; 1990:441–445.

139. Micheletti G. Ulcers of the lower extremities. In: Gogia PP, ed. *Clinical Wound Management.* Thorofare, NJ: Slack; 1995:100–101.

140. Porter JM, Moneta GL. International Consensus Committee on Chronic Venous Disease. Reporting standards in venous disease: An update. *J Vasc Surg.* 1995;21:635–645.

4

Wound Measurements and Prediction of Healing

Carrie Sussman

CHAPTER OBJECTIVES

At the completion of this chapter, the reader will be able to:

1. Explain the importance of wound measurement accuracy and reliability.
2. Describe the benefits and disadvantages of each of the three most commonly used methods of wound measurement: linear, tracing, and photography.
3. Use the linear method to measure a wound surface area (SA), undermining/tunneling, and depth.
4. Use wound measurements to calculate and track the rate of wound healing.
5. Use wound healing rates to predict the effectiveness of therapeutic interventions.
6. Describe new technologies for measuring and reporting wound healing.

Wound measurement looks quantitatively at four wound assessment components: SA, undermining/tunneling, depth, and volume. These components are directly associated with the phases of wound healing and are therefore direct indicators of healing. As new granulation tissue develops, wound depth and volume decrease, the wound contracts, new epithelium covers the wound, and the area decreases in size. This chapter discusses common methods of wound measurement, including linear ruler measurements, tracings, and photography. Each has its advantages, disadvantages, and level of reliability, which are discussed in this chapter. Step-by-step procedures for measuring wounds and the surrounding tissues, along with user-friendly hints and clinical "words of wisdom," are provided.

INITIAL CONSIDERATIONS IN WOUND MEASUREMENT

Before we discuss the three methods for measuring wound size, we explore some initial considerations regarding frequency and documentation of measurements. We also discuss the issues of consistency, completeness, accuracy, and reliability of measurements.

Frequency of Baseline and Subsequent Measurements

Measurement taken at the beginning of care establishes a baseline wound size; subsequent measurements are then performed at regular intervals depending on the health-care setting. For example, wound measurements are required weekly for the first

4 weeks in long-term care, usually every 48 hours in acute care, and at every visit in home care. The rationale for measurement is to quantify and measure the progression of wound healing and aid in predicting the treatment outcome.[1] A number of studies have found that baseline wound size, when accompanied by other risk factors for healing, is a significant predictor of response to treatment and 100% healing.[2–5] As we discussed in Chapter 3, larger ulcers were less likely than smaller ones to heal rapidly, even with optimal therapy; in the former case, the prognosis of the need for a longer time to heal should be documented, or a referral could be triggered.[4]

A policy and procedure (P&P) document concerning the frequency and method of wound measurement is necessary to set the standard for a particular facility and improve consistency across practitioners and disciplines. Comparison of wound measurements is only valuable if they are taken under the same conditions using the same methods. A standard for wound measurement also has legal and regulatory implications, since the baseline measurement and changes in wound size are the basis for judging changes in wound status and compliance with regulation.

A section of the P&P can address the issue of who should perform baseline and subsequent measurements. For example, the policy could dictate that the baseline measurement be taken by a health-care professional and that, after training, a family member in the home could take subsequent wound measurements and report to the health-care professional at a specified interval, such as weekly. Linear measurement of the size of the open SA of a wound is an example of a type of measure that might be delegated to a family member. The significance of changes in wound size would be interpreted by the professional case manager.

TABLE 4.1	Common Locations of Chronic Wounds by Etiology		
Arterial Ulcers	**Pressure Ulcers**	**Neuropathic Ulcers**	**Venous Ulcers**
Lower leg dorsum	Bony prominences:	Plantar surface of foot	Above the ankle
Foot	Occiput	Metatarsal heads	Medial lower leg
Malleolus	Ears	Heel	
Toe joints	Shoulder	Lateral border of foot	
Lateral border of foot	Scapulae	Midfoot deformities	
	Sacrum		
	Coccyx		
	Trochanter		
	Ischial tuberosity		
	Knees—condyles, patella		
	Tibia/fibula		
	Malleolus		
	Heel		
	Metatarsal heads		
	Toes		

Documenting the Wound Location

Documenting the anatomic location of the wound is the first step in being able to reproduce measurements at that site. Record the anatomic name that clearly describes the wound location at the time of the wound measurement. For example, *trochanter* is a more precise descriptor than *hip* and signifies that the wound lies over the bony prominence. A circle over the anatomic site on the body diagram gives quick, easy identification of wound location on the completed wound measurement form.

The wound's anatomic location can be an indication of the wound etiology (Table 4.1). For example, wounds located over bony prominences are usually pressure wounds, wounds on the soles of the feet are often due to pressure and insensitivity (diabetic wounds), and wounds over the medial side of the ankle are often venous ulcers. Location also provides important information about the expected wound healing. Wounds in areas of diminished blood flow, such as over the tibia, heal slowly.

If several wounds are clustered close together in a location, they should be identified by either different letters or references such as *outer, inner, upper,* and *lower.* It is important to keep the same reference location ID for all of the wounds by name throughout the course of care. If one of the wounds in the cluster heals, this fact should be documented, and the same reference names for the remaining wounds should be retained for further documentation. If several wounds join together to become one, this information should be recorded, with a new ID name given to the revised wound site. Exhibit 4.1 shows an example of how to document wound location for multiple wounds.

Using Measurement Forms

Measurements of wound size, extent, and changes are important to the interdisciplinary team, payers, and regulators, as well as to the patient and the family. Well-documented wound measurements can also be used as the best legal defense. The changes and progress toward recovery can also provide positive feedback to the clinician, who can review the measurements and feel a sense of accomplishment. Alternatively, measurements can serve as the red flag that all is not well, triggering reevaluation of the wound, patient, and treatment interventions.

Because the information gathered is so important, the documentation must be complete and accurate. In addition, the language used requires uniform and consistent terminology to encourage good communication among the team members; such terminology is also beneficial for reimbursement.

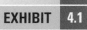

EXHIBIT 4.1

Documenting Wound Location

Documenting Wound Location with Narrative Note

Example:
1. Single wound location: coccyx
2. Multiple wounds at a location:

Initial note: *Three wounds are located upper, middle, and outer side on the right trochanter.*

The upper and middle wounds merge. Since they are upper to the outer wound, the same term upper is retained and the merger noted as in this example:

Follow-up note: *The upper and middle wounds have merged and will in the future be referred to as the upper wound on the right trochanter.*

One way to promote uniformity, consistency, and completeness is with the use of forms. Forms guide the examiner in a logical sequence and assist in organizing the information gathered. Forms can be paper-and-pencil instruments or electronic templates. They save time, because one simply completes the appropriate information on the preprinted form, which becomes a part of the documentation record.

There are numerous forms in use for documenting wound measurements. Exhibit 4.2 is a sample completed form for performing a wound measurement examination. A new form is used each week, and the forms are "tiled" onto pages of note paper with tape in the chart for easy reference to prior measurements or in paperless facilities the data can be recorded on a computer template designed for this purpose. Keeping the measurements together in one place facilitates regular monitoring of the size changes. The sample form uses the clock method (see below) for monitoring wound depth and undermining and includes the following items:

- Wound anatomic location (called the *wound ID*)
- Size, including length-by-width open area, length-by-width area of erythema (color change), depth, undermining/tunneling, and overall wound size estimate (explained below)
- Period of the wound assessment: initial, interim observation week number (OB), and discharge(DC)
- Information about the wound healing phase (initials are inserted next to *wound phase* to identify the current wound phase—*I* for inflammatory, *P* for proliferative, and *E* for epithelialization, as described in Chapters 2 and 3)
- Discharge outcome status (healed or not healed)

The sample form works well when used in conjunction with the Sussman Wound Healing Tool (SWHT),[6] described in Chapter 5. Data can be entered into a computer database and program outcomes monitored.

Promoting Accuracy and Reliability of Wound Measurements

The accuracy and consistency of measurements are critical to the objective evaluation of wounds in clinical practice and for research. Many studies of the best way to measure wounds to achieve a reliable result have been published; however, no method reported is completely reliable.[7,8] In other words, at this time, there is no gold standard for wound measurement. This fact presents a dilemma for the wound care provider: Accurate measurements are required to establish a wound diagnosis, plan treatment, and document results. If the measurements are not reliable, how can the clinician ensure that the wound is healing and responding to the treatment interventions in a timely fashion?

Fortunately, you can maximize the accuracy of wound measurements by using the following strategies:

- Define the specific procedures you used to determine the wound edge, total wound area, and description of areas of necrotic tissue (i.e., percentage of wound area).
- Be consistent. Take the measurement the same way each time from a noted reference point on the body. Meaningful comparisons can only be made if a standardized measurement system is used.
- Use the same terminology and units of measure for each measurement.

EXHIBIT 4.2

Completed Wound Measurement Form

Wound Measurements

Initial ___X___
Discharge _____
OBWK#: ___0___
DC Status: _____

Date: ___01/23/08___   Patient Name: ___G. Lucky___

Wound ID: ___R Trochanter___   Med Rec#: ___0397___

Wound Phase: ___Chronic inflammation___
(all measurements in cm)

Linear Size: L(12:00–6:00) ___4.4___ X   W (3:00–9:00) ___3.3___ = ___14.52 cm²___
Undermined: 12:00 (A1) ___0___   6:00 (A2) ___0.5___   3:00 (B1) ___1.5___   9:00 (B2) ___0___
Overall Undermined
    Estimated Area   L + A1 + A2   X W + B1 + B2   = UEA
    (UEA):   (a) ___4.9 (overall length)___   X (b) ___4.8 (overall width)___   = ___23.52 cm²___

Depth   12:00 ___0___
_____   3:00 ___0.3___
         6:00 ___0___
         9:00 ___0___

Erythema   12:00–6 :00 ___6.5 cm___   X   3:00–9:00 ___4.5 cm___   area = ___29.25 cm²___
    (measured across wound surface)

Examiner: ___B Sweet, PT___   (OBWK = the observation week # since start of care)

- When possible, have the same person take repeat measurements.
- Record even small changes indicating improved or deteriorated wound status.
- When possible, use an assistant to record measurements as they are taken and help position the patient.
- Use a prepared form, and fill in a measurement number at each space indicated on the form. This form can be pre-printed or handwritten so nothing is forgotten. Record as soon as each parameter is measured; memory is not accurate.
- If a characteristic is assessed and found absent, record a zero to confirm that you observed the characteristic and assessed it. For example, partial-thickness wounds are superficial, so a zero should be written next to the depth measure spaces. A blank space does not show that this characteristic was assessed.

Comparing the Three Methods of Wound Measurement

Table 4.2 provides an overview of the three commonly used methods for measuring wounds and monitoring wound healing.[9] The table identifies the purpose, requirements, and information derived from each method. All are discussed in this chapter, but not all will be useful in all settings. Different skills and interests will determine the methods and measurements used.

Table 4.3 is a guide to the frequency with which the different wound measurement techniques are used clinically. For example, a measurement of length by width is always performed, but a video is rarely used. This table will become more useful to you as you learn about each technique.

Most clinical wound measurements are approximations rather than precise measurements. Although sophisticated

---

TABLE 4.2	**Monitoring Recovery of Chronic Wounds: Photo, Tracing, Measurements**		
Purpose	**Photo**	**Tracing/Planimetry**	**Measurements**
Objective	Establishes baseline wound status and tracks changes throughout recovery	Records shape and size changes at baseline and throughout recovery	Linear: estimates size
	Wound size measurement	Wound size area	Perimeter: estimates boundary
	Records change in recovery phase or wound stage		Digitization: approximates surface area
Treatment planning	Validates overall treatment plan	Demonstrates short-term response to treatment plan	Demonstrates rate of recovery
Frequency	Baseline, weekly, or change in phase/condition, discharge	Baseline, weekly, or change in phase/condition, discharge	Baseline, weekly, or change in phase/condition, discharge
Time reference	Prospective	Prospective	Prospective
	Ongoing/interim	Ongoing/interim	Ongoing/interim
Requirements	**Photo**	**Tracing**	**Measurements**
Conditions	Correct light, body position, and device to indicate relative size; adjust for curvature and position	Use of standard anatomic landmarks and method to transfer tracing to medical record	Use of standard anatomic landmarks
Equipment	Camera and digital recording card or film	Tracing kit or digital recording	Measurement tool and recording form
		Graph paper or grid	
Information	**Photo and Flash**	**Tracing**	**Measurements**
Type	Displays full-color picture	Gives black-and-white picture of size and shape	Provides numeric information
Comparison	Provides color comparison of phase, size, and tissue attributes	Represents topographic effects, size, and change	Summarizes quantitative changes for use in a graph
Use	Clinical medical review, program management, referral source, reports, survey team, legal, patient compliance	Clinical medical review, program management, referral source, reports, survey team, legal, self-care, patient compliance	Clinical medical review, program management, referral source, reports, survey team, legal, self-care, patient compliance

TABLE 4.3	Frequency of Usage for Different Wound Measurement Techniques			
Always	**Often**	**Sometimes**	**Rarely**	**New**
L and W L × W = area	Clock L × W area	Depth—greatest	Polaroid grid photo	Depth—four points of clock
Tracing shape	Undermining —longest and "mapping"	Digital photography with computer technology	Stereophotography	Undermining/Tunnelling—four points of clock
	Digital photo with flash	Planimetry	Video	Undermined estimate
				Area of erythema or discoloration in darkly pigmented skin
				Digital Tracing "wound map" with computed measurements

computer-assisted technologies can increase precision, information about measuring with such equipment has been omitted from this chapter because these devices are usually research tools and are not commonly available in clinical practice settings.

WOUND MEASUREMENT: LINEAR METHODS

This section describes linear measurements, which you will use to track changes in wound size over time. These include SA measurements (length multiplied by width), undermining or tunnels, and depth. At the conclusion of this section, we will briefly discuss measurements of volume.

Measuring the Surface Area

The most common wound measurements are length and width, which are measured from wound edge to wound edge, and are used to calculate SA. Other terms used for edge may be border, or margin. It is extremely important to identify the wound edge before you start. Edges may be indistinct and diffuse; there are areas where the normal tissues blend into the wound bed. Well-defined edges are clear and distinct, and can easily be outlined on a transparent piece of plastic. Therefore, the determination of the wound edge is based on the perception of the examiner. Thus during repeated measurements, identical measurement points for the wound edge cannot be guaranteed, and this accounts for most variations in SA measurements reported by different observers.[8] Edges that are not attached to the base of the wound imply a wound with some depth of tissue involvement. The wound edge can be described as nonadvancing or undermined.[10] Figure 4.1 shows an example of a wound with all of these attributes. Chapters 3 and 5 have pictures and more fully describe wound edges and their significance.

Choose a Consistent Method

Two SA measurement methods are commonly used in clinical practice. Figure 4.2 illustrates the two measuring methods.

The *greatest length and greatest width method* refers to measurement across the diameter of the greatest length and greatest width of the wound. Multiplying the length by the width gives the estimated SA of the wound in centimeters squared. This product is a single number that can be easily monitored for change in size. Length, width, and SA are always measured

and sometimes are the only linear measurements recorded (see Table 4.3).

The *clock method* is another way to measure the SA of wounds. In this method, you imagine the wound as the face of a clock. Select a 12:00 reference position on the wound; this position is usually toward the patient's head. Then, take the measurement from 12:00 to 6:00 and from 3:00 to 9:00. The four steps of the procedure are as follows:

1. Establish the 12:00 position by choosing an anatomic landmark that is easy to identify and document it for all following measurements (e.g., 12:00 toward head).
2. Mark 12:00 with arrow on the skin. Repeat with marks at 6:00, 3:00, and 9:00.
3. Measure from wound edge at 12:00 to wound edge at 6:00 position.
4. Measure from wound edge at 3:00 to wound edge at 9:00 position.

In situations such as severe contractures of the trunk and lower extremities, it may be more convenient and easier to reproduce the measurements if another convenient anatomic landmark is selected as the 12:00 reference point; for example, measurements in the foot may use the heel or toes. In a person whose body is contracted in the fetal position, a trochanteric pressure ulcer may be more easily tracked if the 12:00 reference point is toward the knee.

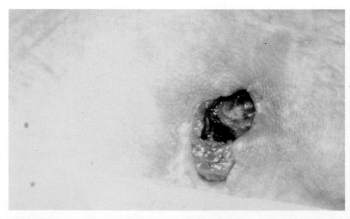

FIGURE 4.1 Wound edges are not attached to the wound bed and the wound edge is not advancing and is undermined. (Copyright © B.M. Bates-Jensen).

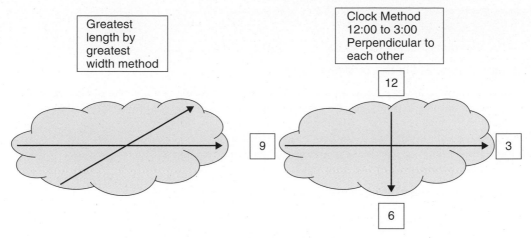

FIGURE 4.2 Two wound measurement methods.

Both of these measurement methods are acceptable and widely used. It is important to bear in mind two things when using them:

1. The geometric formula for the area of a rectangle (length times width) gives only an approximation of a wound's SA. In fact, it has been estimated to inflate the size of the wound by as much as 44% if the wound is irregularly shaped and large.[10]
2. All wound shapes are irregular, so assume that this measurement will be inflated.

In short, the goal is not to make a precise measurement, but rather to make consistent measurements that can be used to monitor healing. So choose a method that you are comfortable with and record which method is used. Then, use this method *consistently*. Exhibit 4.3 lists advantages and disadvantages of the clock method and the greatest length and greatest width method.

Gather Your Supplies
Assemble the supplies needed for wound measurement in advance to improve efficiency and reduce patient fatigue. If wound measurements are taken frequently, assemble a kit made up of these supplies. Keep it with you in a small plastic carrier. These supplies include

- Pen or pencil
- Disposable, plastic straight-edge ruler with linear measure ruled in centimeters
- Disposable gloves
- Normal saline
- Disposable syringe with 18-gauge needle or angiocatheter (for cleaning)
- Gauze paper, pocket-sized notebook, or wound measurement form to record data (see Exhibit 4.4)

Follow a Step-by-Step Procedure
Before measuring, the wound should be cleaned and examined closely. Look carefully at the edges to determine whether they are distinct so that you can measure from wound edge to wound edge. You may wish to use an assistant to help you position and comfort the patient, control wound "sagging" (see Step 6), record measurements, or seek additional supplies or assistance. Take the following steps:

1. Position the patient. It is easier for everyone if the patient is comfortable during the procedure. Some patients and some

wounds are difficult to position for accurate measurement. Once a convenient and comfortable position is found, record the position that works best. This will save time and effort and improve the uniformity of measurements over time.

Example: Coccyx wound—position: right side-lying; heel wound—position: left side-lying.

2. Don gloves and remove wound dressing and packing.
3. Place dressing and packing in disposable infectious waste bag.
4. Clean wound with normal saline and syringe with 18-gauge needle or angiocatheter (see Chapter 17 for wound cleansing procedure).
5. Take measurements with disposable wound measurement ruler.

EXHIBIT 4.3

Comparison of Two Wound Measurement Methods
Greatest Length by Greatest Width Method
Advantages
- Simple and easy to learn and use
- Most common method
- Reliable

Disadvantages
- Diameters change as size and shape change, so different diameters are measured each time
- Wound open area will be larger than in clock method

Clock Method
Advantages
- Simple and easy to learn and use
- Tracks same place on the wound over time
- More conservative measure of area

Disadvantages
- Requires more steps to perform
- More precision required to line up wound points along the clock "face"
- Less commonly used

EXHIBIT 4.4

Calculating Percentage Rate of Change in Wound Size

One interesting way to determine how a wound is progressing is to look at the percentage rate of change. This is also an effective way to measure and predict successful outcomes. Percentage rate of change is a simple statistical calculation that uses the following formula:

1. Baseline (week 0) wound size (0A or overall 0A size) measurement is used as the original size.
2. Subtract the next wound size 0A or overall 0A size measurement (interim) taken from the baseline.
3. Divide by baseline wound measurement and multiply by 100%.

Formula for computing rate of change in wound open area:

$$\frac{\text{Baseline open area (OA)} - \text{Interim open area (OA)}}{\text{Baseline open area}} \times 100\%$$

Example:

Wound open area (OA) baseline week 0	= 30 cm^2
Wound open area (OA) week 1 (interim)	= 28 cm^2
OA baseline – OA week 1 (interim)	= 30 − 28 = 2
Divide the remainder by the baseline OA	= 2/30 = 0.066
Multiply 0.066 × 100% = 6.6%	= Percentage rate of change

Note: A weekly percentage of change would use the prior week's size measurement instead of baseline. Wound size often changes significantly from week to week in the early phases of healing, and then the rate slows. Referring to the percentage rate of change on a weekly or biweekly basis is a reliable measure of how the wound is healing.

6. Measure the wound using one of the three methods just described. If measurements are always taken in the same order, the tracking of wound size will be more consistent.

Take the length first and the width second. If the clock method is used, take measurements from 12:00 to 6:00 then from 3:00 to 9:00 for consistency. While measuring, control sagging wounds. Full-thickness wounds with undermining can sag from lack of subcutaneous support and the pull of gravity. Try to keep sagging to a minimum and maintain uniform tension for accurate length and width measurements.

7. Record each measurement *as it is taken*.
8. Dispose of measurement instrument and gloves in infectious waste container.
9. Dispose of syringe with 18-gauge needle in sharps container.

CLINICAL WISDOM

Using a Template to Improve Measurement Accuracy

To improve accuracy and better align the measurements, cut a circle from paper folded in half twice and mark the four clock points at the four paper folds. Place the circle over the wound to use as a template or guide, taping it to the periwound skin to keep it from shifting.[11] Take all measurements with the template in place to uniformly track the same wound locations for SA, undermining, and depth (Fig. 4.3).

10. Apply fresh dressing.
11. Calculate wound SA.
12. Repeat weekly or more frequently, if indicated.

Measuring Undermining and Tunneling

Measurements of undermining (erosion under the wound edge) and tunneling (a sinus) indicate the extent of wound damage into surrounding deep tissue. Undermining/tunneling is often the consequence of wound debridement: when a body of necrotic tissue is removed, the fascial planes can separate during the probing action. Tunneling can progress to become a sinus tract and a pathway for infection. For this reason, any measurement of undermining and tunneling requires careful, gentle probing to avoid further separation of the fascial planes. A measurement of extensive tunneling is a red flag that indicates the urgent need to contact the physician and report the finding.

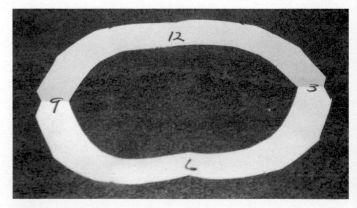

FIGURE 4.3 Using a template to improve measurement accuracy.

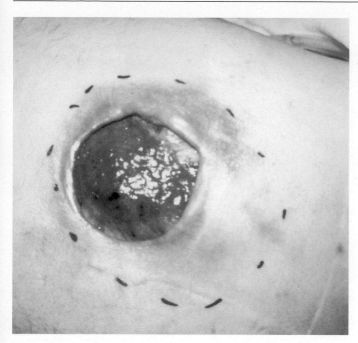

FIGURE 4.4 Mapping undermining around the entire wound perimeter. (Courtesy of Evonne Fowler, MN, RN, CETN.)

Some wound experts claim that the true extent of a wound is not known unless undermining/tunneling is measured.[12] Figure 4.4 shows the larger perimeter of a wound when undermining is mapped, and Figure 4.5 compares measurements over time of

the total wound area when undermining is calculated, compared with measurement of the SA alone. Figures 4.6 and 4.7 demonstrate the extent of the tunneling process in a trochanteric pressure ulcer.

In a principal component analysis of the Pressure Ulcer Scale for Healing (PUSH) (see Chapter 5), the addition of a tunneling measurement was not found to improve the validity and reliability of that tool; therefore, the measurement is not part of the tool components.[12] Facilities and healthcare organizations need to determine if the measurement of undermining and tunneling should be part of wound documentation and thus included in the wound care policies and procedures.

Choose a Consistent Method

Three methods for measuring undermining and tunneling are described below. Choose one and use it consistently (see Figs. 4.8 and 4.9).

Method 1

1. Map undermining around the *entire* wound perimeter by inserting a moist, cotton-tipped applicator into the length of the undermined/tunneled space and continuing around the perimeter. Dip the cotton tip into normal saline before insertion, so it slides in easier and is less likely to cause tissue trauma (Fig. 4.4).

2. At the end point, *do not force* further entry, but gently push upward until there is a bulge in the skin. Mark the points on the skin with a pen and connect them. Measure the length

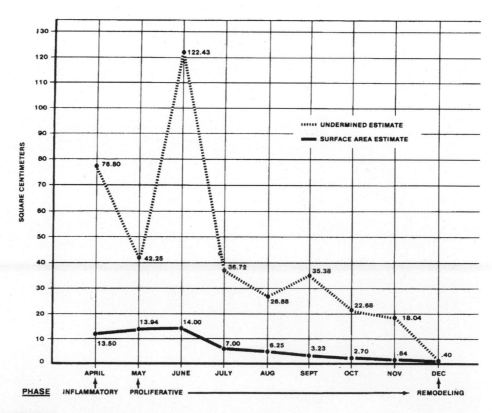

66-YEAR-OLD FEMALE
WOUND TYPE: PRESSURE WOUND
LOCATION: LEFT HIP

FIGURE 4.5 Wound healing trajectory: recovery of a pressure wound.

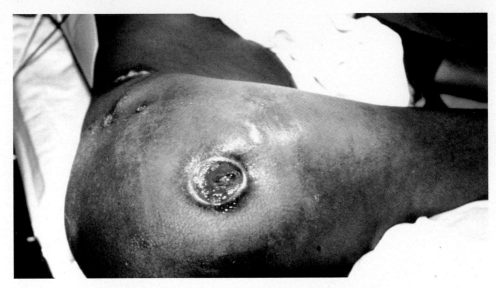

FIGURE 4.6 Unobservable tunneling. (Copyright © J. Wethe.)

and width, and multiply these measurements to calculate the *overall undermined estimate* (explained below).

Method 2

1. The Sussman method for wound measurement applies the four cardinal points of the clock method to measurement of undermining and tunneling.[9] The 12:00 position is toward the head unless otherwise noted.

2. Wet the cotton-tipped applicator with normal saline and insert gently into tunnel. Mark the place on the skin where the cotton tip causes a bulge, and withdraw the cotton-tipped applicator.

3. Grip the cotton-tipped applicator at the point at which the skin and wound edge meet, and withdraw it. This is the length of the tunnel.

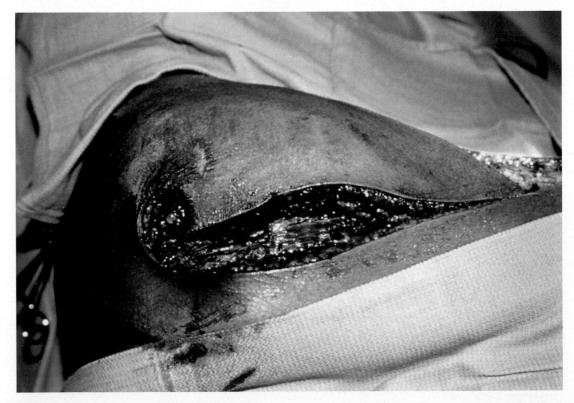

FIGURE 4.7 Same wound as in Figure 4.6 with surgical dissection demonstrating the extent of the tunneling process, forming a sinus tract. (Copyright © J. Wethe.)

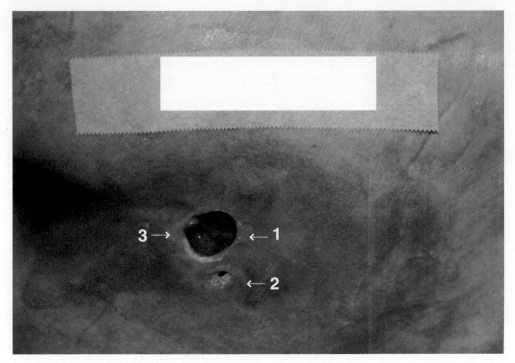

FIGURE 4.8 Wound with tunneling before insertion of a cotton-tipped applicator. Note: (1) Ulcer reoccurrence at site of old scar tissue; (2) Skin bridge between two open ulcers; (3) Surrounding skin has unblanchable erythema; wound edges rolled under demonstrate chronic inflammatory phase. (Copyright © B.M. Bates-Jensen.)

4. Place the length of the cotton-tipped applicator up to the withdrawal point against a centimeter ruler or measure from wound edge to mark on skin as in method 1. Record the length measurement.

Method 3

1. Test the perimeter for undermining with a cotton-tipped applicator, and then select the longest tunnel to measure.
2. Use the clock method to identify the location(s) on the wound perimeter where tunneling is present, and then track the tunnel over time.

Calculating the Overall Undermined Estimated Size

To derive an estimate of the *overall undermined estimated size* of the wound area, add the measurements of undermining/

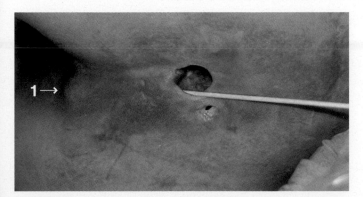

FIGURE 4.9 Same wound as in Figure 4.8. The wound's overall size is much larger than the surface open area. Tunneling is present. Note the bulge from the end of the cotton-tipped applicator. (Copyright © B.M. Bates-Jensen.)

tunneling to the SA length and width to derive the overall length and overall width. Next, multiply the overall length by the overall width.[9] For example, using the clock method:

12:00–6:00 length + 12:00 undermining + 6:00 undermining = overall length

3:00–9:00 width + 3:00 undermining + 9:00 undermining = overall width

Overall length × overall width = overall estimated area

RESEARCH WISDOM

Accuracy and Reliability of Wound Undermining Measurements

Taylor[11] studied the variability of measurements of wound undermining among physical therapists trained in the Sussman wound undermining measurement method. Her findings show that the most significant variation occurred when the 12:00 position coincided with the greatest length of the wound's open SA, which inflated the area measurements.

The results of studying measurements by 39 physical therapists over a 4-week period demonstrated several interesting findings. Three common errors occurred: misreading the measuring device, transferring the numbers, and calculating. As would be expected, there were more errors in measurement when the wounds were smaller. Overall, the variation was 10.5% or less. Validation of the measuring technique was proven highly reliable, suggesting that this measurement can be used to document progress in the healing of undermined wounds.[11]

The product is a single number that can be monitored and graphed to show the trajectory of healing over time, as indicated by the dashed line in the graph in Figure 4.5. This figure also shows how the overall undermined estimated size compares with the SA estimate.[9] If only the open SA is monitored for change in size, the wound appears significantly smaller than it actually is, and information about incremental changes in size is lost.

Graphing the Trajectory and Percentage of Healing

Wound SA and undermining measurements can be plotted on a graph to show a *trajectory of healing* that identifies those patients whose wounds are on track to heal and those whose wounds are not healing. The points on the trajectory can be used as end points to compare results, rather than complete healing.[13] Graphs showing the wound healing trajectory, such as the one shown in Figure 4.10, are a very useful visual method for monitoring healing over time. Graphing is recommended for tracking the scores obtained using the Pressure Ulcer Scale for Healing (PUSH) tool (see Chapter 5). Recently, the wound healing trajectory has been suggested as a method for tracking significant points along the continuum of healing, rather than a single end point, when determining the efficacy of treatment interventions.[13]

Controlled clinical trials of many types of wound healing products use reduction in ulcer SA as the dependent variable, and results are reported as a percentage of reduction in unit area per unit time (cm^2/mm^2 or %/day/week).[14] *Percentage of healing per unit of time (PHT)* refers to the decrease in wound area from the baseline to the day of measurement for each reevaluation period (e.g., per week) as a percentage of the wound size. PHT rates have been used to calculate the linear daily or weekly healing rates analyzed for different wound etiologies (pressure ulcers, venous ulcers, and diabetic ulcers). (Refer to Part II for information about different wound etiologies.) These rates are now becoming the standard predictor of whether the wound will heal, and are also useful for comparing the results and costs of different interventions.[2-4,15-17]

Steps for Graphing the Trajectory and Percentage of Healing

Creating a trajectory of healing involves the following basic steps. Note that the graph can be generated as part of a database program or manually drawn on graph paper:

1. Perform the size measurements following a defined protocol.
2. Calculate the total wound area (cm^2) or the percentage change in size. Methods of calculating the PHT vary. See Exhibit 4.4 for an example. Plot the wound healing curve on a graph. This requires two axes: horizontal and vertical. The horizontal axis represents time, and the vertical axis represents size in square centimeters or percentage of change. Time should be graphed at consistent intervals (e.g., weekly, with the baseline week 0). See Figure 4.10 for example.

Using the Trajectory Graph to Determine Phase of Healing

A great deal of information can be gleaned from trajectory graphs. For instance, consider again the simple trajectory graph in Figure 4.5. Note the significant variations in the extent of the wound between May and July. However, notice the linear reduction in wound extent from September to December. As the wound healed, undermined/tunneled spaces closed, tissue integrity was restored, and the overall size was reduced.

Graphing can also show how changes in the undermined estimate parallel the changes in wound phase. For example, notice the abrupt jump in wound overall undermined estimate from 42.25 cm to 122.43 cm; this frequently coincides with the early proliferative phase. The expansion of the wound extent reflects the effects of wound debridement on loss of subcutaneous tissue integrity (the separation of fascial planes), producing tunneling. Loss of subcutaneous tissue integrity produces increased risk of infection, but subcutaneous tissue integrity is restored as the wound progresses through the proliferative phase to the remodeling phase.

Using the PHT to Predict Healing and Nonhealing

As you can see, percentage reduction in wound size—rather than the actual size measurements—is a valid and useful method for predicting wound healing rates and tracking the healing of pressure ulcers, venous ulcers, and diabetic ulcers.[16,18,19]

FIGURE 4.10 Trajectory of healing for healing and nonhealing diabetic ulcers. (Source: Robson MC, Hill D, Woodske M, et al. Wound healing trajectories as predictors of effectiveness of therapeutic agents. *Arch Surg.* 2000;135(7):773–777.)

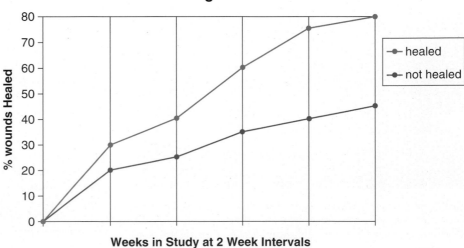

The conclusion supported by a number of studies is that pressure ulcers and leg ulcers (venous and diabetic) that do not reduce in size between 30% and 50% in a 2- to 4-week period are not on a healing trend and are less likely to heal than ulcers that do reduce by these amounts.[5,15,16,19–21]

Healing trajectories are significantly different for healers and nonhealers (see Fig. 4.10)[13]. By plotting the percentage of change on a graph, you will create a trajectory that you can then use to compare against these numbers. This will indicate whether the wound is following a course for healing or for nonhealing.

In addition, review of the PHT at clinical decision points can be extremely valuable in helping you identify early on the patients who require more aggressive and possibly more expensive interventions.

It can also help you identify those who are likely to heal with standard care. Shifting of the wound healing trajectory from an impaired course to a more ideal course can also be one way to evaluate the efficacy of the treatment plan.

It is clear that the precision of wound measurement and the method of calculating the rate of change can and should influence clinical decision making. Clinicians today are responsible for setting the goals of treatment and differentiating wounds that will go on to heal with standard care from those that should be triaged to adjunctive therapy.

Limitations of PHT Calculations

The calculation method presented in Exhibit 4.4 is commonly used to measure healing. However, this method can exaggerate the progress made by larger wounds relative to smaller ones, and the percentage of reduction in area can minimize the actual progress made by large wounds relative to the progress made in small wounds.[19] Wounds of different sizes and shapes present special problems. To compensate for these problems, Gilman[22] proposed a formula for measuring the wound perimeter change over time (Exhibit 4.5). Tallman et al.[3] found that using initial wound size as the baseline for percentage of change in size calculation to determine the weekly healing rate gave healing rate instability from week to week, which decreased the ability to predict complete healing. They created another method to compare healing rates, which takes the mean of all previous healing rates between each visit (which becomes the mean adjusted healing rate) and uses that rate as the baseline size to calculate the percentage of change. This method improved healing rate stability from week to week and allowed prediction of complete healing as early as 3 weeks from start of therapy ($p < 0.001$).[3]

CLINICAL WISDOM

Healing Rates

Healing rates should not be used to predict a specific anticipated healing date because factors that affect healing cannot be controlled. The rates should be used to help clinical decision making and identify effective and ineffective treatments. Accurate measurement of wound size is the basis for reliable predicting.

EXHIBIT	4.5

Gilman Method of Measuring Wound Healing Using the Wound Perimeter

$$\bar{d} = \Delta A \bar{p}$$

$\bar{d}$ = units of distance; $\bar{d}$ represents the average distance of advance of the wound margin over the study time T, in a direction toward the wound center

ΔA = the difference in area of the wound before and after the study time T

$\bar{p}$ = the average perimeter before and the wound perimeter after time T

Reprinted with permission from T.H. Gilman, Parameter for Measurement of Wound Closure, *Wounds: A Compendium of Research and Practice*, 1990;2(3):95–101. Health Management Publications.

Comparing Healing Rates

Venous ulcers that healed in 4 weeks or more had an initial healing rate of 0.049–0.065 cm per week, and diabetic ulcers had a rate of 0.063 cm per week, suggesting that there may be a fairly uniform rate of healing for chronic ulcers, regardless of etiology.[23] Because repairing wounds appear to heal at the same rate, there should be no correlation between initial ulcer size and the rate of healing. By using the 0.062 cm per week rate of healing for full-thickness chronic ulcers, a 4-week period could be sufficient to establish a healing trend.[23] Before this recommendation can be used as a standard for all chronic wounds, consider the findings that the trajectory for healing differs for partial-thickness and full-thickness ulcers. Linear advancement of the wound margin was 0.056 mm per day (0.0392 cm per week) for partial-thickness ulcers and 0.021 mm per day (0.0147 cm per week) for full-thickness ulcers. Median time is the time by which at least one-half of the patients have healed. Median time to healing for the partial-thickness ulcers was 28 days, and it was 56 days for full-thickness ulcers. These findings suggest that norms for duration and rate of healing are specific to the level of tissue injury (Exhibit 4.6). Polansky and vanRijswijk suggest using the *median* time of healing for study groups, rather than

EXHIBIT	4.6

Factors that Significantly Affect Healing Outcomes

- Initial SA size: Larger ulcers take longer to heal.[4,16]
- Duration: Ulcers of short duration are most likely to heal.[4]
- Healing rate: A 30% to 50% reduction in area size in the first 2 to 4 weeks predicts healing.[4,15,16,19]
- Circulation: Moderate arterial insufficiency (ankle-brachial index (0.5–0.8) increases risk of delayed healing.[2]
- Nutrition: Full-thickness pressure ulcers heal faster with proper nutrition.[16]

the *mean (midpoint)* time to plot healing time curves.[14] The healing time curve provides a "moving picture" of healing and is developed using the Kaplan-Meir method called *survival analysis*. This methodology is particularly useful when there is a large study population and a significant number of patients who do not complete the entire study course; it may also be useful for prediction of healing of individual wounds.[13] These healing time curves provide more information about healing than looking at the proportion of the population healed at the end of a study. More research on the rate of healing of a large population sample with chronic wounds is needed to substantiate the trend before using these numbers as benchmarks for the rate of healing for all chronic wounds. Robson et al. showed that healing trajectories are significantly different for healers and nonhealers with diabetic ulcers (see Fig. 4.10).[13] Shifting of the wound healing trajectory from an impaired course to a more ideal course can be one way to evaluate the efficacy of the treatment plan. For more information about the measurement methods involved in doing survival analysis for wound healing in a clear and relatively easy-to-understand way, readers are encouraged to read the Polansky and vanRijswijk article.[14]

The healing rates for chronic wounds can be put into perspective when they are compared with the healing rates for acute wounds. Ramirez et al. looked at the rate of healing of acute surgical wounds in normal adults in 1969.[24] The average surgical wound size was 10 cm², and there was a 50% reduction in wound size in 13 days, for an estimated healing rate of 0.37 cm² per day. Wound closure was achieved in 21 days. Gilman calculated that this healing rate is about six times faster than chronic wounds make when making good progress.[25]

Measuring Wound Depth

Wound depth is defined as the distance from the visible skin surface edge to the wound bed.[29] Initially, wound depth is correlated with the depth/extent of tissue damage, and several staging systems use depth to categorize wound severity (see Chapter 3). As the wound heals, measurement of wound depth is a crude method of tracking the growth of granulation tissue in the wound base of deep wounds. It is also a way to measure early healing progress that may otherwise be missed, since depth reduction usually precedes the reduction in wound SA.[30,31] Reduction in wound depth is accomplished through the formation of scar tissue that does *not* represent replacement of the tissue destroyed. Recently, another rationale for considering a change in wound depth was proposed: this is the observation that "pocketing" at the bottom of a wound is a clinical indicator of critical wound colonization or infection.

Accuracy of Depth Measurements

When measuring wound depth, it is common practice to try to find the deepest site in the wound bed. This method is difficult

---

RESEARCH WISDOM

Healing rate during the first 4 weeks of observation has been validated as a predictor of healing outcome and is steady over the course of healing for venous, diabetic, and pressure ulcers.[3,4,15,16,18,23,26–28]

---

to reproduce from measurement to measurement because the wound bed fills in irregularly; what is the deepest spot one time may not be the same spot at the next measurement. There is controversy, especially among researchers, about the usefulness of depth measurements because of the inaccuracies recorded.[32]

The Clock Method

Depth measurement accuracy is limited, regardless of how this measurement is made; however, the clock method allows for consistency in the measurement site that can be more closely reproduced at subsequent tests than the use of a single "deepest spot" method. Using the clock method for measuring wound depth is also suggested as a method of tracking changes in depth at specific locations around the wound bed; however, reliability for this use has not been validated.[9] Steps for measuring depth using the clock method are as follows:

1. Cleanse the wound thoroughly before measuring.
2. Take depth measurements at the 12:00, 3:00, 6:00, and 9:00 positions.
3. Insert a cotton-tipped applicator perpendicular to the wound edge.
4. Hold the stick of the applicator with fingers at the wound skin surface edge.
5. Holding this position on the applicator stick, place applicator stick along a centimeter-ruled edge. Record for each of the four positions.
6. These depth measurements may or may *not* be at the deepest area of the wound.
7. A separate measurement may be taken and noted at the deepest area.

Partial-thickness wounds have a depth of less than 0.2 cm. Wounds with greater than 0.2 cm depth are difficult to measure and should be recorded as greater than 0.2 cm. Measure the depth of full-thickness wounds of greater than 0.2 cm depth. When a wound is undergoing debridement of nonviable tissue, the wound depth usually increases; as the wound bed fills with granulation tissue, the depth decreases. Reduction in wound depth is a measurement of progression through the proliferative phase of healing.

Numeric Score Method

Instead of a quantitative measurement of wound depth, some wound measurement tools observe the layers of tissue lost and rank the loss by an increasing numeric score that corresponds to greater depth of tissue lost. For example, a superficial ulcer may have a score of 1. A full-thickness wound with tissue loss to the bone may have a score of 4 or 5.

Measuring Wound Volume

Wound volume measurements present special challenges. Although advances in technology may improve their reliability, currently they are too costly to implement in most wound care settings. However, they are used in research studies for quantifying research results more accurately than is possible with standardized measurements; thus, to help you appreciate the direction that wound measurement is taking, we introduce you here to two currently available volume measurement technologies.

One method involves filling the wound with a measured amount of normal saline from a syringe. This works best for wounds that can be positioned horizontally so the liquid does not spill out. Still, accuracy is questionable because the amount of fluid absorbed by wound tissue or left in the wound cannot be measured.[33]

Another method involves the use of Jeltrate, an alginate hydrocolloid used by dentists. By pouring the rapidly setting plastic into the wound, a mold of the wound is made. Jeltrate is reported to be well tolerated by the wound tissue.[32]

Regardless of which method of measuring wound volume is used, there are significant inaccuracies. Use of this parameter of measurement appears to be most appropriate in the research arena and of less value to the clinician.[32] Some studies appear to support the idea that measurement of depth or volume may be superfluous, since percentage of change calculations based on SA have demonstrated validity for tracking healing.

Measuring Surrounding Skin Erythema

Erythema of the skin surrounding a wound can be a measure of the inflammation phase of healing or a sign of infection. Chronic wounds often show a halo of erythema but lack the other signs of inflammation. As discussed in Chapter 3, the periwound erythema can be identified as unblanchable redness (see Figs 4.11 and 4.12). The "Clinical Wisdom" below addresses measurement of erythema in darkly pigmented skin. Streaking or significant signs of erythema projecting out a distance from the wound can indicate cellulitis, and medical measures are warranted. Measurement can be taken using the greatest length and greatest width method or the clock method.

Gather Your Supplies
Assemble all supplies needed:
- Two acetate measuring guides or one each plastic wrap over wound, topped by measuring guide
- Two pieces of plastic wrap, cut in approximately 6 inches × 8 inches pieces or larger, if wound plus periwound erythema is larger
- Fine-point transparent film-type marking pen, so that ink would not bead up on the plastic (dark Pentel™ or Vis-a-Vis™)
- Paper towel, folded in half lengthwise
- Paper or graph form
- Transparent tape

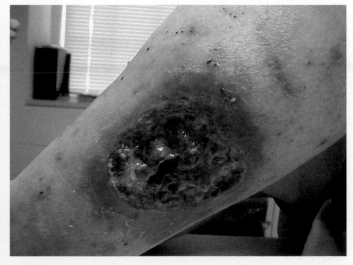

FIGURE 4.11 Periwound erythema or, in darkly pigmented skin, a darkening of the skin.

CLINICAL WISDOM

Measurement of Erythema in Darkly Pigmented Skin

Skin color changes reported by clinicians and in the literature[27] indicate that, when inflamed, the skin color of darkly pigmented individuals darkens to an eggplant/purplish color (see Fig. 4.12). It can be difficult to differentiate darkening of inflammation from hemosiderin staining. When this is the case, proceed with temperature and edema examinations. For a full description of the assessment of darkly pigmented skin, see Chapter 3.

The following are guidelines for measuring the extent of inflammation/trauma in darkly pigmented skin:

- Use natural light or halogen light, not fluorescent light.
- Outline the margins of color change on the surrounding skin with a marking pen.
- Select a reference point for future measures.
- Measure using the greatest length and the greatest width or the clock method.
- Calculate the area of color change (as described for all length-by-width measurements).

How to Measure Using the Clock Method
1. Measure across the wound SA from the 12:00 to the 6:00 position and to the outer margin of the periwound erythema.
2. Measure across the wound SA from the 3:00 to the 9:00 position and to the outer margin of the periwound erythema.
3. Compute the periwound area of erythema: 12:00 to 6:00 length × 3:00 to 9:00 width = _____ cm².

Example: 9:0 cm × 6.0 cm = 54 cm²

WOUND MEASUREMENT: WOUND TRACINGS

Making a *wound tracing*, also known as the *acetate method*, is a popular and practical method for measuring wound area. A tracing is a drawing of the wound shape. It can be made on acetate measuring sheets supplied by manufacturers for this

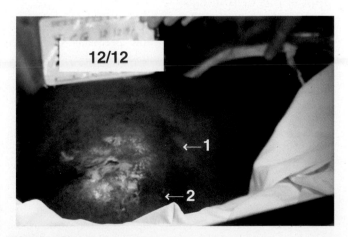

FIGURE 4.12 Suspected deep tissue injury pressure ulcer. Note: (1) Line of demarcation between healthy tissue and hemorrhagic or erythematous tissue in darkly pigmented skin; (2) Note small areas of tissue break down.

RESEARCH WISDOM

Measuring Wounds of Different Shapes

A comparison of the standard error of measurement for wounds of different shapes using four techniques: linear ruler length and width, planimetry, stereophotogrammetry (SPG) length and width, and SPG area showed that linear ruler length and width measurements best measured circular wounds, tracing worked best for pear-shaped wounds, and SPG had the lowest standard error of measurement for L-shaped wounds.[34] SPG incorporates the use of enhanced digital photography with a computer system using wound measurement software.

purpose or household plastic wrap with a plastic transparency marking pen (the ink does not bead up). These can then be transferred to graph paper to determine size by counting the squares (centimeters). This is called *planimetry*. Using 1 cm graph paper to count squares has been reported to be quick, efficient, and realiable.[34,35] Compared with linear measurements with a ruler, there is less overestimation of the real wound area. This method is most useful on wounds that are on flat surfaces, and it has limited usefulness for full-thickness wounds. Accuracy of measurement with the tracing method depends on how carefully the wound edges are followed as the tracing is drawn. Greater reliability using planimetry has been found for wounds with edges that begin to approximate over a bed of granulation tissue.[34] The method of measuring the wound area from transparency tracings and placing it on graph paper to determine size by counting the centimeters has shown high intratester and intertester reliability (0.99).

Repeated tracings show changes in the size and shape of a wound over the course of recovery. Tracing is easy to learn, inexpensive, readily available, and requires minimal training.[36]

Clean tracings taped to a sheet of paper can be stored in the patient record. However, because these tracings can come loose or become ragged, the tracing and form can be photocopied, with the photocopy stored in the chart.

Applications of Tracings

Following are ways that tracings can be used:

- Tracings show change in the wound perimeter shape over time. Wound shape is a helpful indicator of the rate of healing. As described in Chapter 2, linear wounds contract rapidly, square or rectangular wounds contract at a moderate pace, and circular wounds contract slowly.[35]
- When placed on a metric graph form (planimetry), tracings show the wound size, as well as the shape of the healing wound (Exhibit 4.7).
- A tracing can become a "wound map," showing features of the wound bed, such as necrotic tissue, and adjacent tissue characteristics, such as erythema (see Exhibit 4.7). Household plastic wrap is better than a grid sheet for this because it is clear.
- When placed on metric graph paper, features such as the actual amount of undermining/tunneling around the wound perimeter can be drawn on the wound map using the actual measurements and a ruler.

- The wound map tracing becomes the document on which assessment findings of tissue attributes are recorded. A map key at the bottom of the graph form assigns letters to each tissue attribute, making this an easy way to describe the tissue in the drawing. The tracing is a paper-and-pencil instrument to track wound healing over time. Note: The tissue attributes on the wound recovery form[37] are the same as those represented in the SWHT described in Chapter 6.
- The wound tracing can be scanned into a computer, making a digitized measurement of the wound. The area can be calculated, and the tracing can be stored on the computer.

Steps for Making a Wound Tracing

1. Place two acetate measuring guides or two pieces of plastic wrap over the wound, so that the bottom piece fits across the wound from 3:00 to 9:00, and the top piece fits from 12:00 to 6:00. This arrangement helps when separating the top layer from the bottom layer. Smooth each piece of plastic to remove wrinkles. Two layers are used to prevent contamination of the layer on which the tracing is made. The layer that was in contact with the wound is discarded with infectious waste after the tracing is completed.
2. Draw an arrow on the plastic wrap in the location and direction of the 12:00 position.
3. Trace the wound edges.

Optional Additions to Tracings

1. Draw any notable features within or around the wound SA, such as an outline of the necrotic tissue or exposed bone. Label the features with a letter from the wound recovery form key.[26]
2. Mark areas of erythema or darkened darkly pigmented skin with broken lines around the wound SA.
3. Mark areas of necrotic tissue or eschar with diagonal lines.
4. Mark other features with circles and dots, and label them with letters.
5. Place the tracing so that the 12:00 arrow is in the conventional 12:00 position on the graph form, and tape it onto the graph form. Make sure the plastic is taut and free of wrinkles. (See instructions for completing the wound recovery form below.)
6. Photocopy the wound tracing to create a permanent record. Discard the graph with the plastic tracing.
7. Mark wound features with lines drawn at right angles to the feature and label.

CLINICAL WISDOM

Tracings on Plastic Sandwich Bags

A plastic sandwich bag can be placed over the wound and a tracing can be made on the top layer, with the bottom layer of the bag acting as a wound barrier. Slit the bag in half and discard the contaminated layer with infectious waste. The top layer can be put on a graph form or placed in a zippered sandwich bag to keep for comparison measurements. This method is very useful for home care.

EXHIBIT 4.7

Wound Recovery Form with Tracing

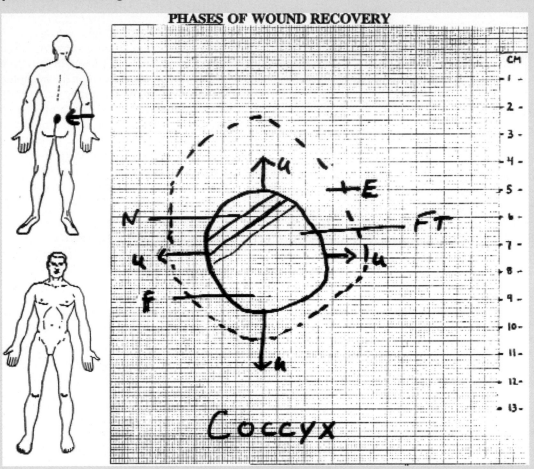

NAME: _G. LUCKY_   DATE: _4/20/08_   _B Sweet_

WOUND I.D. (1) _____COCCYX_____ (2) _____ (3) _____

INFLAMMATION   PROLIFERATION   EPITHELIALIZATION
   X

B = BLISTER	F = FIBROPLASIA	EP = EPITHELIALIZATION
E = ERYTHEMA	C = CONTRACTION	M = MACERATION
H = HEMORRHAGIC	FT = FULL THICKNESS	R = REMODELED
SB = SCAB	PT = PARTIAL THICKNESS	I = INTACT
N = NECROSIS	U = UNDERMINING	

DRAINAGE: DRAINAGE: DRAINAGE:
 V = VISCOUS   S = SEROUS   S = SEROUS
PU = PURULENT   SS = SEROSANGUINEOUS   DY = DRY

Adapted with permission from Sussman CA. Physical therapy choices for wound recovery. *Ostomy/Wound Management*. 1990;20:20–28, Health Management Publication, Inc., Wayne, PA.

HELPFUL HINTS

Tracings

A grid printed on acetate film that peels off a plastic backing sheet can be used to make wound tracings. The sheet acts as a barrier to infection and is discarded. The tracing is then ready to place in the medical record.

Using a Wound Recovery Form

The wound recovery form[37] is a paper-and-pencil instrument that consists of a centimeter graph sheet, a linear measure aligned with the graph coordinates to show size, and anatomic figures (front and back) to mark location. The tissue characteristics are listed by phase: inflammation, proliferation, and epithelialization. You can use this key in evaluating and developing the wound phase healing diagnosis and in tracking the recovery of the wound by phase and wound characteristics. A completed form is shown in Exhibit 4.7.

The supplies needed for the wound recovery form include

- Wound recovery form
- Wound tracing
- Transparent tape
- Fine-tip marking pen
- Photocopier (optional)

The steps in creating a wound recovery form include the following:

1. Prepare wound tracing (see above).
2. Place tracing on wound recovery graph with the arrow aligned with lines at the 12:00 position.
3. Tape tracing in place unless it is adhesive backed.
4. Draw lines that are exactly the same length as the length measurements taken from the undermining at clock points around the wound perimeter, starting at wound edges and moving outward.
5. Draw lines from the tissue characteristics out to the side of the graph and label with letter from key.

CLINICAL WISDOM

Using the Wound Tracing for Positive Reinforcement

The wound tracing can also be a positive reinforcement for wound patients. Two wound tracings are made on acetate film or plastic wrap. A date is placed on the tracing next to the wound edge. One copy is placed in the patient records, and the other is given to the patient. The next assessment day, the patient brings in his or her copy, and the copy from the chart is presented. The wound is redrawn on both pieces of film and dated, so the size change can be visually compared. Patients receive positive reinforcement for their efforts by seeing their wounds get smaller (N. Elftman, *personal communication*).

6. Print wound location at the bottom of the picture. Mark its location on anatomic figures.
7. This "wound map" is also a tissue assessment report.

WOUND MEASUREMENT: WOUND PHOTOGRAPHY

"A picture is worth a thousand words." This adage certainly applies to wound photography. As discussed below, photographs of wounds serve many important clinical functions. In addition, they can be extremely valuable in preventing litigation, allowing us to put a new twist on the old adage: "A picture of a wound is worth thousands of dollars."[7] That's because serial photographs serve as a permanent record of the wound at baseline and throughout the patient's course of care. In fact, in many facilities, the photographs of wounds are part of the patient's medical record; wound photographs were reported to be part of the documentation procedures in 75% of the home health-care agencies in the United States.[38]

Use of Serial Photographs

Any wound present upon admission should be photographed promptly. Wounds that develop during the patient stay should be photographed when acquired and at discharge, as well. In long-term care settings, wounds should be photographed.

Serial color photographs are useful for many reasons. First, they document wound tissue characteristics. For instance, they can show color, streaking. However, the type of lighting affects the color: flash photography and fluorescent lighting tend to give a blue tone to the photograph, and incandescent light gives a yellow tone.

Photographs are used also to measure the wound size; however, the accuracy of wound measurements derived from photographs is compromised by the problem caused by measuring wound area on curved surfaces.[36]

Serial photographs can also be used to validate the overall treatment outcome. Serial photos are also effective teaching tools for in-services, referral sources, reimbursement, and patient encouragement.

Choosing the Equipment

Photographs can be taken with simple point and shoot digital cameras or with more complex camera equipment. However, with lower end equipment, color and image quality may not accurately represent the wound. For instance, resolution with low-priced digital cameras like those found in cell phones is not high enough to assure a quality image. Fortunately, better resolution is now available using moderate-priced digital cameras, so this technology is now widely available.

Digital photography has many real benefits. For instance, with a digital camera, you can view the photo instantly to determine if it is a good representation of the wound. If not, you can quickly and easily retake it. Also, you can use the dating feature to help you maintain accurate records. Moreover, digital photographs can be downloaded into a computer where the records can be stored, and you can quickly print the photos on inexpensive photo printers. You can also add to each photo identification information that protects patient privacy while still allowing for accurate record keeping. Obviously, in order to maintain the validity of the original, digital photos should not be retouched.

Digital photography can be combined with computerized planimetry. This noncontact method of photography and measurement eliminates the risk of wound bed contamination and trauma, and avoids procedural pain.[31] The photograph is uploaded to the computer and analyzed using computer software that is also designed to be used as a database of wound information. Unfortunately, these systems are not yet available in many facilities.

Scanning is yet another method for digitally storing photographs. Again, the quality of photograph and scanner influence the quality of the computer image.

More complex camera equipment and computer systems are typically limited to use by researchers, but their availability to clinicians may increase as the standards for recording and documenting wounds are revised and use of telemedicine expands.

Taking a High-Quality Photograph

Unless consent for patient photography is part of the facility admission package, consent should be obtained before photography is used. The following are suggestions for taking high-quality photographs:

- Use a good light source.
- Position patient and wound carefully, ensuring that the patient's private areas are screened from the camera.
- Position a linear measure (ruler) in the photo to show relative size.
- Use a string of known length to measure distance from the camera to the wound for consistency of photos over time.
- Use an identification sign with patient ID, wound location, and date in the photograph (unless dated by the camera).
- Select a camera with a zoom and/or macro feature, if possible, to take close-up views of the wound.
- If you are using an SLR-type camera, use a ring flash attachment on a 35-mm close-up lens to eliminate shadows.
- Use an assistant to help maintain the patient's position and perhaps to position the marker.
- Record wound and patient position for repeated photographing sessions (e.g., "right side-lying").

Using a Photographic Wound Assessment Tool

The Photographic Wound Assessment Tool (PWAT) is a modified version of the Bates-Jensen Wound Assessment Tool (BWAT) (see Chapter 5). It makes use of six domains of the BWAT that can be determined from photographs alone and do not require bedside assessment.[38] Each domain item of the PWAT is scored numerically, and a total score is calculated by adding the scores assigned to each of the six domains (Exhibit 4.8). The range of possible total PWAT scores is between 0 and 24, with zero representing a healed ulcer.[38]

The PWAT was applied and tested with pressure ulcers and leg ulcers and found to have high intertester and intratester reliability among experienced wound clinicians. It was also found to have high concurrent validity, based on the degree of agreement between SA calculations obtained from the wound photograph (n = 46), as compared to wound tracings and linear measurements. Researchers were able to divide the ulcers into "healers" and "nonhealers," based on the changes in wound SA, as measured by the PWAT. A comparison of PWAT scores revealed that there were almost statistically significant differences between the

two groups ($p = 0.07$). The highest reliability was achieved when the PWAT was applied to pressure ulcers, compared with leg ulcers, probably reflecting its derivation from the BWAT, which was designed for assessment of pressure ulcers.

Drawbacks to its use are the added costs associated with wound photography, the need for consent before taking photographs, and the impact on the decision-making process by the clinician.[38] However, the PWAT may play an important role in the field of wound telemedicine. A tool that gives you a reliable and easy-to-use method of quantifying the status of wounds from photographs could potentially improve the quality of outpatient wound care. Trials of telemedicine using digital photography show that wound evaluation on the basis of viewing digital images is comparable to standard wound examination and results in similar diagnoses, most of the time.[39]

Use of Video Teleconferencing

Interactive video teleconferencing has also been pilot tested on patients with wounds.[40] Video teleconferencing offers the benefit over still photography and digital imaging alone of allowing visualization of the wound from a variety of angles and positions with immediate feedback from the clinician, other health-care practitioners, patient, and family.[40] It is especially beneficial for patients with wounds who are unable to travel to health-care centers. Additional benefits to the health-care system includes more time efficient use of skilled personnel.[40]

A number of challenges to implementation of this type of service do exist. These include the difficulty of providing proper lighting and a private space designated for the teleconference, as well as the need to secure funding for purchase of the equipment and telecommunication services, and for operator training. Still,

---

HELPFUL HINTS

Making an Identification Marker for Photographs

1. Tape plastic measuring sheet to a 3 inches × 5 inches index card.
2. Put card into a plastic sandwich bag.
3. Put two strips of white tape on the plastic sandwich bag.
   - Write patient ID and wound location on the first strip (e.g., W.J., coccyx).
   - Write date on second strip (e.g., 01/23/2010).
4. Throw away the plastic bag.
5. Reuse the card.

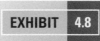

EXHIBIT   4.8

Six Domains of PWAT

1. Edges
2. Necrotic tissue type
3. Necrotic tissue amount
4. Skin color surrounding skin
5. Granulation tissue
6. Epithelialization

this technology holds potential for enhancing patient access to quality health-care services. Patients who experience telemedicine report being "very satisfied" with the telemedicine visit.[40] It is clear that telemedicine consult for wounds is increasing.

REFERRAL CRITERIA AND SOURCES

As you and your colleagues perform serial wound measurements, you may discover that a wound is not progressing or is on a downward course. In this case, a prompt referral for alternative or adjunctive treatment is necessary. The availability of advanced technologies for treatment, such as growth factors and tissue-engineered products, has made it very important to be able to recognize and understand the criteria for referral. To do that, you must have a valid and reliable way of measuring the efficacy of standard care. The standard care for chronic wounds has been well developed and includes pressure relief off-loading or compression, debridement, moisture balance, bacterial balance, and proper nutrition.

Consider referral when one or more of the following four criteria are met[41]: Initial ulcer size and duration indicates that standard care is likely to fail (e.g., large, deep ulcer of longer than 1-year duration):

- Rate of healing with standard care predicts failure (>30% healing)
- Wound fails to heal in predicted time, based on guideline of 30% to 47% reduction in size in 2 to 4 weeks
- Special circumstance exists, such as unusual diagnosis or patient demand
- Emergent referral is warranted when:
  - The extent of wound involves bone and/or deep subcutaneous spaces—may indicate osteomyelitis or other infection.
  - There is an impending exposure of a named anatomic structure—wound extent should be evaluated medically.
  - There are black holes or tunnels that cannot be measured—high-risk situation.
- Wound tunneling may perforate the peritoneal cavity in either the abdomen or rectum.
- Wound size is enlarging more than expected.

Many health-care practitioners have experience in complex wound management. If any of the referral criteria listed above is met, contact one or more of these professionals for follow-up management. Some choices are shown in Table 4.4.

SELF-CARE GUIDELINES

In today's health-care environment, family members and other at-home caregivers commonly measure and monitor the wound size parameters discussed in this chapter, reporting their findings to the expert clinician for interpretation. The most successful results occur when step-by-step instructions and repeated demonstrations are given to the designated data collector. Prepare an instruction sheet for measuring and/or tracing wounds and create a record such as that shown in Exhibit 4.9 for recording the data. The patient or caregiver can then send the record via e-mail or fax to the wound case manager.

Before beginning instruction, assess the individual's ability to follow directions. If the patient or a lay caregiver is going to perform the measurements, teach only the simple length-by-width method. It is helpful if you teach measurement methods in the same sequence each time (e.g., first length then width). If the person monitoring the wound is a paraprofessional, physical therapist assistant, or licensed practical nurse, you can teach additional wound measurements.

Both lay caregivers and paraprofessionals may also be capable of making wound tracings. Doing so can help them see that the wound is getting smaller as the report number decreases, or that the wound is changing in shape and size. This reinforces both the caregiver's and the patient's feeling of success. If the wound is not decreasing in size, this fact will be more obvious, triggering a change in treatment planning.

Instructions for Measuring a Wound at Home
Gather the following supplies
- Disposable wound measurement ruler (provided)
- Nonsterile disposable gloves
- Measurement form
- Waste disposal container

Follow these instructions
Wound measurements are taken once a week or biweekly.

1. Note the position of the patient (e.g., side-lying on right side)
2. Note the date.
3. Measure the longest diameter of the wound in each direction, head to toe (length) and side to side (width). Do in the same order each time.
4. Record the length and width in the appropriate boxes on the form as the measurements are taken.

TABLE 4.4	Referral Sources	
Physicians	**Nurses**	**Other Providers**
Dermatologist	Dermatology nurse	Physical therapist
Orthopedic surgeon	Wound ostomy continence nurse	Vascular technician
Plastic surgeon	Registered nurse	Podiatrist
Vascular surgeon	Geriatric nurse practitioner	
	Vascular nurse	

EXHIBIT 4.9

Wound Measurement Record
Name: _____   Medical Record #: _____

Date	Length (cm)	Width (cm)	Total (cm²)
4/30/14	5	3	15
5/15/14	4.5	2.5	11.25
5/30/14	4.0	1.75	8.8
6/15/14	2.5	1.25	3.13

Instructions for Making a Wound Tracing at Home
Gather the following supplies
- Plastic measuring sheet (provided), clear kitchen plastic wrap, or plastic sandwich bag
- Fine-point transparent film-type marking pen so that ink won't bead up on the plastic (dark Pentel™ or Vis-a-Vis™)
- Nonsterile disposable gloves

Follow these instructions
1. Use either two pieces of clear plastic wrap, or a plastic sandwich bag.
2. Place one layer of plastic against the clean wound. Place the second layer on top of the first. If the plastic becomes foggy, lift a corner of the plastic to allow the heat and moisture to escape, and the fog will go away.
3. When you can see the edges of the wound, use a fine point felt-tip marking pen to draw around the wound edges. Mark the date of the drawing beside the wound drawing.
4. After the ink is dry (about 10 seconds), lift the top layer of plastic wrap or cut off the top layer of the plastic bag.
5. Save the piece with the wound tracing in another clean plastic sandwich bag.
6. Discard the dirty plastic sheet.

CONCLUSION

This chapter described several measurement strategies for monitoring wound extent and healing by tracking change in six parameters of size: length, width, SA, undermining/tunneling, depth, and volume. Obviously, performing all of the above measurements on all wounds is not realistic. Hold a team meeting to decide on the method that meets the needs of the majority of practitioners and conveys the desired information. There is enough similarity among methods that the information communicated through the continuum of care can and will be readily interpreted. The keys to successful measurements are consistency and accuracy. Once a method is selected, incorporate it into the facility policies and procedures and then make sure it is used consistently by all clinicians.

REVIEW QUESTIONS

1. What is the most important consideration when taking wound measurements?
   A. Choosing the longest length
   B. Choosing the widest part
   C. Choosing a consistent method of taking measurements
   D. Choosing who will take the measurements
2. What anatomic feature of the wound needs to be identified for reliable wound measurements?
   A. Undermined area
   B. Wound edge
   C. Granulation tissue
   D. Wound depth
3. What is the healing rate expected for a wound that is on a healing trajectory?
   A. 15% to 25% in 2 to 4 weeks
   B. 10% to 15% in 2 to 4 weeks
   C. 30% to 50% in 2 to 4 weeks
   D. 75% to 80% in 2 to 4 weeks
4. To maximize the accuracy of wound measurements,
   A. Record even small changes
   B. Encourage all staff to participate
   C. Position the patient however they are comfortable
   D. Have a variety of terminology and units of measurement
5. When utilizing the clock method to measure a wound,
   A. Length is the longest measurement
   B. Width is the smallest measurement
   C. Length and width are added to determine SA
   D. Select a 12:00 reference position

RESOURCES

- Plastic/acetate measuring sheets are available from many wound care product manufacturers.

REFERENCES

1. vanRijswijk L. Frequency of reassessment of pressure ulcers: National Pressure Ulcer Advisory Panel Proceedings. *Adv Wound Care.* 1995:19–24.
2. Marston W, Carlin R, Passman M, et al. Healing rates and cost efficacy of outpatient compression treatment for leg ulcers associated with venous insufficiency. *J Vasc Surg.* 1999;30(3):491–498.
3. Tallman P, Muscare E, Carson P, et al. Initial rate of healing predicts complete healing of venous ulcers. *Arch Dermatol.* 1997;133(10):1231–1234.
4. Phillips T, Machado F, Trout R, et al. Prognostic indicators in venous ulcers. *J Am Acad Dermatol.* 2000;43(4):627–630.
5. Arnold T, Stanley J, Fellows E, et al. Prospective multicenter study of managing lower extremity venous ulcers. *Ann Vasc Surg.* 1994;8(4):356–362.
6. Sussman C, Swanson, GH. The utility of Sussman wound healing tool in predicting wound healing outcomes in physical therapy. Paper presented at National Pressure Ulcer Advisory Panel Fifth Biennial Conference, Washington, DC; 1997.
7. Salcido R. The future of wound measurement. *AdvSkin Wound Care.* 2000;13(2):54,56.

8. Van Poucke S, Nelissen R, Jorens P, et al. Comparative analysis of two methods of wound bed area measurement. *IntWounds*. 2010;7(5):366–77.

9. Sussman C, Swanson GH. A uniform method to trace and measure chronic wounds. Paper presented at Symposium for Advanced Wound Care, San Francisco, CA; 1991.

10. Schultz GS, Romanelli M, Claxton K. Wound healing and TIME: new concepts and scientific applications. *Wound Repair Regen*. 2005;13(4):S1–S11.

11. Taylor DR. Reliability of the Sussman method of measuring wounds that contain undermining. Paper presented at American Physical Therapy Association Scientific Meeting; April, San Diego, CA; 1997.

12. Maklebust J. PUSH tool reality check: audience response. *Adv Wound Care*. 1997;10(5):102–106.

13. Robson MC, Hill D, Woodske M, et al. Wound healing trajectories as predictors of effectiveness of therapeutic agents. *Arch Surg*. 2000;135(7):773–777.

14. Polansky M, vanRijswijk L. Utilizing survival analysis techniques in chronic wound healing studies. *Wounds: A Compendium of Clinical Research and Practice*. 1994;6(5):15–58.

15. vanRijswijk L. Full-thickness pressure ulcers: patient and wound healing characteristics. *Decubitus*. 1993;6(1):16–21.

16. vanRijswijk L, Polansky M. Predictors of time to healing deep pressure ulcers. *Ostomy Wound Manage*. 1994;40(8):40–48.

17. Kantor J, Margolis DJ. Expected healing rates for chronic wounds. *Wounds: A Compendium of Clinical Research and Practice*. 2000;12(6):155–158.

18. Pham HT, Falanga V, Sabolinski ML, et al. Healing rate measurement can predict complete wound healing rate in chronic diabetic foot ulceration. Paper presented at Symposium for Advanced Wound Care and Medical Research Forum on Wound Repair; May, Las Vegas, NV; 2001.

19. Sheehan PJP, Caselli A, Gurini JM, et al. Percent change in wound area of diabetic foot ulcers over a 4-week period is a robust predictor of complete healing in a 12-week prospective trial. *Diabetes Care*. 2003;26:1879–1882.

20. vanRijswijk L. Full-thickness leg ulcers: patient demographics and predictors of healing. Multi-center leg ulcer study group. *J Fam Pract*. 1993;36(6):625–632.

21. vanRijswijk L. Group M-CLUS. Full-thickness leg ulcers: patient demographics and predictors of time to healing. *J Fam Pract*. 1993;36(6):625–632.

22. Gilman TH. Parameter for measurement of wound closure. *Wounds: A Compendium of Clinical Research and Practice*. 1990;2(3):95–101.

23. Margolis DJ, Gross EA, Wood CR, et al. Planimetric rate of healing in venous ulcers of the leg treated with pressure bandage and hydrocolloid dressing. *J Am Acad Dermatol*. 1993;28(3):418–421.

24. Ramirez AT, Soroff HS, Schwartz MS, et al. Experimental wound healing in man. *Surg Gynecol Obstet*. 1969:283–293.

25. Gilman TH. Calculating healing rate of acute surgical wounds. In: Sussman C, ed. Torrance; 2001: email messages.

26. Pecoraro RE, Ahroni JH, Boyko EJ, et al. Chronology and determinants of tissue repair in diabetic lower extremity ulcers. *Diabetes*. 1991;40:1305–1313.

27. Cherry GW, Hill D, Poore S, et al. Initial healing rate of venous ulcers: are they useful as predictors and comparators of healing? Paper presented at Symposium for Advanced Wound Care and Medical Research Forum on Wound Repair; May, Las Vegas, NV; 2001.

28. Cukjati DRS, Karba R, Miclavici D. Modelling of chronic wound healing dynamics. *Med Biol Eng Comput*. 2000;38:339–347.

29. Hess CT. *Nurse's Clinical Guide, Wound Care*. Springhouse, PA: Springhouse; 1995.

30. Flanagan M. Wound measurement: can it help us to monitor progression to healing? *J Wound Care*. 2003:189–194.

31. Keast DH, Bowering CK, Evans AW, et al. CS MEASURE: a proposed assessment framework for developing best practice recommendations for wound assessment. *Wound Repair Regen*. 2004;12:1–17.

32. Gentzkow G. Methods for measuring size in pressure ulcers. National Pressure Ulcer Advisory Panel Proceedings. *Adv Wound Care*. 1995:43–45.

33. Banks PBK, Washington MO, Stubblefield AM, et al. Fluid volume measurements: the gold standard? Paper presented at 15th Annual Meeting and Exposition of the Wound Healing Society, Chicago, IL; 2005.

34. Langemo DK, Melland H, Hanson D, et al. Two-dimensional wound measurement: comparison of 4 techniques. *Adv Wound Care*. 1998;11(7):337–343.

35. Majeske C. Reliability of wound surface area measurement. *Phys Ther*. 1992;72:138–141.

36. Harding K. Methods for assessing change in ulcer status. *Adv Wound Care*. 1995:37–42.

37. Sussman C. Physical therapy choices for wound recovery. *Ostom Wound Manage*. 1990; 29:20–28.

38. Houghton PE, Kincaid CB, Campbell K, et al. Photographic assessment of the appearance of chronic pressure and leg ulcers. *Ostom Wound Manage*. 2000;46(4):20–30.

39. Wirthlin D, Buradagunta S, Edwards R, et al. Telemedicine in vascular surgery: feasibility of digital imaging for remote management of wounds. *J Vasc Surg*. 1998;27(6):1089–1099.

40. Ratliff CR. Telehealth for wound management in long-term care. *Ostom Wound Manage*. 2005;51(9):40–45. www.hmpcommunications.com

41. Eaglstein W. What is standard care and where should we leave it? Paper presented at Evidence Based Outcomes in Wound Management; March, Dallas, TX; 2000.

SUGGESTED READINGS

Gilman TH. Parameter for measurement of wound closure. *Wounds*. 1990;2(3):95–101.

Polansky M, vanRijswijk L. Utilizing survival analysis techniques in chronic wound healing studies. *Wounds*. 1994;6(5):15–58.

CHAPTER 5

Tools to Measure Wound Healing

Barbara M. Bates-Jensen and Carrie Sussman

CHAPTER OBJECTIVES

At the completion of this chapter, the reader will be able to:

1. Identify the criteria used to evaluate wound healing tools.
2. Identify the wound characteristics commonly included in wound healing assessment tools.
3. Describe the development and use of three wound healing tools:
   - Sussman Wound Healing Tool (SWHT)
   - Pressure Ulcer Scale for Healing (PUSH)
   - The Bates-Jensen Wound Assessment Tool (BWAT)
4. Describe wound healing tools developed for specific needs or populations.

Most clinical standards and practice guidelines require assessment of wounds to determine healing at least weekly. Clearly, this demonstrates agreement on the importance of frequent evaluation; however, the best method for evaluating wound healing has not been agreed on.

As you learned in Chapter 3, classification or staging systems—which assess wound tissue appearance—are appropriate for determining the initial severity of damage but are inadequate for measuring wound healing. Use of a single wound characteristic has not been helpful in monitoring healing, determining treatment response, or prescribing therapy. Thus, there is general agreement on the need for assessment of multiple wound characteristics to monitor and measure healing. In addition, although limited data exist to demonstrate improved outcomes by using a standardized, research-based tool, use of a systematic approach promotes effective communication among those involved in the wound care plan and is recommended in clinical practice guidelines.

Several such tools have been proposed;[1-9] this chapter focuses on the SWHT,[5] the PUSH,[2] and the BWAT,[1] which are currently in use for clinical practice or research in the United States and internationally. All are standardized tools that assess multiple wound characteristics to enable the clinician to evaluate healing. This chapter describes these tools, exploring how each was developed, its attributes, and its use in clinical practice. Three additional tools that focus on specific needs or populations are also presented including the Photographic Wound Assessment Tool (a derivation of the BWAT),[6] The Wound Bed Score,[8] and the Spinal Cord Injury-Pressure Ulcer Monitoring Tool (SCI-PUMT). Table 5.1 shows the wound characteristics and scoring systems used by these tools.

CRITERIA FOR EVALUATING WOUND HEALING TOOLS

Before deciding on which tool to use in your clinical practice, it may be helpful to understand the psychometric properties of the tool. Psychometric properties of validity and reliability provide important information on how useful a tool is likely to be when used by different clinicians and with various patient populations. Criteria to evaluate the appropriateness and utility of a tool include validity, reliability, responsiveness, and clinical practicality. We hope this basic discussion will help you to understand better the use of an evidence-based instrument for measuring wound healing.

Validity

Validity is the accuracy with which an instrument or test measures what it purports to measure.[10] Validity is *context specific*, meaning that a tool that is valid in one study or clinical setting may not be valid for another study or clinical setting. For instance, a tool that is valid for measuring healing in pressure ulcers in elders may not be valid for measuring healing in lower extremity vascular ulcers or in persons with spinal cord injury. Validity, as it relates to tool development, is a cyclical process. When indicated, information from validity testing may be used to change a tool to increase validity, and then the newly revised tool is retested. There are three main qualities in validity:

- *Content validity* is the degree to which an instrument measures an intended content area. For example, if the tool is intended to measure wound healing in lower extremity ulcers, are the areas that are important in healing of lower extremity ulcers actually included on the tool? Content validity is often determined

TABLE 5.1	Comparison of Wound Healing Tools

Wound Characteristics and Format	SWHT	PUSH	BWAT, previously PSST	PWAT	WBS	SCI-PUMT
Size	X	X	X	X		X
Depth or stage	X		X	X	X	X
Necrotic tissue	X	X	X	X	X	X
Granulation tissue	X	X	X	X	X	
Epithelial tissue	X	X	X	X	X	
Surrounding tissue Characteristics	X		X	X	X	
Exudate		X	X	X	X	X
Undermining and tunneling	X		X	X		X
Scoring Methods						
Likert scale			X	X	X	X
Subscales with total score	X	X	X		X	X

using an expert panel whose members rate, in some manner, the items on the tool and the tool's ability to measure the objective. Guidelines are available for interpreting content validity but, in clinical practice, evaluation of how the tool was developed, who was involved, where knowledge of the content was obtained, and the outcome of the expert panel is usually enough information. Ratings of the content specialists are only as good as their levels of expertise in the area measured.

- *Criterion validity* evaluates the relationship between the instrument and some other criterion. Criterion validity is concerned with the pragmatic issue: is the tool a useful predictor? Two types of criterion validity are concurrent and predictive. *Concurrent validity* tests the tool against present performance or status on a criterion. An example of concurrent validity for wound healing tools is the ability of a tool to separate partial- and full-thickness wounds, based on their scores on the tool. *Predictive validity* tests the tool against future performance or status on a criterion. An example is the ability of a tool to predict wound closure. Predictive validity can be either positive or negative; for instance, a tool would be equally beneficial if it predicted those wounds that would not heal as it would if it predicted wounds that would heal. It also includes the characteristics of sensitivity and specificity, both of which involve precision and accuracy of the instrument. For example, a sensitive wound healing assessment tool should be able to determine all of the wounds that have improved. And in an ideal world, a tool should be 100% specific to the condition being measured.
- *Construct validity* focuses on the tool's ability to function in accordance with the purpose for which it is being used. For instance, tools to measure wound healing should function by identifying wounds that are healing or nonhealing (the purpose for which the wound healing tool is being used).[11]

Reliability

Our next criterion for evaluating wound healing assessment tools is *reliability*, a tool's ability to be used with minimal random error. Reliability reflects the consistency of the measure obtained and is concerned with accuracy, dependability, consistency, and comparability of the tool. Note that a tool can be very reliable and still not meet the criteria for validity, but it is not possible to have a tool that is valid and not reliable. In other words, reliability is also an essential component of validity.

As with validity, reliability estimates are specific to the population in the sample being tested. In clinical practice, this means that a wound healing tool that works for one type of organization may not work for another type of organization, or another type of clinician user. For example, a tool may be reliable when used by physicians but nurse aides may be unable to use the same tool with reliability. Each organization may have to test the tools to determine which work most reliably for the clinician users and the organization.

There are three aspects of reliability:

- *Stability reliability* or *intrarater reliability* is the consistency of the tool with repeated measures. Ideally in this type of reliability, the same clinician gets the same score when observing the same wound repeatedly at different times. This is often difficult to demonstrate with wound healing tools as wounds themselves change over time, thus scores from a wound healing tool would also change.
- *Equivalence or interrater reliability* is concerned with different clinicians getting the same score on the tool when evaluating the same wound. This is essential as there is no benefit to using a wound assessment tool that cannot be accurately used by different clinicians equally well.
- *Homogeneity* is the similarity or "sameness" of items within an instrument. That is, all items on a tool should consistently measure the same objective. For example, the presence or absence granulation tissue and the amount of exudate both contribute to measuring aspects of wound healing.

Responsiveness

Responsiveness, or sensitivity to change, is another criterion for evaluating a tool. An appropriate tool must be able to detect changes in the condition of the wound over time with repeated administrations, and to respond with a change in tool score.

In other words, responsiveness is the ability of the tool to respond quickly to changes in the wound status.

Clinical Practicality

Clinical practicality, our final criterion, means that the tool must be simple, easy to learn, and easy to use, with clear instructions. It must be time-efficient. The tool must also provide data that are meaningful enough to warrant the additional time and energy required to complete the assessment. In a clinically practical tool, the level of the language used, the understandability of the items, the scoring mechanisms, and any mathematical calculations required must be appropriate for the intended user.

WOUND CHARACTERISTICS ASSESSED IN WOUND HEALING MEASUREMENT TOOLS

This section provides a brief description of wound characteristics commonly included in wound assessment instruments. More comprehensive descriptions of wound characteristics are found in Chapter 3. The precise characteristics included in any given tool vary according to the purpose of the instrument (prediction of healing, assessment of wound status, prescription of treatment, etc.) and the philosophy of the instrument developers.

Location

Assess the location of the wound by identifying where the lesion occurs on the patient's anatomy. As discussed in Chapter 3, body diagrams are typically used to document wound location. Location may also be identified by choosing the anatomic site from a list. Specific wound locations beneficial or detrimental to healing are still to be determined.

Shape

Some assessment tools measure wound shape. Wound shape, which also helps to determine the overall size of the wound, is determined by evaluating the perimeter of the wound. Shape of the wound is related to wound contraction: as wounds heal, they often change shape and may begin to assume a more regular, circular/oval shape. Compare Figures 5.1 to 5.3 to see the onset and progression of contraction and epithelialization. It is identified by a change in wound open area size as well as a change in wound shape (e.g., from irregular to symmetric, such as the circular or oval formation and rounding off of the edges of the wound). One wound shape deserves mention, the butterfly shape or mirror image pressure ulcer on the sacrum. This shape is important because it has been associated with rapid evolution and mortality. The butterfly shape as seen in Figure 5.4 has been suggested as a characteristic of terminal pressure ulcers related to skin failure.[12,13]

Size

Most tools include some measure of size. Size can be determined by measuring (in cm) the longest and perpendicularly widest aspect of the wound surface that is visible. Determine surface area by multiplying the length by the width. It can be difficult to determine where to measure size on some wounds, because the edge of the wound may be hard to visualize or the edge may be irregular. This is a skill that takes practice. Use of the same reference points for determining size improves the reliability and meaningfulness of the measures. In clinical practice, one of two reference points are used; the longest aspect of

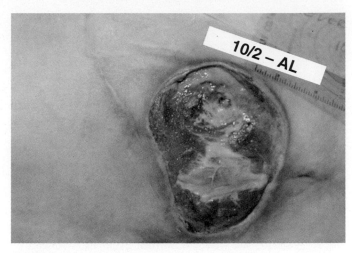

FIGURE 5.1 Stage IV pressure ulcer on sacrum with stringy yellow slough evident. Note the epidermal ridge formation. (Copyright © C. Sussman.)

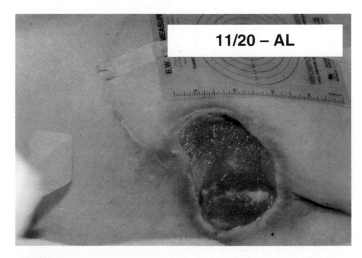

FIGURE 5.2 Same wound as in Figure 5.1. The wound shows evidence of contraction with a smaller surface area. Healthy granulation tissue present throughout wound bed. (Copyright © C. Sussman.)

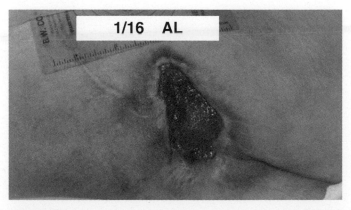

FIGURE 5.3 Same wound as in Figures 5.1 and 5.2. The wound is now 100% filled with healthy granulation tissue. Note sustained wound contraction and evidence of epithelialization. (Copyright © C. Sussman.)

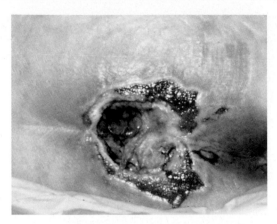

FIGURE 5.4 Butterfly-shaped pressure ulcer on the sacrum. Note also soft, soggy black eschar present. (Copyright © B.M. Bates-Jensen.)

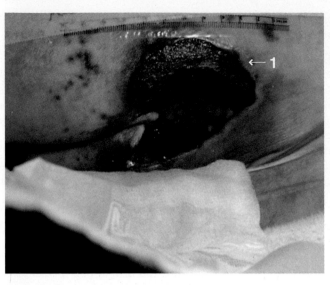

FIGURE 5.6 Full-thickness pressure ulcer that is bowl or crater-shaped. The wound has edges that are not attached to the wound base. (Copyright © C. Sussman.)

the wound and perpendicular widest aspect of the wound or the length of the wound from head to toe (or using a clock face to represent the body, 12 o'clock—the head to 6 o'clock—the feet) and the width of the wound from side to side (or 3 o'clock to 9 o'clock). (Chapter 4 has step-by-step procedures for measuring size, depth, and undermining.)

Depth

Measure the depth of the wound as explained in Chapter 4. Multiple measures of depth within the wound can increase reliability of depth evaluation. Some tools evaluate wound depth using description of tissues involved instead of numeric measurements.

Edges

The edges of the wound reflect some of the most important characteristics of the wound. When assessing edges, consider the following qualities:

- *Distinctness.* Look for how clear and distinct the wound outline appears. If the edges are indistinct and diffuse, there are areas where the normal tissues blend into the wound bed. Well-defined edges are clear and distinct and can be outlined easily on a transparent piece of plastic.
- *Attachment.* Edges that are even with the skin surface and the wound base are edges that are attached to the base of the wound. This means that the wound is flat, with no appreciable

depth. Edges that are not attached to the base of the wound imply a wound with some depth of tissue involvement (see Fig. 5.5). The wound that is a crater or has a bowl/boat shape is a wound with edges that are not attached to the wound base as shown in Figure 5.6. The wound has walls or sides. There is depth to the wound.

- *Thickness.* As the wound ages, the edges become rolled under and thickened to palpation. Wounds of long duration may continue to thicken, with scar tissue and fibrosis developing in the wound edge, causing the edge to feel hard, rigid, and indurated. Hyperkeratosis is the callus-like tissue that may form around the wound edges, especially with diabetic ulcers (see Chapters 3 and 12).
- *Color.* The edge achieves a unique coloring with time. The pigment turns a grayish hue in both dark- and light-skinned persons.

Evaluate the wound edges by visual inspection and palpation. Figures 5.5 to 5.7 show wounds with different edges.

Undermining/Tunneling

Some wound assessment tools include an evaluation of undermining or pocketing and tunneling. As explained in Chapters 3 and 4,

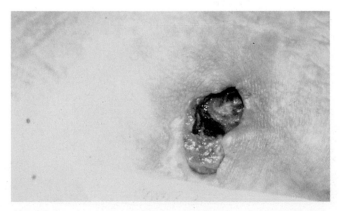

FIGURE 5.5 Full-thickness pressure ulcer with wound edges that are not attached to the base of the wound. The edges are rolled and thickened. (Copyright © B. M. Bates-Jensen.)

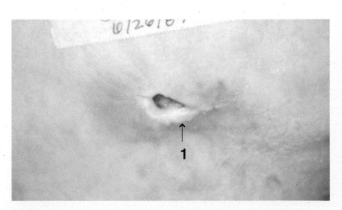

FIGURE 5.7 Pressure ulcer with chronic fibrosis and scarring at the wound edge. The edge is rolled and thickened and indurated to palpation. (Copyright © B.M. Bates-Jensen.)

CLINICAL WISDOM

Tips for Assessing Wound Edges

Definitions for help in assessing wound edges:

- Indistinct, diffuse—unable to distinguish wound outline clearly
- Attached—even or flush with wound base, no sides or walls present, flat
- Not attached—sides or walls are present; floor or base of wound is deeper than edge
- Rolled under, thickened—soft to firm and flexible to touch
- Hyperkeratosis—callus-like tissue formation around wound and at edges
- Color—intensified color, increased pigmentation with grey hue at edge

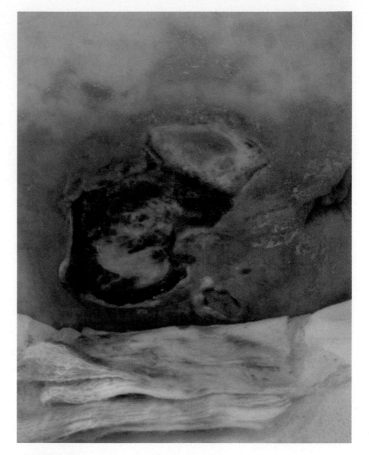

FIGURE 5.8 Sacral pressure ulcer with yellow slough and black necrotic areas present. Large amount of serosanguineous exudate present, the dressing is saturated. (Copyright © B.M. Bates-Jensen.)

undermining and tunneling represent the loss of tissue underneath an intact skin surface. Typically, instruments measure undermining and tunneling as either present or absent or with measurements of the extent of the processes. If measurements are used, the percent of the wound edge involved in the process and the distance the process extends from the edge are evaluated.

Necrosis

Necrosis is dead, devitalized tissue. Characteristics of necrotic tissue included in most wound healing measurement tools include *presence, amount, color, consistency or moisture content,* and *adherence to the wound bed.* In most cases, the clinician is asked to choose the predominant characteristic present in the wound. For additional information on necrosis, see Chapters 3 and 17 and Figures 5.4 and 5.8.

The amount of necrotic tissue present in the wound is evaluated by one of two methods. One method involves using clinical judgment to estimate the percentage of the wound covered with necrosis. Picture the wound as a pie and divide it into four (25%) quadrants. Look at each quadrant and judge how much necrosis is present. Add up the total percentage from judgments of each quadrant; this determines the percentage of the wound involved. A second method involves actual linear measurements of the necrotic tissue. Measure the length and width of the necrosis and multiply to determine surface area of necrosis.

Exudate/Drainage

Most wound healing measurement tools require evaluation of exudate or drainage type and amount. Evaluating exudate type can be tricky because of the moist wound healing dressings used on most wounds. Some dressings interact with wound drainage to produce a gel or fluid, and others may trap liquid and drainage at the wound site. Before assessing exudate type, gently cleanse the wound with normal saline or water and evaluate fresh exudate. Additionally, observe the wound dressing for exudate prior to discarding it. Pick the exudate type that is predominant in the wound, according to color and consistency.

To judge the amount of exudate in the wound, observe two areas: the wound itself and the dressing used on the wound. Observe the wound for the moisture present. Are the tissues dry and desiccated? Are they swimming in exudate? Is the drainage spread throughout the wound? Use clinical judgment to determine how wet the wound is. Evaluate the dressing used on the wound for how much it interacts with exudate. (See also Chapter 18 for management of exudate and infection.) Figures 5.9 to 5.12 show different characteristics of exudate.

Surrounding Skin Characteristics

The tissues surrounding the wound are often the first indication of impending further tissue damage. Some wound healing assessment tools include evaluation for

- Color, including erythema
- Edema
- Induration
- Maceration
- Hemorrhage or hematoma

Information on assessing for these characteristics of surrounding skin was provided in Chapter 3.

Granulation Tissue

Most wound-measurement tools include assessment of the wound bed for granulation tissue. As presented in Chapter 2, the presence of granulation tissue signals the proliferative phase

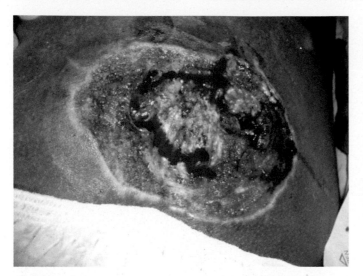

FIGURE 5.9 Wound with bleeding or sanguineous exudate. (Copyright © B.M. Bates-Jensen.)

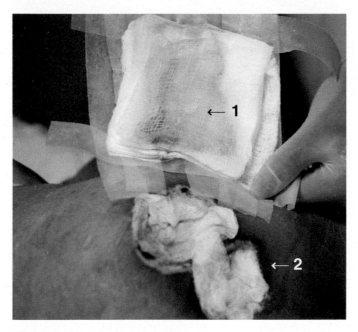

FIGURE 5.10 Wound with packing still present, note the moderate amount of serous exudate on dressing. The green color suggests possible infection. (Copyright © C. Sussman.)

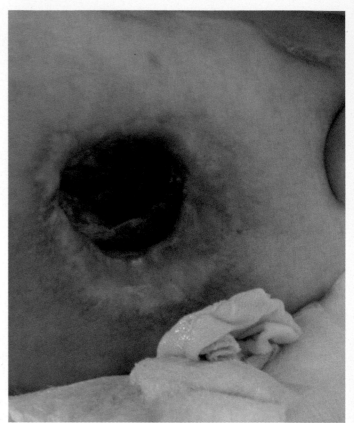

FIGURE 5.11 Full-thickness stage IV pressure ulcer with moderate amount of serous exudate. (Copyright © B.M. Bates-Jensen.)

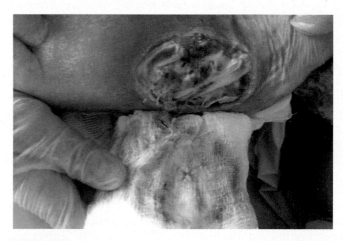

FIGURE 5.12 Wound with moderate amount of purulent exudate. (Copyright © B.M. Bates-Jensen.)

of wound healing. It is present in full-thickness wounds only. Partial-thickness wounds do not require granulation tissue formation for wound healing. Granulation tissue is healthy when it is bright, beefy red, shiny, and granular with a velvety appearance. The tissue looks bumpy and may bleed. Well-vascularized granulation tissue can be seen in Figures 5.13 and 5.14.

Epithelialization

As discussed in Chapter 2, epithelialization is the process of epidermal resurfacing and appears as pink or red skin. Figures 5.15 to 5.17A–D show the process of epidermal resurfacing. In partial-thickness wounds, the epithelial cells migrate from islands on the wound surface as well as from the wound edges. In full-thickness wounds, epidermal resurfacing occurs

from the edges only. Use of a transparent measuring guide can be helpful to determine percentage of the wound involved in resurfacing and to measure the distance that the epithelial tissue extends into the wound from proliferative edges.

Use of Wound Characteristics Assessment in Specific Measurement Tools

The wound healing measurement tools discussed in this chapter include assessments of some combination of the foregoing characteristics. All evaluate tissue attributes of the wound, and several evaluate surrounding skin. Methods of assessment,

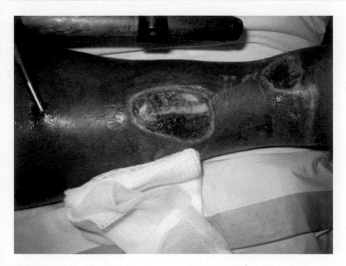

FIGURE 5.13 Traumatic wound with healthy granulation tissue present. Note bumpy appearance.

format, and scoring differ. Copies of the SWHT, PUSH, and BWAT tools and instructions for their use are found in this chapter's appendixes.

SUSSMAN WOUND HEALING TOOL

The SWHT was developed by Sussman and Swanson[5] to monitor and track the effectiveness of physical therapy technologies used for pressure ulcer healing. The monitoring and tracking of healing and treatment outcomes are essential for clinical decision making and triage. In addition, they improve utilization management for payers and providers. The SWHT is based on the acute wound healing model and can be applied to chronic wounds, such as pressure ulcers, as well.

Development of the SWHT
The basis for the SWHT is the acute wound healing model (see Chapter 2) that describes the changes in tissue status and size over time as the wound progresses through the physiologic

phases of wound healing. Chronic wounds heal by the same process but much slower due to complicating factors as described in Chapter 3. Some attributes of the wound that are observed during each phase are considered to be related to failure to heal or "not good for healing," and others are considered to be indicators of improvement or "good for healing." For example, necrosis is thought to be negative or not good for healing, whereas granulation tissue is considered good for healing. The concept of the SWHT is to benchmark the wound attributes as it recovers and progresses throughout the healing phases. For example, the "not good" attribute, necrosis, should change over time from present to absent, thus moving from "not good for healing" to "good for healing." The "good for healing" attribute, granulation, significant reduction in depth should be observed as the wound heals and changes from absent to present, which indicates improved tissue status.

SWHT is a qualitative instrument, meaning that a wound would be described as having certain tissue attributes. It is composed of 10 wound and periwound skin attributes,

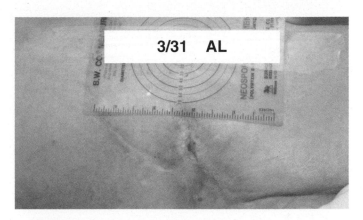

FIGURE 5.15 Same wound as in Figures 5.1 to 5.3 fully resurfaced with epithelial tissue. (Copyright © C. Sussman.)

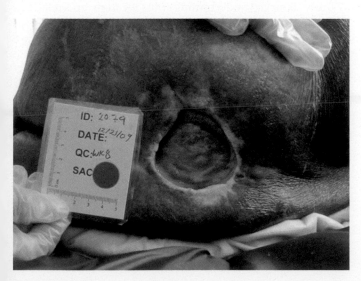

FIGURE 5.14 Stage IV pressure ulcer with pale initial granulation tissue. (Copyright © B.M. Bates-Jensen.)

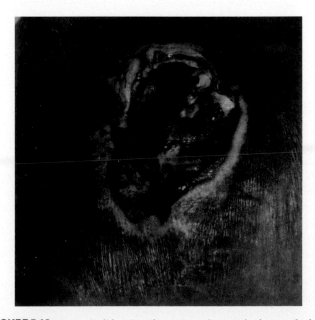

FIGURE 5.16 Acute proliferative phase. Note the attached wound edges from the 12:00 to 6:00 positions and how well vascularized granulation tissue fills up one side of the ulcer. A new pink border of epithelium surrounds the granulation tissue. (Copyright © B.M. Bates-Jensen.)

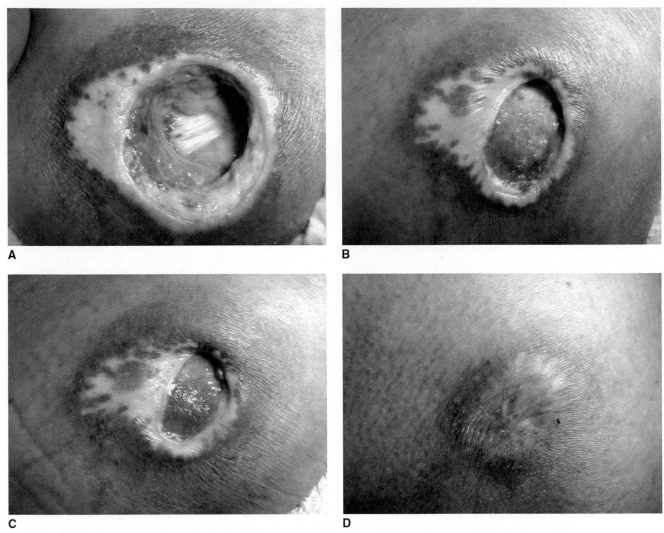

FIGURE 5.17   A–D Series with same wound showing contraction and epithelialization process. **A.** Pressure ulcer in early stages of proliferative phase of wound healing. Minimal epithelialization present. **B.** Ulcer is now clean with evidence of re-epithelialization noted at the wound edge. New epithelial tissue appears as bright pink tissue at edge of wound. **C.** 50% of original wound is now reepithelialized. **D.** Wound closed and fully resurfaced with epithelial tissue. (Copyright © B.M. Bates-Jensen.)

CLINICAL WISDOM

Appearance of Unhealthy Granulation Tissue

Unhealthy granulation tissue due to poor vascular supply appears as pale pink or blanched to dull, dusky red color. Usually, the first layer of granulation tissue to be laid down in the wound is pale pink; as the granulation tissue deepens and thickens, the color becomes the bright, beefy red color. Try to judge what percentage of the wound has been filled with granulation tissue. This is much easier if there is history with the wound. If the same person follows the wound over multiple observations, it is simple to judge the amount of granulation tissue present in the wound. If the initial observation of the wound was done by a different observer or if the data are not available, simply use best judgment to determine the amount of tissue present.

combined with 9 descriptive attributes of depth, and extent of tissue damage (undermining) plus location, and relationship to the acute wound healing phase, which are not measurable. All wound depth and undermining attributes are each assigned a score, as in Part I, of present or absent but are not ranked. It has been suggested that the tracking of tunneling in addition to undermining would be useful to show wound extent. That can be added to the tool without significantly changing its descriptive qualities. Since undermining and tunneling changes occur more slowly than change in tissue attributes, another suggestion is to evaluate the tissue attributes as in Part I weekly and those attributes in Part II at 2- to 4-week intervals.

Use of the SWHT

Appendix 5A shows the two parts of the long version of the SWHT with definitions for each of the attributes and the procedure for using the SWHT. Part I is the collection form for 10 wound and surrounding tissue attributes. Part II is the list of

11 other attributes, including extent, location, and wound healing phase. All items on the SWHT are scored present (1) or absent (0) except location and the wound healing phase. Omission of a score indicates that the assessment of the attribute was not completed.

Scoring begins at baseline, week 0. This reporting format is readily compatible with computer technology and simplifies using the tool to build a database.

Completion of the form requires understanding of the definitions for each of the scored items. This is discussed next. Notice that the assessment process is visual except for determining the presence of undermining/tunneling, which cannot be seen at the surface, and measurement of the open surface area of the wound. Assessment of tissue attributes is described in more detail in Chapter 3 and reviewed earlier in this chapter. Chapter 4 teaches how to measure wounds and use this information for wound prognosis.

Explanations of SWHT Attributes
Part I: Tissue Attributes

The first five attributes listed in Part I of the SWHT are hemorrhage, maceration, undermining/tunneling, erythema, and necrosis. Of these five attributes, hemorrhage present at *baseline* was ranked as the most statistically significant attribute for prediction of nonhealing and was followed at *week 1* by maceration, undermining, erythema, and necrosis.[6] Therefore, these are all classified as attributes "not good for healing". These items require a brief explanation. As you learned in Chapter 3, hemorrhagic tissue appearance can signify deep tissue injury and maceration indicates very friable tissue that is easily traumatized and subject to breakdown with subsequent wound enlargement. Undermining, or the excavation of subcutaneous tissues, as recently discussed, occurs in full-thickness wounds, and is an indicator of wound severity. On the SWHT Part I, it is recorded if present at any one or more of four locations corresponding to the four quadrants of the clock around the wound perimeter. The extent of undermining is not recorded or included as part of the assessment; only the presence or absence of this attribute if it is greater than 0.2 cm. This attribute should be measured as described in Chapter 4. Erythema, as used in this tool, refers to redness or darkening of the skin in darkly pigmented skin, in the periwound skin and is usually accompanied by heat. Necrosis as used here includes all types of necrotic tissue from eschar to slough.

Figure 5.18 shows an ulcer with hemorrhagic tissue, maceration, erythema, necrosis, and undermining. On the SWHT, all five items would be recorded as present and scored as "1."

The second five attributes—adherence at wound edge, granulation tissue, contraction, sustained contraction, and epithelialization—are all classified as good for healing. These items also require a brief explanation.

Adherence at the wound edge means that there is continuity of the wound edge and the base of the wound at *any* location along the wound perimeter (refer to Figs. 5.1–5.3). By definition, a partial-thickness wound will be adhered at all the wound edges (see Fig. 5.19). A full-thickness or deeper wound will have closed by either granulation or contraction to the point where some area of the wound edge will be even with the skin surface (see Fig. 5.1).

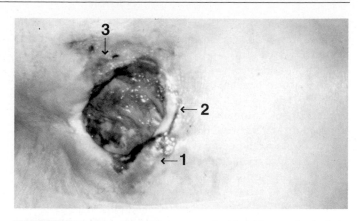

FIGURE 5.18 Pressure ulcer shows a wound with (*1*) hemorrhagic tissue at the wound edge, (*2*) maceration from wound fluid, (*3*) new superficial damage with signs of inflammation. (Copyright © B.M. Bates-Jensen.)

Granulation tissue is evaluated by measuring wound depth, with a significant reduction in depth indicating proliferation of granulation tissue formation. A significant reduction in depth is defined as at least 0.2 cm change in linear depth measurements since the prior assessment. Figures 5.1 to 5.3 show a significant reduction in depth.

Contraction is assessed as being present when the open surface area size of the wound reduces. This item is scored at subsequent assessments as the contraction continues or if it has stopped. If the wound enlarges, however, this item would change from present to absent, and a new appearance of contraction would be required to have a score of "present" again.

Sustained contraction means there is a continued drawing together of the wound edges that is measured by a reduction

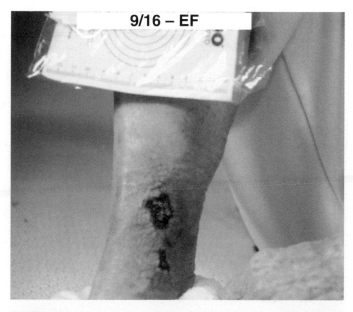

FIGURE 5.19 Wound edges are attached to the wound base; there is evidence of wound contraction. The edges are soft, irregular with evidence of new epithelialization. The wound is in an epithelialization phase. (Copyright © C. Sussman.)

in wound surface open area size. It is usually accompanied by a change in wound shape. (Again refer to Figs. 5.1–5.3.) These figures show the same wound as it goes through wound contraction. Sustained contraction is scored 0 at the appearance of the contraction benchmark, then scored 1 at *subsequent* reassessment (see Figs. 5.2 and 5.3), following the appearance of contraction. Occasionally, something interferes with the wound contraction, and the wound does not reduce in size or increases. This attribute would be marked 0—absent—if the wound size does not reduce or enlarges after the appearance of contraction.

Notice that the not-good-for-healing attributes are all related to attributes that are commonly observed when the wound is in a chronic inflammatory phase of healing as presented in Chapter 3. The attributes that are good for healing are related to the acute proliferative and epithelialization phases of healing. Thus, indicating that the wound is progressing through the phases corresponding to those of acute wound healing.

Part II: Size Location and Wound Healing Phase Measures

Wound depth and undermining indicate extent of wound. If a wound has a depth less than 0.2 cm, it is scored as 0 at all four points and at general depth. Greater depth and undermining means that the wound has extended into subcutaneous tissues and the wound is now full thickness, which are two indicators of "not good for healing."

11–15: Wound Depth

Five items on Part II of the SWHT are related to presence of depth of at least 0.2 cm, both in general depth and at the four points of the clock—the 12, 3, 6, and 9 o'clock positions. Depth is measured as described in Chapter 4, and if it is at least 0.2 cm, it is recorded as present. Extent of depth is not reported for this assessment as long as it is at least 0.2 cm. Figure 5.20 has greater than 0.2 cm and is classified as full-thickness depth.

16–19: Undermining/Tunneling

Undermining and tunneling are measured at all four points of the clock, like depth. Likewise, the indication used to report this attribute is present or absent at each point The more points

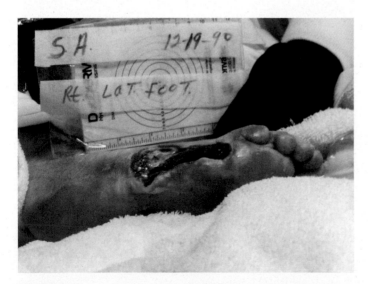

FIGURE 5.20 Soft, soggy necrosis and bruising often referred to as "purple" ulcer. Food shows signs of cellulitis and edema. Acute inflammatory phase. (Copyright © C. Sussman.)

of undermining and tunneling measured the greater the risk for slower healing and the larger the wound extent.

Additional Descriptive Attributes
Wound Location

A blank line is provided to note the wound location. Indicate the region most closely related to the wound site as follows: *UB* for upper body, *C* for coccyx, *T* for trochanter, *I* for ischial, *H* for heel, and *F* for foot. Wounds in other locations can be added to the list if they are commonly seen in the practice setting by using letters on the form and adding a location descriptor to the key (e.g., *K* = knee, *A* = abdomen, *Th* = thigh). Be sure to include the side of the body where the wound is located—right or left—by putting an *R* or an *L* next to the location letter.

Wound Healing Phase

The wound healing phase refers to the four biologic phases of wound healing. Letters are used to represent the current wound healing phase: *I* for inflammatory, *P* for proliferative, *E* for epithelialization, and *R* for remodeling. As described in Chapter 3, the wound healing phase may be chronic, acute, or absent. Placing the letter *C* before the phase indicates chronic. No letter before the phase indicates the acute. You may use the letter *L* for lacking or absent. A change in phase over time is an expected outcome. Chronicity of a phase should change to an active state of the phase, followed by progression to the next phase in the trajectory. Absence of a phase indicates need for investigation as to why the phase has not been achieved. This item is listed but unscored.

SWHT Reliability and Practicality

The SWHT has been clinically tested for reliability and clinical practicality by physical therapists (PTs) and PT assistants working in long-term care facilities. It has been found to be very reliable for monitoring and tracking healing and nonhealing of pressure ulcers. Its clinical practicality is high. It relies primarily on visual observation skills. No linear measurements, arithmetic calculations, or estimates of amount of tissue characteristic present are required. To health-care professionals who treat wounds, the SWHT information communicates wound progress or risk. Documentation is simple, and outcomes are visual. For example, it takes the clinician about 5 minutes to complete the assessment. In a trial educational session, a group of 10 PTs and PT assistants, who received 1 hour of classroom training followed by 1 hour of clinical practice on pressure ulcer patients, learned to use it well.

Assessment of Treatment Outcomes

The initial reason for development of the SWHT was to assess treatment outcome. Most patients are referred to the PT by the nurse for treatment after conventional treatments fail to heal the wound. To qualify for an intervention by the PT, the patient and the wound often need to meet a criterion of no progress, regression, or a halt of healing. Once the patient has been referred, the PT would use the SWHT to set target outcomes, and then for reporting wound outcomes associated with the interventions, such as biophysical agents discussed in Part IV of this book. Response to treatment with these interventions should demonstrate consistent change in tissue status that corresponds to the biologic model for acute wound healing. A change in tissue status benchmarks the healing process and becomes a target functional outcome for reporting purposes, such as the wound will be hemorrhage free, undermining free, necrosis free, and so forth. Clinicians can quickly determine a change in wound tissue status during the course of care because, as already described, the wound attributes should change from those that are not good for healing to those that are good for healing.

SWHT Forms
Form A

There are two forms of the SWHT (see Appendix 5A). Form A, Part I contains the 10 tissue attributes, listed in descending order of severity, next to an explanation of each s, followed by a column listing the rating option for the attribute as present or not present. The next column ranks the relationship to healing as not good or good. The last column is where the rating is listed as a score of present or absent. Part II lists measures and extent. The same scoring system of present or absent for 19 attributes of extent is applied. The attributes are the general depth of greater than 0.2 cm, the depth at the four clock points, and undermining at the four clock points. Date and week of care should be noted on the form. The benefit of this form is having the definitions on the form. This would be helpful to a nurse or PT learning the system or for medical reviewers and surveyors looking for information about the rating system used for documentation.

Form B of the SWHT is the same as Form A, except that in this version the form lacks the explanations printed on the form. Form B lists only the attributes and has columns to record data for multiple weeks as shown in Exhibits 5.1A and 5.1B.

CASE STUDY

Using SWHT Form B

Patient History

Bed and wheelchair bound 90-year-old female with a recurrent pressure ulcer in the left scapular region as a secondary complication of a significant kyphoscoliosis of the thoracic spine. Scar tissue is present in this area and there is a prior history of pressure ulceration at that location. The SWAT is used to record wound progress with physical therapy wound management over the course of a 4-week period. Since this wound is a partial-thickness ulcer, there were no scores for depth or undermining and there is adherence from baseline. Debridement of the necrotic tissue left appearance of a thin layer of granulation tissue. Tables 5.2 and 5.3 show how the SWHT reflected the wound's progress.

Case Study Source: Rujita Dhere, MSPT, WCC 2010

TABLE 5.2 — Patient with Upper Back Pressure Ulcer

SWHT Part I: Wound Tissue Attributes

Week	0	1	2	3	4
Date: 2010					
1. Hemorrhage	0	0	0	0	0
2. Maceration	0	0	0	0	0
3. Undermining	0	0	0	0	0
4. Erythema	1	1	1	1	0
5. Necrosis	1	1	0	0	0
6. Adherence	1	1	1	1	1
7. Granulation (decreased depth)	0	1	1	1	1
8. Appearance of contraction (reduced size)	0	0	1	1	1
9. Sustained contraction (more reduced size)	0	0	0	1	1
10. Epithelialization	0	0	0	0	1
Total "Not Good"	2	2	1	1	0
Total "Good"	1	2	3	4	5

Key: Present = 1. Absent = 0.

TABLE 5.3

SWHT Part II: Size, Location, Wound Healing Phase Measures, and Extent

Week	0	1	2	3	4
Date:					
11. General depth > 0.2 cm	0	0	0	0	0
12. Depth @ 12:00 > 0.2 cm	0	0	0	0	0
13. Depth @ 3:00 > 0.2 cm	0	0	0	0	0
14. Depth @ 6:00 > 0.2 cm	0	0	0	0	0
15. Depth @ 9:00 > 0.2 cm	0	0	0	0	0
16. Underm @ 12:00 > 0.2 cm	0	0	0	0	0
17. Underm @ 3:00 > 0.2 cm	0	0	0	0	0
18. Underm @ 6:00 > 0.2 cm	0	0	0	0	0
19. Underm @ 9:00 > 0.2 cm	0	0	0	0	0
Location	UB	UB	UB	UB	UB
Wound healing phase	I	P	P	E	E

Key: Present = 1. Not present = 0. Location choices: upper body (UB), coccyx (C), trochanter (T), ischial (I), heel (H), and foot (F); add right or left (R or L). Wound healing phase: inflammation (I), proliferation (P), epithelialization (E), remodeling (R).

CLINICAL WISDOM

Use of Forms for Wound Measurement Along with the SWHT

Because wound measurement and tissue assessment or reassessment are usually done at the same time, it makes sense to record the information at the same time using a companion form. Chapter 4 has examples of a sample wound measurement form designed to fit this model.

Part I can be printed on one side of a page and Part II on the other. Printing the forms as a pad punched with a hole pattern to match the notebook or chart where a paper form is kept makes it easy and convenient to keep forms on hand. A set of the explanations and scoring can be printed on the same size paper, and then kept in the notebook for reference. An additional benefit of Form B is that it is easy to see a complete history of the change in tissue status over multiple weeks of assessment. Reading the report over time provides a quick and clear evaluation to monitor wound healing progress. The entire SWHT can become part of the patient's electronic record by creating a template of the form for completion by the clinician on the computer.

EXHIBIT 5.1A

SWHT Short Form Part I: Wound Tissue Attributes

Name: _____ Med Rec # _____ Examiner: _____

Week	0	1	2	3	4
1. Hemorrhage					
2. Maceration					
3. Undermining					
4. Erythema					
5. Necrosis					
6. Adherence					
7. Granulation (decreased depth)					
8. Appearance of contraction (reduced size)					
9. Sustained contraction (more reduced size)					
10. Epithelialization					
Key: Present = 1. Not present = 0.					
Total not good					
Total good					

Source: Copyright © 1997, Sussman Physical Therapy, Inc.

EXHIBIT 5.1B

SWHT Short Form Part II: Size, Location, Wound Healing Phase Measures, and Extent

Date	0	1	2	3	4
11. General depth > 0.2 cm					
12. Depth @ 12:00 > 0.2 cm					
13. Depth @ 3:00 > 0.2 cm					
14. Depth @ 6:00 > 0.2 cm					
15. Depth @ 9:00 > 0.2 cm					
16. Underm @ 12:00 > 0.2 cm					
17. Underm @ 3:00 > 0.2 cm					
18. Underm @ 6:00 > 0.2 cm					
19. Underm @ 9:00 > 0.2 cm					
Location					
Wound healing phase					

Key: Present = 1. Not present = 0. Location choices: upper body (UB), coccyx (C), trochanter (T), ischial (I), heel (H), and foot (F); add right or left (R or L). Wound healing phase: absent (A), chronic (C), inflammation (I), proliferation (P), epithelialization (E), remodeling (R).
Source: Copyright © 1997, Sussman Physical Therapy, Inc.

Case Example 2 Using the SWHT

Exhibits 5.2A and 5.2B show an example of a case where wound healing was monitored over a 5-week course of care, as reported on Form A of the SWHT, Parts I and II. A summary (see Exhibit 5.3) of the case example shows how the SWHT can be used to document a change in wound tissue status from a predominance of not-good-for-healing attributes to a predominance of good attributes. Exhibits 5.2A and 5.2B reflect the following:

- At baseline, week 0, the patient had the presence of hemorrhage, necrosis, and erythema, and absence of any attributes good for healing. The presence of these attributes at baseline is an indication that this wound will need aggressive intervention to improve.
- At week 2, there were multiple attributes that were indicators that this patient would be in the risk-for-not-healing group, including undermining and depth at all four clock points, further indicating the medical necessity for aggressive intervention to put the wound on a course of healing.
- Following aggressive intervention undertaken at week 2, the improvement in the wound tissue status from not good to good is significant by week 4.

SWHT Database

The SWHT can be used to create a wound database on a computer. The scoring system of using a 1 or a 0 is computer compatible for data management and data entry. The SWHT forms are printed on the computer as screens, and data are entered

EXHIBIT 5.2A

SWHT Part I: Wound Tissue Attributes

Week	0	1	2	3	4
Date: 2010	1/7	1/14	1/21	1/28	2/4
1. Hemorrhage	1	0	0	0	0
2. Maceration	0	0	0	0	0
3. Undermining	0	0	1	1	1
4. Erythema	1	1	1	0	0
5. Necrosis	1	1	1	0	0
6. Adherence	0	0	0	1	1
7. Granulation (decreased depth)	0	0	1	1	1
8. Appearance of contraction (reduced size)	0	0	1	1	1
9. Sustained contraction (more reduced size)	0	0	0	1	1
10. Epithelialization	0	0	0	1	1
Total "Not Good"	3	2	3	1	1
Total "Good"	0	0	2	5	5

Key: Present = 1. Absent = 0.
Source: Copyright © 1997, Sussman Physical Therapy, Inc.

EXHIBIT 5.2B

SWHT Part II: Size, Location, Wound Healing Phase Measures, and Extent

Week	0	1	2	3	4
Date:	1/7	1/14	1/21	1/28	2/4
11. General depth > 0.2 cm	0	1	1	1	1
12. Depth @ 12:00 > 0.2 cm	0	1	1	1	1
13. Depth @ 3:00 > 0.2 cm	0	1	1	1	1
14. Depth @ 6:00 > 0.2 cm	0	1	1	1	1
15. Depth @ 9:00 > 0.2 cm	1	1	1	1	1
16. Underm @ 12:00 > 0.2 cm	0	0	1	1	0
17. Underm @ 3:00 > 0.2 cm	0	1	1	0	0
18. Underm @ 6:00 > 0.2 cm	0	1	1	1	0
19. Underm @ 9:00 > 0.2 cm	0	0	1	1	1
Location	RT	RT	RT	RT	RT
Wound healing phase	I	I	I	P	P

Key: Present = 1. Not present = 0. Location choices: upper body (UB), coccyx (C), trochanter (T), ischial (I), heel (H), and foot (F); add right or left (R or L). Wound healing phase: inflammation (I), proliferation (P), epithelialization (E), remodeling (R).
Source: Copyright © 1997, Sussman Physical Therapy, Inc.

either prospectively or retrospectively. Data reports can be printed, and the captured data can be analyzed for each individual patient or by group.

PRESSURE ULCER SCALE FOR HEALING

The PUSH is a tool originally developed for measuring the healing of pressure ulcers.

Development of the PUSH

In 1996, the National Pressure Ulcer Advisory Panel (NPUAP) convened a task force to address the practice of reverse staging of pressure ulcers in long-term care facilities in the United States. At the time, the practice had been encouraged by Medicare documentation requirements using the Minimum Data Set (MDS) system. The Panel's objective was to develop a biologically accurate and easy-to-use instrument to replace reverse staging. The task force developed and tested a tool to measure pressure ulcer healing,[14] and the PUSH tool was presented in 1997 at the NPUAP biennial conference[2,15] (see Appendix 5B).

Use of the PUSH

The PUSH tool was first developed as a way to measure healing of pressure ulcers,[2,14,15] and has since been evaluated as an instrument to assess progress of venous and diabetic foot ulcer healing.[16–18]

The PUSH tool involves assessment of three wound characteristics: surface area measurements, exudate amount, and surface appearance. Use of the tool therefore involves measuring size, evaluating exudate, and categorizing tissue type. The clinician measures the size of the wound, using length and width to calculate surface area (length × width) and chooses the appropriate size category on the tool (there are 10 size categories, from 0–10). Exudate is evaluated as none (0), light (1), moderate (2), or heavy (3). Tissue type choices include closed (0), epithelial tissue (1), granulation tissue (2), slough (3), and necrotic tissue (4). The three subscores are then summed for a total score and can be plotted on a graph.

The PUSH tool was designed for use as a trigger to identify when goals of treatment are being met and when patients may need to be reevaluated. In short, it is best used as a method of quantitatively reporting the direction of healing over time. The PUSH scores can be monitored with an ulcer healing record form and a graph that allows for recording of subscores and total score on a periodic basis.

Utility of the PUSH tool

Utility of the PUSH tool has been demonstrated most with pressure ulcers in long-term care settings.[19–21] Total PUSH score and change in PUSH scores over time can be used as outcome measures for a variety of interventions targeted at wound healing. For example, PUSH score change was used as the outcome measure for evaluating a set of clinical decision trees to guide multidisciplinary interaction and collaboration in long-term

EXHIBIT	5.3	

Summary of Wound Attribute Change over a 5-Week Course of Care

Week 0	Week 2	Week 4
"NOT GOOD" for healing	*"NOT GOOD" for healing*	*"NOT GOOD" for healing*
Hemorrhage	Necrosis	Undermining
Undermining	Undermining	Depth 12, 3, 6, 9:00
Erythema	Erythema	Undermining 9:00
Necrosis	Depth 12, 3, 6, 9:00	
Depth 9:00	Undermining 12, 3, 6, 9:00	
"GOOD" for healing	*"GOOD" for healing*	*"GOOD" for healing*
None	Fibroplasia	Fibroplasia
	Appearance of contraction	Appearance of contraction
		Sustained contraction
		Adherence
		Epithelialization
Wound healing phase	*Wound healing phase*	*Wound healing phase*
Inflammatory phase	Inflammatory phase	Proliferative phase

Source: Copyright © 1997, Sussman Physical Therapy, Inc.

care facilities.[19] Total PUSH scores have been used to evaluate pressure ulcer healing among residents in nursing homes.[20,21] PUSH scores are responsive to change in ulcer status and can differentiate between ulcers that heal and those that do not.[20,21] In prospective studies using the PUSH tool weekly to measure pressure ulcer healing, PUSH scores:

- Were significantly lower among pressure ulcers that healed compared with unhealed ulcers[20,21]
- Decreased significantly over time among healed ulcers but did not among unhealed ulcers[21]
- Differentiated between healing and nonhealing ulcers starting with the first week[20]
- Were highly correlated with scores on the Pressure Sore Status Tool (PSST [now the BWAT]) and surface area measurements[21]

Use of the PUSH tool does not necessarily correlate with traditional nursing observations and documentation in long-term care settings.[22] In 370 observations for 48 nursing home residents with pressure ulcers where both PUSH scores and traditional nursing assessment (primarily ulcer

size documented weekly) were recorded in medical records, when traditional assessment determined an ulcer "improved" (n = 212 observations), there were only 42% "better" or concordant PUSH scores. Further, of the 212 observations of improved ulcers, 47% received PUSH scores indicating no change and 11% had scores indicating worsening ulcer status. In ulcers that were noted by traditional nursing assessment to have deteriorated (n = 48), only 25% of PUSH scores also indicated worsening status.[22]

Pompeo[23] revised the way PUSH tool data were collected in order to capture system wide wound outcome information. The same methodology and components of the original PUSH tool were kept intact. The revisions involve how the data were aggregated and used for determining organizational outcomes. The data used to determine organizational outcomes included

- Combining total PUSH scores for multiple wounds on the same patient to obtain a wound burden score
- Identifying the initial or admission and end of stay or discharge total PUSH score
- If available, use of monthly summed PUSH scores
- Noting change in total PUSH score from admission or initial assessment to discharge or end of stay assessment
- Calculating healing rate (PUSH score/total days of stay)

Appendix 5C is a copy of the Pompeo form.

The PUSH tool has also been validated for use in monitoring healing in diabetic foot ulcers and venous ulcers.[16–18] PUSH score was used as an outcome measure to evaluate a community-based "Leg Club" support group on venous leg ulcer healing and demonstrated responsiveness to change in ulcer status for ulcers that healed with the intervention.[18] Feasibility of using the PUSH tool with venous ulcers has also been positively evaluated in a clinic setting with venous leg ulcers.[16] As with PUSH tool use with pressure ulcers, when the PUSH tool is used to monitor healing in diabetic foot ulcers and venous leg ulcers, it demonstrates responsiveness to change with significant differences in PUSH scores between healing diabetic foot ulcers and venous ulcers compared to nonhealing diabetic foot ulcers and venous ulcers.[17]Aspects of the PUSH tool have been incorporated into several standardized patient assessment documents for various health-care organizations including the OASIS for home healthcare, the MDS 3.0 for long-term care, and the proposed CARE tool for transitions across health-care settings. To summarize, PUSH is a valid tool for monitoring pressure ulcer, leg ulcer, and diabetic foot ulcer healing or deterioration over time and enhancing communication among health-care providers regarding changing wound status.

THE BATES-JENSEN WOUND ASSESSMENT TOOL

BWAT is a measuring instrument used to assess and monitor healing in pressure ulcers and other chronic wounds.

Development of the BWAT

In 1990, Bates-Jensen[1] developed the PSST, which was revised in 2001 as the BWAT. The original PSST was developed as a wound assessment tool for both clinical and research use.

Over the years, BWAT use has evolved to include measuring and predicting wound healing and is used in a wide variety of wounds beyond pressure ulcers. The BWAT has provided a basis for many other wound assessment tools and is the most widely used of the instruments presented. Only minor changes were made to the PSST to create the second generation tool, the BWAT.

Use of the BWAT

The BWAT is recommended for use to assess and monitor healing in pressure ulcers and other chronic wounds. It uses a numerical scale to rate wound characteristics from best to worst possible (see Appendix 5D). Two items are nonscored: location and shape. The remaining 13 are scored items. These are: size, depth, edges, undermining or pockets, necrotic tissue type, necrotic tissue amount, exudate type, exudate amount, surrounding skin color, peripheral tissue edema, peripheral tissue induration, granulation tissue, and epithelialization. Each scored item appears with characteristic descriptors rated on a scale (1 indicating best for that characteristic and 5 indicating worst). Once a lesion has been assessed for each item on the BWAT, the 13 item scores can be summed to obtain a total score for the wound. The total score can then be plotted on the wound continuum at the bottom of the tool to "see at a glance" healing or degeneration of the wound. Total scores range from 9 (wound closure) to 65 (profound tissue degeneration). The tool has a one-page sheet of instructions for use, in addition to the item descriptions (Appendix 5D). There is also a pictorial guide for training health professionals in use of the BWAT.[24,25] The BWAT Pictorial Guide includes 102 photographs of a variety of wound types, not just pressure ulcers, illustrating each descriptor for each of the BWAT items. Validation of the photographic content was accomplished in a three-stage consensus process working with nurses specializing in wound care.[24] Figure 5.21 provides an example of a page from the pictorial guide.

Wounds should be scored with the BWAT initially for a baseline assessment and at regular intervals (i.e., at least weekly) to evaluate intervention effectiveness.

Validity and Reliability of the BWAT

The original items on the BWAT were developed using a modified Delphi process that involved use of a multidisciplinary panel of experts in pressure ulcers and wound healing. The expert panel reviewed and developed consensus on the items and descriptors of each item on the tool, format of the tool, and scoring mechanisms. Once developed, the tool was validated through the use of a second expert panel, which established content validity for each individual item on the tool and for the total tool.[1] Concurrent validity was established in a study with nursing home residents by comparing total tool scores and the depth item scores with the NPUAP's staging classification system.[26]

Reliability of the BWAT was demonstrated on adult patients in an acute care hospital with enterostomal therapy (ET) nurses or nurses with special training in wound care and demonstrated excellent reliability with correlation coefficients greater than 0.90.[1] Reliability with practitioners who did not have education or experience in wound assessment and management

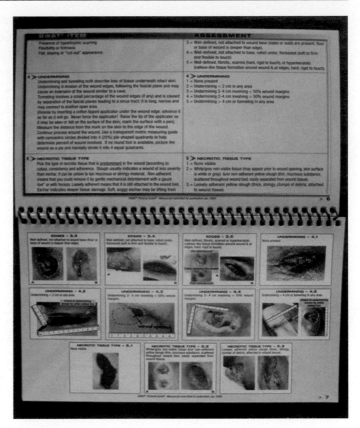

FIGURE 5.21 A page from the Bates-Jensen Wound Assessment Pictorial Guide. (Copyright © B.M. Bates-Jensen.)

resulted in lower reliability than the tool's use by specialists, but still within an acceptable range.[27] Predictive validity has also been evaluated. This study involved assessments of 143 pressure sores over 6 weeks, with a minimum of three assessments per ulcer during the study period.[28] The main outcome measure of the study was time to 50% healing, as measured by surface area. The results showed that changes in the BWAT score at 1 week plus changes in surface area measurements were predictive of those wounds that achieved 50% healing during the 6 weeks compared to those that did not. A 1-week net decrease (improvement) in total BWAT score plus a decrease in surface area was the best predictor of time to 50% wound closure. The positive predictive value of a net improvement in total PSST score at 1 week was 65%, whereas the positive predictive value of a net deterioration in PSST score at 1 week was only 31%. Sensitivity in this sample was 61%, and specificity was 52%.[28] Thus, the total BWAT score may provide a method of predicting outcomes. More research is needed in this area.

Converting BWAT Scores into PUSH Scores

A PUSH score can be calculated from the BWAT tool and the two tools are highly correlated.[21] The following guidelines will enable you to convert BWAT subscale scores into PUSH subscale scores. Table 5.4 provides an example of conversion.

1. Wound size: It is best to use actual surface area measurements, length by width, to determine which PUSH size

TABLE 5.4	Example of PUSH Score Derivation from BWAT Scores		
BWAT Items	**BWAT Scores**	**PUSH Items**	**PUSH Scores**
1. Size	*4* (6.5 × 6.0 cm = 39 cm²)	*1. Size* **(724 cm²)**	*10*
2. Depth	3		
3. Edges	2		
4. Undermining	1		
5. Necrotic Tissue Type	3		
6. Necrotic Tissue Amt.	4		
7. Exudate Type	4		
8. Exudate Amt.	5	2. Exudate Amt. (Heavy)	*3*
9. Skin Color	4		
10. Edema	1		
11. Induration	2		
12. Granulation	*3*	Tissue Type[a] (Slough)	*3*
13. Epithelialization	4		
Total Score	**40**	Total Score	**16**

[a]Note that necrotic tissue is item 5 on BWAT and 3 on PUSH, where slough is not classified as necrotic tissue if all necrotic tissue is absent.

category is appropriate. If actual measurements are not available, the following guide may be helpful:

- If BWAT size category = 1, then PUSH size category score = 0, 1, 2, 3, 4, 5, or 6.
- If BWAT size category = 2, then PUSH size category score = either 7 or 8.
- If BWAT size category = 3, then PUSH size category score = either 9 or 10.
- If BWAT size category = 4 or 5, then PUSH size category score = 10.

2. Exudate amount:
   - If BWAT exudate amount score = 1, then PUSH exudate amount score = 0.
   - If BWAT exudate amount score = 2 or 3, then PUSH exudate amount score = 1.
   - If BWAT exudate amount score = 4, then PUSH exudate amount score = 2.
   - If BWAT exudate amount score = 5, then PUSH exudate amount score = 3.

3. Tissue type:
   - If BWAT Total Score = 13, then PUSH Type Score = 0.
                    OR
   If Granulation = 1 and Epithelialization = 1, then PUSH Type Score = 0.
   - If Necrotic Tissue Type = 4 or 5, then PUSH Type Score = 4.
   - If Necrotic Tissue Type = 2 or 3, then PUSH Type Score = 3.
   - If Epithelialization < 5, then PUSH Type Score = 1.
   - If Granulation < 5 AND Epithelialization = 5, then PUSH Type Score = 2.

Utility of the BWAT

An additional benefit associated with the assignment of numeric values to items on the BWAT is that it assists you in setting realistic goals. Clinical experience shows that not all wounds heal and certainly not always in the same setting. The BWAT allows for more realistic goal setting as appropriate to the health-care setting and the individual patient and wound. For example, the patient with a large, necrotic, full-thickness wound in acute care will probably not be in the facility long enough for the wound to heal completely. However, the tool enables clinicians to set intermediate or secondary goals, such as "Necrotic tissue in the wound will decrease in amount and type."

As already noted, the BWAT allows for monitoring of improvement or deterioration in individual characteristics, as well as the total score. This in turn enables you to assess the patient's response to specific treatments. For example, the characteristics of necrotic tissue type and amount may be tracked with exudate type and amount to evaluate

---

CLINICAL WISDOM

Realistic Goal Setting

In some instances, a wound may never heal because of host factors or other contextual circumstances. In this case, an example of a goal might be to maintain the total BWAT score between 20 and 22.

the response to debridement or infection management. The ability to track wound symptoms such as exudate allows you to evaluate outcomes of interventions designed to alleviate distressing wound symptoms and may be useful for palliative care, wound-related complaints, and when symptoms affect the patient's quality of life.[29]

Use of BWAT Scores to Identify Severity State and Guide Treatment

The severity of a wound, as well as overall health status of the patient, can determine the appropriate management approach for healing. Severity states are a measure of the degree of the tissue insult or wound burden on the patient. The goals of wound care are to decrease the overall severity status and to make this decrease in a timely fashion. You can use the BWAT to help you identify a wound's severity state, and thereby guide your care planning.

As shown in Figure 5.22, BWAT scores can be divided into four suggested severity states: total scores of 13–20 indicate minimal severity; 21–30 indicates mild severity; 31–40 is moderate severity; and 41–65 is extreme severity. An example of a treatment algorithm for one wound in each of these severity states is presented below. These treatment algorithms are derived from clinical practice guidelines.

BWAT Minimal Severity Scores 13–20

Wounds with a BWAT total score of 13–20 are generally shallow partial-thickness wounds. Figure 5.23 presents a generic algorithm for treatment for wounds in this severity state. The main goals for wounds in this severity state are to prevent further damage and to provide a moist wound environment for healing.

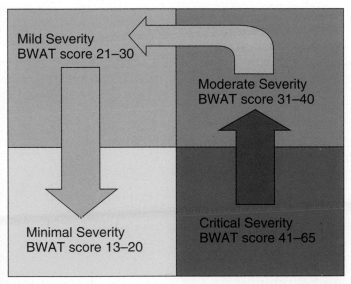

FIGURE 5.22 Severity states based on BWAT scores. The goals of therapy are (1) to decrease the overall severity state of the wound and, thus, the BWAT score and (2) to make the decrease in a timely fashion. There is equal concern regarding severity of the wound and the duration of time that the wound spends in any severity state. (Copyright Barbara Bates-Jensen.)

BWAT Mild Severity Scores 21–30

Wounds with mild severity include both partial-thickness and full-thickness wounds. Figure 5.24 presents a general treatment algorithm for partial-thickness wounds with mild severity scores. The goals of care for partial-thickness wounds with mild severity scores are to absorb excess wound exudate, maintain a clean wound bed, and maintain a moist environment. Full-thickness wounds with mild severity scores offer more options for treatment because the wound can present as a clean, full-thickness wound or as a wound filled with necrotic debris.

BWAT Moderate Severity Scores 31–40

Figure 5.25 is a care plan for a full-thickness wound with necrotic tissue present. The goals of care for full-thickness wounds with moderate severity scores are to obtain/maintain a clean wound bed, provide a moist environment, absorb excess exudate, prevent premature closure, and reduce wound dead space. Wounds with moderate (and mild) severity scores have the most diverse presentations clinically, so choices regarding treatment are numerous.

Figures 5.26 to 5.28 demonstrate general treatment algorithms. These algorithms can be used to determine appropriate care for a variety of chronic wounds with moderate to extreme BWAT severity scores. Wounds in the moderate severity state are predominantly full-thickness wounds such as stage III or IV pressure ulcers. Figure 5.26 presents the case of the full-thickness wound with necrotic debris and large amounts of exudate. Treatment is focused on debridement and absorbing exudate. Figure 5.27 presents the case of the full-thickness clean wound with undermining or dead space, and the treatment focus is on eliminating the dead space and prevention of premature wound closure. The goals of care for wounds in this severity state are to obtain/maintain a clean wound bed, absorb excess exudate, eliminate dead space to prevent premature wound closure, and provide a moist wound environment.

BWAT Critical Severity Scores 41–65

Wounds with BWAT total scores between 41 and 65 are generally deep full-thickness wounds with more critical clinical manifestations, including undermining and necrosis. Figure 5.28 presents an algorithm for treatment of a wound with necrotic eschar. The goals of care for wounds in this severity state are to identify and treat infection, obtain a clean wound bed, absorb excess exudate, eliminate dead space to prevent premature wound closure, and provide a moist wound environment.

Considerations in Using the BWAT Scores to Guide Treatment

The use of the BWAT score for determining severity state and guiding treatment offers one approach to managing wounds. This approach may be useful in designing broad generic treatment guidelines; however, you must still use your clinical judgment to individualize the care plan. Moreover, the treatment plans presented based on the BWAT severity scores focus only on topical wound care. Attention to nutrition, use of

Assessment:

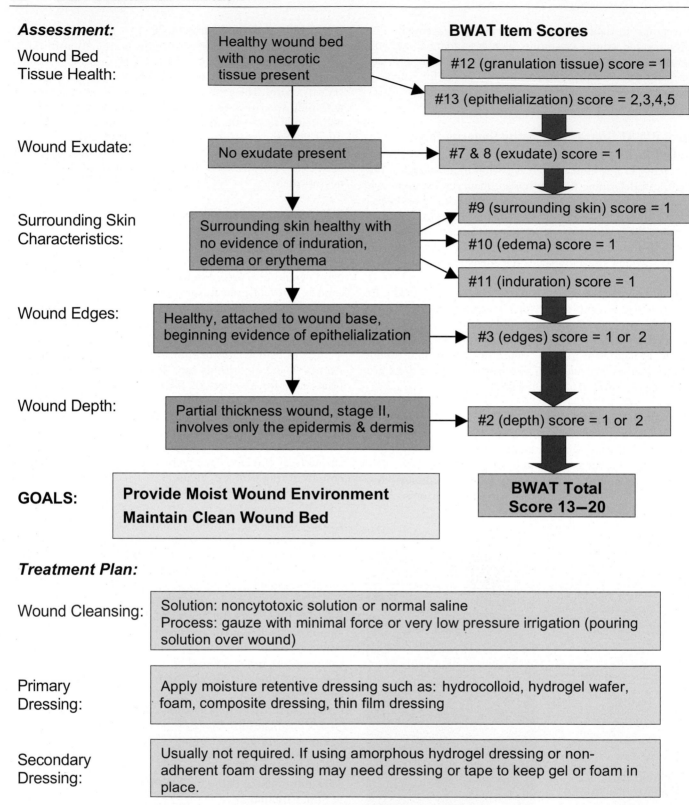

FIGURE 5.23 Minimal BWAT severity score treatment algorithm for mild, dry, partial-thickness wound. (Adapted from ConvaTec, with permission.)

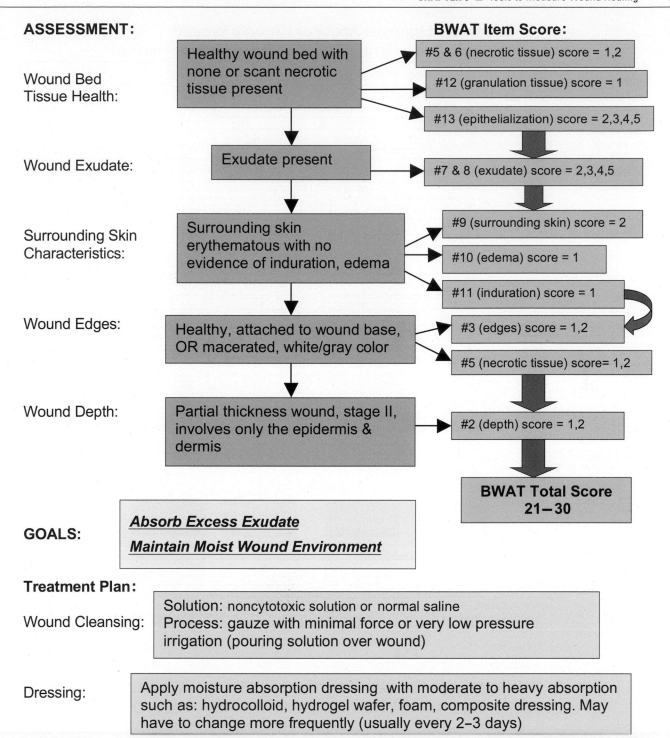

ASSESSMENT:

Wound Bed Tissue Health:

Wound Exudate:

Surrounding Skin Characteristics:

Wound Edges:

Wound Depth:

BWAT Item Score:

Healthy wound bed with none or scant necrotic tissue present

Exudate present

Surrounding skin erythematous with no evidence of induration, edema

Healthy, attached to wound base, OR macerated, white/gray color

Partial thickness wound, stage II, involves only the epidermis & dermis

#5 & 6 (necrotic tissue) score = 1,2

#12 (granulation tissue) score = 1

#13 (epithelialization) score = 2,3,4,5

#7 & 8 (exudate) score = 2,3,4,5

#9 (surrounding skin) score = 2

#10 (edema) score = 1

#11 (induration) score = 1

#3 (edges) score = 1,2

#5 (necrotic tissue) score= 1,2

#2 (depth) score = 1,2

BWAT Total Score 21—30

GOALS:

Absorb Excess Exudate
Maintain Moist Wound Environment

Treatment Plan:

Wound Cleansing:

Solution: noncytotoxic solution or normal saline
Process: gauze with minimal force or very low pressure irrigation (pouring solution over wound)

Dressing:

Apply moisture absorption dressing with moderate to heavy absorption such as: hydrocolloid, hydrogel wafer, foam, composite dressing. May have to change more frequently (usually every 2–3 days)

OUTCOMES:

Wound edges healthy with no maceration
Wound partially to fully resurfaced with new epithelium

FIGURE 5.24 Partial-thickness wound with mild BWAT severity score treatment algorithm. (Adapted from ConvaTec, with permission.)

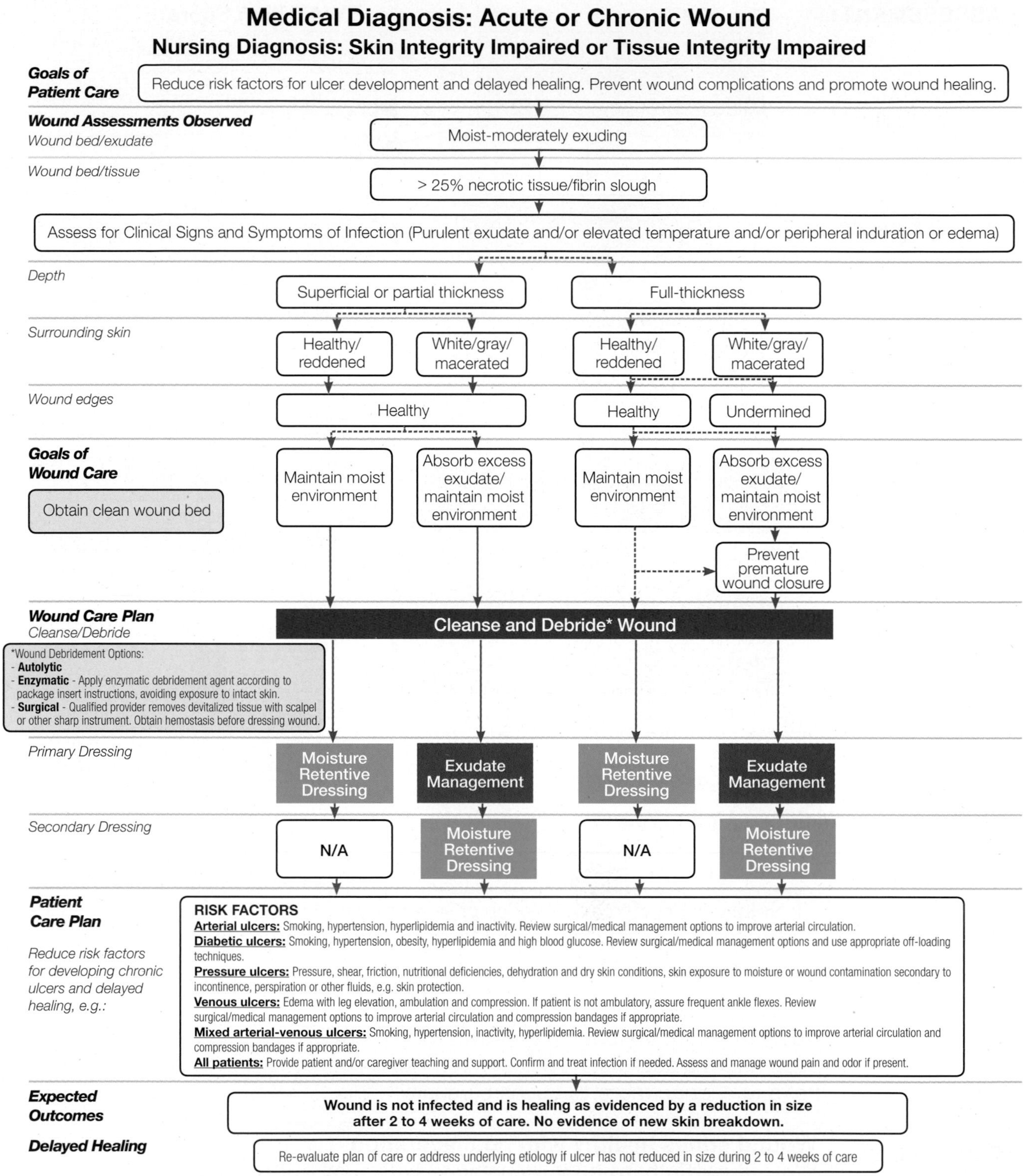

Medical Diagnosis: Acute or Chronic Wound
Nursing Diagnosis: Skin Integrity Impaired or Tissue Integrity Impaired

Goals of Patient Care
Reduce risk factors for ulcer development and delayed healing. Prevent wound complications and promote wound healing.

Wound Assessments Observed

Wound bed/exudate
Moist-moderately exuding

Wound bed/tissue
> 25% necrotic tissue/fibrin slough

Assess for Clinical Signs and Symptoms of Infection (Purulent exudate and/or elevated temperature and/or peripheral induration or edema)

Depth
Superficial or partial thickness | Full-thickness

Surrounding skin
Healthy/reddened | White/gray/macerated | Healthy/reddened | White/gray/macerated

Wound edges
Healthy | Healthy | Undermined

Goals of Wound Care
Obtain clean wound bed

Maintain moist environment | Absorb excess exudate/maintain moist environment | Maintain moist environment | Absorb excess exudate/maintain moist environment

Prevent premature wound closure

Wound Care Plan
Cleanse/Debride

Cleanse and Debride* Wound

*Wound Debridement Options:
- **Autolytic**
- **Enzymatic** - Apply enzymatic debridement agent according to package insert instructions, avoiding exposure to intact skin.
- **Surgical** - Qualified provider removes devitalized tissue with scalpel or other sharp instrument. Obtain hemostasis before dressing wound.

Primary Dressing
Moisture Retentive Dressing | Exudate Management | Moisture Retentive Dressing | Exudate Management

Secondary Dressing
N/A | Moisture Retentive Dressing | N/A | Moisture Retentive Dressing

Patient Care Plan

Reduce risk factors for developing chronic ulcers and delayed healing, e.g.:

RISK FACTORS
Arterial ulcers: Smoking, hypertension, hyperlipidemia and inactivity. Review surgical/medical management options to improve arterial circulation.
Diabetic ulcers: Smoking, hypertension, obesity, hyperlipidemia and high blood glucose. Review surgical/medical management options and use appropriate off-loading techniques.
Pressure ulcers: Pressure, shear, friction, nutritional deficiencies, dehydration and dry skin conditions, skin exposure to moisture or wound contamination secondary to incontinence, perspiration or other fluids, e.g. skin protection.
Venous ulcers: Edema with leg elevation, ambulation and compression. If patient is not ambulatory, assure frequent ankle flexes. Review surgical/medical management options to improve arterial circulation and compression bandages if appropriate.
Mixed arterial-venous ulcers: Smoking, hypertension, inactivity, hyperlipidemia. Review surgical/medical management options to improve arterial circulation and compression bandages if appropriate.
All patients: Provide patient and/or caregiver teaching and support. Confirm and treat infection if needed. Assess and manage wound pain and odor if present.

Expected Outcomes
Wound is not infected and is healing as evidenced by a reduction in size after 2 to 4 weeks of care. No evidence of new skin breakdown.

Delayed Healing
Re-evaluate plan of care or address underlying etiology if ulcer has not reduced in size during 2 to 4 weeks of care

FIGURE 5.25 Full-thickness stage III or stage IV pressure ulcer with a moderate BWAT severity score treatment algorithm. (Adapted from ConvaTec, with permission.)

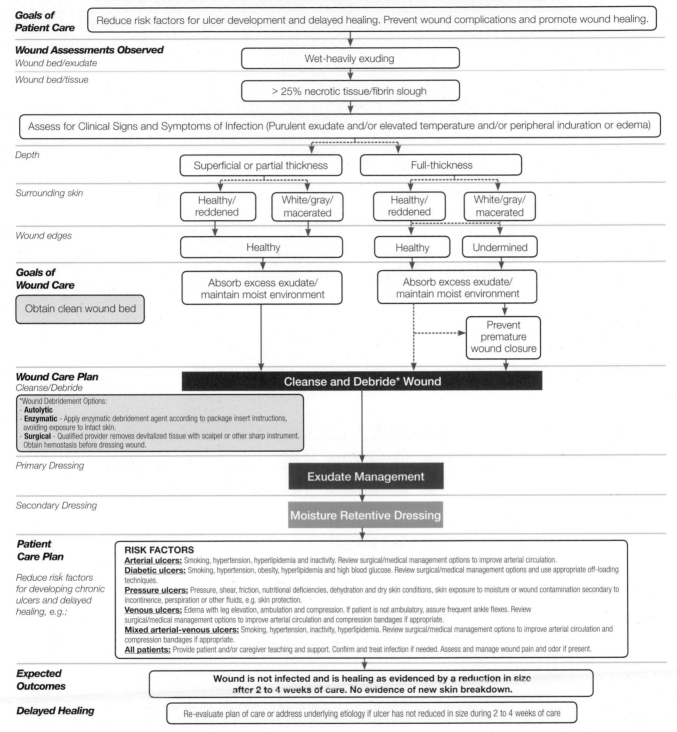

Medical Diagnosis: Acute or Chronic Wound
Nursing Diagnosis: Skin Integrity Impaired or Tissue Integrity Impaired

Goals of Patient Care

Reduce risk factors for ulcer development and delayed healing. Prevent wound complications and promote wound healing.

Wound Assessments Observed

Wound bed/exudate — Wet-heavily exuding

Wound bed/tissue — > 25% necrotic tissue/fibrin slough

Assess for Clinical Signs and Symptoms of Infection (Purulent exudate and/or elevated temperature and/or peripheral induration or edema)

Depth — Superficial or partial thickness | Full-thickness

Surrounding skin — Healthy/reddened | White/gray/macerated | Healthy/reddened | White/gray/macerated

Wound edges — Healthy | Healthy | Undermined

Goals of Wound Care

Obtain clean wound bed

Absorb excess exudate/maintain moist environment | Absorb excess exudate/maintain moist environment

Prevent premature wound closure

Wound Care Plan
Cleanse/Debride

Cleanse and Debride* Wound

*Wound Debridement Options:
- **Autolytic**
- **Enzymatic** - Apply enzymatic debridement agent according to package insert instructions, avoiding exposure to intact skin.
- **Surgical** - Qualified provider removes devitalized tissue with scalpel or other sharp instrument. Obtain hemostasis before dressing wound.

Primary Dressing

Exudate Management

Secondary Dressing

Moisture Retentive Dressing

Patient Care Plan

Reduce risk factors for developing chronic ulcers and delayed healing, e.g.:

RISK FACTORS
Arterial ulcers: Smoking, hypertension, hyperlipidemia and inactivity. Review surgical/medical management options to improve arterial circulation.
Diabetic ulcers: Smoking, hypertension, obesity, hyperlipidemia and high blood glucose. Review surgical/medical management options and use appropriate off-loading techniques.
Pressure ulcers: Pressure, shear, friction, nutritional deficiencies, dehydration and dry skin conditions, skin exposure to moisture or wound contamination secondary to incontinence, perspiration or other fluids, e.g. skin protection.
Venous ulcers: Edema with leg elevation, ambulation and compression. If patient is not ambulatory, assure frequent ankle flexes. Review surgical/medical management options to improve arterial circulation and compression bandages if appropriate.
Mixed arterial-venous ulcers: Smoking, hypertension, inactivity, hyperlipidemia. Review surgical/medical management options to improve arterial circulation and compression bandages if appropriate.
All patients: Provide patient and/or caregiver teaching and support. Confirm and treat infection if needed. Assess and manage wound pain and odor if present.

Expected Outcomes

Wound is not infected and is healing as evidenced by a reduction in size after 2 to 4 weeks of care. No evidence of new skin breakdown.

Delayed Healing

Re-evaluate plan of care or address underlying etiology if ulcer has not reduced in size during 2 to 4 weeks of care

FIGURE 5.26 General full-thickness wound with critical BWAT severity score treatment algorithm. (Reprinted from ConvaTec, with permission.)

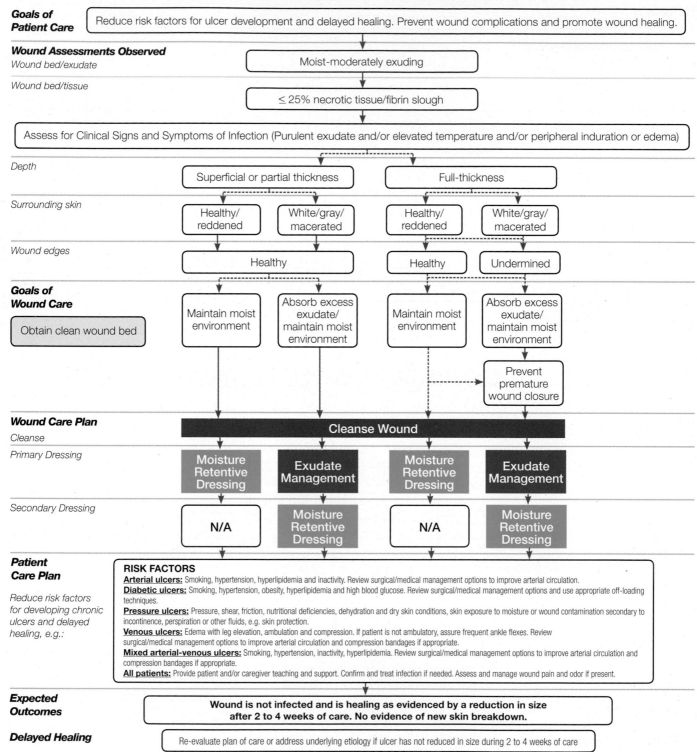

FIGURE 5.27 General full-thickness wound with undermining or pocketing with moderate BWAT severity score treatment algorithm. (Reprinted from ConvaTec, with permission.)

Medical Diagnosis: Acute or Chronic Wound
Nursing Diagnosis: Skin Integrity Impaired or Tissue Integrity Impaired

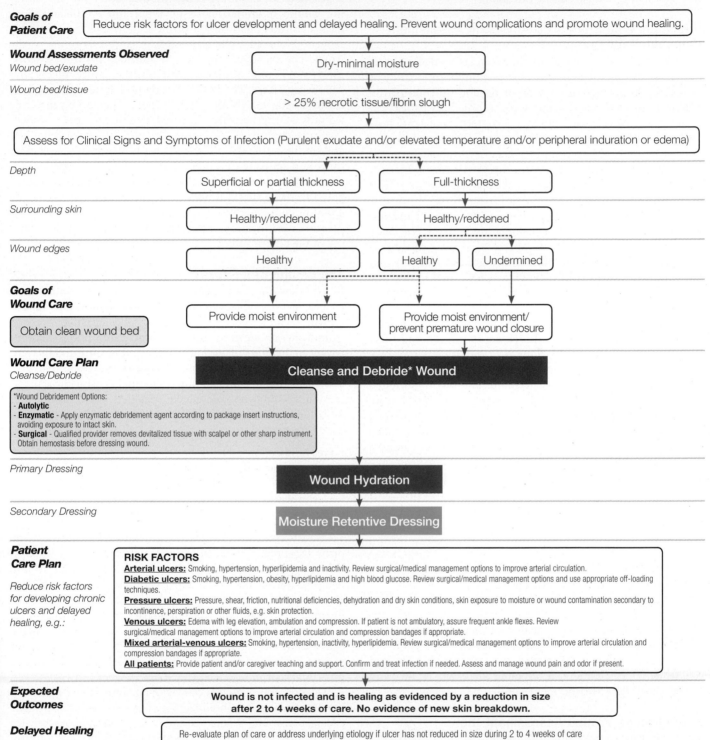

Goals of Patient Care

Reduce risk factors for ulcer development and delayed healing. Prevent wound complications and promote wound healing.

Wound Assessments Observed

Wound bed/exudate

Dry-minimal moisture

Wound bed/tissue

> 25% necrotic tissue/fibrin slough

Assess for Clinical Signs and Symptoms of Infection (Purulent exudate and/or elevated temperature and/or peripheral induration or edema)

Depth

Superficial or partial thickness | Full-thickness

Surrounding skin

Healthy/reddened | Healthy/reddened

Wound edges

Healthy | Healthy | Undermined

Goals of Wound Care

Obtain clean wound bed

Provide moist environment | Provide moist environment/prevent premature wound closure

Wound Care Plan

Cleanse/Debride

Cleanse and Debride* Wound

*Wound Debridement Options:
- **Autolytic**
- **Enzymatic** - Apply enzymatic debridement agent according to package insert instructions, avoiding exposure to intact skin.
- **Surgical** - Qualified provider removes devitalized tissue with scalpel or other sharp instrument. Obtain hemostasis before dressing wound.

Primary Dressing

Wound Hydration

Secondary Dressing

Moisture Retentive Dressing

Patient Care Plan

Reduce risk factors for developing chronic ulcers and delayed healing, e.g.:

RISK FACTORS
Arterial ulcers: Smoking, hypertension, hyperlipidemia and inactivity. Review surgical/medical management options to improve arterial circulation.
Diabetic ulcers: Smoking, hypertension, obesity, hyperlipidemia and high blood glucose. Review surgical/medical management options and use appropriate off-loading techniques.
Pressure ulcers: Pressure, shear, friction, nutritional deficiencies, dehydration and dry skin conditions, skin exposure to moisture or wound contamination secondary to incontinence, perspiration or other fluids, e.g. skin protection.
Venous ulcers: Edema with leg elevation, ambulation and compression. If patient is not ambulatory, assure frequent ankle flexes. Review surgical/medical management options to improve arterial circulation and compression bandages if appropriate.
Mixed arterial-venous ulcers: Smoking, hypertension, inactivity, hyperlipidemia. Review surgical/medical management options to improve arterial circulation and compression bandages if appropriate.
All patients: Provide patient and/or caregiver teaching and support. Confirm and treat infection if needed. Assess and manage wound pain and odor if present.

Expected Outcomes

Wound is not infected and is healing as evidenced by a reduction in size after 2 to 4 weeks of care. No evidence of new skin breakdown.

Delayed Healing

Re-evaluate plan of care or address underlying etiology if ulcer has not reduced in size during 2 to 4 weeks of care

FIGURE 5.28 Critical BWAT severity score with dry eschar treatment algorithm. (Reprinted from ConvaTec, with permission.)

an adequate support surface, determining need for more advanced wound care, and consideration of the status of the whole patient is also part of the care plan.

Outcomes with Standardized Wound Assessment Using the BWAT

The BWAT was evaluated as part of a standardized assessment and treatment program in a prospective multicenter study of wound healing outcomes.[30] Wound healing outcomes from March 26 to October 31, 2001 were recorded on patients in three long-term care facilities, one long-term acute care hospital, and 12 home care agencies for wounds selected by staff to receive care based on computer-generated validated wound care algorithms, which were based on BWAT scores. Most of the 767 wounds selected to receive the standardized protocols of care based on BWAT scores were stage III to IV pressure ulcers (n = 373; mean healing time 62 days) or full-thickness venous ulcers (n = 124; mean healing time 57 days). The study provides data on use of BWAT scores to identify treatments and measure healing. In addition to being used to identify specific wound treatments, the BWAT has been used to describe characteristics of recurrent pressure ulcers in persons with spinal cord injury as these ulcers have not been well described. Because the BWAT evaluates multiple wound characteristics it is particularly well suited for describing specific wound characteristics in special populations or wounds. For example, recurrent pressure ulcers in persons with spinal cord injury tend to occur at the same anatomic location as the original ulcer, present as full-thickness ulcers with a mean BWAT score of 33.63, minimal exudate, and with nearly half presenting with undermining (48%) and necrotic slough (50%).[31] The BWAT has also been used as an outcome measure examining use of negative pressure wound therapy for pressure ulcers in a long-term acute care setting.[32] The BWAT is incorporated into several health-care organizational electronic medical records (EMR) and lends itself well to EMR in terms of data entry and data access for reports.

WOUND HEALING ASSESSMENT TOOLS DEVELOPED FOR SPECIFIC NEEDS OR POPULATIONS

Several wound healing assessment tools have been developed to address specific needs or populations. In this section, we present three such instruments: the Photographic Wound Assessment Tool (PWAT), the Wound Bed Score (WBS), and the Pressure Ulcer Measurement Tool.

Photographic Wound Assessment Tool

To this point, we have discussed wound healing assessment tools that have been developed to be used at the point of care, in the presence of the patient and wound. In many cases, the expert clinician is not present with the patient and wound. This is particularly true in home health and rural areas, where photos and telemedicine are often used for documentation of wound status and delivered to expert clinicians or consultants for determining wound treatment and judging treatment response. To assess wounds from photographs,

Houghton et al.[6] adapted the BWAT. The PWAT includes six items that can be evaluated from a photograph: wound edges, necrotic tissue type and amount, skin color surrounding wound, granulation tissue type, and epithelialization. Each item was rated on a 5-point scale where a score of "0" reflects the best for the characteristic and a score of "4" the worst. The six items can then be summed for a total score. The PWAT was validated with both pressure ulcers and venous leg ulcers. The PWAT has demonstrated a strong correlation with the BWAT as performed in person on the same wounds at the bedside.[6] Trained health-care professionals demonstrated excellent intrarater and interrater reliability and similar to the BWAT, the PWAT is responsive to changes in wound status with scores significantly greater (better) for wounds (pressure ulcers and venous ulcers) that healed compared to those that did not heal.[6] The PWAT has been used as an outcome measure to evaluate electrical stimulation for pressure ulcer healing in persons with spinal cord injury living in the community.[33]

The Wound Bed Score

In today's wound care treatment options, there are many high technology and advanced therapies such as topically applied growth factors, bioengineered skin, and negative pressure wound therapy devices. Future wound care options may see advanced therapies including genetic modification and therapy. In order to effectively use these advanced therapies for maximal benefit, wound bed preparation is essential as using these therapies on a wound not adequately prepared will result in poor outcomes at a high price. Adequate wound bed preparation means the wound is

- Free of infection
- Well vascularized
- Free of fibrinous material
- Free of scarring
- With minimal exudate

To assist clinicians in assessing wound bed preparation prior to application of advanced high technology therapy, Falanga[8,34] developed the WBS to specifically address wound bed preparation. The WBS consists of a score for wound bed appearance (includes items evaluating granulation tissue, fibrinous tissue, and presence of eschar) and a wound exudate score (includes items evaluating extent of exudate control, exudate amount, and dressing requirements).[6,34] The score for wound bed appearance and wound exudate can be summed for a total score.

The WBS was revised in 2006 with additional items relating to the surrounding skin (healing edges, black eschar, wound depth, edema, periwound dermatitis, and callus).[35] Each item receives a score from 0 (worst score) to 2 (best score) with all items summed for a total score. The modified WBS is presented in Exhibit 5.4. The WBS has been used in venous ulcers and correlated with healing.[35] The instrument can be used at the bedside to determine the likelihood that wound closure will occur. The higher the score, the more favorable the wound outcome and total scores are divided into four quartiles: scores up to 9; scores of 10 and 11; scores of 12 and 13; and scores of 14 to 16. For each quartile increase, there is an increased chance of healing of 22.8%.[35]

EXHIBIT	5.4			

Modified Wound Bed Score

Wound bed score Characteristics	0	1	2
Healing edges	None	25%–75%	>75%
Black eschar	>25% of wound surface area	0%–25%	None
Greatest wound depth/granulation tissue	Severely depressed or raised when compared to periwound skin	Moderate	Flushed or almost even
Exudate amount	Severe	Moderate	None/mild
Edema	Severe	Moderate	None/mild
Periwound dermatitis	Severe	Moderate	None or minimal
Periwound callus fibrosis	Severe	Moderate	None or minimal
Pink wound bed	None	50%–75%	>75%
Wound duration prior to treatment	≥1 year		<1 year

1. The total WBS adds each individual score for each characteristic to give a total score.

2. The maximum possible score (best score) is 18.

3. The minimum possible score (worst score) is 0.

Copyright V. Falanga, used with permission

The Spinal Cord Injury Pressure Ulcer Monitoring Tool (SCI-PUMT)

Thomason and Colleagues[9] developed a tool to monitor pressure ulcer healing over time, in persons with spinal cord injury (SCI). Expert panels developed a 31-item pool of SCI-specific variables for monitoring pressure ulcer healing, which included items from the BWAT and the PUSH (see Exhibit 5.5). Sixty-six participants with a history of SCI for at least 1 year and at least one pressure ulcer were assessed weekly for each of the 31 variables over a 12-week period. A panel of experts identified a pool of items designed to gauge pressure ulcer healing and a second group of experts established content validity of the items. Based on exploratory factor analysis and clinical judgment, seven items were identified and included in the final version of the SCI-PUMT. The seven-item SCI-PUMT demonstrated predictive validity explaining 65% of the variance of surface area and volume of the ulcers at baseline and the total score was associated with the measure of area/volume across the 12-week follow-up period of the study. Interrater reliability was 0.79. Because the item pool included items from the PUSH and BWAT, comparisons were made of predictive validity and sensitivity to change over time of these tools to those of the SCI-PUMT. At baseline, the BWAT accounted for 49% and the PUSH accounted for 46% of the variance in surface area and volume variables compared to 65% for the SCI-PUMT. In the mixed model analysis for sensitivity, the SCI-PUMT model accounted for a reduction of 55% of unexplained variance, while the models with the BWAT and PUSH scores reduced unexplained variance by 33% and 27%, respectively. This seven-item tool is being tested for use in monitoring pressure ulcers in persons with SCI. The SCI-PUMT Quick Reference Guide is presented in Exhibit 5.6.

CONCLUSION: CLINICAL UTILITY OF WOUND HEALING ASSESSMENT TOOLS

Wound healing assessment tools provide a framework for assessment and documentation of wound healing, with an attempt at quantification of aspects of multiple wound attributes. Thus, their use should promote more meaningful communication among health-care professionals involved in wound care. An objective method of assessing wound healing and monitoring changes over time also allows for evaluation of the therapeutic plan of care and may be used to guide and direct therapy. For example, if a specific treatment modality is in use and the patient's wound status, as determined with the wound healing tool, has not changed in 2 weeks, reevaluation of the plan of care is warranted. Use of wound healing tools may uncover other outcome criteria that will help to identify critical attributes during the course of healing.

Use of a research-based wound healing tool, such as those described in this chapter, can also allow discrimination in studies dealing with treatment modalities, and may help to improve our overall understanding of wound healing. It can provide increased sensitivity as well, for example, allowing greater precision and clarity in studies related to the treatment of pressure ulcers. Overall, an instrument that is sensitive to changes in wound status helps us develop improved guidelines for wound care and helps us evaluate individual patient's progress more effectively.

EXHIBIT 5.5

SPINAL CORD IMPAIRMENT PRESSURE ULCER MONITORING TOOL (SCI-PUMT)

Patient _____   SS#_____   Ulcer # _____

Pressure Ulcer

Site: ☐ Sacrum-Coccyx   ☐ Trochanter   ☐ Ischium   ☐ Heel   ☐ Other _____

Body Side: ☐ Right   ☐ Left   ☐ Midline

Orientation: ☐ Medial   ☐ Lateral

Positioning

Upper Leg *Flexed* When Turned: ☐ Yes   ☐ No

Surface Turned *Onto*:   ☐ Right   ☐ Left   ☐ Back   ☐ Abdomen

Variables	Scoring Options					Variable Score
Geometric Factor						
Surface Area (L x W)	**1** ≤ 1 cm^2	**2** $>1-\leq 2.5$ cm^2	**3** $>2.5-\leq 5$ cm^2	**4** $>5-\leq 10$ cm^2	**5** $>10-\leq 15$ cm^2	
	6 $>15-\leq 25$ cm^2	**7** $>25-\leq 35$ cm^2	**8** $>35-\leq 55$ cm^2	**9** $>55-\leq 85$ cm^2	**10** >85 cm^2	
Depth	**0** 0 cm	**1** $>0-\leq 1$ cm	**2** $>1-\leq 2$ cm	**3** $>2-\leq 3$ cm	**4** >3 cm	
Edges	**1** • Indistinct, diffuse, none clearly visible • Distinct, outline clearly visible, attached, even with ulcer base • Well-defined, not attached to ulcer base		**2** • Well-defined, not attached to base, rolled under, thickened • Well-defined, fibrotic, scarred, or hyperkeratotic			
Tunneling	**0** None	**1** ≤ 2 cm	**2** $> 2-\leq 4$ cm	**3** >4 cm		
Undermining	**0** None	**1** ≤ 2 cm	**2** $> 2-\leq 4$ cm	**3** >4 cm		
Sub-total Score Geometric Factor						
Substance Factor						
Exudate Type	**0** None	**1** Serous/Sanguineous	**2** Green/Purulent			
Necrotic Tissue Amount	**0** None	**1** $\leq 25\%$	**2** $>25\%$			
Sub-total Score Substance Factor						
TOTAL SCORE (Total of Geometric and Substance Sub-totals)						

Maximum score = **26**   The HIGHER the score, the more severe the ulcer.

Evaluator: _____   Date:_____

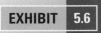

EXHIBIT   5.6

SCI-PUMT Quick Reference Guide

Specificity
- The SCI-PUMT is specific *only* to pressure ulcers.
- Reliability and validity of the SCI-PUMT have not been established to track the healing of dermatitis, excoriations, macerations, skin tears, or neuropathic, venous, and arterial ulcers.

Scoring
- Determine the geometric subtotal scores (i.e., surface area, depth, edges, tunneling, undermining).
- Determine the substance subtotal scores (i.e., exudate type, necrotic tissue amount).
- Add geometric and substance subtotals to obtain the total score (maximum score is 26).
- The HIGHER the score, the more severe the ulcer.

General Guidelines
- **Pressure Ulcer Location:**   Indicate the location of the pressure ulcer being assessed: sacrum, coccyx, trochanter, ischium, heel, other.
- **Pressure Ulcer Body Side:**   Document the body side of the ulcer: left side, right side, midline.
- **Positioning:**   Use consistent patient positioning to obtain accurate measurements. Two or more clinicians are often required to position the patient to optimize ulcer visualization and measurement. Use safe patient handling and movement techniques (e.g., use a sling to position the body to the side or lift the leg). Document the position to which the patient is turned *onto* during the assessment: left side, right side, prone, supine.
- **Hip/Leg Flex:**   Flex the upper leg if the patient is turned to the side to maximize the ulcer's surface area and visualization.

Supplies
- Use separate supplies for each ulcer to avoid cross contamination.
- Supplies include:
  - *Personal protective equipment (e.g., gloves)*
  - *Biohazardous bag*
  - *Linear guide in centimeters*
  - *Measurement grid with blocks and/or marked into 4 quadrants*
  - *Cotton-tipped applicators (1–2)*

SCI-PUMT Assessment Variables—Geometric	
Surface Area	
Instruction	**Key Points**
Measure the length as the greatest distance head-to-toe (12 o'clock to 6 o'clock)	Measure the distance inside the ulcer bed using a non-stretch linear guide with centimeters; use the patient's head as 12 o'clock and the feet as 6 o'clock
Measure the width as the greatest distance side-to-side (9 o'clock to 3 o'clock)	Measure the width perpendicular to the length
Multiply the length × width Score 1–10 (Variable: ≤1 to >85 cm²)	Only measure open, uninterrupted, continuous areas; avoid measuring over "islands" of intact skin that are within the ulcer bed

Depth	
Instruction	**Key Points**
Place a cotton-tipped applicator horizontally across the ulcer edges.	Establish a reference point for the periulcer skin surface.
Place a disposable ruler perpendicular to the horizontal applicator.	Measure the depth from the deepest point of the ulcer bed, excluding tunnels.
Measure the distance from the skin surface (i.e., horizontal applicator) to the *deepest aspect* of the ulcer base. Score 0–4 (Variable: 0 to >3 cm²)	Use a second applicator to measure vertical distance if a disposable ruler is unavailable. Use a pen to mark the vertical applicator where the two applicators intersect. Place the vertical applicator beside a linear guide to measure.

(continued)

EXHIBIT **5.6 (*continued*)**

Edges[a]	
Instruction	**Key Points**
Identify the *worse case* with *any* of the following descriptions:	The edge is where *intact skin contacts the ulcer bed;* the edge is sometimes known as the ulcer margin.
Variable 1	
• Indistinct, diffuse, none clearly visible	
• Distinct, outline clearly visible, attached, even with ulcer base	
• Well defined, not attached to ulcer base	
Variable 2	
• Well-defined, not attached to base, rolled under, thickened	
• Well-defined, fibrotic, scarred, or hyperkeratotic	
Score the edges based upon the *edge appearance* and *ulcer depth*.	Edge integrity facilitates or impedes epithelialization.
Score 1–2	*Score 1*: Edges are not rolled/thickened and are even with the ulcer base; sides/walls are not present. *Score 2*: Edges are rolled and are typically higher than the ulcer base.

Tunneling	
Instruction	**Key Points**
Measure only the longest tunnel.	A tunnel is a space that extends laterally, obliquely, or vertically from the ulcer bed or epithelium; a tunnel is sometimes known as a sinus tract or channel.[b]
Insert a ruler to measure the distance from the ulcer bed to the most distal aspect of the tunnel.	The Clinician *should not* be able to visualize skin elevation of the distal tip of an applicator when it is inserted into a tunnel.
Never force the ruler or applicator into a tunnel if resistance is encountered.	Use an applicator if a disposable ruler is unavailable or the tunnel is too narrow. Use a pen to mark the proximal part of the applicator where it contacts the ulcer bed. Place the applicator beside a linear guide to measure.
Score: 0–3 (Variable: None to >4 cm²)	Tunnels inhibit granulation of full-thickness ulcers and may result in abscesses.

Undermining	
Instruction	**Key Points**
Measure only the greatest undermined distance.	Undermining is an opening that begins at the ulcer edge and extends beneath the skin either parallel or tangential to the skin surface.[b] Undermining is under intact skin adjacent to the open ulcer.
Insert a ruler to measure the distance from the ulcer edge to the most distal aspect of undermined area.	The clinician *should be* able to visualize skin elevation of the distal tip of an applicator when it is inserted into an undermined area.

EXHIBIT 5.6 (*continued*)

Never force the ruler or applicator into an undermined area if resistance is encountered.	Use an applicator if a disposable ruler is unavailable or the undermined area is too narrow. Use a pen to mark the proximal part of the applicator where it contacts the ulcer edge. Place the applicator beside a linear guide to measure.
Score: 0–3 (Variable: None to >4 cm²)	Undermining negatively impacts the circulation of the intact epidermis and dermis.

SCI-PUMT Assessment Variables—Substance

Exudate Type	
Instruction	**Key Points**
Assess drainage on the *soiled dressing*, not the ulcer bed.	Exudate is the fluid that drains from tissues due to inflammation or injury.[b]
Assess the presence and type of drainage.	Serous drainage is clear.
Variable 0	Sanguineous drainage is bloody.
• No drainage	Green or purulent drainage is opaque.
Variable 1	
• Serous	
• Sanguineous	
Variable 2	
• Green	
• Purulent	
Score 0–2	Green or purulent drainage may indicate infection that may inhibit the healing process.

Necrotic Tissue Amount[a]	
Instruction	**Key Points**
Use a transparent metric measuring guide divided into 4 (25%) pie-shaped quadrants to determine the percent of the ulcer that has necrotic tissue.	Necrosis is the pathological death of tissues or cells resulting from irreversible damage.[b]
	Devitalized collagen may present as *slough* or *eschar* that may be relatively thick or thin.
	• *Slough* is devitalized tissue that may involve a portion or all of the ulcer bed. Slough is typically yellow but may be green or brown. It is often stringy.
	• *Eschar* is dark, leathery tissue that may involve a portion or all of the ulcer bed. It is typically dry but may be moist.
Score 0–2 (Variable: None to >25%)	Necrosis inhibits granulation tissue in full-thickness ulcers.

[a]Variables of Edges and Necrotic Tissue Amount were adapted from the Bates-Jensen Wound Assessment Tool.
[b]Consortium for Spinal Cord Medicine (2000). Pressure ulcer prevention and treatment following spinal cord injury: From *A Clinical Practice Guideline for Health-Care Professionals*. Washington, DC: Paralyzed Veterans of America.

REVIEW QUESTIONS

1. Predictive validity is best described as follows:
   A. It tests the tool against present performance or status on a criterion.
   B. It tests the tool against future performance or status on a criterion.
   C. It tests scores from one rater against a second rater.
   D. It tests the tool against a gold standard.

2. Which are wound characteristics commonly included in instruments to evaluate wound healing?
   A. Size, shape, necrotic tissue characteristics, exudate
   B. Size, granulation tissue characteristics, exudate, necrotic tissue characteristics
   C. Size, stage, necrotic tissue characteristics, surrounding skin characteristics
   D. Size, depth, necrotic tissue characteristics, exudate

3. Which is a recommended method of measuring wound size?
   A. Measure the longest length and the perpendicular widest width in centimeters.
   B. Measure the wound circumference.
   C. Measure the length from 12 o'clock to 6 o'clock and multiply by 2.
   D. Measure the head-to-toe length and the side-to-side length.

4. Interrater reliability is best defined by which statement?
   A. The consistency of the tool with repeated measures.
   B. It is concerned with different clinicians getting the same score on the tool when evaluating the same wound.
   C. It is the accuracy of the tool.
   D. It is concerned with all items on a tool consistently measuring the same objective.

5. The ability of the tool to respond quickly to changes in the wound status is the definition of
   A. intrarater reliability
   B. predictive validity
   C. responsiveness
   D. sensitivity

REFERENCES

1. Bates-Jensen BM, Vredevoe, D, Brecht ML. Validity and reliability of the Pressure Sore Status Tool. *Decubitus.* 1992;5(6):20–28.
2. Thomas DR, Rodeheaver GT, Bartolucci AA, et al. Pressure ulcer scale for healing: Derivation and validation of the PUSH tool. *Adv Wound Care.* 1997;10(5):96–101.
3. Krasner D. Wound healing scale, version 1.0: a proposal. *Adv Wound Care.* 1997;10(5):82–85.
4. Ferrell BA, Artinian BM, Sessing D. The Sessing scale for assessment of pressure ulcer healing. *J Am Geriatr Soc.* 1995;43:37–40.
5. Sussman C, Swanson G. The utility of Sussman Wound Healing Tool in predicting wound healing outcomes in physical therapy. *Adv Wound Care.* 1997;10(5):74–77.
6. Houghton PE, Kincaid CB, Campbell K, et al. Photographic assessment of the appearance of chronic pressure and leg ulcers. *Ostomy Wound Manage.* 2000;46(4):20–30.
7. Wagner FEW. The dysvascular foot: a system for diagnosis and treatment. *Foot Ankle.* 1981(2):64–122.
8. Falanga, V. Classifications for wound bed preparation and stimulation of chronic wounds. *Wound Rep Reg.* 2000;8(5):347–352.
9. Thomason SS, Nelson AL, Luther SL, Harrow JJ. Monitoring Pressure Ulcer Healing in Persons with Spinal Cord Impairment. 2009. Department of Veteran Affairs, Veterans Health Administration, Health Services Research and Development Service, Nursing Research Initiative (NRI 03-245-4 (IRB#104145).
10. Burns N, Grove SK. The concepts of measurement. In: Burns N, ed. *The Practice of Nursing Research: Conduct, Critique & Utilization.* 4th ed. Philadelphia, PA: WB Saunders; 2000:389–410.
11. Waltz CF, Strickland OL, Lenz ER. Reliability and validity of criterion-referenced measures. In: Waltz CF, Lenz ER, ed. *Measurement in Nursing Research.* 2nd ed. Philadelphia, PA: FA Davis; 1991:229–257.
12. Kennedy K. The prevalence of pressure ulcers in an intermediate care facility. *Decubitus.* 1989;2(2):44–45.
13. Sibbald RG, Krasner DL, Lutz JB, et al. The SCALE expert panel: skin changes at life's end. *Final Consensus Document.* 2009.
14. Bartolucci AA, Thomas DR. Using principal component analysis to describe wound status. *Adv Wound Care.* 1997;10(5):93–95.
15. Stotts NA, Thomas DR, Frantz R, et al. An instrument to measure healing in pressure ulcers: Development and validation of the Pressure Ulcer Scale for Healing (PUSH). *J Gerontol A: Med Sci.* 2001;56(12):M795–M799.
16. Ratliff CR. Use of the PUSH Tool to measure venous ulcer healing. *Ostomy Wound Manage.* 2005;51(5):58–63.
17. Hon J, Lagden K, McLaren AM, et al. A prospective, multicenter study to validate use of the Pressure Ulcer Scale for Healing (PUSH(c)) in patients with diabetic, venous, and pressure ulcers. *Ostomy Wound Manage.* 2010;56(2):26–36.
18. Edwards H, Courtney M, Finlayson K, et al. Improved healing rates for chronic venous leg ulcers: pilot study results from a randomized controlled trial of a community nursing intervention. *Int J Nurs Pract.* 2005;11(4):169–176.
19. Posthaur ME. Nutrition: A key link in clinical decision trees. *Adv Skin Wound Care.* 2004;17(9):474,476.
20. Gunes, UY. A prospective study evaluating the Pressure Ulcer Scale for Healing (PUSH Tool) to assess stage II, stage III, and stage IV pressure ulcers. *Ostomy Wound Manage.* 2009;55(5):48–52.
21. Gardner SE, Frantz RA, Bergquist S, et al. A prospective study of the Pressure Ulcer Scale for Healing (PUSH). *J Gerontol A: Med Sci.* 2005;60A(1):93–97.
22. George-Saintilus E, Tommasulo B, Cal CE, et al. Pressure ulcer PUSH score and traditional nursing assessment in nursing home residents: do they correlate? *J Am Med Dir Assoc.* 2009;10(2):141–144.
23. Pompeo M. Implementing the PUSH tool in clinical practice: Revisions and results. *Ostomy Wound Manage.* 2003;49(8):32–46.
24. Harris C, Bates-Jensen B, Parslow N, et al. Bates-Jensen wound assessment tool: pictorial guide validation project. *J Wound Ostomy Continence Nurs.* 2010;37(3):253–259.
25. Harris C, Bates-Jensen B, Parslow N, et al. The Bates-Jensen Wound Assessment Tool (BWAT): development of a pictorial guide for training nurses. *Wound Care Canada.* 2009;7(2):33–38.
26. Bates-Jensen BM, McNees, P. The wound intelligence system: Early issues and findings from multi-site tests. *Ostomy Wound Manage.* 1996;42(suppl 7A):1–7.
27. Bates-Jensen B, McNees, P. Toward an intelligent wound assessment system. *Ostomy Wound Manage.* 1995;41(suppl 7A):80–88.

28. Bates-Jensen B. A quantitative analysis of wound characteristics as early predictors of healing in pressure sores. *Dissertation Abstracts International*, Vol. 59, No. 11, Los Angeles: University of California, 1999.

29. De Laat EH, Scholte OP, Reimer WH, et al. Pressure ulcers: diagnostics and interventions aimed at wound-related complaints: a review of the literature. *J Clin Nurs.* 2005;14(4):464–472.

30. Bolton L, McNees P, Van Rijswijk L, et al. Wound-healing outcomes using standardized assessment and care in clinical practice. *J Wound Ostomy Continence Nurs.* 2004;31(2):65–71.

31. Bates-Jensen BM, Guihan M, Garber SL, et al. Characteristics of recurrent pressure ulcers in veterans with spinal cord injury. *J Spinal Cord Med.* 2009;32(1):34–42.

32. De Leon JM, Barnes S, Nagel M, et al. Cost-effectiveness of negative pressure wound therapy for postsurgical patients in long-term acute care. *Adv Skin Wound Care.* 2009;22(3):122–127.

33. Houghton PE, Campbell KE, Fraser CH, et al. Electrical stimulation therapy increases rate of healing of pressure ulcers in community-dwelling people with spinal cord injury. *Arch Phys Med Rehabil.* 2010;91(5):669–678.

34. Falanga V. Measurements in wound healing. *Int J Low Extrem Wounds.* 2008;7(1):9–11.

35. Falanga V, Saap LJ, Ozonoff A. Wound bed score and its correlation with healing of chronic wounds. *Dermatol Ther.* 2006;19:383–390.

Sussman Wound Healing Tool (SWHT)
WOUND ASSESSMENT FORM

NAME: _____   MEDICAL RECORD NO.: _____

DATE: _____   EXAMINER: _____

CIRCLE WEEK OF CARE: B   1   2   3   4   5   6   7   8   9   10   11   12

SWHT Variable	Tissue Attribute	Attribute Definition	Rating	Relationship to Healing	Score
1	Hemorrhage	Purple ecchymosis of wound tissue or surrounding skin	Present or absent	Not good	
2	Maceration	Softening of a tissue by soaking until the connective tissue fibers are soft and friable	Present or absent	Not good	
3	Undermining	Includes both undermining and tunneling	Present or absent	Not good	
4	Erythema	Reddening or darkening of the skin compared to surrounding skin; usually accompanied by heat	Present or absent	Not good	
5	Necrosis	All types of necrotic tissue, including eschar and slough	Present or absent	Not good	
6	Adherence at wound edge	Continuity of wound edge and the base of the wound	Present or absent	Good	
7	Granulation (Fibroplasia—significant reduction in depth)	Pink/red granulation tissue filling in the wound bed, reducing wound depth	Present or absent	Good	
8	Appearance of contraction (reduced size)	First measurement of the wound drawing together, resulting in reduction in wound open surface area	Present or absent	Good	
9	Sustained contraction (more reduced size)	Continued drawing together of wound edges, measured by reduced wound open surface area	Present or absent	Good	
10	Epithelialization	Appearance and continuation of resurfacing with new skin or scar at the wound edges or surface	Present or absent	Good	

MEASURES AND EXTENT (Depth and Undermining: Not Good)

Depth/ Location			SCORE	Undermining/ Location	SCORE	Other	Letter
11	General depth >0.2 cm			16	Underm @ 12:00	Location	
12	General depth @ 12:00 >0.2 cm			17	Underm @ 3:00	Wound healing phase	
13	General depth @ 3:00 >0.2 cm			18	Underm @ 6:00	Total "Not Good"	
14	General depth @ 6:00 >0.2 cm			19	Underm @ 9:00	Total "Good"	
15	General depth @ 9:00 >0.2 cm						

Key: Present = 1. Absent = 0. Location choices: upper body (UB), coccyx (C), trochanter (T), ischial (I), heel (H), foot (F); add right or left (R or L). Wound healing long phase: inflammation (I), proliferation (P), epithelialization (E), remodeling (R).

Source: Copyright © 1997, Sussman Physical Therapy Inc.

Location _____

Wound healing phase _____

Total "Not Good" _____

Total "Good" _____

Procedure for Using the SWHT

Completion of the SWHT is by observation and physical assessment, as follows:

1. Each wound of each patient needs its own SWHT attributes form.
2. The patient's name, medical record number, and date of assessment are written at the top of the form.
3. The examiner signs the document.
4. As the wound is assessed, the rater marks a 1 or a 0 to signify present or absent on the form next to each of the 19 attributes. The squares in the column must be marked with one of the two scores.
5. The wound location and the current wound healing phase are marked with the appropriate letter. Choose the appropriate letter to represent the anatomic location of the wound and place it in the square at the time of the initial assessment and subsequent reassessments. The location will not change.
6. Letters are also used to represent the current wound healing phase: mark an *I* for inflammatory, *P* for proliferative, *E* for epithelialization, and *R* for remodeling. In the appropriate box, the phase is noted initially and at each reassessment. The wound healing phase should change as the wound heals.
7. Undermining and depth require some physical assessment to determine presence or absence.
8. Open area measurements are made and listed on a separate form (see Chapter 4), then compared with subsequent measurements of these characteristics to determine contraction and sustained contraction, measured as reduction in linear size.
9. Scoring part I. Add the number of "not good for healing" attributes and the number of "good for healing" attributes listed. The score of "not good for healing" should diminish as the wound heals, and the score of "good for healing" attributes should increase.
10. A summary of the change is shown in Exhibit 5.4.

PUSH Tool 3.0

Patient Name: _____   Patient ID#: _____

Ulcer Location: _____   Date: _____

DIRECTIONS:

Observe and measure the pressure ulcer. Categorize the ulcer with respect to surface area, exudate, and type of wound tissue. Record a subscore for each of these ulcer characteristics. Add the subscores to obtain the total score. A comparison of total scores measured over time provides an indication of the improvement or deterioration in pressure ulcer healing.

Length	0	1	2	3	4	5	
	0 cm²	<0.3 cm²	0.3–0.6 cm²	0.7–1.0 cm²	1.1–2.0 cm²	2.1–3.0 cm²	
× Width		6	7	8	9	10	**Subscore**
		3.1–4.0 cm²	4.1–8.0 cm²	8.1–12.0 cm²	12.1–24.0 cm²	>24 cm²	
Exudate Amount	0	1	2	3			**Subscore**
	None	Light	Moderate	Heavy			
Tissue Type	0	1	2	3	4		**Subscore**
	Closed	Epithelial tissue	Granulation tissue	Slough	Necrotic tissue		
							Total Score

Length × Width: Measure the greatest length (head to toe) and the greatest width (side to side) using a centimeter ruler. Multiply these two measurements (length × width) to obtain an estimate of surface area in square centimeters (cm²). Caveat: Do not guess! Always use a centimeter ruler and always use the same method each time the ulcer is measured.

Exudate Amount: Estimate the amount of exudate (drainage) present after removal of the dressing and before applying any topical agent to the ulcer. Estimate the exudate (drainage) as none, light, moderate, or heavy.

Tissue Type: This refers to the types of tissue that are present in the wound (ulcer) bed. Score as a "4" if there is any necrotic tissue present. Score as a "3" if there is any amount of slough present and necrotic tissue is absent. Score as a "2" if the wound is clean and contains granulation tissue. A superficial wound that is reepithelializing is scored as a "1." When the wound is closed, score as a "0."

4—Necrotic Tissue (Eschar): black, brown, or tan tissue that adheres firmly to the wound bed or ulcer edges and may be either firmer or softer than surrounding skin.
3—Slough: yellow or white tissue that adheres to the ulcer bed in strings or thick clumps, or is mucinous.
2—Granulation Tissue: pink or beefy red tissue with a shiny, moist, granular appearance.
1—Epithelial Tissue: for superficial ulcers, new pink or shiny tissue (skin) that grows in from the edges or as islands on the ulcer surface.
0—Closed/Resurfaced: the wound is completely covered with epithelium (new skin).

Version 3.0: 9/15/98
©National Pressure Ulcer Advisory Panel

Source: Copyright © National Pressure Ulcer Advisory Panel.

PRESSURE ULCER HEALING CHART
(To Monitor Trends in PUSH Scores over Time)
(Use a separate page for each pressure ulcer)

Patient Name: _____   Patient ID#: _____

Ulcer Location: _____   Date: _____

Directions: Observe and measure pressure ulcers at regular intervals using the PUSH Tool. Date and record PUSH subscale and total scores on the pressure ulcer healing record below.

PRESSURE ULCER HEALING RECORD

DATE													
Length × Width													
Exudate Amount													
Tissue Type													
Total Score													

Graph the PUSH total score on the pressure ulcer healing graph below (see Exhibit 5.4)

PUSH Total Score	PRESSURE ULCER HEALING GRAPH												
17													
16													
15													
14													
13													
12													
11													
10													
9													
8													
7													
6													
5													
4													
3													
2													
1													
Healed 0													
DATE													

PUSH Tool Version 3.0: 9/15/98

Instructions for Using the PUSH Tool

To use the PUSH Tool, the pressure ulcer is assessed and scored on the three elements in the tool:

- Length × Width → scored from 0 to 10
- Exudate Amount → scored from 0 (none) to 3 (heavy)
- Tissue Type → scored from 0 (closed) to 4 (necrotic tissue)

Ensure consistency in applying the tool to monitor wound healing, definitions for each element are supplied at the bottom of the tool.

Step 1: Using the definition for length × width, a centimeter ruler measurement is made of the greatest head-to-toe diameter. A second measurement is made of the greatest width (left to right). Multiply these two measurements to get square centimeters, then select the corresponding category for size on the scale and record the score.

Step 2: Estimate the amount of exudate after removal of the dressing and before applying any topical agents. Select the corresponding category for amount and record the score.

Step 3: Identify the type of tissue. Note: if there is ANY necrotic tissue, it is scored a 4. If there is ANY slough, it is scored a 3, even though most of the wound is covered with granulation tissue.

Step 4: Sum the scores on the three elements of the tool to derive a total PUSH Score.

Step 5: Transfer the total score to the Pressure Ulcer Healing Graph. Changes in the score over time provide an indication of the changing status of the ulcer. If the score goes down, the wound is healing. If it gets larger, the wound is deteriorating.

Unmodified Version 3.0: 9/15/98

©National Pressure Ulcer Advisory Panel

Reprint Permission granted. Further reprint requests should be directed to: NPUAP online at: www.npuap.org

Patient:	Admit Date: DC Date:		# of Days:
Hosp. #:			

Patient Discharges for Month of:		Scoring Completed by:	

Identifiers: (circle if wound acquired)		Admit PUSH Scores				Discharge PUSH Scores			
		Initial Sub-Scores			Total	Final Sub-Scores			Total
	Wound Location	Size	Exudate	Tissue		Size	Exudate	Tissue	
A									
B									
C									
D									
E									
F									
G									
H									
I									
J									
		Sum of initial Total ↓ PUSH Scores				Sum of final Total ↓ PUSH Scores			

Length	0 0 cm²	I < 0.3 cm²	2 0.3-0.6 cm²	3 0.7-1.0 cm²	4 1.1-2.0 cm²	5 2.1-3.0 cm²	
x Width		6 3.1–4.0 cm²	7 4.1–8.0 cm²	8 8.1–12.0 cm²	9 12.1–24.0 cm²	10 >24.0 cm²	Sub-score
Exudate Amount	0 None	I Light	2 Moderate	3 Heavy			Sub-score
Tissue Type	0 Closed	I Epithelial Tissue	2 Granulation Tissue	3 Slough	4 Necrotic Tissue		Sub-score
							Total score

Number of Acquired wounds: _____

Change in PUSH = ⬜PUSH = PUSH initial – PUSH final = _____
                              (HEALING Score)

Healing Rate = ⬜PUSH/Total Days = _____/_____ =   _____

Form 1: Individual Patient Pressure Ulcer Scale for Healing
(may be reproduced without permission)

Instructions for use

General Guidelines

Fill out the attached rating sheet to assess a wound's status after reading the definitions and methods of assessment described below. Evaluate once a week and whenever a change occurs in the wound. Rate according to each item by picking the response that best describes the wound and entering that score in the item score column for the appropriate date. When you have rated the wound on all items, determine the total score by adding together the 13-item scores. The HIGHER the total score, the more severe the wound status. Plot total score on the Wound Status Continuum to determine progress. If the wound has healed/resolved, score items 1, 2, 3, and 4 as = 0.

Specific Instructions

1. **Size:** Use ruler to measure the longest and widest aspect of the wound surface in centimeters; multiply length × width. Score as = 0 if wound healed/resolved.

2. **Depth:** Pick the depth, thickness, most appropriate to the wound using these additional descriptions, score as = 0 if wound healed/resolved:

   1 = tissues damaged but no break in skin surface.
   2 = superficial, abrasion, blister or shallow crater. Even with, and/or elevated above skin surface (e.g., hyperplasia).
   3 = deep crater with or without undermining of adjacent tissue.
   4 = visualization of tissue layers not possible due to necrosis.
   5 = supporting structures include tendon, joint capsule.

3. **Edges:** Score as = 0 if wound healed/resolved. Use this guide:

Indistinct, diffuse	=	unable to clearly distinguish wound outline.
Attached	=	even or flush with wound base, *no* sides or walls present; flat.
Not attached	=	sides or walls *are* present; floor or base of wound is deeper than edge.
Rolled under, thickened	=	soft to firm and flexible to touch.
Hyperkeratosis	=	callous-like tissue formation around wound and at edges.
Fibrotic, scarred	=	hard, rigid to touch.

4. **Undermining:** Score as = 0 if wound healed/resolved. Assess by inserting a cotton tipped applicator under the wound edge; advance it as far as it will go without using undue force; raise the tip of the applicator so it may be seen or felt on the surface of the skin; mark the surface with a pen; measure the distance from the mark on the skin to the edge of the wound. Continue process around the wound. Then use a transparent metric measuring guide with concentric circles divided into four (25%) pie-shaped quadrants to help determine percent of wound involved.

5. **Necrotic Tissue Type:** Pick the type of necrotic tissue that is *predominant* in the wound according to color, consistency, and adherence using this guide:

White/gray nonviable tissue	=	may appear prior to wound opening; skin surface is white or gray.
Nonadherent, yellow slough	=	thin, mucinous substance; scattered throughout wound bed; easily separated from wound tissue.
Loosely adherent, yellow slough	=	thick, stringy, clumps of debris; attached to wound tissue.
Adherent, soft, black eschar	=	soggy tissue; strongly attached to tissue in center or base of wound.
Firmly adherent, hard/black eschar	=	firm, crusty tissue; strongly attached to wound base *and* edges (like a hard scab).

6. **Necrotic Tissue Amount:** Use a transparent metric measuring guide with concentric circles divided into four (25%) pie-shaped quadrants to help determine percent of wound involved.

7. **Exudate Type:** Some dressings interact with wound drainage to produce a gel or trap liquid. Before assessing exudate type, gently cleanse wound with normal saline or water. Pick the exudate type that is *predominant* in the wound according to color and consistency, using this guide:

Bloody	=	thin, bright red
Serosanguineous	=	thin, watery pale red to pink
Serous	=	thin, watery, clear
Purulent	=	thin or thick, opaque tan to yellow or green may have offensive odor

© 2001 Barbara Bates-Jensen

8. **Exudate Amount**: Use a transparent metric measuring guide with concentric circles divided into four (25%) pie-shaped quadrants to determine percent of dressing involved with exudate. Use this guide:

None	=	wound tissues dry.
Scant	=	wound tissues moist; no measurable exudate.
Small	=	wound tissues wet; moisture evenly distributed in wound; drainage involves ≤25% dressing.
Moderate	=	wound tissues saturated; drainage may or may not be evenly distributed in wound; drainage involves >25% to ≤75% dressing.
Large	=	wound tissues bathed in fluid; drainage freely expressed; may or may not be evenly distributed in wound; drainage involves >75% of dressing.

9. **Skin Color Surrounding Wound**: Assess tissues within 4 cm of wound edge. Dark-skinned persons show the colors "bright red" and "dark red" as a deepening of normal ethnic skin color or a purple hue. As healing occurs in dark-skinned persons, the new skin is pink and may never darken.

10. **Peripheral Tissue Edema and Induration**: Assess tissues within 4 cm of wound edge. Nonpitting edema appears as skin that is shiny and taut. Identify pitting edema by firmly pressing a finger down into the tissues and waiting for 5 seconds, on release of pressure, tissues fail to resume previous position and an indentation appears. Induration is abnormal firmness of tissues with margins. Assess by gently pinching the tissues. Induration results in an inability to pinch the tissues. Use a transparent metric measuring guide to determine how far edema or induration extends beyond wound.

11. **Granulation Tissue**: Granulation tissue is the growth of small blood vessels and connective tissue to fill in full thickness wounds. Tissue is healthy when bright, beefy red, shiny and granular with a velvety appearance. Poor vascular supply appears as pale pink or blanched to dull, dusky red color.

12. **Epithelialization**: Epithelialization is the process of epidermal resurfacing and appears as pink or red skin. In partial thickness wounds it can occur throughout the wound bed as well as from the wound edges. In full thickness wounds it occurs from the edges only. Use a transparent metric measuring guide with concentric circles divided into four (25%) pie-shaped quadrants to help determine percent of wound involved and to measure the distance the epithelial tissue extends into the wound.

© 2001 Barbara Bates-Jensen

BATES-JENSEN WOUND ASSESSMENT TOOL   NAME _____

Complete the rating sheet to assess wound status. Evaluate each item by picking the response that best describes the wound and entering the score in the item score column for the appropriate date. If the wound has healed/resolved, score items 1, 2, 3, and 4 as = 0.

Location: Anatomic site. Circle, identify right (**R**) or left (**L**) and use "**X**" to mark site on body diagrams:

_____ Sacrum and coccyx   _____ Lateral ankle
_____ Trochanter   _____ Medial ankle
_____ Ischial tuberosity   _____ Heel
_____ Buttock   _____ Other site:

Shape: Overall wound pattern; assess by observing perimeter and depth. Circle and *date* appropriate description:

_____ Irregular   _____ Linear or elongated
_____ Round/oval   _____ Bowl/boat
_____ Square/rectangle   _____ Butterfly   _____ Other Shape

Item	Assessment	Date Score	Date Score	Date Score
1. Size*	*0 = Healed, resolved wound 1 = Length × width <4 cm^2 2 = Length × width 4 to <16 cm^2 3 = Length × width 16.1 to <36 cm^2 4 = Length × width 36.1 to <80 cm^2 5 = Length × width >80 cm^2			
2. Depth*	*0 = Healed, resolved wound 1 = Nonblanchable erythema on intact skin 2 = Partial thickness skin loss involving epidermis and/or dermis 3 = Full thickness skin loss involving damage or necrosis of subcutaneous tissue; may extend down to but not through underlying fascia; and/or mixed partial and full thickness and/or tissue layers obscured by granulation tissue 4 = Obscured by necrosis 5 = Full thickness skin loss with extensive destruction, tissue necrosis or damage to muscle, bone or supporting structures			
3. Edges*	*0 = Healed, resolved wound 1 = Indistinct, diffuse, none clearly visible 2 = Distinct, outline clearly visible, attached, even with wound base 3 = Well-defined, not attached to wound base 4 = Well-defined, not attached to base, rolled under, thickened 5 = Well-defined, fibrotic, scarred or hyperkeratotic			
4. Undermining*	*0 = Healed, resolved wound 1 = None present 2 = Undermining <2 cm in any area 3 = Undermining 2–4 cm involving <50% wound margins 4 = Undermining 2–4 cm involving >50% wound margins 5 = Undermining >4 cm or Tunneling in any area			

5. **Necrotic Tissue Type**	1 = None visible 2 = White/grey nonviable tissue and/or nonadherent yellow slough 3 = Loosely adherent yellow slough 4 = Adherent, soft, black eschar 5 = Firmly adherent, hard, black eschar			
6. **Necrotic Tissue Amount**	1 = None visible 2 = <25% of wound bed covered 3 = 25%–50% of wound covered 4 = >50% and <75% of wound covered 5 = 75%–100% of wound covered			
7. **Exudate Type**	1 = None 2 = Bloody 3 = Serosanguineous: thin, watery, pale red/pink 4 = Serous: thin, watery, clear 5 = Purulent: thin or thick, opaque, tan/yellow, with or without odor			
8. **Exudate Amount**	1 = None, dry wound 2 = Scant, wound moist but no observable exudate 3 = Small 4 = Moderate 5 = Large			
9. **Skin Color Surrounding Wound**	1 = Pink or normal for ethnic group 2 = Bright red and/or blanches to touch 3 = White or grey pallor or hypopigmented 4 = Dark red or purple and/or nonblanchable 5 = Black or hyperpigmented			
10. **Peripheral Tissue Edema**	1 = No swelling or edema 2 = Nonpitting edema extends <4 cm around wound 3 = Nonpitting edema extends >4 cm around wound 4 = Pitting edema extends <4 cm around wound 5 = Crepitus and/or pitting edema extends >4 cm around wound			
11. **Peripheral Tissue Induration**	1 = None present 2 = Induration, <2 cm around wound 3 = Induration 2–4 cm extending <50% around wound 4 = Induration 2–4 cm extending >50% around wound 5 = Induration >4 cm in any area around wound			
12. **Granulation Tissue**	1 = Skin intact or partial thickness wound 2 = Bright, beefy red; 75%–100% of wound filled and/or tissue overgrowth 3 = Bright, beefy red; <75% and >25% of wound filled 4 = Pink, and/or dull, dusky red and/or fills ≤25% of wound 5 = No granulation tissue present			

13. **Epithelialization**	1 = 100% wound covered, surface intact
	2 = 75% to <100% wound covered and/or epithe-
	    lial tissue extends >0.5 cm into wound bed
	3 = 50% to <75% wound covered and/or epithe-
	    lial tissue extends to <0.5 cm into wound bed
	4 = w25% to < 50% wound covered
	5 = <25% wound covered			

TOTAL SCORE				
SIGNATURE				

WOUND STATUS CONTINUUM

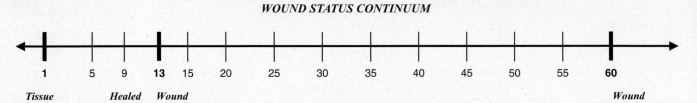

| 1 | 5 | 9 | **13** | 15 | 20 | 25 | 30 | 35 | 40 | 45 | 50 | 55 | **60** |

Tissue   *Healed*   *Wound*   *Wound*

Health   Regeneration   Degeneration

Plot the total score on the Wound Status Continuum by putting an **"X"** on the line and the date beneath the line. Plot multiple scores with their dates to see-at-a-glance regeneration or degeneration of the wound.

© 2001 Barbara Bates-Jensen

Gregory K. Patterson

CHAPTER OBJECTIVES

At the completion of this chapter, the reader will be able to:

1. Identify the areas of the medical history and the physical examination techniques important for assessing patients for vascular disease.
2. Compare and contrast techniques for noninvasive arterial testing.
3. Explain the technique for obtaining an ankle brachial index.
4. Describe the most common type of invasive arterial study.
5. Discuss the physiologic and anatomic tests for evaluating venous insufficiency.

Many of the patients referred to wound care specialists have wounds with a vascular etiology. These include arterial, venous, and diabetic wounds. Despite modern wound care therapies, few of these wounds will heal unless the underlying cause is assessed and treated or confirmed to be not significant. Wounds that do heal without treatment of their etiology exhibit a high rate of recidivism. This is especially true for venous ulcers with underlying chronic venous insufficiency. For these reasons, the initial evaluation of the wound care patient should always contain a thorough vascular assessment. This is the subject of this chapter.

PROCEDURE FOR VASCULAR EVALUATION

The procedure for conducting a thorough vascular assessment consists of three steps: a medical history focusing on vascular-related events, a targeted physical examination, and specific vascular testing.

Past Medical History

Exhibit 6.1 lists areas of the medical history used to identify risk factors for vascular disease, both arterial and venous. Notice that it goes beyond the general medical history discussed in Chapter 1 and focuses on specific vascular-related events. The medical history should include questions about diagnoses of peripheral vascular disease (PVD), atherosclerotic cardiovascular disease, diabetes mellitus, renal disease, prior deep vein thrombosis, varicose veins, chronic venous insufficiency, and elevated cholesterol and triglycerides. A thorough surgical history should include all previous operations, especially vascular procedures, including peripheral arterial and venous procedures. Cardiac procedures should also be included, because the greater

saphenous vein is often utilized for bypass procedures. This can cause significant wounds, especially in the diabetic population, and can aggravate any long-standing venous insufficiency.

It is also essential to review the patient's use of medications. Especially significant are the use of steroids, rheologic agents, antihypertensive medications, anticoagulants, antiplatelet agents, and aspirin.

Critical evaluation of the patient's symptoms can help you distinguish the cause of the wound. In the patient with suspected arterial problems, pay attention to reports of pain, including the following:

- *Claudication.* Typical **claudication** (from the Greek for "to limp") is pain in the calf upon walking some distance. It is due to inadequate perfusion to the calf muscles. The pain rapidly diminishes after the activity is stopped. If this symptom disappears for long periods of time or if the pain is helped by positional changes, a neurologic cause, such as spinal stenosis or disk problems, should be entertained. This is the so-called pseudoclaudication or neuroclaudication.
- *Rest pain.* **Rest pain** is pain across the forefoot, mainly associated with positional elevation. It occurs with inadequate blood supply to the foot. Patients may state that, to relieve the pain at night, they will "hang" their feet over the side of the bed. This enables gravity to increase blood flow, thus relieving pain.
- *Fatigue and/or swelling.* Often patients with vascular disease will experience a sensation of "tiredness" in the limbs. They may also experience swelling that increases during the day or during long periods of standing.

With female patients, elicit an obstetrical history focusing on the development of varicosities during pregnancy. The varicosities

EXHIBIT 6.1

Past Medical History

Risk Factors for Peripheral Vascular Disease[1]

Cardiac history

- Heart disease (cardiac catheterization? results?)
- Heart attack (date of last event)
- Chest pain (note location of the pain, how is pain relieved? onset?)
- Stroke (date of event, note location of weakness or speech deficit)

Hypertension (severity, medications, age at onset, highest blood pressure reading)

Hyperlipidemia (last cholesterol level, medication, number of years)

Smoking history (number of packs per day × years smoked = number of pack-years) (For example: a patient smoking two packs per day for 20 years has a 40-pack-year smoking history.) (quit? year quit)

Diabetes (number of years, medications)

Concomitant illnesses (renal disease, collagen vascular disease, arthritis, pulmonary disease, malignancy [type of malignancy], back [spine] problems, etc.)

Family history of arterial disease

Risk Factors for Venous Disease

Trauma (type, date)

Deep vein thrombosis (date, anticoagulants)

Prolonged inactivity or standing activity

Multiple pregnancies

Family history of venous disease or varicose veins

Obesity

Clotting disorders

Past Surgical History

Vascular surgery (date of procedure, indication)

Angiogram/venogram (dates, indication, intervention?)

General surgery (date of procedure, indication)

---

occur secondary to the effect of high levels of estrogen on the vein walls or pelvic congestion from the gravid uterus "pressing" on the iliac veins.

Physical Examination

The general physical examination is extremely important for patients with suspected or known vascular disease. It includes techniques of inspection, palpation, and auscultation that can help you identify objective signs of vascular insult. To perform the examination and interpret the findings appropriately, you need a thorough understanding of the anatomy and physiology of the cardiovascular and lymphatic systems. Use Table 6.1 to help you differentiate between inspection and palpation findings due to arterial insufficiency and those due to venous insufficiency.

Inspection should include the size and symmetry of the limb in question. Compare it with the contralateral limb.

TABLE 6.1   Comparison of Arterial and Venous Disease

	Arterial Insufficiency	Venous Insufficiency
Pain	Intermittent claudication. May progress to rest pain; chronic, dull aching pain. Progressive throughout the day.	
Color	Pale to dependent rubor, a dull to bright, reddish color. More common with advanced disease.	Normal to cyanotic. More common with advanced disease.
Skin temperature	Poikilothermic, taking on the environmental temperature. Much cooler than normal body temperature.	Usually no effect on temperature.
Pulses	Diminished to absent without Doppler stethoscope.	Usually normal. May be difficult to palpate. Secondary to significant edema.
Edema	Usually not present unless combined disease or can be related to cardiac disease and congestive heart failure.	Present from mild to severe pitting edema. Can have weeping edema fluid from open wounds.
Tissue changes	Thin and shiny. Hair loss. Trophic changes of the nails. Muscle wasting.	Stasis dermatitis with flaky, dry, and scaling skin. Hemosiderin deposits—brownish discoloration. Fibrosis with narrowing of the lower legs, "bottle legs."
Wounds	Distal ulceration, especially on toes and in between in the web spaces. May develop gangrene and severe tissue loss.	Shallow ulcers in the gaiter distribution of the foot and ankle, usually the medial surface.

CLINICAL WISDOM

Trophic Changes

Trophic changes are skin changes that occur over time in patients with chronic arterial insufficiency. Trophic changes include absence of leg hair; shiny, dry, pale skin; and thickened toenails. These symptoms are due to the chronic lack of nutrition from an inadequate blood supply to the extremity. Some of these changes occur naturally in elderly patients.

CLINICAL WISDOM

The pulse exam includes locating and grading bilateral femoral, popliteal, dorsalis pedis, and posterior tibial artery pulses. The following system should be used to grade pulses:

- 0 = No pulse
- 1+ = Barely felt
- 2+ = Diminished
- 3+ = Normal pulse (easily felt)
- 4+ = Bounding, aneurysmal ("pulse hits you in the face")

Observe for edema or swelling. Check the color and texture of the skin, including the nail beds and capillary refill. Also assess for the absence of hair, which is highly suggestive of arterial disease, and for muscle wasting. Determine the overall venous pattern, and document the presence and location of all varicose veins. Scars, rashes, and pigmentation changes, such as hemosiderin deposits seen in chronic venous insufficiency, should be noted.

The palpation step of the physical exam begins with palpation of all major pulse points. Palpate the radial and brachial pulses in the arm, the carotid pulse in the neck, and the femoral pulse in the groin (Fig. 6.1). Although the popliteal pulse can be difficult to assess, you should check it routinely, as a bounding popliteal pulse could indicate popliteal artery aneurysm. The popliteal pulse can be assessed from an anterior approach with the patient supine (Fig. 6.2); however, it is easier to palpate with the patient in the prone position, using the posterior approach (Fig. 6.3). The dorsalis pedis and posterior tibial arteries are also assessed (Figs. 6.4 and 6.5).

Auscultation includes assessment for any audible harsh sounds, called *bruits*. This can be done with a regular stethoscope and is performed typically over the larger vessels, the carotids, the aorta, renal arteries, and iliac arteries. Auscultation for bruits occurs after palpation of the pulses. The bell of the stethoscope is placed over the artery, and you should listen for a blowing or rushing sound. A bruit may be a sign of arterial narrowing. Finally, assessment of any visible wounds should be completed as with all wound patients (see Chapter 3).

Vascular Testing

If findings from the standard history and physical suggest that further investigation of a patient's vascular status is needed, vascular testing should be obtained. Many vascular tests are noninvasive, using some form of external imaging or measurement method to gather data on the structure and functioning of the vessels in a given region. The most commonly used noninvasive techniques employ ultrasound and its many derivatives. As part of your vascular evaluation, you should be prepared to conduct a variety of noninvasive tests.

Other vascular evaluation techniques are invasive; they are performed by vascular labs or radiology departments and may be recommended if noninvasive testing indicates problems that require more in-depth examination. Those involving injection of contrast media and data acquisition, usually in the form of radiographs, are the most commonly employed.

As a wound care professional, you should become familiar with the various tests, their benefits, and their limitations. These are the subject of the remainder of this chapter. We first discuss noninvasive tests of the arterial system. We then discuss briefly the invasive tests—mainly angiography—that require the care of a vascular surgeon. We then explore tests conducted to evaluate chronic venous insufficiency.

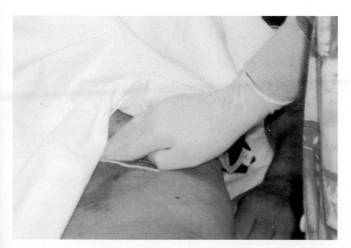

FIGURE 6.1 Palpation of femoral artery. (Courtesy of Archbold Wound Care Center, Thomasville, Georgia.)

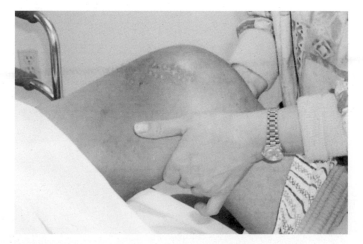

FIGURE 6.2 Palpation of popliteal artery (anterior approach). (Courtesy of Archbold Wound Care Center, Thomasville, Georgia.)

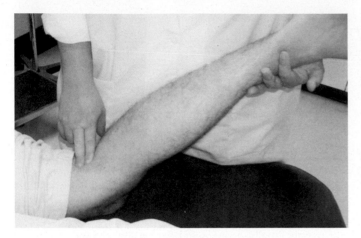

FIGURE 6.3 Palpation of popliteal artery (posterior approach). (Courtesy of Archbold Wound Care Center, Thomasville, Georgia.)

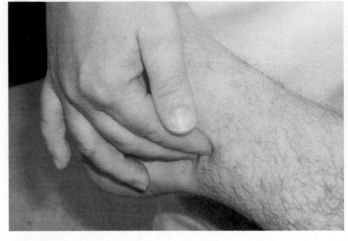

FIGURE 6.5 Palpation of posterior tibial artery. (Courtesy of Archbold Wound Care Center, Thomasville, Georgia.)

NONINVASIVE ARTERIAL STUDIES

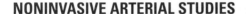

Noninvasive tests of the arterial system include those employing ultrasound as well as measurements of transcutaneous oxygen and skin perfusion, and magnetic resonance imaging (MRI) and computed tomography (CT) scans.

Continuous Wave Doppler Ultrasound and the Ankle Brachial Index

In 1842, Christian Johann Doppler, a physicist, discovered the Doppler effect. This principle states that when a sound source and a reflector are moving toward one another, the sound waves are spaced closer to one another. When the two are moving apart, the sound waves are farther apart. A modern example of this principle is that as a train approaches, the whistle's pitch rises (because the sound waves are closer together), and as it passes, the pitch becomes lower (because the sound waves are farther apart). By using this principle today, we can determine the velocity and direction of blood flow. This is the basis of many of the modern noninvasive vascular tests.

The most widely used noninvasive test is the continuous wave Doppler ultrasound. This instrument consists of a crystal

embedded in a handheld probe (Fig. 6.6). The crystal emits a sound wave that is reflected by the red blood cells traveling in the vessel of interest. This sound wave is reflected back to the probe and is transformed into an audible signal, which you can evaluate subjectively or record on a graphic analyzer.

The continuous wave Doppler gives us a phasic flow pattern. The normal flow is triphasic: The first sound represents forward flow during systole. The second sound represents a reversal of flow during diastole. The third and smallest sound represents a return of forward flow, caused by elastic recoil of the artery. As vascular disease progresses, this triphasic flow diminishes to a biphasic flow. This is due initially to the loss of elastic recoil caused by "hardening" of the arteries. If the disease progresses further, the flow will decrease to a monophasic signal; that is, the flow will lose its pulsatile nature altogether (Fig. 6.7).

The phasic flow patterns are mainly a subjective test in which the data are interpreted in a subjective manner by the clinician. When we apply a blood pressure cuff and occlude the flow in the artery, and then use the Doppler to access the return of flow as the pressure is decreased in the blood pressure cuff, we have obtained a Doppler blood pressure. In vascular assessment,

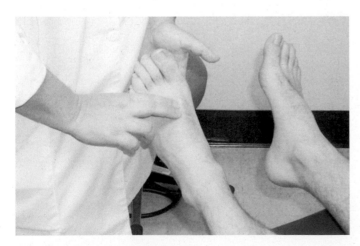

FIGURE 6.4 Palpation of dorsalis pedis artery. (Courtesy of Archbold Wound Care Center, Thomasville, Georgia.)

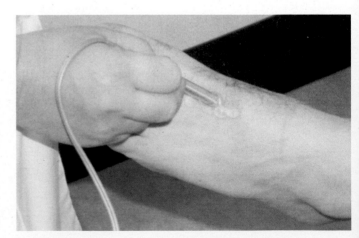

FIGURE 6.6 Continuous wave Doppler probe assessing dorsalis pedis artery. (Courtesy of Archbold Wound Care Center, Thomasville, Georgia.)

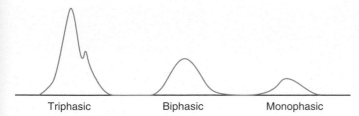

FIGURE 6.7 Phasic flow patterns.

the most common use of this is the **ankle brachial index (ABI)**. This compares (or indexes) the blood pressure in the arm to the blood pressure in the ankle. This value is obtained by first assessing the systolic arm pressure, then placing the blood pressure cuff just above the ankle, and measuring the systolic pressure with the Doppler probe. Conduct the test at both the posterior tibial artery and the dorsalis pedis artery. The ankle systolic pressure is then divided by the arm systolic pressure, giving a percentage value. In a normal patient, this value is equal to 1.0. In diabetic patients, the ABI may be greater than 1 due to microvessel inelasticity, and these patients should be referred to a vascular specialist for more specific testing. There is some disease present when the number falls below 0.90 to 0.95. However, the patient usually becomes symptomatic (with claudication pain) at around 0.70. Rest pain usually occurs at 0.4 to 0.5. Tissue loss occurs at 0.3 and below. Table 6.2 presents ABI data on prediction of wound healing, and the ABI values and their significance are presented in Exhibit 6.2.

Bear in mind that patients experience claudication pain when walking. If a patient's symptoms are consistent with claudication and the ABIs are not, this may be because they were obtained at rest. Therefore, to test for claudication, you should begin by having the patient exercise by walking, thus increasing

CLINICAL WISDOM

The ABI in Diabetic Patients

The ABI can be falsely elevated in patients with diabetes. This is due to calcification of the inner layer of the artery, that is, the cuff is unable to compress calcified distal vessel(s). This phenomenon is referred to as *noncompressible vessels*. Instead of ABI, one should measure systolic pressure in the digital arteries of the toes, as discussed shortly.

vascular demand, decreasing vascular resistance, and decreasing overall relative blood flow. Utilizing this exercise testing will uncover some marginal patients.[1] Some of the flaws in obtaining ABIs are operator error, placing the cuff too high on the lower leg, and dividing the arm pressure by the foot pressure, instead of vice versa.

Segmental and Digital Plethysmography

An expansion of the standard ABI is the **segmental plethysmography** (or *lower extremity arterial study*). This utilizes either a three- or a four-cuff system to obtain blood pressures along the entire leg: from the high thigh, low thigh, below the knee, and above the ankle. All pressures are indexed again to the brachial artery blood pressure. A significant decrease between two cuff measurements indicates an arterial lesion between these two locations. This allows you to localize arterial disease and can be seen in Figure 6.8A. However, such measurements may be somewhat difficult to interpret if there is multifocal disease.

TABLE	6.2	Table of ABI Values

Dopplex® Ankle Pressure Index (API) Guide

Ankle Pressure (mmHg)

Brachial Pressure (mmHg)

	30	35	40	45	50	55	60	65	70	75	80	85	90	95	100	105	110	115	120	125	130	135	140	145	150	155	160	165	170	175	180	185	190	195	200	
180	.16	.19	.22	.25	.27	.30	.33	.36	.38	.41	.44	.47	.50	.52	.55	.58	.61	.63	.66	.69	.72	.75	.77	.80	.83	.86	.89	.92	.94	.97	1.00					180
175	.17	.20	.22	.25	.28	.31	.34	.37	.40	.42	.45	.48	.51	.54	.57	.60	.62	.65	.68	.71	.74	.77	.80	.82	.85	.88	.92	.94	.97	1.00						175
170	.17	.20	.23	.26	.29	.32	.35	.38	.41	.44	.47	.50	.52	.55	.58	.61	.64	.67	.70	.73	.76	.79	.82	.85	.89	.91	.94	.97	1.00							170
165	.18	.21	.24	.27	.30	.33	.36	.39	.42	.45	.48	.51	.54	.57	.60	.63	.66	.69	.72	.75	.78	.81	.84	.87	.90	.94	.96	1.00								165
160	.18	.21	.25	.28	.31	.34	.37	.40	.43	.46	.50	.53	.56	.59	.62	.65	.68	.71	.75	.78	.81	.84	.87	.90	.93	.96	1.00									160
155	.19	.22	.25	.29	.32	.35	.38	.41	.45	.48	.51	.54	.58	.61	.64	.67	.70	.74	.76	.80	.83	.87	.90	.93	.96	1.00										155
150	.20	.23	.26	.30	.33	.36	.40	.43	.46	.50	.53	.56	.60	.63	.66	.70	.73	.76	.80	.83	.86	.90	.93	.96	1.00											150
145	.20	.24	.27	.31	.34	.37	.41	.44	.48	.51	.55	.58	.62	.65	.69	.72	.75	.79	.82	.86	.90	.93	.96	1.00												145
140	.21	.25	.28	.32	.35	.39	.42	.46	.50	.53	.57	.60	.64	.67	.71	.75	.78	.82	.85	.89	.92	.96	1.00													140
135	.22	.26	.29	.33	.37	.40	.44	.48	.51	.55	.59	.62	.66	.70	.74	.77	.81	.85	.88	.92	.96	1.00														135
130	.23	.27	.30	.34	.38	.42	.46	.50	.53	.57	.61	.65	.69	.73	.77	.80	.84	.88	.92	.96	1.00															130
125	.24	.28	.32	.36	.40	.44	.48	.52	.56	.60	.64	.68	.72	.76	.80	.84	.88	.92	.96	1.00																125
120	.25	.29	.33	.37	.40	.45	.50	.54	.58	.62	.66	.70	.75	.79	.83	.87	.91	.95	1.00																	120
115	.26	.30	.34	.39	.43	.48	.52	.56	.60	.65	.69	.74	.78	.82	.86	.91	.95	1.00																		115
110	.27	.31	.36	.40	.45	.50	.54	.59	.63	.68	.72	.77	.81	.86	.90	.95	1.00																			110
105	.28	.33	.38	.42	.47	.52	.57	.61	.66	.71	.76	.80	.85	.90	.95	1.00																				105
100	.30	.35	.40	.45	.50	.55	.60	.65	.70	.75	.80	.85	.90	.95	1.00																					100

GREATER THAN 1.00

Huntleigh Healthcare, a world leading manufacturer of pocket Dopplers, offers an extensive range of bi-directional pocket Dopplers with visual flow and rate display, together with a wide range of interchangeable probes for both vascular and obstetric applications.

WARNING: False high readings may be obtained in patients with calcified arteries because the sphygmomanometer cuff cannot fully compress the hardened arteries. Calcified arteries may be present in patients with history of Diabetes, Arteriosclerosis and Atherosclerosis.

Courtesy of Huntleigh Diagnostics Ltd., Cardiff, United Kingdom.

EXHIBIT 6.2

Significance of Ankle Brachial Index Values

ABI ≤ 0.5	Referral to vascular specialist (compression therapy contraindicated)
ABI = 0.5–0.8	Referral to vascular specialist. Intermittent claudication indicating peripheral arterial occlusive disease (compression therapy contraindicated)
ABI = 0.8–1.00	Mild peripheral arterial occlusive disease (compression therapy with caution)
ABI = 1.00	Normal vascular flow
ABI ≥ 1.00	Referral to vascular specialist. Indicates calcified vessels if diabetic.

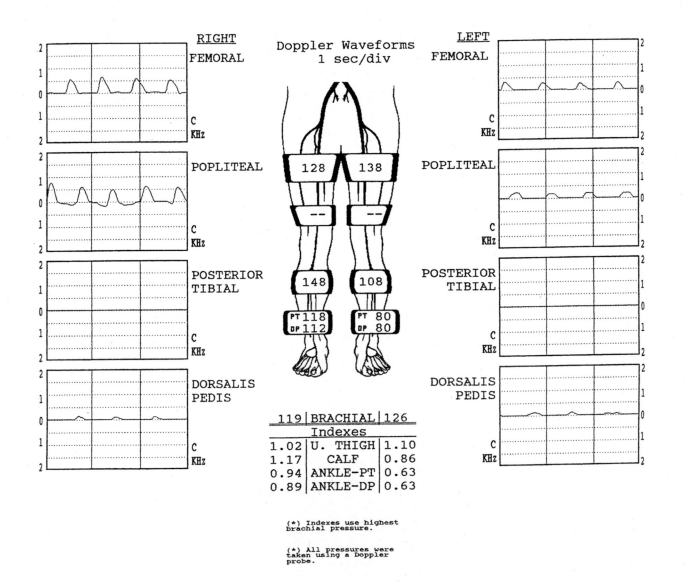

EVIDENCE FOR MILD OCCLUSIVE DISEASE ON RIGHT AT REST.   SEVERE ON LEFT.

PROBABLY SUPERFICIAL FEMORAL ARTERY IN NATURE.   ABNORMAL TBI BILATERALLY.

FIGURE 6.8 Segmental pressure study with PVRs. (A) shows severe occlusive disease on the left leg, which is seen just with the pressure reading alone.

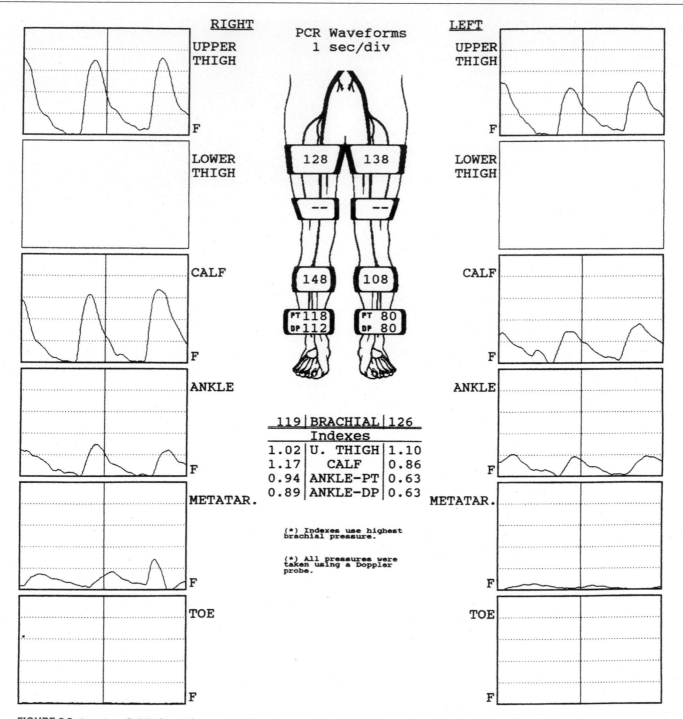

FIGURE 6.8 (*continued*) **(B)** shows decrease in the artery upstroke for the femoral, popliteal, and dorsalis pedis arteries; there is also decrease in volume under the curve evident in the waveforms for the left leg. Both findings indicate severe occlusive disease.

Segmental plethysmography measurements, or *segmental pressures*, as they are also known, are typically accompanied by **pulse volume recordings (PVRs)**. PVRs show the volume of change in the limb with each pulse beat. These are obtained with the same equipment, including the blood pressure cuffs, as with the segmental pressures. The cuffs are inflated to occlude arterial flow, and then deflated to just below systolic pressure, so that only arterial flow is maintained in the limb. The readings are then obtained. These readings usually have a sharp upstroke, indicating systolic flow. They also have a

corresponding dicrotic notch, a small downward deflection seen on the downstroke of an arterial pressure waveform, indicating elastic recoil of the artery wall. With mild disease, there is loss of the dicrotic notch. With moderate to severe disease, there is decrease in the upstroke of the waveform. With severe disease, there is loss of the volume beneath the curve noticeable when the right and left leg waveforms are compared in Figure 6.8B.

Digital plethysmography measurements, or "toe pressures," are the same as segmental pressures, except that a special, small-sized cuff is used and placed on the toe, usually the great hallux. Because of the small-sized digital arteries and the increase in vascular resistance through these arteries, these pressures are reduced. When indexed to the brachial pressure as a *toe brachial index* (TBI), the normal value is greater than or equal to 0.75. TBIs are extremely useful with diabetic patients because of the process of medial calcific stenosis (MCS), which is a process where the tunica media of the vessel wall is calcified. This causes a standard segmental pressure study to have values that are falsely elevated (>1.2) as the vessels become noncompressible because the vessel in question cannot be occluded to obtain a true systolic blood pressure. MCS does not affect digital arteries; therefore, they will be more indicative of arterial disease in diabetic patients.

Arterial Duplex Scanning

Duplex scanning is a combination of two scanning methods: ultrasound scanning is used to reveal anatomic details, and pulsed Doppler is used to show blood direction. When there is a blockage within a vessel, the resulting reversal of flow appears as a mosaic color pattern. The Doppler signal can be set to analyze the interior of the vessel only, so that the readings are not confused with other surrounding structures. Duplex scanning can reveal arterial stenosis, because the velocity or speed of the blood increases through the stenosis. A good example of this is when you place your finger over the end of a water hose. The more of the opening you cover, the faster the water will come out. Velocity measurements are recorded in centimeters per second (cm/s).[2-4]

Transcutaneous Oxygen Measurements

The primary concern of all vascular studies is adequate delivery of blood to the tissues, but, in reality, the actual measurement of oxygen at the tissue level mirrors the delivery on the cellular level. Thus, measurement of transcutaneous oxygen levels—skin oxygenation—provides data about cellular oxygenation.

In **transcutaneous oxygen ($tcPO_2$) measurement,** an airtight fixation ring is affixed to the site in question. An electrode inside the ring is then heated above body temperature to 41°C. This allows diffusion of oxygen from the capillary level to the skin level, and a measurement in millimeters of mercury (mm Hg) is made.

Transcutaneous oxygen measurements have been shown to be predictive for healing of ulcers and amputation wounds[5] and for determining the extent of chronic ischemia in limbs with and without wounds.[6,7] If the $tcPO_2$ is less than 20 mm Hg, the wound or ulcer will not heal. If the $tcPO_2$ is greater than 30 mm Hg, the wound or ulcer should heal without problems. This is also true of an ulcer that needs to be debrided. Safe debridement

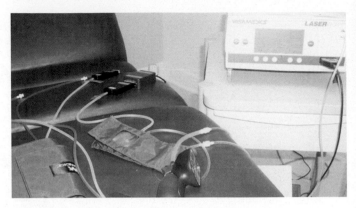

FIGURE 6.9 Laser Doppler unit with transducer cuffs. (Courtesy of Archbold Wound Care Center, Thomasville, Georgia.)

may be carried out if the $tcPO_2$ is greater than 30 mm Hg. In the case of amputation, less than 5 mm Hg indicates insufficient levels of oxygen for healing.[8]

As mentioned earlier, the diabetic patient with PVD presents some difficulty in evaluating because of MCS. Toe pressure of digital plethysmography is the test of choice, but, as is often the case, if the toes are involved, extensively calloused, or have been amputated, $tcPO_2$ measurements are very useful.

Transcutaneous oxygen measurements do have disadvantages. The reproducibility of the test can be questioned. Also, the test is time-consuming: it takes approximately 30 minutes to perform.

Skin Perfusion Pressures and the Laser Doppler

The skin in many vascular patients seems to become the "first victim" of critical limb ischemia. With this in mind, the actual **skin perfusion pressure (SPP)** has been looked at for a prediction of critical ischemia. Traditionally, SPP had a variety of drawbacks: it required special equipment; the patient had to keep the limb in question immobile for at least 20 minutes; and the procedure could be painful, necessitating analgesics.

Fortunately, new techniques of measuring SPP with a laser Doppler (Fig. 6.9) have been developed in the past several years. The laser Doppler uses a low-energy laser probe, secured in the bladder of a blood pressure cuff. These cuffs come in a variety of sizes, from large cuffs for thigh measures to tiny cuffs for toe digital SPP measurements (Fig. 6.10). The cuff is inflated to stop skin perfusion; after an adequate baseline is obtained, the cuff

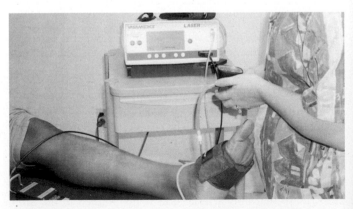

FIGURE 6.10 Patient undergoing laser Doppler exam. (Courtesy of Archbold Wound Care Center, Thomasville, Georgia.)

CLINICAL WISDOM

Accuracy of $tcPO_2$ Measurements

Transcutaneous oxygen measurements are not reliable in patients with swelling or infection! Do not test these patients. The patient can be tested when the infection is clear and the swelling is gone.

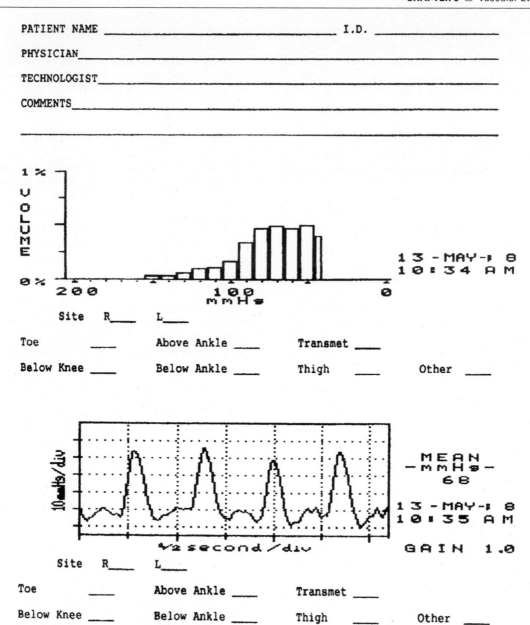

FIGURE 6.11 Normal laser Doppler exam with SPP = 90 to 100 mm Hg and normal PVR waveforms.

is slowly deflated. The skin perfusion is measured in volume percent units (LDFU or laser Doppler flow units); the SPP is the reading that increases at least 40% over baseline (Fig. 6.11). The laser Doppler can also obtain PVRs of skin perfusion, thus allowing for further assessment of a patient's vascular status. Newer machines often have both a laser Doppler and a tcPO$_2$.

The laser Doppler has been shown to be 80% accurate at predicting critical limb ischemia.[9,10] In a study of use of SPP in the diagnosis of critical limb ischemia, patients with an SPP greater than 45 mm Hg were shown to have a 100% healing rate. Those patients with SPP of 25 mm Hg, exhibited a 50% healing rate.[9] SPP has also been shown to be a good predictor of healing of amputation wounds.[11]

Magnetic Resonance Angiography

Magnetic resonance angiography (MRA) is a vascular study that uses MRI technology. MRA can visualize all of the same vessels and hemodynamically significant stenoses seen with more invasive techniques such as contrast angiography (discussed shortly).

MRA has several advantages over traditional contrast angiography. As just noted, it is essentially noninvasive. If contrast is used, it is a nonionic contrast, which does not cause any nephrotoxicity. Also, cortical bone does not show up on MRA, so it does not affect findings as much as seen in traditional contrast angiography where cortical bone is reduced in digital subtraction angiography, but it has not been completely eliminated. Probably the single greatest advantage of MRA is that it can readily identify those vessels of concern or the targeted recipient vessels not always identified on conventional contrast angiography.[12] This problem of contrast "washout" before the vessels of concern have been visualized on the angiography may increase amputation rates before vascular reconstruction is attempted. This is a significant advantage of MRA over conventional contrast angiography. MRA is also comparable in overall cost to contrast angiography.

MRA does have some disadvantages. Successful testing and interpretation require experienced radiologists and surgeons. With inexperienced clinicians, "overreading" or overcalling the severity of the stenoses is common. It also needs the availability of an MRI unit, including specialized software and coils. Despite this, it is replacing angiography in some centers.

Computed Tomography Angiography

One of the newer applications of an existing radiologic test is that of **computed tomography (CT) angiography**. This test employs ultrafast helical CT scanners to obtain multiple serial images enhanced with contrast. These images are then reconstructed into a three-dimensional projected image. Many of the newer generation CT scanners and the available software allow for some of the most "contrast-enhanced angiogram"–like pictures, when compared with true angiography.

The acquisition of CT angiography images is quick and noninvasive for the patient, but the reconstruction of these images requires highly sophisticated computer software and hardware that has only recently become more widely available. Future computer and reconstructive developments will undoubtedly move CT angiography to the forefront of all noninvasive vascular imaging techniques.

INVASIVE ARTERIAL STUDIES

Invasive arterial studies require some type of invasive intervention. The most common is **contrast angiography**, which usually requires a femoral artery puncture or brachial artery cutdown where a small incision is made in the skin and the artery is accessed. A catheter is then inserted and advanced. During the manipulation of the catheter, complications can occur such as plaques breaking off with resultant embolization or damage to the vessel wall itself. Serious complications can occur from the procedures, including heart failure, contrast-induced renal heart failure, and even death (0.05%).[13–15] Despite these complications, angiography remains the "gold standard" for vascular evaluation. If angiography is entertained, the patient should be in the care of a general or vascular surgeon.

Angiography does have advantages over other types of arterial studies. These include easier anatomical approaches that lead to better localization of vessels in question. Smaller incisions and more direct approaches during revascularization can be used because of the better anatomic approach and resulting improved identification of vessels for repair. Endoluminal interventions, such as angioplasty, can also be done during the procedure. This is a significant advantage beyond pure diagnostic tests, as it expands the role of angiography to include a therapeutic modality.

Angiography is all about visualization of vessels by observing contrast media flow through the vasculature. It is the ability to actually visualize blood flow through vessels of concern that makes it so advantageous as a diagnostic test. One technically significant disadvantage of angiography is nonvisualization of distal runoff vessels. The inability to observe blood flow through runoff vessels is of concern as these vessels may provide for collateral blood flow to an area. The problems with visualization relate to dilution and washout of the contrast media before reaching the distal runoff vessels. Several studies have shown that up to 70% of patients have failure to opacify the small distal runoff vessels during angiography.[12–19] Therefore, the vessels should be explored before amputation is considered or before patients undergo "on-table" intraoperative angiography and, in some cases, MRA.[18–21]

STUDIES OF VENOUS INSUFFICIENCY

Chronic venous insufficiency also known as **chronic venous disease** is a condition that occurs when the veins cannot pump blood back to the heart effectively. The primary purpose of evaluation studies is to look for two underlying problems, venous obstruction and reflux. Obstruction can be due to a previous thrombosis, a congenital malformation, or external compression from something such as a tumor or a scar. Reflux, which is categorized by abnormal flow back through the valves within veins, is usually caused by incompetent valves.

Before we describe the various tests, a brief review of venous circulation may be helpful. Recall that the heart pumps blood inferiorly through the systemic arteries to the legs. Obviously, this is a high-pressure system. The return of blood to the heart occurs as blood is transported by the superficial veins to the deep venous system via perforator veins at a much lower pressure. It would seem, therefore, that this situation would result in a significant build-up of blood pressure at the ankle level. But normally, this increased pressure does not occur because the venous valves maintain just the pressure in the isolated column of the vein between two subsequent valves. If, however, there is an obstruction such that a valve cannot open to allow blood to flow superiorly, then pressure will build up in the region of the vein inferior to the obstruction. On the other hand, if a valve becomes incompetent (cannot shut tightly), the column of blood superior to it will flow backward into the next column of blood, increasing the pressure in that column significantly. With more than one obstruction or incompetent valve, such problems can occur throughout the leg, causing ambulatory venous hypertension, the main pathophysiologic problem associated with chronic venous insufficiency. Again, the above-mentioned tests evaluate both for obstruction of blood flow and for reflux from incompetent valves.

The tests can be divided into two main types:

- Physiologic tests provide some type of quantitative measure of the overall venous hemodynamics that occur. They include ambulatory venous pressure monitoring, photo plethysmography (PPG), string gauge plethysmography, and air plethysmography (APG). These tests can be useful both prior to treatment and after treatment to quantify the overall improvement of the venous hemodynamics.
- Anatomic tests provide a qualitative assessment of the overall function or dysfunction of the venous system. Duplex ultrasound is the most commonly used anatomic test.

Ambulatory Venous Pressure Monitoring

Ambulatory venous pressure monitoring records the pressure in the veins while the patient ambulates. The test is typically performed using a small butterfly needle, such as a 20- or 21-gauge needle, which is placed in a superficial vein on the foot, and is then connected to a pressure transducer and recording device. First, static pressure measurements are obtained while the patient is still. Then, the patient is asked to perform provocative maneuvers such as dorsiflexion of the foot up on the "tip toes," and dynamic pressure is recorded. In addition, the overall time for the pressure to return to a resting level can also be calculated.

Interpret the findings of this test as follows: Active dorsiflexion of the foot normally causes blood to be pumped out of the lower leg, so you should see a drop in venous pressure. When the activity is stopped, the pressure will slowly rise as the arterioles fill through the capillary system back into the venous system. This usually takes approximately up to 2 to 5 minutes but typically can be seen in 1 minute. If the pressure returns to baseline much more quickly, for example, in less than 30 seconds, there is some evidence of reflux through the veins. This is considered abnormal. Also, a resting ambulatory venous pressure of greater than 30 mm Hg is considered abnormal. Overall, the greater the extent of chronic venous insufficiency, the higher the venous ambulatory pressure found. Studies have also shown a correlation between increased ambulatory venous pressure and increased incidence of ulceration.

Photoplethysmography

Photoplethysmography (PPG) essentially measures the venous refill time; that is, the time that it takes for the vein to refill through the normal arterial capillary system. In a situation of reflux, refill time decreases, reflecting the backward flow of blood through the veins. PPG measures the light reflected from the skin as it changes color with filling of microvasculature. A light-emitting diode is placed approximately 10 to 15 cm from the medial malleolus. The machine is calibrated and zeroed, and then the patient is asked to perform passive dorsiflexion of the foot to cause venous pumping through the calf sinusoids, emptying the lower leg veins. After approximately eight passive dorsiflexions, the foot is relaxed. Utilizing both paper tracing and an audible change in tone emitted by the machine, the examiner can measure the rapidity in which the veins refill, again obtaining a quantitative venous refill time.

Interpretation of the findings is as follows: Refill times greater than 24 seconds are considered normal. Rapid refill times can be quantified on the overall severity of chronic venous insufficiency (Table 6.3).[22] False negatives can occur if there is any significant arterial inflow disease, as this may hamper normal filling of the vessels through the arterial circuit. Also, a significant decrease in ankle mobility can decrease calf-muscle pumping of venous blood out of the venous circuit.[23]

TABLE 6.3	Venous Refill Times and Levels of Venous Disease	
	Normal	>25 s
Level 1	Mild	20–24 s
Level 2	Moderate	10–19 s
Level 3	Severe	<10 s

These correlate with the overall severity of chronic venous insufficiency.

Light reflective rheography (LRR) is a variation of PPG that uses infrared light and three light diodes. This reduces the overall effect of external light and surface reflection, in theory giving a much more accurate study.

Both PPG and LRR have been discussed at national wound care meetings as screening tools for large scale wound care populations. Both versions have been shown to be effective.

String Gauge Plethysmography

String gauge plethysmography is a variation of PPG that also studies venous refill times, as well as overall venous emptying. It uses a string gauge to encircle the leg and sense tension changes caused by the calf with exertion. A small, specialized blood cuff can also be used to occlude superficial venous structures and help in isolating superficial disease. String gauge plethysmography is not widely used anymore as newer techniques such as APG have come to replace it.

Air Plethysmography

Air plethysmography (APG) uses air cuffs to show volumetric changes in the leg that can be quantified to reveal venous reflux times. Again, the patient is instructed to repeatedly dorsiflex the foot so that the calf pumps blood out of the venous circuit. Refill times are obtained through the air chambers in the cuff, which are connected to a pressure transducer and a computerized recorder. Tourniquets may be placed above the ankle, below the ankle, below the knee, and above the knee to stop abnormal refill times and show corrected refill times. This can isolate disease, both to the superficial system differentiating between the greater saphenous and lesser saphenous vein, as well as the perforator system, and finally on to the deep system.

Outflow obstruction can also be evaluated by changing the patient's position. Doing so may reveal evidence of a more proximal occlusion from a previous clot or anatomic abnormality.

Venous Duplex Scanning

Duplex scanning, which we defined earlier as combining ultrasound scanning to reveal anatomic details and pulsed Doppler to show blood direction, is the gold standard in detecting reflux in the outpatient setting. The test can also detect the presence of a clot from deep vein thrombosis, as well as sluggish blood flow, indicating engorgement of the vessels. The test can also assess for vessel compressibility. Normally, a vein is easily compressible; if a thrombosis is present, it will be noncompressible. A complete venous duplex ultrasound should show not only the patency of the vessels, but any anatomic abnormalities, accessory vessels, and vessels with reflux, and should isolate these to what system of veins is involved. A full assessment should include all the deep veins, including the common femoral vein, superficial femoral vein, profunda femoral vein, popliteal vein, posterior tibial and peroneal veins, and occasional isolation of the anterior tibial veins. Superficial veins should include not only the greater saphenous vein and lesser saphenous vein but also accessory pathways such as the vein of Giacomini. Perforator vessels should be elicited as well with the standard criteria being if reflux is not visualized, then reflux may be present in a dilated perforator greater than 3 mm in size. Perforators should be typically identified in relationship to a known anatomic spot, such as the medial malleolus, and distance from the top of the medial malleolus should be given in centimeters so that isolation of these areas is obtained.

Duplex testing can also be used to evaluate an ulcer bed, but caution should be taken to protect the transducer head from contamination by covering it with a commercially available sterile bag or a sterile glove in which ultrasound gel has been placed. Additional sterile gel is placed in the wound, and the wound is then scanned with the covered transducer ultrasound probe. Veins running underneath the ulcer or within 2 cm of the periphery are considered the damaged veins responsible for development of the ulcerated area and generally correspond to known anatomic vessels. Typically, medial lower leg wounds above the medial malleolus are drained by branches from the greater saphenous vein, the posterior arch system, the posterior tibial veins, and potentially the peroneal veins. Laterally placed ulcers correspond to the short saphenous vein and peroneal veins and anteriorly placed ulcers to the anterior arch of the greater saphenous vein and anterior tibial system. Other ulcer locations correspond to other vessels.

Other Studies of Venous Insufficiency

Invasive tests for chronic venous insufficiency include **venography**, which is similar to contrast angiography. Ascending venography evaluates for obstruction, and descending venography is used to assess for valvular function. Typically, these tests are performed on separate days because contrast loads can be nephrotoxic. In addition, multiple superficial points must be accessed for ascending venography, whereas access points are usually in the deep femoral vessels in descending venography.

Other noninvasive studies may include magnetic resonance venography or CT venography. However, it can be difficult to obtain accurate data from these tests because of problems in timing contrast injections so that only the venous phase is obtained and there are no arterial vessels present causing "arterial contamination" of the results.

Intravascular ultrasound (IVUS) is a new method initially employed in arterial evaluation but is gaining more favor in venous evaluation. IVUS can be used during invasive venous procedures such as bedside placement of inferior vena cava filters where the filter is placed with the assistance of an IVUS catheter without typical x-ray studies. Typically, the IVUS catheter has either a tiny rotating vascular ultrasound head at the end of the catheter or multiple arrays in a circumferential pattern that give a full picture of the vessel wall. IVUS provides information on vessel stenoses by evaluating the vessel diameter and any changes in diameter. Obstructive processes can be determined with IVUS. IVUS can present data on general anatomy including vessel branches for visualization of smaller veins and to identify anatomic landmarks for use in performing interventions.

Lymphoscintigraphy

Lymphoscintigraphy is a test requiring injection of a radioactive tracer, technetium-99m–sulfur colloid. It is used to diagnose **lymphedema**, which can be caused by lymphatic obstruction or overwhelming venous obstruction. A portion of technetium-99m–sulfur colloid is administered through an intradermal and subcutaneous injection at the first web space of each foot. A picture is obtained with a gamma camera n of both the legs and pelvis at certain times: 10, 20, 30, and 60 minutes. The patient walks before, during, and in between the examinations to provide venous return.

Findings are interpreted as follows: Normally, radioactive material should flow superiorly from the foot and be visualized in the groin lymph nodes faintly at 10 minutes and well at 20 minutes. If the groin lymph nodes can be visualized at 10 and 20 minutes, further study can be concluded as essentially normal. Abnormal studies show faint or delayed uptake at 30 minutes. No uptake at 60 minutes indicates absence of lymphatic activity.

REFERRAL CRITERIA

The following indicators guide referral to a vascular surgeon or the vascular lab:

1. ABI greater than 1.0, $tcPO_2$ measurement greater than 30 mm Hg: semi-urgent vascular appointment
2. Gangrene present: urgent vascular appointment
3. ABI
   a. Greater than 0.8: routine vascular appointment
   b. Between 0.5 and 0.8: semi-urgent vascular appointment
   c. Below 0.5: urgent vascular appointment
4. Exposed bone or tendon at the base of ulcer: urgent vascular appointment
5. Gross infection or cellulitis: urgent vascular appointment
6. ABI less than 1.0 with diminished or absent pulses: semi-urgent vascular appointment
7. Nonhealing wounds despite 3+ pulses and good wound care: semi-urgent vascular appointment

When in doubt, refer to vascular lab for further evaluation

SELF-CARE TEACHING GUIDELINES

The key to preventing vascular diseases is patient education. Patients need to learn how to reduce stress to their circulatory system, and they must understand the signs and symptoms that should prompt them to contact their physician immediately.

Self-Care Teaching Guidelines Specific to Arterial Insufficiency

1. Do not smoke! Even one cigarette a day can decrease circulation.
2. Follow your physician's directions for controlling blood pressure, diabetes, and high cholesterol.
3. Inspect your legs and feet daily, and report any signs of redness, pain, or ulceration immediately. Be sure to inspect between your toes.
4. Wash and dry your feet every day.
5. Lubricate your skin to avoid cracks.
6. The first thing to go into your shoes in the morning should be your hand! Check to make sure there are no protrusions or foreign objects inside your shoes that could injure the foot.
7. Cut your toenails straight across. If possible, have a podiatrist cut your toenails.

8. Do not wear tight shoes.
9. Test your bath water with a hand or thermometer (<98°F) to avoid burns.
10. Do not walk barefoot at any time, either inside or outside the home.
11. Wear comfortable, wide-toed shoes that cause no pressure (orthotics, if necessary).
12. Do not wear constricting clothes.
13. Wear clean cotton socks with smooth seams or without seams.

Self-Care Teaching Guidelines Specific to Venous Insufficiency

1. Do not smoke!
2. Wear support stockings as prescribed.
3. Avoid crossing legs.
4. Elevate legs when sitting.
5. Inspect legs and feet daily, and report any increased swelling, new or larger ulcers, increased pain, redness, or infection.

6. Avoid trauma to legs, such as bumping or scratching.
7. Keep legs and feet clean.
8. Eat a well-balanced nourishing diet that is low in sodium.

CONCLUSION

Since vascular disease underlies many wounds, all wound care patients should undergo a targeted history and physical examination. Once a major etiology is considered, you'll need to obtain further data by noninvasive vascular testing. As a wound care specialist, you should be familiar with and ready to apply the ABI. You should also familiarize yourself with the more sophisticated testing that is available at your institution and determine the institution's accuracy for this testing. If you are considering referring the patient for invasive testing such as angiography, consultation with a general or vascular surgeon will be needed.

REVIEW QUESTIONS

1. Taking segmental pressures is a noninvasive diagnostic test for arterial competence. In a comparison of lower extremity pressures with upper extremity pressures, which of the following is associated with a poor prognosis in terms of lower leg wound healing?
   A. Ankle brachial index of 1.1
   B. Ankle brachial index of 0.9
   C. Ankle brachial index of 0.8
   D. Ankle brachial index of 0.5
2. Which of the following descriptions is MOST characteristic of venous ulcers?
   A. Commonly occur on the tips of toes or over the malleolar head, with minimal exudate.
   B. Usually pale ulcer base, with necrotic tissue present.
   C. Wound edges are punched out and regular in appearance, and wound is usually painful.
   D. Commonly occur superior to the inner or outer malleolus with irregular wound edges and moderate exudate.
3. Which of the following best reflects adequate tissue perfusion and oxygenation to support wound healing?
   A. Capillary refill time greater than 35 seconds
   B. Transcutaneous oxygen tension greater than 40 mm Hg

   C. Albumin levels greater than 2.5
   D. Palpable dorsalis pedis and posterior tibial pulses
4. In evaluating PVRs from segmental pressure studies, evidence of moderate to severe occlusive disease is evident when
   A. there is a sharp upstroke in the waveform
   B. the dicrotic notch is evident on the downstroke
   C. volume under the curve is reduced
   D. both a and b
5. In venous duplex scanning the goal is to
   A. visualize the deep venous system and any occlusions that may be present
   B. visualize only superficial venous system as well as collateral accessory vessels
   C. determine location of any occlusions
   D. visualize deep, superficial, and perforator venous systems; determine presence of any occlusions; and view any anatomic abnormalities, accessory vessels, and vessels with reflux.

REFERENCES

1. Yao ST. Haemodynamic studies in peripheral arterial disease. *Br J Surg.* 1970;57(10):761–766.
2. Kohler TR, Nance DR, Cramer NM, et al. Duplex scanning for diagnosis of aortoilliac and femoropopliteal disease: a prospective study. *Circulation.* 1987;76(5):1074–1080.
3. Edwards JM, Coldwell DM, Goldman ML, et al. The role of duplex scanning in the selection of patients for transluminal angioplasty. *J Vasc Surg.* 1991;13(1):69–74.
4. Malone JM, Anderson GG, Lalka SG, et al. Prospective comparison of noninvasive techniques for amputation level selection. *Am J Surg.* 1987;154(2):179–184.

5. Wyss CR, Matsen FA III, Simmons CW, et al. Transcutaneous oxygen tension measurements on limbs of diabetic and nondiabetic patients with peripheral vascular disease. *Surgery.* 1984;95(3):339–345.
6. Ballard JL, Eke CC, Bunt TJ, et al. A prospective evaluation of transcutaneous oxygen measurement of diabetic foot problems. *J Vasc Surg.* 1995;22:485–492.
7. Franzeck UK, Talke P, Bernstein EF, et al. Transcutaneous PO$_2$ measurements in health and peripheral arterial occlusive disease. *Surgery.* 1982;91(2):156–163.
8. Wagner WH, Keagy BA, Kotb MM, et al. Noninvasive determination of healing of major lower extremity amputation: the continued role of clinical judgment. *J Vasc Surg.* 1988;8:703–710.

9. Castronuovo JJ Jr, Adera HM, Smiell JM, et al. Measurement is valuable in the diagnosis of critical limb ischemia. *J Vasc Surg*. 1997;26(4):629–637.

10. Castronuovo JJ. Diagnosis of critical limb ischemia with skin perfusion pressure measurements. *J Vasc Technol*. 1997;21(3):175–179.

11. Adera HM, James K, Castronuovo JJ Jr, et al. Prediction of amputation wound healing with skin perfusion pressure. *J Vasc Surg*. 1995;21(5):823–828.

12. Owen RS, Carpenter JP, Baum RA, et al. Magnetic resonance angiography of angiographically occult runoff vessels in peripheral arterial occlusive disease. *N Engl J Med*. 1992;326:1577–1578.

13. Shehadi WH, Toniolo G. Adverse reactions to contrast media: a report from the Committee on Safety of Contrast Media of the International Society of Radiology. *Radiology*. 1980;137:299–302.

14. Hessel SJ, Adams DF, Abrams HL. Complications of angiography. *Radiology*. 1981;138:273–281.

15. Waugh JR, Sacharias N. Arteriographic complications in the DSA era. *Radiology*. 1992;182:243–246.

16. Carpenter JP, Owen RS, Baum RA, et al. Magnetic resonance angiography of peripheral runoff vessels. *J Vasc Surg*. 1992;16(6):807–815.

17. Edelman RR, Mattle HP, Atkinson DJ, et al. MR angiography. *Am J Roentgenol*. 1990;154:937–946.

18. Patel KR, Semel L, Clauss RH. Extended reconstruction rate for limb salvage with intraoperative prereconstruction angiography. *J Vasc Surg*. 1988;7:531–537.

19. Ricco JB, Pearce WH, Yao JS, et al. The use of operative prebypass arteriography and Doppler ultrasound recordings to select patients for extended femoro-distal bypass. *Ann Surg*. 1983;198:646–653.

20. Scarpato R, Gembarowicz R, Farber S, et al. Intraoperative prereconstruction arteriography. *Arch Surg*. 1981;116:1053–1055.

21. Flanigan DP, Williams LR, Keifer T, et al. Prebypass operative angiography. *Surgery*. 1982;92:627–633.

22. Sarin S, Shields DA, Scurr JH, et al. Photo plethysmography: a valuable non-invasive tool in the assessment of venous dysfunction? *J Vasc Surg*. 1992;16:154–162.

23. Schroeder PJ, Dunn E. Mechanical plethysmography and Doppler ultrasound diagnosis of deep vein thrombosis. *Arch Surg*. 1982; 117:300–303.

Assessment and Treatment of Nutrition

Mary Ellen Posthauer

CHAPTER OBJECTIVES

At the completion of this chapter, the reader will be able to:

1. Identify the guidelines for completing a nutritional screening and assessment.
2. Screen patients at risk for nutrition deficiency, using a nutritional screening tool.
3. Describe the role of nutrients in the process of wound healing.
4. Identify nutrients of particular importance to wound healing.
5. Discuss the nutritional implications of pressure ulcers, surgical wounds, burns, skin tears, leg ulcers, and dermatitis.
6. Demonstrate appropriate documentation of medical nutrition therapy in the patient's medical record.

With the spotlight on elaborate diagnostic tests, high-tech surgeries, and complex drug prescriptions, it is easy to lose sight of the basic importance of nutrition. Indeed, nutrition is often the forgotten factor in wound healing. The identification of a patient's nutritional status begins with a nutrition screen, followed by an assessment. A plan of care is then developed, based on the data derived from the assessment process.

As defined by the American Dietetic Association (ADA) Nutrition Care Process and Model, **medical nutrition therapy (MNT)** begins with a screening and referral system for identifying risk factors, which leads to the nutrition assessment. The assessment includes review and analysis of a patient's food and nutrition-related history, biochemical data, tests and procedures, anthropometric measurements, nutrition-focused physical findings, and patient history.[1] Based on the assessment, the nutrition modalities most appropriate to manage the condition or treat the illness or injury are chosen. The registered dietitian (RD) analyzes and interprets the data using evidence-based standards and documents the use of these standards. A plan of care including nutrition interventions follows the assessment.

NUTRITIONAL SCREENING

Nutritional screening is the process of identifying characteristics known to be associated with nutritional problems. Its purpose is to pinpoint individuals who are malnourished or at nutritional risk. A screening involves interdisciplinary collaboration and can be completed by a member of the health-care team, such as the RD, dietetic technician, registered nurse (RN), physician (MD), or other qualified health-care professional.

Nutritional Screening Guidelines

The Centers for Medicare and Medicaid Services (CMS), which regulates long-term care facilities in the United States, has targeted pressure ulcers, inadequate nutrition, and inadequate hydration as key survey issues. Surveyors at both the federal and the state level utilize an Investigative Pressure Ulcer Protocol to determine whether pressure ulcers are avoidable or unavoidable. As part of a facility's pressure ulcer prevention and treatment strategies, the Protocol investigates assessment, including nutritional screening and assessment.

The National Pressure Ulcer Advisory Panel and the European Pressure Ulcer Advisory Panel published the 2009 Pressure Ulcer Prevention and Treatment Clinical Practice Guideline.[2] These guidelines provide evidence-based recommendations that can be used by health-care professionals around the world. The nutrition guidelines assist dietetic practitioners to assess and develop action plans for the nutritional care of patients with pressure ulcers. The Braden Scale for Predicting Pressure Sore Risk (see Chapter 9) includes a nutrition subscale, which provides information about the patient's nutritional status.

Risk Factors Important in Nutritional Screening

There are several valid, reliable, and practical tools for nutrition screening. The Malnutrition Screening Tool (MST), Short Nutritional Assessment Questionnaire (SNAQ), or the

CLINICAL WISDOM

Ensuring Optimal Nutrition for Residents of Long-Term Care Facilities

Maintaining or improving the nutritional status of elderly individuals in long-term care settings presents a challenge for the health-care team. Identification of risk factors that contribute to undernutrition or malnutrition in long-term care facilities is essential. Federal regulations mandate that nursing facilities provide care that maximizes the resident's quality of life. Protein-energy undernutrition has been associated with the development of pressure ulcers, cognitive problems, infections, and increased mortality. Optimizing nutrition screening and intervention helps to achieve positive outcomes for the resident. Often, reimbursement rates do not cover the cost of care. Oral nutritional supplements or fortified foods are not reimbursable under state or federal regulations but fall under the daily rate of care.

Mini Nutrition Screening Form (MNA) consists of questions that are most predictive of malnutrition.[3,4] The MNA screening tool designed for adults 65 years and above has an 80% sensitivity and specificity and correlates with the full MNA assessment form.[5] Screening tools consider current weight status (e.g., weight versus usual weight, percent of weight lost), food/appetite intake, and severity of disease. If the nutrition screen indicates an individual is at risk for skin breakdown, undernourished, or at nutritional risk, a comprehensive nutritional assessment should be completed. See Appendix for sample screening and assessment forms.

NUTRITIONAL ASSESSMENT

Nutritional status should be assessed at minimum every 3 months for those patients at low risk and monthly for those at high risk or who are already undernourished. Nutritional assessment includes the interpretation of data from the screening process, as well as a review of data from other disciplines (e.g., physical therapy and occupational therapy), which can affect the assessment process.

Functional limitations affect the patient's ability to ingest adequate calories and fluids. Chewing and swallowing problems can result in poor oral intake and lead to undernutrition. Edentulous patients or those who have loose dentures as a result of weight loss often avoid foods high in protein—such as meat or meat alternates—that are difficult to chew. This restricts their overall intake, thus increasing the chance for weight loss. If untreated, patients with dysphagia become dehydrated, lose weight, and may develop pressure ulcers. Loss of dexterity is another functional limitation with nutritional implications: difficulty manipulating eating utensils can result in poor oral intake. Furthermore, reduced mobility can affect a person's ability to shop, prepare meals, or travel to a dining room. Sensory losses, such as reduced hearing and vision, compromise a patient's communication skills and can result in poor intake at meals. The saying, "We eat with our eyes," is obvious when poor vision reduces appetite or hampers self-feeding.

A diminished sense of taste and/or smell, thus decreasing appetite, can also result in poor intake.

Altered mental status can limit a patient's ability to feed himself or herself, or to comprehend the importance of consuming a balanced diet. Advanced dementia often results in weight loss, dysphagia, undernutrition, and pressure ulcers. The probability of developing pressure ulcers increases among clients who can no longer respond to their caregivers' attempts to assist in their nourishment.

Depression has been linked to weight loss and poor nutritional status especially among older adults.[6] Any decline in nutritional status places patients at risk for pressure ulcer development and hampers the healing process. An antidepressant may result in increased food intake.

Specific medical conditions can also put patients at nutritional risk. For example, chronic hyperglycemia impairs the body's ability to eliminate bacteria, leading to an increase in infections. Soft tissue infections of the lower extremities and gangrene are serious complications.[7] Disorders involving gastrointestinal function, including atrophic gastritis, GI cancers, liver disease, and malabsorption disorders such as celiac disease, can dramatically increase the risk of malnutrition. Hip fractures and spinal cord injuries that restrict a client's mobility often result in increased pain and the functional limitations mentioned above that interfere with eating.

Drug therapy can often cause side effects, such as nausea and gastric disturbances, which limit food and fluid intake. Corticosteroids inhibit protein synthesis; cause depletion of vitamin A from the liver, plasma, adrenals, and enzymes; and interfere with collagen synthesis and resistance to infection, increasing the risk of wound complications.[8]

Nutritional assessment precedes development of a care plan, intervention, and evaluation. *The Prevention of Pressure Ulcers: Nutrition Decision Tree* (Fig. 7.1) can be used as guidelines for performing a nutritional assessment. See MNA Screening and Full Assessment form.

The RD reviews the screen and assessments from the various therapies to determine a nutritional care plan. The speech therapist determines the diet texture, including the need for any special feeding techniques, to be implemented by the dietary department. As an example, patients may require thickened liquids to prevent dehydration or aspiration. The occupational therapist determines the need for self-help feeding devices, which promote eating independence. The RD is then responsible for ensuring that this special equipment is provided at meal time. Physical therapy sessions often result in the need for both increased calories and fluid, for which the RD will calculate and arrange provision at appropriate times.

Poor Nutritional Status

The RD and other health-care professionals should examine the patient for physical signs of malnutrition, a condition of inadequate nutrition. The term *malnutrition* or undernutrition refers to an excess or imbalance of energy, protein, and other nutrients that cause adverse effects on tissues, body structures, body function, and clinical outcomes. Undernutrition has been defined as pure protein and energy deficiency, which is reversed solely by the administration of nutrients.[9] Finally, poor nutritional status also encompasses evidence that a patient's nutritional status may be deteriorating over time. Such evidence can

Algorithm for Prevention of Pressure Ulcers: Nutrition Guidelines [≠]

Trigger Conditions:

- Unintended wt. loss ≥5% in 30 days; ≥10% in 180 days
- BMI [§] < 18.5 (weight (lb) / (height (in) x height (in)) x 703 **or** weight (kg) / (height (m) x height (m))
- Swallowing Problems /dysphagia
- Receiving enteral or parenteral nutrition
- Poor oral intake
- At risk of developing pressure ulcer (i.e., low score on Braden Scale [Δ])
- Immobility
- Infections (i.e., respiratory, urinary tract, gastrointestinal)
- Decline in ADLs (activities of daily living)
- Other selected conditions per facility

[§] Body Mass Index
[Δ] Braden BJ & Bergstrom N. *Decubitus* 1989;2(3):44

Refer to dietitian to Assess & Document:
` **RD follows the Nutrition Care Process**

At Nutrition Risk?

No → **Monitor Status as needed or following a change in condition**

Yes → **Provide Nutrition Therapy**

Re-assess & Document as needed

Dietitian Assessment: [1]

- Current weight/height
- Determine deviation from Usual Body Weight.
- Body Mass Index (BMI)
- Interview for food preferences/intolerances
- Determine nutritional needs
  1. Calories (30-35 kcal/kg body wt (BW)s
  2. Protein (1.25-1.5 g/kg)
  3. Fluid (1 mL fluid per calorie intake/d or minimum of 1500 mL/day or per medical condition)
- Compare nutrient intake with nutritional needs: assess adequacy
- Laboratory values (within 30 days)
  1. Serum protein levels may be affected by inflammation, renal function, hydration and other factors and do not reflect nutritional status
  2. Consider lab values as one aspect of the assessment process. Refer to facility policy for specific labs
- Risk factors for pressure ulcer development
  1. Medical history
  2. Validated risk assessment (i.e., Braden Scale)
  3. Malnutrition (use screening tool, e.g. Mini Nutritional Assessment (MNA® for ≥65 years located at www.mna-elderly.com)
  4. Medical Treatments
  5. Medications (review type of medications)
  6. Ability to meet nutritional needs orally (if inadequate, consider alternative method of feeding) consistent with individual's wishes
  7. Oral Problems (e.g. chewing, swallowing) EAT-10: A Swallowing Assessment Tool available through Nestlé Nutrition Institute

Considerations:

- Incorporate fortified foods at meals for weight gain
- Provide supplements between meals as needed
- Vary the type of supplements offered to prevent taste fatigue
- Provide preferred food/food substitutions
- At admission weigh weekly x 30 days and then monthly
- Monitor acceptance of food and/or supplements offered
- Monitor tolerance of oral nutritional supplements, e.g. diarrhea
- Provide a vitamin/mineral supplement, if intake is poor
- Provide assistance at meal time if needed
- Encourage family involvement
- Offer food/fluid at appropriate texture for condition
- Liberalize restrictive diets
- Consult with Pharmacist and provide food and drugs at appropriate times and amounts
- Consider alternative method of feeding and if consistent with individual's wishes and goals of therapy:
  1. Provide tube feeding to meet needs per assessment
  2. Monitor tolerance, if needed recommend a specialty formula
  3. Provide parenteral nutrition when gut is non-functioning

© 2010 Nestlé. All rights reserved.
[1] National Pressure Ulcer Advisory Panel and European Pressure Ulcer Advisory Panel. Prevention and treatment of pressure ulcers: clinical practice guideline. Washington DC: National Pressure Ulcer Advisory Panel; 2009.
[≠] These are general guidelines based on various clinical references and are not intended as a substitute for medical advice or existing facility guidelines. An individual assessment is recommended.

FIGURE 7.1 Algorithm for prevention of pressure ulcers: nutrition guidelines.

be derived from objective clinical signs and responses to direct, specific questions about diet and nutrition (even if complaints are not volunteered), and reliable observations from third parties (family, friends, caregivers, aides, social workers).[10]

Assessment of Physical Conditions Related to Nutritional Status

Observe the client's skin condition, looking for signs of skin breakdown and nonhealing wounds, purpura, or bruises.[11] Older adults are particularly prone to pressure ulcers as a result of decreased mobility and loss of muscle mass, multiple contributing diagnoses, and poor nutrition. Nutritional factors that contribute to skin breakdown include protein deficiency, creating a negative nitrogen balance; anemia, inhibiting the formation of red blood cells; and dehydration, causing dry, fragile skin. Dehydration can also increase the blood glucose level and slow the healing process.[12]

Make a visual scan for dry, flaky skin, and skin that "tents." These signs suggest dehydration. The loss of skin elasticity and moisture, coupled with reduced sensation in susceptible areas, place older clients at risk for impaired skin integrity.

CLINICAL WISDOM

The Link Between Poor Nutritional Status and Pressure Ulcer Development

Warning Signs

The following are signs that an individual is at risk for or suffering from pressure ulcers (Table 7.1):

- Subject to incontinence
- Needs help
  - Moving arms, legs, or body
  - Changing position when sitting
- Loses weight
- Eats less than half of meals/snacks served
- Is dehydrated
- Has discolored, torn, or swollen skin over bony area

Report and Take Action

Below are some action steps to help individuals who are at risk for or suffering from pressure ulcers.

- Report observations and warning signs to nurse and dietitian.
- Check and change linens as appropriate.
- Handle/move the resident with care to avoid skin tears and scrapes.
- Reposition the resident frequently and properly.
- Use "unintended weight loss action steps" so the patient gets more calories and protein.
- Use "dehydration action steps" so the patient gets more to drink.
- Record meal/snack intake.

Adapted with permission from the Nutrition Screening Initiative, a project of the American Academy of Family Physicians, the American Dietetic Association, and the National Council on the Aging, Inc., and funded in part by a grant from Ross Products Division, Abbott Laboratories Inc.

Loose skin can be evidence of weight loss. Question the client about his or her usual weight. (Also see anthropometry, discussed shortly.)

Look for edema and/or ascites, which can be indicative of protein deficiency, renal disease, or hepatic disease. For other physical manifestations of malnutrition (see Table 7.1).

Anthropometry

Anthropometry is the measurement of body size, weight, and proportions. These measurements are used to evaluate a patient's nutritional status. For example, low body weight, when associated with illness or injury, increases the risk of morbidity. Obesity is common among nonambulatory patients whose caloric expenditure is low. In addition, the natural process of aging causes changes in body composition, including a decrease in lean body mass (sarcopenia), loss of height, and increased body fat.

Height and Weight

Measure the patient's height and weight. Weight tends to peak in the sixth decade of life, plateau, and then gradually decrease beyond the seventh decade. Height also normally decreases with advanced age as intervertebral disks compress; however, significant loss of height suggests osteoporosis.[13] Body composition shifts as well: the proportion of lean body mass (LBM) declines by 40% from age 20 to 80.[14] LBM contains smooth muscles, collagen (skin and tissue and cell structure). Preservation of LBM is critical to would healing since its functions include structure of bone and muscles, digestion, energy production, regulating metabolism, body's defense system (immune cells), and the movement of nutrients such as protein through the body.

Body Mass Index

Use the height and weight measurements to calculate the patient's **body mass index**, or **BMI**. BMI is a weight-to-height ratio representing a person's body weight in kilograms divided by the square of his or her height in meters:

$$BMI\,(kg/m^2) = \frac{weight\,(kg)}{height\,(m)^2}$$

It is generally agreed that a normally hydrated person with a BMI of 30 or more is obese, and a person with a BMI of more than 27 is at major risk for obesity.[15] A BMI of 25 or above is overweight, and a BMI between 18.5 and 24.9 is normal weight. A BMI at or below 21 with involuntary weight loss places a client at risk for developing pressure ulcers.[16]

Although BMI is highly correlated with body fat throughout the general population, increased lean body mass or a large body frame can also increase the BMI. For example, athletes commonly have a BMI above 25. In addition, the BMI standards are based on middle-aged adults and do not adequately reflect age-related changes in adults over 65 years, or muscle and bone growth in children.

Unintentional Weight Loss

Unintentional weight loss has a significant impact on overall health, and the degree of a person's weight loss positively correlates with the severity of the impact. When evaluating significant and severe weight loss, it is important to determine possible causes, such as recent surgery or any recently initiated treatments (e.g., radiation or diuretic therapy) that can affect weight status.

| TABLE 7.1 | **Physical Signs of Malnutrition (Bundled Item)** |

Signs	Possible Nutrition-Related Causes
Hair	
Dull, dry; lack of natural shine, easily plucked	Protein-energy deficiency
	Essential fatty acid deficiency (EFA)
Thin, sparse; alopecia	Zinc, biotin, protein deficiency
Color changes, depigmentation, lack luster	Other nutrient deficiencies: manganese, copper
Easily plucked with no pain	Protein deficiency, seen in kwashiorkor and occasionally in marasmus
Corkscrew hair; unemerged, coiled hairs	Vitamin C deficiency
Eyes	
Small, yellowish lumps around eyes	Hyperlipidemia
White rings around both eyes	
Angular inflammation of eyelids, "grittiness" under eyelids, superficial vascularization, ulcerations of cornea	Riboflavin deficiency
Pale eye and mucous membranes	Vitamin B_{12}, folate, and/or iron deficiency
Night blindness, dry membranes, dull or soft cornea	Vitamin A, zinc deficiency
Redness and fissures of eyelid corners; red and inflamed conjunctiva, swollen and sticky eyelids	Niacin deficiency riboflavin/pyridoxine deficiency
Ring of fine blood vessels around cornea	General poor nutrition
Bitot spots (white spots in eyes)	Vitamin A deficiency
Ophthalmoplegia	Thiamin, phosphorus deficiency
Lips	
Redness and swelling of mouth, stomatitis	Niacin, riboflavin, iron, and/or pyridoxine deficiency
Angular fissures, scars at corner of mouth (cheilosis)	Niacin, riboflavin, iron, and/or pyridoxine deficiency
Soreness, burning lips, pallor	Riboflavin deficiency
Gums	
Spongy, swollen, bleeds easily, redness (swollen, bleeding gums; retracted gums with teeth)	Vitamin C deficiency
Gingivitis	Folate, pyridoxine, vitamin C, zinc deficiency
	Vitamin A excess
Mouth	
Cheilosis, angular scars	Riboflavin, iron, pyridoxine, niacin deficiency
Soreness, burning	Riboflavin deficiency
Tongue	
Sores, swollen, scarlet, raw, "beef tongue"	Folate, niacin deficiency
Smooth, beefy red tongue	Vitamin B_{12}, niacin deficiency
Soreness, burning tongue	Riboflavin deficiency
Purplish/magenta color	
Smooth with papillae (small projections)	Riboflavin, vitamin B_{12}, pyridoxine, niacin, folate, protein, iron deficiency
Glossitis	Riboflavin, iron, zinc, pyridoxine deficiency

(continued)

TABLE 7.1	**Physical Signs of Malnutrition (*continued*)**
Taste	
Sense of taste diminished	Zinc deficiency
Teeth	
Gray-brown spots; mottling	Increased fluoride intake
Missing or erupting abnormally	General poor nutrition
Face	
Skin color loss, dark cheeks and eyes; enlarged parotid glands, scaling of skin around nostrils	Protein-energy deficiency; specifically niacin, riboflavin, and pyridoxine deficiencies
Pallor	Iron, folate, vitamin B_{12} and vitamin C deficiencies
Hyperpigmentation	Niacin deficiency
Neck	
Thyroid enlargement	Iodine deficiency
Symptoms of hypothyroidism	Iodine deficiency
Nails	
Fragility, banding	Protein deficiency
Spoon shaped; concave	Iron deficiency
Skin	
Slow wound healing, decubitus ulcers	Zinc, vitamin C, protein deficiency; kwashiorkor
Psoriasis	Biotin deficiency
Eczema; lesions	Riboflavin, zinc deficiency
Scaling of the scalp, dandruff, oiliness of the scalp, lips, and nose	Biotin deficiency, pyridoxine, zinc, riboflavin, essential fatty acids deficiency; vitamin A excess or deficiency
Purple or red spots due to skin bleeding	Vitamin C and/or K deficiency
Dryness, mosaic, sandpaper feel, flakiness	Increased or decreased vitamin A
Dark, dry, scaly skin	Niacin deficiency
Lack of fat under skin, cellophane appearance	Protein-energy deficiency, vitamin C deficiency
Bilateral edema	Protein-energy, vitamin C deficiency
Yellow colored	Beta carotene excess, vitamin B_{12} deficiency
Cutaneous flushing, desquamation	Niacin
Body edema; round swollen face	Protein, thiamin deficiencies
Pallor, fatigue, depression, apathy	Iron, folic acid deficiencies
Gastrointestinal	
Anorexia, flatulence, diarrhea	Vitamin B_{12} deficiency
Muscular System	
Weakness	Phosphorus or potassium deficiency, vitamin C deficiency, vitamin D deficiency
Wasted appearance	Protein-energy deficiency
Calf tenderness, absent knee jerks, foot and wrist drop	Thiamin deficiency

TABLE 7.1	Physical Signs of Malnutrition (*continued*)
Peripheral neuropathy, tingling, "pins and needles"	Folate, pyridoxine, pantothenic acid, phosphate, thiamine deficiencies, vitamin B_{12} deficiency
Muscle twitching, convulsions, tetany	Magnesium or pyridoxine excess or deficiency; calcium, vitamin D deficiencies
Muscle cramps	Chloride decreased, sodium deficiency; calcium, vitamin D, magnesium deficiencies
Muscle pain	Biotin deficiency
Skeletal System	
Demineralization of bone	Calcium, phosphorus, vitamin D deficiencies
Epiphyseal enlargement of leg and knee, bowed legs	Vitamin D deficiency
Bone tenderness	Vitamin D deficiency
Nervous System	
Listlessness	Protein-energy deficiency
Loss of position and vibratory sense, decrease and loss of ankle and knee reflexes, depression, inability to concentrate, defective memory, confabulation, delirium	Thiamin, pyridoxine, vitamin B_{12} deficiencies
Seizures, memory impairment, and behavioral disturbances	Magnesium, zinc deficiencies
Peripheral neuropathy, dementia	Pyridoxine deficiency
Dementia	Niacin, vitamin B_{12} deficiencies

Resources
1. Chernoff R. *Geriatric Nutrition: The Health Professional's Handbook.* Jones & Bartlett; 2006
2. *Journal of the American Medical Association*, February 11, 2004.
3. Hetzel BS, Clugston GA. Iodine. In: Shils M, Olson JA, Shike M, Ross AC, eds. *Nutrition in Health and Disease.* Vol. 9. Baltimore, MD: Williams & Wilkins; 1999:253–264.
4. The Merck Manual. Available at http://www.merck.com/pubs/mmanual_ha/tables/tb17_1.html. Accessed August 26, 2009.
Table adapted from Pocket Resource for Nutrition Assessment 2009, rev. Dietetics in Health Care Communities a dietetic practice group of the American Dietetic Association, pp. 65–69, with permission.

Undernutrition or poor nutritional status impairs the wound healing process in a self-perpetuating cycle: undernutrition, dehydration, or unintentional weight loss, whether secondary to poor appetite or other disease processes, increases a patient's risk for tissue breakdown. When a wound develops, the patient is stressed, which further depletes nutrient stores. Hypermetabolism, a responsive increase in metabolic rate, is triggered by injury, trauma, and/or infection. For example, during wound healing, the metabolic rate increases. Hypermetabolism, a catabolic reaction, breaks down glycogen, triglycerides, and protein stores energy stress factors. Catecholamines and cortisol increase glycogen breakdown, mobilize free fatty acids from triglyceride stores, and accelerate glucose production from visceral protein stores. Protein from the skeletal muscle, gut, and connective tissues supplies glucose and amino acids necessary for the synthesis of stress factors and immune cells. As a result of these processes, body stores of glycogen, triglycerides, and protein decline (Fig. 7.2).[17]

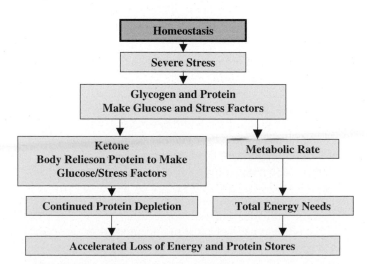

FIGURE 7.2 Metabolic response to severe stress. (Reprinted from Mary Ellen Posthauer, RD, CD, LD. Published in *Advances in Skin and Wound Care*, September 2005, with permission.)

Therapeutic Diets

A highly restrictive diet order, especially when it denies patients their favorite foods, can contribute significantly to reduced food intake and a marked decline in nutritional status. It can also diminish a patient's quality of life. Food is not nutritious unless eaten. Certain medical conditions require diet modifications, but these can often be met with simple adjustments and minimal restrictions.[18] It is important for the nursing staff to communicate with the RD when a patient refuses to eat or eats very little. If after evaluating the patient's intake of a therapeutic diet and food preferences, it is determined that the restrictions hinders the intake of nutrients the RD recommends the appropriate individualized meal plan. For example, a patient with diabetes may consume a consistent carbohydrate diet with the carbohydrate containing foods balanced throughout the day. Nutrition goals for patients with wounds should focus on adequate intake of nutrients rather than strict limitations that may compromise the healing process. An obese patient should not be placed on a low calorie diet below 1500 kcal, which would not have adequate vitamins or minerals.[19] The primary goal for the obese patient is wound healing not weight reduction.

Role of Medications in Nutritional Risk

Many of the drugs designed to calm or reduce agitation can, in turn, reduce a client's mobility and activity levels, resulting in decreased food intake. The common side effects of some drugs, such as gastric disturbances, affect the intake of food and fluid. Radiation therapy, chemotherapy, and renal dialysis can result in increased nausea and vomiting, as well as decreased activity.

Medication should be checked for possible effects on nutritional intake, as well as any effect on the client's mental and physical status. Constipation and diarrhea are medication-related risk factors that should be addressed in a nutritional assessment. In addition, laxative abuse, which is common with some older adults, can induce a state of malabsorption. Chronic diarrhea can lead to dehydration and weight loss, which increase the risk for malnutrition and pressure ulcers.

Lab Values

Laboratory indexes are one aspect of a nutrition assessment but there is not one test that can specifically identify nutritional status. Hepatic proteins such as albumin, prealbumin (transthyretin), or transferrin have been linked to nutritional status. However, research indicates serum hepatic protein levels correlate with severity of illness.[20] Serum albumin, prealbumin, and transferrin decrease with acute changes in clinical status such as infection, injury, trauma, cytokine-induced inflammatory state, and dehydration. Levels increase when the body recovers from these conditions.[20] Age and declining liver function also affect the ability of the body to synthesize albumin. Levels are shown with implications in Table 7.2. Other lab values of significance include serum cholesterol and hemoglobin/hematocrit. A serum cholesterol level of less than 160 mg per dL with poor intake and weight loss places a client at risk for undernutrition. A hemoglobin level less than 12 mg per dL and hematocrit level less than 33% may indicate iron deficiency anemia or anemia of chronic disease.[21]

Biochemical assessment data must be used with caution because they can be altered by hydration, medication, and changes in metabolism. Parameters for evaluating hydration status include assessing urine output (I/O), weight, blood urea nitrogen (BUN)/creatinine ratio (>10 to 1), and skin turgor (Table 7.3).

THE ROLE OF NUTRIENTS IN WOUND HEALING

More than just food, nutrition encompasses the six classes of nutrients—carbohydrates, proteins, fats, vitamins, minerals, and water—all of which are vital to the healing of wounds.

Carbohydrates

Carbohydrates are energy nutrients consisting of molecules of carbon, hydrogen, and oxygen atoms arranged in simple ring shapes or more complex chains. Plants synthesize the most abundant form of dietary carbohydrate, glucose, using sunlight, in the process called photosynthesis. Carbohydrates provide 4 kcal per g.

CLINICAL WISDOM

Unintended Weight Loss

Warning Signs

- Needs help eating or drinking
- Eats less than half of meal/snack served
- Has mouth pain
- Has dentures that don't fit
- Has a hard time chewing or swallowing
- Coughs or chokes while eating
- Has sadness, crying spells, or withdrawal from others
- Is confused, wanders, or paces
- Has diabetes, chronic obstructive pulmonary disease (COPD), cancer, HIV, or other chronic disease

Report and Take Action

Below are some action steps to increase food intake, create a positive dining environment, and help individuals consume adequate calories:

- Report observations and warning signs to other members of the health-care team.
- Encourage the resident to eat.
- Honor food likes and dislikes.
- Offer many kinds of foods and beverages.
- Help individuals who have trouble feeding themselves.
- Allow enough time to finish eating.
- Notify nursing staff if the resident has trouble using utensils.
- Record meal and snack intake.
- Provide oral care before meals.
- Position individual correctly for feeding.
- If the resident has had a loss of appetite and/or seems sad, ask what's wrong.

Adapted with permission from the Nutrition Screening Initiative, a project of the American Academy of Family Physicians, the American Dietetic Association, and the National Council on the Aging, Inc., and funded in part by a grant from Ross Products Division, Abbott Laboratories Inc.

TABLE 7.2	Selected Laboratory Values for Adults*	
Test	**Normal Values**	**Some Implications**
Albumin Serum ALB	3.5–5.0 g/dL (35–50 g/L SI units) >60 y 3.4–4.8 g/dL (34–48 g/L SI units)	**Function:** Maintain colloidal osmotic pressure; transport molecule for enzymes, fatty acids, hormones, bilirubin, and some drugs. **Site of synthesis:** Liver **Half Life:** 12–18 d **Increased:** Dehydration; also diarrhea, Hodgkin disease, metastatic carcinomatosis, non-Hodgkin lymphoma, ulcerative colitis, uremia, and vomiting. **Decreased:** Overhydration; also acute infection and chronic inflammation, alcohol abuse, ascites, beriberi, burns, cholecystitis, CHF, cirrhosis, Crohn's, Cushing's, cystic fibrosis, dementia, diabetes mellitus, essential HTN, liver disease, leukemia, lymphoma, malabsorption syndrome, malnutrition, meningitis, myasthenia, myeloma, MI, neoplasms, nephrotic syndrome, nephrosis, osteomyelitis, peptic ulcer, pneumonia, pregnancy, protein-losing enteropathies and protein-losing nephropathies, rheumatic fever, rheumatoid arthritis, sarcoidosis, scleroderma, sprue, steatorrhea, stress, surgery, systemic lupus erythematosus, thyrotoxicosis, trauma, tuberculosis, and ulcerative bowel disease. Is this correct that the same conditions can cause either an increase or a decrease? Many repeats between these two sections. This was corrected by CP.
Blood Urea Nitrogen BUN Blood Urea Nitrogen, BUN, cont.	10–20 mg/dL 3.6–7.1 mmol/L (SI units) >60 y: 8–21 mg/dL 2.9–7.5 mmol/L (SI units)	**Function:** End product of protein metabolism converted in the liver to form urea. **Site of synthesis:** Liver **Increased:** Addison disease, allergic purpura, amyloidosis, anabolic steroid use, analgesic abuse, blood transfusions, burns, cachexia, cardiac failure, congenital hypoplastic kidneys, CHF, dehydration, DM with diabetic ketoacidosis, Fanconi syndrome, excessive fluids, excessive protein intake, GI bleed, glomerulonephritis, Goodpasture syndrome, gout, heavy-metal poisoning, hemoglobinurias, hypovolemia, infection, intestinal obstruction, MI, nephritis, nephropathy, nephrosclerosis, nephrotoxic drugs, pancreatitis, peritonitis, pneumonia, polyarteritis nodosa, polycystic disease, postsurgical state, pregnancy, protein catabolism, pyelonephritis, renal arterial stenosis or thrombosis, renal insufficiency or failure, scleroderma, sepsis, shock, sickle cell anemia, starvation, stress, subacute bacterial endocardititis, suppuration, systemic lupus erythematosus, thyrotoxicosis, tumor necrosis, uremia, and urinary tract obstruction. **Decreased:** Acromegaly, alcohol abuse, amyloidosis, celiac, cirrhosis, hemodialysis, hepatitis, insufficient protein intake, overhydration, liver damage or failure, malabsorption, malnutrition, nephrotic syndrome, pregnancy (advanced), and syndrome of inappropriate antidiuretic hormone.
Cholesterol—blood Total Chol	<200 mg/dL <5.2 mmol/L (SI units) 200–239 mg/dL Borderline high >239 mg/dL High	**Function:** Used to form bile acids and hormones; component of brain and nerve cells and cell membranes throughout the body. μ: Liver and intestines **Increased:** Aplastic anemia, anorexia nervosa, atherosclerosis, bile duct obstruction, biliary cirrhosis, carbon disulfide exposure (textile workers), CHD, CHF, celiac, cholestasis, Cushing's, DM (uncontrolled), excessive cholesterol, saturated or trans fat consumption, Forbes disease, glycogen storage diseases, *H. pylori*, hypercholesterolemia, hyperlipidemia, hyperlipoproteinemia, hypertension, hypothyroidism, jaundice, leukemia, lipoidosis, MI, nephrosis, nephrotic syndrome, obesity, oophrectomy, pancreatectomy, pancreatitis (chronic), pregnancy, smoking, stress, and xanthomatosis. **Decreased:** Acanthocytosis, amylopectinosis, Andersen disease, anemia (hemolytic or pernicious), Bassen-Kornzweig syndrome, brancher deficiency, cancer, cholesterol lowering drugs, chromium enhanced diet, cirrhosis, depression, epilepsy, absent cholesterol esters, gastric bypass surgery, Gaucher disease,

(continued)

TABLE 7.2	Selected Laboratory Values for Adults* *(Continued)*	

Test	Normal Values	Some Implications
		Hansen disease, hepatic disease, hepatitis, hyperthyroidism, hypolipoprotein-emias (Abeta and hypobeta), infections(severe), intestinal obstruction, jaundice, leprosy, liver necrosis, malnutrition, MI (up to 90 days), pancreatic carcinoma, porphyria, premenstrual time phase, steatorrhea, suicidal behavior, Tangier disease, TB, glycogen deposition diseases, and uremia.
Creatinine Serum	Male: 0.6–1.2 mg/dL 53–106 μmol/L (SI units) Female: 0.5–1.1 mg/dL 44–97 μmol/L (SI units) Elderly: may be lower	**Function**: Nitrogenous by-product in the breakdown of muscle creatinine phosphate for energy metabolism. **Site of synthesis**: N/A **Increased**: Acromegaly, allergic purpura, amyloidosis, analgesic abuse, azotemia, congenital hypoplastic kidneys, CHF, DM, dehydration, high meat intake, gigantism, glomerulonephritis, Goodpasture syndrome, gout, hemoglobinuria, high dietary intake, hypovolemic shock, hypothyroidism, intestinal obstruction, Kimmelstiel-Wilson syndrome, microalbuminemia, metal poisoning, multiple myeloma, muscle destruction, nephritis, nephropathy, nephrosclerosis, nephrotoxic drugs, pancreatitis (necrotizing), polyarteritis nodosa, polycystic disease, preeclampsia, pyelonephritis, renal artery stenosis or thrombosis, renal failure, rhabdomyolosis, rheumatoid arthritis, scleroderma, sickle cell anemia, subacute bacterial endocarditis, systemic lupus erythematosus, testosterone therapy, toxic shock, uremia, urinary obstruction, and vomiting. Values are significantly higher later in the day. Decreased: DKA (artifactual), overhydration, muscular dystrophy, myasthenia gravis, severe muscle wasting.
Prealbumin Serum PAB	15–36 mg/dL 150–360 mg/L (SI units)	**Function**: Transport protein that carries thyroxine and retinol in the body. **Site of synthesis**: Liver Half-Life: 2–4 d **Increased**: Adrenal hyperfunction, CKD, dehydration, Hodgkin disease, nephrotic syndrome, pregnancy, shigellosis. **Decreased**: Abdominal peritoneal dialysis, burns, cirrhosis, chronic illness (with concomitant subnormal nutritional status), CF, DM, disseminated malignant disease, epithelial ovarian carcinoma, hereditary amyloidosis, infection, inflammation, liver damage, overhydration, protein and calorie malnutrition, salicylate poisoning.
Total lymphocyte count (TLC)	2500–3300 cells/mm³ 2500–3300 × 10⁶	**Function**: Fight infection and fight against foreign bodies (both bacterial and viral). Site of synthesis: Bone marrow stem cells Increased: Chronic bacterial infection, infectious hepatitis, infectious mononucleosis, lymphocytosis, lymphocytic leukemia, multiple myeloma, mumps, rubella, and radiation. **Decreased**: Adenocorticosteroid therapy, antineoplastic therapy, HIV (late stage), immunodeficiency diseases, leukemia, lymphocytopenia, radiation therapy, sepsis, systemic lupus erythematosus. cancer, chemotherapy, radiotherapy, surgery, lymphopenia, malnutrition, AIDS, bone marrow failure, Cushing syndrome, renal failure.

* Each laboratory may use different standards to establish normal values; therefore, figures may vary among different sources.
Adapted from Pocket Resource for Nutrition Assessment, 2009, Dietetics in Health Care Communities a dietetic practice group of the American Dietetic Association, pp. 71–85 with permission.

Simple carbohydrates are single sugar rings—glucose, fructose, or galactose—or double rings composed of two simple sugars joined together—lactose, maltose, or sucrose. Simple carbohydrates are the natural sugars contained in fruits, vegetables, honey, table sugar, and milk. Added sugars in desserts, soft drinks, and many other processed foods also provide simple carbohydrates in the diet.

Complex carbohydrates are generally long chains of glucose. They are supplied by starches in the form of grains, legumes (peas, beans, and lentils), and tubers (potatoes and yams). They are of course also supplied by products made from these staples, such as breads. Fiber is a nonnutrient complex carbohydrate that passes through the digestive tract without being metabolized or absorbed; however, it absorbs water and provides bulk that aids in the elimination of feces.

Carbohydrates serve several functions:

- Provide 4 kcal per g of energy
- Serve as the most readily available source of energy for the body and the preferred energy source for brain and blood cells

TABLE 7.3	Useful Lab Values to Screen for Hydration Status		
Lab Test	**Normal Values**	**Dehydration**	**Over-hydration**
Osmolality	280–303 mOsm/kg	> 303 mOsm/kg (critical)	> 320 mOsm/kg
Serum sodium	135–145 mEq/L	> 145 mEq/L	< 130 meEq/L
Albumin	3.4–5.4 g/dL	Higher than normal	Lower than normal
Blood urine nitrogen (BUN)	7–20 mg/dL	> 35 mg/dL	< 7mg/dL
BUN/creatinine ratio	10:1	> 25:1	< 10:1
Urine specific gravity	1.002–1.028 g/mL	> 1.028 g/mL	< 1.002 g/mL

Medline Plus Medical Encyclopedia
Reprinted from *Healing Solutions, Hydration Care for Wound Prevention and Healing, Novartis Medical Nutrition;* 2004:25, with permission.

- Spare protein for its primary use: building and maintaining tissues
- Provide cellular components for regulating metabolism
- Provide fiber to help maintain bowel function
- Provide flavor, color, and variety to the diet

Protein

Proteins are energy nutrients consisting of carbon, hydrogen, oxygen, and nitrogen atoms. Like carbohydrates, they provide 4 kcal per g. All proteins contain nitrogen, and some also contain phosphorus and sulfur. Proteins molecules are long chains of subunits called *amino acids*. Of the 20 amino acids in the body, 9 are indispensable; that is, the body cannot synthesize them and they must be obtained in the diet. The remaining 11 amino acids can be manufactured by the body and are dispensable amino acids.

Dietary proteins that provide all nine of the indispensable amino acids are considered *complete proteins*. Food sources of complete protein include meat, poultry, fish, eggs, milk products, and soybeans. Other legumes, grains, and vegetables provide dispensable protein; however, if eaten in complementary combinations (e.g., rice with vegetables, or pasta with beans), the meal provides complete protein.

The body utilizes proteins in numerous ways:

- Provide 4 kcal per g of energy
- Provide amino acid building blocks for the growth, repair, and maintenance of tissues
- Act as enzymes to facilitate chemical reactions throughout the body
- Are components of antibodies and essential to immune system functioning
- Act as hormones and serve in important regulatory functions
- Help maintain fluid and electrolyte balance and acid-base balance
- Help transport lipids and other substances in the blood and across cell membranes

Adequate protein is also essential for wound healing. For example, proteins are required for cell multiplication, for the synthesis of collagen and connective tissue, and for enzymes involved in wound healing. Protein is also a component of the antibodies necessary for proper immune system function, and thus is important to prevent and fight infection.

Earlier, we mentioned that dispensable amino acids can be synthesized by the body and do not need to be consumed in food; however, under conditions of physiologic stress, arginine, cysteine, glycine, proline, tyrosine, and glutamine become conditionally indispensable amino acids. Arginine, which is 32% nitrogen, stimulates the insulin-like growth factor that promotes healing. This stimulation of insulin secretion promotes the transport of amino acids into tissue cells and supports the formation of protein in the cells. Arginine is also the substrate for nitric acid and a regulator of nucleic acid synthesis. As discussed in Chapter 2, nitric acid production activates wound macrophages, which are rich sources of growth factors, cytokines, bioactive lipid products, and proteolytic enzymes necessary for the healing process.[22,23] In addition, an increased level of arginine promotes the conversion of arginine to ornithine, which is a precursor to proline, which is incorporated into collagen.[22,23]

Given the contributions of protein to wound healing, it's not surprising that increased protein levels are linked to improved wound healing in patients with pressure ulcers.[24,25] The NPUAP/EPUAP guideline recommends a protein range of 1.25 to 1.5 g of protein a day per kilogram of body weight when compatible with goals of care.[2]

Patients with chronic kidney disease may not be candidates for receiving high levels of protein. Renal function should be assessed to ensure tolerance of higher protein levels.[26]

Nutritional supplements formulated for wound care are often fortified with arginine, cysteine, and glutamine, as well as β-hydroxy-β-methylbutyrate (HMB), the metabolite of the amino acid leucine, which has a role in supporting immune function. HMB serves as a precursor to cholesterol, which is a component of all cell membranes, and enhances the integrity of cells and reduces cell rupture under stress. Thus, lean body mass and muscle integrity are preserved.[27] Clinical judgment should be used when recommending the use of supplements with arginine alone or combined and other nutrients for pressure ulcer healing.[28]

Patients with chronic kidney disease who are not on dialysis and require limited protein should be offered foods with complete protein, such as eggs, meat, poultry, fish, milk, and cheese. The RD evaluates the appropriate quality and type of protein that will meet the diet order for these patients. Patients who are obese or those on low-cholesterol diets should select foods low in saturated fat, such as skim milk, lean fish, and low-fat cheese.

CLINICAL WISDOM

Tips for Adding Protein and Calories

- Add dry milk to cream soups, mashed potatoes, casseroles, puddings, and milk-based desserts.
- Add one-third cup of nonfat dry powdered milk to each cup of regular milk.
- Add cheese to vegetables, salads, potatoes, rice, noodles, and casseroles.
- Mix commercial supplements with ice cream or sherbet.
- Add yogurt to fruit and cereal.
- Add nuts, seeds, or wheat germ to casseroles, breads, muffins, pancakes, and cookies.
- Sprinkle nuts, seeds, or wheat germ on fruit, cereal, ice cream, and yogurt, or use in place of bread crumbs.
- Add peanut butter to sandwiches, toast, crackers, or muffins; use as a dip for vegetables and fruit; or add to milk and blend.
- Add dry beans to soups or casseroles.

Modular protein supplements can be added to the diets to increase the amino acid intake. This type of supplement provides the necessary protein to promote healing in a moderate amount of calories and is a good choice for patients who are obese.

Fats

Fats are energy nutrients made up of carbon, hydrogen, and oxygen. They provide 9 kcal per g. Triglycerides, which are composed of three fatty acid chains attached to a molecule of glycerol, are the most common fats in both the diet and the body. Saturated fats are provided largely from animal sources such as meat, poultry, fish, eggs, and dairy products (e.g., milk, butter, cream). They exert negative effects on blood lipids and increase the risk for heart disease. Unsaturated fats are provided mostly from vegetable oils, nuts, and some fruits, such as olives and avocados. They exert beneficial effects on blood lipids and, in moderation, reduce the risk for heart disease.

The functions of fats include the following:

- Provide the most concentrated source of energy, 9 kcal per g
- Are the body's main source of energy during rest, sleep, and long periods of food deprivation
- Are a major energy source during exercise
- Maintain normal cell membrane function
- Permit the absorption of the fat-soluble vitamins (A, D, E, and K) and allow other fat-soluble substances to move in and out of the cell
- Insulate the body from heat and cold
- Cushion the kidneys, bones, and other organs from shock and injury
- Provide flavor, texture, and variety to foods

Micronutrients: Vitamins

Vitamins and minerals are micronutrients that are essential in small amounts for the body. The Institute of Medicine (IOM) and National Academy of Sciences (NAS) Dietary Reference Intakes indicate the level of each micronutrient needed at each stage of life for healthy individuals.[29]

A **vitamin** is an organic compound that the body requires in small amounts for proper functioning. Except for vitamins D and K, the body cannot produce vitamins, so they must be obtained from food and beverages or from synthetic supplements. Vitamins facilitate various chemical reactions in the body, with different vitamins performing different functions. For example, although vitamins do not themselves provide energy, they support the cell's ability to break down the energy nutrients and build the energy molecule, ATP. Vitamins also participate in protein synthesis and cell replication. The functions of specific vitamins are best known by the results of their deficiencies.

Vitamin supplements are recommended if a patient's diet is poor or limited in calories, or if a vitamin deficiency is suspected. A daily high-potency multiple vitamin and mineral supplement is necessary if vitamin and mineral deficiencies are confirmed or suspected. In addition, supplement-medication interactions are not uncommon: a pharmacist or physician can determine the appropriate time to take a vitamin supplement in relationship to other medications.

Vitamins are divided into two groups, according to whether they are soluble in fat or water.

Fat-Soluble Vitamins

Vitamins A, D, E, and K are derived from the fatty and oily parts of certain foods. They remain in the liver and fat tissue of the body until they are used. Because the body does not excrete excess fat-soluble vitamins, there is some risk of toxicity from overdose resulting from overaccumulation. On the other hand, deficiencies of the fat-soluble vitamins can occur if the diet is extremely low in fat, or in the presence of malabsorption disorders.

Vitamin A is required for the inflammatory response, and deficiencies of vitamin A have been associated with retarded epithelialization and decreased collagen synthesis. Fortunately, because vitamin A is a fat-soluble vitamin and not excreted from the body, deficiencies are rare.

Vitamin D is essential for calcium regulation and bone health, as well as for cell differentiation and healthy immune function. Although it can be synthesized by the body in response to exposure to adequate sunlight, many people, especially elderly residents of long-term care facilities, lack sufficient sun exposure to avoid deficiency. Vitamin D is also available from fortified milk and breakfast cereals, a few fatty fish such as salmon and sardines, and from supplements.

Vitamin E is an antioxidant that protects cell membranes from oxidation, and by protecting white blood cells, enhances immune function. It is widespread in the diet, especially in plant oils.

Vitamin K is important in bone health as well as in blood clotting, and thus is important for effective wound healing. It is produced in our large intestine and is available from green leafy vegetables and some plant oils.

Water-Soluble Vitamins

Water-soluble vitamins include the vitamin B family and vitamin C and are derived from the water components of foods. They are distributed throughout the water compartments of the body and, for the most part, are carried in the bloodstream.

Unlike fat-soluble vitamins, they are not stored but are excreted in the urine when their concentration in the blood becomes too high.

B vitamins are necessary for the production of energy from glucose, amino acids, and fat. Vitamin B_6 (pyridoxine) helps maintain cellular integrity and form red blood cells. Thiamine and riboflavin are needed for cross-linking and collagenation.

Deficiency of vitamin C (ascorbic acid) is associated with impaired fibroblast function and decreased collagen synthesis, resulting in delayed healing, capillary fragility, and breakdown of old wounds. Vitamin C increases the activation of leukocytes and macrophages to a wound site, and deficiency is associated with impaired immune function, decreasing the individual's ability to resist infection.[30] Because vitamin C is a water-soluble vitamin and cannot be stored in the body, deficiencies can develop quickly if adequate intake is not maintained. Thus, if a patient's diet is deficient in good sources of vitamins, a multivitamin may be appropriate. Vitamin C supplementation in mega doses has not been demonstrated to accelerate wound healing.[31,32]

Minerals

Minerals are inorganic elements that are needed by the cells to build and maintain body tissues, maintain fluid balance, and activate enzyme systems. Once ingested, mineral salts usually dissolve in body fluids and form ions. The skeletal system depends on the minerals calcium, magnesium, and phosphorus for its structural rigidity.

Various minerals play a role in wound healing. These include iron, which is essential for oxygen transport, and copper, which is required for cross-linking of collagen fibers in rebuilding tissue. Zinc is an essential cofactor for formation of collagen and for protein synthesis. Zinc deficiencies have been associated with delayed healing, and appear to act by reducing the rate of epithelialization and fibroblast proliferation.[33] Good sources of zinc include high protein foods such as meat, liver, and shellfish. Zinc supplementation (above the upper tolerable limit of 40 mg per day) is not recommended.[29] High serum zinc levels may inhibit healing, interfere with copper metabolism, and induce a copper deficiency, resulting in anemia. Copper and zinc compete for binding sites on the albumin molecule.[34,35] Copper deficiency may be harmful as copper is crucial for collagen cross-linking.[3]

Water

Water, which constitutes about 60% of an adult's body weight, is the most critical nutrient. It is distributed in the body in three fluid compartments: intracellular, interstitial, and intravascular. Water serves many vital functions in the body:

- Acts as a solvent for vitamins, minerals, amino acids, and glucose, enabling them to diffuse in and out of cells
- Transports vital substances to cells and carries away wastes
- Serves as a lubricant and cushion for joints, the brain, the spinal cord, the lungs, and other organs
- Helps to maintain body temperature
- Accounts for blood volume
- Aids in hydration of wound site and oxygen perfusion

Fluid requirements are met with 30 mL per kg of body weight or 1 mL per kcal, or a minimum of 1500 mL per day (1.5 L)

CLINICAL WISDOM

Nutritional Strategies

Once you have performed a nutritional assessment, you can devise an appropriate individualized nutrition plan for the patient. Some patients will be able to maintain their nutritional status by oral intake of a balanced diet, supplemented with a multivitamin/mineral. But for other patients, such as those with pressure ulcers, the concurrent challenges of weight gain and wound healing may make greater nutrient demands. For these patients, the following interventions may be appropriate:

- Provide calorically dense supplement between meals with a protein profile of 8 g or higher and 200 to 250+ kcal per serving.
- Determine the client's flavor preferences and offer those preferred flavors. Clients often prefer a fruit-based product rather than the traditional milk-based products.
- Offer 2 fl oz of a nutrient-dense supplement three to four times daily, followed by 4 fl oz of water.
- Serve juice and/or fruit with meals to increase vitamin C intake.
- Offer supplements at least 1 hour before the next meal so the patient is hungry for the meal.
- Liberalize the diet when possible, as restrictive diets often reduce food intake. The American Dietetic Association has stated that the quality of life and nutritional status of older adults residing in heal care communities can be enhanced by individualization to the least restrictive diet appropriate.[36]
- Consider nutritional support (enteral or parenteral) when the patient cannot meet nutritional needs orally.
- Inform the patient and/or caregivers of the risks and benefits of nutritional support. Ensure that nutritional support achieves the desired goals and is compatible with the wishes of the client and family.

---

unless medically contraindicated. Clients with end-stage renal disease or severe congestive heart failure may require slightly less fluid intake, calculated at 20 to 25 mL per kg body weight. In contrast, additional fluids are needed for clients with heavily draining wounds, emesis, diarrhea, elevated temperature, and increased perspiration. Nutritional Needs and Assessment is a guide for calculating energy and fluid requirements (Table 7.4). Signs and symptoms of dehydration include

- Weight loss (2% mild, 5% moderate, 8% severe)
- Dry skin
- Cracked lips
- Thirst (may be diminished in the elderly)
- Poor skin turgor (may be an unreliable test in the elderly)
- Either fever or low body temperature
- Altered sensation
- Loss of appetite
- Nausea
- Dizziness
- Increased confusion

TABLE 7.4	Nutritional Needs and Assessment: Shortcut Method for Estimating Adult Energy Needs per Kilogram

	kcals Required
Nonobese population	25–35 kcal/kg body weight
Obese, critically ill population	21 kcal/kg body weight
Paraplegics[a]	28 kcal/kg/d
Quadriplegics[a]	23 kcal/kg/d

[a]Estimated energy needs for paraplegics and quadriplegics are adjusted by reducing calculated desirable body weights because immobilized patients lose muscle.

Indirect Calorimetry

Indirect calorimetry (IC) is considered the gold standard for energy expenditure estimation. IC determines resting metabolic rate (RMR) by measuring respiratory gas exchange. Measured RMR is preferred to the use of prediction equations because such equations fail by more than 10% in up to one-third of patients. Because IC quantifies stress due to injury, illness, and other idiosyncratic medical conditions, including the affects of medications, the dietitian only needs to apply the appropriate activity factor.

Pros: Advances in technology make IC accurate, affordable, accessible, and easy to administer with minimal staff training.

Cons: Food, ethanol, stimulants, physical activity, and ambient conditions affect RMR; therefore, adherence to pretest protocol is necessary to obtain accurate results.

Costs: IC units range in price from $4000 to $20,000. Insurance reimbursement for IC ranges from $10 to $130.

"Because energy expenditure is difficult to predict on the basis of conventional equations, patients in long-term acute care facilities routinely are overfed and underfed, with only 25% receiving calories within 10% of required needs. Measuring a patient's energy requirement at least once by IC is important, because the degree of metabolism predicts how easily a patient will be underfed or overfed. "—McClave, S, Are patients fed appropriately according to their caloric requirements?, JPEN, Nov-Dec 1998; vol. 22, pp. 375–381.

References Indirect Calorimetry

1. Compher, C., et.al., Best Practice Methods to Apply to Measurement of Resting Metabolic Rate in Adults: A Systematic Review, J Am Diet Assoc, February 2006.

2. Schoeller, D., Making Indirect Calorimetry a Gold Standard for Predicting Energy Requirements for Institutionalized Patients, J Am Diet Assoc, March 2007.

3. Manual of Clinical Dietetics, 6th edition, 2000, p 31.

Protein Needs:

Another method of calculating protein needs is as a ratio of nonprotein calories to grams of nitrogen (6.25 g protein = 1 g N).

Patient Conditions	Ratio of Nonprotein kcal: 1 g N
Adult Medical	125–150:1
Minor Catabolic	125–180:1
Severe Catabolic	150–250:1
Hepatic or Renal Failure	250–400:1

Adult Fluid Requirements

Hydration status as a part of nutritional status is often overlooked. This can affect interpretation of biochemical measurements, anthropometry, and the physical exam. Assessment of hydration is quick and easy and should include assessment of fluid intake.

Method I:	Wt (kg) × 30 mL = Daily Fluid Requirement Fluid requirements may differ for those clients with cardiac problems, renal failure, dehydration, or for those requiring fluid restrictions

TABLE 7.4	Nutritional Needs and Assessment: Shortcut Method for Estimating Adult Energy Needs per Kilogram (*continued*)

	kcals Required
Method II:	100 mL/kg for first 10 kg body weight +50 mL/kg for second 10 kg body weight +15 mL/kg for remaining kg body weight
Shortcut Method II:	(kg body weight − 20) × 15 + 1500 = mL fluid requirement

Serum Osmolality

Osmolality measures the concentration of particles in solution. Osmolality increases with dehydration (loss of water without loss of solutes) and decreases with overhydration.

Greater than normal levels may indicate: dehydration, diabetes insipidus, hyperglycemia, hypernatremia, uremia.

Lower than normal levels may indicate: hyponatremia, overhydration, inappropriate ADH secretion.

Serum Osmolality = $(2 \times (Na + K)) + (BUN/2.8) + (glucose/18)$. Normal range is 285–295 mOsm/kg.

Factors That May Alter Fluid Requirements

The following may INCREASE fluid needs:

• Anabolism	• Diarrhea	• Hemorrhage	• Medications
• Burns	• Emesis	• Hot or dry environments	• Nasogastric Suctioning
• Constipation	• Fever[a]	• Hyperventilation	• Polyuria[b]
• Dehydration	• Fistulas/drains	• Hypotension	

[a]Fluid needs increase 7% for each °F above normal; 13% for each °C.
[b]Poor glucose control; excess alcohol, caffeine; osmotic diuresis.

The following may DECREASE fluid needs:

• Cardiac disease (especially CHF)

• Edema

• Fluid overload

• Hepatic failure with ascites

• Medications

• Renal failure

• SIADH

• Significant hypertension

• "Third spacing" of fluid

Adapted with permission from Pocket Resource for Nutrition Assessment, 2009 Edition. Dietetics in Health Care Communities, a dietetic practice group of the American Dietetic Association, pp. 22–24.

• Increased serum creatinine hematocrit, BUN, K⁺, CL⁻, osmolarity (sodium can be increased, normal, or decreased depending on the underlying cause of the dehydration)
• Decreased blood pressure
• Increased pulse
• Constipation (may be due to recent diarrhea)
• Concentrated urine

Daily body weight measurements can indicate large fluid losses or gains. For example, a weight loss of 2 kg in 48 hours indicates a corresponding loss of 2 L of fluid. Health-care providers should offer hydration more frequently to elderly patients whose sense of thirst is declining.

NUTRITION BASED ON WOUND ETIOLOGY

Pressure Ulcers

Refer to PU guidelines. As previously noted, nutrition plays a key role in the prevention and treatment of pressure ulcers. The 2009 NPUAP/EPUAP Pressure Ulcer Nutrition Prevention and Treatment Guidelines offer recommendations that are a resource for practitioners when developing nutrition interventions for individual patients (Table 7.5). The Guideline was developed following a systematic, comprehensive review of the peer-reviewed, published research on pressure ulcer treatment. The guidelines have a cumulative strength of evidence

TABLE 7.5	International Guideline Prevention and Treatment of Pressure Ulcers: Quick Reference Guide

International Guideline

Prevention and Treatment of Pressure Ulcers:

Quick reference Guide

Specific Recommendations: Nutrition Prevention

1. Offer high-protein mixed oral nutritional supplements and/or tube feeding, in addition to the usual diet, to individuals with nutritional risk and pressure ulcer risk because of acute or chronic diseases, or following surgical intervention. (Strength of Evidence = A.)

    1.1. Administer oral nutritional supplements (ONS) and/or tube feeding (TF) in between the regular meals to avoid reduction of normal food and fluid intake during regular mealtimes. (Strength of Evidence = C.)

Role of Nutrition in Pressure Ulcer Healing

1. Screen and assess nutritional status for each individual with a pressure ulcer at admission and with each condition change and/or when progress toward pressure ulcer closure is not observed. (Strength of Evidence = C.)

    1.1. Refer all individuals with a pressure ulcer to the dietitian for early assessment and intervention of nutritional problems. (Strength of Evidence = C.)

    1.2. Assess weight status for each individual to determine weight history and significant weight loss from usual body weight ($\geq$ 5% change in 30 d or $\geq$ 10% in 180 d). (Strength of Evidence = C.)

    1.3. Assess the individual's ability to eat independently. (Strength of Evidence = C.)

    1.4. Assess the adequacy of total nutrient intake (food, fluid, oral supplements, enteral/parenteral feedings). (Strength of Evidence = C.)

2. Provide sufficient calories. (Strength of Evidence = B.)

    2.1. Provide 30–35 kcal/kg body weight for individuals under stress with a pressure ulcer. Adjust formula based on weight loss, weight gain, or level of obesity. Individuals who are underweight or who have had significant unintentional weight loss may need additional kilocalories to cease weight loss and/or regain lost weight. (Strength of Evidence = C.)

    2.2. Revise and modify (liberalize) dietary restrictions when limitations result in decreased food and fluid intake. These adjustments are to be managed by a dietitian or medical professional. (Strength of Evidence = C.)

    2.3. Provide enhanced foods and/or oral supplements between meals if needed. (Strength of Evidence = B.)

    2.4. Consider nutritional support (enteral or parenteral nutrition) when oral intake is inadequate. This must be consistent with individual's goals. (Strength of Evidence = C.)

3. Provide adequate protein for positive nitrogen balance for an individual with a pressure ulcer. (Strength of Evidence = B.)

    3.1. Offer 1.25–1.5 g protein/kg body weight daily for an individual with a pressure ulcer when compatible with goals of care, and reassess as condition changes. (Strength of Evidence = C.)

    3.2. Assess renal function to ensure that high levels of protein are appropriate for the individual. (Strength of Evidence = C.)

4. Provide and encourage adequate daily fluid intake for hydration. (Level of Evidence = C.)

    4.1. Monitor individuals for signs and symptoms of dehydration: changes in weight, skin turgor, urine output, elevated serum sodium, or calculated serum osmolality. (Strength of Evidence = C.)

    4.2. Provide additional fluid for individuals with dehydration, elevated temperature, vomiting, profuse sweating, diarrhea, or heavily draining wounds. (Strength of Evidence = C.)

5. Provide adequate vitamins and minerals. (Strength of Evidence = B.)

    5.1. Encourage consumption of a balanced diet that includes good sources of vitamin and minerals. (Strength of Evidence = B.)

    5.2. Offer vitamin and mineral supplements when dietary intake is poor or deficiencies are confirmed or suspected. (Strength of Evidence = B.)

Adapted from European Pressure Ulcer Advisory Panel and National Pressure Ulcer Advisory Panel. *Prevention and Treatment or Pressure Ulcers: Quick Reference Guide.* Washington, DC: National Pressure Ulcer Advisory Panel; 2009, with permission.

Dehydration

Patients who are at risk of dehydration must be monitored carefully.

Watch for Warning Signs

The following are signs that an individual may be at risk for or suffering from dehydration:

- Drinks less than six cups of liquid daily
- Has one or more of the following: dry mouth cracked lips sunken eyes dark urine
- Needs help drinking from a cup or glass
- Has trouble swallowing liquids
- Has frequent vomiting, diarrhea, or fever
- Is easily confused/tired

Report and Take Action

Most individuals need at least six cups of liquid to stay hydrated. Below are some action steps to help residents get enough to drink:

- Report observations and warning signs to nurse and dietitian.
- Encourage the residents to drink every time you see him or her.
- Offer 2 to 4 oz of water or liquids frequently.
- Record fluid intake and output.
- Offer ice chips frequently (unless the patient has a swallowing problem).
- Check swallowing precautions; if appropriate, offer sips of liquid between bites of food at meals and snacks.
- Drink fluids with the residents, if allowed.
- Make sure pitcher and cup are near enough and light enough for the residents to lift.
- Offer the appropriate assistance, as needed, if the resident cannot drink without help.

Adapted with permission from the Nutrition Screening Initiative, a project of the American Academy of Family Physicians, the American Dietetic Association and the National Council on the Aging, Inc., funded in part by a grant from Ross Products Division, Abbott Laboratories Inc.

supporting each recommendation. The Clinical Practice Guideline (CPG) summarizes recommendations and supporting evidence for the guidelines. The Algorithm for Treatment of Pressure Ulcers: Nutrition Guideline (Fig. 7.3) offers suggestions for implementing the guidelines. The RD should use clinical judgment when applying any guideline, as the specific recommendation may not be appropriate in all circumstances.

Surgical Wounds

Acute surgical wounds result from operative procedures and typically progress in a timely fashion along the healing trajectory, with at least external manifestations of healing apparent early in the postoperative period. Key factors influencing healing include the systemic state of the client; nutritional status; presence of underlying medical conditions or malignancies; management of postoperative therapies such as wound care; and skin prep/type of suture material used.

Burns

Major burns result in severe trauma. In this state, energy requirements can increase as much as 100% above resting energy expenditure, depending on the extent and depth of the burn. This hypermetabolism is accompanied by exaggerated protein catabolism (i.e., breaking down of amino acids for energy) and increased urinary nitrogen excretion. Clients suffering from burns are in negative nitrogen balance because their bodies are using protein for energy (Fig. 7.4). Protein is also lost through the burn wound exudate. Metabolic needs are reduced slightly by the practice of covering wounds as early as possible to reduce evaporative and nitrogen losses and prevent infection.

Skin Tears

Lacerations resulting from falls, bumps, or shearing forces due to poor lifting technique are often found in the frail elderly. Their skin is less elastic, has limited subcutaneous fat stores, is more susceptible to medication reactions, and is prone to tearing away. A skin tear that shows only limited improvement in 7 to 14 days may require the initiation of more aggressive nutrition therapy, such as the addition of protein, calories, and fluid. The RD should assess the current diet for adequacy prior to initiating additional nutrients.

Leg Ulcers

Many chronic, nonhealing ulcers occur on the lower legs and feet, particularly those of vascular origin. Management of lower extremity ulcers is complex and is discussed in detail in Chapter 11. It is extremely important to provide support for possible alterations in life style (e.g., weight loss, proper diet, and smoking cessation).

Oral Candidiasis

The yeast-like fungus *Candida albicans* lives with the normal flora of the mouth, vaginal tract, and gut. In the adult, oral candidiasis occurs for several reasons. It may occur among diabetic clients with depressed cell-mediated immunity, the elderly, and those with cancer, particularly leukemia. Prolonged

Tips to Increase Fluids

- Hydration carts—offer fluids, such as juices, flavored water, or lemonade three times a day
- Popsicles
- Gelatin cubes
- Soups
- Sorbet/sherbet
- Ice cream
- Milk and milkshakes
- Ice chips
- Offer 4 oz of water between meals

Algorithm for Treatment of Pressure Ulcers: Nutrition Guidelines

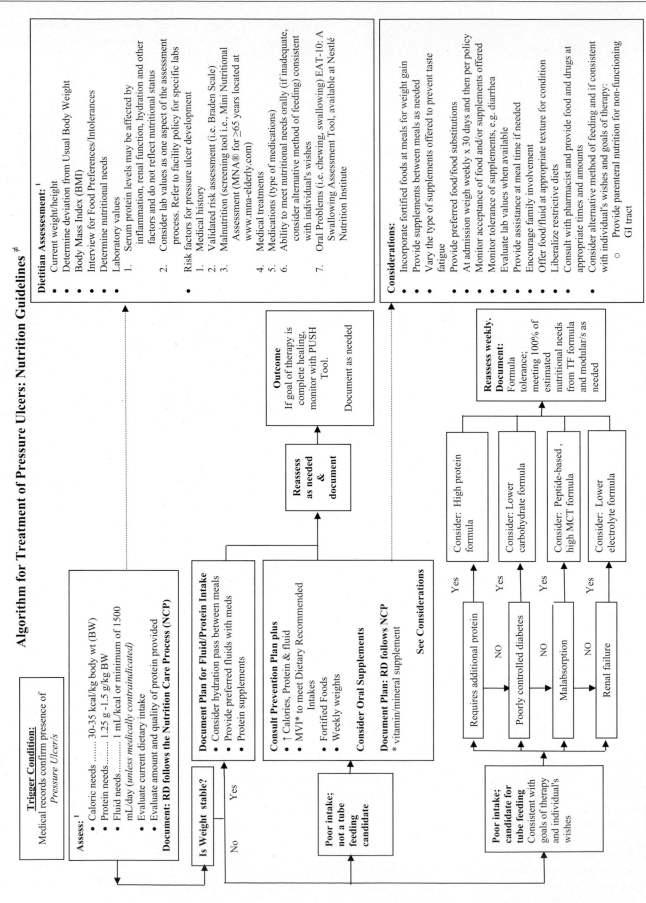

Dietitian Assessment: [1]

- Current weight/height
- Determine deviation from Usual Body Weight
- Body Mass Index (BMI)
- Interview for Food Preferences/Intolerances
- Determine nutritional needs
- Laboratory values

1. Serum protein levels may be affected by inflammation, renal function, hydration and other factors and do not reflect nutritional status
2. Consider lab values as one aspect of the assessment process. Refer to facility policy for specific labs

- Risk factors for pressure ulcer development

1. Medical history
2. Validated risk assessment (i.e. Braden Scale)
3. Malnutrition (screening tool i.e., Mini Nutritional Assessment (MNA® for ≥65 years located at www.mna-elderly.com)
4. Medical treatments
5. Medications (type of medications)
6. Ability to meet nutritional needs orally (if inadequate, consider alternative method of feeding) consistent with individual's wishes
7. Oral Problems (i.e. chewing, swallowing) EAT-10: A Swallowing Assessment Tool, available at Nestlé Nutrition Institute

Considerations:

- Incorporate fortified foods at meals for weight gain
- Provide supplements between meals as needed
- Vary the type of supplements offered to prevent taste fatigue
- Provide preferred food/food substitutions
- At admission weigh weekly x 30 days and then per policy
- Monitor acceptance of food and/or supplements offered
- Monitor tolerance of supplements, e.g. diarrhea
- Evaluate lab values when available
- Provide assistance at meal time if needed
- Encourage family involvement
- Offer food/fluid at appropriate texture for condition
- Liberalize restrictive diets
- Consult with pharmacist and provide food and drugs at appropriate times and amounts
- Consider alternative method of feeding and if consistent with individual's wishes and goals of therapy:
  - Provide parenteral nutrition for non-functioning GI tract

Trigger Condition:
Medical records confirm presence of *Pressure Ulcer/s*

Assess: [1]

- Caloric needs ...... 30-35 kcal/kg body wt (BW)
- Protein needs........ 1.25 g -1.5 g/kg BW
- Fluid needs........... 1 mL/kcal or minimum of 1500 mL/day (*unless medically contraindicated*)
- Evaluate current dietary intake
- Evaluate amount and quality of protein provided

Document: RD follows the Nutrition Care Process (NCP)

Is Weight stable?

No   Yes

Document Plan for Fluid/Protein Intake

- Consider hydration pass between meals
- Provide preferred fluids with meds
- Protein supplements

Consult Prevention Plan plus

- ↑ Calories, Protein & fluid
- MVI* to meet Dietary Recommended Intakes
- Fortified Foods
- Weekly weights

Consider Oral Supplements

Document Plan: RD follows NCP
* vitamin/mineral supplement

See Considerations

Poor intake; not a tube feeding candidate

Reassess as needed & document

Outcome
If goal of therapy is complete healing, monitor with PUSH Tool.

Document as needed

Poor intake; candidate for tube feeding
Consistent with goals of therapy and individual's wishes

Requires additional protein   Yes → Consider: High protein formula

NO

Poorly controlled diabetes   Yes → Consider: Lower carbohydrate formula

NO

Malabsorption   Yes → Consider: Peptide-based, high MCT formula

NO

Renal failure   Yes → Consider: Lower electrolyte formula

Reassess weekly.
Document:
Formula tolerance; meeting 100% of estimated nutritional needs from TF formula and modular/s as needed

FIGURE 7.3 Algorithm for treatment of pressure ulcers: nutritional guidelines.

© 2010 Nestlé. All rights reserved. [1] National Pressure Ulcer Advisory Panel and European Pressure Ulcer Advisory Panel. Prevention and treatment of pressure ulcers: clinical practice guideline. Washington DC: National Pressure Ulcer Advisory Panel; 2009. #These are general guidelines based on various clinical references and are not intended as a substitute for medical advice or existing facility guidelines. An individual assessment is recommended.

corticosteroid, immunosuppressive, and broad-spectrum anti-biotic therapy, as well as inhalant steroids, can also cause infection. Nutritional therapy includes.

NUTRITIONAL SUPPORT

The term nutritional support is commonly used to describe a variety of techniques available for use when patients are unable or unwilling to meet their nutrient needs by normal ingestion of food. The goal of nutritional support is to place the patient into positive nitrogen balance (i.e., the body maintains the same amount of protein in its tissues from day to day), in accordance with the goals of care and compatibility with the patient's and family's wishes.

The technique chosen for nutritional support can be quite simple. For example, in addition to the client's usual oral diet, a liquid nutritional supplement or high calorie pudding, or frozen dairy products can be provided between meals. The diet may include fortified foods such as cereal, mashed potatoes, or soups.

A more complex form of nutritional support is *enteral nutrition*, feeding by way of a tube placed into the gastrointestinal tract. Enteral feeding can be initiated when the ability to chew, swallow, and absorb nutrients through the normal gastrointestinal route is compromised by conditions such as stroke, Parkinson disease, cancer, and dysphagia, or when clients cannot meet their nutritional needs orally. Most enteral tube feeding formulas are nutritionally complete and designed for a specific purpose.

Even more invasive is total parenteral nutrition (TPN, which is a form of feeding that administers nutrients directly into the venous system, bypassing the GI tract). TPN is initiated when enteral feeding is contraindicated—for example, when the gastrointestinal tract is not functional—or when enteral feeding is insufficient to maintain nutritional status or has led to serious complications. The *Prevention of Pressure Ulcers Nutrition Decision Tree* (see Fig. 7.1) can be used to determine when enteral and parenteral feeding should be considered.

DOCUMENTATION OF MEDICAL NUTRITION THERAPY

Documentation of medical nutrition therapy in the medical record should include

- Amount or % of meals consumed. If applicable, type and amount (ounces) of supplements consumed
- Average fluid consumed daily (mL), related to amount required
- Ability to eat: assisted, supervised, or independent
- Acceptance or refusal of diet, meals, and/or supplements
- Current weight and percent gained or lost
- New conditions affecting nutritional status, such as introduction of thickened liquids or new diagnosis
- New medications affecting nutritional status
- Current laboratory findings (past 3 months)
- Condition and/or stage of wounds; for example, healing stage IV pressure ulcers
- Current calorie, protein, or fluid requirements
- Recommendation for new interventions if current treatment plan is not achieving the desired outcome

CONCLUSION

Undernutrition impedes healing of both chronic and acute wounds. Indeed, the development of a pressure ulcer or the failure of any type of wound to heal can be an indicator of undernutrition or poor nutritional status. Reduced food intake, unintended weight loss, hydration deficits, and the impaired ability to eat independently are known risk factors for pressure ulcer development, and unless these deficits are reversed, wound healing is delayed.[16,37,38]

Medical nutrition therapy can provide the means to meet these challenges. A diet that allows the client to enjoy favorite foods using oral nutrition supplements (if needed) or enteral and parenteral nutrition support can achieve optimal nutrition, thereby exerting a positive impact on wound healing.

CASE STUDY

Clinical Data

Mrs. T, 85 years old, has dementia and a nonhealing, draining stage IV pressure ulcer on her coccyx. She is 5′6″ and weighs 120 lb, having lost 10 lb (8%) in 30 days. The staff reports that she consumes only 50% of her 2 g sodium diet, or about 900 calories. Because she prefers liquids to solid food, most of these calories come from beverages; her protein intake averages only 16 to 20 g per day. Mrs. T is very distracted when she eats in the dining room with other patients.

One week later, neither Mrs. T's weight nor her pressure ulcer shows any sign of improvement. She has lost another 5 lb and continues to refuse meat or vegetables. Her body is clearly under stress and in a catabolic state. She requires increased

energy, in the form of carbohydrate calories to promote anabolism and preserve her lean body mass. In addition, she needs to consume additional sources of high-quality protein to advance the healing process. Unfortunately, the traditional intervention of enhancing her meals with fortified foods is failing to achieve a positive nitrogen balance because Mrs. T refuses to eat them.

1. Based on the NPUAP Nutrition Guidelines, how many calories should Mrs. T receive daily?
   a. 2010–2210 kcal
   b. 1568–1829 kcal
   c. 1640–1909 kcal
   d. 1772–2069 kcal
   Answer: b

CASE STUDY

2. Based on the NPUAP Nutrition Guidelines, how many grams of protein should Mrs. T receive daily?
   a. 65–79 g
   b. 80–89 g
   c. 75–86 g
   d. 79–104 g
   Answer: a.

3. Based on her current clinical condition, Mrs. T should receive
   a. 220 mg zinc sulfate bid
   b. 500 mg ascorbic acid bid
   c. Multivitamin/minerals q daily
   d. 50 mg elemental zinc
   Answer: c.

4. Mrs. T's current BMI is
   a. 19
   b. 21
   c. 24
   d. 18
   Answer: a

5. The current plan of action for Mrs. T should include
   a. Weekly prealbumin
   b. Request liberalized diet
   c. Initiate a tube feeding
   d. Weekly electrolytes
   Answer: b

6. Strategies should include
   a. Supplements with meals
   b. Two eggs per day
   c. Supplements between meals
   d. Six meals
   Answer: c

7. Minimum fluid requirements are
   a. 30 mL/kg/body wt
   b. 40 mL/kg/body wt
   c. 1 mL/kcal
   d. 2 mL/kcal
   Answer: c

8. The registered dietitian should
   a. Assess adequacy of total nutrient intake
   b. Reassess caloric requirements, if decline continues
   c. Recommend Mrs. T dine in a quiet area
   d. All of the above
   Answer: d

REVIEW QUESTIONS

1. Albumin levels are decreased with
   A. acute inflammation
   B. surgery
   C. infection
   D. all of the above
   E. both C and A

2. The Center for Medicare and Medicaid Services (CMS) defines significant weight loss as
   A. 7% in 60 days
   B. 5% in 30 days
   C. 3% in 14 days
   D. 10% in 180 days
   E. both B and D

3. A client who weighs 140 lb with a stage IV pressure ulcer has a protein requirement of
   A. 80–95 g of protein per day
   B. 64–74 g of protein per day
   C. 51–74 g of protein per day
   D. 76–86 g of protein per day
   E. 95–127 g of protein per day

4. Identify the factor(s) associated with the body's metabolic response to severe stress:
   A. Metabolic rate slows
   B. Conservation of energy per protein stores
   C. Protein is the prime source for glucose
   D. Accelerated loss of energy and protein stores
   E. Both C and D

REFERENCES

1. American Dietetic Association. *International Dietetics and Nutrition Terminology (IDNT) Reference Manual: Standardized Language for the Nutrition Care Process.* 2nd ed. Chicago, IL: The American Dietetic Association; 2009.
2. National Pressure Ulcer Advisory Panel and European Pressure Ulcer Advisory Panel. *Pressure Ulcer Prevention and Treatment: Clinical Practice Guideline.* Washington, DC: National Pressure Ulcer Advisory Panel; 2009.
3. Ferguson M, Capra S, Bauer J, et al. Development of a valid and reliable malnutrition screening tool for adult acute hospital patients. *Nutrition.* 1999;15:458–464.
4. Kruizenga HM, Seidell JC, de Vet HC, et al. Development and validation of a hospital screening tool for malnutrition: the short nutritional assessment questionnaire (SNAQ). *Clin Nutr.* 2005;24:75–82.
5. Kaiser MJ, et al. Validation of the Mini-Nutritional Assessment Short Form (MNA-SF): a practical Tool for identification of Nutritional Status. *JNHA.* 2009;13:782–788.

6. Woods, NF, LaCroix AZ, Gray SL, et al. Fraility: emergence and consequences in women aged 65 and older in the Women's Health Initiative Observational Study. *J Am Geriatr Soc.* 2005;53(8):1321–1330.

7. Schaberg DS, Norwood JM. Case study: infections in diabetes mellitus. *Diabetes Spectr.* 2002;15:37–40.

8. Maklebust J, Sieggreen M. *Pressure Ulcers: Guidelines for Prevention and Nursing Management.* 3rd ed. Springhouse, PA: Springhouse Corporation; 2001:356.

9. ASPEN Board of Directors and the Clinical Guidelines Task Force. Guidelines for the use of parenteral and enteral nutrition in adult and pediatric patients. *J Parenter Enteral Nutr.* 2002;26:22SA–24SA.

10. Nutrition Screening Initiative, a project of the American Academy of Family Physicians, ADA, and the National Council on the Aging, and funded in part by a grant from Ross Products Division, Abbott Laboratories, Inc. Washington, DC: Nutrition Screening Initiative; 1993:2.

11. Niedert K, Dorner B. *Nutrition Care of the Older Adult.* Chicago, IL: American Dietetics Association; 2004:125.

12. Maklebust J, Sieggreen M. *Pressure Ulcers: Guidelines for Prevention and Nursing Management.* 3rd ed. Springhouse, PA: Springhouse Corporation; 2001:37.

13. Dwyer JT. *Screening Older Americans' Nutritional Health: Current Practices and Future Possibilities.* Washington, DC: Nutrition Screening Initiative; 1991.

14. Thomas DR. Loss of skeletal muscle mass in aging: examining the relationship of starvation, sarcopenia and cachexia. *Clin Nutr.* 2007;26(4):389–399.

15. Report of the Dietary Guidelines Advisory Committee on Dietary Guidelines for Americans, 2000. Washighton DC: US Department of Agriculture, Agricultural Research Service; 2000:3.

16. Horn SD, Bender SA, Bergstrom N, et al. Description of the National Pressure Ulcer Long-Term Care Study. *J Am Geriatr Soc.* 2002;50:1816–1825.

17. MacIntosh C, Morley JE, Chapman IM. The anorexia of aging. *Nutrition.* 2000;16:983–995.

18. Position of the American Dietetic Association: Individualized Nutrition Approaches for Older Adults in Health Care Communities. *J Am Diet Ass.* 2010;110:1549–1553.

19. van Staveren W, de Groot C. Disturbance of the energy balance in elderly people: frequent cause of a insufficient diet, leading to frailty. *Nederlands Tijdschrift voor Geneeskunde.* 1998;142:2400–2404.

20. Myron Johnson A, Merlini G, Sheldon J, et al. Clinical indications for plasma protein assays: transthyretin (prealbumin) in inflammation and malnutrition. *Clin Chem Lab Med CCLM/FESCC.* 2007;45(3):419–426.

21. Litchford MD. *Practical Applications in Laboratory Assessment of Nutritional Status.* Greensboro, NC: Case Software; 2010.

22. Albina JE, Mills CD, Barbul A. Arginine metabolism in wounds. *Am J Physiol.* 1988;254:E459–E467.

23. Kirk JS, Barbul A. Role of arginine in trauma, sepsis, immunity. *J Parenter Enteral Nutr.* 1990;14:226S–229S.

24. Lee SK, Posthauer ME, Dorner B, et al. Pressure ulcer healing with a concentrated, fortified, collagen protein hydrolysate supplement: a randomized controlled trial. *Adv Skin Wound Care* 2006;19(2):92–96.

25. Pompeo M. Misconceptions about protein requirements for wound healing: results of a prospective study. *Ostomy/Wound Manage.* 2007;53(8):30.

26. Clinical practice guidelines for nutrition in chronic renal failure. K/DOQI, National Kidney Foundation. *Am J Kidney Dis.* 2000;35 (6 suppl 2):S1–S140.

27. Nissen S, Aumbrad N. Nutritional role of leucine metabolite β-hydroxy-β-methylbutyrate (HMB). *J Nutr Biochem.* 1997;8:300–311.

28. Langer G, Schloemer G, Knerr A, et al. Nutritional interventions for preventing and treating pressure ulcers. *Cochrane Database Syst Rev.* 2007;1.

29. Institute of Medicine. *National Academy of Sciences (NAS): Dietary Reference Intakes: The Essential Guide to Nutrient Requirements.* Washington, DC: National Academies Press; 2006.

30. Ronchetti IP, Quaglino D, Bergamini G. *Ascorbic Acid and Connective Tissue. Subcellular Biochemistry, Volume 25: Ascorbic Acid: Biochemistry and Biomedical Cell Biology.* New York, NY: Plenum Press; 1996.

31. Vilter RW. Nutritional aspects of ascorbic acid: uses and abuses. *West J Med.* 1980;133:485–492.

32. ter Riet G, Kessels AG, Knipschild PG. Randomized clinical trial of ascorbic acid in the treatment of pressure ulcers. *J Clin Epidemiol.* 1995;48(12):1453–1460.

33. Stephens P, Thomas D. The cellular proliferate phase of the wound repair process. *J Wound Care.* 2002;11:253–261.

34. Reed BR, Clark RA. Cutaneous tissue repair: practical implications of current knowledge. II. *J Amer Acad Dermatol.* 1985;13:919–941.

35. Thomas DR. The role of nutrition in prevention and healing of pressure ulcers. *Clin Geriatr Med.* 1997;13:497–511.

36. Position of the American Dietetic Association: Older Adults in Health Care Communities Benefit form Less Restrictive Diets. *J Am Diet Ass.* 2010 (in publication)

37. Gilmore SA, Robinson G, Posthauer ME, et al. Clinical indicators associated with unintentional weight loss and pressure ulcers in elderly residents of nursing facilities. *J Am Diet Assoc.* 1995;95(9):984–992.

38. Lyder C, Yu C, Stevenson D, et al. Validating the Braden Scale for the prediction of pressure ulcer risk in blacks and Latino/Hispanic elders: a pilot study. *Ostomy Wound Manage.* 1998;44(suppl 3A): 42S–49S.

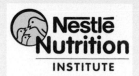

Mini Nutritional Assessment
MNA®

Last name:		First name:		
Sex:	Age:	Weight, kg:	Height, cm:	Date:

Complete the screen by filling in the boxes with the appropriate numbers. Add the numbers for the screen. If score is 11 or less, continue with the assessment to gain a Malnutrition Indicator Score.

Screening

A Has food intake declined over the past 3 months due to loss of appetite, digestive problems, chewing or swallowing difficulties?
0 = severe decrease in food intake
1 = moderate decrease in food intake
2 = no decrease in food intake ☐

B Weight loss during the last 3 months
0 = weight loss greater than 3kg (6.6lbs)
1 = does not know
2 = weight loss between 1 and 3kg (2.2 and 6.6 lbs)
3 = no weight loss ☐

C Mobility
0 = bed or chair bound
1 = able to get out of bed / chair but does not go out
2 = goes out ☐

D Has suffered psychological stress or acute disease in the past 3 months?
0 = yes   2 = no ☐

E Neuropsychological problems
0 = severe dementia or depression
1 = mild dementia
2 = no psychological problems ☐

F Body Mass Index (BMI) (weight in kg) / (height in m²)
0 = BMI less than 19
1 = BMI 19 to less than 21
2 = BMI 21 to less than 23
3 = BMI 23 or greater ☐

Screening score
(subtotal max. 14 points) ☐☐

12 points or greater: Normal – not at risk – no need to complete assessment

11 points or below: Possible malnutrition – continue assessment

Assessment

G Lives independently (not in nursing home or hospital)
1 = yes   0 = no ☐

H Takes more than 3 prescription drugs per day
0 = yes   1 = no ☐

I Pressure sores or skin ulcers
0 = yes   1 = no ☐

J How many full meals does the patient eat daily?
0 = 1 meal
1 = 2 meals
2 = 3 meals ☐

K Selected consumption markers for protein intake
• At least one serving of dairy products (milk, cheese, yoghurt) per day   yes ☐   no ☐
• Two or more servings of legumes or eggs per week   yes ☐   no ☐
• Meat, fish or poultry every day   yes ☐   no ☐
0.0 = if 0 or 1 yes
0.5 = if 2 yes
1.0 = if 3 yes ☐.☐

L Consumes two or more servings of fruit or vegetables per day?
0 = no   1 = yes ☐

M How much fluid (water, juice, coffee, tea, milk...) is consumed per day?
0.0 = less than 3 cups
0.5 = 3 to 5 cups
1.0 = more than 5 cups ☐.☐

N Mode of feeding
0 = unable to eat without assistance
1 = self-fed with some difficulty
2 = self-fed without any problem ☐

O Self view of nutritional status
0 = views self as being malnourished
1 = is uncertain of nutritional state
2 = views self as having no nutritional problem ☐

P In comparison with other people of the same age, how does the patient consider his / her health status?
0.0 = not as good
0.5 = does not know
1.0 = as good
2.0 = better ☐.☐

Q Mid-arm circumference (MAC) in cm
0.0 = MAC less than 21
0.5 = MAC 21 to 22
1.0 = MAC 22 or greater ☐.☐

R Calf circumference (CC) in cm
0 = CC less than 31
1 = CC 31 or greater ☐

Assessment (max. 16 points) ☐☐.☐

Screening score ☐☐.☐

Total Assessment (max. 30 points) ☐☐.☐

Malnutrition Indicator Score

17 to 23.5 points   ☐   at risk of malnutrition

Less than 17 points   ☐   malnourished

Ref.   Vellas B, Villars H, Abellan G, et al. *Overview of MNA® - Its History and Challenges.* J Nut Health Aging 2006; 10: 456-465.
Rubenstein LZ, Harker JO, Salva A, Guigoz Y, Vellas B. Screening for Undernutrition in Geriatric Practice: *Developing the Short-Form Mini Nutritional Assessment (MNA-SF).* J. Geront 2001; 56A: M366-377.
Guigoz Y. The Mini-Nutritional Assessment (MNA®) *Review of the Literature – What does it tell us?* J Nutr Health Aging 2006; 10: 466-487.
® Société des Produits Nestlé, S.A., Vevey, Switzerland, Trademark Owners
© Nestlé, 1994, Revision 2006. N67200 12/99 10M
For more information: www.mna-elderly.com

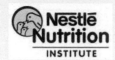

Mini Nutritional Assessment
MNA®

Last name:		First name:		
Sex:	Age:	Weight, kg:	Height, cm:	Date:

Complete the screen by filling in the boxes with the appropriate numbers. Total the numbers for the final screening score.

Screening

A Has food intake declined over the past 3 months due to loss of appetite, digestive problems, chewing or swallowing difficulties?
0 = severe decrease in food intake
1 = moderate decrease in food intake
2 = no decrease in food intake ☐

B Weight loss during the last 3 months
0 = weight loss greater than 3 kg (6.6 lbs)
1 = does not know
2 = weight loss between 1 and 3 kg (2.2 and 6.6 lbs)
3 = no weight loss ☐

C Mobility
0 = bed or chair bound
1 = able to get out of bed / chair but does not go out
2 = goes out ☐

D Has suffered psychological stress or acute disease in the past 3 months?
0 = yes   2 = no ☐

E Neuropsychological problems
0 = severe dementia or depression
1 = mild dementia
2 = no psychological problems ☐

F1 Body Mass Index (BMI) (weight in kg) / (height in m²)
0 = BMI less than 19
1 = BMI 19 to less than 21
2 = BMI 21 to less than 23
3 = BMI 23 or greater ☐

IF BMI IS NOT AVAILABLE, REPLACE QUESTION F1 WITH QUESTION F2.
DO NOT ANSWER QUESTION F2 IF QUESTION F1 IS ALREADY COMPLETED.

F2 Calf circumference (CC) in cm
0 = CC less than 31
3 = CC 31 or greater ☐

Screening score ☐☐
(max. 14 points)

12-14 points: Normal nutritional status
8-11 points: At risk of malnutrition
0-7 points: Malnourished

For a more in-depth assessment, complete the full MNA® which is available at **www.mna-elderly.com**

Ref.   Vellas B, Villars H, Abellan G, et al. *Overview of the MNA® - Its History and Challenges.* J Nutr Health Aging 2006;10:456-465.
Rubenstein LZ, Harker JO, Salva A, Guigoz Y, Vellas B. *Screening for Undernutrition in Geriatric Practice: Developing the Short-Form Mini Nutritional Assessment (MNA-SF).* J. Geront 2001;56A: M366-377.
Guigoz Y. *The Mini-Nutritional Assessment (MNA®) Review of the Literature - What does it tell us?* J Nutr Health Aging 2006; 10:466-487.
® Société des Produits Nestlé, S.A., Vevey, Switzerland, Trademark Owners
© Nestlé, 1994, Revision 2009. N67200 12/99 10M
For more information: www.mna-elderly.com

Medical Nutrition Therapy Quarterly/MDS Progress Note

MEDICAL NUTRITION THERAPY QUARTERLY / MDS PROGRESS NOTE (MR#_____)

NAME:_____ GENDER: ❑ M ❑ F

TARGET WEIGHT _____ lb HEIGHT:_____ AGE:_____ years

1ST QUARTER			2ND QUARTER	3RD QUARTER
DIET ORDER:			Changed ❑ Y ❑ N	Changed ❑ Y ❑ N
SUPPLEMENT:			Changed ❑ Y ❑ N	Changed ❑ Y ❑ N
FORTIFIED FOODS:			Changed ❑ Y ❑ N	Changed ❑ Y ❑ N
TUBE FEEDING FLUSH			Changed ❑ Y ❑ N	Changed ❑ Y ❑ N
FOOD/FLUIDS % Intake	_____ B _____ L _____ S	_____ HS _____ Fluids _____ Supplement	____B ____HS ____L ____Fluids ____S ____Supp	____B ____HS ____L ____Fluids ____S ____Supp
FEEDING ABILITY	❑ Dependent ❑ Limited Assist ❑ Self-Help Devices	❑ Independent ❑ Set-up Only ❑ Type_____	Changed ❑ Y ❑ N	Changed ❑ Y ❑ N
ORAL STATUS	❑ Normal ❑ Requires modification to swallow solid foods and liquids, puree and thickened liquids ❑ Combined Oral and Tube Feeding ❑ No Oral Intake	❑ Mechanical Soft	Changed ❑ Y ❑ N	Changed ❑ Y ❑ N
MEAL LOCATION	❑ DR ❑ Restorative DR	❑ Room ❑ Other_____	Changed ❑ Y ❑ N	Changed ❑ Y ❑ N
COGNITIVE STATUS	❑ Alert/Oriented ❑ Cog. Impaired ❑ Combative ❑ Comatose	❑ Depressed ❑ Disoriented / Confused ❑ Wanders ❑ Other _____	Changed ❑ Y ❑ N	Changed ❑ Y ❑ N
CURRENT WEIGHT: _____ LBS ____% Change ❑ 30 days ❑ 90 days ❑ 180 days			____Wt ____% change ❑ 30 ❑ 90 ❑ 180	____Wt ____% change ❑ 30 ❑ 90 ❑ 180
PLANNED WEIGHT CHANGE: ❑ Yes ❑ No			❑ Yes ❑ No	❑ Yes ❑ No
CALORIC / HYDRATION REQUIREMENT:	_____ Calories _____ Protein _____ Fluid		Changed ❑ Y ❑ N	Changed ❑ Y ❑ N
SKIN CONDITION	❑ Intact ❑ Edema ❑ Surgical Wounds ❑ Open Lesion/Infections _____	❑ Burns 2nd/3rd degree ❑ Reddened Areas ❑ Other: _____	❑ Intact ❑ Burns 2nd/ 3rd degree ❑ Edema ❑ Reddened Areas ❑ Surgical Wounds ❑ Open Lesion/Infections ❑ Other:_____	❑ Intact ❑ Burns 2nd/ 3rd degree ❑ Edema ❑ Reddened Areas ❑ Surgical Wounds ❑ Open Lesion/Infections ❑ Other:_____
PRESSURE ULCER(S) ❑ YES ❑ NO STAGE: 1 2 3 4 LOCATION:_____ SIZE:_____			❑ YES ❑ NO STAGE: 1 2 3 4 LOCATION:_____ SIZE:_____	❑ YES ❑ NO STAGE: 1 2 3 4 LOCATION:_____ SIZE:_____
MEDICATIONS: Note new medications since last review				

Source: Mary Ellen Posthauer, RD,LD,CD

Monthly Medical Nutrition Therapy Tube Feeding Progress Note

Monthly Medical Nutrition Therapy Tube Feeding Progress Note F–74 (11/00)		
NAME:_____	GENDER: ❑ M ❑ F	
TARGET WEIGHT_____lb	HEIGHT:_____	AGE:_____years
Date:_____	Date:_____	Date:_____
TUBE FEEDING ORDER:	Changed Yes/No	Changed Yes/No
FLUSH:	Changed Yes/No	Changed Yes/No
FORMULA PROVIDES: Calories:_____ Free H2O:_____ Protein:_____ Flush:_____ Total Water:_____	Changed Yes/No Changed Yes/No	Changed Yes/No Changed Yes/No
DIET:_____ PUMP:_____ NPO:_____ BOLUS:_____	Changed Yes/No	Changed Yes/No
TOTAL CALORIES PER TUBE: ❑ 1%–25% ❑ 51%–75% ❑ 26%–50% ❑ 76%–100%		
NUTRIENT NEEDS: BEE_____ Activity Factor_____ Injury Factor_____ Total Calories_____ Protein_____g/kg Total Protein_____g Fluid_____cc/kg Total Fluids_____mL	Changed Yes/No	Changed Yes/No
SIGNIFICANT LAB VALUES: LABS	LABS	
WEIGHT:		
CURRENT WEIGHT:_____ % CHANGE:_____ ❑ Intact	Weight:_____ % Change:____ ❑ Intact	Weight:_____ % Change:____
SKIN CONDITION: ❑ Edema ❑ Intact ❑ Open Lesion/Infections ❑ Edema _____ ❑ Reddened Areas ❑ Pressure Ulcer Stage:_____	❑ Edema ❑ Red Areas ❑ Open Lesion/Infections ❑ PU Stage:____	❑ Red Areas ❑ Open Lesion/Infections ❑ PU Stage:_____
RECOMMENDATIONS: RD SIGNATURE: _____ _____ _____		

Mary EllenPosthauer, RD,CD,LD

Management by Wound Etiology

Barbara M. Bates-Jensen

Determining the etiology of a wound is a critical task in creating a comprehensive treatment plan for patients with wounds. Expanding your knowledge of wound etiology will empower you to provide quality comprehensive care in clinical practice. The chapters in Part II focus on management by wound etiology with specific information on acute surgical wounds, pressure ulcers, vascular ulcers, and neuropathic ulcers. In these chapters, we'll discuss the pathophysiology involved in the wound type, assessment methods, and prevention and management of specific wound types.

Chapter 8 presents management of the acute surgical wound. Chapters 9 and 10 describe issues related to the pathophysiology, detection, and prevention, of pressure ulcers. Chapter 11 provides an in-depth analysis of the diagnosis and management of vascular ulcers. Chapters 12 and 13 continue the examination of lower extremities with a focus on the neuropathic foot and management of common foot problems, including those involving the skin and nails of the foot.

Chapter 14 describes management of malignant wounds and fistulas, which are often complex and difficult to manage. Palliative care and the role of wound care clinicians when faced with wounds with little or no healing potential are emphasized in this chapter. Finally, Chapter 15—which is new to this edition—discusses management of burn wounds.

Although similarities exist in the treatment of any wound, the treatment approach varies depending on wound etiology. The chapters in Part II form a foundation of knowledge that should provide you with a more individualized and more effective approach to caring for the patient with a wound.

Management of Acute Surgical Wounds

Barbara M. Bates-Jensen and John Williams

CHAPTER OBJECTIVES

At the completion of this chapter, the reader will be able to:

1. Discuss factors affecting healing of acute surgical wounds.
2. Describe assessment and management of the acute surgical wound, including care of the surgical dressing.
3. Identify circumstances in which a surgical wound may be left to heal by secondary or tertiary intention.
4. Discuss outcome measures for acute surgical wounds during the preoperative, intraoperative, and postoperative periods.
5. Identify referral criteria for patients with surgical wounds.

As you learned in Chapter 2, acute wounds are disruptions in the integrity of the skin and underlying tissues that progress through the healing process in a timely and uneventful manner. The acute surgical wound is an example of a healthy wound in which healing can be maximized. However, not all surgical wounds are uncomplicated. Acute surgical wounds can occur in unhealthy tissues, in a compromised host, or as a result of unexpected or significant trauma.

Surgical wounds are most commonly allowed to heal by **primary intention**. Wounds that heal by primary intention are wounds with edges that are approximated and closed as shown in Figure 8.1. The acute surgical incision wound healing by primary intention is the focus of this chapter; however, we also discuss special situations requiring healing by secondary (see Fig. 8.2A–D) and tertiary intention later in this chapter. Table 8.1 provides definitions of the three types of acute wound healing. A surgical incision healing by primary intention could be described as the ideal wound for healing. The wound is controlled with attention to tissue handling and proper use of surgical instruments by the surgeon, and the wound edges are apposed and aligned immediately to decrease the risk of infection. In general, such a wound should complete the proliferative phase of wound healing in 4 weeks; that is, the incision line should have filled with granulation tissue and be resurfaced with epithelial tissue. Acute surgical wounds that progress at a slower pace or fail to progress can be considered chronic.

FACTORS AFFECTING HEALING IN ACUTE WOUNDS

Healing in acute surgical wounds involves the interaction of extrinsic and intrinsic factors. Extrinsic factors relate to those agents outside the person, whereas intrinsic factors are those influencing the person internally or systemically.

Extrinsic Factors

The physical environment before and during surgery, surgical preparation, surgical techniques, and types of sutures are all examples of extrinsic factors that can affect acute wound healing. Thus, for the surgical wound, evaluation of the perioperative period is important, because it plays a role in the wound outcome. Wound infection is the major cause of surgical wounds failing to progress through the healing process in a timely and uneventful manner and can be caused by extrinsic factors. Surgical site infections (SSIs) both greatly increase a patient's length of stay and costs and contribute to morbidity and mortality.[1,2] An estimated 2.6% of nearly 30 million operations are complicated by SSIs each year.[2] Organizations such as the Institute of Medicine and the Institute for Healthcare Improvement have pushed for patient safety to be a higher priority for health-care personnel, and preventing SSIs is a facet of this undertaking. SSIs are caused by either external (from the operating room environment or personnel) or internal (from the patient's own body) microbial contamination. Operating

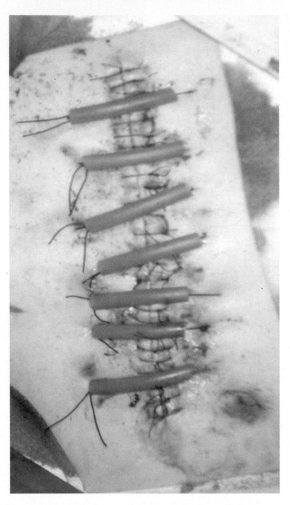

FIGURE 8.1 Surgical incision healing by primary intention. Wound edges are well approximated and closure materials remain in place. (Courtesy of Dr. M.A. Treadwell, Eastland, Texas.)

TABLE 8.1	Types of Surgical Wound Healing
Wound Healing Type	**Definition**
Primary intention	Wound edges approximated and closed at time of surgery
Secondary intention	Wound left open after surgery and allowed to heal with scar tissue replacing the tissue defect
Tertiary or delayed primary closure	After surgery, wound left open initially and after short period of time, wound edges are approximated and wound is closed

Preoperative Period

The length of time a patient spends in the hospital prior to surgery influences the rate of surgical wound infection. As the length of the hospital stay increases prior to surgery, the risk of wound infection increases, though length of stay is more likely a surrogate for disease severity and comorbidities.[2,3] Preparation of the operative site also influences the risk of wound infection. The use of a systematic approach for preoperative skin preparation can decrease SSI rates by sustaining a greater and longer preparation time.[3] Although showering with a hexachlorophene or 4% chlorhexidine gluconate prior to surgery is common practice, there is limited evidence showing any benefit of showering or bathing with chlorhexidine over bar soap or other products in reducing SSIs.[1,4,5] Further, there are mixed findings comparing bathing with chlorhexidine with no preoperative washing.[5]

Shaving the operative area and the method used to shave the area have also been implicated in surgical wound infection,[6] because shaving causes skin aberrations that can become infected by proliferating microorganisms.[7]

Preoperative prophylactic antibiotic administration is more strongly supported for most surgeries and is specifically recommended for clean surgery, when a prosthetic or implant is placed, clean-contaminated, and contaminated surgery

room protocols, attention to instrumentation, and appropriate surgical technique are all means of decreasing the risk of infection and ensuring optimal healing from the outset for the surgical wound.

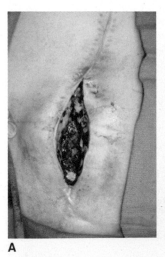
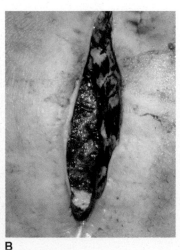
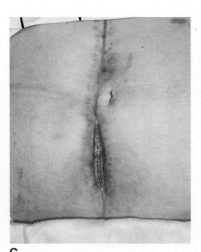
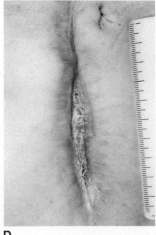

A   B   C   D

FIGURE 8.2 Surgical incision healing by secondary intention. **A:** Wound has been left open after surgery with a tissue cavity that must be filled with scar tissue (granulation tissue). **B:** Wound appearance postoperatively. **C,D:** Wound 8 weeks later showing complete closure and wound resurfaced with epithelium. (Courtesy of Dr. M.A. Treadwell, Eastland, Texas.)

RESEARCH WISDOM

Operative Site Preparation

Body hair is regularly removed prior to surgery, but there is insufficient evidence to suggest that this practice reduces SSI rates and hair should only be removed if it will interfere with the procedure.[7] Use of depilatory creams, electric razors, or clippers is associated with reduced wound infection rates when compared with the use of nonelectric razors to shave the operative area. It is still unclear whether it is best to remove hair on the day of surgery or the day prior.[7]

(see Table 8.2).[1,6,8,9] When indicated, prophylactic antimicrobial agents have been found to effectively reduce SSIs.[10] Antibiotics should be administered by an intravenous route and timed in such a manner that therapeutic concentrations of the drug are perfused to the tissues by the time the incision is made.[9] This means that most antibiotics should be given within 1 hour of surgery and intraoperatively when anesthesia is administered to ensure that the drug is present in the tissue until after the incision is closed.[8,9,11] If possible, all infection remote to the surgical site should be treated prior to elective surgery.

Intraoperative Period

Limiting the infection rate intraoperatively is largely under the control of the surgeon. Sometimes, infection control is difficult to achieve. For example, the surgeon has limited power over the nature of the problem for which the surgery is performed, the operative site, and the general condition of the patient; all are complex factors that are not easily controlled. The type of surgical procedure also influences the risk of infection.[12] Table 8.2 shows the classification of surgical procedures according to the risk of infection.[13]

The National Nosocomial Infections Surveillance (NNIS) System Basic Surgical Site Infections (SSI) Risk Index is another method for determining the risk of infection.[14] The NNIS system scores surgical procedures by including the American Society of Anesthesiologists (ASA) classification perioperatively, whether the procedure is contaminated or dirty infected, and the duration of the surgical procedure. The NNIS Basic SSI Index is a multivariate index for wound classification that compensates for the limitation of the traditional wound classification system, which does not take into account a patient's intrinsic risk of developing a surgical wound infection.[14]

In addition to the degree of wound classification and ASA score, the duration of the surgical procedure has been found to be independently associated with surgical wound infections.[6] Strict adherence by operating room personnel to an infection control protocol has also resulted in decreased wound infection rates.[15] Data comparing use of hand antisepsis using alcohol scrubs with additional active ingredients to aqueous scrubs (such as povidone iodine and chlorhexidine) by surgical personnel to reduce SSIs have shown mixed findings, although aqueous scrubs with chlorhexidine were more effective in reducing the amount of bacteria on the hands compared to aqueous scrubs with povidone iodine.[16]

Other factors such as obesity or increased tension on the surgical incision site and specific comorbidities have also demonstrated increased risk for surgical wound infection. Some degree of mechanical stress on tissue during surgery is inevitable; however, excess trauma from this stress can lead to a prolonged inflammatory phase of healing, decreased tensile strength, and increased risk of infection. Surgeons must be concerned with wound tension, vascular supply, and proper surgical technique. If the wound cannot be closed without a significant amount of tension or if the vascular supply is poor, there is increased risk of dehiscence, necrosis, and infection.[9,10]

TABLE 8.2	Surgical Wound Classifications		
Wound Classification	**Surgical Label**	**Definition**	**Procedure Type**
I	Clean	• Nontraumatic injuries • No inflammation found during procedure • No break in sterile technique	• Exploratory laparotomy • Mastectomy • Total hip replacement • Vascular surgeries
II	Clean-contaminated	• Procedures involving GI or respiratory tract • No significant contamination	• Bronchoscopy • Small bowel resection • Whipple pancreaticoduodenectomy
III	Contaminated	• Major break in sterile technique • Gross spillage from GI tract	• Appendectomy for inflamed appendicitis • Bile spillage during cholecystectomy • Diverticulitis
IV	Dirty or infected	• Acute bacterial inflammation found • Pus encountered • Devitalized tissue encountered	• Excision and drainage of abscess • Perforated bowel • Peritonitis

RESEARCH WISDOM

Operation Environment

Traffic in and out of the operating room should be minimized in order to reduce the microbial level of the air and the room should be at a positive pressure relative to surrounding areas. Operating room doors should be kept closed except as needed for passage of personnel, equipment, and the patient.[8]

For example, Australian investigators developed a preoperative scoring system to better predict sternal SSIs as a result of coronary artery bypass graft (CABG) surgical procedures that incorporates obesity as a risk factor. The Australian Clinical Risk Index assigns 1 point for diabetes mellitus, 1 point for body mass index (BMI) of 30 or greater but less than 35, and 2 points for BMI of greater than 35. Each point in the scoring system represents approximately a doubling of risk for infection.[17] The Australian Clinical Risk Index performed better than the NNIS system in predicting risk for SSI and can stratify patients into discrete groups associated with increased risk of SSIs.[18] There are several methods to predict risk for SSI.

Methods of reducing infection risk and optimizing wound healing outcomes include attention to suturing technique. Use of buried sutures and primary layered anatomic closure can improve primary wound healing by decreasing the potential for hematoma formation in dead space under the incision, giving tensile support in the first 2 to 4 months while the wound is still weak, and decreasing tension on the apposed wound edges.[9,19] Surface sutures can negatively impact optimal healing because they provide additional "wounds" to heal alongside the incision. In some cases, tissue adhesives may be used to close wounds. In general, there are no differences between use of tissue adhesives and sutures for most outcomes. Some evidence exists that wounds breakdown more frequently when stitches/sutures are used compared to tissue adhesives, and tissue adhesives are more time-consuming to use than other methods.[20]

Postoperative Period

The stress response associated with surgery can impair wound healing.[21] The stress of surgery stimulates the sympathetic nervous system, with a resultant sympathetic nervous system–mediated vasoconstriction. High levels of circulating catecholamines in the immediate postoperative period cause vasoconstriction, with factors that trigger the sympathetic nervous system, including hypoxia, hypothermia, pain, and hypovolemia.[21,22] Measures of subcutaneous tissue wound oxygenation are lower after extensive, more complex surgical procedures.[22] Attempts to restore tissue and wound oxygen deficits minimize the risks of hypothermia, pain, hypovolemia, and hypoxia simultaneously in the immediate postoperative period.

Fluid replacement occurs simultaneously with rewarming efforts. Correcting hypovolemia with adequate fluid infusion prevents the continuing vasoconstriction caused by hypovolemia. Administration of supplemental intravenous fluids until hemodynamic balance is reached is beneficial.

CLINICAL WISDOM

Maximizing Wound Healing

Critical measures to maximize wound healing in the immediate postoperative period include keeping the patient

- Warm
- Well hydrated, intravenously or orally
- Pain free by use of patient-controlled analgesia, if possible
- Well oxygenated by use of supplemental oxygen, if needed

Thermoregulatory responses are diminished in surgical patients because of their prolonged exposure to the cold operating room environment. Patients treated with active rewarming by use of heated blankets during the recovery period experience a faster return of normal tissue and wound oxygen levels than do those allowed to return to normothermia without rewarming interventions.[22] The routine use of measures to actively warm the patient during the surgical procedure, such as warming blankets and warmed intravenous fluids, along with active monitoring, also helps to prevent thermoregulatory problems.[8,9] It is easier to prevent thermoregulatory problems than to remedy them. Normothermia and absence of hypoxia increase tissue perfusion that assists in wound healing and prevention of SSIs.[9]

Providing adequate oxygenation to the tissues may require supplemental oxygen for the patient. Patients should be given sufficient oxygen during major surgery and in the recovery period to ensure that a hemoglobin saturation of more than 95% is maintained.[8] As pain increases the stress response and causes vasoconstriction, management of pain is recommended to ensure optimal wound healing.[15,21,22]

Intrinsic Factors

Intrinsic factors that affect healing of the acute surgical wound are those that influence the patient systemically. Intrinsic factors include age, concurrent conditions, nutritional status, and oxygenation and tissue perfusion.

Age

The physiologic changes that occur with aging place the older individual at higher risk for poor wound healing outcomes.[9,23–25] The healing process for older adults proceeds more slowly and this population is more likely to present with comorbidities.[9] Aging causes skin changes, including decreased elastin in the skin with thinning of the dermoepidermal junction and decreased collagen and elastin content of the skin.[25] Cellular senescence occur as well. Cellular senescence is the decline in the ability of cells to multiply and divide and this is most evident when the skin of an elder is challenged with wound healing.[25] Neutrophils and macrophages demonstrate decreased growth factor production, migration, and phagocytosis. Growth factors are less responsive, and their amounts are decreased.[26] A decreased rate of migration by keratinocytes affects the rate of wound healing and, in particular, reepithelialization of the skin.[26] Finally, older adults demonstrate decreased ability to replace collagen after abdominal surgery.[27]

CLINICAL WISDOM

Risk of Delayed Wound Resurfacing in the Older Adult

Delays in wound resurfacing put older patients at risk for wound infection. Daily wound assessments and use of topical dressings for protection may be required for a longer period of time than is necessary for younger patients. However in healthy older patients, clinicians can expect the final outcome to be consistent with that of younger individuals despite the age-related changes in older adults.[23,24]

Several aging-related changes have been shown to be reversible. For example, estrogen hormone replacement therapy can increase healing capacity in wounds with normal older adults.[28] Some have suggested that estrogen alone is the major regulator of delayed wound healing in elders.[29] Much of the delayed healing response in elders has been attributed to an inappropriately prolonged and excessive inflammatory response, and research has demonstrated that the decline in sex steroid hormones with aging may play a major role on the inflammatory response. Further, topical and systemic estrogen and progesterone treatments have shown an increased rate of healing by reducing inflammation and stimulating matrix deposition and reepithelialization.[30,31]

The normal decline in immune system function with age may account for the increased risk of infection in older adults. The diminished immune response allows microorganisms to proliferate in the wound before they can be removed. Older adults may also present with chronic diseases, circulatory changes, and nutritional problems, all of which increase the risk for poor or delayed wound healing. Decreased motor coordination and diminished sensory function increase the potential for injury, wound complications, and repeated wounding at the same site.[23]

Concurrent Conditions

The presence of certain diseases, conditions, and treatments can influence surgical wound healing outcomes. Diabetes mellitus is associated with small vessel disease, neuropathy, and problems specific to glucose control—all of which predispose the individual to impaired wound healing.[32] Wound healing problems related to diabetes include increased risk of infection, delayed epithelialization,[33] impaired or delayed collagen synthesis with decreased or delayed quantity of granulation tissue,[33] and slowed wound contraction and closure. There may be a delayed response or impaired functioning of the leukocyte and fibroblast cells, decreased or impaired growth factor production,[33] and imbalance between the accumulation of extracellular matrix components and their remodeling by metallomatrix proteinases (MMPs) all of which are essential for wound repair.[32–34]

The effect of surgery on patients with diabetes can be dramatic. Patients with diabetes respond to the stress of surgery by releasing a series of hormones: epinephrine, glucagon, cortisol, and growth hormone. These stress hormones reduce the amount of circulating insulin while increasing circulating glucose. Elevated glucose levels can reduce the effectiveness of neutrophils' phagocytotic function and alter the deposition of collagen by fibroblasts, leading to a decrease in wound tensile strength.[35] Elevated glucose levels can also lead to cellular malnutrition, because insulin is the key for allowing nutrient use in cells. When glucose cannot be used as energy, proteins and fats are used as fuel, depleting the necessary substrates for wound healing. Maintaining serum glucose levels of 120 to 180 mg/dL is recommended for postoperative patients with diabetes to decrease their risk for wound infection.[35] Careful monitoring of blood glucose levels and insulin administration as necessary can promote optimal healing.[9,35]

Immunocompromised patients are another group at risk for poor healing outcomes. As just noted, the immune system plays a significant role in wound healing, and any impairment (e.g., aging, malnutrition, cancer, and HIV infection) can result in serious sequelae for patients with surgical wounds.[9]

Treatments that affect wound healing include steroids, anti-inflammatory drugs, antimitotic drugs, and radiation therapy. Steroids inhibit all phases of wound healing, affecting phagocytosis, inflammation, collagen synthesis, and angiogenesis. Steroid doses should be minimized before wounding and during wound healing.[9] The effects of steroids can be diminished with the use of topical vitamin A; when applied directly to a wound, it acts as an inflammatory agent. Vitamin A is appropriate to apply to open wound beds. However, wounds healing by primary intention that are closed with well-approximated edges may not be appropriate candidates for topical vitamin A.

Other anti-inflammatory drugs also inhibit wound healing, with effects seen predominantly during the inflammatory phase. Cancer therapies, including antimitotic medications and radiation therapy, impede the normal cell cycle in rapidly dividing cells. The antimitotic activity interferes with new tissue generation in wounds. In addition, radiation therapy has both acute effects on cellular function and long-term sequelae for healing. Its long-term effects are caused by hypoperfusion of tissues in the irradiated field due to damage, deterioration, and fibrosis of the vasculature. Measures to maximize the time between neoadjuvant and adjuvant therapy and surgery are encouraged.[9] Cancer patients may also present with malnutrition, or cancer cachexia. Providing enteral nutritional supplementation (not intravenous supplementation) improves healing in cancer patients.[9]

It is especially important to take comorbidities into account when caring for surgical wounds in older adult populations because risk for chronic illness rises with age and many older adults suffer from conditions such as cardiovascular disease, cancer, and diabetes. Ischemic states due to heart disease and diabetes may contribute to prolonged inflammation and wound dehiscence, as well as impaired angiogenesis.

CLINICAL WISDOM

Vitamin A Use for Wounds

The usual dose of topical vitamin A is 1,000 IU applied three times a day to the open wound bed for 7 to 10 days.

Nutritional Status

As discussed in detail in Chapter 4, adequate nutrition is essential for wound healing. In healthy surgical patients, malnutrition may not be an issue. However, with the population aging and more procedures being performed on older adults, nutritional status is increasingly a concern for wound healing. Adequate amounts of calories, proteins, fats, carbohydrates, vitamins, and minerals are all required for wound repair. Inadequate amounts of any nutrients negatively influence wound healing.[32] Chapter 4 provides a full discussion of the role of specific nutrients in wound healing.

Malnutrition in older adults is a significant impediment to the healing of wounds; it has been estimated that up to 60% of residents of long-term care facilities suffer from malnutrition, a condition that both impairs healing as well as increases susceptibility to infection.[36] Prior to surgery, older adults should consume sufficient calories, supplementing with protein if necessary.

Oxygenation and Perfusion

As discussed in Chapter 3, adequate wound oxygenation and tissue perfusion is essential for healing of any wound, including surgical wounds. Thus, postoperative interventions to improve the circulatory and oxygen-carrying capacity of the tissues and blood (the oxygen saturation of tissues) can enhance wound healing.

Problems related to tissue perfusion and oxygenation can be due to hypovolemia. Thus, maintaining vascular volume is critical for ensuring adequate tissue perfusion. It is essential, therefore, to balance fluid replacement to prevent both underhydration and overhydration. Excess hydration can lead to hypervolemia and edema, which can decrease tissue oxygenation.

Decreased oxygenation and perfusion can also be caused by concurrent cardiovascular or pulmonary disease. To optimize oxygenation in the presence of adequate tissue perfusion, use of pulmonary hygiene interventions, assessment and monitoring of tissue oxygen levels, and low-flow supplemental oxygen may be warranted.[37] Pulmonary hygiene, including incentive spirometry, deep breathing and coughing, and postural drainage, improves the pulmonary toilet and increases the likelihood of adequate oxygenation of the wound. Low-flow oxygen can saturate hemoglobin so that the supply to the tissue is ample. Promoting activity, such as repositioning and early ambulation, can also be beneficial for peripheral tissue perfusion and oxygenation.[37]

Stress and Pain

Pain and stress are complex and interrelated processes that can slow wound healing. Pain alone has been found to increase healing time and can increase stress.[40,41] Stress that involves

CLINICAL WISDOM

Immune Enhancing Supplements

Supplementing the diets of older adult patients with L-arginine and omega-3 fatty acids can help to strengthen the immune system and promote faster recovery. Additionally, maintaining glucose levels below 200 mg/dL should be maintained in the period prior to surgery.[8]

RESEARCH WISDOM

Smoking and Wound Healing

Because nicotine causes adrenergic vasoconstriction, tissue perfusion is decreased. A study of patients undergoing head and neck surgery found that those patients who had abstained from smoking for longer than 3 weeks prior to surgery had fewer incidences of impaired wound healing than those who smoked within the 3 weeks prior to surgery.[38] Refraining from smoking for 3 to 4 weeks prior to surgery and during the postoperative period has been shown to decrease incidence of SSIs but not wound dehiscence or improve healing.[39]

physical components, such as pain and exhaustion, and psychological factors, such as anxiety and anger, raises cortisol levels that, when prolonged, can decrease immune and inflammatory responses.[42] It is therefore important that both be regularly assessed and appropriately managed.

ASSESSMENT AND MANAGEMENT OF THE ACUTE SURGICAL WOUND

Assessment of the acute surgical wound involves physical examination of the wound site and surrounding wound tissues in relation to the wound healing process. This examination includes

- Anatomic location of the incision
- Linear measurement of the length of the incision (in centimeters)
- Observation of the wound tissues for epithelial resurfacing, wound closure, wound exudate, and health of surrounding tissues
- Palpation of the incision for collagen deposition and health of surrounding tissues

Observation and palpation of the incision line provide insight into the healing process taking place in the underlying tissues. Healing proceeds in the surgical incision as it does in other wounds with inflammation, proliferation of new tissues, and remodeling. In the surgical incision, the wound healing processes are not always visible. Thus, the standard for assessment of healing may be best based on time since the surgical injury. It is important to track the postoperative time, because the healing progress of the wound can be measured against the standard time expectations for acute wound repair.

Knowledge of the wound healing process, described in Chapter 2, provides a critical foundation for assessment of the acute surgical incision. During the inflammatory phase, assessment focuses on identification of signs and symptoms of inflammation, evaluation of wound closure materials and wound dressings, and appraisal of epithelial resurfacing. The central point during the proliferation phase of wound healing is evaluation of collagen deposition, wound exudate, and tissues surrounding the incision. Assessment during the remodeling phase is directed toward examination of collagen remodeling at the incision site.

CLINICAL WISDOM

Signs of Inflammation

It is normal to observe signs of inflammation, such as warmth, erythema or discoloration, pain, and edema, at the incisional wound site during the first few days after surgery.

CLINICAL WISDOM

Incisional Color Changes

As new epithelial tissue migrates across the incision, the color of the incision can change from bright red to pink; although this change is not observed in all patients, it is a useful clinical sign that demonstrates maturing epithelial tissue.

The Inflammatory Phase

Signs of inflammation are expected and normal during the first 4 postoperative days. The surgical incision may feel warm to the touch, and there may be surrounding erythema and edema at the incision site.

Patients who are immunocompromised may not be able to mount an effective inflammatory process; in such cases, the signs of inflammation at the incision would not be visible. In fact, lack of inflammation at the incision site is itself an indication of immune system compromise. Again, an incision with no indication of inflammation is an abnormal finding during the first 4 days after surgery.

The process of epithelial resurfacing also occurs during the inflammatory phase of wound healing. In the acute surgical incision, new epidermal tissues are generated quickly because of the presence of intact hair follicles and sebaceous and sweat glands, as well as the short distance the epithelial cells must travel to resurface the incision. The surgical incision is resurfaced with epithelium within 72 hours postsurgery. The new epidermis provides a barrier to bacterial organisms and, to a small degree, external trauma. The tensile strength of the incision is relatively weak, however, and the incision is not able to withstand force, thus the need for sutures and other closure materials to provide external support.

Astute clinicians can observe changes in the new incision that indicate the presence of new epithelial tissue. The incision is evaluated for close approximation of the wound edges and color of the incision line. Wound edges should appear well aligned, with no tension observed (see Fig. 8.1).

Once epithelial resurfacing has occurred, a wound dressing is no longer necessary to prevent bacterial contamination of the incision. However, wound dressings provide other benefits at this stage. Some clinicians suggest that the presence of a dressing at this point can be a reminder of the wound's presence and the need to use care in the wound area. The dressing also provides a physical barrier to rough edges of clothing to limit local irritation. Moreover, a dressing can promote patient adaptation to the wound: by allowing more gradual viewing, it can help patients include the wound in their new body image.

Assess wound closure materials for the reaction of the surrounding incisional tissues. The use of sutures of any type to approximate the wound edges creates small wounds alongside the incision wound. The suture wounds increase inflammation at the wound site and can cause ischemia if the sutures are pulled taut with increased tension, either from poor technique or postoperative wound edema. Although the continued presence of sutures or staples provides additional tensile strength for the wound, sutures can also increase the risk of infection and potential for wound ischemia. Use of Steri-Strip tapes for wound closure or early removal of sutures with Steri-Strip tape replacement can decrease the problems associated with sutures. Removal of the wound sutures or staples in a timely manner is a proactive healing intervention. Removal of sutures in healthy surgical patients in 7 to 10 days postoperatively can be used as a general guideline, depending on surgical site.

The Proliferative Phase

Evaluation of the incision healing ridge, wound exudate, and surrounding incisional tissues provides information on the progress of wound healing during the proliferative phase.

Palpation of the surgical incision reveals the underlying process of collagen deposition. New collagen tissues can be palpated as a firmness or stiffness along the incision, extending 1 cm on either side of the incision.[15] This firmness to the tissues, caused by new collagen deposition in the wound area, is called the *healing ridge*. The healing ridge should be palpable along the entire length of the incision between day 5 and day 9 postoperatively; if it is not palpable in this time frame, the wound is at risk for dehiscence or infection.[15,21]

Evaluation of surgical incision wound exudate requires knowledge of the expected changes to the characteristic and amount of wound exudate during the course of healing. The wound exudate immediately after surgery is bloody. Within 48 hours, the wound drainage becomes serosanguineous in nature and, finally, the exudate is serous. The amount of wound exudate should gradually decrease throughout the healing period. An increase in wound exudate usually indicates compromised wound healing caused by infection. New drainage from a previously healed incision forewarns of wound dehiscence, infection, and, in some cases, fistula formation.

Observe and palpate the tissues immediately surrounding the incision for the presence of edema and induration, and for color changes. The presence of edema retards the wound healing process because excess fluid in the tissues provides an obstacle to angiogenesis and increases the potential for wound ischemia. Skin color changes can indicate bruising or hematoma formation caused by surgery. The skin color will appear dark red or purple. Skin color changes can also indicate impending infection. Signs of erythema, warmth, and edema, as well as increased pain at the incision wound, are indicators of possible wound infection.

The Remodeling Phase

The remodeling phase of wound healing can last 1 to 2 years. In the surgical incision in the remodeling phase, assess wound healing by evaluating the color of the incision. As the scar tissue is remodeled and reorganized structurally, the color of the tissue changes. Throughout the first postoperative year, the color of the incision gradually changes from bright red or pink to a silvery gray or white.

The tensile strength of the wound also gradually increases over the first year, eventually achieving approximately 80% of the original strength of the tissues. The focus of interventions at this stage is to limit force and tension on the wound site, including teaching the patient to avoid heavy lifting, bending, and straining at the site.

Care of the Surgical Dressing

Management of the surgical incision includes attention to factors that affect wound healing, as addressed earlier, as well as dressing care. The surgical dressing includes the primary and secondary dressings.

The primary, or first, surgical dressing is the dressing that is in direct contact with the wound. The direct wound contact requires that the primary dressing be nontraumatic to the wound. The primary dressing absorbs drainage, maintains a sterile wound environment, and serves as a physical barrier to further wound trauma. It should be nonadherent to the wound site. In contrast, a traditional gauze dressing adheres to new incisions and, upon removal, can cause new tissue injury.

The primary dressing absorbs wound exudate and wicks it away from the wound site, allowing the exudate to be absorbed into the secondary dressing. Secondary wound dressings provide increased absorptive capacity or hold the primary dressing in place. Secondary wound dressings are applied on top of the primary dressing and can be composed of the same materials. The secondary dressing is important when increased amounts of wound exudate are anticipated, because it absorbs drainage from the primary dressing and wicks the exudate away from the wound bed and into the absorbent material of the dressing. There is no evidence that providing a dressing on a clean surgical incision in the immediate postoperative period decreases SSIs but it is prudent to protect the incision from harm.[8] There is no robust evidence to support the use of one dressing over another. However, one practice guideline recommends use of a semipermeable film membrane with or without an absorbent island dressing in the majority of cases.[8] There is scattered consensus that the use of gauze as a primary dressing should be avoided because of its association with pain and disruption of healing tissues at the time of dressing change. However, these beliefs have not always been upheld by the evidence.[8,43,44]

Tape is usually used to secure wound dressings. Premature and frequent dressing changes can damage the tissues surrounding the incisional wound and interfere with wound healing. Use of Montgomery straps, skin sealants, or hydrocolloid frames around the wound and underneath the tape can eliminate skin stripping around incision wounds, a problem that can develop from frequent dressing changes. However, frequent dressing changes are more likely to be a problem with draining wounds and with wounds that are healing by secondary intention or tertiary intention, discussed next. (See Chapter 19 for more information about wound dressings.)

SURGICAL WOUND HEALING BY SECONDARY AND TERTIARY INTENTION

Secondary intention wounds are wounds that are left open after surgery. Their healing involves scar tissue replacement during the proliferative phase; that is, the tissue defect must fill with new collagen tissue. Figure 8.2A–D shows a surgical incision healing by secondary intention.

Tertiary intention healing, or delayed primary closure, involves aspects of both primary and secondary wound healing. In tertiary intention healing, the wound is left open initially; after a short period of time, the edges are approximated, and the wound is closed. Tertiary wound healing is designed for specialized wounds in which primary intention is preferred but not possible at the time of wounding. The delay in primary closure can be necessary to clear infection, allow for some wound contracture, or create a healthy granulation base for a graft.

Most surgical wounds that are left to heal by secondary or tertiary intention are those in which the risk of infection is increased. Often, the inflammatory phase of wound healing becomes prolonged because of wound contamination. Assessment of the wound for signs and symptoms of infection includes evaluation of the character and amount of wound exudate, and examination of the wound and surrounding tissues for erythema, edema, induration, heat, and pain. In addition, the administration of systemic antibiotics, when appropriate, can lessen the infection risk.

Surgical wounds left to heal by secondary or tertiary intention often show extensive tissue loss such that the wound edges cannot be approximated without unacceptable tension on the incision. You can promote reversal of tissue loss in the early weeks following surgery with careful wound assessment and care. The primary wound dressing becomes critically important in the care of these wounds. Nonadherent, absorptive dressings optimize healing. However, clinical evidences supporting the choice of moisture-retentive dressings or gauze are based on education of clinical providers (most are educated with gauze as the dressing of choice), case series, small cohort studies, small methodologically flawed randomized trials, and systematic reviews that tentatively suggest that gauze is more labor intensive and painful than moisture-retentive dressings. There is no evidence to suggest that there are any differences in wound healing time or duration of hospital stay between gauze dressings and moisture-retentive dressings for surgical wounds.[43,44]

Overall, surgical wounds that are left open to heal by secondary or tertiary intention have a reparative trajectory similar to that of chronic wounds. Thus, you should evaluate healing using the same parameters used for chronic wounds. Evaluate the wound size and depth, presence or absence of necrotic tissue, characteristics and amount of exudate, condition of the surrounding tissues, and presence of the healing characteristics of granulation and epithelialization.

RESEARCH WISDOM

Surgical Incisional Dressings

The majority of primary intention surgical wound dressings continue to be gauze. Conversion to moisture-retentive dressings in the immediate postoperative period has not been shown to improve wound healing and data are equivocal in relation to moisture-retentive dressings providing for less pain during dressing changes compared to traditional gauze dressings in surgical wounds.[43,44]

RESEARCH WISDOM

Wound Dressing

Primary incision wounds should be protected with a sterile dressing for 24 to 48 hours after surgery. The nurse should perform hand hygiene before and after any contact with the surgical site, and, in contrast to chronic wounds, sterile technique should be used while performing dressing changes. It is important to inform the patient and the family on proper incision care, the symptoms of infection and the importance of reporting possible infection.

OUTCOME MEASURES

Outcome measures for acute surgical incisions relate to healing progress according to time frame since injury, as described below.

Postoperative Days 1 Through 4

The following signs and symptoms represent measures of positive outcomes for acute surgical incision wounds. During the first 4 days after surgery, the presence of an inflammatory response, including erythema or skin discoloration, edema, pain, and increased temperature at the incision site, is a sign of normal healing. Lack of inflammation at a new surgical incision is a negative outcome.

Wound exudate should be bloody in character initially; toward days 3 and 4, it should change to serosanguineous exudate. The amount of wound exudate should gradually decrease from moderate to scant by day 4. Many surgical wounds, especially facial wounds, have no exudate past days 2 or 3. Failure of the wound exudate to decrease in amount and to change in character from bloody to serosanguineous is a negative indicator for healing.

Epithelial resurfacing should be complete by day 4. The incision will appear bright pink, as opposed to its initial red color. The lack of epithelial resurfacing of the surgical incision indicates delayed healing and less than optimal outcomes.

One negative outcome that can occur at any time during the postoperative course of the patient is the development of a hematoma. External evidence of hematoma formation includes swelling or edema at the site; a soft or boggy feel to the tissues initially, which may be followed by induration at the site; and color change of the skin (similar to bruising).

Postoperative Days 5 Through 9

The major healing outcome in the surgical incision on days 5 through 9 is the presence of a healing ridge along the entire length of the incision. A healing ridge indicates new collagen deposition in the wound site. Lack of development or incomplete development of a healing ridge can be prodromal to wound dehiscence and wound infection. A deficient or nonexistent healing ridge is a negative outcome measure for wound healing.

Wound exudate character should change from serosanguineous to serous and gradually disappear over days 4 to 6. The exudate amount should diminish from a minimal amount to none. Any increase in the amount of wound exudate during days 5 to 9 is considered a negative outcome and heralds probable wound infection.

Suture materials should begin to be removed from the incisional site during days 5 through 9. Adhesive tape strips or Steri-Strips can be used to provide additional wound tensile strength. Failure to remove any of the wound suture materials during days 5 to 9 can indicate a negative outcome for the wound.

Continued signs of inflammation at the incision site during days 5 to 9 are indicative of delayed wound healing. Signs of erythema or edema, extensive pain, and increased temperature at the incision wound during this time frame indicate that wound healing is not normal. Prolonged inflammation can occur as a result of underlying infection, compromised immunity, or continued trauma at the wound site.

Documentation of all characteristics of the incision and healing is important for continuity of care throughout the wound recovery period, but especially during this time period, because the patient will likely be changing health-care settings and communication between health-care providers during the transition is important. For example, surgical patients are often discharged from an acute care hospital to the home setting very soon after surgery, typically between days 5 and 9.

Postoperative Days 10 Through 14

The major outcome measure for days 10 through 14 is the removal of external incision suture materials. Internal or "buried" sutures remain in place. Failure to remove external suture materials during this time period will prolong incision healing. Healing is delayed by increasing the risk of infection from the suture microwounds and the continued insult to the tissues by the presence of the foreign objects (the suture materials), prolonging the inflammatory response.

Postoperative Day 15 Through 1–2 Years

During the end of the proliferative phase of wound healing and throughout the remodeling phase, characteristic changes occur in the incisional scar tissue. The collagen deposited alongside the incision is gradually realigned, restructured, and strengthened. The outcome measure for this time period is predominantly based on changes in the color of the incisional scar tissue. The color of the incision changes from a bright pink after the initial epithelial resurfacing, gradually fading to pink and, eventually, turning a pearly gray or silvery white color. In addition, the noticeable induration and firmness associated with the healing ridge gradually softens. Finally, recovery of functional ability with the scar tissue becomes a key outcome measure for many surgical incisional wounds.

Negative outcomes include reinjury of the incisional line, such as herniation of the wound site, and complications associated with scarring, such as keloid formation and hypertrophic scarring. Loss of or reduction in functional ability is also a negative outcome.

At 1 year, positive outcome measures include lack of significant hypertrophic scarring and wound herniation, maximal functional ability with the new scar, and acceptable cosmetic results of healing, with a silvery white or gray scar line. Tables 8.3 and 8.4 present the positive and negative outcome measures for time frames from the point of surgery to the end of remodeling. Chapter 22 discusses management of scars.

TABLE 8.3	Positive Outcome Measures for Incisional Wound Healing			
Outcome Measure	Days 1–4: Inflammation	Days 5–9: Proliferative	Days 10–14: Proliferative	Day 15–Years 1–2: Proliferative Remodeling
Incision color	Red, edges approximated	Red, progressing to bright pink	Bright pink	Pale pink, progressing to white or silver in light-skinned patients; pale pink, progressing to darker than normal skin color in darkly pigmented skin
Surrounding tissue inflammation	Edema, erythema, or skin discoloration; warmth, pain	None present	None present	None present
Exudate type	Bloody or sanguineous, progressing to serosanguineous and serous	None present	None present	None present
Exudate amount	Moderate to minimal	None present	None present	None present
Closure materials	Present, may be sutures or staples	Beginning to remove external sutures/staples	Sutures/staples removed, Steri-Strips or tape strips may be present	None present
Epithelial resurfacing	Present by day 4 along entire incision	Present along entire incision	Present	Present
Collagen deposition (healing ridge)	None present	Present by day 9 along entire incision Present along entire incision	Present	

CLINICAL WISDOM

Documentation of Incisional Wound Healing

Documentation should include all of the following:

- Time since surgery in days
- Location
- Size in centimeters
- Closure materials present
- Color of the incision
- Type and amount of exudate
- Presence or absence of epithelial resurfacing
- Presence or absence of collagen deposition or healing ridge
- Actions taken for follow-up or referral, as necessary
- Primary and secondary dressings, as appropriate

Example: *Postoperative day 6 for a 12-cm midline abdominal incision with Steri-Strips present. Incision is completely reepithelialized, with no exudate present. Incision is bright pink, with healing ridge palpable along anterior 10 cm of incision. Posterior 2 cm of incision is soft and boggy to touch, with no healing ridge palpable and erythema present. Physician notified of possible impaired healing. Dry gauze 2 × 2-inch dressing applied to posterior aspect of incision for protection of site.*

REFERRAL CRITERIA

Refer patients meeting any of the following descriptions to a physician or advanced practice nurse for evaluation and intervention for complications of wound healing.

- Patients with markedly increased bloody drainage during the immediate postoperative period may be at risk of hemorrhage from undetected leaking blood vessels in the surgical field.
- Patients with exudate that changes from bloody or serosanguineous to purulent should be evaluated for wound infection or abscess formation and treated with appropriate antimicrobial therapy.
- Patients with an increase in the amount of exudate after postoperative day 4. This situation is indicative of wound infection or abscess formation and requires evaluation by the primary-care provider and appropriate antimicrobial therapy.
- Patients with a wound showing the absence of a healing ridge along the entire length of the incision by postoperative day 9. This situation indicates impaired healing and, often, abscess formation. Prompt referral to the primary-care provider usually results in drainage of the abscess area, antimicrobial therapy, and a wound left to heal by secondary intention.
- Patients with signs and symptoms of wound infection, including erythema, edema, elevated temperature, and increased pain along the incision after day 4, *and/or* signs of systemic

TABLE 8.4 **Negative Outcome Measures for Incisional Wound Healing**

Outcome Measure	Days 1–4: Inflammation	Days 5–9: Proliferative	Days 10–14: Proliferative	Day 15–Years 1–2: Proliferative Remodeling
Incision	Red, edges approximated but tension evident on incision line	Red, edges may not be well approximated; tension on incision line evident	May remain red, progressing to bright pink	Prolonged epithelial resurfacing, keloid or hypertrophic scar formation
Surrounding tissue inflammation	No signs of inflammation present: *no* edema, *no* erythema or skin discoloration, *no* warmth, and minimal pain at incision site; hematoma formation	Edema, erythema, or skin discoloration; warmth, pain at incision site; hematoma formation	Prolonged inflammatory response with edema, erythema, or skin discoloration; warmth and pain; hematoma formation	If healing by secondary intention, may be stalled at a plateau (chronic inflammation or proliferation), with no evidence of healing and continued signs of inflammation
Exudate type	Bloody or sanguineous, progressing to serosanguineous and serous	Serosanguineous and serous to seropurulent	Any type of exudate present	Any type of exudate present
Exudate amount	Moderate to minimal	Moderate to minimal	Any amount present	Any amount present
Closure materials	Present, may be sutures or staples	No removal of any external sutures/staples	Sutures/staples still present	For secondary intention healing, failure of wound contraction or edges not approximated
Epithelial resurfacing	Present by day 4 along entire incision	Not present along entire incision	Not present along entire incision, dehiscence evident	Not present or abnormal epithelialization, such as keloid or hypertrophic scarring
Collagen deposition (healing ridge)	None present	Not present along entire incision	Not present along entire incision, dehiscence evident	Abscess formation with wound left open to heal by secondary intention

---

CASE STUDY

Lack of Inflammatory Response Postoperatively

M.J., a 71-year-old Caucasian woman, was admitted for bowel surgery with resection of the descending colon and low anterior anastomosis. M.J.'s history included long-term steroid therapy for rheumatoid arthritis. On postoperative day 1, her midline incision primary dressing showed evidence of bright red bleeding. The wound edges were well approximated, with staples as the closure material. Assessment of the incision on postoperative days 2 and 3 revealed no evidence of edema, warmth, erythema, or discoloration at the incision site. Exudate was moderate and serosanguineous to seropurulent in nature. By postoperative day 4, the incision was not fully resurfaced with new epithelial tissue. Signs of inflammation, although now present, were diminished, and the exudate remained seropurulent and moderate in amount. M.J. showed signs of confusion and agitation (signs of infection in older adults), and lab tests confirmed the presence of wound infection. In this case, the absent signs of inflammation were early warning signs of impaired healing and wound infection.

infection, including elevated temperature, elevated white blood cell count, and confusion in the older adult, require evaluation. These signs and symptoms suggest a wound infection, and the primary-care provider should evaluate and treat the patient appropriately.

- Patients with frank wound dehiscence or fistula formation require evaluation by the primary-care provider, usually the surgeon, and may warrant a referral to a certified wound nurse (a nurse specializing in management of draining wounds) for management.

SELF-CARE TEACHING GUIDELINES

General self-care teaching guidelines for patients with acute surgical incisions are provided in Exhibit 8.1. However, every patient's and caregiver's instruction in self-care must be individualized to the type of surgical incision and the patient's wound, the specific incisional dressing management routine, the individual patient's learning style and coping mechanisms, and the ability of the patient/caregiver to perform procedures.

CASE STUDY

Incisional Wound Healing

P.L., a 78-year-old African American man, was admitted for radical prostatectomy surgery for prostate cancer. P.L. has a history of diabetes mellitus, hypertension, obesity, and peripheral vascular disease. His diabetes is managed with oral hypoglycemic agents and an 1,800-calorie diabetic diet (with which he is noncompliant). P.L. lives alone on a small pension and fixed income. He is a smoker. He was admitted with a random blood sugar of 198 mg/dL.

Preoperatively

Assessment of P.L. revealed several risk factors for impaired healing: uncontrolled diabetes mellitus, obesity, advanced age, hypertension, and peripheral vascular disease. Control of blood sugar level was identified as a goal in the preoperative period, and P.L. was started on sliding-scale insulin therapy with blood glucose monitoring. P.L.'s history of hypertension and peripheral vascular disease put him at risk for poor tissue perfusion; thus, in the immediate postoperative period (days 1 and 2), he was put on supplemental oxygen by nasal cannula to optimize tissue oxygenation. Obesity is a risk factor for excess incision wound tension, which increases the potential for poor perfusion of the incision wound due to the presence of excess subcutaneous tissue.

Postoperative Day 4

P.L.'s 15-cm midline abdominal incision showed evidence of inflammation with edema, skin discoloration, and warmth at the site. There was evidence of epithelial resurfacing, and the incision line was bright pink. There was a continued minimal amount of serous drainage, and staples remained in place. The primary gauze dressing was changed daily. Blood sugars ranged from 110 to 132 mg/dL on insulin therapy. Oxygen was administered the first 2 days postoperatively at 2 L by nasal cannula.

Postoperative Day 9

P.L. was discharged from the hospital to his home with home-health nursing follow-up. Upon discharge from the hospital, P.L.'s incision was bright pink with no exudate present. The incision was completely resurfaced with new epithelial tissue present along the entire incision, and half of the staples had been removed. A healing ridge was palpable along the anterior 13 cm of the wound, but not palpable at the posterior aspect of the wound.

Postoperative Day 10

The home-health nurse evaluated P.L.'s incision and found surrounding skin discoloration, increased pain, and edema present at the posterior aspect of the wound. No healing ridge was palpable at the posterior aspect of the wound, although collagen deposition was evident along the anterior 13 cm of the wound. Half of the original staples were still present in the incision line. The physician was notified, and P.L. was referred to the physician's office for evaluation of the incision.

CASE STUDY *(continued)*

Postoperative Day 12

The physician removed the remaining staples, performed an incision and drainage (I&D) of the posterior aspect of the incision in the office, started P.L. on systemic antibiotics, and left the posterior aspect of the wound open to heal by secondary intention, using moist saline gauze dressings.

Postoperative Day 15

P.L.'s posterior incision was 75% filled with granulation tissue, and there is minimal serous exudate present. The anterior aspect of the incision was well healed and pale pink. P.L.'s incision wound went on to heal uneventfully by secondary intention over the next 10 days.

CONCLUSION

A variety of strategies are available for use to optimize wound healing in patients with an acute surgical incision. The measures described in this chapter will help you reduce the risk of complications, identify delayed or impaired healing, and provide for a supportive healing environment. The key to successful intervention for the patient with an acute surgical incision is knowledge of normal healing mechanisms and temporal expectations, knowledge of factors that impair wound healing, and vigilant attention to both. The case study presented earlier helps to demonstrate the interaction between knowledge of normal healing and normal healing times, and factors that interfere with normal healing.

EXHIBIT 8.1

Self-Care Teaching Guidelines

Self-Care Guidelines Specific to Acute Surgical Incisions	Instructions Given (Date Initials)	Demonstration or Review of Material (Date Initials)	Return Demonstration or States Understanding (Date Initials)

1. Type of incisional wound and specific cautions required
  a. No heavy lifting and other measures to prevent hernia formation
  b. Showering or bathing area
  c. Importance of adequate nutrition for wound healing			

2. Significance of wound exudate, incision wound tissue color, surrounding tissue condition, and presence of healing ridge			

3. Wound dressing care routine
  a. Wash hands, then remove old dressing and discard
  b. Clean wound with normal saline
  c. Apply primary dressing to wound
  d. Apply secondary dressing if appropriate
  e. Secure dressing with tape
  f. Universal precautions and dressing disposal
  g. Frequency of dressing changes			

4. Expected change in wound appearance during healing process
  a. Scheduled removal of closure materials
  b. Incision color change as wound heals (bright red or pink to pale pink and finally to silvery white or gray)			

5. When to notify the health-care provider
  a. Signs and symptoms of wound infection (erythema, edema, pain, elevated temperature, change in exu date character or amount, discoloration in tissues surrounding incision wound)
  b. Absent or incomplete healing ridge along incision after postoperative day 9			

6. Importance of follow-up with health-care provider			

REVIEW QUESTIONS

1. Which of the following provides the best example of the acute surgical wound?
   A. Surgical wound healing by secondary intention
   B. Dehisced surgical wound
   C. Pressure ulcer
   D. Surgical incision

2. Which of the following statements best describes the effects of age as an intrinsic factor affecting wound healing?
   A. Aging decreases elastin in the skin; affects collagen replacement; decreases the rate of replacement of cells, delaying reepithelialization; and causes a decline in immune function.
   B. Aging decreases protein synthesis, causes lower levels of serum albumin, and causes a decline in immune function.
   C. Aging causes collagen weakness, leading to poor binding with ground substances, and causes a decrease in fibroblast function and poor white blood cell function.
   D. Aging increases blood glucose levels, leading to poor leukocyte function and inadequate protein synthesis.

3. Factors affecting wound healing in the immediate postoperative period include which of the following?
   A. Hydration, pain management, and protein intake
   B. Tissue perfusion, pain management, and temperature
   C. Tissue perfusion, protein intake, age, and concurrent conditions
   D. Volume status, pain management, tissue perfusion, and temperature

4. A clinician assessing a client's abdomen 3 days post abdominal-perineal resection surgery notes erythema, slight edema, and a slight increase in temperature at the abdominal incision site. These findings are most consistent with which of the following?
   A. These are normal signs of the inflammatory phase of wound healing.
   B. The wound is exhibiting early signs of impending infection.
   C. The wound is in the proliferative phase of wound healing.
   D. The wound is exhibiting signs of abscess formation.

5. A clinician is evaluating a client's status post abdominal surgery on postoperative day 8. In assessing the midline abdominal incision, the clinician should be aware of which of the following?
   A. Signs of inflammation, including redness, warmth, pain, and edema are expected signs of normal healing at this time.
   B. A moderate amount of serous to serosanguineous drainage is expected during this phase of healing.
   C. A healing ridge or collagen matrix deposition should be palpable along the incision line.
   D. The wound edges should begin to show signs of approximation by this time.

REFERENCES

1. Mangram AJ, Horan TC, Pearson ML, et al. Guideline for prevention of surgical site infection. *Infect Control Hosp Epidemiol.* 1999;27:94–134.
2. Malone DL, Gunit T, Tracy JK, et al. Surgical site infections: analysis of risk factors. *J Surg Res.* 2002;103:89–95.
3. Seal LA, Paul Cheadle D. A systems approach to preoperative surgical patient skin preparation. *Am J Infect Control.* 2003;32:57–62.
4. Edwards P, Lipp A, Holmes A. Preoperative skin antiseptics for preventing surgical wound infections after clean surgery (review). *Cochrane Libr.* 2009;(3).
5. Webster J, Osborne S. Preoperative bathing or showering with skin antiseptics to prevent surgical site infection (review). *Cochrane Libr.* 2009;(3).
6. Cruse PJE, Foord F. The epidemiology of wound infection: a ten-year prospective study of 62,939 wounds. *Surg Clin North Am.* 1980;60:27–40.
7. Tanner J, Woodings D, Moncaster K. Preoperative hair removal to reduce surgical site infection (review). *Cochrane Libr.* 2008;(4).
8. National Institute of Health and Clinical Evidence. Surgical site infection: prevention and treatment of surgical site infection. Clinical Guideline No. 74. October 2008. http://www.nice.org.uk/nicemedia/live/11743/42378/42378.pdf, last accessed July 24, 2010.
9. Frantz MG, Robson MC, Steed DL, et al. Guidelines to aid healing of acute wounds by decreasing impediments of healing. *Wound Rep Reg.* 2008;16:723–748.
10. Bratzler DW, Houck PM. Antimicrobial prophylaxis for surgery: an advisory statement from the national surgical infection prevention project. *Clin Infect Dis.* 2004;38:1706–1715.
11. Prevention of surgical site infections. In: Betsy Lehman Center for Patient Safety and Medical Error Reduction, JSI Research and Training Institute, Inc. Prevention and control of healthcare-associated infections in Massachusetts. Part 1: Final recommendations of the Expert Panel. Boston, MA: Massachusetts Department of Public Health; 2008:61–68.
12. Burns JL, Mancoll JS, Phillips LG. Impairments to wound healing. *Clin Plast Surg.* 2003;30(1):47–56.
13. Narong MN, Thongpiyapoom S, Thaikul N, et al. Surgical site infections in patients undergoing major operations in a university hospital: using standardized infection ratio as a benchmarking tool. *Am J Infect Control.* 2003;31:274–279.
14. Gaynes RP, Culver DH, Horan TC, et al. Surgical site infection (SSI) rates in the United States, 1992–1998: the National Nosocomial Infections Surveillance System basic SSI risk index. *Clin Infect Dis.* 2001;33(suppl 2):S69–S77.
15. Phillips SJ. Physiology of wound healing and surgical wound care. *Am Soc Artif Intern Organ J.* 2000;46:S2–S5.
16. Tanner J, Swarbrook S, Stuart J. Surgical hand antisepsis to reduce surgical site infection. *Cochrane Database Syst Rev.* 2008;(1). Art. No.: CD004288. DOI: 10.1002/14651858. CD004288.pub2.
17. Friedman ND, Bull AL, Russo PL, et al. An alternative scoring system to predict risk for surgical site infection complicating coronary artery bypass graft surgery. *Infect Control Hosp Epidemiol.* 2007;28(10):1162–1168. Epub 2007 Aug 3.
18. Chen LF, Anderson DJ, Kaye KS, et al. Validating a 3-point prediction rule for surgical site infection after coronary artery bypass surgery. *Infect Control Hosp Epidemiol.* 2010;31(1):64–68.
19. Shelton RM. Repair of large and difficult to close wounds. *Dermatol Clin.* 2001;19:535–553.

20. Coulthard P, Esposito M, Worthington HV, et al. Tissue adhesives for closure of surgical incisions. *Cochrane Database Syst Rev*. 2010, Issue 5. Art. No. CD004287. DOI: 10. 1002/14651858. CD004287. Pub 3.

21. Lee CK, Hansen SL. Management of acute wounds. *Surg Clin North Am*. 2009;89(3):659–676.

22. Whitney JD, Heitkemper MM. Modifying perfusion, nutrition, and stress to promote wound healing in patients with acute wounds. *Heart Lung*. 1999;28(2):123–133.

23. Gosain A, DiPietro LA. Aging and wound healing. *World J Surg*. 2004;28:321–326.

24. Stotts NA, Hopf HW. Facilitating positive outcomes in older adults with wounds. *Nurs Clin North Am*. 2005;40:267–279.

25. Pittman J. Effect of aging on wound healing. *J Wound Ostomy Continence Nurs*. 2007;34(4):412–415.

26. Xia YP, Zhao Y, Tyrone JW, et al. Differential activation of migration by hypoxia in keratinocytes isolated from donors of increasing age: implications for chronic wounds in the elderly. *J Invest Dermatol*. 2001;116:50–56.

27. Lenhardt R, Hopf HW, Marker E, et al. Perioperative collagen deposition in elderly and young men and women. *Arch Surg*. 2000;135:71–74.

28. Ashcroft GS, Mills SJ, Ashworth JJ. Aging and wound healing. *Biogerontology*. 2002;3:337–345.

29. Hardman MJ, Ashcroft GS. Estrogen, not intrinsic aging, is the major regulator of delayed human wound healing in the elderly. *Genome Biol*. 2008;9(5):80.

30. Son ED, Lee JY, Lee S, et al. Topical application of 17beta-estradiol increases extracellular matrix protein synthesis by stimulating tgf-beta signaling in aged human skin in vivo. *J Invest Dermatol*. 2005;124:1149–1161.

31. Routley CE, Ashcroft GS. Effect of estrogen and progesterone on macrophage activation during wound healing. *Wound Rep Reg*. 2009;17:42–50.

32. Greenhalgh DG. Wound healing and diabetes mellitus. *Clin Plast Surg*. 2003;30:37–45.

33. Falanga V. Wound healing and its impairment in the diabetic foot. *Lancet*. 2005;366:1736–1743.

34. Brem H, Tomic-Canic M. Cellular and molecular basis of wound healing in diabetes. *J Clin Invest*. 2007;117(5):1219–1222.

35. Hoogwerf BJ. Postoperative medical complications: postoperative management of the diabetic patient. *Med Clin North Am*. 2001;85:1213–1228.

36. Williams JZ, Barbul A. Nutrition and wound healing. *Surg Clin North Am*. 2003;83(3):571–596.

37. Gottrup F. Oxygen in wound healing and infection. *World J Surg*. 2004;28:312–315.

38. Kuri M, Nakagawa M, Tanaka H, et al. Determination of the duration of preoperative smoking cessation to improve wound healing after head and neck surgery. *Anesthesiology*. 2005;102:892–896.

39. Sorensen LT, Gottrup F. Smoking and postsurgical wound healing—an update on mechanisms and biological factors. In: Sen C, ed. *Translational Medicine: From Benchtop to Bedside to Community and Back. Advances in Wound Care*, Vol. 1. 2010 Yearbook of the Wound Healing Society. New Rochelle, NY: Mary Ann Liebert, Inc.; 2010:83–87.

40. McGuire L, Heffner K, Glaser R, et al. Pain and wound healing in surgical patients. *Ann Behav Med*. 2006;31(2):165–172.

41. Woo K, Sibbald G, Fogh K, et al. Assessment and management of persistent (chronic) and total wound pain. *Int Wound J*. 2008;5(2):205–215.

42. Ebrecht M, Hextall J, Kirtley L, et al. Perceived stress and cortisol levels predict speed of wound healing in health male adults. *Psychoneuroendocrinology*. 2004;29:798–809.

43. Vermeulen H, Ubbink DT, Goossens A, et al. Systematic review of dressings and topical agents for surgical wounds healing by secondary intention. *Br J Surg*. 2005;92:665–672.

44. Ubbink DT, Vermeulen H, Goossens A, et al. Occlusive vs Gauze dressings for local wound care in surgical patients: a randomized clinical trial. *Arch Surg*. 2008;143(10):950–955.

Pressure Ulcers: Pathophysiology, Detection, and Prevention

Barbara M. Bates-Jensen

CHAPTER OBJECTIVES

At the completion of this chapter, the reader will be able to:

1. Describe the epidemiology of pressure ulcers in various health-care settings and with a variety of populations.
2. Explain the role of physical forces and tissue tolerance on the pathophysiology of pressure ulcer development.
3. Define each category in the National Pressure Ulcer Advisory Panel's pressure ulcer classification system.
4. Identify risk factors contributing to the development of pressure ulcers.
5. Explain pressure ulcer risk screening and pressure ulcer risk assessment.
6. Describe the Braden Scale for Predicting Pressure Sore Risk and the Norton Scale.
7. Describe three methods of detecting pressure-induced tissue damage.
8. Outline, describe, and explain components of pressure ulcer prevention programs.
9. Identify and describe strategies for implementing pressure ulcer prevention guidelines into practice.
10. Identify the most appropriate outcome measures to evaluate the effectiveness of pressure ulcer prevention programs.

Pressure ulcers are areas of local tissue trauma, usually developing where soft tissues are compressed between bony prominences and any external surface for prolonged time periods. Thus, they are most commonly found over bony prominences subject to external pressure. A pressure ulcer is a sign of local tissue necrosis: The skin may be involved or there may be major muscle and subcutaneous fat tissue destruction underneath intact skin.

PRESSURE ULCER SIGNIFICANCE

Pressure ulcers are a highly complex, multifactorial, and costly global health problem common in all health-care settings. The Joint Commission estimates that 2.5 million patients in United States acute care hospitals are treated for pressure ulcers each year[1] and this number is likely to increase as the population ages. *Prevalence is the number of all persons with the condition at one particular point in time.* Thus, prevalence includes both facility-acquired cases and those admitted with the condition.

- Among hospitalized elders of all ages, the prevalence of pressure ulcers has been estimated at 15%.[2]

- Critical care units are of special concern with prevalence rates as high as 23% among critical care patients.[3]
- Prevalence among nursing homes is 11% based on the 2004 National Nursing Home Survey, a continuous cross-sectional survey of a nationally representative sample of US nursing homes.[4]
- Hispanic and non-Hispanic blacks have a higher prevalence of pressure ulcers than non-Hispanic whites (7.6%, 9.7%, and 12.1%, respectively).[5] In a separate study of black and white nursing home residents, pressure ulcer prevalence was 18.2% for black residents compared to 13.8% for whites.[6]
- In home health-care settings, the prevalence of pressure ulcers has been estimated to be 6% to 9%.[7,8]
- In outpatient settings, the prevalence of pressure ulcers is estimated to be 1.6%.[9]
- Pressure ulcer prevalence in palliative care settings ranges from 9% to 38%.[7]
- Rehabilitation facilities present special concerns related to pressure ulcer development because patients in rehabilitation facilities have conditions that limit mobility, such as spinal cord injury, traumatic brain injury, cerebral vascular accident, burns, multiple trauma, or chronic neurologic disorders.

Prevalence rates are reported between 11%–12%[10,11] and 25%.[12]

- Among persons with spinal cord injury, pressure ulcer prevalence rates are as high as 40% during acute rehabilitation, 15% at the first annual examination, and 29% to 32% at 20 years post discharge.[13,14]
- Prevalence of recurrent pressure ulcers among veterans with spinal cord injury over 3 years has been reported at 39%, with most ulcers occurring over the pelvic area (sacrum, ischium, trochanters) and at stage IV (e.g., full thickness involving muscle, bone) severity.[15]

Incidence is the number of new cases developing over a period of time. Incidence includes only facility-acquired conditions and, as such, can reflect the effectiveness of the prevention program in the organization.

- Patients with a stay in critical care units are twice as likely to develop pressure ulcers as those without.[16] Hospital-acquired pressure ulcer (HAPU) rates in critical care units are reported from 9% to 12%.[3,16]
- Palliative care incidence varies from 3% to 13%, the majority of which are stage I or II ulcers.[17,18]
- African Americans demonstrate a higher incidence of pressure ulcers compared to Caucasians in long-term care facilities with incidence rates reported as 0.56 per person year compared to 0.35 per person year for Caucasians in nursing homes.[19]
- Rehabilitation facility incidence rates over 2 months have been reported at 4%.[20]
- Incidence of pressure ulcer development for nonhospice, pressure ulcer–free older adults during their home health-care period has been reported as ranging from 6.3% to 9.2%, with 20% of the pressure ulcers developing in the first week after admission.[21]
- Pressure ulcer incidence reportedly increases 10% each week of home care services through week 4. Of home care patients who developed a pressure ulcer, 50% developed the ulcer within 24 days after admission.[21]
- Individuals with spinal cord injury are at higher risk for pressure ulcer development, with incidence rates reported at 20% for those undergoing spinal surgery[22] to 31% over 1 year's time.[23]
- The incidence of pressure ulcers among acutely ill pediatric patients has been reported at 27%,[24] for those undergoing cardiac surgery 17%,[25] and for neonates in intensive care units 19%.[26]

The Department of Health and Human Services' Agency for Healthcare Research and Quality (AHRQ) data show the number of pressure ulcers in acute care hospitals increased by 63% during the period 1993 to 2003.[2] Clearly, pressure ulcers are a significant problem in all health-care settings and there is evidence that the condition has not improved as data from the Healthcare Cost and Utilization Project report point out.[2] From 1993 to 2006, hospitalizations increased by 15%. During this same time period, there was an 80% increase in hospital stays with pressure ulcers for a total of 503,300 hospital stays in 2006. Hospital stays with a secondary diagnosis of pressure ulcers increased by 86.4% during this period, while stays principally for pressure ulcers increased by 27.2%. Adult hospital stays noting a diagnosis of pressure ulcers totaled $11.0 billion in 2006. This suggests that hospitals did not improve in pressure ulcer prevention during this time period. Stays principally for pressure ulcers were slightly longer than those with a secondary pressure ulcer diagnosis (14.1 days versus 12.7 days).[2] Furthermore, the length of stay for hospitalizations principally for pressure ulcers was nearly three times longer than hospitalizations with no diagnosis of pressure ulcers (14.1 days versus 5.0 days). Though stays principally for pressure ulcers were longer than stays with a secondary diagnosis of pressure ulcers and those with no pressure ulcer diagnosis, the average cost per day ($1,200) was lower—nearly $400 less than secondary pressure ulcer stays ($1,600 per day) and $800 less than stays for all other conditions ($2,000 per day).[2]

Data from other sources suggest that the progress is more positive. The National Database of Nursing Quality Indicators (NDNQI) is national project established by the American Nurses Association in 1998 to monitor quality indicators in hospitalized patients that are nursing sensitive. In 2000, the NDNQI added HAPUs as one of the patient safety and quality of care indicators to monitor in participant hospitals. Hospital sites in 2011 include 1,721 hospitals in 50 states. Participating institutions collect data by medical record abstraction and direct skin assessments and enter it into a secure website. Comparing HAPU data from 2010 (first and second quarter) to 2004 (quarters 2 and 3) and 2006 (quarter 4) to 2007 (quarter 1) shows a decrease in stages I to IV and unstageable pressure ulcers with a rate of 3.8% in 2010 compared to 6.4% in both 2004 and 2006–2007.[27]

Pressure ulcers are costly. In 1999, the cost of treating pressure ulcers ranged from $5 to $8.5 billion annually.[28] Factoring in a 7% per year increase to account for health-care inflation, costs for treating pressure ulcers can be estimated at $10.5 to $17.8 billion dollars for 2010. The cost for managing a single full-thickness pressure ulcer is as much as $70,000.[1] One study reports the average hospital-associated costs for managing one full-thickness stage IV ulcer and related complications for one hospital admission at $129,248 and costs for managing a community-acquired stage IV ulcer over an average of four hospital admissions at $124,327.[29] The Centers for Medicare/Medicaid Services (CMS) reports the cost of treating a pressure ulcer in acute care (as a secondary diagnosis) is $43,180.00 per hospital stay.[28] Contributing cost factors include increased length of stay due to pressure ulcer complications such as pain, infection, high-tech support surfaces, and decreased functional ability.[30] The AHRQ reported that pressure ulcer–related hospitalizations ranged from 13 to 14 days and cost $16,755 to $20,430 compared to the average stay of 5 days and costs approximately $10,000.[2] Health-care utilization and costs of caring for persons with SCI who experience the complication of a severe (stage III/IV) pressure ulcer are high (in excess of $100 k annually).[31] Clearly, there are considerable financial repercussions related to pressure ulcers.

Pressure ulcers are significant in terms of morbidity and mortality.[32–34] Sepsis is the most serious complication of pressure ulcers. There are 3.5 episodes of pressure ulcer–associated bacteremia per 10,000 discharges. Of these episodes of pressure ulcer–associated bacteremia, the pressure ulcer is the probable source in nearly half of the cases. When the pressure ulcer is the source of bacteremia, the in-hospital mortality is nearly

60%. Clinicians should be aware that transient bacteremia occurs after débridement of pressure ulcers in as many as 50% of patients. In-hospital mortality is higher for pressure ulcer–related hospitalizations, especially among those hospitalizations with a secondary diagnosis of pressure ulcers. In-hospital death occurred in 11.6% of stays with pressures ulcers noted as a secondary diagnosis, as compared to 4.2% of stays principally for pressure ulcers and 2.6% of stays for all other conditions. Development of a hospital-acquired pressure ulcer is associated with greater risk of death at 1 year, with one study reporting 59% of patients developing a pressure ulcer dying within 1 year compared to 38% of patients without pressure ulcers.[34] Each year 60,000 persons die from pressure ulcer complications.[2]

Pressure ulcers have also received attention in the courtroom. Health-care organizations have been prosecuted for negligence related to pressure ulcer care and development.[35,36] One report reviewed 54 nursing home law suit cases from September 1999 to April 2002 involving pressure ulcers. The average monetary recovery was more than $13.5 million and included awards of up to $312 million in one case, when determined by a verdict or settlement.[36] In a landmark case, a care-home operator was found guilty of manslaughter for a resident's death related to improper care for her pressure ulcers.[37] In a New Mexico case, the jury awarded $10.3 million to the estate of a man who sued a Medical Center after he developed pressure ulcers.[38] Of the total awarded, $595,000 was designated as compensatory damages and $9.75 million as punitive damages. The patient spent a week at the hospital after undergoing hip surgery, then spent a week at a nursing home before returning to the hospital for 2 more weeks. He developed serious pressure ulcers on his heels because the hospital failed to follow its system of screening for and protecting against pressure ulcers.[38] Pressure ulcers are a significant costly problem in all health-care settings.

PRESSURE ULCER PATHOPHYSIOLOGY

Pressure ulcers are the result of mechanical injury to the skin and underlying tissues. Traditionally, pressure (stress), shear, and friction were considered the primary external factors involved in pressure ulcer development.[39–43] More recently, deformation (strain),[44–52] heat,[53] reperfusion injury,[54–56] and impaired lymphatic function[57] have been considered as additional primary forces involved in pressure damage.[58,59] Four hypotheses for the pathophysiology behind pressure ulcer development include

1. Ischemia caused by capillary occlusion
2. Impairment in lymphatic flow with increase in metabolic waste products
3. Reperfusion injury (damage that occurs because of the inflammatory response that occurs when blood flow resumes to the ischemic tissues)
4. Deformation of tissue cells

There are probably aspects of each of these hypotheses that play a role in pressure ulcer development. Pressure (stress) and deformation (strain) are involved in all four pressure ulcer development hypotheses. Pressure is the perpendicular force or load exerted on a specific area, causing ischemia and hypoxia of the tissues. The gravitational pull on the skeleton causes loading and deformation of the soft tissue between the bony prominence and external support surface. High-pressure areas in the supine position are the occiput, sacrum, and heels. In the sitting position, the ischial tuberosities exert the highest pressure, and the trochanters are affected in the side-lying position.[40,60] The mechanical physical forces of shear, which is force applied against a surface as it moves or slides in an opposite but parallel direction stretching tissues and displacing blood vessels laterally, and deformation, which stretches and pulls cells, are also key factors in pressure ulcer development. Friction, which is the resistance to motion or rubbing of one object or surface against another in a parallel direction, and moisture, which macerates tissues and increases the coefficient of friction between surfaces, are major forces in superficial damage over bony prominences, abrading the epidermal surface and increasing the risk for infection.

Pathophysiology of Pressure Ulcer Formation

The triggering event in pressure ulcer formation is development of a pressure gradient. With perpendicular pressure, as the amount of soft tissue available for compression decreases and the deformation increases, the pressure gradient increases. Likewise, as the tissue available for compression increases, the pressure gradient decreases. Thus, most pressure ulcers occur over bony prominences where there is less tissue for compression and the pressure gradient within the vascular network is altered.[42] Figure 9.1 demonstrates this relationship.

Pathophysiology at the Tissue Level

Over time, pressure occludes blood and lymphatic circulation, causing deficient tissue nutrition and buildup of waste products. If pressure is relieved before a critical time period is reached, reactive hyperemia, a normal compensatory mechanism, restores tissue oxygenation and compensates for compromised circulation. If pressure is not relieved before the critical time period is reached, then the increased pressure gradient leads to vascular network changes first in the venous system followed by arterial changes. Initially, the interstitial fluid pressure increases, exceeding and inhibiting venous flow. The increased interstitial fluid pressure and the increase in venous pressure increase the pressure gradient throughout the vascular network impeding arteriolar circulation. Increased capillary arteriole pressure leads to fluid loss through the capillaries, tissue edema, and subsequent autolysis. The capillaries collapse and thrombosis occurs. Lymphatic flow is also decreased, increasing tissue edema and contributing to tissue necrosis.[39–41] The tissues are deprived of oxygen, nutrients, and waste removal. In the absence of oxygen, cells use anaerobic pathways for metabolism and produce toxic byproducts. The toxic byproducts lead to tissue acidosis, increased cell membrane permeability, edema, and eventual cell death.[39] Muscle tissue is more sensitive to ischemia and hypoxia likely due to the increased vascularization and higher metabolic demand compared to the skin and subcutaneous tissue.[61]

It is not just the hypoxia and ischemia that cause damage. Deformation of tissues is a key factor in the damage seen in deep tissue injury (DTI) and full-thickness pressure ulcers and may be the force that initiates cell death. Tissues are deformed due to the bone's compression of the soft tissue against the external surface. How the tissues are deformed depends on the tissues (i.e., size and shape of the different tissue layers), the mechanical properties of the involved tissues (e.g., stiffness, strength), and the magnitude and distribution of the external mechanical force applied to the tissues. The tissue's ability

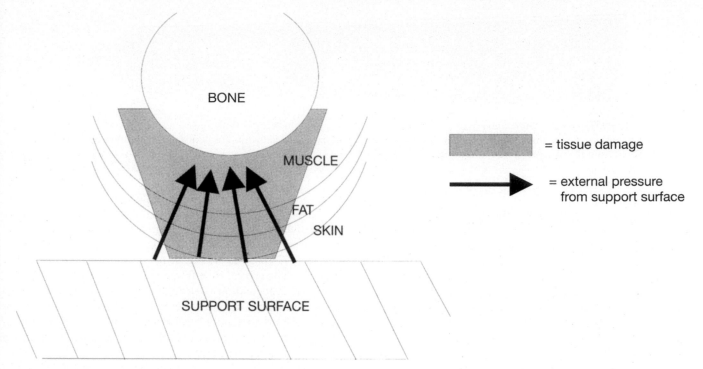

FIGURE 9.1 Pressure gradient at the bony prominence. (Source: Barbara M. Bates-Jensen.)

to withstand deformation can change with time due to aging, lifestyle changes, injury, or disease. The sustained mechanical deformation damages cells directly and also obstructs blood flow.[48–52] In fact, it is likely that tissue deformation is the major underlying factor in muscle damage. Several investigators have examined the reaction of cells to deformation. Observing single muscle cells has demonstrated that deformations exceeding 80% have consistently ruptured cell membranes, causing immediate and irreversible damage.[49] Observations of an entire muscle have demonstrated similar findings; 2 hours of sustained deformation at strains higher than 50% inflicted irreversible damage to muscle tissue.[48] As with hypoxia and ischemia, muscle tissue is more sensitive to deformation forces and irreversible damage may be present at the muscle layer without such damage occurring in the skin or subcutaneous layers. The cell death and local tissue necrosis change the geometry and characteristics of the tissues that further increases the deformation force exacerbating the pressure injury.

Heat accumulation or increased skin temperature intensifies the effects of ischemia and hypoxia on tissues.[53] Increased skin temperature causes an increase in metabolic rate, which increases the need for oxygen in the tissues.[53] Normal skin temperature ranges from 90°F to 95°F. When skin temperature approaches 95.5°F the perspiration threshold is reached and local sweating occurs to cool the skin. The sweat increases moisture on the skin. Thus, the increase in heat increases metabolic activity of the tissues and may increase moisture on the skin creating a microclimate that places the tissues at increased risk for breakdown.

When prolonged pressure is finally relieved, the damage does not end. As the vascular network is relieved of pressure, the tissues are reperfused and reoxygenated. The sudden entry of oxygen into previously ischemic tissues releases oxygen-free radicals known as *superoxide anions, hydroxyl radicals,* and *hydrogen peroxide,* all of which induce new endothelial damage and decrease microvascular integrity causing postischemic

or reperfusion injury.[55,58,60–66] These cellular changes result in inflammation and edema *locally* at the site of injury.[56,60–66] These inflammatory changes exist in the tissues before any damage is fully visible on the skin surface.[44,45,47,67] This is the *nonvisible spectrum of pressure-induced tissue damage,* the preclinical stage of disease in the physiology cascade leading to frank ulceration. These inflammatory changes with tissue edema can occur from 3 to 10 days before visible skin breakdown[44,45,67] (see Fig. 9.2).

Pathophysiology at the Cellular Level

Ischemia results in hypoxic injury to the cell. Lack of oxygen results in a rapid decrease in mitochondrial phosphorylation with subsequent insufficient adenosine triphosphate (ATP) production. The lack of ATP leads to increased anaerobic metabolism and causes the plasma membrane's sodium-potassium pump and sodium-calcium exchange to fail, which leads to an intracellular accumulation of sodium and calcium, and diffusion of potassium out of the cell.[68] Sodium and water can then enter the cell freely and cellular swelling results. The movement of water and ions into the cell causes dilation of the endoplasmic reticulum, which causes ribosomes to detach with subsequent reduced protein synthesis. The cell becomes more swollen and with continued hypoxia, the accumulation of calcium in the cell activates multiple enzyme systems. The result is cytoskeleton disruption, membrane damage, activation of inflammation, DNA degradation, and eventual cell death.[68] The activation of inflammation leads to vascular dilation, increased membrane permeability, and movement of fluid from the vascular space to the interstitial space.[68] The end result is increased water and fluid in the tissues or subepidermal moisture (SEM) at the site of injury. The tissue edema resulting from inflammation is subclinical disease or preclinical pressure damage (pre-stage I) that is invisible on the skin.

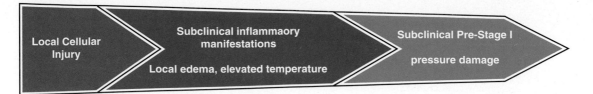

FIGURE 9.2 Local cellular injury occurs as a result of vascular changes which trigger inflammation and release of inflammatory mediators. Inflammatory mediators cause vascular dilation, increased membrane permeability and movement of fluid from the vascular space to the interstitial space. This results in *local* tissue edema from inflammation. This is subclinical disease or pre-stage I pressure damage that is *invisible* on the skin. (Source: Barbara M. Bates-Jensen.)

Intensity and Duration of Pressure

Ischemia and hypoxia of body tissues are produced when capillary blood flow is obstructed by localized pressure. How much pressure and what amount of time is necessary for ulceration to occur has been a subject of study for many years. In 1930, Landis,[69] using single-capillary microinjection techniques, determined normal hydrostatic pressure to be 32 mm Hg at the arteriole end and 15 mm Hg at the venule end. His work has been the criterion for measuring occlusion of capillary blood flow. Generally, a range from 25 to 32 mm Hg is considered normal capillary blood flow and is used as the marker for adequate relief of pressure on the tissues. We now know that it is not just the pressure that is at work but also the forces of deformation of cells.

Pressure is most intense at the bony prominence and soft tissue interface and gradually lessens in a cone-shaped gradient to the periphery.[54,70–73] Thus, although tissue damage apparent on the skin surface may be minimal, the damage to the deeper structures can be severe. Recall that damage at the cellular level with resultant edema and tissue damage exist prior to visible skin damage and that significant muscle death can be present even with intact nondamaged skin. In addition, subcutaneous fat and muscle are more sensitive than the skin to ischemia. Muscle and fat tissues are more metabolically active and, thus, more vulnerable to hypoxia with increased susceptibility to pressure damage. The vulnerability of muscle and fat tissues to deformation and pressure forces explains DTI lesions and pressure ulcers where large areas of muscle and fat tissue are damaged with undermining or pocketing due to necrosis, yet the skin opening is relatively small.[44,45,74]

Pressure intensity also differs according to body position. Pressures are highest (70 mm Hg) on the buttocks in the lying position, and in the sitting position can be as high as 300 mm Hg over the ischial tuberosities.[71] These levels are well above the normal capillary closing pressure and are capable of causing tissue ischemia. Further, deformation forces are most intense in the sitting position with ischial tuberosities compressing gluteal muscle tissue. Deformation forces over 200 mm Hg are associated with irreversible and nearly immediate damage to muscle tissue.[50–52]

It is also important to understand the relationship between intensity and duration of pressure in pressure ulcer development. The most recent work on pressure-time curves views the curve as a sigmoid curve that is supported with cell studies and animal research where muscle tissue has a finite tolerance to high levels of pressure and finite load limits that can be borne over very long time periods.[50] This failure strength of the tissue is estimated at about 240 mm Hg.[49,73] Some pressures lower than those that cause immediate tissue damage when present over a long period of time are as capable of producing tissue damage as are higher pressures for a short period of time.[70–73] The critical time frame is 1 to 3 hours for both pressure and deformation. Deformations below 65% (of normal tissue formation) are only tolerated by muscle cells for periods of time less than 1 hour.[50] Moreover, when tissues have been compressed for prolonged periods, tissue damage continues to occur, even after the pressure is relieved. This continued tissue damage relates to changes at the cellular level that lead to difficulties with restoration of perfusion as discussed earlier and to increased muscle stiffness (from muscle cell death) that widens the area of loading, changing the strain and stress distributions, and increasing tissue damage.[48,50,73]

CLINICAL PRESENTATION OF PRESSURE ULCERS

Four levels of skin breakdown occur, depending on the amount of time tissue is exposed to unrelieved pressure.[72,74] Hyperemia can be observed within 30 minutes or less; it is manifested as redness of the skin and dissipates within 1 hour after pressure is relieved. Ischemia occurs after 2 to 6 hours of continuous pressure; the erythema is deeper in color and may take 36 hours or more to disappear after pressure is relieved. Necrosis is the third level and occurs after 6 hours of continuous pressure. The skin may take on a blue or gray color and become indurated. Damage that has progressed to this level may take longer periods to disappear and the time to recovery is variable. Ulceration is the fourth and final level and may occur within 2 weeks after necrosis with potential infection; it resolves on a variable basis.[74]

Two types of pressure ulcers exist; superficial and deep tissue ulcers. Superficial ulcers are those caused by friction and shearing forces and involve the epidermis and part of the dermis. Deep tissue ulcers start at the bony tissue interface, involve muscle damage and over a period of time, involve the skin structures. Pressure ulcers are commonly classified by the level of *visible* tissue damage, where stage I pressure ulcers exhibit nonblanchable erythema (i.e., redness) on intact skin, stage II pressure ulcers are partial-thickness ulcers, and stages III and IV ulcers involve full-thickness damage. The visible spectrum of pressure-induced tissue damage often begins with *blanchable* erythema or redness of the skin. Ability of the tissues to blanch indicates sufficient perfusion of the tissues for capillary refill to occur. More severe pressure damage is observed as *nonblanchable* erythema. Nonblanchable erythema may appear as red, maroon, dark red, or purple discoloration

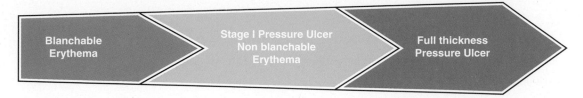

FIGURE 9.3 Beginning visible clinical indicators of pressure ulcers all relate to the signs of inflammation in the tissues. The first visible sign of damage is *Blanchable* erythema. *If detected*, this beginning stage of damage may be transient if pressure is relieved. If pressure is not relieved, the damage can progress to a stageable pressure ulcer or *nonblanchable* erythema (Stage I). Stage I pressure ulcers are also thought to be reversible, although tissues may take 1 to 3 weeks to return to normal. If pressure is not relieved, and in cases where initial pressure was intense, damage may present as a full thickness ulcer. (Source: Barbara M. Bates-Jensen.)

on the skin depending on the individual's skin color and the severity of the damage. Without intervention, and sometimes even with aggressive intervention, blanchable and nonblanchable erythema can progress to full-thickness ulceration (see Fig. 9.3). The classic clinical signs of pressure ulcer formation are discussed next.

Early Pressure-Induced Tissue Damage

The immediate response of the tissues to a sustained period of pressure are related to the inflammatory response and are manifest as elevated temperature, subepidermal edema, and erythema. Skin temperature and subepidermal edema are reflections of the nonvisible spectrum of pressure-induced tissue damage. Elevated skin surface temperature, as compared with that of healthy tissues can be evaluated by palpation, skin thermistors, or thermography. Subepidermal edema can be assessed using ultrasound and surface electrical capacitance methods. These are discussed in more detail later.

If pressure is not relieved, pressure-induced tissue damage progresses to the visible spectrum. The first visible indicator of pressure damage is blanchable erythema. Erythema presents as redness of a flat, nonraised area of the skin larger than 1 cm. The discoloration varies in intensity from pink to bright red in persons with light skin tones. In persons with dark skin tones, the discoloration appears as a deeper than normal pigmentation or a purple or blue-gray hue to the skin.

In light-skinned patients, the severity of the tissue insult can be evaluated by testing for blanchability of tissues. After finger pressure is applied to the area, complete blanching of the skin occurs, followed by quick return of redness from capillary refill, once the finger is removed. In patients with dark skin tones, the blanch response is not visible. Increased tissue damage is observed when pressure and other mechanical forces continue to assault the skin and tissues. To enhance communication about this visible pressure-induced tissue damage, the National Pressure Ulcer Advisory Panel (NPUAP) developed a six category system for classifying pressure ulcers by visible tissue damage. The NPUAP classification system is used throughout the United States in all health-care organizations.[75] Exhibit 9.1 presents the pressure ulcer categories.

Stage I Pressure Ulcers

If pressure is not relieved, the damage progresses to stage I category, with additional temperature, coloration, and texture changes seen.[76–78] As the tissues become more disturbed, the

temperature may decrease, signaling underlying tissue damage. Nonblanchable erythema develops, in which the color of the skin becomes more intense, varying from dark red to purple or cyanotic in both light- and dark-skinned patients (Fig. 9.4). Persons with dark skin tones may show a deepening of normal skin color, a purple, blue or grey color to the skin.[79,80] In light-skinned patients, nonblanchable erythema is detected by testing for capillary refill of tissues. Increased damage to tissues is indicated by the inability of the tissues to blanch.

In addition, skin texture changes. The skin may feel hard and indurated, and observation may reveal heightened skin features or an orange-peel appearance.[79,80] This stage of tissue destruction is also reversible, although tissues may take 1 to 3 weeks to return to normal.[81] Additionally, the patient may report pain at the site.

Stage II Pressure Ulcers

Stage II category pressure ulcers are superficial ulcers most often the result of the mechanical force of friction on the epidermis. Stage II pressure ulcers involve damage to the epidermis and part of the dermis, they are partial-thickness lesions. The ulcer is superficial, with indistinct margins and a red pink, shiny base (Fig. 9.5). It is usually surrounded by blanchable or nonblanchable erythema. If not dealt with aggressively, stage II ulcers can progress to involve deeper tissues. Still, if properly treated, the situation may resolve in 2 to 4 weeks.[81]

Stage III and IV Pressure Ulcers

Whereas superficial or partial-thickness ulcers such as stage II ulcers begin at the skin surface and progress to deeper layers, deep, full-thickness ulcers do not originate at the skin surface; they begin at the bony prominence–soft tissue interface at the muscle tissue layer and spread to involve the skin structures.

The chronic deep ulcer usually has a dusky red wound base and does not bleed easily (Fig. 9.6). It is surrounded by blanchable or nonblanchable erythema or deepening of normal skin tone, induration, possible edema, change in temperature compared to healthy tissues, and possible mottling with or without hemosiderin staining. Undermining and tunneling may be present with a large necrotic cavity.

Unstageable Pressure Ulcers

Pressure ulcers that present covered with devitalized necrotic tissue are classified as unstageable because the depth of tissue destruction is not visible. The necrotic tissue may be slough or

EXHIBIT	9.1

National Pressure Ulcer Advisory Panel Pressure Ulcer Staging Classifications

Stage	Definition
Stage I	• Intact skin with nonblanchable redness of a localized area usually over a bony prominence. Darkly pigmented skin may not have visible blanching; its color may differ from the surrounding area. • **Further description:** The area may be painful, firm, soft, warmer or cooler as compared to adjacent tissue. Stage I may be difficult to detect in individuals with dark skin tones. May indicate "at risk" persons (a heralding sign of risk).
Stage II	• Partial-thickness loss of dermis presenting as a shallow open ulcer with a red pink wound bed, without slough. May also present as an intact or open/ruptured serum-filled blister. • **Further description:** Presents as a shiny or dry shallow ulcer without slough or bruising.[a] This stage should not be used to describe skin tears, tape burns, perineal dermatitis, maceration or excoriation.
Stage III	• Full-thickness tissue loss. Subcutaneous fat may be visible but bone, tendon or muscle are not exposed. Slough may be present but does not obscure the depth of tissue loss. May include undermining and tunneling. • **Further description:** The depth of a stage III pressure ulcer varies by anatomical location. The bridge of the nose, ear, occiput and malleolus do not have subcutaneous tissue and stage III ulcers can be shallow. In contrast, areas of significant adiposity can develop extremely deep stage III pressure ulcers. Bone/tendon is not visible or directly palpable.
Stage IV	• Full-thickness tissue loss with exposed bone, tendon or muscle. Slough or eschar may be present on some parts of the wound bed. Often include undermining and tunneling. • **Further description:** The depth of a stage IV pressure ulcer varies by anatomical location. The bridge of the nose, ear, occiput and malleolus do not have subcutaneous tissue and these ulcers can be shallow. Stage IV ulcers can extend into muscle and/or supporting structures (e.g., fascia, tendon or joint capsule) making osteomyelitis possible. Exposed bone/tendon is visible or directly palpable.
Unstageable	• Full-thickness tissue loss in which the base of the ulcer is covered by slough (yellow, tan, gray, green, or brown) and/or eschar (tan, brown, or black) in the wound bed. • **Further description:** Until enough slough and/or eschar is removed to expose the base of the wound, the true depth, and therefore stage, cannot be determined. Stable (dry, adherent, intact without erythema or fluctuance) eschar on the heels serves as "the body's natural (biologic) cover" and should not be removed.
Suspected DTI	• Purple or maroon localized area of discolored intact skin or blood-filled blister due to damage of underlying soft tissue from pressure and/or shear. The area may be preceded by tissue that is painful, firm, mushy, boggy, warmer or cooler as compared to adjacent tissue. • **Further description:** DTI may be difficult to detect in individuals with dark skin tones. Evolution may include a thin blister over a dark wound bed. The wound may further evolve and become covered by thin eschar. Evolution may be rapid exposing additional layers of tissue even with optimal treatment.

[a]Bruising indicates suspected DTI.
Source: National Pressure Ulcer Advisory Panel and European Pressure Ulcer Advisory Panel. Prevention and treatment of pressure ulcers: Clinical practice guideline. Washington DC: National Pressure Ulcer Advisory Panel; 2009.

eschar. Eschar is the formation of an acellular dehydrated compressed area of necrosis, usually surrounded by an outer rind of blanchable or nonblanchable erythema (Fig. 9.7). Eschar formation indicates a full-thickness loss of skin and may be the result of both pressure and shear forces. Slough is devitalized tissue with a higher water content than eschar. Slough appears as yellow or tan material that is thickly adherent to wound bed tissues (Fig. 9.8). Slough also indicates full-thickness tissue damage.

Suspected Deep Tissue Injury

Pressure-induced skin damage that manifests as purple, blue, or black areas of intact skin may be suspected DTI areas.[44–48,73,75] These lesions commonly occur on the sacrum and heels and signal more severe tissue damage below the skin surface (Fig. 9.9). DTI lesions reflect tissue damage at the bony tissue interface and may progress rapidly to large tissue defects.[62,82]

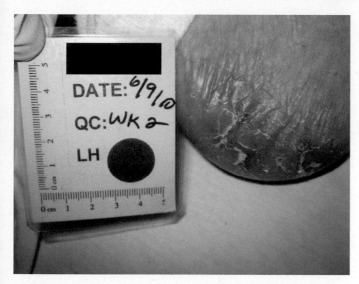

FIGURE 9.4 Stage I pressure ulcer of the heel exhibiting nonblanchable erythema. The color is an intense, dark red in light skinned persons. (©B. M. Bates-Jensen.)

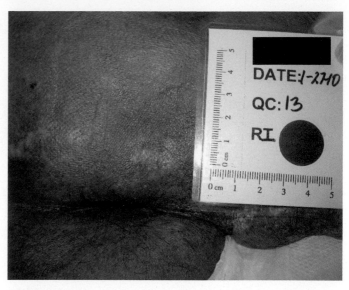

FIGURE 9.5 Stage II pressure ulcer presents as a superficial shallow abrasion with a pink-red clean base. (©B. M. Bates-Jensen.)

Location

The great majority of pressure ulcers occur on the lower half of the body; more than 95% develop over five classic locations: sacral/coccygeal area, greater trochanter, ischial tuberosity, heel, and lateral malleolus. Several multisite prevalence surveys of pressure ulcers in hospitals have found the sacrum the most common location, followed by the heels.[83–85] In the spinal cord–injured population, the sacral/coccygeal area and ischial tuberosities are the most common locations.[86,87] While the prevalence of pressure ulcers is low (4%) in the pediatric population, 66% are facility-acquired lesions and the most common locations are the head area (31%), seat area (20%), and foot area (19%).[88] Correct anatomic terminology is important for communicating the location of the pressure ulcer to other health-care professionals. For example, many clinicians document pressure ulcers as being located on the patient's hip. The hip, or iliac crest, is not a common location for pressure ulcers. The iliac crest is located on the front of the patient's body and is rarely subject to pressure forces. The area that these clinicians typically are referring to is the *greater trochanter*. This is the bony prominence located on the side of the body, just above the proximal, lateral

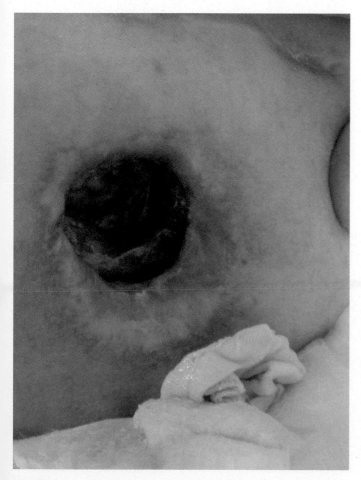

FIGURE 9.6 Full thickness Stage IV pressure ulcer presents with extensive loss of tissue. The wound bed appears dusky and the head of the trochanter can be seen at the base of the wound. (©B. M. Bates-Jensen.)

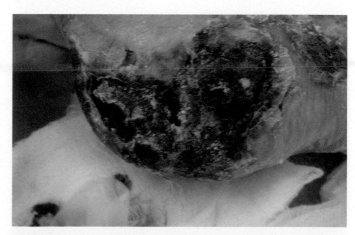

FIGURE 9.7 Unstageable pressure ulcer on the heel of a patient. The ulcer is covered with necrotic black eschar such that the depth of the wound cannot be determined. The ulcer is full thickness but we are unable to determine if deep structures are involved until debridement occurs. (©B. M. Bates-Jensen.)

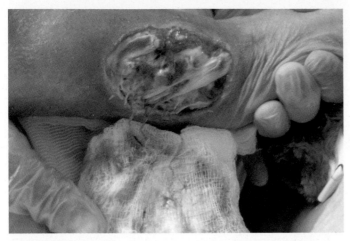

FIGURE 9.8 This full thickness pressure ulcer presents with areas of yellow slough. The slough is dead necrotic material. (©B. M. Bates-Jensen.)

aspect of the thigh or "saddle-bag" area. Figure 9.10 presents the typical locations of pressure ulcer development with correct anatomic terminology.

Although pressure ulcers most commonly occur over bony prominences, they can develop at any site where tissues have been compressed, causing tissue ischemia and hypoxia. Patients with contractures are at special risk for pressure ulcer development because of the internal pressure of the bony prominence and the abnormal alignment of the body and its extremities. (Refer to Chapter 10 on Therapeutic Positioning.) Other locations of concern are body areas under or around medical devices.[89] In the case of medical devices, individuals are at special risk due to the pressure on tissues caused by the medical device itself.[90] In many instances, the medical device cannot be removed and it may not be possible to reduce the pressure on the tissues from the device.[89,90] This is particularly true if the device is applied when edema is present. One study found that patients with medical devices were 2.4 times more likely to develop a pressure ulcer.[90]

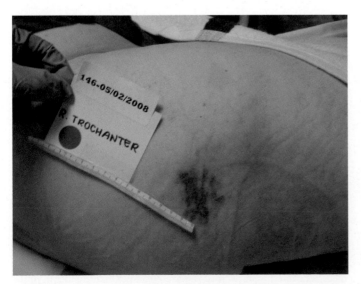

FIGURE 9.9 The pressure area presents as suspected deep tissue injury which is identified by the deep purple discoloration of the tissues. (©B. M. Bates-Jensen.)

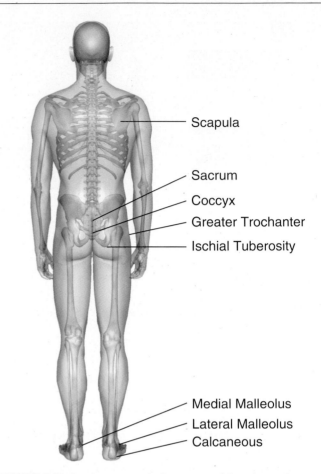

FIGURE 9.10 Correct anatomical names and locations of common pressure ulcer sites.

CLINICAL WISDOM

Managing Medical Devices

Use of soft silicone foam under tracheostomy tubes and oxygen tubing may help reduce pressure. For CPAP masks, alternating use with full face devices has been successfully applied as a prevention strategy.

PRESSURE ULCER DETECTION

Stage I pressure ulcers account for up to 47% of all pressure ulcers in the elderly,[83] many of which progress to more severe ulcers. In hospitalized patients, 22% to[91] 26% of stage I pressure ulcers deteriorate to more severe ulcers in as little as 7 days.[92] Nursing homes report pressure ulcer deterioration among residents with stage I pressure ulcers range from 9%[89] to 58% in as short as 2 weeks.[93,94] Thus, *detection* of subclinical pressure-induced tissue damage is important because early intervention may prevent decline to stage I pressure ulcers and more severe pressure ulcers.

The standard method of detecting early pressure damage is visual skin assessment observing for blanchable and non-blanchable erythema. While this method has some reliability for individuals with light skin tones,[94] by the time nonblanchable erythema is evident, tissue damage has already occurred. In fact,

CLINICAL WISDOM

Monitoring for Deterioration of Erythema

One method of monitoring existing erythema for progression of tissue damage is to test capillary refill every 8 hours. When capillary refill is not present, it indicates an increase in tissue damage.[45]

blanchable erythema alone has been suggested as a strong predictor of later stage ulcers among nursing home residents and can be viewed as visible prestage I pressure damage.[94–96] In addition, evidence suggests that visual skin assessment fails to detect skin color changes in darkly pigmented skin, missing both prestage I pressure damage and stage I pressure ulcers.[32,82,97] Use of a plastic or glass disc pressed into the tissues to evaluate capillary refill and blanching has been shown to be more effective than use of finger pressure alone.[92] There are several nonvisual methods of detecting pressure damage: ultrasound, thermography, spectroscopy, and surface electrical capacitance.

Ultrasound Evaluation of Pressure-Induced Skin and Tissue Damage

High-resolution ultrasound is a noninvasive method of visualizing skin and soft tissues that provides echogenic images of skin and deeper tissues. Ultrasound has been used for evaluating skin structure and thickness,[98] chronic wound healing,[99] differentiating benign skin lesions from melanoma,[100] detecting skin involvement in systemic sclerosis,[101] and to determine pathogenesis of pressure ulcer development.[102] High-resolution ultrasound is portable, noninvasive, and provides visual images of microscopic inflammatory changes in the skin and deeper tissues. Researchers found that over 50% of ultrasound images obtained from nursing home residents indicated abnormal findings with tissue edema present compared to ultrasound images obtained from healthy volunteers.[102] Nearly 80% of those with abnormal ultrasound images did not have documentation of erythema suggesting that ultrasound technology can detect tissue damage before clinical signs occur.[102] Researchers at Georgia Institute of Technology also conducted field trials on the use of ultrasonic imaging devices to detect early stage pressure ulcers and underlying tissue damage and to age bruises as a method of diagnosing neglect among elders.[103] Others have shown high-resolution ultrasound's ability to identify edema in the tissues, which precedes palpable skin involvement.[100,101] Advantages of ultrasound technology for detecting early pressure ulcer development include (1) reproducibility, (2) noninvasiveness, and (3) objective and quantitative data on tissue damage below skin surface.

Temperature as a Method of Detecting Pressure-Induced Skin and Tissue Damage

The NPUAP includes skin temperature as a nonvisual method of early pressure ulcer detection yet it is not clear whether increased or decreased temperature, or both, or the pattern of temperature over time is the critical element. Both increased and decreased skin temperature (compared to adjacent normal tissue) is associated with stage I pressure ulcers in rehabilitation

patients with pressure-induced erythema.[77] Skin temperature variability also differentiates between nursing home residents at high and low risk for pressure ulcer development and between those residents who do and do not develop pressure ulcers.[104] In a study using a hand-held thermistor to measure skin surface temperature, temperatures for sacral and buttocks sites with erythema or stage I pressure ulcers were significantly higher than for normal skin. Skin surface temperature was responsive to visual changes in the skin, with higher temperatures associated with any change in the skin: deterioration or improvement. Further, a decrease in skin surface temperature by 4°F predicted stage I pressure ulcers that were visible on the skin the following week.[105] This is also true for predicting diabetic foot ulcers. Patients with diabetes were able to use a hand-held infrared skin temperature probe to monitor foot temperatures and informed to seek healthcare when temperatures were elevated from the contralateral foot by 4°F. Those patients not using the infrared thermometer to monitor for impending ulcers were 10 times more likely to develop a foot complication compared with patients using the hand-held infrared thermometer to assess skin temperature.[67] In the case of predicting diabetic foot ulcers, it is the pattern of skin temperature that is important as simply using temperature as an initial screening method has not been successful.[106] The same is likely to be true in predicting pressure-induced damage. Others have not been able to show a direct relationship between skin temperature and pressure ulcer severity.[107] It may be that temperature is best used with specific populations such as elders and those with neurologic impairment. For example, older tissue may be more at risk for pressure damage due to accumulated dysfunction with impaired pressure-induced vasodilation and associated skin temperature dysfunction.[78,108] In persons with spinal cord injury or other neurologic impairment, increased

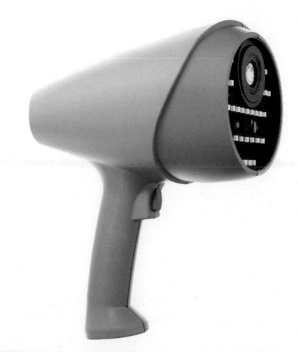

FIGURE 9.11 The thermography device records both a photograph of the ulcer and a thermograph scan showing temperature variation in the tissues indicating underlying tissue damage. (Courtesy of Wound-Vision, 410 South College Ave, Suite 100 | Indianapolis, IN 46203.)

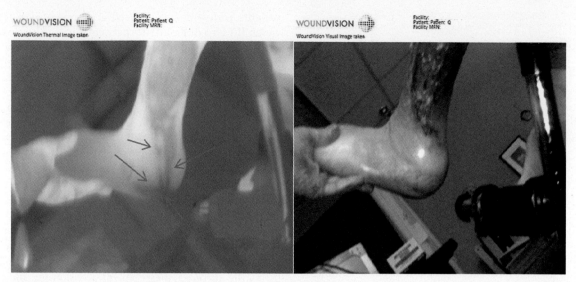

FIGURE 9.12 Thermography image demonstrates extent of tissue damage below intact skin surface. In the thermography image (**left**) the deep tissue damage is indicated by *arrows*. This is a thermal image of a pressure ulcer on a patient's left heel. This particular patient was being treated for a venous stasis ulcer on both legs but developed a pressure ulcer on their left heel due to no preventative care plan. The right heel did have a preventative care plan and proper offloading which resulted in no pressure ulcer. To confirm the imaging a physical evaluation of the left heel could not detect an existing DTI with pending pressure ulcer development. (Courtesy of WoundVision, 410 South College Ave, Suite 100 | Indianapolis, IN 46203.)

temperature may be a predictor of pressure ulcer development; a 1.2°C increase in skin temperature may occur 24 to 96 hours before sacral pressure ulcer development.[109]

Temperature has also been employed to predict healing of existing ulcers and as an intervention to limit pressure-induced tissue damage. When a patient lies in a supine position for a period of time, heat is generated at the sacral bony prominence. The metabolic needs of the tissues are increased due to the increased temperature thus further compromising the tissues. Mild cooling of the skin may provide protection from pressure damage.[110] Temperature has been examined as a method of limiting pressure-induced tissue damage (specifically cooling) where local cooling of tissues resulted in reduced postischemic reactive hyperemia, thus providing a protective effect.[111] Thermography has also been used to predict delayed healing in persons with existing pressure ulcers. More ulcers with low skin temperatures at the wound margins healed compared to those ulcers that healed with higher temperatures.[112] Higher temperatures surrounding the ulcers may be indicative of increased inflammatory response or undetected clinical infection.[112] Devices that perform thermography and temperature screening range from simple hand-held thermistors to thermography cameras. (Fig. 9.11 shows an example of a thermography camera and Fig. 9.12 shows the results of a thermography image for detecting deep tissue damage.)

Tissue Reflectance Spectroscopy as a Method of Detecting Pressure-Induced Skin and Tissue Damage

The dermatology field has used tissue reflectance spectroscopy (TRS) as a method of examining changes in skin color during and after skin treatments. TRS is a noninvasive measurement approach that uses the characteristic absorption of light by hemoglobin and melanin in the skin layers to measure the amount of these substances present in the tissue. Briefly, light passes through the epidermis (and the melanin present in the epidermis), then passes through blood vessels in the dermis (and the hemoglobin present) to the collagen layer in the lower dermis and then is reflected back.[113] The technology is based on the tissue chromophores: melanin, hemoglobin, and oxyhemoglobin. In the visible portion of the spectrum, light is absorbed by melanin and hemoglobin and reflected off the collagen layer. Oxygenated hemoglobin has absorption peaks at 542 and 574 nm; deoxygenated hemoglobin has an absorption peak at 545 nm.[114] Melanin has a linear decreasing absorption function with the wavelength and absorption related to the amount of melanin present.[113] Detection of subcutaneous hemoglobin is likely in the green portion of the spectrum and the near-infrared spectrum. In general terms, light at the red and green end of the spectrum are directed through the tissues and the reflected light data is captured in an image and interpreted using an algorithm. Use of TRS entails a light-emitting apparatus directed to the skin area of concern; an image and data are collected and an algorithm is used to interpret collected data. Algorithms have been tested[113] with several demonstrating good sensitivity and specificity for erythema detection.[76,113] A variety of devices and techniques are used for spectroscopy evaluation. One method, multispectral imaging, has demonstrated excellent sensitivity and specificity for erythema detection significantly enhancing contrast of erythema over that observed with digital photographs.[115] Use of TRS has also been used to characterize of reactive hyperemia[116] and detect erythema in persons with dark skin tones.[115] Near infrared imaging is another method of spectroscopy for detecting erythema in persons with dark skin tones.[114] Many of the devices used in TRS are not yet clinically practical; however, as invention and research in this area continues, it is likely that equipment will become more useful to clinicians.[115] These techniques, as well as studies using laser Doppler perfusion imagers, have shown that there is a significant difference between the blood flow in normal tissues compared to tissues with erythema, both blanching and nonblanching, supporting the importance of clinical identification of erythema as a precursor to pressure damage.[76,117]

Subepidermal Moisture as a method of Detecting Pressure-Induced Skin and Tissue Damage

Measurement of water content of skin and tissue has been used to assess the maturity of the epidermal barrier function of the skin,[118–126] measure edema in irritant exposed skin,[119,120] and is related to development and healing of wounds.[121,124,126] Measurement of the hydration or water content of the skin and underlying tissue can be accomplished using capacitive devices. These devices detect and measure water *below* the stratum corneum (the uppermost layer of skin and the most influenced by outside surface moisture). While the stratum corneum of the epidermis is influenced by environmental moisture, the lower epidermal layers contain water generated from within the tissues and are not as affected by environmental moisture. The ability to measure water content in the lower epidermal layers, dermis, and subcutaneous fat allows for evaluation of SEM without significant interference by surface moisture such as occurs with incontinence. These devices determine hydration with electrical methods using two approaches, capacitive and impedance-based capacitive parameters or dielectric parameters. Both approaches share similarities in technique but differ in measurement values and how values are calculated. SEM is measured by electrical properties based on different water contents of skin layers. Both capacitive and conductive properties of tissues are related to the water content. When measuring skin using dielectric parameters with an electromagnetic field penetrating through the skin, the uppermost layer is predominantly capacitive, while the deeper layers are conductive.[118,122] The dry stratum corneum acts like a dielectric medium. Addition of water in the tissues makes the stratum corneum responsive to an electrical field.

Using dielectric parameters, high-frequency low-power electromagnetic waves of 300 MHz are transmitted via a device that is manually placed on the skin. In the skin, the induced electrical field interacts mainly with water molecules closest to the probe with depth of interaction depending on the diameter of the circular probe.[122,123] The portion of the electromagnetic energy that is not absorbed by tissue water is reflected and measured by the same electrode as used for wave transmission. From the properties of the reflected wave, the dielectric properties of the site are determined and displayed in the measuring unit. Among dielectric properties, a dielectric constant is calculated and is directly proportional to the free and bound water (total water) in the skin and tissues.[122] Depending on the device used, SEM values are displayed in pico Farads (pF) or relative dielectric constant units. The dielectric constant is a dimensionless physical quantity and it is directly proportional to the water content in the measured tissue. The measured value increases when water content increases. Dielectric constant of water molecules depends on the used radiofrequency. Free and bound water behave electrically differently with different frequencies. At around 300 MHz, the electrical properties of free and bound

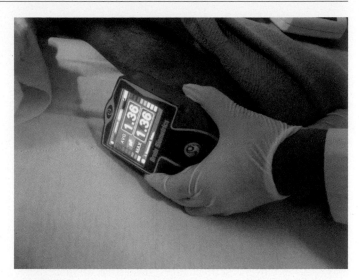

FIGURE 9.13 Use of a dermal phase meter, the SEM Scanner (Bruin Biometrics, LLC) to evaluate the heel of a patient. These devices typically require light skin touch and provide a reading of the moisture in the skin and tissues in 3 to 5 seconds. Higher readings reflect increased moisture in the skin and tissue as a result of local inflammatory response to tissue damage. (©B. M. Bates-Jensen.)

water are nearly identical and thus, the measure is reflective of total water content in the tissue.[122,123] Pure water has a dielectric constant of 78.5, the dielectric constant of air is 1, and normal skin is approximately 40.[118,122,123] For devices that measure in pF the range of readings is 0 to 4.096 pF with normal skin values between 0.9 and 2 pF.

At the cellular level, SEM indirectly measures the action potential of sodium and potassium across cell membranes. When tissues and cells are injured such as that occurs with early pressure-induced tissue damage, cellular permeability increases and the action potential across the cell membrane is decreased allowing quick/high electrical charges to pass through the tissues (e.g., SEM increases). Devices to measure SEM are small, hand-held dermal phase meters that require light skin touch with readings available within 3 to 8 seconds (Fig. 9.13).

SEM measures have been used to quantify wound healing in burn patients[124] and lymphedema presence in mastectomy patients,[125] and to examine erythema and stage I PUs.[126–129] In nursing home residents, SEM has detected inflammatory changes in the tissues, identifying prestage I and stage I pressure ulcers on the sacrum and buttocks.[127–129] In addition, SEM was higher (e.g., increased edema and inflammation) when residents exhibited no visible skin damage at the time but a stage I pressure ulcer was visible on the skin 1 week later. SEM values have identified 26%[127] and 30%[128] of the stage I pressure ulcers the following week, *25% more than with expert visual assessment.* SEM has also been used to detect erythema and stage I pressure ulcers in nursing home residents with dark skin tones.[129]

DIFFERENTIAL DIAGNOSIS

Clinical diagnosis of pressure ulcers can be complicated. Superficial stage II pressure ulcers and incontinence associated dermatitis (IAD) are often confused. Differentiating between skin failure and a terminal pressure ulcer is also difficult.

Superficial Stage II Pressure Ulcers and IAD

Assess the patient's skin for signs of IAD. IAD is inflammation of the skin that happens when the perineal area is subject to prolonged contact with urine or stool.[130] Objective signs of IAD include erythema, swelling, vesiculation, oozing, crusting, and scaling, with subjective symptoms of tingling, itching, burning, and pain[130,131] (Figs. 9.14 and 9.15). In persons with dark skin tones, IAD presents with white, dark red, purple, or yellow skin discoloration.[130,132,133] The condition can occur anywhere in the perineal region, which is broadly defined as the perineum (area between the vulva or scrotum and anus), buttocks, perianal area, coccyx, and upper/inner thigh regions. The clinical presentation is variable and may be dependent on the frequency of incontinence episode, rapidity and efficacy of postepisode hygiene, and duration of incontinence.[131,132]

IAD may present with manifestations characteristic of acute episodes, or chronic skin changes suggestive of more long-standing incontinence. In acute episodes, the skin characteristics most predominant are erythema, papulovesicular reaction, frank erosions and abrasions, and, in some cases, evidence of monilial infection, due to the moist warm environment. In general, a diffuse blanchable erythema is present involving buttock areas, coccyx area, perineum, perianal area, and upper/inner thighs. The extent of the erythema varies, and the intensity of the reaction may be muted in immunocompromised and some elderly patients. A papulovesicular rash is particularly evident in the groin and perineum areas (upper/inner thigh, vulva/scrotal area). Secondary skin changes include crusting and scaling, and are usually evident at the fringes of the reaction. Erosions and frank denudation of the skin may be more common with incontinence associated with feces. The distribution of the dermatitis differs in men and women, as might be expected. Typically, the more severe damage in male patients

occurs on the posterior aspect of the penile shaft and the anterior aspect of the scrotum. More damage is seen in the lower perineal regions, such as the inner thighs and low buttocks, than in the higher perineal regions, such as the sacral/coccygeal area or groin. In women, the skin damage usually involves the vulva and groin areas and spreads distally from those sites.

Chronic skin changes in patients with long-standing incontinence include a thickened appearance of skin where moisture is allowed to maintain skin contact, and increased evidence of scaling and crusting. The thickened appearance of the skin is due to urine or stool pooling on the skin. This skin is overhydrated and easily abraded, with minimal friction. The reaction is notable at the coccyx, scrotum, and vulva. Excoriation from patients' scratching at affected sites may also be present.[95] In many cases of long-standing incontinence, partial-thickness ulcers are present over the sacral/coccygeal area and medial buttocks region, close to the gluteal fold. Although these lesions present in a typical pressure ulcer location, some characteristics of these partial-thickness ulcers differ from characteristics seen with superficial pressure-induced skin trauma as shown in Table 9.1. First, the lesions tend to be multiple. The lesions may or may not be directly over a bony prominence, the lesions are typically surrounded by other characteristics of IAD (e.g., diffuse blanchable erythema), they may present as copy lesions, or "kissing" ulcers, where one lesion on the buttocks mirrors a second lesion on the opposite buttock and they may present in the gluteal cleft itself.

When caring for patients who are incontinent of urine and feces, you are faced with the challenge of preventing IAD and pressure ulceration as a result of the decreased tissue tolerance to trauma. As we have seen, superficial stage II pressure ulcers result from friction forces abrading the epidermis. When moisture, urine, and feces have caused maceration and

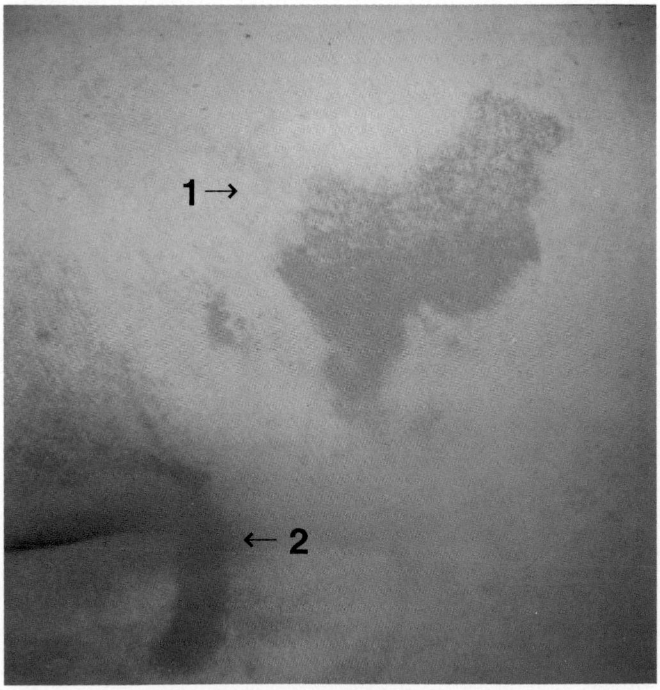

FIGURE 9.14 Superficial partial thickness ulcers caused by incontinence. Note the location of the damage is not over the bony prominence. (©B. M. Bates-Jensen.)

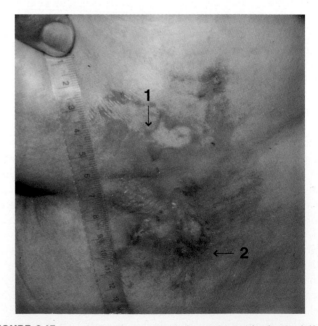

FIGURE 9.15 Incontinence associated dermatitis with classic differentiating characteristics of diffuse erythema across the buttocks and perineal area, and partial thickness skin loss. Note there are multiple, partial thickness ulcers with irregular wound edges and the ulcers occur across the area singly and in groups and not necessarily over the bony prominence. (©B. M. Bates-Jensen.)

TABLE 9.1	Characteristics of Pressure Ulcers and IAD				
	Pathologic Factors	**Incontinence**	**Location**	**Acute/Early Skin Signs**	**Chronic/Late Skin Signs**
Pressure ulcers	Any disease or condition that leads to limited mobility or immobility such that pressure/compression in association with • Friction • Shearing • Moisture over a bony prominence leads to skin and tissue damage	May or may not be present; if present, is a risk factor as moisture increases the coefficient of friction (i.e., less friction necessary to damage skin)	Pelvic locations: Sacrum, coccyx, buttocks, and ischial tuberosities No gender differences	• Progression from less severe, blanchable erythema to more severe, nonblanchable erythema • In dark-skinned individuals, purple-bluish color • Progression from increased temperature to cool temperature of the skin • Slight edema • Progression from intact skin to partial-thickness skin loss shallow crater (epidermis, dermis, or both)	• Full-thickness skin loss surrounded by blanchable or nonblanchable erythema • Progression to a deep crater (subcutaneous tissue to the fascia) to exposure of the muscle, bone, or supporting structures (i.e., tendon) • Surrounding skin may appear with deepening of ethnic skin tone or erythema, induration, warmth, possible mottling
Incontinence associated dermatitis	Moisture macerates the skin and the excess moisture in the skin tissues makes the epidermis friable. Urine and especially stool change the pH of the skin increasing the risk for skin infection and damage from friction.	Fecal or urinary incontinence must be present	Buttocks, coccyx, perineum, perianal area, and upper/inner thighs Male: • Common on the posterior side of the penile shaft and the anterior side of the scrotum • More damage typically on the lower perineal areas (i.e., inner thighs and low buttocks) Female: • Common on the vulva and groin areas and spreads distally out from those areas	Primary: • Diffuse, blanchable erythema • Papulovesicular reaction (specifically, in the groin and perineum areas) • Tingling, itching, burning, and pain • Frank erosions and abrasions • Monilial infection, in some cases Secondary: • Scaling and crusting at edges of papulovesicular reaction • Erosions and frank denudation especially with fecal incontinence	• Thickened appearance of the skin • Increased amount of scaling and crusting • Overhydrated • Easily abraded with minimal friction • Some evidence to support the presence of itching • Multiple lesions • Partial thickness • May or may not be over a bony prominence • Surrounded by other characteristics of incontinence associated dermatitis

overhydration of the epidermis, the skin and tissues are less tolerant of friction forces. Further moisture increases the coefficient of friction, which increases damage to the epidermis with less friction force applied. Stage II partial-thickness skin lesions, such as abrasions, are most commonly attributed to friction and shearing forces and it is likely that incontinence plays a critical role in the development of superficial pressure ulcers.[134]

Skin Failure and Terminal Pressure ulcers

Persons at life's end, during an acute critical illness or with severe trauma may experience skin failure or terminal pressure ulcers. Skin failure is defined as an acute episode where the skin and subcutaneous tissues die (become necrotic) due to hypoperfusion that occurs concurrent with severe dysfunction

or failure of other organ systems.[135] It is the hypoperfusion that creates an extreme inflammatory reaction along with severe dysfunction or failure of multiple organ systems that compromises the skin. The skin, the largest organ of the body, is no different from other organs, and also can become dysfunctional. Skin compromise, including changes related to decreased perfusion and hypoxia, can occur at the tissue, cellular, or molecular level resulting in decreased oxygen availability and reduction in nutrient use by the tissues.[136–138] These changes weaken the skin making it less tolerant of mechanical forces such as pressure, shear, and friction. Skin failure may present anywhere on the body (not just bony prominences) but often occurs over bony prominences.

One manifestation of skin failure may be a terminal pressure ulcer. One of the first clinical descriptions of terminal ulcers was

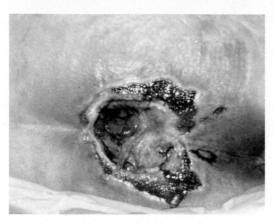

FIGURE 9.16 Suspected terminal pressure ulcer in a nursing home patient. The ulcer progressed rapidly even with intervention. The ulcer is butterfly–shaped with each buttock mirroring the ulceration on the opposite buttock. (©B. M. Bates-Jensen.)

by Kennedy in 1989.[139] Kennedy described a specific subgroup of pressure ulcers that some individuals developed as they were dying. They present typically over the sacrum and are shaped like a pear, butterfly, or horseshoe (Fig. 9.16).[139] The ulcers are a variety of colors including red, yellow, or black, are sudden in onset, typically deteriorate rapidly, and usually indicate that death is imminent with just over half (55.7%) dying within 6 weeks of discovery of the ulcer. Others have also reported terminal pressure ulcers occurring in the 2 weeks prior to death.[140]

PRESSURE ULCER RISK SCREENING

Pressure ulcers are physical evidence of multiple causative influences, and our discussion of etiology and pathophysiology would not be complete if we failed to identify these. Understanding the factors that make an individual susceptible to pressure ulcer development is an essential component of prevention programs and includes risk screening and risk assessment. Risk screening and assessment are strategies for targeting interventions to those persons most in need of protection. Pressure ulcer risk screening involves identification of individuals for whom a more complete risk assessment is needed. Risk assessment is a method of determining the specific factors that place an individual at increased risk of developing a pressure ulcer. Risk assessment should include use of a risk assessment scale or tool to identify specific factors that place an individual at increased risk for pressure ulcer development, skin assessment to determine existing skin condition, and clinical judgment based on specialty-specific indicators related to a person's risk status.[141] We first discuss risk factors in general, then provide guidance on risk screening and finally review risk assessment tools and assessment for specialty-specific factors and skin assessment.

Risk Factors for Pressure Ulcer Development

It may be helpful to classify risk factors into two general groups: those that increase the pressure force over the bony prominence, and those that reduce the tolerance of the tissues to pressure. Figure 9.17 illustrates Braden and Bergstrom's conceptual framework, which divides factors into these two categories according to the role they play in pressure ulcer development.

Immobility, inactivity, and sensory loss increase pressure. Extrinsic factors (shear, friction, and moisture) and intrinsic factors (poor nutrition, advanced age, and reduced arteriolar pressure) reduce tissue tolerance. Several additional areas may influence pressure ulcer development: concurrent medical conditions, emotional stress, temperature, smoking, and interstitial fluid flow.[141,142]

Immobility, Inactivity, and Sensory Loss

Any disease process leading to immobility and limited activity levels, whether a spinal cord injury, dementia, Parkinson disease, severe congestive heart failure, or lung disease, increases the risk of pressure ulcers. Immobility or severely restricted mobility is the most important risk factor for all populations and a necessary condition for the development of pressure ulcers. Mobility is the state of being movable. Thus, the immobile patient cannot move, or facility and ease of movement is impaired. Exton-Smith and Sherwin[143] demonstrated that 90% of individuals with 20 or fewer spontaneous nocturnal body movements developed a pressure ulcer, whereas none of the persons with greater than 50 movements per night developed a pressure ulcer.

Closely related to immobility is limited activity. Often defined clinically as the ability of the individual to ambulate and move about, activity is more generally the production of energy or motion. Patients who are bed or chair bound and are thus inactive are at greater risk for pressure ulcer development.[144–146] A sudden reduction in activity level may signal a deterioration in health status and increased potential for pressure ulcer development.

Sensory loss increases the risk for compression of tissues and pressure ulcer development because the normal mechanism for translating pain messages from the tissues is dysfunctional. Patients with intact nervous system pathways feel continuous local pressure, become uncomfortable, and change their position before tissue ischemia occurs. These responses are reduced or absent in patients with spinal cord injury and many patients with altered mental status. Thus, these patients have a higher incidence and prevalence of pressure ulcers.[147,148] Specifically, patients with paraplegia or quadriplegia are unable to sense increased pressure, and if their body weight is not shifted, pressure ulceration develops. Further, denervation of the muscle tissue changes the functional nature of the tissue making it more susceptible to mechanical forces of deformation and pressure. Likewise, patients with changes in mental status functioning may not feel the discomfort from pressure, not be alert enough to move spontaneously, not remember to move, be too confused to respond to commands to move, or be physically unable to move.

RESEARCH WISDOM

Immobility

Immobility or severely restricted mobility is the most important risk factor for all populations and a necessary condition for the development of pressure ulcers.

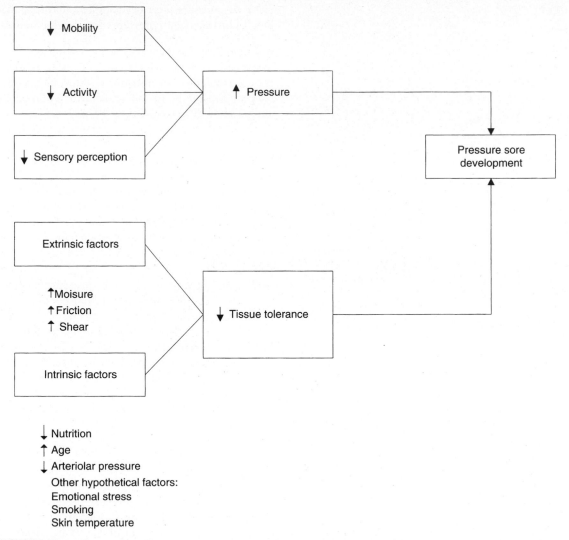

FIGURE 9.17 Factors contribution to the development of pressure ulcers. (Reprinted from Braden, B. (1987), a conceptual schema for the study of the etiology of pressure sores. Rehabilitation Nursing, 12(1), 9 with permission of the Association of Rehabilitation Nurses. Copyright © 1987 by the Association of Rehabilitation Nurses.)

Extrinsic Factors

Extrinsic risk factors are those external forces that make the tissues less tolerant of pressure. Extrinsic forces include shear, friction, and moisture (see Fig. 9.17).

Shear

At the beginning of this chapter, we noted that, whereas pressure acts perpendicularly to cause ischemia, shear is a parallel force that causes ischemia by displacing blood vessels laterally, thereby impeding blood flow to tissues.[134,149,150] Shear acts to stretch and twist tissues and blood vessels at the bony tissue interface and, as such, affects the deep blood vessels and deeper tissue structures. Further, eschar formation may be a result of larger vessel damage below the skin surface from shearing forces. Shear forces are those responsible for deformation of tissues (both the strain—relative deformation and the stress—force transferred per unit area).[141] Figure 9.18 shows the effect of shearing and friction on the tissues when the head of the bed is raised.

Shear is caused by the interplay of gravity and friction. The most common circumstance for shear occurs in the bed patient in a semi-Fowler position (semisitting position with knees flexed and supported by pillows on the bed or by elevation of the head of the bed). The patient's skeleton slides down toward the foot of the bed, but the sacral skin stays in place (with the help of friction against the bed linen). This produces stretching, pinching of cells and occlusion of the underlying vessels, resulting in ulcers with large areas of internal tissue damage at the muscle level and less damage at the skin surface.

Friction

Friction and moisture, although not direct factors in pressure ulcer development, have been identified as contributing to the problem by reducing tolerance of tissues to pres-sure.[134] Friction occurs when two surfaces move across one another. Friction acts on the tissue tolerance to pressure

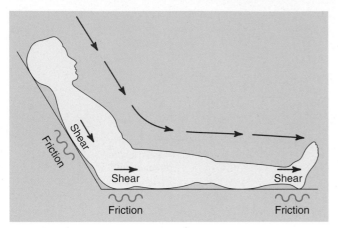

FIGURE 9.18 Mechanical forces contribute to pressure ulcer development. As the person slides down or is improperly pulled up in bed, friction resists this movement. Shear occurs when one layer of tissue slides over another, disrupting microcirculation of skin and subcutaneous tissue. (Reprinted from Smeltzer SC, Bare BG. *Brunnar & Suddarth's Textbook of Medical -Surgical Nursing.* 9th ed. Philadelphia, PA: Lippincott Williams & Wilkins; 2000, with permission.)

by abrading and damaging the epidermal and upper dermal layers of the skin. Additionally, friction acts with gravity to cause shear. Friction abrades the epidermis, which may lead to superficial pressure ulcer development by increasing the skin's susceptibility to pressure injury and increases the risk for infection. Pressure combined with friction produces ulcerations at lower pressures than does pressure alone.[134] Friction acts in conjunction with shear to contribute to development of sacral/coccygeal superficial pressure ulcers on patients in the semi-Fowler position.

Moisture

Moisture contributes to pressure ulcer development by removing oils on the skin, making it more friable and less tolerant of mechanical forces, as well as by interacting with body support surface friction. Constant moisture leads to maceration of the epidermis. Once it is eroded, there is increased likelihood of further tissue breakdown. Moisture also alters the resiliency of the epidermis to external forces. Both shearing force and friction increase in the presence of mild to moderate moisture.

Excess moisture may be due to wound drainage, diaphoresis, and fecal or urinary incontinence. In fact, urinary and fecal incontinence are common risk factors associated with pressure ulcer development. Incontinence contributes to pressure ulcer formation by creating excess moisture on the skin and by chemical damage to the skin.[151] Fecal incontinence has an added detrimental effect: the presence of bacteria in the stool, which can contribute to infection as well as to skin breakdown. Enzymes in stool also contribute to skin breakdown.[151–154] In the presence of both urinary and fecal incontinence, the pH in the perineal area is increased by the fecal enzymes' conversion of urea to ammonia. The elevated pH increases the activity of proteases and lipases found in stool, which, in turn, cause increased permeability of the skin, leading to irritation by other agents, such as bile salts.[152–154] Inadequately managed incontinence poses a significant risk

factor for pressure ulcer development, and fecal incontinence is highly correlated with pressure ulcer development.[130,141]

Intrinsic Risk Factors

The major intrinsic risk factors affecting tissue tolerance to pressure include poor nutritional status, increased age, reduced oxygenation and perfusion, and concurrent medical conditions and psychological factors (Fig. 9.17).

Nutrition

Weight loss, cachexia, and malnutrition are all commonly identified as risk factors predisposing patients to pressure ulcer development.[155,156] In addition, individuals with low serum albumin levels (hypoalbuminemia) are at increased risk for pressure ulcers. Measures of nutritional intake[157,158] and weight[159] are also predictive of pressure ulcer development.

Age

Advanced age is a risk factor for pressure ulcer development with several studies identifying that persons over age 70 are more susceptible to pressure ulcers.[145,157–162] The skin and support structures undergo changes in the aging process. There is a loss of muscle, a decrease in serum albumin levels, diminished inflammatory response, decreased elasticity, and reduced cohesion between the dermis and epidermis.[163] These changes combine with other changes related to aging to make the skin less tolerant of pressure forces, shear, and friction.

Reduced Oxygenation and Perfusion

Factors that reduce oxygenation and perfusion of the skin and tissues increase the likelihood of pressure ulcer development. Reduced arteriolar pressure produces hypoperfusion of the tissues leading to compromised oxygenation and hypoxia of the skin. Hypoperfusion of the tissues decreases the tolerance of the tissues for mechanical forces. Reduction in arteriolar flow and the resultant skin compromise typically occurs in critically ill patients with cardiovascular instability or norepinephrine use and these persons are at higher risk for pressure ulcers.[146,157,160,164–166] Persons with low blood pressure[146,157,160] and diabetes mellitus[145,157] also experience decreased oxygenation and perfusion of tissues increasing risk for pressure ulcer development.

Concurrent Medical Conditions and Psychological Factors

Certain medical conditions or disease states are also associated with pressure ulcer development. Orthopedic injuries specifically hip fractures and spinal cord injury[11–14] (in addition to the sensory loss) are such conditions.[167] Others have examined psychological factors that may increase risk for pressure ulcer development.[168] These include poor self-concept, depression, and chronic emotional stress.[167] General health status has also been associated with pressure ulcer development. Higher illness severity scores or increased acuity,[146,157,164–166] acute versus elective admission to the hospital,[157] mechanical ventilation specifically in pediatric patients,[166] and length of stay all increase risk for pressure ulcer development.

Risk Screening

Certain risk factors can be easily identified and used to quickly screen individuals in order to place them immediately on a general prevention program. For these individuals, a more complete risk assessment is necessary to identify specific factors that are amenable to more targeted prevention strategies. Screening is particularly useful for acute care hospitals and specific populations. Screening factors range from individual factors such as age to factors that are more related to procedures or medical conditions such as emergent admission to the hospital or prolonged surgical time. Some factors that might be used as a screen for pressure ulcer risk include the following:

- Demographic characteristics: female gender, African American race, and advanced age (over 75 years old).[169,170]
- As a general screen, individuals of all ages who have limited mobility or for whom movement is not possible without staff or caregiver assistance should be considered at risk. This includes persons who are unable to move due to sedation.[170]
- Persons admitted to the hospital from a nursing home. These individuals are already frail as they require nursing home care and they are acutely ill.[171]
- Persons admitted to the critical care unit from the emergency department.[172]
- Persons over 65 years old admitted to the acute care hospital who are scheduled for a surgical procedure anticipated to be 4 hours or longer.
- Patients who experience intraoperative hypotensive episodes.[89,141]
- Elders admitted to the hospital from the community who were found down for a prolonged time.
- Patients undergoing special therapy, for example, oncology patients admitted for bone marrow transplant or with graft versus host disease.
- Patients with hospital transport times greater than 1 hour.
- Patients readmitted to a nursing home from the hospital.
- All persons who have had a previous pressure ulcer and especially persons with spinal cord injury or dysfunction with prior pressure ulcers.[170]
- Patients admitted to the acute care hospital with any diagnosis affecting skin integrity (besides obvious open wounds this includes gangrene, nutritional deficiencies, diabetes, anemia).[169]
- Patients admitted to the acute care hospital with system failure including paralysis, senility, respiratory failure, acute renal failure, cerebral vascular accident, and nonhypertensive congestive heart failure.[169,170]
- Patients admitted to the acute care hospital with infection: sepsis, osteomyelitis, pneumonia, bacterial infections, and urinary tract infections.[169]
- Intensive care unit patients with sepsis, surgery times greater than or equal to 8 hours, or long-term vasopressor therapy (consider at high risk).[173–175]

Pressure ulcer risk screening should not take the place of risk assessment but rather mobilize you to complete a more comprehensive pressure ulcer risk assessment.

Risk Assessment Tools

For practitioners to intervene cost-effectively, a method of evaluating persons for the presence of risk factors is necessary. Risk assessment tools promote prevention by distinguishing patients who are at risk for pressure ulcer development from those who are not. The use of a risk assessment tool also enables you to allocate resources effectively, targeting interventions to specific risk factors for specific patients. Selection of which risk assessment instrument to use is determined by reliability of the tool for the intended raters, predictive validity of the tool for the population, sensitivity and specificity of the instrument under consideration, and ease of use and time required for completion. The most common risk assessment tools are the Norton Scale[176,177] and the Braden Scale for Predicting Pressure Sore Risk.[142,178,179] We also discuss two risk assessment scales developed for specific populations, the Braden Q scale for use in infants and children[24,180] and a supplement to the Braden Scale for evaluating high-risk critical care patients.[173]

The Norton Scale

The Norton Scale is the oldest risk assessment instrument. Developed in 1961, it consists of five subscales: physical condition, mental state, activity, mobility, and incontinence.[176] Each parameter is rated on a scale of 1 to 4, with 4 being normal. The sum of the ratings for all five parameters yields a total score ranging from 5 to 20. Scores of 17 to 20 are considered low risk. A score of 13 to 16 indicates "onset of risk," and scores 12 and below indicating high risk for pressure ulcer formation.[177]

The Braden Scale for Predicting Pressure Sore Risk

The Braden Scale was developed in 1987 and is composed of six subscales that conceptually reflect degrees of sensory perception, moisture, activity, mobility, nutrition, and friction and shear.[178,179] All subscales are rated from 1 to 4, except for friction and shear, which is rated from 1 to 3. The subscales may be summed for a total score, with a range from 6 to 23 (see Exhibit 9.2).

Lower scores indicate lower function and higher risk for developing a pressure ulcer. The cutoff score for hospitalized adults is considered to be 18, with scores of 18 and below indicating at-risk status.[96,142] In older patients, some have found cutoff scores of 17 or 18 to be better predictors of risk status.[160,179] Levels of risk are based on the predictive value of a positive test. Scores of 15 to 16 indicate mild risk, with a 50% to 60% chance of developing a stage I pressure ulcer; scores of 12 to 14

CLINICAL WISDOM

Pressure Ulcer Risk Assessment in Nursing Homes

The only risk assessment tool recognized by the CMS is the Resident Assessment Protocol (RAP) for Pressure Ulcers. Pressure ulcer risk screening occurs in nursing homes with the use of the Minimum Data Set (MDS), which must be completed within 7 days of admission. This is then followed by completing the pressure ulcer RAP for risk assessment.

EXHIBIT 9.2

Braden Scale for Predicting Pressure Sore Risk

Patient's Name—————— Evaluator's Name—————— Date of Assessment

Sensory Perception	1. Completely Limited:	2. Very Limited:	3. Slightly Limited:	4. No Impairment:
Ability to respond meaningfully to pressure-related discount	Unresponsive (does not moan, flinch, or grasp) to painful stimuli, due to diminished level of consciousness or sedation. OR limited ability to feel pain over most of body surface.	Responds only to painful stimuli. Cannot communicate discomfort except by moaning or restlessness. OR has a sensory impairment that limits the ability to feel pain or discomfort over 1/2 of body.	Responds to verbal commands, but cannot always communicate discomfort or need to be turned. OR has some sensory impairment that limits ability to feel pain or discomfort in one or two extremities.	Responds to verbal commands. Has no sensory deficit which would limit ability to feel or voice pain or discomfort.
Moisture	**1. Constantly Moist:**	**2. Very Moist:**	**3. Occasionally Moist:**	**4. Rarely Moist:**
Degree to which skin is exposed to moisture	Skin is kept moist almost constantly by perspiration, urine, etc. Dampness is detected every time patient is moved or turned.	Skin is often, but not always moist. Linen must be changed at least once a shift.	Skin is occasionally moist, requiring an extra linen change approximately once a day.	Skin is usually dry, linen only requires changing at routine intervals.
Activity	**1. Bedfast:**	**2. Chairfast:**	**3. Walks Occasionally:**	**4. Walks Frequently:**
Degree of physical activity	Confined to bed.	Ability to walk severely limited or nonexistent. Cannot bear own weight and/or must be assisted into chair or wheelchair.	Walks occasionally during day, but for very short distances, with or without assistance. Spends majority of each shift in bed or chair.	Walks outside the room at least twice a day and inside room at least once every 2 h during waking hours.
mobility	**1. Completely Immobile:**	**2. Very Limited:**	**3. Slightly Limited:**	**4. No Limitations:**
Ability to change and control body position	Does not make even slight changes in body or extremity position without assistance.	Makes occasional slight changes in body or extremity position but unable to make frequent or significant changes independently.	Makes frequent though slight changes in body or extremity position independently.	Makes major and frequent changes in position without assistance.
NUTRITION	**1. Very Poor:**	**2. Probably Inadequate:**	**3. Adequate:**	**4. Excellent:**
Usual food intake pattern	Never eats a complete meal. Rarely eats more than 1/3 of any food offered. Eats 2 servings or less of protein (meat or dairy products) per day. Takes fluids poorly. Does not take a liquid dietary supplement. OR is NPO and/or maintained on clear liquids or IVs for more than 5 d.	Rarely eats a complete meal and generally eats only about 1/2 of any food offered. Protein intake includes only 3 servings of meat or dairy products per day. Occasionally will take a dietary supplement. OR receives less than optimum amount of liquid diet or tube feeding.	Eats over half of most meals. Eats a total of 4 servings of protein (meat, dairy products) each day. Occasionally will refuse a meal, but will usually take a supplement if offered. OR is on a tube feeding or TPN regimen that probably meets most of nutritional needs.	Eats most of every meal. Never refuses a meal. Usually eats a total of 4 or more servings of meat and dairy products. Occasionally eats between meals. Does not require supplementation.
FRICTION AND SHEAR	**1. Problem:**	**2. Potential Problem:**	**3. No Apparent Problem:**	
Requires moderate to maximum assistance in moving. Complete lifting without sliding against sheets is impossible. Frequently slides down in bed or chair, requiring frequent repositioning with maximum assistance. Spasticity, contractures, or agitation leads to almost constant friction.	Moves feebly or requires minimum assistance. During a move skin probably slides to some extent against sheets, chair, restraints, or other devices. Maintains relatively good position in chair or bed most of the time but occasionally slides down.	Moves in bed and in chair independently and has sufficient muscle strength to lift up completely during move. Maintains good position in bed or chair at all times.		

Total Score

Source: Copyright © 1988, Barbara J. Braden and Nancy Bergstrom.

indicate moderate risk, with a 65% to 90% chance of developing a stage I or II lesion; and scores below 12 indicate high risk, with a 90% to 100% chance of developing a stage II or deeper pressure ulcer.[96,179]

The Braden Scale has been tested in acute care and long-term care settings with several levels of nurse raters and demonstrates high interrater reliability with registered nurses. The Braden scale offers the best balance between sensitivity and specificity and the best risk estimate.[181] Validity has been established by expert opinion, and predictive validity has been studied in several acute care settings, with good sensitivity and specificity demonstrated.[96,160] The Braden Scale has a firm evidence base and is the most widely used instrument in the United States. However, it is not the ideal risk assessment tool for pediatrics, critically ill patients, or for persons with spinal cord injury. For use with infants and children, the Braden scale has been adapted by altering the subscales slightly to reflect developmental needs of the pediatric population. In critically ill patients, it may require supplemental assessment to identify those at highest risk. In the spinal cord–injured population, the risk factors may not be different, rather it is a matter of range restriction or a floor effect as everyone with a spinal cord injury is at risk for pressure ulcer development.

The Braden Q Scale

Risk assessment for pressure ulcer risk in pediatrics is targeted at acutely ill infants and children. Immobility and hemodynamic instability present the same concerns in the pediatric population that they do in the adult population. Quigley and Curley adapted the Braden Scale for use in the pediatric population.[180] The Braden Q scale adaptations involved changing subscale definitions to reflect developmental needs of pediatric patients, the prevalence of tube feedings in this population, and the availability of laboratory and other noninvasive diagnostic tests for acutely ill pediatric patients. Modifications include the following:

- Mobility: changed "2 very limited" to unable to completely turn self independently.
- Activity: all patients unable to walk based on developmental age are scored a "4, walks frequently."
- Sensory perception: refined definition, ability to respond in a developmentally appropriate way to pressure-related discomfort.
- Moisture: changed frequency of definitions of linen changes.

RESEARCH WISDOM

Does Risk Assessment Matter?

Yes, it does! A systematic review of risk assessment scales for pressure ulcer prevention, which included 33 studies on risk assessment scale validation and 3 studies on clinical judgment alone, found that use of either the Braden or Norton Scale are more accurate than nurses' clinical judgment in predicting pressure ulcer risk. Further, use of a scale increases the intensity and effectiveness of prevention interventions.[181]

- Friction and Shear: added additional category at the low end to account for different pediatric patient groups and refined operational definitions of each choice.
- Nutrition: added feedings to the definitions, defined as adequate or not for age, and added albumin levels.
- Added a new category, "Tissue Perfusion and Oxygenation": this subscale quantifies tissue perfusion and uses arterial pressure readings, oxygen saturation, hemoglobin levels, capillary refill, and/or serum pH, all of which are commonly available in a pediatric acute care setting.[143]

Each subscale on the Braden Q is rated from 1 to 4 with 1 indicating high risk and 4 indicating less risk. The range of scores is from 7 to 28 points and persons with scores less than 23 are considered at risk for pressure ulcer development.[180] Generally, scores of 25 to 21 are considered at mild risk, those with scores of 16 to 21 moderate risk, and scores below 16 high risk. In a study of patients in pediatric intensive care units using a cutoff score of 16 for determining risk resulted in sensitivity of 0.88 and specificity of 0.58.[24] The performance of the Braden Q scale with pediatric patients is similar to the performance of the Braden Scale in adults. Risk assessment with the Braden Q scale should occur on admission to the pediatric intensive care unit as most pressure ulcers develop within 24 hours after an infant or child is admitted.[24] Although, some subscales on the Braden Q scale require trending information, determining risk quickly in this high-risk population is essential.

High-risk Critical Care Patient Risk Assessment

Patients in critical care settings often experience uncontrollable risk factors placing them at very high risk for pressure ulcers. While use of the Braden Scale is helpful in identifying patients at risk in most health-care settings, additional factors may increase risk for patients in intensive care, thus a method of further assessment may be helpful. Essentially, the goal of pressure ulcer risk assessment in critically ill patients is to target more aggressive prevention strategies to the "sickest of the sick."[173] Uncontrollable factors specific to intensive care that increase risk for critically ill patients include multiple surgical procedures, mechanical ventilation, sedation or paralytics, traction and/or external fixators, weeping anasarca, shock, multiorgan dysfunction syndrome, cardiac arrest, multiple vasopressors, drive lines, and nitric oxide ventilation.[173–175] To identify these high-risk patients, Brindle developed a supplement to the Braden Scale for use with critically ill patients.[173] The high-risk identifier tool is designed to target patients for immediate prevention actions. Two groups of criteria are identified: automatic action criteria and summary criteria. Automatic action criteria are factors that, if any single factor is present, require prevention actions. Summary criteria are a second group of factors that are actionable if five or more are present. The automatic action criteria include

1. Surgical procedure greater than 8 hours (may be cumulative surgeries = 8 hours)
2. Cardiac arrest during current admission
3. Vasopressors greater than 48 hours
4. In shock, SIRS, MODS

If five of the summary criteria are present, the clinician should initiate additional prevention actions and these criteria include

- Weeping edema/anasarca
- Traction
- Morbid obesity
- Age greater than 65 years old
- Diabetes Mellitus
- Bedrest
- Liver failure
- Malnutrition (prealbumin <20, albumin <2.5, or NPO >3 days)
- Sedation/paralytics greater than 48 hours
- Mechanical ventilation greater than 48 hours
- Quadriplegia or spinal cord injury
- Nitric oxide ventilation
- Restraints
- Drive lines (LVAD, RVAD, Balloon pump)
- Past history of pressure ulcers

Use of a supplement to the Braden Scale such as developed for critically ill patients is an approach that may be beneficial for other risk groups. For example, if other general major risk factors are present such as fever, poor dietary intake of protein, diastolic pressure less than 60 mm Hg, or hemodynamic instability, then advance the patient to the next level of risk regardless of their total Braden Scale score:

- Mild risk: 15 to 18
- Moderate risk: 13 to 14
- High risk: 10 to 12
- Very High risk: ≤ 9

Conducting a risk assessment using a scale or tool and identifying specialty-specific risk factors are only the first steps in pressure ulcer risk assessment. It should be followed by a comprehensive skin assessment.

Skin Assessment

A complete skin assessment is a critical part of risk assessment as persons with existing pressure ulcers or other skin damage are at higher risk for pressure ulcer development. Key areas for skin assessment are the common bony locations for pressure ulcer development: sacrum, coccyx, ischial tuberosities, trochanters, buttocks, ankles, heels. Medical devices should be removed and the skin examined for wounds, abrasions, or signs of pressure damage. Other areas for examination include the occiput of the head, shoulder blades, elbows,

> ### CLINICAL WISDOM
>
> #### Skin Assessment
>
> Use of technology and devices such as ultrasound, skin temperature measurement, spectroscopy, or SEM to better detect pressure-induced tissue damage is recommended as a part of skin assessment.

> ### CLINICAL WISDOM
>
> Handle the skin gently to prevent skin tears, especially in older patients. The epidermis and dermis junction is lessened with age, making older patients at higher risk for skin tears.

hips, and knees. Observe for open wounds, abrasions, evidence of friction, signs of early pressure damage, IAD, skin tears, and rashes.

General skin assessment parameters are discussed in Chapter 3. Briefly, examine the skin for moisture, temperature, sensory deficits, edema, and induration. Evaluate the patient's skin for dryness and cracking. Skin texture should be smooth and elastic. Dehydration is present if the skin is dry, wrinkled, withered, and has poor turgor. Older adults are at higher risk for dry skin, and dry skin may decrease tissue tolerance to external forces. To check for turgor in older adults, check the forehead or sternum and gently lift the skin, if the skin "tents" or hangs in the shape you lifted it before resuming normal position, the patient may be dehydrated. Lack of moisture in the air may contribute to dry skin and can be counteracted by use of a humidifier in the room.

Skin should be warm to touch. The dorsal aspect of the hand is more sensitive to temperature changes than the palm of the hand; thus, clinicians should use the dorsal aspect of the hand to judge skin temperature. Two-point discrimination is used to evaluate skin sensation. The patient should be able to distinguish sharp, dull, or pressure sensations against the skin surface. Diminished sensation may be generalized or localized to a specific area, such as the lower extremities. Edema causes the skin to appear taut and shiny and may present as pitting or nonpitting. Induration is an abnormal stiffness or firmness to the tissues. Both edema and induration may indicate underlying tissue damage. Observe for coloration changes over bony prominences and areas subject to pressure forces. If skin color is altered, check for blanching. It is essential that the skin assessment be documented in the medical record on

> ### CLINICAL WISDOM
>
> #### Who Can Conduct Skin Assessments?
>
> The skin assessment must be performed by registered nurses or physicians. Direct care providers can be taught to inspect the skin for characteristics may indicate a problem. Caregivers can monitor the wound by taking digital photographs and transmitting them to health-care providers for evaluation. Thus, caregivers can *inspect* and *monitor* the skin for changes indicating a potential problem and notify licensed providers of areas of concern, but they cannot assess the skin.

admission to the health-care facility. This ensures that areas of concern and areas with existing damage are communicated to the health-care team. Skin assessment should be conducted daily at a minimum. Additionally, in acute care hospitals skin assessment of major pressure areas (sacrum, buttocks, ischial tuberosities, and heels for adults, occiput and buttocks for pediatrics) should be conducted whenever a change in provider occurs; at the change of shift as part of the handoff to the nurse taking over the care, whenever the patient is transferred to a new unit or different level of care and prior to discharge from the facility.

Risk Assessment Frequency

Persons admitted to general medical–surgical units of hospitals should have risk assessment conducted on admission and if the risk assessment indicates "at risk," every 48 hours after admission. Those persons admitted to critical care units should have a risk assessment that includes specialty-specific risk factors conducted on admission and at least daily thereafter.[182]

In long-term care, conduct pressure ulcer risk assessment on admission to the facility and if the risk assessment score indicates "at risk" then weekly for 4 weeks, and for all residents quarterly or whenever a change in status occurs.[182] The MDS is the mandated resident assessment for all persons admitted to nursing homes and this must be completed within 7 days of admission to the facility. However, completing the pressure ulcer risk assessment within 24 hours of admission is recommended. For home care patients, assess risk on admission to home healthcare, weekly for the first 4 weeks, and every other week thereafter until day 62 depending on patient condition and frequency of home visits.[20]

Of course, regardless of health-care setting, risk assessment should be performed whenever a significant change occurs in the patient's general health and status. A registered nurse should perform risk assessment. However, in many instances, a registered nurse will need input from the direct-care provider, such as a family member or a nursing attendant.

Specific prevention strategies should be targeted to risk factors identified in individual patients. In those persons in whom prevention is not successful, the continued monitoring of risk status may prevent further tissue trauma at the wound site and development of additional wound sites. Exhibit 9.3 presents a flow diagram for determining prevention strategies based on risk factor assessment.

Risk Stratification

Risk stratification is a method of arranging data related to quantifiable outcomes, resource utilization, or other phenomena associated with pressure ulcer prevention or treatment by level of risk. For example, using the Braden Scale for Risk Assessment instrument, patients can be stratified, or grouped, according to their levels of risk, as follows:

- Mild risk = 15 to 18 Braden Score
- Moderate risk = 13 to 14 Braden Score
- High risk = 10 to 12 Braden Score
- Very high risk= ≤9 Braden Score

EXHIBIT 9.3

Determining Prevention Strategies Based on Risk Factor Assessment

Presence of tissue trauma over bony prominence? (usual locations: sacral/coccygeal, trochanter, ischial tuberosity, malleolus, heel)

NO	YES, provide for wound assessment and treatment plus prevention strategies

Patient NOT chair or bed bound and thus at no or low risk?
(patient scores a 1 or 2 on Braden Scale activity subscale)

NO, complete full risk assessment	YES, do not need further risk assessment at this time

Pressure ulcer risk factors present?

Immobility	Inactivity	Decreased Sensory Perception	Nutrition	Friction and Shear	Moisture Urinary and Fecal Incontinence

Prevention interventions by risk factors:

Immobility, Inactivity, and Decreased Sensory Perception		Malnutrition	Friction and Shear	Moisture Incontinence
passive repositioning, pillow bridging, pressure-reducing/relieving support surfaces		provide nutrition supplement: protein, calorie, vitamin C, zinc, iron	cornstarch, lubricants, pad protectors, transparent film, thin hydrocolloid dressings, turning, and draw sheets	absorbent products, diagnosis of incontinence, general skin care

Risk stratification can give a more realistic picture of a facility's progress in prevention of pressure ulcers. It can also supply a more realistic means of comparison between different institutions' outcomes. Risk stratification can also provide a tool to see where strengths and weaknesses in the program of prevention might exist.

PRESSURE ULCER PREVENTION STRATEGIES

Pressure ulcer prevention includes actions to reduce pressure effects, maintain skin integrity, and address nutritional status. Early interventions to prevent the development of pressure ulcers should focus on eliminating specific risk factors. Prevention interventions should also be appropriate to the patient's *level* of risk. For example, the risk factor of immobility is managed very differently for the comatose patient versus the spinal cord–injured patient. The comatose patient requires that you educate the caregiver, especially about repositioning. The spinal cord–injured patient requires self-care education and may be able to perform self-repositioning. Thus, the intervention for the risk factor of immobility is very different for these two patients.

Reduce Pressure Effects

Patients with impaired ability to reposition and who cannot independently change body positions must have local pressure alleviated by scheduled repositioning performed by the caregiver and use of pressure redistribution support surfaces for chair and bed. Additional strategies include measures to increase mobility and activity and to decrease friction and shear.

Scheduled Repositioning

Scheduled repositioning is part of all pressure ulcer clinical practice guidelines as a key intervention for patients with immobility risk factors. Scheduled repositioning is a costly prevention strategy as it involves significant use of staff time and it is difficult to implement on a consistent continual basis. Typically, repositioning schedules are based on event or time. Event-based schedules relate to typical events during the day, for example, repositioning the patient after each meal. If time based, repositioning schedules are usually interpreted as every 2 hours for full-body change of position and more often for small shifts in position. Full-body change of position involves turning the patient to a new lying position, for example, turning the patient from the right side-lying position to the left side-lying position or the supine position.

How often should repositioning occur? Frequency of repositioning should be based on the individual's tissue tolerance, level of mobility and activity, medical condition, skin integrity, treatment goals, and support surface use.[141,170] Use of 4-hour repositioning schedules in conjunction with use of viscoelastic support surfaces has been shown to reduce the frequency and time to occurrence of stage II or greater pressure ulcers compared to standard care (no turning schedule), those on standard hospital mattresses who were turned every 2 and every 4 hours and to persons on a viscoelastic support surface

who were turned every 6 hours.[183] Further, there was no significant difference in the incidence of stage II or greater pressure ulcers between patients on a viscoelastic support surface who were placed in a lateral position for 2 hours and those who were allowed to remain in a lateral position for 4 hours, thus supporting use of a 4-hour repositioning frequency when used in conjunction with a viscoelastic pressure-redistributing support surface.[183,184] In general, for patients on a standard hospital mattress repositioning should occur every 2 hours. Persons with acute spinal cord injury may require more frequent repositioning because of the microvascular dysfunction that occurs.[109]

In what position should patients be placed? Use the 30-degree side-lying position as shown in Figure 9.19 alternating with the supine position and prone position (if the patient can tolerate proning). When the side-lying position is used in bed, avoidance of direct pressure on the trochanter is recommended. Transcutaneous oxygen and blood flow measures at the trochanter are decreased in the 90-degree side-lying position, even if the patient is placed on a pressure-redistributing support surface.[185–187] Interface pressures also have been shown to be higher in the 90-degree side-lying position and although interface pressures are an intermediate outcome measure, the use of the 90-degree side-lying position is not recommended. To avoid placing pressure on the trochanter, position the patient in a 30-degree laterally inclined side-lying position instead of the 90-degree side-lying position. The 30-degree side-lying position allows for distribution of pressure over a greater area (see Fig. 9.19). However, in studies evaluating the use of the 30-degree side-lying position, many participants (30% to 60%) are noted to have changed their positions from the 30-degree side-lying position to a supine position in-between repositioning events.[184,187] This suggests that use of the 30-degree side-lying position may not be comfortable for patients, it may be an unnatural position, and that it may be difficult to maintain the position.

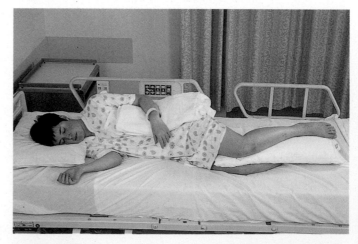

FIGURE 9.19 Sidelying position. Note the pillow between the knees. Pillows can also be placed between the ankles to alleviate pressure. One pillow is placed behind the back for the patient to lean back against, leaving the patient in a 30 degree side lying position. (From Smeltzer SC, Bare BG. *Brunnar & Suddarth's Textbook of Medical -Surgical Nursing.* 9th ed. Philadelphia, PA: Lippincott Williams & Wilkins; 2000.)

When positioning patients in the supine position the issue is elevation of the head of the bed. Maintain the head of the bed at or below 30 degrees. Elevations above 30 degrees increase pressure at the sacrum and increase friction and shearing forces between the skin and the support surface.[188,189] Elevating the knees and feet at 30 degrees as well as the head of the bed elevation of 30 degrees results in lower pressures at the sacrum.[189] Positioning patients in a semi-Fowler position increases the sacral interface pressures compared to other positions regardless of type of redistribution support surface in use.[190] Keeping the head of the bed below 30° is problematic for patients who are on ventilators as elevations below 30° are associated with ventilator-associated pneumonia. For these patients, it is necessary for infectious disease and wound care nurses to meet and decide which approach is in the best interests of the individual patient. This decision may change as the patient's condition changes. Small shifts in position involve moving the patient but keeping the same lying position,[191] for example, changing the angle of the right side-lying position or changing the lower extremity position in the right side-lying position. Pillows or foam wedges can be used to change the angles of legs or the body to achieve small shifts in position. Small shifts in position are helpful in achieving reperfusion of compressed tissues, but *only full-body change of position completely relieves pressure.*

There are techniques to make turning patients easier and less time consuming. Turning sheets, draw sheets, and pillows are essential for passive movement of patients in bed. Turning sheets are useful in repositioning the patient to a side-lying position, and draw sheets are used for pulling the patient up in bed. Both help to prevent dragging the patient's skin over the bed surface. Two-person repositioning is a simple task with the turning sheet and can be accomplished in a very small amount of time with little risk of producing shearing:

1. Position one person on each side of the bed.
2. Bend the patient's knees and fold the patient's arms across the chest.
3. Roll up the draw sheet next to the patient's body and grasp firmly.
4. On a prearranged verbal cue, both persons lift and move the patient up in bed.
5. Next, one person pulls on the turn sheet to roll the patient passively toward the side.
6. The person on the other side of the bed immediately places pillows behind the patient's back for support.
7. Additional pillows are then used for easing pressure on other bony prominences.

Turning patients (nonbariatric) with one person takes, on average, 5 minutes to complete.[192] There are devices available to assist with turning and repositioning that decrease the time and physical effort required to reposition patients. One example is shown in Figure 9.20. This system offloads the sacrum, includes a method of managing moisture due to incontinence, minimizes friction and shear, and assists in positioning the patient at the 30-degree angle with use of two small foam wedges. It includes a low-friction material that has one side that holds the body

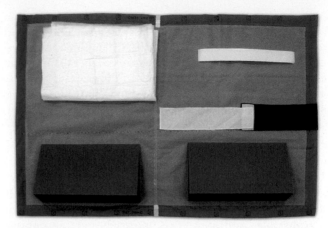

FIGURE 9.20 The Prevalon® Turn and Position device includes two 30-degree wedge shaped foam cushions, a breathable low friction sheet (side toward the bed is ripstop nylon), with a full body disposable pad that wicks away moisture and incontinence from the skin and allows air flow through the pad, and an anchor strip that affixes to the head of the bed so the device stays with the patient's body and does not slide down the bed. (Courtesy of Sage Products, Inc.)

pad in place under the patient and one side that is ripstop nylon that slides easily across the bed linens. The ripstop nylon decreases friction and helps the sheet move with the patient to make turning easier. Both the device and the pad are breathable, allowing air circulation, and can be used on any support surface. There are also therapeutic beds that include turn assistance built into the support surface. For example, the P500 (Hill-Rom Services, Inc.) support surface features a turn assist bladder that allows the patient to be turned with the push of a button and inflation of the surface itself. Further, the device includes a reminder feature that can be used to schedule repositioning episodes. Devices such as this can decrease the time and effort required to reposition a patient increasing the likelihood that repositioning actions will occur.

Repositioning in Special Populations

There are special considerations for repositioning pediatric and bariatric patients, patients in critical care units, and patients receiving palliative care.

Pediatric Patients

Repositioning schedules for pediatric patients may include the prone position as this position is often easier to

---

CLINICAL WISDOM

Repositioning Schedules in the Critical Care Unit

Many patients in the critical care unit can tolerate a repositioning program and for those who cannot the nurse must continually reassess the patient to determine when the patient recovers some stability and can safely resume some level of repositioning.

implement and tolerated better in infants and children. Prone position in critically ill infants and children with acute lung injury does not result in difficulties with airway management, mechanical ventilation, enteral nutrition, pain, sedation management, or staff utilization of the position compared to the supine position.[193] Two other groups may use the prone position, persons with spinal cord injury and patients in the operating room undergoing specific surgical procedures.

Critical Care Patients

Repositioning in critically ill patients sometimes must be avoided because of hemodynamic instability or other medically unstable conditions. Two approaches are appropriate when critically ill patients are so unstable such that repositioning is contraindicated. First, these patients should be placed on a high-level redistribution support surface to help compensate for the lack of repositioning. Second, these patients must be reassessed very frequently during the period of time when repositioning is not possible. Reassessment is focused on determining when the patient is more stable from a hemodynamic status and thus, able to resume some level of repositioning and detection and monitoring of any skin areas with erythema or early pressure ulcer damage. For critical care patients who are not hemodynamically unstable repositioning can and should occur as with other patients at risk for pressure ulcer development. In fact, several investigators have evaluated 2 hour repositioning using the 30-degree side-lying position in patients early after heart surgery and showed no influence from the repositioning on cardiac index, antihypertensive or inotropic/vasopressor therapy, or practical issues even with intraaortic balloon pumps.[194] Further, measurements of pulmonary artery and pulmonary wedge pressures obtained in the 30-degree side-lying position and supine positions have been found to be clinically interchangeable, supporting use of repositioning in critical care patients.[195] Of note, when repositioning critical care patients, attention must be focused on making sure that the patient is not positioned on tubing or a medical device.[141]

Palliative Care patients

Repositioning for persons receiving palliative care is an important part of the pressure ulcer prevention program for this population. As with critical care patients, most palliative care patients can be placed on a repositioning program. The goal of scheduled repositioning for persons who are receiving palliative care is to prevent or minimize pressure-induced skin damage. Repositioning may be painful for palliative care patients yet often this can be managed with adequate pain management. Premedicate patients with systemic pain medication at least 30 minutes prior to repositioning the patient. Because of increased risk for pressure ulcers and the pain associated with routine repositioning, palliative care patients may benefit from high-level pressure redistribution support surfaces. Near death, patients may have a position of most comfort. This is the time when repositioning may be postponed or eliminated from the care plan. Small shifts in position may be less painful and most appropriate during this time.

Bariatric Patients

There are unique concerns for repositioning bariatric patients. The patient must be placed on an appropriate bed frame that allows enough room for safe repositioning. The bed must be large enough to allow for the patient's body to fit easily in a side-lying position. Bariatric patients present additional risk for pressure ulcer development and placement on a high-level pressure redistribution support surface specific for bariatric patients is recommended. Repositioning requires the proper equipment and adequate staff to safely (for staff and the patient) move the patient to the new position. When positioning patients with a large abdominal pannus in a side-lying position, the pannus should be lifted away from the underlying skin and supported with pillows, foam wedges, or other off-loading devices.[141,196]

Scheduled Repositioning in Chairs

Similar approaches are useful for patients in chairs. Full-body change of position for persons in chairs involves standing the patient and resitting him or her in the chair. Small shifts in position for those in chairs might be changing lower extremity position or tilting the chair. For the chair-bound patient, if the patient's feet do not touch the floor it is helpful to use a footstool to help reduce the pressure on the ischial tuberosities and to distribute the pressure over the wider surface of the thigh.[141,170,197] Attention to proper alignment and posture is essential. Yet, this must be matched by maintaining the person's functional abilities.[141] Individuals at risk for pressure ulcer development should avoid uninterrupted sitting in chairs and should be repositioned every hour. Limiting chair sitting to 2 hours or less per session may result in fewer pressure ulcers in patients after fracture or orthopedic surgery compared to sitting in a chair for unlimited periods.[198] Limiting the sitting time and allowing for a rest period of at least 1 hour is recommended for acutely ill patients.[199] The rationale behind the shorter time frame is the extremely high pressure, shear and deformation generated on the ischial tuberosities in the seated position.

Patients with spinal cord injury have amplified issues regarding chair repositioning as they spend considerable time up in a chair. Thus, they are better served by high-level pressure redistribution support surfaces for the chair. Patients with upper body strength should be taught to shift weight every 15 minutes to allow for tissue reperfusion. Weight shifting can occur with chair push-ups, backward chair tilts, leaning side to side, or forward leans.[200–202] Forward leans, side-to-side leans and backward tilts may be more achievable for patients compared to chair push-ups.[200] Forward leans demonstrate the most effective pressure relief compared to the other methods.[201] Again, pillows or foam wedges may be used to help position the patient in proper body alignment. Physical therapy and occupational therapy can assist in body alignment strategies with even the most contracted patient. (See Chapter 10 for

CLINICAL WISDOM

Positioning Pillows

Five pillows can overcome repositioning pressure point difficulties. Use the pillows in the following positions:

Pillow 1: under legs to elevate the heels
Pillow 2: between the ankles
Pillow 3: between the knees
Pillow 4: behind the back
Pillow 5: under the head

further discussion on Management of Pressure by Therapeutic Positioning.)

Pillow Bridging

Pillow bridging involves the use of pillows to position patients with minimal tissue compression. The use of pillows can help to prevent pressure ulcers from occurring on the medial knees, the medial malleolus, and, to a lesser degree, on the heels. Pillows should be placed between the knees, between the ankles, and under the heels to completely offload them from the support surface.
(Use a small pillow for comfort under the arm in side-lying position.)

Pillow use is especially important for reducing risk of development of heel ulcers, regardless of the support surface in use. The best prevention strategy for eliminating pressure ulcers on the heels is to keep the heels off the surface of the bed. Use of pillows under the lower extremities, if they remain in place, can keep the heel from making contact with the support surface of the bed. Pillows help to redistribute the pressure over a larger area, thus reducing high pressure in one specific area; however, it can be difficult to keep them appropriately positioned under the legs with the heels floated off the end.[203] Position the pillows to support the entire calf making sure the heel and the Achille's tendon are both free of pressure. Pillows are best used for patients with little or no movement of extremities. Patients that move will often dislodge the pillow reducing the effective off-loading of the heels. Some specialized heel pressure-redistributing devices are effective in reducing pressure on heels and completely off-load the heel. Many of these devices also prevent foot drop. These devices are appropriate

RESEARCH WISDOM

Donut Pillow Devices

One type of pillow device is not recommended for use. Use of a donut type or ring cushion device is contraindicated. Donut ring cushions cause venous congestion and edema, and actually increase pressure to the area of concern.

for patients who are able to move their lower extremities. Many can be worn when ambulating and provide for low friction when extremities are moved in bed. Look for devices that are easy to apply and remove to assure compliance.

Pressure Redistribution Support Surfaces

The use of support surfaces to prevent and manage pressure ulcers is important; however, regardless of the type of support surface in use with the patient, the need for scheduled repositioning remains an important component of the prevention program.[170] The support surface serves as an adjunct to strategies for positioning and careful monitoring of patients. The NPUAP defines a support surface as a specialized device for pressure redistribution developed for managing tissue loads, microclimates, or other therapeutic functions.[204] Pressure redistribution support surfaces assist in pressure ulcer risk reduction by managing tissue loading either by reducing the load or duration of loading.[205] The type of support surface chosen is based on a multitude of factors, including clinical condition of the patient, type of care setting, ease of use, maintenance, cost, characteristics of the support surface, and whether or not the patient can tolerate scheduled repositioning. The primary concern should be the therapeutic benefit associated with the surface. Support surfaces are used to redistribute pressure in bed and chairs, over the heels, and during operative procedures.

Support Surfaces for Beds

There are two basic types of pressure redistribution support surfaces, nonpowered and powered. Nonpowered devices do not move; they reduce pressure by spreading the load over a larger area, and do not require electricity or a battery to function. Pressure redistribution nonpowered support surfaces increase the body surface area that comes in contact with the support surface to decrease the interface pressure (pressure between the body and the support surface interface). Increasing the body surface area that comes in contact with the support surface is accomplished by immersion and envelopment (i.e., the body sinks into or is engulfed by the surface). Examples of nonpowered support surfaces are high-specification foam, air, or gel mattress overlays and water-filled mattresses. Mattress overlays are devices that are applied on top of the standard mattress. Most overlays require a one-time charge, setup fee, daily rental fee, or a combination of fees. Most are single-use items and may present environmental issues for disposal. When using mattress overlays, the height of the bed is increased, so transfers and linen fit may be complicated.

When considering high-specification foam support surfaces, you should consider stiffness of the foam and the density and thickness of the foam. Indentation load deflection (ILD) is a measure of the stiffness of the foam; generally, the ILD should be 25% for 30 lb. The density and thickness of the foam relate to the foam's ability to deflect the pressure and redistribute the pressure over a wider area. Typically, the density and thickness of a foam product should be 1.3 lb per cubic foot and 3 to 4 inches, respectively.[206] High-specification foam surfaces have difficulties with retaining moisture and heat, and typically do not reduce shear. Air and water surfaces also have difficulties associated with retaining moisture and heat. Use of high-specification foam or specialized sheepskin overlays reduce pressure ulcer incidence compared with standard hospital mattresses.[207,208] There is no difference between different high-specification foam mattresses.

Powered active support surfaces require a motor or pump and electricity or batteries to operate. Powered redistribution support surfaces work by sequentially altering the parts of the body that bear load and so reduce the duration of loading on the tissues at any given anatomic location.[141,205] Examples are alternating pressure air mattresses and overlays. Most use an electric pump alternately to inflate and deflate air cells or air columns, thus the term *alternating* pressure air mattress. The air cells in alternating pressure air mattresses need to be greater than 10 cm in order to be sufficiently inflated to ensure pressure relief over the deflated cells.[141] These devices may also include physical features that allow for envelopement and immersion as well as alternating pressure. Powered support surfaces may also have difficulties with moisture retention and heat accumulation. Some powered active support surfaces are equipped to help reduce skin temperature and moisture and maintain the microclimate. Most use air flow to the skin to maintain the microclimate. Use of alternating pressure powered support surfaces reduces incidence of pressure ulcers in hospitalized patients compared to standard hospital mattresses and may also be effective in critical care units.[207,209–212] Alternating pressure active support surfaces should be used for patients at higher risk of pressure ulcer development when repositioning is not possible.[141] There is no evidence of any difference between alternating pressure active support surface overlays or mattresses although patients may prefer mattresses to overlays.[141,212]

Table 9.2 provides intrinsic and extrinsic factors to consider when deciding on a support surface. One additional factor to consider when choosing a support surface is the microclimate at the skin and surface interface. The microclimate is the local temperature and moisture at the body support surface interface. Heat is a risk factor for pressure ulcer development as it contributes to superficial ulcerations. Heat accumulates at the skin surface over time. So, the longer the patient is in one position, the more likely the local temperature is of the skin and tissue is elevated. Controlling the microclimate can be accomplished with thermal mass, low-air-loss devices, and regular repositioning. Support surface coverings that wick moisture away from the body or those that have continual air flow at the skin-surface interface reduce local temperature and control the microclimate.

High-end powered support surfaces include low-air-loss therapy beds and overlays, air-fluidized beds, and kinetic therapy. Low-air-loss therapy is a bed frame with a series of connected air-filled pillows with surface fabrics of low-friction material. The amount of pressure in each pillow can be controlled and can be calibrated to provide maximum pressure relief for the individual patient. They provide pressure redistribution in any position, and most models have built-in scales.

Fluidized air or high-air-loss therapy consists of a bed frame containing silicone-coated glass beads. The design incorporates both air and fluid support: the beads become fluid when air is pumped through, making them behave as a liquid. High-air-loss therapy has bactericidal properties because of the alkalinity of the beads (pH 10), the higher temperature, and entrapment of microorganisms by the beads. High-air-loss therapy relieves pressure and reduces friction, shear, and moisture (due to the drying effect of the bed). However, the increased air flow can increase evaporative fluid loss, leading to dehydration. Also, it is difficult to transfer patients in these devices because of the height of the bed frame in relation to the support surface itself. Finally, if the patient is able to sit up, a foam wedge may be required, thus limiting the beneficial effects of the bed on the patient's upper back.

Kinetic therapy beds or continuous lateral rotation therapy beds are designed to counter the effects of immobility by continuous passive motion. Multiple body systems are involved in the therapy, which is believed to improve respiratory function and oxygenation, prevent urinary stasis, and reduce venous stasis. Generally, the patient must have a stable spine. The beds usually are of two types: Either the bed frame itself moves or the air cushions inflate or deflate, rotating the patient from side to side or pulsating. Pressure relief and low-friction surfaces are provided with repositioning. Most models include built-in scales for obtaining weight of patients. Conscious patients may not tolerate the movement of the bed.

How can you tell if the support surface is working? One problem with support surface mattress overlays is inadequate support or "bottoming out." Bottoming out occurs when the patient's body sinks down, the support surface is compressed beyond function, and the patient's body lies directly on the hospital mattress. When bottoming out occurs, there is no pressure redistribution for the bony prominence of concern. Bottoming out typically happens when the patient is placed on a support surface that is not appropriately filled with air or when the patient has been on a foam support surface for extended periods of time. The health-care provider can monitor for bottoming out by inserting a flat, outstretched hand between the overlay and the patient's body part at risk. If less than an inch of support material is felt, the patient has bottomed out. It is important to check for bottoming out when the patient is in various body positions and to check at various body sites. For example, when the patient is lying supine, check the sacral/coccygeal area and the heels; when the patient is side-lying, check the trochanter and lateral malleolus.

The method most commonly used to examine efficacy of support surfaces is interface pressure measurements and pressure mapping. Interface pressure is a measurement obtained

---

CLINICAL WISDOM

Recommendations for Bed Support Surfaces

- Use a high-specification foam mattress or overlay instead of standard hospital mattress for persons determined at risk for pressure ulcer development.
- Use alternating pressure active support surface overlays or mattresses for persons at high risk for pressure ulcer development and those who cannot be repositioned.

TABLE 9.2	Intrinsic and Extrinsic Criteria for Selection of Support Surfaces

Intrinsic Criteria	Considerations
Wound burden	Tissue history—previous ulcers, surgical repair, stress, duration of pressure ulcer, number of pressure ulcers present
Body build	Obese, thin, contractures present[a]
Magnitude and distribution of pressures	Location of highest pressures

Extrinsic Criteria	Considerations
The number of hours spent on the support surface daily	Will product be needed for short- or long-term use?[b]
Shear and friction effects	Is the patient agitated? Are they exhibiting continual body movements?
Environmental factors	What is the temperature, humidity, continence, and moisture of the environment?
Micro-climate factors	Will the support surface allow for maintaining normal skin surface temperature and moisture?
Living arrangements	Will the patient be in a long-term care or home care setting? If patient sleeps with a significant other, can the support surface be used on half of the bed? Is the patient on a standardized mattress or does the surface need to be placed on top of a nonhospital mattress?
Self-care deficits	Is the risk of pressure ulcer development likely to increase or decrease?
Ease of transition and weaning to other products or other health-care settings	Movement off support surface can promote patient independence if patient able. Transitioning to less costly surfaces can reduce financial burden if clinically appropriate.
Ease of use and manageability	How can independence be promoted? Is the support surface feasible for the home environment? Can the home caregiver maintain and provide care with the device?
Initial cost level	Is the patient expected to recover or improve?[c]
Service and warranty of the surface	Evaluate product services to achieve optimal efficiency and efficacy.
Availability of product	What options are accessible? Consider patient needs and economic versus clinical benefits.
Scientific validity	What does the research show?

[a]Patients with severe contractures may not require a support surface that has good heel pressure readings (with contraction of the legs, the heels do not reach the bottom of the mattress).
[b]The patient who uses the support surface only at night and spends most of the day in the chair will require an aggressive approach to seating support surfaces, and a lesser support surface can be chosen for the bed. If the patient spends most of the day in bed, the support surface chosen will be different.
[c]If the patient is expected to recover or improve, a lower-cost support surface may be appropriate. If the patient is expected to decline in function, choosing a support surface that will meet future, as well as present, skin care needs may be best.

by placing a sensor between the skin and the resting support surface. It is usually obtained with some type of electropneumatic pressure sensor connected to an inflation system and gauge or a mat composed of many sensors connected to or read by a computer. Instrumentation (size of sensor, shape of sensor, position of sensor, number and density of sensors in a pad system) greatly affects values of pressure readings, so it is difficult, if not impossible, to make comparisons between studies. In addition to variability in accuracy of measurements, another problem with interface pressures is that due to a patient's weight and body type, interface pressures alone are not sufficient to evaluate the efficacy of a particular device or class of devices.[207,210,213] Interface pressures are only an indirect indication of the actual pressure and deformation of the tissues at the bony tissue interface. Pressure on subcutaneous tissues may be three to five times higher than skin interface pressure. Typically, interface pressures are evaluated by comparing the values obtained to capillary closing pressure (generally considered to be 12–32 mm Hg). Capillary closing pressure values vary by individual. Other factors that should be considered include

- Skin tension
- Shear force
- Temperature
- Humidity
- Magnitude and duration of pressure
- Pressure and blood flow distribution

New pressure mapping devices have been introduced that provide real time monitoring of pressure magnitude and duration of pressure. These devices use multiple sensors that provide data on interface pressure both the magnitude of pressure at specific sites and the duration of that pressure. The data are presented as a real-time color map of bony prominences with pressure magnitude and duration of pressure displayed. Figure 9.21 presents an example of such a device. This type of technology may be helpful in providing more information on pressure magnitude and duration to clinicians allowing for more individualized repositioning programs. However, it is not known if devices that provide additional information on pressure assist clinicians in preventing pressure ulcers.

Two populations require additional considerations related to support surfaces, bariatric and pediatric patients. For bariatric patients, it is important that surfaces designed for bariatric patients be utilized. These support surfaces are designed to provide pressure reduction for the severely obese patient and can accommodate extreme loading. Bariatric devices have features similar to the other support surfaces described. Generally, the bed frame is larger and many have a feature that can raise the patient to a sitting and standing position while positioned in the bed. There are also chair devices for bariatric patients.

In the pediatric population, use of low air loss support surfaces is not recommended as most were not designed for use with infants and children. Pressure redistribution support surfaces such as nonpowered high-specification foam mattress overlays or gel pillows are alternatives.[213,214] Further, use of powered alternating pressure support surfaces may not be sized appropriately for infant and children body size; the

child's extremities and buttocks may fall into gaps between the air cells.[214]

Throughout the decision-making process, one thought should prevail: it is important to promote patient independence, not dependent behavior. Patient mobility out of bed and off of the support surface is important for those patients who are able, and you should encourage and support this whenever appropriate.

Seating Support Surfaces

Providing pressure redistribution for chair-bound patients is critical because of the high pressures across the ischial tuberosities when sitting upright. Most pressure-redistributing support surfaces for chairs are nonpowered overlays, such as those made out of foam, gel, air, or some combination. Positioning chair-bound individuals includes evaluation of body contours, postural alignment, weight distribution, and balance/stability in addition to pressure redistribution. The use of a chair support surface can help lessen the burden of wheelchair push-ups or side leans, but does not eliminate the need for reperfusion of the tissues. This is difficult as few people can actually consistently sustain the rigor associated with maintaining a schedule of weight changes. Use of a timer or alarm may be helpful in reminding patients and/or caregivers of the need for body movement. Chapter 10 provides additional information on Therapeutic Positioning.

Patients with spinal cord injury need special attention to chair support surfaces because of long-term limited mobility. Routine maintenance and evaluation of chair support surfaces

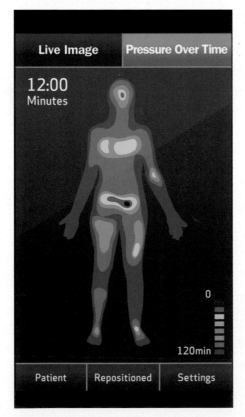

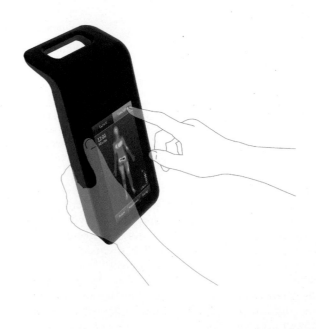

FIGURE 9.21 The handheld M.A.P ® System collects data from the sensor pad coverlet placed over the support surface of the bed. The device provides bedside pressure mapping and gives clinicians real-time pressure distribution data on the location, magnitude, and duration of pressure across the body. These types of systems provide feedback on off-loading and may assist in repositioning patients off bony prominences of concern. The system can be programmed with pre-set reminders for repositioning schedules.
Source: WellSense USA, Inc. 2416 21st Avenue South Nashville, TN. 37212.

RESEARCH WISDOM

Evaluating Studies Using Interface Pressures

- Look for interface pressures stated as a percentage against a standard surface, usually a hospital mattress. Standard hospital mattress interface pressures for sacrum = 36 to 48 mm Hg and for trochanter = 62 to 97 mm Hg.[215] For example, a support surface that reports tissue interface pressure readings of 25 mm Hg for the sacrum has approximately 30% lower pressures than the standard hospital mattress pressures for the sacrum ($25/36$ mm Hg $\times 100 = 69.44$; $100-70 = 30\%$ of hospital mattress pressures).

- Look for standard deviations (SD) reported in the study—95% of measurements lie within 2 SD of the mean (average). So, the larger the standard deviation, the less reproducible the pressure measurements and the more variable the results with the product. For example, a study reports mean tissue interface pressures of 25 mm Hg with standard deviation of 8.2. So, 95% of all the measurements were between 8.6 and 41.4 mm Hg. This is not so bad at the 8.6 end, but what about the 41.4 mm Hg? That figure is far higher than standard capillary closing pressure of 32 mm Hg.

- To interpret the study results, consider these issues:
  1. Range and number of pressure readings obtained for each site. How was site placement determined? (The bony prominence is usually larger than the pressure probe. Was it placed in the center of the bony prominence? Was the site marked so subsequent readings were taken at the same location?) Was a full-body or partial-body pressure mapping system used?
  2. Procedure used to acquire the pressure readings should be described as well as the training procedures for those conducting the testing.
  3. Who were tested and how do they compare with the patients you care for?
  4. How were they tested?
  5. How often was equipment recalibrated? (The equipment is fragile and subject to malfunction.)

is essential for the spinal cord–injured patient. In choosing a chair support surface for spinal cord–injured patients, it is helpful to use pressure mapping to identify areas of high pressure. Pressure mapping can also identify changes in pressures over time as the patient ages and determine when a new support surface is needed.

Pressure Redistribution Support Surfaces for Heels

The heels are particularly prone to pressure ulcer formation because of the lack of soft tissue to redistribute pressure forces, the large calcaneus bone, and the small surface area of the heel. The heels should not be in contact with the support surface. Support surfaces fail to redistribute the pressure by increasing the contact area with the support surface or by decreasing the duration of pressure over the small area of the heel.[203] There are some data suggesting patients on viscoelastic nonpowered pressure redistribution support surfaces develop more heel ulcers compared

CLINICAL WISDOM

Additional Considerations for Choosing a Support Surface

The following examples help to illustrate other considerations in choosing a support surface:

- Patients who undergo surgical operative repair of an existing pressure ulcer may need to be placed on air fluidized therapy postoperatively.
- Patients with multiple ulcers involving more than one turning surface need to be placed on pressure-redistributing support surfaces, such as low-air-loss therapy.
- Patients with severe contractures may not require a support surface that has good heel pressure readings (with contraction of the legs, the heels do not reach the bottom of the mattress).
- If the bony prominence of concern is the greater trochanter, the support surface chosen must adequately reduce pressure over the trochanter.
- The patient who uses the support surface only at night and spends most of the day in a chair will require an aggressive approach to seating support surfaces, and a lesser support surface can be chosen for the bed. If the patient spends most of the day in bed, the support surface chosen will be different.
- A support surface's ability to handle shearing and friction may be critical for agitated patients (particularly those with continual body motions), and good choices may involve evaluation of the support surface covering.
- If the patient is at home, with no air conditioning, is incontinent of urine, and lives in a humid environment, the ability of the support surface to breathe and handle moisture are essential to positive outcomes.
- Evaluation of the patient's prognosis is helpful in support surface choice. Is the patient expected to recover and improve? If so, a pressure redistribution nonpowered support surface may be appropriate. However, if the patient is expected to decline in function, choosing a support surface that will meet future, as well as present, skin care needs may be prudent.

As these case examples illustrate, the clinician must evaluate the individual patient's needs.

CLINICAL WISDOM

Reimbursement of Bed Support Surfaces

Support surfaces are reimbursed in home care under Medicare Part B benefits. Medicare requirements for reimbursement include the following:

- Must be stage III or IV pressure sore
- Must have pressure sore located on trunk of body
- Must have current Medicare Part B coverage
- Must be in permanent residence (own home, long-term care facility, etc.)

to those placed on alternating pressure air mattress support surfaces.[216] As previously discussed, pressure can be relieved completely from the heels by elevating them off the support surface with pillows placed under the calves.[141] Use of standard pillows has been compared to foam wedge cushions for off-loading heels and patients treated with the foam wedge cushions had lower incidence of heel pressure ulcers.[217] Heel protection support surfaces may offload the heel by redistributing the pressure along the calf of the leg. When high-specificity foam, medical grade sheepskin, and air-filled heel protection support surfaces have been compared, the results have demonstrated no difference in heel pressure ulcer development.[212] When devices have been compared to use of standard pillows, the incidence of pressure ulcers has not been significantly different although time to ulcer development was shorter with pillows use for off-loading.[203]

There are several considerations for choosing a heel pressure redistribution support surface. Use of foam wedges that span the width of the end of the bed and keep the legs cradled in place do successfully suspend the heels off the bed surface. However, these devices may limit mobility and do not address foot drop. Heel pressure redistribution boots stay in place and do address foot drop issues. Those that incorporate a brace should be properly fitted by a physical therapist for proper attention to foot drop and leg alignment. Boots without a brace are made of foam, air cushions, fiber filled, or medical grade sheepskin. Those made of high-specificity foam may be warm and limit ease of movement in bed because of friction; however, they are relatively inexpensive. Air-filled cushions address friction and shear, they are light and do not limit bed mobility. They do require monitoring to be sure sufficient inflation is present. Fiber-filled boots can be washed, and they wick moisture and heat from the foot. Sheepskin boots may increase temperature.[203] Additional questions to address in deciding on a heel support surface include

- Foot drop addressed by device?
- Moisture and temperature issues?
- Able to ambulate with device?
- Ability to remain in place?
- Shear and friction addressed?
- Bed mobility issues?
- Able to wash device?[203]

Use of Pressure Redistribution Support Surfaces in the Operating Room

Pressure redistribution support surfaces should be used on the operating table for persons determined at risk for pressure ulcers and those undergoing prolonged procedures or at risk of hypotensive episodes during surgery.[170,218–221] Use of high-specification foam or medical grade sheepskin on the operating table as a pressure-redistributing support surface can reduce the incidence of operative acquired pressure ulcers.[170] More specifically, use of a viscoelastic support surface on the operating table compared to the standard operating table resulted in a relative reduction in incidence of postoperative pressure ulcers of 47% for those persons undergoing elective major general, gynecologic, or vascular surgery.[218] Alternating pressure air support surfaces used during surgery and postoperatively have also demonstrated lower pressure ulcer incidence.[219,220] In addition to use of pressure redistribution support surfaces on the operating table, padding bony prominences after positioning for

surgery and assessing heels and off-loading if possible may also be helpful.[141] It is also important to continue use of pressure redistribution support surfaces during the immediate postoperative recovery period. Positioning the patient in a different position following the surgery, if possible, is also recommended.[222]

In summary, effective use of support surfaces requires the following actions: choosing support surfaces for patients based on multiple factors, use of a multidisciplinary team to finalize selections, and periodic reevaluation of products and patient/institution needs based on baseline pressure ulcer prevalence and incidence data. These steps are critical as limited evidence exists to support use of one specific device versus another.

Measures to Increase Mobility and Activity

Overhead bed frames with trapeze bars are helpful for patients with paraplegia, stroke patients with upper body strength, and obese patients, and may increase mobility and independence with body repositioning.[141,170] Wheelchair-bound patients with upper body strength can be taught and encouraged to do wheelchair push-ups and body tilts/leans to relieve pressure and allow for reperfusion of the tissues at the ischial tuberosity. For patients who are weak from prolonged inactivity, providing support and assistance for reconditioning and increasing strength and endurance will help to prevent future disability and dysfunction. Setting goals for increased mobility and activity may be helpful. Progressive sitting plans are helpful for patients with spinal cord injury, especially following operative repair of existing pressure ulcers. Mobility plans for each patient should be individualized, with the goal of attaining the highest level of mobility and activity individually possible. Mobility plans are the responsibility of nurses and physical therapists working together in all health-care settings. Even frail elder nursing home patients are capable of improving mobility and activity levels; one study showed nursing home residents could successfully participate in an incontinence and exercise intervention conducted every 2 hours from 8 AM to 5 PM 5 days a week and that walking distance and walking time improved as did other measures of mobility.[221]

It is essential to train and observe home caregivers in the mobility plan and, in particular, repositioning techniques. Caregivers in the home are often left to fend for themselves for prevention interventions and may be frail and have health problems themselves. A return demonstration of a repositioning procedure or performance of a mobility exercise can be very informative, revealing a need to coach, improvise, or think of creative strategies for caregivers to use in the home setting in order to meet the patient's need for movement, activity, and tissue reperfusion.

Reducing Friction and Shearing

Measures to reduce friction and shear relate to passive or active movement of the patient. To reduce friction, two interventions are generally appropriate: Provide topical preparations to eliminate or reduce the surface tension between the skin and the bed linen or support surface and use appropriate techniques when moving patients so that skin is never dragged across linens. Patients who exhibit voluntary or involuntary repetitive body movements (particularly of the heels or elbows) are at higher risk for damage to the skin from friction.

Reducing Surface Tension Between the Skin and the Support Surface

To help eliminate the surface contact of the area and decrease the friction between the skin and the linens, consider using any of the following: cornstarch to decrease skin resistance; a protective film, such as a transparent film dressing or a skin sealant; a protective dressing, such as a thin hydrocolloid[223]; a soft silicone or sheet hydrogel dressing[173]; hyperoxygenated fatty acid preparations[224]; hexachlorophene lotion[170]; or protective padding. Hydrocolloid dressings have been shown to be effective in reducing shear force on heels in elder hospitalized patients.[223] Soft silicone sheets have been effective in reducing sacral pressure ulcers on patients in critical care units.[173] Transparent film dressings have been used on the face of patients undergoing noninvasive ventilation to protect the skin from face mask pressure and friction damage.[225] New textiles and materials that have a low coefficient of friction may be useful to decrease friction over the heels and sacrum.[226] One such garment fits over pressure redistribution support surfaces on the heels as shown in Figure 9.22 and has been shown to reduce friction with lower skin damage outcomes.[226] It is not known if these garments aid in reducing the incidence of pressure ulcers. Avoid vigorous massage over bony prominences as this creates friction damage from the repetitive parallel rubbing or sanding of the epidermis.[170] Pay special attention to elbows and skin areas that are macerated as moisture increases the friction coefficient and results in damage more readily.[141,170]

Techniques for Moving Patients

Use of lift sheets, draw sheets, or devices to turn and transfer patients will assist in avoiding dragging or pulling that can result in friction on the skin. Use of devices such as the Prevalon Turn and

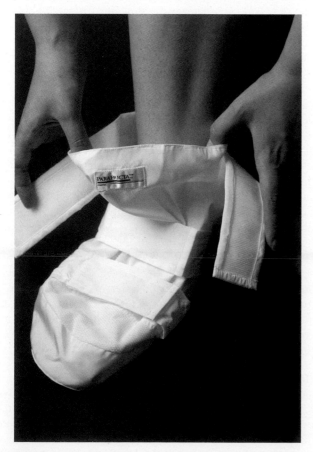

FIGURE 9.22 These garments are placed over the pressure redistribution support surface on the heels and provide for a low coefficient of friction reducing the friction forces between the skin and the underlying bed support surface and making movement easier. (Courtesy of APA Parafricta LTD, Medical INVISTA, Kennesaw, GA 30144.)

Position System® (see Fig. 9.21) helps reduce friction by maintaining a low coefficient of friction between the patient and the bed linens. The low friction between the device and the bed linens makes moving the patient easier and minimizes dragging. Maintaining the head of the bed at or below 30 degrees (if consistent with the medical condition of the patient) to prevent sliding and shear injury.[170] Lowering the head of the bed 1 hour after meals or tube feedings if possible to prevent pressure damage to the sacrum. Use of transfer boards with low-friction surfaces is helpful for moving from bed to wheelchair for patients with spinal cord injury. Even though heel, ankle, and elbow protectors do nothing to reduce or relieve pressure, they can be effective aids against friction.

Most shear injury can be eliminated by proper positioning, such as avoidance of the semi-Fowler position and limiting use of the upright position (positions over 30 degrees inclined). Use of footboards and knee gatches (or pillows under the lower leg) to prevent sliding and to maintain position can also help reduce shear effects on the skin when in bed. Observation of the patient when sitting is also important, because the patient who slides down in the chair is at equally high risk for shear injury. Use of footstools and the foot pedals on wheelchairs, and appropriate 90-degree flexion of the hip (which may be achieved with pillows, special seat cushions, or orthotic devices) can help prevent chair sliding.

Moisture

Moisture can macerate the skin decreasing the tolerance of the tissues to pressure and friction forces. Further, moisture removes the oils on the skin, which makes it friable and softens the skin's connective tissue leading to erosion of epidermis. To minimize skin exposure to excessive moisture, assess for excessive moisture by determining the cause; for example, urine, feces, perspiration, wound exudate, saliva. If urinary and/or fecal incontinence is the main contributing factor to moisture, establish a bowel and bladder regimen for patients. Since most, but not all, moisture concerns in patients at risk for pressure ulcers is related to incontinence, we focus this discussion on management of incontinence. In this chapter, we can only briefly address the strategies for managing incontinence most pertinent to the patient at high risk of developing a pressure ulcer.[127,170]

The etiology and type of incontinence should be determined and if the incontinence is reversible or transient, the cause should be eliminated. Management strategies for incontinence are grouped into three main areas for this discussion: behavioral management, containment strategies, and skin protection guidelines.

Behavioral Management Strategies

Patients at risk for pressure ulcer development are not candidates for all methods of behavioral management. The most successful behavioral management strategies for frail, cognitively impaired patients at risk of pressure ulcer development include scheduled toileting and prompted voiding programs. Both strategies are caregiver dependent and require a motivated caregiver to be successful. Scheduled intake of fluid is an important underlying factor for both strategies.

Scheduled toileting (also called *habit training*) is toileting on a planned basis. The goal is to keep the person dry by assisting him or her to void at regular intervals. Try to match the interval to the patient's natural voiding schedule: avoid attempting to motivate patients to delay voiding or to resist the urge to void. Scheduled

CLINICAL WISDOM

Reducing Friction

Sprinkling cornstarch on the bed linen or use of skin lubricants is helpful in reducing overall friction.

toileting may be based on the clock (toilet the patient every 2 hours) or based on activities (toilet the patient after meals and before transferring to bed). Like scheduled toileting, *prompted voiding* involves use of a toileting schedule (every 2 hours); however, this is supplemented with teaching the incontinent patient to discriminate their continence status and to request toileting assistance. Three additional elements in prompted voiding include monitoring the incontinent patient routinely, prompting the patient to use the toilet, and praising the patient for maintenance of continence. Prompted voiding results in 40% to 50% reduction in frequency of daytime incontinence, and between 25% and 33% of urinary incontinent patients in nursing homes respond to the therapy.[227,228] Prompted voiding has also been shown to be effective in dependent and cognitively impaired nursing home incontinent patients.[227,228]

Both of these behavioral management strategies have the added benefit of moving the patient at routine intervals. This relieves pressure over bony prominences and reduces the risk of pressure ulcer development by allowing reperfusion of the tissues.

Containment Strategies

Underpads and briefs may be used to protect the skin of patients who are incontinent of urine or stool. These products are designed to absorb moisture, wick the wetness away from the skin, and maintain a quick-drying interface with the skin. Studies with both infants and adults demonstrate that products designed to present a quick-drying surface to the skin and to absorb moisture do keep the skin drier and are associated with a lower incidence of dermatitis. It is important to note that the critical feature is the ability to absorb moisture and present a quick-drying surface, not whether the product is disposable or reusable. Regardless of the product chosen, containment strategies imply the need for a check and change schedule for the incontinent patient, so that wet linens and pads may be removed and the skin cleansed in a timely manner.

Underpads are not as tight or constricting as briefs. Kemp[229] suggests alternating the use of underpads and briefs if the skin irritation is thought to be related to the occlusive nature of the brief. Her recommendations echo the early work of Willis[230] on warm water immersion syndrome, who found that the effects of water on the skin could be reversed and tempered by simply allowing the skin to dry out between wet periods. Use of briefs when the patient is up in a chair, ambulating, or visiting another department and use of underpads when the patient is in bed is one suggestion for combining the strengths of both products.

External collection devices may be more effective with male patients. External catheters or condom catheters are devices applied to the shaft of the penis to direct the urine away from the body to a collection device. Newer models of external catheters are self-adhesive and easy to apply. A key concern with use of external collection devices is routine removal of the product and inspection and hygiene of the skin.

There are special containment devices for fecal incontinence, as well. Fecal incontinence collectors consist of a self-adhesive skin barrier attached to a drainable pouch. Application of the device is somewhat dependent on the skill of the clinician, and the patient should be put on a routine for changing the pouch prior to leakage to facilitate success. The skin barrier provides a physical obstacle to the stool on the skin and helps to prevent dermatitis and associated skin problems. In fact, skin barrier wafers without an attached pouch can be useful in protecting the skin from feces or urine.

There are also indwelling bowel catheters for managing fecal incontinence but they are not a long term care option and data are limited regarding effect on skin health.

Incontinence Skin Hygiene

After an incontinence episode, the skin should be cleansed with pH-balanced cleansers.[170] Special perineal cleansers are more effective at preventing IAD than soap and water.[229] Bar soap tends to dry the skin and creates an alkaline pH resulting in increased risk for tissue damage. Cleansing should be gentle as vigorous cleansing can strip the surface epidermis. Use of smooth woven disposable clothes is preferred over washcloths as they create less surface friction on the skin.[133] Use of solutions designed for incontinence care cleansing can be protective of the skin and can decrease the time and energy involved in postepisode cleansing. These commercially available cleansers include surfactants as ingredients. The surfactants make the removal of urine and stool residue easier, with less abrasiveness. Every attempt should be made to cleanse the perineal skin immediately after an incontinent episode to limit the amount of contact time between the urine or stool and the skin.

Moisture barriers protect the skin from the effects of moisture. The success of the particular product is linked to its formulation and hydrophobic properties. Generally, pastes are thicker and more repellent of moisture than are ointments. A quick evaluation is the ease with which the product can be removed with water during routine cleansing. If the product comes off the skin with just routine cleansing, it probably is not an effective barrier to moisture. Mineral oil for cleansing some of the heavier barrier products, such as zinc oxide paste, will ease removal from the skin. Products with humectants (e.g., urea, glycerin, alpha hydroxyl acids, and lactic acid) should be avoided as they retain water in the skin and with incontinence the problem is too much water retained in the skin.[133] Dimethicone (3%) skin protectants have been shown to decrease pressure ulcer incidence at the sacrum and buttocks in incontinent long-term care patients.[230]

General Skin Care

Basic skin care should begin with daily skin inspections with specific attention toward identifying reddened areas. Neither reddened areas nor bony prominences should be massaged as noted earlier as this can further damage fragile blood vessels. Discovery of dry and cracked skin should also be regarded with concern as these areas indicate diminished skin integrity and increase risk for the occurrence of pressure ulcers. Exhibit 9.4 presents a skin observation form that can be used with caregivers.

EXHIBIT 9.4

Skin Observation Form for Direct Caregivers

Instructions: Observe skin daily and record if condition is present

Name:_____ Month:_____ Year:_____

Body Location	Day:	1	2	3	4	5	6	7	8	9	10	11	12	13	14	15	16	17	18	19	20	21	22	23	24	25	26	27	28	29	30	31
	Skin Condition																																
Sacrum or Tailbone	Redness																																
	Bruise																																
	Open Wound																																
Right Buttock	Redness																																
	Bruise																																
	Open Wound																																
Left Buttock	Redness																																
	Bruise																																
	Open Wound																																
Right Ischium (At gluteal fold)	Redness																																
	Bruise																																
	Open Wound																																
Left Ischium (At gluteal fold)	Redness																																
	Bruise																																
	Open Wound																																
Right Hip	Redness																																
	Bruise																																
	Open Wound																																
Left Hip	Redness																																
	Bruise																																
	Open Wound																																
Right Heel	Redness																																
	Bruise																																
	Open Wound																																
Left Heel	Redness																																
	Bruise																																
	Open Wound																																
Other Locations:	Redness																																
	Bruise																																
	Open Wound																																
Other Locations:	Redness																																
	Bruise																																
	Open Wound																																

Skin hygiene interventions involve daily skin hygiene and skin cleansing after fecal or urinary incontinent episodes. The older adult's skin is less tolerant of the drying effects of soap and hot water. Use of warm water and a mild soap (if any soap at all) can limit skin drying. For older adults, daily bathing is not necessary for skin health.. Daily cleansing of the feet, axilla, and perineal areas is appropriate, but daily showers or baths can be damaging to the skin. Use of a schedule of twice weekly or every other day bathing or showering is sufficient. Use of moisturizers and emollients for dry skin and lubricants for reduction in friction injuries is recommended.[141] The use of hyperoxygenated fatty acids has been shown to result in a reduction in pressure ulcer development when compared to a placebo and shows promise as an emollient of choice for pressure ulcer prevention.[224]

Skin maintenance interventions involve actions to prevent skin breakdown and actions to promote healthy skin. Maintaining skin lubrication is essential. Use of moisturizers on a routine basis can prevent skin drying and cracking. Application of moisturizers immediately after bathing or showering helps to remoisturize and lubricate the skin.

There are three main types of moisturizers—lotions, creams, and ointments. Lotions have the highest water content and, therefore, must be reapplied more frequently to be effective. Creams are mixtures of oil and water and, for best results, should be applied four times a day. Ointments (generally lanolin or petrolatum bases) have the lowest water content, are the most occlusive, and have the longest duration of moisturizing action. Special attention to moisturizing the lower legs and feet is often needed to compensate for decreased perfusion and diminished skin health in these areas.

Nutrition

In Chapter 4, we discussed the importance of a nourishing diet in maintaining healthy skin and tissues. So it is not surprising that there is a strong relationship between nutrition and pressure ulcer development.[155] The severity of ulceration is also correlated with the severity of the nutritional deficits, especially low protein intake or low serum albumin levels.[155,156,166,231–240] Thus, nutritional assessment should be performed on all patients determined to be at risk for pressure ulcer formation at routine intervals. However, the role of nutrition in the prevention of pressure ulcers is controversial, the relationship is assumed but there is limited evidence to support it.[241–243] While multiple studies have demonstrated a relationship between different markers of malnutrition (e.g., serum albumin level, dietary protein intake, inability to feed self, and weight loss) and pressure ulcer formation and severity, defining a causal relationship between malnutrition and pressure ulcer development, something that seems so logical, has proven difficult. Data supporting a prophylactic effect of nutritional supplements on pressure ulcer development are not so clear. See Chapter 4 for more information on General Assessment of Nutrition.

The following findings suggest malnutrition:

- Hypoalbuminemia (serum albumin levels below 3.5 mg/dL). This finding has been associated with pressure ulceration,[149,228] although some have found no relationship and little prognostic value for pressure ulcer healing.[233–235] When protein intake is insufficient, the serum albumin decreases. Serum

CLINICAL WISDOM

When to Consult the Dietitian

General parameters for consultation with the dietitian for a thorough nutritional assessment are

- Inadequate dietary intake (e.g., <50% of most meals consumed)
- Drop in body weight of 5%, *or*
- Serum albumin level below 3.5 mg/dL
- Patients with previous or existing pressure ulcer
- Patients at risk for pressure ulcers

albumin contributes to the amino acid pool, and amino acids are essential building blocks for new tissue development. It is also essential for maintaining oncotic pressure in the vascular fluid compartment and thus avoiding edema.

- Total lymphocyte count less than 1,800 mm. Malnutrition impairs the immune system, and total lymphocyte counts are a reflection of immune competence.
- A decrease in body weight by more than 15%.

If the patient is diagnosed as malnourished, nutritional supplementation may be indicated to help achieve a positive nitrogen balance. Examples of appropriate oral supplements are assisted oral feedings and dietary supplements. The goal of care is to provide approximately 30 to 35 kcal/kg of weight per day and 1.25 to 1.5 g of protein per kg of weight per day. Patients should be encouraged to improve their own dietary habits, and education should focus on maintaining a varied diet with adequate caloric and protein intake.

It may be difficult for a pressure ulcer patient or an at-risk patient to ingest enough protein and calories necessary to maintain skin and tissue health. Oral supplements can be very helpful in boosting calorie and protein intake. Liquid nutritional supplements are designed to be used as an adjunct to regular oral feedings.

Monitoring nutritional indexes is essential to determine effectiveness of the care plan. Serum albumin, protein markers, body weight, dietary intake, and nutritional assessment should be performed at least every 3 months in long-term care and more frequently in acutely ill patients to monitor for changes in nutritional status.

IMPLEMENTING PRESSURE ULCER PREVENTION PROGRAMS: WHAT WORKS?

One of the struggles in preventing pressure ulcers is implementing and maintaining a prevention program within an organization.[244] Facilities often fail to show an improvement in pressure ulcer outcomes such as incidence because attention has not been focused on the process of implementing new interventions in an organization. Successful pressure ulcer prevention requires a comprehensive multipronged approach that is designed by a staff from multiple disciplines. Further, we know that a single approach to implementing programs is generally not successful and that use of multiple implementation strategies is more likely to succeed. What strategies should you employ as you work to implement a pressure ulcer prevention program? Here we outline approaches that have demonstrated achievement.

An interdisciplinary approach is fundamental in the pressure ulcer prevention.[244] One of the commonalities prevalent in recent successful quality improvement efforts in hospitals and in nursing homes is the multiapproach structure of pressure ulcer care that includes the collaboration of multiple disciplines. By drawing on the expertise of interdisciplinary members, care that is both current and evidence based can be delivered. Stakeholders that can be included in the pressure ulcer team are wound care specialists, nurses, nutritionists, physical therapists, social workers, and physicians from a variety of disciplines (e.g., vascular surgery, plastic surgery, geriatricians). The cross disciplinary care can allow for a patient to receive débridement from a certified wound specialist or plastic surgeon, diet and nutritional status evaluation by a nutritionist, wheelchair support surface pressure mapping and mobility conditioning by a physical therapist, and pain management by a physician. Through the coordinated efforts of the multidisciplinary team, effective and efficient care can be successfully achieved. This can be accomplished with skin care rounds. Use of a multidisciplinary team that meets/rounds on patients at risk each week is a strategy that has worked in hospitals as the key clinicians have an opportunity to provide input into the care plan for individual patients. One person, no matter how talented or devoted, can do it alone.

Delivery of care that appreciates the highly interdependent nature of pressure ulcer management and recognizes the importance of communication is of great importance. Under the shared goal of improving clinical outcomes and providing quality care, the health-care team can collaborate to meet the dynamic and individual needs of the patient. So the second recommendation is to incorporate methods of improving communication among the health-care team as part of the implementation plan. Implementation of a standardized means of communication such as SBAR (situation, background, assessment, and recommendation) can facilitate continuity of care. This method of exchange allows for a situational awareness that all stakeholders can understand and appreciate. Under this system, the patient's history and priority problems are made very clear and the report is timely and efficient. Critical language can also be addressed, to ensure that there is little misunderstanding on the severity or meaning of words used. The SBAR concludes with a recommendation that the clinician on the receiving end can then consider when adjusting the patient's plan of care. This standardized means of communicating can ensure that each member of the health-care team has a current understanding of the patient's condition and is aware of the priority goals of care. A critical part of this communication vehicle is use of standard tools for reporting activities. For example, if a hospital uses the Braden Scale for pressure ulcer risk assessment, all clinicians in the hospital should be familiar with it and those nursing homes who routinely receive patients from the hospital should also use the Braden Scale. Use of the same standard tools enhances transitions from one care level to another within and between health-care organizations. Use of the same standard tools facilitates accurate communication about the patient's pressure ulcer risk status, prevention strategies in use, and response to prevention.

Another method of improving communication is to incorporate "Turn on Transfer" and "hand off" protocols. Turn on Transfer protocols require that when a patient is transferred anywhere within an institution that the receiving clinician must turn the patient (unless the medical condition prohibits turning) and check the sacrum, buttocks, and heels prior to accepting the patient. This takes very little time and assures that all are aware of the status of the skin. Change of shift is handled in the same manner, as a part of change of shift "handoff," the patient's risk status, current prevention strategies, and response to prevention strategies is reported and the patient is turned to check the sacrum, buttocks, and heels.

Research has shown that a third approach beneficial in improving patient outcomes has been to bundle a standardized set of interventions necessary to achieving quality care and create an acronym for the bundled care practices.[245–248] Similar to the bundles created for prevention of ventilator associated pneumonia or surgical site infection in the acute care setting, the NO ULCERS and SKIN bundles have been established as a means to prevent the inadvertent omission of any steps in pressure ulcer care. The NO UCLERS bundle, created by the New Jersey Hospital Association is an acronym for Nutrition and fluid status, Observation of skin, Up and walking or turn and position, Lift (don't drag) skin, Clean skin and continence care, Elevate heels, Risk assessment, and Support surfaces for pressure redistribution.[246,247] Similarly, the SKIN (Surface selection, Keep turning, Incontinence management, and Nutrition) bundle acts as an alternative tool kit for standardizing pressure ulcer prevention and management.[246–248] Such bundles serve as a reminder of what procedures of pressure ulcer care are most important and provide clinicians with a consistent set of interventions that can be referenced for improved communication. The acronyms assist in communication and motivation, examples of other acronyms include SOS—save our skin; PUPP—pressure ulcer prevention program. Bundles work because they have built in redundancy; if one aspect of care is missed when the next care practice is delivered, the missed care is caught and corrected.

One of the distinct advantages of bundles is that it allows multiple disciplines to communicate effectively regarding the status of care already received and care that has yet to be performed. Thus, the bundle can clarify when and where to make referrals and ease the continuity of care between disciplines.

The fourth recommendation is to incorporate routine audits of behaviors with prompt feedback on performance to clinicians. Providing feedback on performance communicates the status of the implementation of the new program and demonstrates where improvement is needed. Providing feedback from data based audits is most successful when the feedback is timely and focused. For example, feedback should be provided on a unit or individual level as compared to on an organization as whole. The audit procedure to collect data on clinician behavior needs to be quick and easily conducted or you run the risk of the audit becoming so burdensome and time consuming that it is not performed. This leads to lack of feedback data to clinicians and the disappearance of the program. Audit data provides the information that can be used to further improve the program. Thus, implementation is a continual process that is data driven based on frequent use of audit and feedback approaches. Small experiments to improve the program can be conducted through quality improvement cycles of plan-do-study-act.[244]

The fifth recommendation is to understand the importance of both clinician and administration or leadership involvement in the process. Identification of a skin champion, a clinician that is focused on improving the skin care of patients on a particular unit is a key strategy in successful programs. But involvement of clinicians and direct care providers is not enough. Leadership of the organization must be actively supportive of the program. Administrators can make skin rounds to talk with

- Patients/family members about how often they are being repositioned
- Nurses and direct care providers about barriers or obstacles to implementing the program
- Unit leaders or champions about progress and patient outcomes

The influence that top administration can make on motivating direct care providers in implementing the program cannot be overstated. Ongoing support, commitment, and recognition from all levels of leadership in the organization are critical to success.

A sixth recommendation is to use visual cues such as turning clocks, stickers on medical records, arm bands on patients at risk, pocket-sized reference cards for nurses, or newsletters updating staff on progress. These cues provide a nonverbal method of quickly communicating patient status to all who work in the organization or provide a quick reference for nurses and direct care providers at the bedside.

While these six recommendations do not include all strategies for implementing a pressure ulcer prevention program, they provide some guidance on what has worked in organizations. One of the difficulties in evaluating implementation of pressure ulcer prevention programs is that there is limited data on sustainability of such programs. There are little data available to know what strategies are successful with long-term sustainability of a program, or even if a program can be institutionalized such that it is maintained. These strategies assume that the organization has a person who is knowledgeable about wounds and pressure ulcers. In some areas, access to a knowledgeable wound care clinician is not available. In these cases, use of telehealth may be helpful in implementing a pressure ulcer prevention program and in treating existing pressure ulcers.

TELEHEALTH AND PRESSURE ULCER CARE

Telecommunication technology enables clinicians to deliver care from a remotely based facility and improves continuity of care. While the health-care provider remains at a distance, utilization of a videophone system, video conferencing exchange, or digital image transfer facilitates the assessment of a patient's clinical condition.[249] Telehealth not only provides relief for patients with impaired mobility but for frail elders who consider transport to specialized clinics both a strenuous and stressful event.[250] Telerehabilitation with transmission of still images and audio regarding stage III/IV pressure ulcers as a means of clinical assessment for spinal cord injury patients in home care results in increased wound healing.[201] Further, by including standard wound characteristics such as tunneling, undermining, granulation tissue, necrotic tissue, purulent exudate, induration, and

erythema, several investigators found that communication via a video telecommunications systems could effectively connect the remotely based nurse with wound care experts.[251] This same approach can be used for pressure ulcer prevention and detection of early pressure damage. In particular, several of the devices to detect early pressure ulcer damage are or would be able to transmit data to off-site experts for interpretation, thus aiding remote facilities in early detection of damage.

The use of digital cameras to track pressure ulcer staging is a popular practice advancing the management and treatment of wounds from distant facilities. By transferring digital photographs from the remote environment to expert clinicians' agencies, both economic and clinical benefits emerge. The images provide objective, detailed records capturing changes in a wound's color, size, and depth. This more advanced form of documentation surpasses the traditional written description of pressure ulcers and can result in superior wound healing outcomes for existing ulcers[252] as well as reducing emergency department visits, decreasing hospitalizations, shortening hospital lengths of stay, and lowering cost.[253]

OUTCOME MEASURES

The most appropriate outcome measures to evaluate the effectiveness of pressure ulcer prevention programs are incidence and prevalence rates. When a prevention program is successful, the organization's incidence of pressure ulcer development should decrease or remain at a low level. Incidence and prevalence data should be risk adjusted by using risk-stratification techniques when gathering data. This will allow comparison of data with other health-care facilities for benchmarking and adequate evaluation of prevention programs as case mix of the organization varies over time. For patients who already have a pressure ulcer, a successful outcome for pressure ulcer prevention is no further areas of skin breakdown. Again, risk-stratification techniques should be used so that data can be compared with other facilities and so that severity of pressure ulcers can be evaluated accurately. In addition to patient outcome data such as incidence, process outcomes measures can be useful in evaluating program success. Examples of process outcome measures include

- Percent of patients admitted to the facility who have a risk assessment conducted within 12 hours
- Percent of patients admitted to the facility who have a skin assessment conducted within 4 hours
- Percent of patients determined at high risk who are placed on a support surface within 8 hours

REFERRAL CRITERIA

As we have seen, an interdisciplinary approach is critical to prevention of pressure ulcers. Referrals assist with appropriate management of particular risk factors for developing pressure ulcers. Use referral in the following circumstances:

- Nutritional consultation for patients determined at risk for pressure ulcers, malnutrition, or with nutritional concerns
- Enterostomal therapy or continence nurse (or clinical specialist in this area) consultation for patients with urinary or fecal incontinence

• Physical therapy for assistance with correct positioning in seated individuals and for conditioning and strength training to increase mobility and activity

SELF-CARE TEACHING GUIDELINES

Patient's and caregiver's instruction in self-care must be individualized to specific pressure ulcer development risk factors, the individual patient's learning style and coping mechanisms, and the ability of the patient/caregiver to perform procedures. In teaching prevention guidelines to caregivers, it is particularly important to encourage return demonstration. Observe the caregiver performing repositioning, managing incontinence, and providing general skin care. Your observations will help you not only to evaluate the caregiver's learning, but also to provide individualized support and follow-up education. General education strategies are presented for patients, caregivers, nurse attendants, and nurses in Table 9.3 and Exhibit 9.5 presents a tool for documenting teaching.

TABLE 9.3	Education for the Direct Health-Care Team			
	Nurse	**Nurse Assistant (or Direct Caregiver)**	**Family/Caregiver**	**Patient**
Turning and Repositioning	Recognize and incorporate the following into the patient's plan of care: • The significance of low pressures over long periods of time and high pressures over short periods of time • Areas of highest pressure and greatest risk: i.e., buttocks and ischial tuberosities in seated position, heels and sacrum in lying position • Recognize the influence of support surfaces in relationship to turning and repositioning • Incorporate individual patient factors into determining frequency of repositioning • Coach, improvise, and devise creative strategies for meeting individual patient needs • Educate family/caregiver and patient • Collaborate with multidisciplinary team to optimize pressure ulcer prevention and treatment	• Maintain a 30-degree tilt with a foam wedge • Create schedule for turning and repositioning • Perform return demonstration of a repositioning procedure to the nurse • Understands the purpose of and how to use turning sheets or turning device • Avoid semi-Fowler position and limit the upright position (anything >30 degrees)	• Turn patient as needed and in accordance with devised turning schedule (every 4 h if also on a pressure redistribution support surface; every 2 h if on a standard mattress) • Position pillows under legs to elevate the heels, between the ankles and the knees, behind the back, and under the head • Perform return demonstration to the nurse • Understands the purpose of and how to use turning sheets • Observation of patient when sitting to avoid sliding out of chair	• Use sidebars or an overhead trapeze to aid with movement • Understands necessity for movement (i.e., weight shifting) • Performs self-care measures when appropriate • Wheelchair-bound patients should perform push-ups, side leans, or back tilts a minimum of once every hour • Use footstools and foot pedals on wheelchairs to prevent chair sliding • Ensure that wheelchair seat cushion is in good condition • Minimize exposure to risk factors (i.e., smoking and drinking)
• Support Surfaces	• Understands the importance of support surfaces (i.e., tissue load) • Assess patient for need of support surface • Evaluate and collaborate with family/caregiver and patient in determining support surface to be used (cost, comfort, ease of use, patients condition, powered versus nonpowered, etc.) • Educate family/caregiver and patient on use of selected surface	• Check for bottoming out (refer to text) • Check to make sure the patient is in-place on the wheelchair, chair, or bed • Check to make sure that the surface is functioning properly (i.e., if it's a powered device)	• Communicates with patients and families/caregivers about concerns regarding support surfaces • Monitors condition of the support surface and reports to nurse when problems occur • Ensures that patient is positioned properly on support surface	• Communicates with family/caregiver, nurse, and multidisciplinary team about preferences and concerns regarding support surface • Monitors condition of the support surface and reports to nurse when problems occur

| | | TABLE | 9.3 | **Education for the Direct Health-Care Team (*continued*)** |

	Nurse	Nurse Assistant (or Direct Caregiver)	Family/Caregiver	Patient
Skin Assessments	• Performs routine skin assessments, specifically over bony prominences and under medical devices • Uses appropriate wound assessment and risk assessment tools (i.e., BWAT and Braden Scale) • Plans and implements interventions accordingly • Takes pictures of skin to monitor progression and improvement of skin breakdown • Uses multidisciplinary approach • Uses telehealth services to aid in skin assessments • Educates family/caregiver and patient on how to perform daily skin observations	• Aids in skin observations especially during bathing and over areas of bony prominences • Inspects patient for incontinent episodes and intervenes accordingly • Communicates with nurse new areas of possible skin breakdown • Takes pictures of skin to monitor skin health	• Aids in daily skin observations over bony prominences • Inspects patient for incontinent episodes and intervenes accordingly • Reports to nurse any changes in skin integrity • Takes pictures of skin to monitor skin health	• Performs daily skin observations on areas accessible to the patient (i.e., using a mirror), especially over bony prominences • Reports to nurse any changes in skin integrity or pain at bony prominences
Nutrition	• Routine assessment of patient's nutritional status to detect and monitor for malnutrition • Uses appropriate tool for nutrition assessment • Assess and monitor patient's dietary intake, weight, body mass index, key laboratory values (e.g., serum albumin, prealbumin, total lymphocyte count) • Consult dietician regarding patients nutritional status (serum albumin, transferring, lymphocyte levels) • Educate family/caregiver on appropriate dietary selections including the importance of consuming high-protein foods • For patients in need of nutritional supplementation and/or vitamin supplementation, educates on importance and type of supplementation	• Assists patient with meals • Measures and records weights • Monitors intake and output • Assists with nutritional supplementation • Encourages sufficient fluid intake	• Purchase and prepare nutritionally relevant meals • Assist patient with meals • Provides snacks and nutritional supplements between meals • Offer plenty of fluids to ensure adequate hydration	• Communicates favorite foods to family/caregiver • Reports anorexia, nausea, vomiting, signs of weight loss to the nurse • Maintains adequate fluid intake

(*continued*)

| TABLE 9.3 | Education for the Direct Health-Care Team (*continued*) |

	Nurse	Nurse Assistant (or Direct Caregiver)	Family/Caregiver	Patient
Moisture Management	• Understands the effects of excessive moisture or lack of moisture on skin integrity and skin breakdown • Helps family/caregiver and patient establish a bowel or bladder regimen • Establishes with family/caregiver and patient a bathing schedule • Encourages and educates family/caregiver and patient on how to give a bath (i.e., avoid hot water and irritating cleansers; use pH-balanced, low-acid moisturizers after bathing) • Understands the importance and use of barrier creams and other equipment • Aids family/caregiver and patient on the purchase of appropriate equipment to manage moisture • Identify presence of fungal infections • Assesses patient for poorly managed incontinence and intervenes accordingly (i.e., need for a collection device or absorbent pads)	• Assist with personal hygiene after incontinent episodes when appropriate • Encourages patient participation in personal hygiene • When performing baths, avoid using hot water • Use pH-balanced lotion after bath and as needed to maintain adequate skin moisture • Replaces pads and linens when soiled • Understands and uses topical barrier to protect skin • Implement the bowel and bladder briefs during incontinence care • Applies ointments/barrier creams to protect skin from IAD	• Inspects for wetness and fecal matter and intervenes accordingly • Assist with personal hygiene after incontinent episodes when appropriate • Encourage patient participation in personal hygiene • Replaces pads and linens when soiled • Understands and uses topical barrier to protect skin • Aid patient with toileting needs • Reports problems in controlling excessive moisture or dryness to the nurse	• Participates in personal hygiene • Involved in bowel and bladder regimen, if incontinent • Reports problems with elimination and moisture management to the nurse

BWAT, Bates-Jensen Wound Assessment Tool.

| EXHIBIT 9.5 | |

Self-Care Teaching Guidelines

Self-Care Guidelines Specific to Pressure Ulcer Prevention	Instructions Given (Date/Initials)	Demonstration or Review of Material (Date/Initials)	Return Demonstration or States Understanding (Date/Initials)
1. Identification of specific risk factors for pressure ulcer development			

2. Immobility, inactivity, and decreased sensory perception strategies
  a. Passive repositioning
    (1) Demonstrates one-person turning
    (2) Demonstrates two-person turning
    (3) Frequency of turning/repositioning
    (4) Full shifts in position versus small shifts in position			

EXHIBIT 9.5 *(continued)*			
Self-Care Guidelines Specific to Pressure Ulcer Prevention	**Instructions Given (Date/Initials)**	**Demonstration or Review of Material (Date/Initials)**	**Return Demonstration or States Understanding (Date/Initials)**
(5) Avoidance of 90-degree side-lying position, demonstrates 30-degree side-lying position			
(6) Passive range of motion exercises and frequency			
b. Pillow bridging			
(1) Use of pillows to protect heels			
(2) Pillows between bony prominences			
c. Pressure-reducing/relieving support surface			
(1) Management of support surface in use			
(2) Devices for sitting			
(3) Up in chair for _____ hour(s), _____ time(s) per day			
3. Nutrition strategies			
a. Provide adequate nutrition			
(1) Small frequent (six meals a day) high-calorie/high-protein meals			
(2) Nutritional supplements provided. Give __ _oz of ____ supplement ___ times per day.			
b. Provide adequate hydration			
(1) Eight 8-oz glasses of noncaffeine fluids per day unless contraindicated			
c. Provide general multivitamin as needed			
4. Friction and shear strategies			
a. Use of turning and draw sheets			
b. Use of cornstarch, lubricants, pad protectors, thin film dressings, or hydrocolloid dressings over friction risk sites			
c. General skin care			
(1) Skin cleansing			
(2) Skin moisturizing (Use _____ product on _____ areas of skin, _____ times a day.)			
5. Moisture—incontinence management strategies			
a. Use of absorbent products			
(1) Pad when lying in bed			
(2) Brief or panty pad when up in chair or walking			
b. Use of ointments, creams, and skin barriers prophylactically in perineal and perianal areas (Use _____ product on perineal/perianal areas of skin, _____ times a day.)			
c. Use of behavioral management strategies for incontinence			
(1) Scheduled toileting: toilet every _____ hours			
(2) Prompted voiding			
d. General skin care			
(1) Skin cleansing			
(a) Cleanser: _____			
(b) Soap: _____			
(c) Frequency: _____			
(2) Skin moisturizing (Use _____ product(s) on _____ areas of skin, _____ times a day.)			
(3) Skin inspection daily			
6. Importance of follow-up with health-care provider			

CONCLUSION

Pressure ulcers are the result of multiple interacting factors and require a multifaceted approach for prevention. Development of a pressure ulcer occurs with mechanical forces of pressure, shear, and deformation, and friction. A wide variety of factors place patients at risk for pressure ulcer development. Timely recognition of risk is essential in able to promptly intervene to prevent pressure-induced damage. Pressure ulcer prevention involves attention to risk assessment, skin assessment, management of tissue loads with repositioning and use of pressure redistribution support surfaces, nutrition assessment, and incontinence management. Much of pressure ulcer prevention is routine care that is delivered at intervals 24 hours a day, 7 days a week in the context of other care delivery. Yet, even as the care is routine, it is also necessary to individual pressure ulcer prevention to the individual risk factors for a particular patient. A successful pressure ulcer prevention program is multidisciplinary and multifaceted.

RESOURCES

- NPUAP
  http://www.npuap.org
  Pressure ulcer prevention and treatment clinical practice guidelines, staging information, powerpoints for teaching, some patient education materials, current information on pressure ulcers

- Wound Ostomy Continence Society
  http://www.wocn.org
  Guideline for the prevention and management of pressure ulcers
- Association for the Advancement of Wound Care
  http://www.aawconline.org/
  Patient education materials on basic skin care and wound care, patient support blog for wound patients, family members, caregivers, powerpoints for teaching, professional education materials
- Wound Healing Society
  http://www.woundheal.org/
  Guidelines for the prevention of pressure ulcers, guidelines for the treatment of pressure ulcers.
- CMS
  Tag F314 Guidance to Surveyors: Pressure Ulcers. Interpretive guidelines: Pressure ulcers. CMS Manual System, Pub 100–07 State Operations, Provider Certification. Centers for Medicare & Medicaid Services, Nov. 12, 2004. On-line: www.cms.hhs.gov/manuals/pm_trans/ R4SOM.pdf
- AHRQ
  http://www.ahrq.gov/research/ltc/pressureulcertoolkit/
  Toolkit for how to implement pressure ulcer prevention programs in hospitals
- Institute for Healthcare Improvement (IHI)
  http://www.ihi.org/ihi
  Tools for implementing best practice related to pressure ulcers.

REVIEW QUESTIONS

1. Pressure ulcers are the primary result of which of the following?
   A. Pressure and deformation of tissues
   B. Friction
   C. Moisture
   D. Friction and shear
2. Which of the following are intrinsic risk factors that decrease the tissue tolerance to pressure?
   A. Shear, friction, and moisture
   B. Nutrition, age, psychological issues, and temperature
   C. Immobility, inactivity, and loss of sensation
   D. Time of pressure, duration of pressure, and compression force
3. Which of the following method of early pressure ulcer detection uses transmission of color to determine the status of tissues?
   A. Spectroscopy
   B. Subepidermal moisture measured with capacitance methods
   C. Ultrasound
   D. Surface temperature

4. Clinical manifestations of a stage II pressure ulcer include
   A. nonblanchable erythema on intact skin
   B. shallow pink lesions or abrasions involving only the epidermis and dermis
   C. ulcers with yellow necrotic slough d. ulcers that present with subcutaneous tissue
5. The clinician is asked to recommend a support surface for P.L., who has three pressure sores: one on the sacral/coccygeal area, one on the left greater trochanter, and one on the right ischial tuberosity. The ulcers range in severity from clean, healing stage II on the sacral/coccygeal area to necrotic stage III on the left trochanter and clean stage IV on the right ischial tuberosity. Which of the following is the MOST appropriate support surface choice?
   A. A nonpowered high-specification foam support surface
   B. An alternating pressure air mattress or low-air-loss bed
   C. Standard hospital mattress
   D. A medical grade sheepskin

REFERENCES

1. Strategies for Preventing Pressure Ulcers, Joint Commission Perspectives on Patient Safety, 2008;8(1):5–7(3). http://www.jcrinc.com/Pressure-Ulcers-stage-III-IV-decubitis-ulcers/. Accessed March 23, 2009.

2. Russo, C. Steiner, C, Specter, W. Hospitalizations related to pressure ulcers among adults 18 years and older, 2006. *Healthcare Cost and Utilization Project. December.* 2008. Retrieved August 4, 2010, from www.hcup-us.ahrq.gov/reports/statbriefs/sb64.pdf

3. Jiricka MK, Ryan P, Carvalho MA, et al. Pressure ulcer risk factors in an ICU population. *Am J Crit Care.* 1995;4(5):361–367.

4. Park-Lee E, Caffrey C. Pressure ulcer among nursing home residents: United States, 2004. U.S. Department of Health and Human Services, Centers for Disease Control and Prevention, National Center for Health Statistics, NCHS Data Brief, No. 14, February 2009.

5. Gerardo MP, Teno JM, Mor V. Not so black and white: nursing home concentration of Hispanics associated with prevalence of pressure ulcers. *J Am Med Dir Assoc.* 2009;10:127–132.

6. Cai S, Mukamel DB, Temkin-Greener H. Pressure ulcer prevalence among black and white nursing home residents in New York state: evidence of racial disparity? *Med Care.* 2010;48(3):233–239.

7. Cuddigan J, Ayello E, Sussman C, eds. National Pressure Ulcer Advisory Panel. *Pressure Ulcers in America: Prevalence, Incidence, and Implications for the Future.* Reston, VA: NPUAP; 2001.

8. Bergquist S. Pressure ulcer prediction in older adults receiving home health care: Implications for use with the OASIS. *Adv Wound Care.* 2003;16:132–139.

9. Margolis DJ, Knauss J, Bilker W, et al. Medical conditions as risk factors for pressure ulcers in an outpatient setting. *Age Ageing.* 2003;32(3):259–264.

10. Hunter SM, Langemo DK, Olson B, et al. The effectiveness of skin care protocols for pressure ulcers. *Rehabil Nurs.* 1995;20(5):250–255.

11. Schue RM, Langemo DK. Pressure ulcer prevalence and incidence and a modification of the Braden Scale for a rehabilitation unit. *J Wound Ostomy Continence Nurs.* 1998;25(1):36–43.

12. Eastwood EA, Hagglund KJ, Ragnarsson KT, et al. Medical rehabilitation length of stay and outcomes for persons with traumatic spinal cord injury 1990–1997. *Arch Phys Med Rehabil.* 1999;80(11):1457–1463.

13. Rintala DH, Garber SL, Friedman JD, et al. Preventing recurrent pressure ulcers in veterans with spinal cord injury: impact of a structured education and follow-up intervention. *Arch Phys Med Rehabil.* 2008;89(8):1429–1441.

14. Chen D, Apple DF, Hudson MF, et al. Medical complications during acute rehabilitation following spinal cord injury. *Arch Phys Med Rehabil.* 1999;80:1397–1401.

15. Bours GJJ, de Laat E, Halfens RJG, et al. Prevalence, risk factors and prevention of pressure ulcers in Dutch intensive care units. *Intensive Care Med.* 2001;27(10):1599–1605.

16. Galvin, J. An audit of pressure ulcer incidence in a palliative care setting. *Int J Palliat Nurs.* 2002;8(5):214–220.

17. Henoch I, Gustafsson M. Pressure ulcers in palliative care: Development of a hospice pressure ulcer risk assessment scale. *Int J Palliat Nurs.* 2003;9(11):474–484.

18. Lyder CH, Yu C, Emerling J, et al. The Braden Scale for pressure ulcer risk: Evaluating the predictive validity in Blacks and Latino/Hispanic elders. *Appl Nurs Res.* 1999;12(2):60–68.

19. Baggerly J, DiBlasi M. Pressure sores and pressure sore prevention in a rehabilitation setting: Building information for improving outcomes and allocating resources. *Rehabil Nurs.* 1996;21(6):321–325.

20. Bergquist S, Frantz RA. Braden scale: validity in community-based older adults receiving home health care. *Appl Nurs Res.* 2001;14(1):36–43.

21. Waters RL, Meyer PR Jr, Adkins RH, et al. Emergency, acute, and surgical management of spine trauma. *Arch Phys Med Rehabil.* 1999;80(11):1383–1390.

22. Garber SL, Rintala DH, Hart KA, et al. Pressure ulcer risk in spinal cord injury: Predictors of ulcer status over 3 years. *Arch Phys Med Rehabil.* 2000;81(4):465–471.

23. Bergquist-Beringer S. National database of nursing quality indicators (NDNQI) update. National Pressure Ulcer Advisory Panel 12th National biennial conference: Emerging healthcare issues. February, 2011.

24. Curley MA, Razmus IS, Roberts KE, et al. Predicting pressure ulcer risk in pediatric patients: the Braden Q Scale. *Nurs Res.* 2003;52(1):22–33.

25. Escher Neidig JR, Klieber C, Oppliger RA. Risk factors associated with pressure ulcers in the pediatric patient following open-heart surgery. *Prog Cardiovasc Nurs.* 1989;4:99–106.

26. Huffines B, Logsdon MC. The neonatal skin risk assessment scale for predicting skin breakdown in neonates. *Issues Compr Pediatr Nurs.* 1997;20:103–114.

27. Beckrich K, Aronovitch SA. Hospital-acquired pressure ulcers: a comparison of costs in medical vs. surgical patients. *Nurs Econ.* 1999;17:263–271.

28. Brem H, Maggi J, Nierman D, et al. High cost of stage IV pressure ulcers. *Am J Surg.* 2010;200(4):473–437.

29. Centers for Medicare & Medicaid Services. Proposed Fiscal Year 2009 Payment, Policy Changes for Inpatient Stays in General Acute Care Hospitals. Available at http://www.cms.hhs.gov/apps/media/press/factsheet.asp. Accessed August 4, 2010.

30. Centers for Medicare & Medicaid Services. Medicare Program; Proposed Changes to the Hospital Inpatient Prospective Payment Systems and Fiscal Year 2009 Rates; Proposed Changes to Disclosure of Physician Ownership in Hospitals and Physician Self-Referral Rules; Proposed Collection of Information Regarding Financial Relationships Between Hospitals and Physicians: Proposed Rule. *Fed Regist.* 2008;73(84):23550. Available at http://edocket.access.gpo.gov/2008/pdf/08-1135.pdf. Accessed August 4, 2010.

31. Stroupe K, Manheim LM, Evans CT, et al. Cost of treating pressure ulcers for veterans with spinal cord injury. *Top SCI Rehabilitation,* 2011;16(4):62–73.

32. Graves N, Birrell F, Whitby M. Effect of pressure ulcers on length of hospital stay. *Infect Control Hosp Epidemiol.* 2005;26:293–297.

33. Redelings MD, Lee NE, Sorvillo F. Pressure ulcers: more lethal than we thought? *Adv Skin Wound Care.* 2005;18(7):367–72.

34. Thomas DR, Goode PS, Tarquine PH, et al. Hospital-acquired pressure ulcers and risk of death. *J Am Geriatr Soc.* 1996;44:1435–1440.

35. Voss AC, Bender SA, Ferguson ML, et al. Long-term care liability for pressure ulcers. *J Am Geriat Soc.* 2005;53:1587–1592.

36. Hahn P. *Report and Results of Updated Research on Nursing Home Liability for Pressure Ulcers.* Columbus, OH: Buckingham, Doolittle & Burroughs, LLP; 2002.

37. Waite D. Caregiver guilty in fatal neglect of patient's bedsores. The Honolulu Advertiser, October 28, 2000.

38. Haywood P. Christus St. Vincent Regional Medical Center slapped with $10.3M penalty in bed sore lawsuit, 2/18/2011; The New Mexican.

39. Daniel RK, Priest DL, Wheatley DC. Etiologic factors in pressure sores: An experimental model. *Arch Phys Med Rehabil.* 1981;62(10):492–498.

40. Kosiak M. Etiology and pathology of ischemic ulcers. *Arch Phys Med Rehabil.* 1959;40:62–69.

41. Reuler JB, Cooney TG. The pressure sore: pathophysiology and principles of management. *Ann Intern Med.* 1981;94:661.

42. Seiler WD, Stahelin HB. Recent findings on decubitus ulcer pathology: implications for care. *Geriatrics.* 1986;41:47–60.

43. Witkowski JA, Parish LC. Histopathology of the decubitus ulcer. *J Am Acad Dermatol.* 1982;6:1014–1021.

44. Berlowitz DR, Brienza DM. Are all pressure ulcers the result of deep tissue injury? A review of the literature. *Ostomy Wound Manage.* 2007;53(10):34–38.

45. Farid, KJ. Applying observations from forensic science to understanding the development of pressure ulcers. *Ostomy Wound Manage.* 2007;53(4):26–28, 30, 32 passim.

46. Gefen A. Reswick and Rogers pressure-time curve for pressure ulcer risk. Part 2. *Nurs Stand*. 2009;23(46):40–44.

47. Stekelenburg A, Gawlitta D, Bader DL, et al. Deep tissue injury: how deep is our understanding? *Arch Phys Med Rehabil*. 2008;89(7):1410–1413.

48. Stekelenburg A, Strijkers GJ, Parusel H, et al. Role of ischemia and deformation in the onset of compression-induced deep tissue injury: MRI-based studies in a rat model. *J Appl Physiol*. 2007;102(5):2002–2011.

49. Peeters EA, Oomens CW, Bouten CV, et al. Mechanical and failure properties of single attached cells under compression. *J Biomech*. 2005;38(8):1685–1693.

50. Gefen A, van Nierop B, Bader DL, et al. Strain-time cell-death threshold for skeletal muscle in a tissue-engineered model system for deep tissue injury. *J Biomech*. 2008;41(9):2003–2012.

51. Linder-Ganz E, Yarnitzky G, Yizhar Z, et al. Real-time finite element monitoring of sub-dermal tissue stresses in individuals with spinal cord injury: toward prevention of pressure ulcers. *Ann Biomed Eng*. 2009;37(2):387–400.

52. Linder-Ganz E, Gefen A. The effects of pressure and shear on capillary closure in the microstructure of skeletal muscles. *Ann Biomed Eng*. 2007;35(12):2095–107.

53. Iaizzo PA. Temperature modulation of pressure ulcer formation: using a swine model. *Wounds*. 2004;16:336–343.

54. Salcido R, Donofrio JC, Fisher SB, et al. Histopathology of pressure ulcers as a result of sequential computer-controlled pressure sessions in a fuzzy rat model. *Adv Wound Care*. 1994;7:23–28.

55. Peirce SM, Skalak TC, Rodeheaver GT, Ischemia-reperfusion injury in chronic pressure ulcer formation: a skin model in the rat. *Wound Rep Reg*. 2000;8:68–76.

56. Houwing R, Overgoor M, Kon M, et al. Pressure-induced skin lesions in pigs: reperfusion injury and the effects of vitamin E. *J Wound Care*. 2000;9:36–40.

57. Miller GE, Seale J. Lymphatic clearance during compressive loading. *Lymphology*. 1981;14:161–166.

58. Gefen A. Risk factors for a pressure-related deep tissue injury: a theoretical model. *Med Bio Eng Comput*. 2007;45:563–573.

59. Shabshin N, Zoizner G, Herman A, et al. Use of weight-bearing MRI for evaluating wheelchair cushions based on internal soft-tissue deformations under ischial tuberosities. *J Rehabil Res Dev*. 2010;47(1):31–42.

60. Lindan O, Greenway RM, Piazza JM. Pressure distribution on the surface of the human body. *Arch Phys Med Rehabil*. 1965;46:378.

61. Gefen A. The biomechanics of sitting-acquired pressure ulcers in patients with spinal cord injury or lesions. *Int Wound J*. 2007;4(3):222–231.

62. Herrman EC, Knapp CF, Donofrio JC, et al. Skin perfusion responses to surface pressure-induced ischemia: Implications for the developing pressure ulcer. *J Rehabil Res Dev*. 1999;36(2):109–120.

63. Pack R, Chang DS, Brevetti LS, et al. Correlation of a simple direct measurement of muscle pO₂ to a clinical ischemia index and histology in a rat model for chronic severe hindlimb ischemia. *J Vasc Surg*. 2002;36:172–179.

64. Walker PM. Ischemial reperfusion injury in skeletal muscle. *Ann Vasc Surg*. 1991;5(4):399–402.

65. Hernandez-Maldonado JJ, Teehan E, Franco CD, et al. Superoxide anion production by leukocytes exposed to post-ischemic skeletal muscle. *J Cardiovasc Surg*. 1992;33:695–699.

66. Schubert V, Fagrell B. Local skin pressure and its effects on skin microcirculation as evaluated by laser-Doppler fluxemetry. *Clin Physiol*. 1989;9:535–545.

67. Lavery LA, Higgins KR, Lanctot DR, et al. Home monitoring of foot skin temperatures to prevent ulceration. *Diabetes Care*. 2004;27:2642–2647.

68. Huether SE. The cellular environment: Fluids and electrolytes, acids and bases. In: McCance KL, Huether SE, eds. *Pathophysiology:*

69. Landis EM. Micro-injection studies of capillary blood pressure in human skin. *Heart*. 1930;15:209.

70. Husain T. An experimental study of some pressure effects on tissues, with reference to the bedsore problem. *J Pathol Bacteriol*. 1953;66:347–358.

71. Kosiak M, Kubicek WG, Olsen M, et al. Evaluation of pressure as a factor in the production of ischial ulcers. *Arch Phys Med Rehabil*. 1958;39:623.

72. Edberg EL, Cerny K, Stauffer ES. Prevention and treatment of pressure sores. *Phys Ther*. 1973;53:246–252.

73. Agam L, Gefen A. Pressure ulcers and deep tissue injury: a bioengineering perspective. *J Wound Care*. 2007;16(8):336–342.

74. Shea JD. Pressures sores: Classification and management. *Clin Orthop*. 1975;112:89–100.

75. NPUAP. Pressure ulcer stages revised by NPUAP. 2007. http://www.npuap.org/pr2.htm. Last accessed March 3, 2011.

76. Sprigle S, Linden M, Riordan B. Analysis of localized erythema using clinical indicators and spectroscopy. *Ostomy/Wound Manage*. 2003;49(3):42–52.

77. Sprigle S, Linden M, McKenna D, et al. Clinical skin temperature measurement to predict incipient pressure ulcers. *Adv Skin Wound Care*. 2001;14(3):133–137.

78. Schubert V, Perbeck L, Schubert PA. Skin microcirculatory and thermal changes in elderly subjects with early stage of pressure sores. *Clin Physiol*. 1994;14(1):1–13.

79. Bennett MA. Report of the task force on the implications for darkly pigmented intact skin in the prediction and prevention of pressure ulcers. *Adv Wound Care*. 1995;8(6):34–35.

80. Graves DJ. Stage I in ebony complexion. *Decubitus Letter to the Editor*. 1990;3(4):4.

81. Parish LC, Witkowski JA, Crissey JT, eds. *The Decubitis Ulcer in Clinical Practice*. Berlin, Germany: Springer-Verlag; 1997.

82. Ankrom MA, Bennett RG, Sprigle S, et al.; National Pressure Ulcer Advisory Panel. Pressure-related deep tissue injury under intact skin and the current pressure ulcer staging systems. *Adv Skin Wound Care*. 2005;18(1):35–42.

83. Amlung SR, Miller WL, Bosley LM. The 1999 National Pressure Ulcer Prevalence Survey; a benchmarking approach. *Adv Skin Wound Care*. 2001;14:297–301.

84. VanGilder C, MacFarlane GD, Harrison P, et al. The demographics of suspected deep tissue injury in the United States: an analysis of the international pressure ulcer prevalence survey 2006–2009. *Adv Skin Wound Care*. 2010;23(6):254–261.

85. VanGilder C, MacFarlane GD, Meyer S. Results of nine international pressure ulcer prevalence surveys: 1989–2005. *Ostomy Wound Manage*. 2008;54(2):40–54.

86. Bates-Jensen BM, Guihan M, Garber S, et al. Characteristics of recurrent pressure ulcers in veterans with spinal cord injury. *J Spinal Cord Med*. 2009;32(1):34–42.

87. Garber SL, Biddle AK, Click CN, et al. Pressure ulcer prevention and treatment following spinal cord injury: a clinical practice guideline for health-care professionals. Consortium for Spinal Cord Medicine Clinical Practice Guidelines, Paralyzed Veterans of America; 2000.

88. McLane KM, Bookout K, McCord S, et al. The 2003 national pediatric pressure ulcer and skin breakdown prevalence survey: a multisite study. *J Wound Ostomy Continence Nurs*. 2004;31(4):168–178.

89. Black JM, Edsberg LE, Baharestani MM, et al.; National Pressure Ulcer Advisory Panel. Pressure ulcers: avoidable or unavoidable? Results of the national pressure ulcer advisory panel consensus conference. *Ostomy Wound Manage*. 2011;57(2):24–37.

90. Black JM, Cuddigan JE, Walko MA, et al. Medical device related pressure ulcers in hospitalized patients. *Int Wound J*. 2010;7(5):358–365.

The Biologic Basis for Disease in Adults and Children. 6th ed. St. Louis, MO: Elsevier Mosby; 2010.

91. Allman RM, Goode PS, Patrick MM, et al. Pressure ulcer risk factors among hospitalized patients with activity limitation. *JAMA*. 1995;273:865–870.

92. Halfens RJG, Bours GJJW, van Ast W. Relevance of the diagnosis 'stage 1 pressure ulcer': an empirical study of the clinical course of stage 1 ulcers in acute care and long-term hospital populations. *J Clin Nurs*. 2001;10(6):748–757.

93. Ek A. Prevention, treatment, and healing of pressure sores in long-term care patients. *Scand J Caring Sci*. 1987;1:7–13.

94. Vanderwee K, Grypdonck M, Defloor T. Non-blanchable erythema as an indicator for the need for pressure ulcer prevention: a randomized-controlled trial. *J Clin Nurs*. 2007;16(2):325–35.

95. Schnelle JF, Adamson GM, Cruise PA, et al. Skin disorders and moisture in incontinent nursing home residents: intervention implications. *J Am Geriatr Soc*. 1997;45(10):1182–1188.

96. Bergstrom N, Braden B, Kemp M, et al. Predicting pressure ulcer risk: A multisite study of the predictive validity of the Braden Scale. *Nurs Res*. 1998:47(5):261–269.

97. Lyder CH, Yu C, Emerling J, et al. The Braden Scale for pressure ulcer risk: evaluating the predictive validity in Blacks and Latino/Hispanic elders. *Appl Nurs Res*. 1999;12(2):60–68.

98. Alexander H, Miller DL. Determining skin thickness with pulsed ultra sound. *J Invest Dermatol*. 1979;72(1):17–19.

99. Rippon MG, Springett K, Walmsley R. Ultrasound evaluation of acute experimental and chronic clinical wounds. *Skin Res Tech*. 1999;5(4):228–236.

100. Harland CC, Kale SG, Jackson P, et al. Differentiation of common benign pigmented skin lesions from melanoma by high-resolution ultrasound. *Br J Dermatol*. 2000;143(2):281–289.

101. Akesson A, Hesselstrand R, Scheja A, et al. Longitudinal development of skin involvement and reliability of high frequency ultrasound in systematic sclerosis. *Ann Rheum Dis*. 2004;63:791–796.

102. Quintavalle PR, Lyder CH, Mertz PJ, et al. Use of high-resolution, high-frequency diagnostic ultrasound to investigate the pathogenesis of pressure ulcer development. *Adv Skin Wound Care*. 2006;19(9):498–505.

103. Georgia Tech Research News, Skin Deep: Imaging Technologies May Detect Pressure Ulcers and Deep-tissue Injuries that Healthcare Workers May Miss. *Research Horizons Magazine*. August 3, 2006 http://gtresearchnews.gatech.edu/newsrelease/skin-deep.htm.

104. Rapp MP, Bergstrom N, Padhye NS. Contribution of skin temperature regularity to the risk of developing pressure ulcers in nursing facility residents. *Adv Skin Wound Care*. 2009;22(11):506–513.

105. Bates-Jensen B, McCreath H. Evaluation of skin surface temperature as a method of detecting erythema and stage I pressure ulcers in nursing home residents: a pilot study. National Pressure Ulcer Advisory Panel Consensus Conference abstracts, Las Vegas, NV. February 24–26, 2011.

106. Armstrong D, Lavery L, Wunderlich RP, et al. Stickel Silver Award. Skin temperatures as a one-time screening tool do not predict future diabetic foot complications. *J Am Podiatr Med Assoc*. 2003;93(6):443–447.

107. Anderson ES, Karlsmark T. Evaluation of four non-invasive methods for examination and characterization of pressure ulcers. *Skin Res Technol*. 2008;14(3):270–276.

108. Fromy B, Sigaudo-Roussel D, Gaubert-Dahan ML, et al. Aging-associated sensory neuropathy alters pressure induced vasodilation in humans. *J Invest Dermatol*. 2010;130(3):849–855.

109. Sae-Sia W, Wipke-Tevis DD, Williams DA. Elevated sacral skin temperature (T(s)): A risk factor for pressure ulcer development in hospitalized neurologically impaired Thai patients. *Appl Nurs Res*. 2005;18(1):29–35.

110. Lachenbruch C. Skin cooling surfaces: estimating the importance of limiting skin temperature. *Ostomy Wound Manage*. 2005;51(2):70–79.

111. Tzen YT, Brienza DM, Karg P, et al. Effects of local cooling on sacral skin perfusion response to pressure: implications for pressure ulcer prevention. *J Tissue Viability*. 2010;19(3):86–97.

112. Nakagami G, Sanada H, Iizaka S, et al. Predicting delayed pressure ulcer healing using thermography: a prospective cohort study. *J Wound Care*. 2010;19(11):465–466, 468, 470 passim.

113. Riordan B, Sprigle S, Linden M. Testing the validity of erythema detection algorithms. *J Rehabil Res Dev*. 2001;38(1):13–22.

114. Leachtenaur J, Kell S, Turner B, et al. A non-contact imaging-based approach to detecting stage I pressure ulcers. Proceedings of the 28th IEEE, 2006; EMBS Annual International Conference, New York City, NY, August 30–September 3, 2006:6380–6383.

115. Sprigle S, Zhang L, Duckworth M. Detection of skin erythema in darkly pigmented skin using multispectral images. *Adv Skin Wound Care*. 2009;22:172–179.

116. Sprigle S, Linden M, Riordan B. Characterizing reactive hyperemia via tissue reflectance spectroscopy in response to an ischemic load across gender, age, skin pigmentation, and diabetes. *Med Eng Phys*. 2002;24:651–661.

117. Nixon J, Cranny G, Bond, S. Pathology, diagnosis, and classification of pressure ulcers: comparing clinical and imaging techniques. *Wound Rep Reg*. 2005;13:365–372.

118. Boyce ST, Supp AP, Harriger MD, et al. Surface electrical capacitance as a noninvasive index of epidermal barrier in cultured skin substitutes in athymic mice. *J Invest Dermatol*. 1996;107(1):82–87.

119. Palensek J, Morhenn VB. Changes in the skin's capacitance after damage to the stratum corneum in humans. *J Cutan Med Surg*. 1999;3(3):127–131.

120. Miettinen M, Monkkonen J, Lahtinen MR, et al. Measurement of oedema in irritant-exposed skin by a dielectric technique. *Skin Res Technol*. 2006;12: 235–240.

121. Ho DQ, Bello YM, Grove GL, et al. A pilot study of noninvasive methods to assess healed acute and chronic wounds. *Dermatol Surg*. 2000;26(1):42–49.

122. Nuutinen J, Ikaheimo R, Lahtinen T. Validation of a new dielectric device to assess changes of tissue water in skin and subcutaneous fat. *Physiol Meas*. 2004;25:447–454.

123. Alanen E, Nuutinen J, Nicklen K, et al. Measurement of hydration in the stratum corneum with the MoistureMeter and comparison with the Corneometer. *Skin Res Technol*. 2004;10:32–37.

124. Goretsky MJ, Supp AP, Greenhalgh DG, et al. Surface electrical capacitance as an index of epidermal barrier properties of composite skin substitutes and skin autografts. *Wound Rep Reg*. 1995;3:419–425.

125. Mayrovitz HN. Assessing local tissue edema in postmastectomy lymphedema. *Lymphology*. 2007;40(2):87–94.

126. Harrow JJ, Mayrovitz HN. Initial assessment of tissue water content surrounding pressure ulcers in spinal cord injury patients. Abstract, *Symposium on Advanced Wound Care & Medical Research Forum on Wound Repair*; April 2006.

127. Bates-Jensen BM, McCreath HE, Kono A, et al. Sub-epidermal moisture predicts erythema and stage i pressure ulcers in nursing home residents: a pilot study. *J Am Geriatr Soc*. 2007;55:1199–1205.

128. Bates-Jensen BM, McCreath H, Pongquan V, et al. Sub-epidermal moisture differentiates erythema and stage i pressure ulcers in nursing home residents. *Wound Repair Regen*. 2008;16:189–197.

129. Bates-Jensen BM, McCreath HE, Pongquan V. Subepidermal moisture is associated with early pressure ulcer damage in nursing home residents with dark skin tones: pilot findings. *J Wound Ostomy Continence Nurs*. 2009;36(3):277–284. PMID: 19448508.

130. Gray M, Bliss DZ, Doughty DB, ET AL. Incontinence-associated dermatitis: a consensus. *J Wound Ostomy Continence Nurs*. 2007;34:45–54.

131. Brown DS, Sears M. Perineal dermatitis: a conceptual framework. *Ostomy/Wound Manage*. 1993;39(7):20–25.

132. Gray M, Incontinence-related skin damage: essential knowledge. *Ostomy Wound Manage.* 2007;53(12):28–32.

133. Junkin J, Selekof JL. Beyond "diaper rash": incontinence-associated dermatitis: does it have you seeing red? *Nursing.* 2008;38(11 suppl):56hn1-10.

134. Dinsdale JM. Decubitus ulcers: Role of pressure and friction in causation. *Arch Phys Med Rehabil.* 1974;55:147–153.

135. Langemo DK, Brown G. Skin fails too: acute, chronic, and end-stage skin failure. *Adv Skin Wound Care.* 2006;19(4):206–211.

136. Sibbald RG, Krasner DL, Lutz JB, et al. The SCALE expert panel: skin changes at life's end. Final Consensus Document. October 1, 2009.

137. Witkowski JA, Parish LC. Skin failure and the pressure ulcer. *Decubitus.* 1993;6(5):4.

138. Witkowski JA, Parish LC. The decubitus ulcer: skin failure and destructive behavior. *Int J Dermatol.* 2000;39(12):894–896.

139. Kennedy KL. The prevalence of pressure ulcers in an intermediate care facility. *Decubitus.* 1989;2(2):44–45.

140. Hanson D, Langemo DK, Olson B, et al. The prevalence and incidence of pressure ulcers in the hospice setting: analysis of two methodologies. *Am J Hosp Palliat Care.* 1991;8(5):18–22.

141. National Pressure Ulcer Advisory Panel and European Pressure Ulcer Advisory Panel. Prevention and treatment of pressure ulcers: Clinical practice guideline. Washington DC: National Pressure Ulcer Advisory Panel; 2009.

142. Bergstrom N, Demuth PJ, Braden BJ. A clinical trial of the Braden Scale for predicting pressure sore risk. *Nurs Clin North Am.* 1987;22:417–428.

143. Exton-Smith AN, Sherwin RW. The prevention of pressure sores: significance of spontaneous bodily movements. *Lancet.* 1961;2:1124–1126.

144. Allman RM, Goode PS, Patrick MM, et al. Pressure ulcer risk factors among hospitalized patients with activity limitations. *JAMA.* 1995;273:865–870.

145. Brandeis GH, Ooi WL, Hossain M, et al. A longitudinal study of risk factors associated with the formation of pressure ulcers in nursing homes. *J Am Geriatr Soc.* 1994;42:388–393.

146. Lindgren M, Unosson M, Fredrikson M, et al. Immobility—a major risk factor for development of pressure ulcers among adult hospitalized patients: a prospective study. *Scand J Caring Sci.* 2004;18(1):57–64.

147. Curry K, Casady L. The relationship between extended periods of immobility and decubitus ulcer formation in the acutely spinal cord injured individual. *J Neurosci Nurs.* 1992;24:185–189.

148. Hammond MC, Bozzacco VA, Stiens SA, et al. Pressure ulcer incidence on a spinal cord injury unit. *Adv Wound Care.* 1994;7(6):57–60.

149. Reichel SM. Shearing force as a factor in decubitus ulcers in paraplegics. *JAMA.* 1958;166:762–763.

150. Bennett L, Kavner D, Lee BY, et al. Skin stress and blood flow in sitting paraplegic patients. *Arch Phys Med Rehabil.* 1984;65(4):186–190.

151. Bates-Jensen B. Incontinence management. In: Parish LC, Witkowski JA, Crissey JT, eds. *The Decubitus Ulcer in Clinical Practice.* Berlin, Germany: Springer-Verlag; 1997:189–199.

152. Berg RW, Milligan MC, Sarbaugh FC. Association of skin wetness and pH with diaper dermatitis. *Pediatr Dermatol.* 1994;11:18–20.

153. Zimmerer RE, Lawson KD, Calvert CJ. The effects of wearing diapers on skin. *Pediatr Dermatol.* 1986;3:95–101.

154. Buckingham KW, Berg RW. Etiologic factors in diaper dermatitis: the role of feces. *Pediatr Dermatol.* 1986;3:107–112.

155. Pinchcovsky-Devin G, Kaminsky MV Jr. Correlation of pressure sores and nutritional status. *J Am Geriatr Soc.* 1986;34:435–440.

156. Bobel LM. Nutritional implications in the patient with pressure sores. *Nurs Clin North Am.* 1987;22:379–390.

157. Nixon J, Cranny G, Bond S. Skin alterations of intact skin and risk factors associated with pressure ulcer development in surgical patients: a cohort study. *Int J Nurs Stud.* 2007;44(5):655–663.

158. Schoonhoven L, Grobbee DE, Donders ART, et al. Prediction of pressure ulcer development in hospitalized patients: a tool for risk assessment. *Qual Saf Health Care.* 2006;15(1):65–70.

159. Reed RL, Hepburn K, Adelson R, et al. Low serum albumin levels, confusion, and fecal incontinence: are these risk factors for pressure ulcers in mobility-impaired hospitalized adults? *Gerontology.* 2003;49(4):255–259.

160. Bergstrom N, Braden B, Kemp M, et al. Multi-site study of incidence of pressure ulcers and the relationship between risk level, demographic characteristics, diagnoses, and prescription of preventive interventions. *J Am Geriatr Soc.* 1996;44(1):22–30.

161. Allman RM, Laprade CA, Noel LB, et al. Pressure sores among hospitalized patients. *Ann Intern Med.* 1986;105:337–342.

162. Perneger TV, Rae AC, Gaspoz JM, et al. Screening for pressure ulcer risk in an acute care hospital: development of a brief bedside scale. *J Clin Epidemiol.* 2002;55(5):498–504.

163. Jones PL, Millman A. Wound healing and the aged patient. *Nurs Clin North Am.* 1990;25:263–277.

164. Boyle M, Green M. Pressure sores in intensive care: defining their incidence and associated factors and assessing the utility of two pressure sore risk assessment tools. *Aust Crit Care.* 2001;14(1):24–30.

165. Theaker C, Mannan M, Ives N, et al. Risk factors for pressure sores in the critically ill. *Anaesthesia.* 2000;55(3):221–224.

166. Curley MA, Quigley SM, Lin M. Pressure ulcers in pediatric intensive care: incidence and associated factors. *Pediatr Crit Care Med.* 2003;4(3):284–290.

167. Vidal J, Sarrias M. An analysis of the diverse factors concerned with the development of pressure sores in spinal cord patients. *Paraplegia.* 1991;29:261–267.

168. Anderson TP, Andberg MM. Psychosocial factors associated with pressure sores. *Arch Phys Med Rehabil.* 1979;60:341–346.

169. Fogarty M, Abumrad N, Nanney L, et al. Risk factors for pressure ulcers in acute care hospitals. *Wound Repair Regen.* 2008;16:11–18.

170. Stechmiller JK, Cowan L, Whitney JD, et al. Guidelines for the prevention of pressure ulcers. *Wound Repair Regen.* 2008;16:151–168.

171. Baumgarten M, Margolis DJ, Localio AR, et al. Pressure ulcers among elderly patients early in the hospital stay. *J Gerontol A Biol Sci Med Sci.* 2006;61(7):749–754.

172. Baumgarten M, Margolis DJ, Localio AR, et al. Extrinsic risk factors for pressure ulcers early in the hospital stay: a nested case-control study. *J Gerontol A Bil Sci Med Sci.* 2008;63(4):408–413.

173. Brindle CT. Outliers to the Braden Scale: identifying high-risk ICU patients and the results of prophylactic dressing use. *World Counc Enterostomal Ther J.* 2010;30(10):2–8.

174. Price M, Whitney J, King C. Development of a risk assessment tool for intraoperative pressure ulcers. *J Wound Ostomy Continence Nurs.* 2005;32(1):19–30.

175. Walton-Geer P. Prevention of pressure ulcers in the surgical patient. *AORN.* 2009;89(3):538–552.

176. Norton D, McLaren R, Exton-Smith NA. *An Investigation of Geriatric Nursing Problems in Hospitals.* Edinburgh, Scotland: Churchill-Living-stone; 1962.

177. Norton D. Calculating the risk: reflections on the Norton Scale. *Decubitus.* 1989;2(3):24–31.

178. Braden BJ, Bergstrom N. A conceptual schema for the study of etiology of pressure sores. *Rehabil Nurs.* 1987;12(1):8–12.

179. Braden B, Bergstrom N. Clinical utility of the Braden Scale for predicting pressure sore risk. *Decubitus.* 1989;2(3):44–51.

180. Quigley SM, Curley MAQ. Skin integrity in the pediatric population: preventing and managing pressure ulcers. *J Soc Ped Nurses.* 1996;1:7–18.

181. Pancorbo-Hidalgo, et al. Risk assessment scales for pressure ulcer prevention: a systematic review. *J Adv Nurs.* 2006;54(1):94–110.

182. Ayello EA, Braden BJ. How and why to do pressure ulcer risk assessment. *Adv Skin Wd Care.* 2002;15(3):125–131.

183. Defloor T, DeBacquer D, Grydonck MH. The effects of various combinations of turning and pressure reducing devices on the incidence of pressure ulcers. *Int J Nurs Stud.* 2005;42(1):37–46.

184. Vanderwee K, Grypdonck MHF, De Bacquer D, et al. Effectiveness of turning with unequal time intervals on the incidence of pressure ulcer lesions. *J Adv Nurs.* 2006;57(1):59–68.

185. Seiler WO, Allen S, Stahelin HB. Influence of the 30 degrees laterally inclined position and the "super soft" 3-piece mattress on skin oxygen tension on areas of maximum pressure: implications for pressure sores prevention. *Gerontology.* 1986;32:158–166.

186. Colin D, Abraham P, Preault L, Bregeon C, et al. Comparison of 90 degrees and 30 degrees laterally inclined positions in the prevention of pressure ulcersusing transcutaneous oxygen and carbon dioxide pressures. *Adv Wound Care.* 1996;9(3):35–38.

187. Sachse RE, Fink SA, Klitzman B. Multimodality evaluation of pressure relief surfaces. *Plast Reconstr Surg.* 1998;102(7):2381–2387.

188. Peterson M, Schwab W, McCutcheon K, et al. Effects of elevating the head of bed on interface pressure in volunteers. *Crit Care Med.* 2008;36(11):3038–3042.

189. Defloor T. The effect of position and mattress on interface pressure. *Appl Nurs Res.* 2000;13(1):2–11.

190. Sideranko S, Quinn A, Burns K, et al. Effects of position and mattress overlay on sacral and heel pressures in a clinical population. *Res Nurs Health.* 1992;15(4):245–251.

191. Smith AM, Malone JA. Preventing pressure ulcers in institutionalized elders: assessing the effects of small, unscheduled shifts in body position. *Decubitus.* 1990;3(4):20–24.

192. Bates-Jensen BM, Cadogan M, Jorge J, et al. Standardized quality-assessment system to evaluate pressure ulcer care in the nursing home. *J Am Geriatr Soc.* 2003;51:1195–1202.

193. Fineman LD, LaBrecque MA, Shih MC, et al. Prone positioning can be safely performed in critically ill infants and children. *Pediatr Crit Care Med.* 2006;7(5):486–487.

194. De Laat E, Schoonhoven L, Schoonhoven M, et al. Early postoperative 30° lateral positioning after coronary artery surgery: influence on cardiac output. *J Clin Nurs.* 2007;16:654–661.

195. Bridges EJ, Woods SL, Brengelmann GL, et al. Effect of the 30 degree lateral recumbent position on pulmonary artery and pulmonary artery wedge pressures in critically ill adult cardiac surgery patients. *Am J Crit Care.* 2000;9(4):262–275

196. Gallagher S. The challenges of obesity and skin integrity. *Nurs Clin North Am.* 2005;40(2):325–335.

197. Defloor T, Grypdonck MH. Sitting posture and prevention of pressure ulcers. *Appl Nurs Res.* 1999;12(3):136–142.

198. Gebhardt K, Bliss MR. Preventing pressure sores in orthopaedic patients. Is prolonged chair nursing detrimental? *J Tissue Viability.* 1994;4:51–54.

199. Clark M. Guidelines for seating in pressure ulcer prevention and management. *Nurs Times.* 2009;105:16.

200. Michael SM, Tilted seat position for non-ambulant individuals with neurological and neuromuscular impairment: a systematic review. *Clin Rehabil.* 2007;21:1063–1074.

201. Regan M, Teasell R, Wolfe D, et al. A systematic review of therapeutic interventions for pressure ulcers after spinal cord injury. *Arch Phys Med Rehabil.* 2009;90(2):213–231.

202. Whitney J, Phillips L, Aslam R, et al. Guidelines for the treatment of pressure ulcers. *Wound Repair Regen.* 2006;14(6):663–679.

203. Junkin J, Gray M. Are pressure redistribution surfaces or heel protection devices effective for preventing heel pressure ulcers? *J Wound Ostomy Continence Nurs.* 2009;36(6):602–608.

204. National Pressure Ulcer Advisory Panel Support Surface Standards Initiative. Terms and definitions related to support surfaces. Washington, DC. National Pressure Ulcer Advisory Panel; 2007.

205. Cullum N, McInnes E, Bell-Syer SE, et al. Support surfaces for pressure ulcer prevention. *Cochrane Database Syst Rev.* 2004;(3):CD001735.

206. Bergstrom N, Bennett MA, Carlson CE, et al. Treatment of pressure ulcers. Clinical Practice Guideline No. 15. Agency for Health Care Research and Quality (AHRQ), formerly known as the Agency for Health Care Policy and Research (AHCPR) Publication No. 95–0652. Rockville, MD: AHRQ, U.S. Public Health Service (PHS), U.S. Department of Health and Human Services (DHHS); December 1994.

207. McInnes E, Bell-Syer SE, Dumville JC, et al. Support surfaces for pressure ulcer prevention. *Cochrane Database Syst Rev.* 2008;8(4):CD001735.

208. Russell L, Reynolds T, Park C, et al. Randomized clinical trial comparing 2 support surfaces: results of the prevention of pressure ulcers study. *Adv Skin Wound Care.* 2003;16(6):317.

209. Vanderwee K, Grypdonck MH, Defloor T. Effectiveness of an alternating pressure air mattress for the prevention of pressure ulcers. *Age Ageing.* 2005;34(3):261–267.

210. Nixon J, Cranny G, Iglesias C, et al. Randomised, controlled trial of alternating pressure mattresses compared with alternating pressure overlays for the prevention of pressure ulcers: PRESSURE (pressure relieving support surfaces) trial. *Br Med J.* 2006;332(7555):1413.

211. Gebhardt KS, Bliss M, WInright P, Thomas J. Pressure relieving supports in an ICU. *J Wound Care.* 1996;5(3):116–121.

212. Still JM, Wilson J, Rinker C, et al. A retrospective study to determine the incidence of pressure ulcers in burn patients using an alternating pressure mattress. *Burns.* 2003;29:505–507.

213. Wound Ostomy Continence Nurses Society (WOCNS). Guidelines for prevention and management of pressure ulcers. WOCN Clinical Practice Guideline Series, 2010.

214. Baharestani MM, Ratliff CR. Pressure ulcers in neonates and children: an NPUAP white paper. *Adv Skin Wound Care.* 2007;20(4):208–220.

215. Krouskop TA, Garber SL. Interface pressure confusion. *Decubitus.* 1989;2:8.

216. Donnelly J, Kernohan GW, Witherow A. Pressure relieving devices for preventing heel pressure ulcers. *Cochrane Database Syst Rev.* 2008;(2).

217. Heyneman A, Vanderwee K, Grypdonck M, et al. Effectiveness of two cushions in the prevention of heel pressure ulcers. *Worldviews Evid Based Nurs.* 2009;6(2):114–120.

218. Nixon J, McElvenny D, Mason S, et al. A sequential randomized controlled trial comparing a dry visco-elastic polymer pad and standard operating table mattress in the prevention of post-operative pressure sores. *Int J Nurs Stud.* 1998;35(4):193–203.

219. Aronovitch SA, Wilber M, Slezak S, et al. A comparative study of an alternating air mattress for the prevention of pressure ulcers in surgical patients. *Ostomy Wound Manage.* 1999;45(3):34–40, 2–4.

220. Russell JA, Lichtenstein SL. Randomized controlled trial to determine the safety and efficacy of a multi-cell pulsating dynamic mattress system in the prevention of pressure ulcers in patients undergoing cardiovascular surgery. *Ostomy Wound Manage.* 2000;46(2):46–50.

221. Bates-Jensen BM, Alessi CA, Al-Samarrai NR, et al. The effects of an exercise and incontinence intervention on skin health outcomes in nursing home residents. *J Am Geriatr Soc.* 2003;51:348–355.

222. Schoonhoven L, Defloor T, Grypdonck MH. Incidence of pressure ulcers due to surgery. *J Clin Nurs.* 2002;11(4):479–487.

223. Nakagami G, Sanada H. Heterotrophic ossification in the sacral pressure ulcer treated with basic fibroblast growth factor: coincidence or side effect? *J Plast Reconstr Surg.* 2007;60(3):327–329.

224. Torra I, Bou JE, Segovia GT, et al. The effectiveness of a hyperoxygenated fatty acid compound in preventing pressure ulcers. *J Wound Care.* 2005;14:117–121.

225. Weng MH. The effect of protective treatment in reducing pressure ulcers for non-invasive ventilation patients. *Intensive Crit Care Nurs.* 2008;24(5):295–299.

226. Smith G, Ingram A. Clinical and cost effectiveness evaluation of low friction and shear garments. *J Wound Care.* 2010;19(12):535–542.

227. Schnelle JF. Treatment of urinary incontinence in nursing home patients by prompted voiding. *J Am Geriatr Soc.* 1990;38:356–360.

228. Ouslander JG, Schnelle JF, Uman G, et al. Predictors of successful prompted voiding among incontinent nursing home residents. *JAMA.* 1995;273:1366–1370.

229. Beeckman D, Schoonhoven L, Verhaeghe S, et al. Prevention and treatment of incontinence-associated dermatitis: literature review. *J Adv Nurs.* 2009;65(6):1141–1154.

230. Clever K, Smith G, Bowser C, et al. Evaluating the efficacy of a uniquely delivered skin protectant and its effect on the formation of sacral/buttock pressure ulcers. *Ostomy Wound Manage.* 2002;48(12):60–67.

231. Bergstrom N, Braden B. A prospective study of pressure sore risk among institutionalized elderly. *J Am Geriatr Soc.* 1992;40:747–758.

232. Berlowitz D, Wilking S. The short term outcome of pressure sores. *J Am Geriatr Soc.* 1990;38:748–752.

233. Hill DP, Cooper DM, Robson MC. Serum albumin is a poor prognostic factor for pressure ulcer healing in controlled clinical trials. *Wounds.* 1994;6(5):174–178.

234. Stotts N. Nutritional parameters at hospital admission as predictors of pressure ulcer development in elective surgery. *J Parenter Enter Nutr.* 1987;11:298–301.

235. Langer G, Schloemer G, Knerr A, et al. Nutritional interventions for preventing and treating pressure ulcers. *Cochrane Database Syst Rev.* 2003;(4):CD003216.

236. Stratton RJ, Ek AC, Engfer M, et al, Enteral nutritional support in prevention and treatment of pressure ulcers: a systematic review and meta-analysis. *Ageing Res Rev.* 2005;4(3):422–450.

237. Bourdel-Marchasson I, Barateau M, Rondeau V, et al. A multi-center trial of the effects of oral nutritional supplementation in critically ill older inpatients. GAGE Group. Groupe Aquitain Geriatrique d'Evaluation. *Nutrition.* 2000;16(1):1–5.

238. Hartgrink HH, Wille J, Konig P, et al. Pressure sores and tube feeding in patients with a fracture of the hip: A randomized clinical trial. *Clin Nutr.* 1998;17(6):287–292.

239. Houwing RH, Rozendaal M, Wouters-Wesseling W, et al, A randomized, double-blind assessment of the effect of nutritional supplementation on the prevention of pressure ulcers in hip-fracture patients. *Clin Nutr.* 2003;22(4):401–405.

240. Chernoff RS, Milton KY, Lipschitz DA. The effect of very high-protein liquid formula on decubitus ulcers healing in long-term tube fed institutionalized patients. *J Am Diet Assoc.* 1990;90:A–130.

241. Breslow RA, Hallfrisch J, Guy DG, et al. The importance of dietary protein in healing pressure ulcers. *J Am Geriatr Soc.* 1993;41(4):357–362.

242. Thomas DR. Issues and dilemmas in the prevention and treatment of pressure ulcers: a review. *J Gerontol Med Sci.* 2001a;56A(6):M328–M340.

243. Thomas DR. Improving the outcome of pressure ulcers with nutritional interventions: a review of the evidence. *Nutrition.* 2001b;17(2):121–125.

244. Berlowitz D, VanDeusen Lukas C, Parker V, et al. Preventing pressure ulcers in hospitals. Quality improvement implementation toolkit. Agency for Healthcare Research and Quality, 2011; http://www.ahrq.gov/research/ltc/pressureulcertoolkit/. Accessed 4/29/11.

245. Armstrong DG, Ayello EA, Capitulo KL, et al. New opportunities to improve pressure ulcer prevention and treatment: implications of the CMS inpatient hospital care present on admission (POA) indicators/hospital-acquired conditions (HAC) policy. *J Wound Ostomy Continence Nurs Soc.* 2008;35(5):485–492.

246. Ayello E, Lyder C. Protecting patients from harm: preventing pressure ulcers in hospital patients. *Nursing.* 2008;37:36–40.

247. Holmes A, Edelstein T. Envisioning a world without pressure ulcers. *Extended Care Product News.* 2007;122:24–29.

248. Gibbons W, Shanks H, Kleinhelter P, et al. Eliminating facility-acquired pressure ulcers at Ascension Health. *J Qual Patient Saf.* 2006;32:488–496.

249. Galea M, Tumminia J, Garback L. Telerehabilitation in spinal cord injury patients: a novel approach. *Telemed e-Health.* 2006;12(2):160–162.

250. Ratcliff C, Forch W. Telehealth for wound management in long-term care. *Ostomy Wound Manage.* 2005;51(9):49–45.

251. Gardner S, Frantz R, Specht J, et al. How accurate are chronic wound assessments using interactive video technology? *J Gerontol Nurs.* 2001;27(1):15–20.

252. Kinsella A. Advanced telecare for wound care delivery. *Home Healthcare Nurse.* 2002;20(7):457–461.

253. Rees R, Bashshur N. The effects of TeleWound management on use of service and financial outcomes. *Telemed J e-Health.* 2007;13(6):663–674.

Management of Pressure by Therapeutic Positioning

Laurie M. Rappl

CHAPTER OBJECTIVES

At the completion of this chapter, the reader will be able to:

1. Defend the need for therapeutic positioning for patients in sitting and recumbent positions.
2. Initiate and complete an evaluation of a patient with limited mobility in the sitting and recumbent positions.
3. Identify the best positioning and the devices to obtain those positions for both sitting and recumbent patients.
4. Evaluate seating and mattress or support surface products for their effectiveness in distributing pressure therapeutically.
5. Explain the potential healing benefits of proper therapeutic positioning interventions.

Therapeutic positioning is a dynamic and necessary part of the wound care prevention and management program for patients with disabilities. If you fail to properly position a patient in bed or in a sitting position, the vulnerable tissues overlying bony prominences will be damaged by inappropriately high carrying loads. Patients who are more sitting dependent than ambulatory and/or who use the recumbent and sitting positions for the majority of the day are at high risk for tissue breakdown. Approximately 50% of all tissue breakdown occurs on the sacrum, most often associated with recumbent positions, and the ischial tuberosities (ITs), most often associated with the sitting position.[1-3] For patients with existing pressure ulcers, proper positioning in the most active and functional positions possible, both sitting and recumbent, may improve healing rates of the ulcers and help to minimize the likelihood of recurrence.

Technological advances in equipment, the huge variety of equipment now available, and the individual needs of patients requiring specialized equipment have elevated therapeutic positioning to a complex specialty among therapists and medical suppliers. Given this complexity, we cannot cover all seating and positioning topics thoroughly in this chapter; instead, we provide essential information on the following topics:

- Overview of the areas that you should examine to determine the need for intervention
- Basics of therapeutic positioning
- How therapeutic positioning affects body system impairments
- Specifics in positioning patients with existing ulcers, both sitting and recumbent

NEED FOR THERAPEUTIC POSITIONING

Just as pressure ulcers affect patients of all ages, from pediatric to young adult to middle aged and elderly, so does the need for therapeutic positioning cross all age groups. The human body requires support for proper postural alignment in both the sitting and the recumbent positions in order to perform functional activities and maintain healthy tissues. Proper positioning has been identified as important for good health in people of all ages and all occupations. Significant research and resources are devoted to correctly positioning and supporting people who sit in their jobs, such as computer users, truck drivers, and workers in manufacturing. It is reasonable to conclude, then, that wheelchair users and bed-bound patients are also in great need of proper support.

IT ulcers, which are located on the major weight-bearing surfaces of the sitting-dependent patient, are associated with the sitting position.[3] It has been estimated that 75% of the sitting-dependent population will develop an IT or other pressure ulcer. Of these, 75% will have a recurrence.[4-6] Therapeutic positioning, using correctly chosen equipment, plays a direct and critical role in reducing these staggering numbers. Any patient with a disability who is sitting dependent for any part of the day or night should be evaluated by a therapist experienced in positioning to ensure that the optimal position is being attained. Although full-time wheelchair users are often considered the only candidates for therapeutic positioning, part-time wheelchair users who sit for relatively shorter periods of time each day are also candidates.

Sacral wounds are most often associated with the recumbent position. This is not surprising since pressures in recumbent patients are highest (70 mm Hg) on this bony area. All patients who are recumbent with limited mobility are candidates for therapeutic positioning. The more bed dependent the patient is, the more critical the need for proper evaluation and positioning interventions.

A common intervention for nonhealing wounds on the ITs or sacrum is a myocutaneous flap surgery, usually referred to as simply a flap. Literature reports the failure rates for flap surgeries at 76% to 91%.[4,5] In addition, it is standard procedure for plastic surgeons to plan for five more flap donor sites on a client before doing the first one. Treating the symptom does not cure the root problem. Therefore, one strategy to reduce the need for surgical intervention and the risk to the patient is to choose an appropriate therapeutic positioning intervention. Therapeutic positioning, using correctly chosen equipment, plays a direct and critical role in reducing these poor outcomes.

Proper therapeutic positioning redistributes interface pressures off of bony prominences to affect the development or healing of pressure ulcers. Positioning can also enhance mobility to reduce the hazards of immobility. These hazards include cardiorespiratory dysfunction, slowing of the digestive system, and cognitive changes. These are discussed in more detail further in this chapter in the section on bed rest.

The process for evaluating a patient's need for therapeutic positioning is discussed next. Reevaluation should occur when there is a significant change in condition, such as the development of a deformity, significant weight gain or loss, occurrence of tissue breakdown, or change in the patient's mobility status, such as increased weakness that further inhibits mobility. Reevaluation may also be necessary if current equipment breaks or is in disrepair, or if warranties have expired.

EVALUATING PATIENTS FOR THERAPEUTIC POSITIONING

The first step in evaluating patients for therapeutic positioning is to determine the reason for referral. Next, review the patient's medical history and body systems to determine the possible related impairments. These data will help direct your examination strategy. After the examination, analyze the information you've gathered to determine a functional diagnosis related to the need for therapeutic positioning. This in turn will guide your selection of appropriate equipment and positioning interventions. Prognosis and expected outcome complete the process.

Reason for Referral

The reason for referral provides the first clue about the positioning needs of the client. The reason identified by the referring clinician may or may not coincide with the reason the family, caregiver, or patient provides for seeking positioning assistance. In such cases, the reasons of the family, caregiver, and patient should take priority. For example, the goal of the caregiver may be comfort in recumbent positions for an uncommunicative client, whereas the clinician may want to pursue an aggressive program to reverse contractures. The clinician's goal may be viable, but if the caregiver cannot devote the time, interest, or financial resources to an aggressive program, you will have to

consider less aggressive positioning goals. Reasons for a referral for therapeutic positioning commonly include the following:

- Decrease pain
- Increase a specific functional ability
- Increase independent mobility
- Increase ease of care for the caregiver
- Decrease risk of tissue breakdown
- Assist in healing existing tissue breakdown

The reason for referral can also be reevaluation of positioning and/or equipment due to a change in the client's condition. Examples include surgery that changes anatomical alignment such as scoliosis or ischiectomy, weight gain or loss that changes the fit of the wheelchair, and tissue breakdown that is thought to have been caused in part by poor positioning.

During the initial interview, make sure to consider the patient's social situation; for example, factors such as the living situation and the patient's level of independence. These factors are important for selecting the appropriate examination techniques and the level of complexity of interventions and equipment. For example, a patient in a solid, supportive home environment with consistent caregivers may be able to handle more complicated equipment than an individual in a group living situation with multiple caregivers. In addition, as discussed in Chapter 9, the number of hours spent sitting or lying down is correlated to the risk of breakdown. Generally, long time periods in sitting or recumbent positions indicate a high risk of breakdown and the need to be highly specific in equipment selection and thorough in your patient/caregiver training.

Medical History

Review the past and current medical history for information that would affect appropriate positioning. Note any comorbidities, as they will affect your choice of systems to review related to appropriate positioning. For example, pulmonary and cardiac pathologies suggest that the patient may benefit from special positioning that provides for optimal breathing function as well as prevention or healing of pressure ulcers.

Medications also affect positioning choices. For example, antispasmodic medications would indicate that spasticity and abnormal movement synergies have been a problem and need to be accommodated for by the equipment and positioning. Some medications cause lethargy or dizziness that may cause the therapist to consider more supportive equipment. Other classes of medications affect cognition, alertness, and muscle tone, which may affect the choice of nonpowered over powered mobility devices.

Note any past surgeries or orthopedic procedures that would limit the ability of the client to achieve the "ideal" sitting position or require accommodation to help the client maintain that position. For example, spinal fixation can limit range of motion (ROM) in the spine and pelvis; this could necessitate equipment that does not force the body to sit in level planes, but instead accommodates and supports a tilted pelvis or curved back posture. Another example is a report of any flap or graft surgeries on the seating surface; this should prompt you to watch for the condition of the scar tissue in the area, which could predispose the tissue to ulcer development.

Following the history is the systems review, which focuses on identifying pathologies and system impairments that potentially could be addressed with therapeutic positioning. These occur in the neuromuscular system, musculoskeletal system, cardiopulmonary and vascular systems, integumentary system, and psychosocial/cognitive system. Your systems review should also guide your choice of systems examinations. Examples are discussed in the following sections.

Neuromuscular Systems Review and Examinations

Pathology of the central or peripheral nervous system leads to many impairments that affect positioning and the development of pressure ulcers. If sensation is diminished, the skin and soft tissues over bony prominences in the insensate areas of the body that are weight bearing will have an undue susceptibility to pressure ulceration. Equipment selection and positioning must protect and redistribute pressure on tissue over bony prominences in the impaired areas as much as possible. In sitting, these prominences are the ITs, sacrum, and coccyx. Bed-restricted individuals and those with poor self-repositioning abilities often develop tissue breakdown over several bony prominences, including occiput, scapula, sacrum, heels, malleoli (ankles), and trochanters (hips). Both the choice of a support surface or seating system and the instruction in proper positioning are critical in protecting these individuals.

If a patient has suffered an insult to the central nervous system, such as a stroke, brain injury, or spinal cord injury, or has a disease of the central nervous system, such as Parkinson disease, the damage can cause spasticity and/or abnormal movement synergies, both of which can lead to impaired postural alignment. The equipment must support the body so as to distribute pressure and provide safe, secure seating and bed positioning. Proper equipment and positioning also facilitate the patient's visual perception, swallowing, and social interaction and can prevent the development of irreversible muscle and joint contractures, which impair functional activities.

Individuals with degenerative diseases of the central nervous system, such as multiple sclerosis, have different needs. These patients may benefit from therapeutic positioning for postural support of weak muscles, which will prolong functional activities, conserve energy, prevent contractures, and increase comfort and safety. For these patients, you should anticipate that the equipment needs will change as the disease progresses over time.

Most interventions directed to individuals with diabetic neuropathy are focused on protecting the feet from injury, but diabetic neuropathy also affects positioning decisions if the individual is bed bound or wheelchair bound. These patients have an increased risk of trauma to areas that are insensate, such as the feet and hands. Also, many individuals in this group are amputees who have special support surface needs due to weight concentration over smaller body areas.

Neurologic Examination

Central nervous system damage can result in problems of motor control that involve components of the neuromuscular system. These include the inability to sequence movements, recruit muscles in the proper sequence, scale the activities, and adapt motor responses to changing task conditions. The goal of the neurologic examination is to identify the impairments that can be influenced by positioning. It is beyond the scope of this book to provide examination strategies for all of these

> **CLINICAL WISDOM**
>
> Position the individual with a strong ATNR so that he or she can visualize the entrance to the room with ease from a frontal position and does not need to rotate the head. This simple act will eliminate a great deal of fear and agitation and positioning problems.

impairments; however, some examples are presented here. Additional resources are provided at the end of the chapter.

One finding commonly seen in central nervous system pathologies is hyperactive reflexes that affect postural control. These hyperactive reflexes, along with abnormal muscle tone, create abnormal movement synergies. One example of a hyperactive reflex is the asymmetric tonic neck reflex (ATNR). This reflex causes the individual to extend the extremities on the face side and flex the extremities on the occiput side when the head is rotated. Such a reflex can interfere with motor control of the upper extremities when performing functional activities. For example, it can cause the patient driving a motorized wheelchair with a side-mounted joystick to have difficulty controlling the device. A center-mounted joystick may solve this problem. A strong ATNR will make maintaining a side-lying position difficult, since it involves not only the upper extremities, but the trunk and lower extremities as well. The head and trunk will need to be positioned to avoid triggering this hyperactive reflex. Positioning the patient so that he or she can see when someone approaches without having to turn the face to look over the uppermost shoulder will help to compensate.

Another common hyperactive reflex is symmetric tonic neck reflex (STNR), which is also influenced by head position. When the neck is flexed, the arms flex and the legs extend. When the neck is extended, the arms extend and the legs flex. The STNR can be accommodated by limiting the movement of the head so that voluntary control of the body is maintained.

A third hyperactive reflex, extensor thrust, which is described as uncontrolled extension of the trunk, hips, and knees, can be the result of extensor spasticity, an associated reaction, or an *extensor synergy*, composed of hip extension, adduction, and internal rotation, knee extension, plantar flexion and inversion of the ankle, and dorsiflexion of the toes. It can be triggered by common activities, such as talking or reaching. The neurologic examination is used to determine the underlying problem and trigger for this response. Then, you can assess what is needed for the patient to maintain as close to a 90- to 95-degree hip angle as possible. For example, seat and back equipment, hip belts, and lap trays and proper foot support that does not trigger the synergy will help the patient maintain a functional sitting posture.

Contact of the ball of the foot on the footrest or floor can trigger a spastic reaction known as clonus. Positioning of the foot to avoid contact with the ball of the foot on the footrest can decrease this uncontrolled movement.

In the supine position, another reflex, the tonic labyrinthine reflex (TLR), can be hyperactive. In this position, extensor posture is activated. This posture increases the risk of breakdown on the occiput and heels, and its presence indicates the need for repositioning so that there is flexion of the hips and knees. Pillows are not stable enough to do this, and specifically designed foam positioning aids are required. These products are more expensive than pillows, but their effectiveness outweighs the cost. Positioning devices designed for controlling the body position are described later in this chapter.

Sensory Examination

Sensation can be partially or completely impaired by a central nervous system insult. For example, in a complete spinal cord lesion, the patient may have no sensation below the lesion. However, if the lesion is due to a cerebral vascular accident, traumatic brain injury, or a partial injury to the spinal cord, the loss of sensation may be incomplete. A sensory examination is useful to determine the extent and type of sensory loss.

Patients are at increased risk for pressure ulcers if they lack the ability to detect light and deep pressure and pain on all areas of the body that are weight bearing or that may come into contact with equipment. The inability to detect pain or pressure can lead to tissue breakdown because the patient does not know when to shift weight to relieve pressure. For the insensate patient, great care must be taken to search for and prescribe equipment that not only positions the body but also protects insensate skin (see the section on seat cushion categories). Chapter 3 includes information on performing sensory testing and Chapter 22 discusses pain testing.

Another important sensory loss is vision. For example, patients with a visual loss on one side of the body can neglect that side. In such cases, you need to protect the involved limbs and position the patient to provide for maximum environmental interaction.

Musculoskeletal System Review and Examinations

Examination of this system can include a manual muscle test to determine muscle strength, ROM testing to identify contractures and limitations and a functional mobility assessment. Impairments can reduce a patient's ability to self-position, to maintain correct postures, and to perform activities of daily living (ADLs) and other movements. In addition, impairments in ROM and/or muscle strength directly affect the patient's ability to shift weight to relieve pressure. This in turn increases the risk of tissue breakdown. For example, a patient who cannot reach 90 degrees of hip flexion will "sacral sit" on a flexed lumber spine, putting excessive pressure on the sacrum, coccyx, and lumbar spinous processes. Equipment must be chosen that accommodates for the limitations in range by supporting the body at the angle available at the hip with a supportive cushion, possibly an angled seat, and a back rest that can be fixed to open the seat-to-back angle to match achievable hip flexion. This is called an angle-adjustable back or an open seat-back angle. Another example is a patient who eats sitting up in bed or seated in a mobility base; the positioning system must support upright posture for functional use of the upper extremities, safe swallowing, and social interaction. Limitations in strength and mobility are also considered in the selection of a powered device over a manual one.

Patients who have had a cerebrovascular accident resulting in a hemiparesis or hemiplegia have patterns of muscle weakness on one side of the body. This imbalance predisposes the client to sit unevenly, thus overweighting one ischium and the overlying soft tissue. Spinal and pelvic malalignment also add to overload in that location. Uncorrected, spinal joint impairments such as scoliosis can ensue.

Skeletal deformities are either fixed or flexible. A flexible deformity is an impairment that can potentially be corrected by therapy and/or the selection of the proper positioning equipment. A fixed deformity, however, is a disability that is immovable and must be accommodated by the equipment. A curved leg resulting from a traumatic break to the tibia is an example of a fixed deformity that requires accommodation with equipment to compensate. Accommodation would be necessary if the curved lower leg made the level of the knees and lap uneven, causing the curved leg to push against the legrest and cause pressure. Surgical changes to the skeletal system require special positioning attention. For example, a unilateral ischiectomy results in an asymmetric pelvis (pelvic obliquity), which will change the biomechanics of the spine from erect alignment to a curvature, and cause excessive weighting of the intact side of the pelvis. In general, rather than attempting to correct the problem associated with a fixed deformity, you should select equipment that conforms to the deformity and helps to hold the patient in the best functional position as close to "ideal" as possible.

Evaluation or reevaluation for seating needs should be done when there are changes in the patient condition, such as significant weight loss, which can make bony prominences that were once fairly protected much more vulnerable to the effects of pressure and shear. Significant weight gain will result in poorly fitting equipment, possibly limiting mobility and transfers and putting skin at increased risk.

Examination of Joint Range of Motion and Muscle Strength

Assessing the patient's joint ROM and muscle strength can help you to determine the contribution of each to the motor coordination problem affecting postural control. In addition, if you identify reduced ROM or strength early on, you can sometimes prevent problems such as the development of contractures. For patients with long-standing neurologic insults, the exam can help you identify the ROM or muscular strength component that contributes to the problem and to develop a positioning plan to prevent worsening of contractures.

ROM evaluation should include the spine and pelvis, as well as the extremities. Examine the spinal curves for proper alignment in sitting, as shown in Figure 10.1. Common deviations from the normal can include

1. Limitations in the ROM of the spine that affect the client's ability to sit upright easily. These problems should be noted as *fixed*, that is immovable, or *flexible*, that is movable or correctable. Fixed problems need to be accommodated for as a disability, whereas flexible problems should be noted as those which the proper equipment or positioning can help to correct.

2. Limitations in movement and position of the pelvis should be evaluated for ROM in anterior and posterior tilt, and lateral rotation. The anterior/posterior tilt is assessed from the side. The anterior superior iliac spines (ASIS) should be roughly level with the posterior superior iliac spines (PSIS). A posterior tilt in which the PSIS are lower than the ASIS will flex and flatten the lumbar spine, decrease hip flexion, and cause the body to assume a "slouched" position. In this case, weight will be concentrated on the ITs and on the

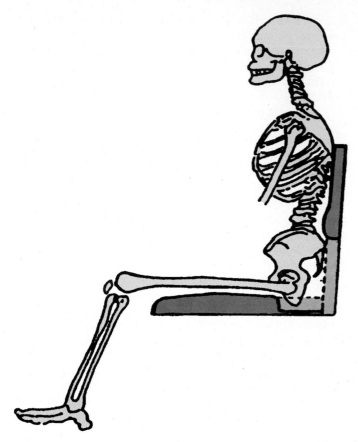

FIGURE 10.1 Ideal sitting position is approximately 95 degrees at hip and knee, and 90 to 95 degrees at the ankle. This is a reference point only; therapists should work to position clients as close to this position as possible. (Courtesy of Span-America Medical Systems, Greenville, South Carolina.)

<table>
<tr><td>

EXHIBIT 10.1

Pelvic Obliquity Evaluation

Pelvic obliquity should be assessed as *fixed* or *flexible*. Examination steps follow:

1. Place the client on a firm seat with knees at 90 degrees and feet supported.
2. Note whether one iliac crest is higher than the other.
3. Note the presence of a lateral curvature of the trunk, both with and without upper extremity support.
4. Place a support under the ischium on the lower side of the pelvis to even the iliac crests.
5. If the trunk curvature remains, and the client becomes more unstable when the arms are raised, the obliquity is fixed.
6. The fixed obliquity should then be accommodated for by building up the cushion under the higher ischium to maintain the pelvic obliquity.
7. If the trunk curvature decreases, and the client is more stable, the obliquity is flexible.
8. The flexible obliquity can be accommodated for in one of two ways:
   a. Putting the client on a firm cushion with both ischials unsupported and both femurs fully supported and at the same height, inducing a level pelvis
   b. Building up the cushion under the lower, supported ischium to even the iliac crests

</td></tr>
</table>

---

coccyx. The thoracic spine will also flex. To shift weight off of the ITs, the patient must be able to shift the weight of the upper body forward by tilting the pelvis forward, extending the lumbar and then the thoracic spine, and raising the neck and head. Document the presence of pelvic rotation, indicated by one iliac crest positioned in front of the other. A tilt to left or right in the frontal plane is called a *pelvic obliquity*. See Exhibit 10.1 for a method of testing for pelvic obliquity.

3. Lack of ROM of hip flexion to 90 degrees that affects the client's ability to be accommodated in a chair with a 90-degree seat-to-back angle. Accommodations will be needed, such as a backrest that is angled back in relation to the seat to open the seat-to-back angle, and a seat cushion that provides enough pelvic stability to keep the hips from sliding forward. A seat that tilts up in front may be helpful if used with a reclining backrest as described.
4. Knee flexion fixed at less than 90 degrees from straight or more than 90 degrees from straight. In either case, the legs will tend to pull the body forward from the back of the seat and out of position. Footrests that support the foot and allow the hip and knee to achieve approximately 90-degree flexion or the specific client's range will help to position the lower body.
5. Limitations in ankle dorsiflexion or plantar flexion or inversion/eversion ROM that affect the support of the lower extremity on the footrest. If the ankle cannot be maintained in a neutral (right angle) position with 0 degree of inversion/eversion, a footrest that can change angulation is necessary to accommodate the position of the foot as closely to ideal as possible.
6. Decreased or imbalanced muscular strength of the trunk and upper extremities. Weakness of the trunk contributes to postural instability and an inability to shift weight off of the IT on the weak side. A hypotonic or weak arm can also affect positioning, because it lacks the ability to provide support from that side.

Mobility Examination—Recumbent

Activities performed in bed should be evaluated for movement impairments that can become the focus of the positioning intervention. Movement impairments to consider include motor coordination, motor planning, and strategies for movement in the recumbent position. Tasks to evaluate include the following:

- Rolling right or left from supine
- Shifting the body from side to side
- Moving from sitting to supine, supine to sitting, sitting to standing (get out of bed), and standing to sitting (get into bed)
- Moving the body toward head of bed and moving the body toward the foot of bed

Assess for the ability and the strategy used by the patient to perform transfers independently, dependently, or assisted in many combinations: bed to chair, chair to bed, commode to bed, bed to commode, and sit to stand. This will impact the choice of support surface for the patient. Firm, stable support surfaces that do not move under the patient make bed mobility much easier to perform for all patients.

For patients with pressure ulcers, functional mobility is often compromised in favor of a less stable surface for improved tissue load management, but this compromise is usually not necessary. There are options within each of the support surface categories: alternating pressure for pressure-related wounds, low–air-loss therapy for patients with excessive perspiration, high–air-loss therapy for patients with both needs, and static pressure redistribution for patients who can utilize a variety of positions that offer the preferred therapy as well as stability for patient mobility. These surfaces can have a firm edge to prevent mattress collapse when the patient rolls or sits on the edge of the mattress.

Mobility Examination—Sitting

The purpose of the sitting evaluation is to determine the best *seating system* to meet the needs of the patient for postural stability, mobility, and safety.

The seat base, the seat cushion, and the back support are the key parts of the seating system. These will be discussed in more detail later in this chapter. The seat base supports the cushion, examples include the sling seat upholstery and a solid board or insert. The cushion is the direct support for the patient. The back support can be solid, flexible, or molded. The system can be configured in a variety of positions depending on the type of backing and seating used and incorporates or attaches to the *mobility base*, the mechanism for moving the patient once in the seating system. For example, the standard wheelchair includes a chair with a sling back, sling seat, and a manual mobility base. Use of a support surface/cushion in the wheelchair would complete this basic seating system.

Many factors go into the decision regarding choice of mobility bases. Some of these include the motor status of the individual; ability to function at the speed afforded by a motorized wheelchair, including such factors as cognition and visual spatial capabilities; required mobility status; cardiovascular status; strength and endurance status; functional goals of the patient or family; and method that will be used to relieve pressure and position the user on the seating surface. Other considerations in choosing the mobility base are the dependent versus independent mobility status of the individual, which includes what is easiest and safest for him or her to use. If the patient does not have the physical, cognitive, or visual perceptive abilities to be safely independently mobile in a manual or power chair, other sitting equipment should be considered.

Some of the considerations in selecting a mobility base include

- Recliner chairs, often called "Geri-chairs," are commonly used in long-term care settings, but they do not provide good support for postural alignment and are not safe for soft tissues without significant extra padding.
- Patients who need one or both feet to propel may best be fitted with a hemi-height wheelchair, which has a lower-than-standard seat-from-floor height. This allows patients to contact the ground firmly with the propelling foot (feet), without having to scoot the pelvis forward on the chair, which

can cause shear and friction to the skin over the ITs when pulling the body forward with the leg. The most efficient foot propulsion can be accomplished if the patient can achieve a heel-toe pattern in forward propulsion.

- A patient who has the functional use of only one arm may be a good candidate for a one-arm-drive chair. However, this equipment is heavy and difficult for some weak patients to operate.
- A patient who is strong and can use both arms but not the feet to propel a wheelchair is a good candidate for a standard-height wheelchair with footrests.
- For patients who have cognitive and perceptive skills, but not physical skills, a powered base, either a power wheelchair or a scooter style, may best meet mobility needs.

Shear and Friction Examination

Friction and shear are two very different forces. These two terms are not synonymous, and their outcomes are not the same. Friction is a one-sided force acting on the surface of the skin. Shear is a two-sided force of an outside pressure pulling the subcutaneous tissues in one direction, while movement of the bony structures beneath the tissues pull in an opposite direction. Friction and shear are two common problems for sitting patients: they can occur during wheelchair propulsion, during postural changes, and during transfers. Proper equipment and positioning can control trunk and pelvic movement in order to limit friction and shearing during these activities. Observe the patient's method of transfer and movement in the wheelchair for potential shear and friction. The best and safest transfer method that reduces risk factors for shear and friction should be determined, and then seating equipment should be selected to meet those requirements. For example, removable or swing-away hardware and positioning pieces can markedly facilitate transfers without shear and friction.

Signs of friction are identified on the skin by elongated, reddened areas on weight-bearing surfaces, similar to what you see on a "skinned knee" or road rash after a motorcycle or bicycle accident. This is in contrast to signs of high vertical pressure, usually round areas of redness or tissue damage over bony prominences in the shape of the object that caused the pressure (Fig. 10.2). Shear causes injury to deep tissues that results in undermining of pressure ulcers or the formation of pockets of fluid or tissue damage deep to the skin (Figs. 10.3 and 10.4).

Activities of Daily Living Evaluation

Evaluate ADLs to determine how they affect movement that puts the patient at risk for tissue breakdown. The more ADLs done in the wheelchair, such as dressing, bathing, eating, and toileting, the more the equipment will need to accommodate

---

CLINICAL WISDOM

Transfer Technique

Poor transfer technique is a major contributor to tissue breakdown, because the skin is dragged across surfaces or subjected to sudden overload when the patient sits down or is seated abruptly.

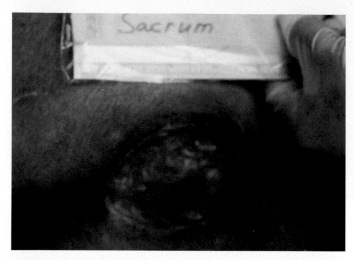

FIGURE 10.2 Wound is in chronic proliferative phase. Note: (1) Trauma to granulation tissue caused hemorrhagic spot that may go on to necrose. (2) Hemosiderin staining from prior bleeding surrounds ulcer. (Copyright © C. Sussman.)

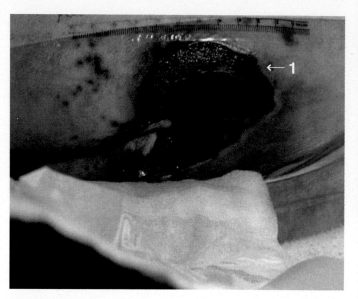

FIGURE 10.4 Undermined wound. Note the shelf. (Copyright © C. Sussman.)

beyond simple positioning. For example, noncontoured seating can assist caregivers with dressing and bathing because the patient can be placed in different positions to pull clothing on and off and to bathe the various body parts. Clothing is easier to pull up using noncontoured seating.

A patient who is able to transfer independently and does so while performing ADLs such as toileting needs a clear path in which to move, so consider the best way to minimize the number of extra devices, such as medial and lateral thigh supports used for positioning. These devices tend to get in the way of independent transfers and are cumbersome for caregivers in dependent transfers.

Interface Pressure Examination

In a study conducted by the University of Pittsburgh, higher interface pressures were directly associated with a higher incidence of pressure ulcers on the sitting surfaces of the body.[7] Using a mathematical approach, Ragan et al. found interface pressures to be good indicators of subcutaneous stress.[8] Research to validate interface pressure mapping measurements such as contact area, percent of force in the IT region, and

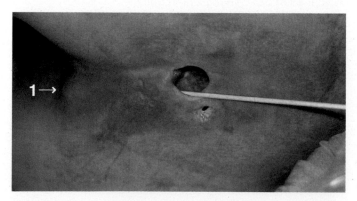

FIGURE 10.3 The wound's overall size is much larger than the surface open area. Tunneling is present. Note the bulge from the end of the cotton-tipped applicator. (Copyright © B.M. Bates-Jensen.)

peak pressure index rather than peak pressure point to quantify differences between cushions and to aid the clinician in the selection process is ongoing.[9,10] Mapping devices give pictorial readouts of the pressure recorded by each cell, the cell with the peak pressure, and many other data points that can help you determine the location and value of peak pressures on a particular client on a particular cushion. High pressures on the most vulnerable prominences (IT, coccyx, sites of previous or current breakdown) can indicate that the cushion and client are not an appropriate match. Figure 10.5 shows an example of interface pressure mapping on two different seat cushions, and Figure 10.6 shows interface pressure mapping on a support surface.

Reducing or eliminating pressure on the ITs and coccyx is the goal of most seat cushion interventions. Reducing pressure by equalizing pressure over the entire sitting surface may be enough intervention for some patients. Other patients may require that the areas of highest risk (i.e., ITs and coccyx) record lower pressures than those at lower risk, such as the femurs; structurally, the femurs tolerate more load and can, therefore, tolerate higher pressures and carry more weight than the vulnerable ITs and coccyx.

Intuitively, it would seem that the better product choice would be the one with the lower peak pressure. However, peak pressure can be recorded by a single, small, aberrant cell that folded or one that recorded a clothing seam rather than a true peak pressure point. Some professionals within the international pressure mapping community have begun to average the readings of the peak pressure cell and the eight cells around it to get a more accurate picture of the pressures in that small area.

Pressure measurements can be taken with single-cell, handheld devices or larger, multiple-cell, computerized mapping devices. The handheld, single-cell monitors are more portable and less expensive, but accurate readings depend heavily on proper placement of the cell under the bony prominence while the client is sitting upright and stable. In contrast, the multiple-cell device gives a better overall picture of the pressures on the entire seating

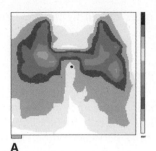 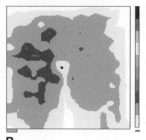

A   **B**

FIGURE 10.5 Pressure mapping uses color and numbers to show areas of high pressure. Red and yellow (warm colors) are areas of high pressure, whereas green and blue (cool colors) are areas of low pressure. Mapping is evaluated by color distribution, not by numbers. Here, the same subject (5′10″ and 175 pounds) was placed on two different seat cushions. Note the different pressure loading patterns of the buttocks on the two cushions. Foam cushion with sized ischial cutout eliminates pressure over the ischial tuberosities and redistributes pressure over the femurs.

surface simultaneously. Pressure mapping uses color and numbers to show area of high pressure. Red and yellow (warm colors) are areas of high pressure, whereas green and blue (cool colors) are areas of low pressure. Mapping is evaluated by color distribution, not by numbers. Figures 10.5 and 10.6 show the results of using mapping devices for sitting and recumbent applications.

With the advent of sophisticated interface pressure mapping devices, many facilities and clinicians are using these measurements as the major factor in determining seat selection. However, pressure is only one of several factors that cause breakdown. You must also consider shearing, friction, heat/moisture buildup, and sitting instability as equally important, even though they are more difficult to measure than interface pressure. Other practical considerations include ease of maintenance and ease of transfers and ADLs with a particular cushion, factors that are subjective and require assessment with the patient and the caregiver. In short, use interface pressure measurements in conjunction with other factors affecting the patient.

CLINICAL WISDOM

The Dangers of Bed Rest

Although sitting-related pressure ulcers can be totally relieved of pressure through bed rest, the hazards of immobility, the increased risk for breakdown on other bony prominences, and the psychological ramifications of an enforced sedentary lifestyle make bed rest a radical treatment recommendation. Clinicians should recommend bed rest only with great caution, forethought, patient preparation, and for as limited a duration as possible.

Cardiopulmonary and Vascular Systems Review and Examinations

Pathology of the cardiopulmonary and vascular systems directly affects the ability of the blood to carry oxygen and nutrients to the integumentary system. Medical diagnoses such as chronic obstructive pulmonary disease, cardiomyopathy, arteriosclerosis, and hypertension are just a few of the pathologies that affect tissue perfusion.

Inactivity and extended bed rest have several negative effects on these systems. Without an active muscle pump or the effects of gravity on the upright body, blood flow and blood diffusion are slowed throughout the body and, therefore, to any wound sites. Increased resting heart rate and decreased maximum oxygen consumption (VO2max) are also potential problems. Immobility promotes fluid stasis in the kidneys, which can lead to kidney stones and infection.[11] Inactivity and bed rest can impair nutrition intake by reducing the appetite. Recumbence also inhibits safe swallowing and facilitates aspiration of food, which can lead to pneumonia. Swallowing occurs 24 hours per day, not just at mealtime. The correct head and neck positions conducive to safe swallowing should be identified and attained in the chair and the bed; consultation with a speech/language pathologist may be necessary for success in this area.

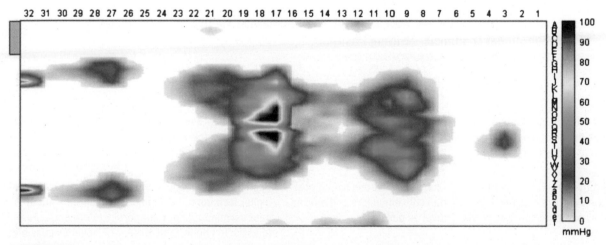

FIGURE 10.6 Four-inch high air-filled cushion takes some of the pressure off the ischials and redistributes it evenly over the surface of the cushion.

Proper upright positioning allows greater diaphragmatic expansion and facilitates breathing, thus improving oxygenation of the blood as well as pulmonary function through better movement of pulmonary secretions.[11,12] Upright positioning in a functional and comfortable position will improve general circulation by encouraging activity and movement. Cardiac function is also improved in the upright position.

Integumentary System Review and Examinations

Skin is more susceptible to breakdown if it is dry, flaky, friable, aged, insensate, prone to excessive sweating, or subjected to incontinence, friction, or shear. Therapeutic positioning can protect the skin over bony prominences, and correct use of the proper equipment can maintain safe postures and reduce tissue loads on those bony prominences. For some people, an equalization of pressure is sufficient to protect skin from breakdown. For others, a maximal reduction in pressure on a certain bony prominence is necessary because the patient's combination of risk factors makes him or her highly susceptible to pressure ulcers. For example, the skin over the coccyx is prone to breakdown because of the shape of the bone, lack of padding over the coccyx, and frequent use as a weight-bearing surface. Equipment that takes pressure completely off the coccyx in the sitting position, when used correctly, can help to avoid or treat this breakdown.

Check the skin and soft tissues over bony prominences for signs of injury; for example, a change in color (red, blue, purple) from the adjacent skin color. If trauma is identified, consider the anatomic location of each area of trauma and its relationship to positioning. Note areas of previous breakdown and any previous surgeries to repair skin, because these areas are at high risk of reopening and must be protected at all costs. Chapter 3 provides more information about skin and wound assessment.

Even if there is no current tissue breakdown, soft tissues covering bony prominences on weight-bearing surfaces can be at risk. Observe and palpate the most prominent, least protected of these tissues, and those that bear the most weight. For example, muscle atrophy of the gluteals and significant weight loss make the ischium or sacrum more prominent than usual and can make protection from breakdown a primary goal in the selection of seat cushions and bed-positioning devices.

Finally, patients who had pelvic irradiation prior to 1980 are at very high risk for tissue breakdown over the sacrum, coccyx, and buttocks, due to tissue changes caused by the irradiation technology in use at that time.

Psychosocial/Cognitive System Review and Examinations

The treatment program for skin ulcers, whether pressure ulcers or vascular ulcers, often entails a decrease in mobility. This can be as minor as occasional brief periods of time elevating the feet higher than the heart to assist blood/lymph flow, or as drastic as 24/7 bed rest for an IT ulcer on a sitting-dependent client. Extended unnatural periods of immobility can lead to many physical and psychological impairments, which are often referred to as *hazards of immobility*. The psychological hazards include subjective sensory distortions after as little as 2.75 hours in bed; this condition persists for a period of time equal to the period of confinement. Other complications are intellectual and perceptual disorders, depression, anxiety, hostility, embarrassment, helplessness, and "learned helplessness."[13] The recumbent position also induces mental and physical lethargy.

Often, a patient who refuses to follow prescribed treatments, including extended bed rest, is labeled "noncompliant" or "nonadherent," that is, having the ability to do a task but willfully not doing it. In many cases, however, he or she may perceive the bed rest as akin to imprisonment and simply cannot "comply" and may be using this behavior as a cry for help in changing the wound management program. If such behavioral signs are observed, the team and the patient should collaborate on finding a solution that will meet the needs of the situation. If this avenue is not available, consider involving psychosocial services for help in coming to a workable solution. The patient with impaired cognitive abilities may be unable to move safely or maintain safe postures independently. The equipment for someone with cognitive impairments is therefore usually more supportive than that for patients who are able to reposition themselves or can request assistance in maintaining safe postures.

Summary

Tables 10.1 and 10.2 list examples of medical and functional diagnoses relating to the need for therapeutic positioning, prognosis, related interventions, and expected functional outcomes for sitting and recumbent patients.

TABLE 10.1 Functional Diagnosis—Sitting Position			
Medical Diagnosis—Functional Diagnosis	**Prognosis**	**Intervention**	**Outcome**
Kyphosis—Client cannot maintain 90-degree hip flexion or keep face vertical due to thoracic kyphosis	Client will sit upright with face vertical and as close to 90-degree hip flexion as possible	Open seat-to-back angle adjustable backrest with stabilizing seat cushion; may need antitippers	Client able to sit stabilized as close to 90-degree back-to-seat angle as possible with face vertical
Scoliosis (fixed)—Client cannot sit with shoulders and hips level due to fixed asymmetric spine or pelvis	Client will maintain sitting position with shoulders and hips as level as possible	Cushion with buildup under higher ischium to accommodate asymmetry; back support to assist in comfortable trunk positioning	Client able to maintain upright sitting with shoulders and hips as close to level as possible

(continued)

TABLE **10.1** Functional Diagnosis—Sitting Position (*continued*)			
Medical Diagnosis—Functional Diagnosis	**Prognosis**	**Intervention**	**Outcome**
Scoliosis (flexible)—Client sits asymmetrically with one shoulder and hip elevated and opposite shoulder and hip depressed, but has potential to sit with shoulders and hips level	Client will maintain upright sitting position with level shoulders and hips without strain	Cushion with pressure elimination at ischials and full femur support or cushion with buildup under lower ischium to raise that side of pelvis; three lateral trunk supports: apex of the curve, and the hip and upper trunk on the contralateral side	Client able to maintain upright sitting with shoulders and hips level and spine straight
<90-Degree hip flexion—Client cannot achieve the 90-degree seat-to-back angle built into the majority of standard wheelchairs	Client will maintain correct sitting position with hips on back of seat	Positioning cushion to stabilize pelvis, with open seat-to-back angle adjustable backrest; angle of recline approximates maximum hip flexion allowed by range of motion limitations	Client will maintain upright sitting as close to 90 degrees as is allowed by range limitations
<90-Degrees knee Flexion available—Client unable to bend knee to 90 degrees to reach standard footrests for support	Provide equipment that supports lower extremity at available range so that client can maintain proper sitting position	Hanger with calf and foot support; angle set at maximum angle allowed at knee	Client will maintain upright sitting with hips on back of seat and lower extremities maintained at allowed knee flexion
>90 degrees Knee Flexion available – Client cannot achieve 90 degrees knee flexion	Provide equipment that supports lower extremity at available range so that client can maintain proper sitting position	Angle adjustable foot/leg support to hold lower leg at comfortable position	Client will maintain upright sitting with hips on back of seat and lower extremities maintained at allowed knee flexion
Foot propeller—Client requires use of feet to mobilize chair; unable to reach floor to propel	Provide equipment that allows efficient heel strike on the floor	Hemi-height chair with cushion or drop seat and cushion, so that total seat-to-floor height is equal to height from bottom of shoe to back of knee of propelling leg; involved leg requires 60 or 70 degrees hangar with thigh supported by wedge	Client will be self-mobile via foot propulsion while maintaining proper seating posture
One-arm driver—Client can use only one arm for self-mobility	Provide equipment designed for propulsion with one arm	One-arm-drive wheelchair	Client will be self-mobile using one arm while maintaining proper seating posture
Above the knee amputee—Client has limited femur length to support body weight; difficult to maintain posture in sitting; may lead to tissue breakdown on ischials due to increased weight on ischials	Provide firm, flat support for femurs and protection for ischials	Stabilizing seat cushion; amputee adapters to move rear wheel axle backward from normal position; antitippers	Client will maintain upright sitting with full protection of ischials and full femur support
Tissue breakdown on sitting surfaces (ischials, sacrum, or coccyx)—Client cannot sit without pressure eliminated at ulcer site	Pressure elimination on ulcer while maintaining correct postural alignment	Cushion with selective pressure elimination	Client will maintain sitting schedule with pressure elimination provided at the site of breakdown
Asymmetric tonic neck reflex (ATNR) influence—Client has difficulty controlling direction of chair with side-mounted joystick when head moves	Change placement of joystick to midline to decrease influence of ATNR	Position joystick in center of lap tray	Client will drive safely and in control despite movement of head

(*continued*)

| TABLE 10.1 | **Functional Diagnosis—Sitting Position** (*continued*) |

Medical Diagnosis—Functional Diagnosis	Prognosis	Intervention	Outcome
Hip fracture—Client cannot sit with full 90-degree hip flexion; may lead to skin breakdown due to ischial and coccyx weight bearing	Provide seating arrangement that allows <90-degree hip flexion with skin protection	Seat cushion that provides ischial/coccyx pressure reduction or elimination with positioning and can be customized with unilateral sloping to accommodate the lack of hip flexion on the involved side; open seat-to-back angle adjustable backrest with sacral protection; solid seat beneath cushion, may require cutout in board.	Client will maintain upright sitting with maximum allowed hip flexion and no pressure on coccyx
Trunk/hip hyperactive extensor tone—Client cannot maintain hips in proper position on seat due to uncontrolled hip extension; may lead to tissue breakdown due to shearing	Provide seating arrangement that best positions the client as close to 90-degree hip flexion as possible; antithrust seat assembly with pre-ischial block	Increase trunk/lower extremity angle past 90 degrees; firm contoured back support; 90-degree positioning belt	Client will maintain proper seated posture with hips on back of seat and trunk upright

Copyright © Laurie Rappl.

| TABLE 10.2 | **Functional Diagnosis Process—Recumbent Position** |

Functional Diagnosis	Prognosis	Intervention	Outcome
Cardiorespiratory or gastrointestinal pathologies requiring elevation of the head of the bed	Client will assume Fowler position with proper positioning and skin protection devices to protect heels and sacrum	Hip aligned at gatch or bend of bed; sacrum protected by lifting under one hip with pillow or foam support; heel protection devices employed; frequent turning/repositioning schedule. Do not substitute elevated head of bed for upright sitting in a supportive chair. Alternately, gatch the knees so that the hips and knees are flexed to 90 degrees and heels are off loaded. Monitor sacrococcygeal area for pressure.	Client will tolerate head of bed elevated without sliding down on the bed causing shear and friction on the sacrococcygeal areas
Less than full hip or knee extension allowed due to joint ROM impairment at the knees; undue susceptibility to pressure ulcers due to potential exposure of heel and sacrum to pressure	Client will assume supine position with foam support devices in place to accommodate hip/knee flexion requirements, and with protection of occiput, heels, and sacrum	Foam positioning devices to protect occiput and heels, and to elevate lower extremities to accommodate flexion contractures; one side of pelvis elevated slightly with towel roll or foam to protect sacrum	Client will maintain supine position with support devices correctly placed
Influence of the asymmetric tonic neck reflex (ATNR) causes involuntary movements into trunk extension and inability to maintain side-lying position	Client will be positioned with strong side down and trunk and upper limbs fully supported		

(*continued*)

TABLE 10.2	Functional Diagnosis Process—Recumbent Position (*continued*)		
Functional Diagnosis	Prognosis	Intervention	Outcome
	OR		
	Client will be positioned with strong side up, body fully supported along full trunk, and the bed situated so that client is not required to turn the face up to view the room	Position with stronger side down and trunk fully supported from shoulder to pelvis; bed is placed so that need for cervical movement is minimized, e.g., against far wall, facing door of the room	30-degree foam wedge fully supporting trunk, pelvis, shoulders, and uppermost arm and leg supported away from midline in abduction; head supported in midline in both frontal and sagittal planes
Venous ulcers on lower extremity with edema	Client will maintain supine or side-lying positions with lower extremity elevated to reduce swelling, and with ulcer and heels pressure-free	Foam device to support leg above the level of the heart in supine position and in 30-degree side-lying position	Client will maintain safe postures with limb elevated and sacrum protected

Copyright © Laurie Rappl.

Based on functional diagnosis, clinicians establish the prognosis and select interventions, with a targeted outcome for each intervention. Interventions include analysis of the most effective forms of equipment required, selection of appropriate equipment to achieve correct therapeutic position, analysis of the patient using the selected equipment, and education of the patient and caregivers in correct use. Therapeutic exercise often is another important component of the total therapy plan of care.

INTERVENTION IN THE SITTING POSITION

Sitting can be regarded as either a cause of tissue breakdown or a part of the solution. In a proactive environment in which educated clinicians have access to the proper equipment and are skilled in the techniques of therapeutic positioning, sitting can and should be part of a prevention program that can improve the quality of life for patients and assist in the healing of tissue breakdown if it occurs. In addition, sitting can decrease medical costs over the course of time. In a study of 30 long-term care residents, Trefler et al. showed that individually fitted wheelchair systems were beneficial in terms of independent mobility, functional reach, quality of life, and satisfaction with an individual's assistive technology.[14] Once equipment is prescribed, follow-up to ensure adequacy of equipment and proper usage is essential. In a study of 42 long-term care residents who used wheelchairs and equipment purchased by Medicaid, 27 were found to have inadequate seat frames, and 24 had inadequate seat cushions. The authors hypothesize that lack of follow-up may have contributed to the frequency of problems discovered.[15]

When the sitting skeleton is viewed from the side, it is apparent that the ITs extend approximately 1.5 inches past the femurs, making the ITs the major weight-bearing points on the sitting surface (see Fig. 10.7). The skin over these points is also

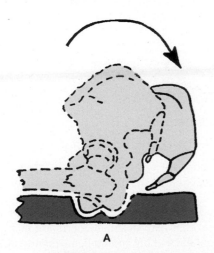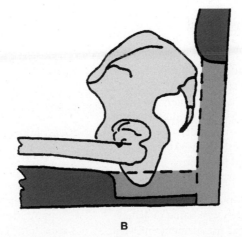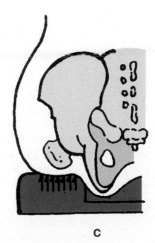

FIGURE 10.7 Pressure equalizing versus pressure eliminating. **A:** Side view of pressure equalizing cushion; loads the ischium, which allows pelvic tilt. **B:** Side view of pressure-eliminating cushion. Note pre-ischial bar limiting forward ischial movement. **C:** Rear view of pressure-eliminating cushion. Note pressure distribution across full width of femur to support the load of the body. (Courtesy of Span-America Medical Systems, Greenville, South Carolina.)

the most vulnerable to tissue breakdown because of their conical shape and poor natural padding. As a patient becomes less mobile and more sitting dependent, muscle atrophy of the gluteal muscles causes the minimal natural padding to deteriorate, making the tissues even more vulnerable to breakdown. The ITs are the fulcrum, or pivot, points for the pelvis. When bearing weight, they cause the pelvis to rock about a horizontal axis through the frontal plane that leads to anterior or posterior pelvic tilt. Most often, people tend to sit in a posterior tilt, or a slouched position. The act of moving into the slouch causes shearing forces on the ITs, and sacral sitting can lead to the formation of pressure ulcers on the sacrum and coccyx, by causing those bones to be weight bearing.

Sitting Posture Examination and Evaluation

The goal in seating a patient is to help maintain a position that is as close to ideal as possible (Fig. 10.1). Orthopedic or neurologic limitations can prevent achievement of the ideal position as a realistic goal, but it is the benchmark position. *Ideal* is the position that the body could be in if ROM, muscle and soft tissue flexibility, neurological integrity, and physical capabilities allowed it to be anatomically aligned to meet four needs:

1. For muscle balance
2. To achieve proper alignment of the bones and joints according to their design
3. To take advantage of the most load-tolerant areas of the body in handling pressure to keep the skin safe from breakdown
4. To maximize safe and functional mobility

An old positioning mantra "90/90/90" referred to 90-degree angles at the hip, knee, and ankle. This is uncomfortable for long-term sitting and has been softened to approximately 95 degrees (with straight being 180 degrees) at the hip and knee, and 90 to 95 degrees at the ankle (see Fig. 10.1 for an approximation of this position). The following points will assist you in evaluating a patient's position and in helping patients to achieve it.

In the "ideal" position:

- The ear should be in line with the acromion process and hip.
- The thigh should be parallel to the ground so that the hip and knee are in line with one another.
- The spine should be supported in its natural curves in the cervical, thoracic, and lumbar regions.
- The face should be vertical.
- Viewed from the front, the trunk and head should be comfortably upright with the shoulders and hips (pelvic crests) level, thighs in neutral position (i.e., not internally or externally rotated), feet flat on the footrests and pointed straight ahead, and arms supported so that the shoulders are not elevated or depressed when the elbows rest on the armrests.
- Dignity issues clearly indicate the need for women to be positioned with their legs together, rather than separated.

Knowledge of the ideal sitting position enables you to evaluate patients to determine how closely they can come to achieving the ideal position comfortably, what impairments prevent them from attaining that position, and then what equipment interventions can assist them in maintaining a position as close to ideal as is possible or functional.[16–22]

Applying the Basic Principles of Seating

Therapeutic positioning has traditionally been considered the realm of physical and/or occupational therapists, and indeed many highly skilled PTs and OTs work in seating clinics for patients with all types of positioning needs. However, specialized seating clinics are not available in all areas, so an understanding of proper seating and positioning must be a priority for all clinicians and caregivers. Your ability to apply the basic principles of seating will benefit the majority of your patients.

Basic principles of proper positioning (Exhibit 10.2) can be learned and applied in the home setting, skilled nursing facility, and rehabilitation facility, by all clinical staff. Of course, some patients need more intervention than just these basic principles. Clinicians and caregivers need to identify when the basic seating principles will not or cannot help the patient, or when equipment needs to accommodate a position that varies from these basic principles, and seek a referral to a skilled outside source.

Interventions Using Additional Seating Concepts

Beyond the basic seating principles are concepts specific to pelvic, thigh, and postural control.

Pelvic Control

Pelvic control is the cornerstone of seating. If the pelvis rolls out of position, the entire sitting posture is difficult to control. Therefore, stabilizing the pelvis is the foundation for stabilizing the entire body. However, the basis of this cornerstone, the ITs, is also the most vulnerable areas for tissue breakdown and the pivot points for pelvic rotation. Most cushions do not address positioning but are flat pads for comfort. Others equalize pressure across the sitting surface, maintain pressure on the ITs, and address pelvic stability by molding around and under the ITs. An alternative way to keep the pelvis in place is to stop the fulcrum action of the ITs by eliminating pressure on them. The pelvis can then be stabilized through the stabilization of the femurs.[22–27]

The femurs are joined to the pelvis at the hips and work together with the pelvis to stabilize the body. Transferring weight onto the femurs unloads the ITs and provides a larger surface area for the cushion to control. The cushion must match the posterior surface of the femurs with firm, flat support, especially for the proximal femur closest to the pelvis. Stabilizing here controls rotation of the entire femur and holds the pelvis

---

EXHIBIT 10.2

Basic Seating Principles

Basic seating principles include the following:

- Level the cushion and seat upholstery (base of support) to keep thighs horizontal to the ground; knees and hips should be even.
- Support the feet so that the knees are even with the hips.
- Support the back so that natural spinal curves are maintained; the ear, shoulder, and hip should be in alignment.
- When the pelvis is properly positioned on the seat, the seat cushion ends 1.5 to 2 inches from the back of the knee.

on the back of the seat. Movement of the pelvis is contained within the pressure elimination area (Fig. 10.7), and the ITs are free of contact. This type of cushion design is contraindicated in patients with unstable hip joints, severe fixed pelvic obliquity, and hip disarticulations.

Any pelvic cushion requires the assistance of a back support. The top of the back of the pelvis must be supported with a back support so that it cannot rock backward. The back support also fills in the lumbar curve for more supported and comfortable sitting and relieves stresses related to back pain by improving the seating ergonomics. Seat cushions are discussed in more detail further in this chapter.

Thigh Control

Except for patients with a strong anterior pelvic tilt, the thighs should be positioned so that they are parallel to the ground. The seat should be flat, with the hips and knees horizontally aligned. If the knees are lower than the hips, the weight of the legs pulls the body forward on the seat and pulls the pelvis into a posterior pelvic tilt, which clinicians work to avoid, and the client slouches. This is the position most commonly seen in settings where generic chairs are used with footrests that are lengthened as much as possible or have been lost.

Conversely, if the knees are higher than the hips, as in the use of a wedge cushion, the natural curve of the lumbar lordosis is lost; the proximal femur, along with the sacrum, coccyx, and ITs, bears an inordinate amount of weight, and the client is put at high risk of tissue breakdown and back pain. This commonly occurs when wedge-type cushions are used in an attempt to keep the client from sliding out of the seat. Wedge cushions cause so many problems that they should be prescribed with extreme caution. These problems can include tissue breakdown on the sacrum and spine due to excessive body weight being forced on those prominences, discomfort in a flexed lumbar spine, difficulties in transferring, and loss of mobility and ADL skills.

Postural Control and Stability

In order for products to help the client as much as possible, they must provide for sitting stability and comfort. The client must be supported in as close to an upright and aligned posture as possible. This will keep pressure on bony surfaces that can tolerate it (femurs) and off of surfaces that are less tolerant (ITs, coccyx, sacrum, and spinous processes). Stability and comfort also make patients as functional as possible and help to prevent further complications, such as contractures and internal organ compression.

CLINICAL WISDOM

Simple Tools

A simple toolbox is a necessity and a relatively inexpensive investment when working with seating equipment. This should include a variety of screwdrivers, wrenches, and a lubrication agent. For example, a simple wrench is usually all that is needed to change the height of a footrest, so that it is the proper height for full foot support.

Interventions Specific to Wheelchairs or Mobility Bases

The major piece of equipment in seating, which carries the highest price tag and serves as the basis for the rest of the seating system, is the mobility base. These can include manual and powered wheelchairs, bedside or living room recliner chairs, collapsible transport chairs, and scooters. Figure 10.8 is an algorithm to guide the clinician through the decision-making process to determine mobility needs.

The appropriate mobility base must be determined along with the seating system. It is often impossible to make any seating system, even the appropriate one for the patient, work on an inappropriate base. For example, many people move their chair by propelling with their feet. If the wheelchair seat is too high to allow the feet to reach the ground, any seat cushion will put the patient even higher and further reduce mobility. "Quick fixes," such as a drop seat, are, at best, only fair compromises.

In the same way, using a seating system on a mobility base for which it is not designed will compromise the effect of the system. Reclining geriatric or Geri-chairs offer little support as mobility bases and are not designed to accept most seating systems. However, these chairs are sometimes the only available alternative to bed rest; therefore, it is necessary to attempt to adapt even these chairs to fit the individual's needs by utilizing the appropriate seat and back cushions, head supports, lateral trunk or hip guides, and lower extremity support.

The standard wheelchair—a folding frame style with adjustable or fixed armrests, a seat 18 inches wide × 16 inches deep, and elevating or adjustable footrests—is designed for temporary transportation, not for mobility and positioning usage all day, every day. The vast majority of users require more support than these chairs can give. There are a multitude of variations on the standard frame:

- Hemi-height wheelchair—The axle for the back wheel is fixed higher on the frame than on standard chairs, thereby lowering the height of the seat and allowing patients who propel with their feet to reach the floor and propel the chair using a heel-toe pattern. Also used for shorter people to facilitate transfers.
- Lightweight wheelchairs—These chairs are useful for individuals such as the frail elderly because they take less energy to propel than standard chairs. Conserving these patients' energy gives them more overall endurance for functional activities.
- Sport or ultra-lightweight—These chairs are for the very active user who needs the lightest frame possible for transporting and maximum mobility.
- Rigid—This is a nonfolding frame style for the very active user; it is less prone to breaking and loosening, and increases stroke propulsion efficiency.
- Pediatric-sized—These chairs are for the child or the child-sized adult.
- Tilt-in-space—Rather than reclining just the backrest and opening up the seat-to-back angle, tilt-in-space maintains the seat-to-back angle of upright sitting and tilts or reclines the entire seat system. Tilt-in-space is favored over reclining back chairs.
- Reclining back chairs—These are adjusted by manual releases, hydraulic releases, ratchet-style fixation, or power. The seat-to-back angle can be changed to accommodate the client who cannot attain upright sitting or who needs to recline for

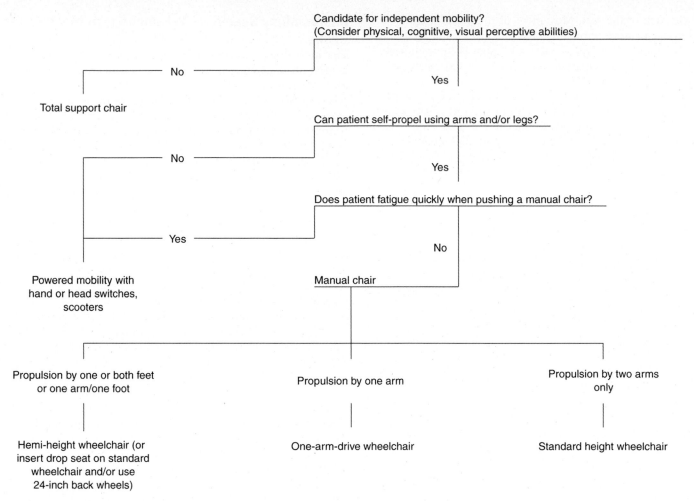

FIGURE 10.8 Algorithm for determining mobility base needs. (Copyright © Laurie Rappl.)

some time during the day, but not necessarily out of the chair. Similarly, upholstered recliners, such as Geri-chairs or living room reclining chairs allow the body to slouch from upright. These chairs cause many positioning problems; for the most part, they have been replaced by tilt-in-space chairs.

• Power chairs—These are available in wheelchair style or as scooters (Fig. 10.9).

Wheelchair Measurement

Comfortable and functional wheelchair seating requires that the seat-to-back angle accommodates the client in approximately a 95-degree hip flexion angle, or as close to that angle as the body will allow. Proper measurements for a wheelchair include (Fig. 10.10)

• *Seat depth.* The seat depth, that is the length of the seat cushion from the backrest to the front edge of the seat upholstery, should be about 1.5 to 2 inches shorter than the distance from the seat back to the back of the knee (Fig. 10.10E). Seats with less depth than this do not take advantage of the weight bearing or support that the posterior femur can give; seats with greater depth than this will pull the body forward on the chair and out of position. Many fleet or institution chairs have very short seat depths, so people tend to slide about on their chairs and slide out of position. Large recliner-style chairs have seat depths that are too deep, causing pressure on the back of the lower legs and pulling the body forward on the seat.

• *Back height.* Measure from the seat cushion to the point on the patient's back that requires needed support without hindering function (Fig. 10.10C). Patients without trunk control often require support up to the upper/mid thoracic regions. Those with active trunk control and who require more mobility will find a lower backrest supporting the lumbar or lower thoracic region is more conducive to daily function and mobility needs.

• *Width.* Measure the width from hip to hip and shoulder to shoulder, kept as close as is comfortable, so that the overall chair is as small as possible (Fig. 10.10D).

• *Footrest adjustment.* The knee should be even with the hip when the foot is flat on the footrest. This foot support measurement

CLINICAL WISDOM

Measurements must include the cushion when measuring the backrest height, seat-to-floor height, and footrest length (Fig. 10.10). Otherwise, the cushion and chair will not work together to position the client successfully.

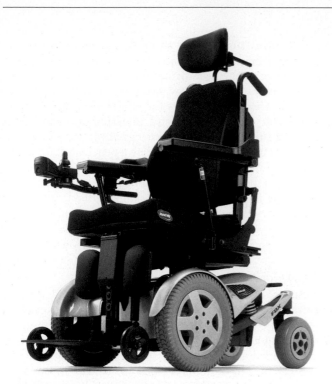

FIGURE 10.9 Power chair with back and seat.

will be the floor-to-seat height in hemi-style chairs, or the footrest selection and setting in a manual or power-propelled chair (Fig. 10.10A).

When choosing equipment, match the needs of the patient with the features of a product. Don't rely strictly on history or manufacturers' claims to determine what products to use; predetermine what features the product should have to fulfill the patient's needs and use clinical decision-making skills, including common sense, to make the product selection with the most benefits for the patient.

Selection of Seat Cushions

The use of appropriate seat cushions is commonly considered to be the primary intervention in positioning patients.[23–25] Products should be evaluated for how well they control physical and physiologic factors that cause skin and seating problems. These factors are pressure, shear, heat and moisture buildup, and postural control and stability (see Exhibit 10.3 and Fig. 10.8).

Pressure

Pressure is considered the major causative factor of tissue breakdown on the body's sitting surfaces, with the greatest effect over bony prominences where high forces are generated on small areas. Large, flat surfaces, such as the posterior femurs, seldom break down because they distribute forces over a larger area. Conversely, the ITs are a common site for tissue breakdown; they are small and

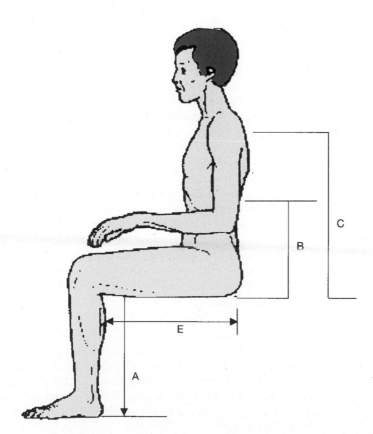
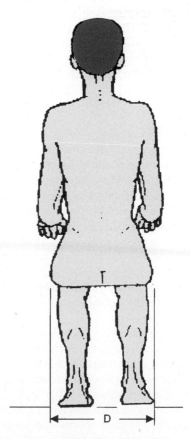

FIGURE 10.10 Measuring for a wheelchair. **A:** Seat-to-foot support height. **B:** Seat to top of sacrum for placement of lumbar support. **C:** Height of backrest needed for back support. **D:** Seat width. **E:** Seat depth, measured from backrest to popliteal fossa less than 1.5 inches (Courtesy of Span-America Medical Systems, Greenville, South Carolina.)

EXHIBIT **10.3**

Seat Cushions are Not Mattresses in Miniature

It is important to understand that the seat cushion is not a mattress in miniature. Consider that a mattress has the advantage of the entire weight-bearing surface of the body over which to spread the load. Because there is more tissue in contact with the bed, the goal of a mattress can be tissue support, that is equalizing pressure across the bony prominences and plateaus such that pressures are not high enough to cause breakdown on any one point. Compare this with the seat cushion, which must bear 75% of the body weight on a small area, average size 18 × 16 inches.

In seating, that body weight is concentrated on two prominences, the ischials, which are the lowermost skeletal points on the sitting surface. The ischials are small, pointed, and unprotected; therefore, they are less load tolerant than the large, flat, padded femurs. With this disparity in load tolerance in mind, it is imperative that the seat cushion be examined for the skeletal support it can provide to protect the skin over these at-risk areas. Then, shift the support to the load-tolerant areas. This is not equalization, but load distribution consistent with tolerances. Equalizing the pressure over the sitting surface causes low-tolerance, high-risk prominences (the ischials) to bear the same weight as the high-tolerance, low-risk areas (the femurs). The skin management principle that dictates removal of pressure at pressure ulcer sites infers that the ischials—on which breakdown occurs most frequently—should bear less weight than the femurs and should not bear any weight in the presence of tissue breakdown. This is also true for those individuals who are identified as being at high risk for tissue breakdown.

pointed, concentrating pressure over the peak of the bony prominence. Thus, the ITs can safely tolerate only one-third to one-half of the amount of pressure that the femurs can tolerate.[26,27]

Any cushion being considered for a sitting client must be assessed for its abilities to reduce pressure under the ITs. This can be done either with a pressure-mapping device or by palpation. To palpate, place the seat cushion on the seat and position the client appropriately on the cushion. Insert one hand, palm up, between the bottom of the seat cushion and the upholstery of the chair, and under the ischium. There should be at least 1 inch of soft support material (e.g., foam, gel, or rubber and air) between the ischium and the seat upholstery to protect the skin from pressure.

Many people believe that a cushion must be 4 in (10 cm) thick to be effective. However, the effectiveness of a cushion depends on many features, not simply thickness. Foams have a wide range of qualities specified by industry standards indentation load deflections (ILDs) and density. However, none of these specifications has been correlated to cushion effectiveness. Ragan et al. found that subcutaneous pressures and stresses decreased with thicker cushions, but almost all of the reduction was obtained with a cushion 8 cm thick; reduction was negligible after this height was reached.[8]

Shear

Many clinicians suspect that shear is underappreciated and even more dangerous to tissues than pressure. Shearing is a tearing force in the deep tissues that causes capillary occlusion, interruption of blood flow, stress in soft tissues, and tissue destruction. Shearing magnifies the effects of pressure, causes increased soft tissue damage and undermining, and makes it more difficult to keep ulcer dressings in place. At this time, shear cannot be measured, nor is there a benchmark for determining "too much shear."

To address shear, the seat cushion must eliminate one of the two opposing forces at work on the skin (i.e., the force coming from the surface onto the pressure-sensitive prominences) or provide inherent movement with significant amplitude in individual cells that can shift with the body and decrease drag on the skin.

Heat and Moisture

Dispersion of heat and elimination of moisture should be prime considerations when selecting seat cushions. Sitting on cushions that depend on immersion or enveloping of the buttocks into the cushion to equalize pressure can allow sweat and heat to be contained around the ITs. This buildup causes maceration or softening from fluid retention in the skin. In this state, the skin is more susceptible to damage from increased friction between the skin and the surface material, which results in shear stresses to the subcutaneous tissues and puts them at risk for pressure damage. Another complication of heat and moisture is loosening of adhesives that keep dressings in place. When this happens, the clinician can be tempted to choose dressings with aggressive adhesives that can damage fragile skin.

Heated tissues can handle less pressure than cooler tissues because heating of the skin increases metabolic demand 6% to 13% per degree Celsius rise in temperature.[28,29] Increased metabolic demands require increased blood perfusion and oxygenation. Higher metabolism will produce more metabolites that need to be removed by the blood stream. At the same time, perfusion is hampered as vessels under pressure are compressed. Cooling the tissues decreases metabolic demand, so that decreased perfusion and blood supply are required for oxygenation. In an integrative review, Lachenbruch estimated that an 8°C reduction in skin temperature would be equivalent to a 29% reduction in interface pressure, and that a 3°C temperature reduction would be equivalent to a 14% pressure reduction.[30]

One way of partially mitigating the heat and moisture problem is to choose cotton or air-exchange covers. These covers help, but they cannot combat total contact around the ischium. The most desirable cushion should provide full ventilation of the IT area with no contact.

Types of Cushions

Cushions can be divided into groups according to their features and abilities to meet various levels of client need for positioning, tissue breakdown risk, and treatment. In 2004, the Centers for Medicare and Medicaid Services (CMS) categorized cushions into six groups based on measurable, physical characteristics of each group:

1. General use
2. Positioning
3. Skin protection

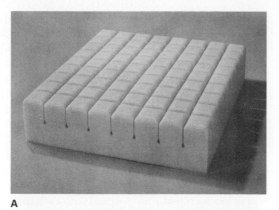

A

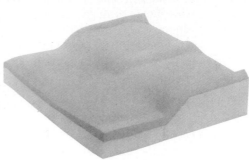

B

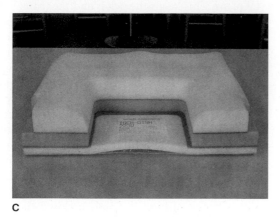

C

FIGURE 10.11 Examples of seat cushions. **A:** Pressure reduction/equalization/redistribution cushion. **B:** A generically contoured or precontoured cushion. **C:** Selective pressure elimination. (Courtesy of Span-America Medical Systems, Greenville, South Carolina.)

4. Skin protection and positioning
5. Adjustable
6. Custom

Each group has specific client criteria that must be met in order for the client to qualify for a cushion from that group.[31]

While the CMS categories are based on physical criteria, in this text, cushions are divided into four groups based on their design philosophy for addressing tissue breakdown:

1. Pressure reduction or equalization/redistribution (Fig. 10.11A)
2. Generically contoured or precontoured (Fig. 10.11B)
3. Selective pressure elimination (Fig. 10.11C)
4. Fully customized contouring

A list of product examples for each group is provided at the end of this chapter.

Pressure-Reduction or Equalization/Redistribution Cushions

These cushions decrease pressure on the ITs and coccyx (compared with no cushion at all) and attempt to equalize or redistribute that pressure across the entire sitting surface (see Fig. 10.11A). This group comprises a wide range of cushions made from flat, noncontoured foam, gel, single- or multiple-cell air bladders, and plastic matrix honeycomb products. The amount of pressure reduction off bony prominences, pressure equalization across the surface, or pressure redistribution depends on the amount of immersion of the body into the surface, the resulting shaping of the cushion around the body, and the prevention of bottoming out. Most of these equalizing cushions do little to address shearing forces, and they may address heat/moisture via cover materials only. These cushions are not all

interchangeable and are appropriate for patients at various levels of risk for tissue breakdown. For many patients, redistributing or equalizing pressure is enough to allow healing.

Many cushions at many price levels satisfy these basic requirements. Assess the patient's risk for tissue breakdown and the pressure-redistributing capabilities of the cushion without regard to price and then balance the capabilities of the product with the cost and acuity of the patient's needs. Most of these products are classified by CMS as General Use or Adjustable Skin Protection cushions, that is, air-filled cushions that equalize pressure, but do not offer positioning features.

Generically Contoured or Precontoured Cushions

These cushions are shaped with a bucketed area under the pelvis to assist with pelvic placement and channels under the femurs to assist in neutral alignment or optimal lower extremity positioning (Fig. 10.11B). They are more sophisticated than pressure equalization cushions because they have some means of actively molding to or mirroring the shape of the body's sitting surfaces to equalize pressure across the ITs and femurs (via air cells, gel or viscous fluids, viscoelastic foam, etc.), while offering contouring for body support. These products are appropriate for patients who are at moderate risk for tissue breakdown and/or require more assistance with positioning than a noncontoured cushion can provide.

It is important to note that the generic contour base is shaped to a muscled bottom, not to the atrophied bottom of a sitting-dependent patient. Therefore, they often do not hold the pelvis as securely as cushions more specifically contoured to fit individual bone structure. Many manufacturers provide optional components, such as medial thigh supports, lateral thigh supports, hip guides, and obliquity wedges that can customize the cushion to control lower extremity positioning even further. These cushions are distributed through four CMS categories: skin protection, positioning, skin protection and positioning, and adjustable, depending on the depth of immersion of the ITs allowed by the cushion and the height of the positioning features of the cushion.

A feasibility study published by the University of Pittsburgh compared the efficacy of generically contoured cushions with simple foam slab cushions. Although no statistically significant differences were seen between the groups for overall pressure ulcer incidence, the generically contoured cushions were more effective in preventing IT pressure ulcers specifically.[7] Generically contoured cushions offer better stability to the user when tested during reaching tasks than air-filled or flat foam, simple pressure reduction cushions.[32]

Selective Pressure Elimination Cushions

These cushions have an area that eliminates pressure on the ITs via a pocket that is sized to the user's IT span—the measurement from the center point of one ischium to the center point of the other (see Fig. 10.11C). They also offer flat support to the full length and width of the posterior femurs, thereby supporting the body on the femurs, not in the elimination area (also see Fig. 10.11B and C). This protects the skin over the ITs through pressure elimination, and the skin over the femurs by pressure redistribution. Although appropriate for the moderate-risk client as well, these products are often used for high-needs patients, who may be characterized by some of the following:

- Sitting dependent
- Minimally ambulatory, if at all
- Insensate
- Limited ability to reposition self to relieve pressure
- Existing or recurrent breakdown on the bony prominences of the sitting surfaces (ITs, sacrum, or coccyx)
- Currently in the granulation or remodeling phases of wound healing
- History of tissue breakdown on those sitting surfaces

Selective pressure elimination at the ITs, shearing elimination, and maximum ventilation puts the skin over the ITs in the healthiest possible environment. These requirements mirror and follow basic medical protocol for pressure ulcer treatment.[6,33–37] Selective pressure elimination cushions are in the CMS category of Skin Protection and Positioning.[38–42]

As with any sitting-dependent client, especially those with tissue breakdown, maintenance of the proper seated position is essential to enhance function and endurance, and to protect the skin under other areas of the sitting surface from breaking down. The pressure elimination cushion positions the pelvis in three ways. First, the ITs are unweighted and cannot act as pivot points for pelvic rotation. Second, the body is controlled by fully supporting the femurs (both length and width) in a nonrotated position such that they are even with each other in the horizontal plane. This keeps the pelvis and the trunk level (rather than obliquely inclined), keeps the pelvis toward the back of the seat, and prevents the pelvis from falling into the cutout area. Third, the walls of the elimination area confine movement of the pelvis to a defined area and keep the ITs from sliding forward with an effective pre-IT block. As with any cushion, the top of the back of the pelvis must also be supported with a back support so that it cannot rock backward. The back support also fills in the lumbar curve for more supported and comfortable sitting.

Do not confuse this time-tested, fitted cushion design with the donut design, which is specifically recommended against by the Agency for Health Care Research and Quality (AHRQ) guidelines.[43] Unlike a true selective pressure elimination cushion, a donut cushion is simply a closed ring of material that cuts off circulation by inducing the tourniquet effect. In addition, the ring forces weight bearing on the area around the ITs, rather than on the femurs, which are the anatomically load-tolerant areas. For these reasons, the donut cushion should never be used, especially by patients with existing breakdown or at high risk for breakdown.

Fully Customized Contouring Cushions

These unique cushions are fashioned specifically for individual patients. Usually they are prescribed for patients with severe structural deformities that cannot be accommodated by off-the-shelf products, or for patients with excessive trunk and lower extremity tone that pulls them out of position on other cushions. The CMS category "Custom" covers these cushions (Fig. 10.12).

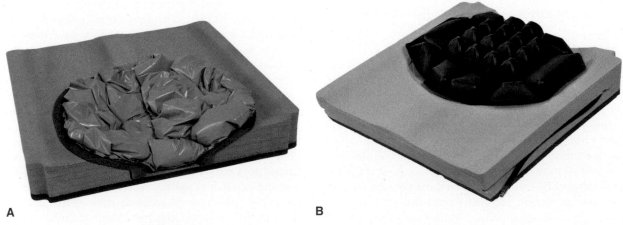

A   B

FIGURE 10.12 A,B: High-end cushion. (Courtesy of Sunrise Medical.)

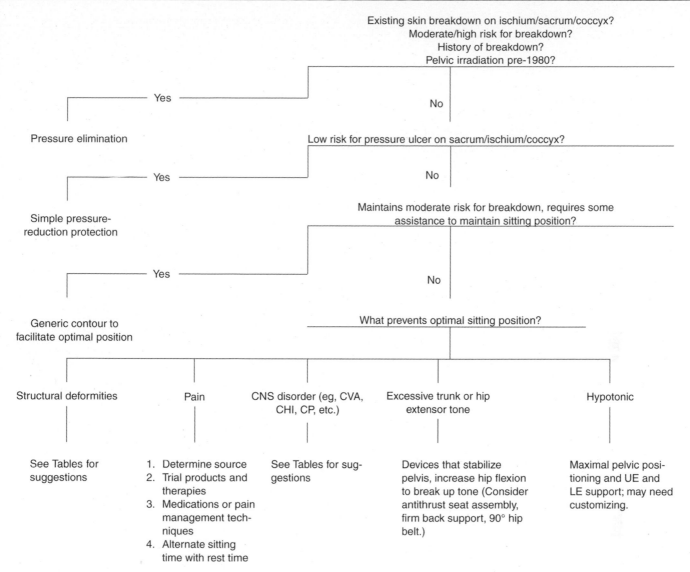

FIGURE 10.13 Algorithm for determining sitting surface. The surface must work with the mobility base to achieve optimal sitting height. CNS, central nervous system; CHI, closed head injury; CP, cerebral palsy; UE, upper extremity; LE, lower extremity. (Copyright © Laurie Rappl.)

Other Cushion Features

Other features to consider when evaluating cushions include urine-proof surface, stability of the sitting surface, washability, weight for portability, leak-proof surface, low maintenance, ease of correct use, cosmesis, durability, and slip resistance. A representative listing of manufacturing sources for these categories of seat cushion is found at the end of this chapter. The algorithm in Figure 10.13 can help you make appropriate seat cushion choices.

Selection of Back Supports

As noted earlier, the seat cushion is only one part of the seating system. To support a body adequately, the proper back support must also be prescribed. Most wheelchairs have a material back that allows the chair to fold. Unfortunately, this material bows in the opposite direction that the back requires. Therefore, almost every patient sitting in a standard folding wheelchair requires an accessory back support to accommodate the lumbar and thoracic curves. The complexity and expense of the back support depends on the needs of the patient and the number of roles that the back support must fill. The algorithm shown in Figure 10.14 can help you choose the appropriate back support for a patient.

A relatively new development in back upholstery is the tension-adjustable back. A series of horizontal Velcro straps between the seat back uprights and under the fold-over upholstery can be tightened or loosened to conform the back to the individual user's body. These backs are not as firm as solid back supports, but weigh less, are easily changed, and can be sufficient for some individuals (Fig. 10.15).

Patients who can maintain the upright ideal position with little or no assistance may require only minimal back support. For these patients, a firm, contoured back that can be slid into the chair with an attachment to the upholstery is often sufficient.

Patients with tissue breakdown on the sacrum need a back support that removes pressure from and ventilates the area.

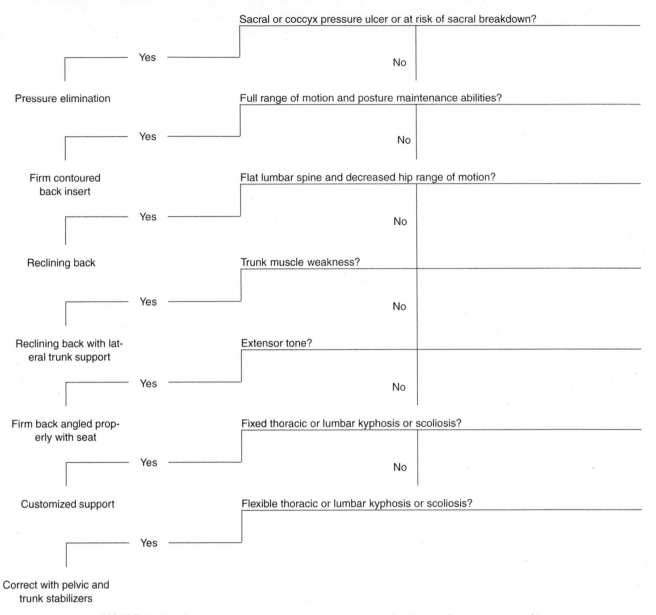

FIGURE 10.14 Algorithm for determining back support needs. (Copyright © Laurie Rappl.)

At the same time, the back support must accommodate natural spinal curves and fixed deformities, as well as correct any flexible deformities. None of these needs can be overlooked when positioning a client with sacral tissue breakdown in a sitting position. Thus, you should look for a commercially available device that is designed to meet all of these goals.

In some patients, including many older adults, the lumbar spine is flattened and the hip ROM is compromised so that it is less than 90 degrees. For these patients, a chair fixed at a 90-degree seat-to-back angle is inappropriate. Instead, select a backrest that can be adjusted to open the seat-to-back angle. This allows the patient to be positioned with the hips all the way back on the seat for full support; the back can be supported at the appropriate degree of recline to facilitate safe swallowing and maximize mobility and function.

Patients with reduced ability to support their trunk can benefit from a backrest that has lateral supports to help maintain the trunk in an upright position. A flexible thoracic or

lumbar kyphosis or scoliosis can be handled by correcting the position of the pelvis and possibly using lateral supports on the trunk. Back supports can also be fully customized to fit the unique contours of an individual. Such a support is indicated for patients with fixed trunk deformities or severe trunk weakness.

Selection of Footrests and Footrest Accessories

Footrests are critical pieces of the seating system that support and position the entire lower half of the body. Since the upper body and lower body are anatomically connected, any action on one affects the function of the other. For instance, if the footrests are too high, the weight is unevenly distributed across the femurs and concentrated on the sacrum and ITs; if they are too low, the weight of the poorly supported legs and lower body pulls the whole body out of position. As a general rule, footrests should support the legs so that the knees are even with the hips and the thighs are parallel to the ground.

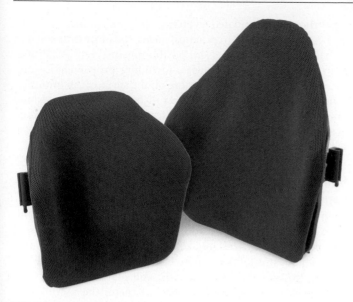

FIGURE 10.15 Back rests.

To keep the thighs parallel to the ground, simply adjust the height of the footrests of the wheelchair. Some footrests also allow adjustment in the sagittal plane to change the angle of the ankle. The pedal or platform of the footrest can be ordered in various sizes to support as much of the foot as possible. Ensure that patients wear the appropriate supportive footwear to protect the feet from trauma, evenly distribute pressures across the entire sole of the foot, and assist in decreasing dependent edema in the feet.

In the past, some clinicians have elevated the height of the foot section of the footrest, so that the foot is level with the knee, believing that this promotes venous return and controls edema. This intervention has little effect on edema, because the extremities must be positioned above the level of the heart for passive edema control; moreover, it can actually pull the body out of position and into the slouched position described earlier, and will also extend the turning radius of the chair, thus limiting mobility.

Selection of Other Accessories

Many patients require the assistance of accessory products, such as head supports, solid seat bases, armrests, back and front wheels, and ancillary devices.

Head Supports

Head supports come in a variety of models, depending on the amount of support needed and the ability of the backrest to support the headrest. Models include flat (attached to the seat back uprights of manually reclining chairs), molded around the neck and occipital regions, adjustable in height and angle, and fixed.

Solid Seat Base

Seat cushions have been discussed above. When cushions are placed on sagging seat upholstery, many of the therapeutic effects are negated. The seat support can be stiffened by adding a solid seat or board to the chair under the seat cushion to eliminate the sling of the upholstery and distribute interface pressure away from the ITs. Another intervention is a drop seat, a solid seat board with hooks that latch onto the side

rails of the mobility base and thereby lowers the user closer to the floor. Be aware that addition of a solid seat can increase the interface pressure over the ITs if the cushion is inadequate in pressure distribution over time; in other words, if the cushion bottoms out, the ITs will press into a solid, unforgiving surface that could then contribute to the formation of a pressure ulcer.

Armrests

Armrests are important in seating because they can be used to stabilize the patient during transfers and weight shifts and can decrease back pain by allowing changes of position. They can also become a hindrance to daily movement if they are not removable or cannot be swung away to facilitate transfers and transportation. Standard armrests on standard wheelchairs come in full length, shortened desk length (allows the chair to be pulled up closer to a table or desk), and height adjustable to accommodate the needs of a wide range of patient heights.

Back Wheels

The back wheels of standard wheelchairs are usually 24 or 26 inches in diameter and come in a variety of widths. Tilt-in-space chairs have 12 to 24 inches wheels, and hemi-height chairs also have smaller diameter wheels. Note that the height of the seat from the floor—a critical factor in the client's mobility—can be affected by changing the diameter of the back wheel.

Wheels are available with solid or inflated tires and treaded or nontreaded tires. For everyday, general use, most people use inflatable tires with moderate tread. Solid tires made with treads are now available for individuals who want to avoid the possibility of flat tires. For mainly indoor use, consider a minimal tread. There are also various tread patterns to benefit various terrains, such as indoor tile, outdoor pavement, and outdoor rough ground.

Front Wheels

The front wheels of wheelchairs (also called "casters") come in almost as many varieties as the back wheels—solid or inflatable, in various widths and diameters. The standard caster is 8 inches in diameter, solid rubber, and minimally treaded, if at all. Sport-type chairs are often seen with casters as small as roller blade wheels for increased turning abilities. Outdoor chairs have more substantial casters with larger diameters and widths (and often treads). Larger diameters are better over rough terrain, whereas smaller diameters are more adaptable to indoor needs.

Ancillary Devices

Ancillary devices include the following:

- Seat belts, lap belts, and anterior pelvic belts are used to help prevent the pelvis and femurs from sliding forward on the wheelchair seat. Lap belts, seat belts, and anterior pelvic belts—usually placed at a 45-degree angle to the seat-to-back angle, but often more effective when secured to the seat side rail, a few inches in front of the seat-to-back junction and crossing the proximal femur at a 90-degree angle, just below the trunk/leg crease. When the wheelchair is transported in a vehicle, installed tie downs and belts are needed to secure

CLINICAL WISDOM

Safe Installation of Vehicle Lap Belts

For safety, lap belts and tie downs for wheelchairs should be installed in the vehicle by a professional installer.

the patient into the vehicle much like standard seat/shoulder harnesses secure a seated passenger in a regular car seat.

- Lap trays—full or partial, clear or solid, padded or unpadded to assist with upper extremity support. These should not be used as a restraint, but as an assist to ADLs, including communication, for support to a flaccid arm, and to help provide a point of stability for hypertonic extremities. Lap trays can also provide trunk support for patients who fatigue over time.
- Antitippers—small wheels that attach to the back of the wheelchair to keep it from tipping over backward. These are usually used as a safety factor. In everyday life, it is necessary to tip wheelchairs backward in order to lift the front of the chair over small bumps and curbs, so antitippers can limit mobility while providing safety for the client. They can be removable.
- Amputee axle adapters—allow the rear wheels to be moved posterior to the seat back upright to keep the patient safe from tipping over backward. Amputees have less weight on the front of the chair, so moving the wheels back provides counterbalance and stability.
- Residual limb support—holds the residual limb of the below-the-knee amputee.
- Chest straps—provide anterior support for the chest and upper trunk. This is useful for patients who lack trunk control, for example those with neurological deficits that impair the ability to sit upright and who need more support than a contoured back or side supports can provide.

Working with Suppliers

Suppliers are important resources on the wound care team. A good supplier will help you keep abreast of new technology and new items on the market; but more importantly, they will help you match equipment to each patient's unique needs. Do not work with a supplier who offers only one or two lines of chairs and other equipment. Look for suppliers who carry multiple lines and are proactive in assisting with selection. Of course, ultimate accountability for this critical aspect of patient care resides with the healthcare team working with the patient, and with the physician, who is responsible for actually prescribing the equipment.

INTERVENTION IN THE RECUMBENT POSITION

The average person spends about one-third of his or her life in bed. Patients who cannot readily maintain standing or sitting positions spend even more time in the recumbent position. Just as with the seated patient, choosing the proper support surface and correctly positioning the recumbent patient are important aspects of humane and holistic treatment. Any patient who depends on the recumbent position for any part of the day or

night should be evaluated to ensure that the optimal positions are being attained.[44–48] In practical terms, the more time spent in bed, the more need there is for positioning intervention. Proper utilization of support surfaces, including proper choice and correct and consistent positioning on the surface, can minimize contractures, minimize the effects of hyperactive reflexes and muscle synergies that positively affect the integrity of the skin, provide restful sleep, and maximize a client's independence in self-mobility.

Effects of Recumbent Position on Pressure Ulcer Formation

No matter how conforming the mattress, when the many contours of the body are placed on a relatively flat surface, tissues over bony prominences are likely to endure high pressures that lead to tissue breakdown. These include the occiput, shoulders, elbows, trochanters, sacrum, heels, and malleoli and all must be protected. Statistics show that, of these, the sacrum and heels are the most likely areas to break down. Oot-Giromini[1] reported incidence rates of up to 48% on the sacrum/coccyx and 14% on the heels, while Cuddigan and Young reported prevalence rates in these same two areas, of 28.3% and 24.1%, respectively.[49] The positioning goals are to support the body, position the major joints in good alignment, and achieve muscular relaxation.

Positioning the Recumbent Patient

The recumbent patient can be positioned in supine, side-lying, or prone positions. Each of these requires special intervention. Throughout this section, the terms "open pack" or "resting position" and "closed-pack" positions are used. The open pack or resting position of a joint refers to the anatomical position in which the joint space is as wide as possible and the tendons and ligaments around that joint are relaxed. Closed pack refers to the position in which the joint spaces are narrow, the joint surfaces are close together, and the tendons and ligaments are tense. Open pack would be preferred because it is the more comfortable position for rest and relief of pain.

Supine Positioning

When the patient is supine, consider the following points:

- The head and neck should be centered, with the cervical and lumbar curves supported.
- The trunk should be aligned and straight.
- The hips and knees should not be fully extended or straight, but bent or flexed 25 to 30 degrees, the open pack position for both the hip and the knee.[44] Maintaining this slight flexion for the hips in the supine position can put increased pressure on the sacrum and heels. Therefore, these prominences should be provided with extra protection if the surface itself is not adequate. Protection for the sacrum can take the form of lifting one side of the pelvis so that the sacrum is not directly bearing weight. The heels can be protected by elevating them with a firm pillow under the calves or with heel protection devices on the feet or under the lower leg (Fig. 10.16A,B). Devices should be chosen that take all weight off of the heel to eliminate pressure, rather than simply putting a layer of padding under the heel.[50]

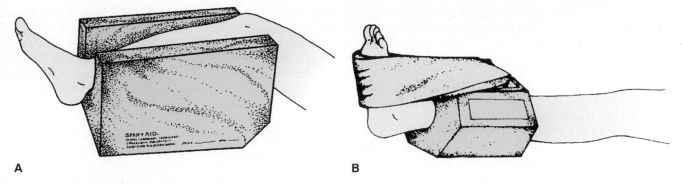

FIGURE 10.16 Protection of sacrum. **A:** limb elevator and **B:** foot drop stop. (Courtesy of Span-America Medical Systems, Greenville, South Carolina.)

- The lower extremities should be maintained in a neutral position, with the knees and toes pointing straight up to the ceiling and about shoulder width apart.
- The ankle/foot angle should be maintained close to 90 degrees (a right angle) if bed rest will be prolonged to prevent the development of foot drop or contractures in the plantar flexors.

Protection in the form of pressure redistributing surfaces or ancillary positioners may be required for the at-risk areas of the occiput, thoracic spinous processes, and elbows.

Side-Lying Positioning

Many people consider side-lying to consist of turning the body, so that it is at a 90-degree angle from supine. However, because this puts the greater trochanter at tremendous risk of breakdown, experts advocate the use of a more moderate 30 degrees incline.[43,51] This position takes direct pressure off the pointed lateral trochanter and distributes weight across flatter areas of the posterolateral femur and the wing of the sacrum. In this position, the head and neck should be centrally aligned, with the cervical curve supported.

Support is needed behind the entire trunk and pelvis to maintain the 30-degree position. Support the uppermost arm as close to the resting position of the shoulder (55 degrees abduction with 30-degree horizontal adduction[48]) as can be achieved comfortably. This will ensure that it does not fall forward across the body or backward, pulling the trunk into a twisted position. The uppermost leg tends to adduct and rest on the bed but should be elevated with pillows or foam positioners, so that it is aligned with the trunk and maintained in a neutral rotation, with slight hip and knee flexion for comfort. Protect the lowermost leg from pressure from the uppermost leg, so that tissue breakdown on the medial knee, malleolus, and foot can be avoided. Protection in the form of pressure-reducing surfaces or ancillary positioners may also be required for the lowermost ear, shoulder, greater trochanter, lateral knee, lateral malleolus, and fifth metatarsal head, as well as the uppermost medial knee and medial malleolus.

Prone Positioning

The prone position *requires* full ROM of the cervical, thoracic, and lumbar spine and since this is not usually the situation, it is not well tolerated by most patients. This position requires full extension at the hip and knee, and full external rotation of the shoulders. The trunk should be centrally aligned, with the head turned to the side. The hips should be in neutral rotation and slight abduction, and the ankles plantar flexed. The bony prominences at risk are the ears, patellas, and dorsum of the feet. The prone position puts the shoulder into its most stressful position of full external rotation with abduction. Because of the ankle position, it can also encourage foot drop. However, the major benefit to this position is that it takes all weight off of sitting weight-bearing surfaces, and is useful for stretching the hips and back into extension, the opposite of their sitting position.

Choosing Equipment

Bed support surfaces were discussed in detail in Chapter 9. Here, we provide a brief review of types of surfaces, focusing on positive and negative features for maintaining position and maximizing mobility.

In 2001, the National Pressure Ulcer Advisory Panel (NPUAP) initiated the Support Surfaces Standards Initiative (S3I), a workgroup tasked with developing uniform terminology and test methods, and reporting standards for support surfaces. The resulting guidelines are intended to provide an objective means for evaluating and comparing support surface characteristics. At the time of this writing, their work is incomplete. Progress and output of this workgroup can be found at the NPUAP Web site at www.npuap.org.

Overlays

As you learned in Chapter 9, overlays are designed to be used on top of mattresses. The term "overlay" is often misused to include any mattress other than a standard hospital or consumer mattress. Overlays are about 1 to 4 inches thick, and thus raise the level of the bed surface. This can make the sit-to-stand movement easier but beware that both moving from standing to sitting and statically sitting on the edge of a bed are safer to accomplish when the height of the surface of the bed is equal to the distance from the back of the knee to the bottom of the foot. Overlays tend to raise this level, making ingress and egress more dangerous. However, overlays are inexpensive, and foam overlays with individual, undercut, and crosscut cells are extremely effective pressure distributors.[52] Therefore, if the level of the height of the bed can be changed or if ingress and egress are not issues, an overlay can be a cost-effective and appropriate choice.

For the most part, overlays are used for prevention of tissue breakdown in patients who are at risk. They are seldom recommended for treatment, as they are, of necessity, too thin to prevent the client from bottoming out onto the very surface they are being protected from.

Mattress and Cushion Replacements

The collapsing edge is a safety concern for both the recumbent and the sitting patient. When patients roll to the side of the mattress, or when they are placed into a sitting position on the edge of the mattress or cushion before or after transfer to a seating system, the edge of the mattress must not collapse under them. Therefore, a stable edge bolster built into the mattress helps to prevent accidental sliding from the sitting position, and prevents entrapment in the side rails of the bedframe or falling to the floor from the recumbent patient.

Types of mattress replacements are next discussed.

Static Mattress Replacements

Static mattress replacements come in a variety of mediums: all foam, foam/air, foam/water, and foam/gel. They are not powered, that is they do not have a motor or plug into the wall. These surfaces replace standard mattresses and are often purchased as permanent equipment, rather than rented. They eliminate the extra height that an overlay entails and offer better redistribution of pressures than overlays or standard mattresses; however, they are more expensive than these two alternatives. Static surfaces generally offer a more stable surface to accomplish bed mobility, ingress, and egress than do alternating pressure or low-air-loss mattresses.

Static mattress replacements are sometimes called "Group I" products, as this is the name for the group of static mattresses that is reimbursable under some Medicare payment scenarios for prevention and first-level ulcer treatment intervention.

Powered Dynamic Mattress Replacements

Powered dynamic mattresses entail some means of moving air through the mattress using electrically powered motors. One technology, *low-air-loss*, uses a porous fabric to wick heat and moisture down into the mattress system and a blower to move the air, heat, and moisture out of the system. The intention is to decrease maceration of the skin and may reduce susceptibility to pressure. In an earlier discussion, you learned that it is estimated that a 3°C drop in skin temperature might equate to a 14% reduction in interface pressure.[30] Another technology, called *alternating pressure*, cyclically moves air through chambers in the mattress to alternately apply and remove pressure from each area of the body at regular intervals. This technology does not remove moisture as the low-air-loss mattresses do.

This group of mattresses is commonly paid for on a rental basis by some Medicare scenarios and by insurance companies during the treatment of tissue breakdown. Since a client should not be positioned on the ulcer, the effectiveness of these surfaces on pressure ulcer healing is questionable. At the very least, they may help to prevent tissue breakdown. Powered surfaces are often referred to as "Group II" surfaces, as this is the name for the group of mattresses that is reimbursable under Medicare for the treatment of pressure ulcers, given certain patient characteristics and settings.

Nonpowered Dynamic Mattress Replacements

This category of mattresses offers the stability of the static mattress replacement for maintaining or changing position, along with the skin protection of a dynamic mattress. Some accomplish this by dynamic air movement via interconnected elasticized reservoirs that accept air from and release air into the support tubes.[53] Others have gel/fluid bladders that conform to the body and claim to reduce shearing. Still others use self-adjusting air valves that maintain constant air pressures within the air cylinders for pressure redistribution. These are included in the Group II category for Medicare reimbursement for the treatment of pressure ulcers, given certain patient characteristics.

Air-Fluidized Surfaces

These are considered to be the best surfaces for equalizing pressures across the body and reducing soft tissue shearing, heat, and moisture on the skin. In a large retrospective study, Ochs et al. found that ulcers on air-fluidized surfaces had significantly faster healing rates for all ulcer stages, particularly stage III and IV pressure ulcers, than did ulcers on powered alternating air or low-air-loss surfaces.[54] However, air-fluidized surfaces are extremely difficult to maintain therapeutic positions on, independent ingress or egress is nearly impossible, independent repositioning is difficult, and many patients complain of pain because the surface is so unstable. These surfaces are referred to as Group III surfaces under certain Medicare reimbursement scenarios.

Effectiveness of Mattress Replacements

Reports in the literature have been inconclusive regarding whether any one of these methods of pressure redistribution is superior to the other in healing tissue breakdown. Many clinicians feel that, because of the constant changes in pressure, temperature, and moisture on any one body part, powered surfaces are safer for the skin than are static surfaces. In a large literature review of randomized controlled trials, Cullum et al. found that the benefits of alternating pressure and low-air-loss for ulcer prevention were unclear.[55] One significant disadvantage of powered mattresses is that the movement in the surface makes maintaining or changing a position more of a challenge than on a static surface. Surfaces that alternate under the client can make transfers and edge-of-bed sitting more dangerous because the bed surface is constantly shifting beneath the client.

Positioning Supplies for Recumbent Patients

Since the resting position of major joints such as the hips, knees, and shoulders is slightly flexed, and bony prominences such as the trochanters require positioning in the 30-degree side-lying position, it is safe to say that all patients require the use of positioning devices to help maintain therapeutic and anatomic

---

CLINICAL WISDOM

Photographs

Photograph a client in position with all appropriate positioning devices and display the photo in a place easily seen by caregivers. This can be the most helpful way to describe positions and use of devices to all caregivers, so that devices are used consistently and appropriately.

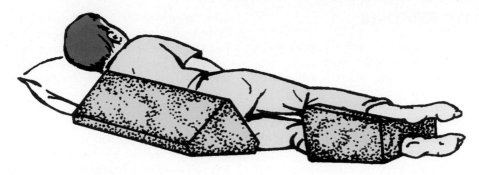

FIGURE 10.17 Thirty-degree Wedge for body alignment in side-lying. (Courtesy of Span-America Medical Systems, Greenville, South Carolina.)

body alignment and protect bony prominences. Pillows are an inexpensive support, but they are only minimally effective. They are puffy rectangles that do not naturally conform to body contours, have a tendency to slide on the surface when body pressure is applied, and are often not readily available for positioning. Foam positioners such as those shown in Figure 10.17 are shaped for supporting specific body contours, do not shift on the surface when pressure is applied, and are less likely to be confiscated for other purposes. The wedge in Figure 10.17

is useful for a variety of recumbent positioning needs—behind the head and neck of a patient with kyphosis, behind the back to maintain a 30-degree side-lying position, between the feet and footboard to prevent foot drop, under the upper arm in side-lying to achieve the open pack position for a painful shoulder. Such devices are often inexpensive to purchase, and they afford the client quality of alignment, positioning, and protection. Table 10.3 describes the use and expected outcomes for commonly used and available positioning supplies.

TABLE 10.3	Positioning Supplies for Recumbent Position	
Device	**Function**	**Action/Outcome**
Abduction pillow	Maintains lower extremities in slight abduction, neutral rotation, and knee extension	Supine—maintains lower extremities (LEs) in neutral positions Side-lying—maintains separation of LEs to protect medial knee and malleolus of upper leg
30-degree incline wedge (see Fig. 10.17)	Supports trunk and pelvis in 30-degree side-lying position	Side-lying—protects lower greater trochanter by maintaining 30-degree incline position
Cradle boot or Heel protector	Keeps heel elevated off surface while maintaining right angle or neutral ankle dorsiflexion	Supine—Protects heel from breakdown by suspending off surface Should also protect malleoli, fifth metatarsal heads, and Achilles tendon Side-lying—suspends lower malleoli and fifth metatarsal head
Limb elevator (see Fig. 10.16A)	Uses wedge with leg trough to put LE in slight hip/knee flexion with ankle elevated above knee	Supine—maintains neutral hip position with slight hip/knee flexion and foot elevation Side-lying—is used with trough side down to cup the lower leg and maintain leg separation for skin protection
Flexion/abduction pillow	Maintains slight knee flexion with separation of medial knee surfaces	Supine—maintains hip/knee flexion while breaking up adduction tone
Cervical pillow	Shaped to support cervical curve while cradling occiput	Maintains cervical curve in supine or side-lying positions
Occipital pillow, head-neck cushion, Occi-Dish	Cradles posterior surface of skull to reduce or eliminate pressure on occiput.	Supine—protects occiput by pressure removal, supports cervical curve, inhibits tonic lab reflex Side-lying—protects lower ear and supports cervical curve

Copyright © Laurie Rappl.

SELF-CARE TEACHING GUIDELINES

Patients and caregivers must be taught as much as possible about the equipment that has been prescribed, including why each piece was chosen, how to use it properly, where it was ordered (for warranty repair), and how to care for it. When changing to a new seat cushion, some patients may need to use a weaning on schedule because new equipment can sit the client differently or put loads on the skin in patterns different from those of the old equipment. A sample of such a schedule follows:

Day 1: 1 hour in morning and afternoon; assess skin response after each session.

Day 2: 1.5 hours in morning and afternoon; assess skin response after each session.

Day 3: 2 hours in morning and afternoon; assess skin response after each session.

Increase the sitting time gradually while checking to see that any redness disappears in a time equivalent to the amount of time sitting. If it takes longer, decrease sitting time to an earlier step in the schedule and continue to monitor the skin. For example, if after 2 hours of sitting on the new cushion morning and afternoon redness is noted that does not go away in 2 hours, decrease sitting time to 1.5 hours morning and afternoon and monitor the skin for a few days. Then increase to 2 hours and monitor again. The goal is to build up the tolerance of the tissues to the new sitting surface, allowing the skin to tell you when it is beyond its tolerance by redness that is slow to remit. Continue this process of gradually increasing sitting time until a full day of safe sitting is achieved.

Similarly, some patients can build skin tolerance to spend a full night in one position. This should be determined carefully, with a gradual increase in time between position changes, and a careful inspection of the skin on the weight-bearing surfaces for redness in a manner similar to that described for increasing sitting tolerance described above.

CONCLUSION

Positioning in the seated and recumbent positions requires constant learning, creativity, and patience. It is up to you to begin and continue the learning process by evaluating new technology as it is developed, determining client needs, assessing features of new products, and matching needs with features to optimally benefit your patients. Because positioning is a dynamic process, reassessment is important. Schedule an appointment for a reassessment, so that you can monitor the fit and functioning of the equipment and modify it to match the patient's changing needs.

CASE STUDY

Therapeutic Positioning for Pressure Ulcer Healing

History

The patient is a long-term resident of a skilled nursing facility. Past medical history includes surgical removal of a benign brain tumor 10 years prior to current therapy intervention. She has paralysis of the lower extremities and significant cognitive deficits (see Fig. 10.18A,B). She sits in a wheelchair for 6 hours, two times per day, for a total of 12 hours daily, and is totally dependent for changing position in bed and sitting. She requires a two-person assist for all transfers. She is totally dependent in all ADLs (feeding, wheelchair propulsion, dental hygiene, dressing).

Reasons for Referral

- Right IT tuberosity pressure ulcer, stage III, increasing in length, width, and depth.
- Hyperactive reflexes, extensor synergy in trunk and hip musculature with mild flexion contractures in knees that make positioning in bed and pressure relief in wheelchair difficult.

Examinations

Neuromuscular

Reflex exam shows hyperactive reflexes of the trunk and hip present in recumbent and sitting positions.

Musculoskeletal

Muscle strength exam. Trunk strength is poor, and upper extremity strength is fair but not functional. The patient has no volitional movement in lower extremities.

ROM exam. All joint ranges of motion are within functional limits with the exception of knee flexion contractures, which measure 20 degrees bilaterally. There is a flexible right pelvic obliquity, 2 inches lower on the right than on the left.

Postural exam. The patient prefers full fetal position with flexion of all major joints in side-lying when recumbent; in supine recumbent position, head and neck are hyperextended into the pillow, and extensor posture dominates at all other major joints. In sitting, she demonstrates trunk, hip, and knee extension with pelvis sliding forward on the seat and into posterior tilt, and the cervical spine is in hyperextension. She is bearing weight on her hands and right hip. The right side of the pelvis is rotated and tilted posteriorly. The right hip is externally rotated, and the left hip is internally rotated. Both knees are flexed (see Fig. 10.18A).

Activities of daily living (ADLs). The patient is unable to move or change positions volitionally in the bed or wheelchair. She is dependent in all transfers, requiring total assistance of two-person transfer. She is dependent for all ADLs, including feeding, hygiene, dressing, and wheelchair propulsion.

Sensory

The patient is unable to detect deep or surface pressure on sitting surfaces and lower extremities.

Integumentary

The patient has a Braden Scale pressure ulcer risk assessment score of 12, which is considered high risk (see Chapter 9).

She presents with a stage III pressure ulcer on the right IT tuberosity, measuring 3 cm × 3 cm × 1 cm deep. The pressure

CASE STUDY *(continued)*

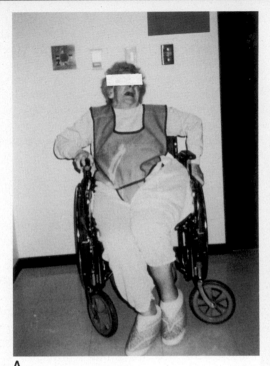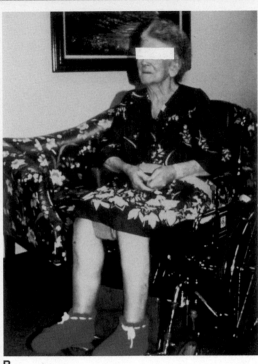

A   B

FIGURE 10.18 Therapeutic positioning for pressure ulcer healing. **A:** Before therapeutic positioning. Note cervical and trunk hyperextension, pelvis/chest restraint, right pelvic obliquity, hips forward on seat, lower extremities unsupported. **B:** After therapeutic positioning. Note that head, neck, and trunk are in good postural alignment and are in a safe and functional position. Shoulders are relaxed and equal, and hands are in clients lap. She is facing forward and able to make eye contact. The knees are level and lower extremities are supported. (Courtesy of Debby Hagler, PT, Cheyenne Mountain Rehabilitation.)

ulcer is 50% yellow slough and 50% granulation tissue. The surrounding skin is pale, and the perimeter is macerated. Drainage is serosanguineous. No undermining or tunneling is present.

Interface pressures over the sacrum, trochanter, heels, and shoulders in the supine and side-lying positions in bed were considered unsafe, as they ranged from 70 mm Hg to greater than 100 mm Hg and were higher than the flat surfaces of the body. Interface pressures over the right IT tuberosity and coccyx in the sitting position in the wheelchair were also considered unsafe, as they were greater than 100 mm Hg and higher than the flatter areas of the sitting surface.

Evaluation

Muscle weakness and joint impairment contribute to her inability to weight shift in the sitting and recumbent positions. She has a learned disuse of her arms and does not demonstrate postural movement strategies to change her position. Her sitting posture puts her at a biomechanical disadvantage to use her weakened muscles, which prevents functional movement. The stage III pressure ulcer over the right IT tuberosity is a consequence of her inability to weight shift off of the bony prominence of the IT. Maceration around the wound site is probably a combination of factors that disrupt

the moisture balance in the area, including heat and moisture build up around her seat cushion, the 6-hour period of time she is seated in her wheelchair twice daily, and possible wound exudate and/or incontinence. Her sensory impairments on the seating surface and impaired cognition contribute to her tissue breakdown.

Functional Diagnosis

Patient is disabled and unable to fulfill functional roles due to her lack of mobility, putting her at risk for pressure ulcers on bony prominences.

Need for Physical Therapist Services

The patient needs intervention by a physical therapist to achieve the following goals:

1. Healing the pressure ulcer
2. Correct postural alignment, including ability to shift weight and redistribute pressures on the seating surface off of bony prominences to tolerant areas
3. Retrain functional movement for weight shifting and use of upper extremities
4. Reduce risk of additional ulcerations

Prognosis

1. The ulcer will heal.
2. The risk of further pressure ulceration will be reduced by positioning intervention to allow restoration of functional mobility.
3. Adaptive support surface and positioning equipment will aid in restoration of function.
4. The patient will sit in a functional upright position in wheelchair with a 90-degree hip-to-back angle with a side-to-side wedged, pressure-eliminating seat cushion and a firm back cushion, with lower extremities supported and protected.
5. In the functional upright position, she will be retrained to use her upper extremities for self-care.
6. The sitting schedule will be changed to 2 hours, three times per day, for a total sitting time of 6 hours; the time up in the wheelchair will be coordinated with the meal schedule to facilitate safe swallowing, improved nutritional intake, and environmental stimulation. Sitting time will be increased gradually according to a prescribed sitting schedule.
7. The patient will be positioned in functional positions in supine and 30-degree side-lying positions on a prescribed support surface in bed, with safe interface pressure readings on all bony prominences in all positions.
8. Staff will demonstrate correct use of all equipment supplied and therapeutic positioning of this patient at all times, whether in bed or in the wheelchair.

Intervention: Therapeutic Positioning

Recommendations for adaptive seating equipment.

1. Wedged seat assembly with 5 inches on one side, decreasing to 3 inches on the other, with full pressure-relief pocket at ITs and coccyx, sized to distribute pressure fully over posterior trochanter and thighs
2. Firm back support to maintain an 85-degree seat-to-back angle to prevent extensor synergy
3. A positioning hip belt secured midway down the seat rail to fasten at a 90-degree angle to the thigh to assist in keeping the pelvis and lower extremities in appropriate position
4. Padded lap tray to provide upper extremity and trunk support
5. Footrests, calf support, and protective footwear to protect and support lower extremities and facilitate appropriate positioning
6. Hip abduction wedge to inhibit adductors and extensors and to facilitate positioning and pressure distribution on the seat assembly
7. Analysis of patient using adaptive equipment for appropriateness and safety
8. Instruction of caregivers in correct use of positioning devices

Recommendations for therapeutic positioning in bed.

1. A self-adjusting, dynamic air/foam mattress replacement to encourage mobility and allow skin protection
2. Positioning in a 30-degree side-lying position to distribute interface pressure away from the trochanter and shoulder
3. Wedges and a pillow placed between the knees to maintain the side-lying position
4. In supine, use of a leg-elevating positioning cushion to facilitate reduction in hip extensor muscle hyperactivity, accommodate for the knee flexion contractures, and position heels off the bed
5. Head-positioning cushion to provide occipital and cervical spine support and prevent excessive cervical extension in supine
6. Over-the-bed trapeze and side rails, and encouragement in their use to assist patient in self-mobility

Assessment of a patient using recumbent positioning and pressure-relief devices for safety and proper pressure relief.
Staff instruction:

1. Instruction in appropriate use of all seating and bed-positioning supplies and equipment
2. Instruction in safe and effective position changes, transfers, and positioning in the bed and wheelchair
3. Provide instruction for two shifts of nursing personnel because of projected sitting schedule of 2 hours, three times per day, coordinated with the meal schedule
4. Provide instruction about monitoring strength, endurance for sitting, and skin tolerance under the new prescribed schedule
5. Follow-up assessment of staff for appropriate and safe use of devices and components of the devices

Functional Outcomes

1. The patient is able to sit in a functional and safe position for a total of 9 hours per 24-hour period (3 hours, three times per day).
2. Interface pressure is eliminated on the ITs and coccyx, and pelvic alignment obliquity is corrected.
3. With corrected postural alignment, movement has been facilitated, and she has learned improved motor control and better use of her weakened muscles in the neck, trunk, hips, and abdomen. She has recovered functional use of her arms and is now using her arms to feed herself and propel the wheelchair.
4. The patient is positioned in a safe and functional position in bed on a nonpowered dynamic air/foam mattress replacement with safe interface pressure on all bony prominences in all positions; in side-lying, using a wedge cushion behind the back, a wedge cushion under the bottom leg, and a pillow between the knees; and in supine, using a leg-positioning cushion and head-positioning cushion.
5. The patient is able to assist in repositioning self from side to side, using the trapeze and side rails. No additional ulcers have developed. The risk assessment score is reduced to 16.
6. The pressure ulcer on the IT tuberosity is healed.

Note: Case study and photographs provided by Debby Hagler, PT, Cheyenne Mountain Rehabilitation.

REVIEW QUESTIONS

1. Healing rates for patients with existing pressure ulcers may improve by proper positioning
   A. in the least active position
   B. in the most functional position
   C. in the sitting position only
   D. in the recumbent position only

2. Which statement is true?
   A. A flexible deformity can potentially be corrected by therapy and/or equipment.
   B. A flexible deformity can potentially be corrected by therapy but not by equipment.
   C. A fixed deformity can potentially not be corrected by therapy or equipment.
   D. A fixed deformity can potentially be corrected by therapy but not by equipment.

3. Which of the following support surfaces is correctly paired for its purpose?
   A. Alternating pressure for patients with pressure ulcers and excessive perspiration
   B. Static pressure for immobile patients
   C. High-air-loss therapy for patients with pressure ulcers and excessive perspiration
   D. Low-air-loss for patients who are mobile

4. The most vulnerable area for tissue breakdown when sitting is
   A. femurs
   B. sacrum
   C. coccyx
   D. ITs

5. When a patient is placed on a relatively flat surface, the tissues over bony prominences most likely to break down are
   A. occiput and sacrum
   B. sacrum and heels
   C. heels and malleoli
   D. shoulders and trochanters

RESOURCES

Motor Control Theory

Shumway-Cook A, Wollacott MH. *Motor Control: Theory and Practical Applications*. 2nd ed. Baltimore, MD: Lippincott Williams & Wilkins; 2001.

The following is a representative listing of manufacturing sources for the categories of seat cushion products discussed in the text. Some manufacturers have products in multiple categories.

Pressure Reduction

AliMed; Ken McRight Supplies - Bye-bye Decubiti; Maddak Skin-Care; Span-America Medical-Geo-Matt

Generic Contour

Cascade Designs–Varilite; Crown Therapeutics-Roho family; Jay Medical-Jay basic, Jay2; Span-America Medical-Geo-Matt Contour, EZ-Dish; Supracor

Selective Pressure Elimination

Span-America Medical-ISCH-DISH; Ride Designs

Customized Contour

Freedom Designs; Invacare–Contour-U; Otto Bock Shape System Signature 2000; Ride Designs

SCI Clinical Practice Guidelines

Paralyzed Veterans of America

Wheelchair Seating Standards

International Standards Organization Working Group-II

Support Surface Standards

Support Surface Standards Initiative (S3I); supported by the National Pressure Ulcer Advisory Panel (NPUAP) found at www.npuap.org

REFERENCES

1. Oot-Giromini B. Pressure ulcer prevalence, incidence and associated risk factors in the community. *Decubitus*. 1993;6(5):24–32.
2. Maklebust J, Sieggreen M. *Pressure Ulcers: Guidelines for Prevention and Nursing Management*. West Dundee, IL: S-N Publications; 1991.
3. Pompeo M, Baxter C. Sacral and ischial pressure ulcers: evaluation, treatment, and differentiation. *Ostomy Wound Manage*. 2000;46(1):18–23.
4. Disa J, Carlton J, Goldberg N. Efficacy of operative care in pressure sore clients. *Plast Reconstr Surg*. 1992;89:272–278.
5. Evans G, Dufresene CR, Manson PN. Surgical correction of pressure ulcers in an urban center: is it efficacious? *Adv Wound Care*. 1994;7(1):40–46.
6. Curtin I. Wound management care and cost: an overview. *Nurse Manage*. 1984;15(2):22.
7. Geyer M, et al. A randomized clinical trial to evaluate pressure reducing seat cushions for at-risk, elderly nursing home residents. *Adv Wound Care*. 2001;14(3):120–129; quiz 131–132.
8. Ragan R, Kernozek TW, Bidar M, et al. Seat-interface pressures on various thicknesses of foam wheelchair cushions: a finite modelling approach. *Arch Phys Med Rehabil*. 2002;83(6):872–875.
9. Sprigle S, Dunlop W, Press L. Reliability of bench tests of interface pressure. *Assist Technol*. 2003;15(1):49–57.
10. Eitzen I. Pressure mapping in seating: a frequency analysis approach. *Arch Phys Med Rehabil*. 2004;85(7):1136–1140.
11. Ross J, Dean E. Integrating physiological principles into the comprehensive management of cardiopulmonary dysfunction. *Phys Ther*. 1989;69:255–259.

12. Gerhart K, Weitzenkamp D, Charlifue S. The old get older: changes over three years in aging SCI survivors. Report from Rehabilitation Research and Training Center on Aging with an SCI, Craig Hospital. *New Mobility.* 1996;7(33):18–21.

13. Norton L, Sibbald G. Is bed rest an effective treatment modality for pressure ulcers? *Ostomy/Wound Manage.* 2004;50(10):40–52.

14. Trefler E, Fitzgerald SG, Hobson DA, et al. Outcomes of wheelchair systems intervention with residents of long-term care facilities. *Assist Technol.* 2004;16(1):18–27.

15. Fuchs RH, Gromak PA. Wheelchair use by residents of nursing homes: effectiveness in meeting positioning and mobility needs. *Assist Technol.* 2003;15(2):151–163.

16. Mooney V, Einbund MJ, Rogers JE, et al. Comparison of pressure distribution qualities in seat cushions. *Bull Prosthet Res.* 1971;10(15):129–143.

17. Engstrom B. *Seating for Independence: Manual of Principles.* Waukesha, WI: ETAC; 1993.

18. Kreutz D. Seating and positioning for the newly injured. *Rehab Manage.* 1993;6:67–75.

19. Manser S, Boeker C. Seating considerations: spinal cord injury. *PT Mag.* 1993;Dec:47–51.

20. Presperin J. Postural considerations for seating the client with spinal cord injury. In: *Proceedings from RESNA Seating Conference*; June 6–11, 1992; Vancouver, BC, Canada.

21. Walpin LA. Posture—the process of body use: Principles and determinants. In: Gelb H, ed. *New Concepts in Craniomandibular and Chronic Pain Management.* St. Louis, MO: Mosby-Year Book; 1994:13–76.

22. Zacharkow D. *Wheelchair Posture and Pressure Sores.* Springfield, IL: Charles C Thomas; 1984.

23. Rappl L. A conservative treatment for pressure ulcers. *Ostomy/Wound Manage.* 1993;39(6):46–48, 50–55.

24. Garber S. Wheelchair cushions for spinal cord injured individuals. *Am J Occup Ther.* 1985;39:722–725.

25. Ferguson-Pell M. Seat cushion selection. *J Rehabil Res Dev.* 1990;(suppl 2):49–73.

26. Key AG, Manley MT. Pressure redistribution in wheelchair cushion for paraplegics: its application and evaluation. *Paraplegia.* 1978–1979;16:403–412.

27. Peterson M, Adkins H. Measurement and redistribution of excessive pressures during wheelchair sitting. *Phys Ther.* 1982;62:990–994.

28. DuBois EF. *Basal Metabolism in Health and Disease.* 3rd ed. Philadelphia, PA: Lea & Febiger; 1936.

29. Ruch RC, Patton HD, eds. *Physiology and Biophysics.* 19th ed. Philadelphia, PA: WB Saunders; 1965:1030–1049.

30. Lachenbruch C. Skin cooling surfaces: estimating the importance of limiting skin temperature. *Ostomy Wound Manage.* 2005;51(2):70–79.

31. Local Coverage Determination for Wheelchair Seating, Palmetto GBA Medicare Region C, L15887. Medical Criteria for Seat Cushions, Original effective date 07/01/2004. http://www.palmettogba.com/palmetto/ lmrps_dmerc.nsf/final/202772596F05D33285256F51006A855 D?Open-Document

32. Aissaoui R, Boucher C, Bourbonnais D, et al. Effect of seat cushion on dynamic stability in sitting during a reaching task in wheelchair users with paraplegia. *Arch Phys Med Rehabil.* 2001;82(2):274–281.

33. Knight A. Medical management of pressure sores. *J Fam Pract.* 1988;27:95–100.

34. National Pressure Ulcer Advisory Panel. Pressure ulcers—Prevalence, cost, and risk assessment: consensus development conference statement. *Decubitus.* 1989;2(2):24–28.

35. Noble PC. The prevention of pressure sores in patients with spinal cord injuries. In: *International Exchange of Information in Rehabilitation.* New York, NY: World Rehabilitation Fund; 1981.

36. Stotts N. The physiology of wound healing. In: Stotts N, Cuzzell J, eds. *Proceedings from the AACCN National Teaching Institute.* Kansas City, MO: Marion Laboratories; 1988.

37. van Rijswijk L. Full thickness pressure ulcers: client wound healing characteristics. *Decubitus.* 1991;6(1):16–21.

38. Ferguson-Pell MW, Wilkie IC, Reswick JB, et al. Pressure sore prevention for the wheelchair-bound spinal injury client. *Paraplegia.* 1980;18:42–51.

39. Perkash I, O'Neill H, Politi-Meeks D, et al. Development and evaluation of a universal contoured cushion. *Paraplegia.* 1984;22:358–365.

40. Reswick JB, Rogers JE. Experience at Rancho Los Amigos Hospital with devices and techniques to prevent pressure sores. In: Kenedi RM, Cowden JM, Scales JT, eds. *Bedsore Biomechanics.* Baltimore, MD: University Park Press; 1976:301–310.

41. Rogers J, Wilson L. Preventing recurrent tissue breakdowns after "pressure sore" closures. *Plast Reconstr Surg.* 1975;56:419–422.

42. Rappl L. Seating for skin and wound management. In: *Proceedings from Thirteenth International Seating Symposium.* Pittsburgh, PA, January 23–25, 1997.

43. Pressure Ulcers in Adults: Prediction and Prevention Clinical Practice Guideline Number 3, AHCPR Pub. No. 92-0047: May 1992. http://www.ahrq.gov/clinic/cpgonline.htm

44. Metzler D, Harr J. Positioning your client properly. *Am J Nurs.* 1996;96:33–37.

45. Plautz R. Positioning can make the difference. *Nurs Homes Long Term Care Manage.* 1992;41:30–34.

46. Cantin JE. Proper positioning eliminates client injury. *Today's OR Nurse.* 1989;11:18–21.

47. Kozier B. *Fundamentals of Nursing: Concepts, Process and Practice.* 4th ed. Redwood City, CA: Addison-Wesley Publishing; 1991.

48. Magee D. *Orthopedic Physical Assessment.* Philadelphia, PA: WB Saunders; 1992.

49. Cuddigan J, Young J. Trends in pressure ulcer prevalence; 1989–2004. *Platform presentation at Wound Ostomy Continence Nurse 2005 Annual Conference*, June 2005, Las Vegas, NV.

50. Pinzur M, et al. Preventing heel ulcers: a comparison of prophylactic body-support systems. *Arch Phys Med Rehabil.* 1991;72:508–510.

51. Seiler WO, Stahelin HB. Decubitus ulcers: preventive techniques for the elderly client. *Geriatrics.* 1985;40(7):53.

52. Day A, Leonard F. Seeking quality care for clients with pressure ulcers. *Decubitus.* 1993;6(1):32–43.

53. Branom R, Rappl L. 'Constant force technology' vs. low-air-loss in the treatment of wounds. *Ostomy Wound Manage.* 2001;47(9):38–46.

54. Ochs R, Horn S, van Rijswijk L, et al. Comparison of air-fluidized therapy with other support surfaces used to treat pressure ulcers in nursing home residents. *Ostomy/Wound Manage.* 2005;51(2):38–68.

55. Cullum N, McInnes E, Bell-Syer SE, et al. Support surfaces for pressure ulcer prevention. *Cochrane Database Syst Rev.* 3:CD001735.

CHAPTER 11

Management and Diagnosis of Vascular Ulcers

William J Ennis, Martin Borhani, and Patricio Meneses

CHAPTER OBJECTIVES

At the completion of this chapter, the reader will be able to:

1. Explain the pathophysiology underlying vascular ulcers of venous and arterial origin attending to both macro- and microvascular dysfunction.
2. Discuss assessment of the patient with vascular ulcers.
3. Identify diagnostic tests appropriate for the patient with vascular ulcers.
4. Describe the general guidelines for treating vascular ulcers of venous and arterial origin.
5. Discuss effective management strategies for vascular ulcers of venous and arterial origin.

One of the most important steps in the process of treating a patient with a nonhealing wound is to obtain an accurate assessment of the vascular supply. Without adequate perfusion, healing is not possible regardless of the dressing selected or modality employed. It is important to assess both inflow (arterial) and outflow (venous and lymphatic) in order to gain a complete understanding of the vascular status of the patient. The clinician must assess these systems at both a macro- and microvascular level.

It is imperative that tissue perfusion is analyzed within the paradigm of both the macro- and microvascular status. Conventional wisdom suggests that when there is adequate circulation at the macro level, the microcirculation should also be sufficient. In fact, both systems need to be assessed independently in order to obtain an accurate assessment of the overall perfusion status. It is important to understand not only the anatomy for each system but also the connections between the systems, interdependencies, and oftentimes similar pathophysiological mechanisms that lead to ulceration and nonhealing. In general, the arterial system delivers blood, oxygen, and nutrients to the tissues. The venous system returns oxygen-depleted blood along with toxic metabolic products back to the central circulation. The lymphatics drain the interstitial spaces and provide an immune function by trapping bacteria and debris in the lymph node network. The lymphatic system is very important but is discussed elsewhere in this textbook (see Chapter 19). Because of the complexity of vascular ulcers and the need to attend to both the macro- and microvascular level of both the arterial and venous system, in this chapter, we present the anatomy, pathophysiology, clinical signs, diagnostic testing/treatment options, and anticipated outcomes for each circulatory system and vascular level separately.

Wound healing is inextricably linked to the vascular system. Without adequate blood flow, with its supply of nutrients and oxygen, the repair process of adult tissue would be impossible. Because of the tremendous growth and interest in the field of vascular medicine, a bias has developed toward the diagnosis and treatment of macrovascular problems. Interventional procedures and surgical techniques have been perfected giving many patients a chance at limb salvage and wound healing that were not available even a few years back. *Macrocirculation* refers to the named vessels that can be seen with the unaided eye and are amenable to interventional or surgical manipulation. As a result of the emphasis placed on the macrovascular system, there is a misconception that the presence of adequate macrovascular flow alone will result in successful healing or limb salvage. Recently wound care clinicians are turning their attention to the status of the microcirculation in order to predict healing. The *microcirculation* refers to an enormous "web" of microscopic vessels and their communications, which the skin and other organs are dependent on for nutrients and oxygen.[1] Studying wound healing along this paradigm requires a refocusing of traditional views from a macro level to the micro or cellular level. At this level, there are many commonalities across tissue types in relation to inflammatory responses and repair processes. Dr. Karl Weber proposed a "common ground" theory as he answered the question: "What characteristics of tissue are common to most organs?"[2] His theory eloquently describes a common ground at the organ (stroma and mesenchymal cells), cellular (fibroblast-like cells), and molecular level (genes that govern phenotypic expression). In this chapter, every effort is made to provide the reader with up-to-date, evidence-based information that can be used in clinical practice.

SIGNIFICANCE

In the United States, the most common cause for leg ulceration is venous disease. While most clinicians have learned to appreciate the importance of compression as a mainstay of therapy, there is still much confusion over the classification of venous disease and how the underlying venous hemodynamics can impact therapeutic decisions. When reviewing the wound care literature, it becomes apparent that most studies have "lumped" all venous ulcers together rather than separating them into groups using accepted classification systems endorsed by vascular surgery societies. This makes both meta-analysis and interstudy comparisons very difficult. Although there has been a tremendous focus in the United States on surgical innovations within arterial surgery, surgical options have, until recently, been limited for venous surgery. Studies report that venous ulcers can take from 6 to 12 months to heal despite an adequate treatment protocol.[3] In addition, up to 70% of venous ulcers are thought to recur within 5 years of closure.[4] Venous ulcers are often painful and are attributed as the cause for up to 2 million work days lost to disability. An estimated 3 billion dollars is spent annually on the treatment of venous disease in the United States.[5] Due to this extreme morbidity and cost to the health-care system, the American Venous Forum has recently published a report targeting a reduction in venous leg ulcerations (VLUs) within 10 years.[6]

While much attention has been given to the treatment of arterial disease, surprisingly little improvement in overall amputation rates have been achieved in the United States. Endovascular procedures are proliferating with little evidence to support long-term outcomes. In addition, there is a poor understanding of the importance of the anatomic distribution of the target vessel for revascularization and the overall final outcome of a healed wound. Lastly, the impact of the microcirculation continues to be frequently overlooked when treating arterial disease. Limb loss is often preceded by a small, painful ischemic ulcer on the foot (see Fig. 11.1).

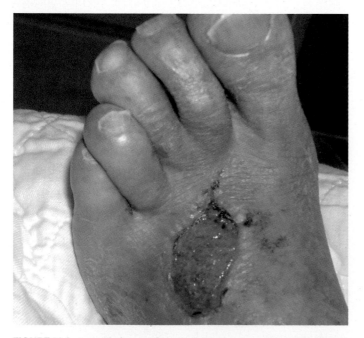

FIGURE 11.1 Arterial ulcer on the top of the foot. (Courtesy of W. Ennis.)

ARTERIAL MACROVASCULAR SYSTEM

The arterial system begins at the ascending aorta as it provides the exit pathway from the left ventricle. The aortic arch, which has several branches, including the brachiocephalic trunk, the left carotid, and the left subclavian artery, is the continuation of the ascending aorta. Further downstream is the thoracic aorta and as this large muscular artery descends through the diaphragm, it becomes the abdominal aorta. The abdominal aorta terminates in a bifurcation (right and left common iliac arteries) at about the level of the umbilicus. The clinician should check for abdominal pulsations at this level and listen with a stethoscope for the presence of bruits, which could be signs of an aneurysm or atherosclerotic narrowing. Each of the common iliac arteries then divides in the pelvis, into an internal and external iliac artery. The internal iliac artery provides the vascular supply to the pelvic viscera and musculature, the gluteal region, medial thigh, and perineum. This vessel cannot be examined through the traditional methods of pulse exam, or handheld Doppler due to its anatomical location and is therefore significantly undervalued during wound care evaluations.

The external iliac artery becomes the common femoral artery as it passes underneath the inguinal ligament. Draw a line in your mind between the anterior superior iliac spine and the pubic tubercle. This is the location of the inguinal ligament. As you palpate the pulse and auscultate the vessel with your stethoscope in the groin, you are feeling and listening to the common femoral vessel. Within a few centimeters from the groin, the common femoral artery divides into the superficial femoral and the profunda artery (Fig. 11.2). The profunda courses laterally into the thigh and is the chief blood supply to the thigh. It is the profunda that allows for healing of an above knee amputation when the superficial

CLINICAL WISDOM

Importance of Internal Iliac Artery in Development of Sacral and Gluteal Ulcers

A patient in the Intensive Care Unit who develops a rapidly expanding area of eschar and necrosis after a vascular surgery procedure is often labeled as having an incident pressure ulcer. Currently, a pressure ulcer that occurs during a hospital stay has clinical, economic, and legal implications for both the hospital and the nursing unit.[7] The more likely scenario is a thromboembolic event involving the internal iliac artery that results in an acute occlusion with subsequent muscle necrosis. The overlying skin eventually fails and the wound looks like a pressure ulcer and is in the correct anatomic location, but the rapid onset and temporal relationship to the surgical procedure should lead the clinician to make this alternate diagnosis.[8] In addition, the failure of a gluteal pressure ulcer to respond to surgical debridement and negative pressure wound therapy can be secondary to an inadequate internal iliac perfusion to allow for tissue growth. These two scenarios point out the importance of understanding the vascular anatomy that supplies any location of the body you are asked to evaluate for a nonhealing wound.

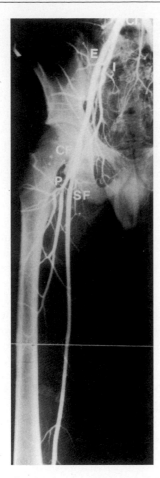

FIGURE 11.2 Normal arterial anatomy in the pelvic region. An angiogram demonstrates the usual course of the right iliac vessels: common iliac (CI), external iliac (E), and internal iliac (I) arteries. The external iliac artery becomes the common femoral artery (CF) when it crosses the inguinal ligament and gives rise to the profunda femoris artery (P) and the superficial femoral artery (SF).

femoral artery is occluded. Through a series of collaterals, the profunda can supply the lower leg and is often patent despite significant proximal atherosclerotic lesions. Lower in the leg, the superficial femoral artery passes through the adductor canal and becomes the popliteal artery. The popliteal artery passes behind the knee to give off the anterior tibial vessel as the popliteal passes deep to the tendinous arch of the soleus (Fig. 11.3). The anterior tibial vessel supplies the anterior compartment of the leg and ultimately becomes the dorsalis pedis as it passes the ankle into the foot. The pulse on top of the foot therefore is a reflection of the patency and flows through the anterior tibial artery. It is also important for the clinician to understand that an ulcer anywhere within the anatomical location of the anterior compartment would primarily be supplied by the anterior tibial artery. Collateral vessels could perfuse this region but would not likely deliver pulsatile flow as would be anticipated with direct axial blood flow from the femoral artery directly into the anterior tibial vessel. The tibioperoneal trunk is the name given to the vessel immediately distal to the anterior tibial takeoff. This vessel then divides into the posterior tibial and the peroneal arteries. The posterior tibial vessel supplies the posterior compartment of the lower leg and foot and is the vessel responsible

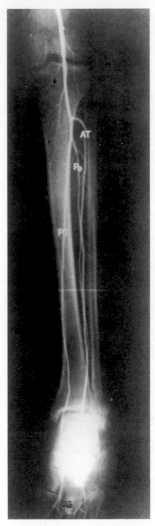

FIGURE 11.3 Normal arterial anatomy in the lower extremity. An angiogram of the left lower extremity demonstrates the usual course of the vessels. The superficial femoral artery traverses the adductor magnus canal to become the popliteal artery (P), which bifurcates into the anterior tibial artery (AT) and a tibioperoneal trunk. The tibioperoneal trunk also bifurcates to give rise to the posterior tibial (PT) and peroneal (Pe) arteries. The peroneal artery terminates at the ankle, and only the anterior and posterior tibial arteries travel into the foot. The anterior tibial artery continues in the foot as the dorsalis pedis artery, and the posterior tibial artery bifurcates into the medial and lateral plantar arteries.

for the pulse you feel behind the ankle on the medial side. The peroneal artery descends obliquely toward the fibula and passes along its medial side. Distally, the peroneal gives rise to a perforating branch and terminal lateral malleolar and calcaneal branches. The diabetic patient frequently has only a patent peroneal artery remaining below the knee, giving rise to the term "diabetic peroneal leg." Since the peroneal artery terminates at the level of the ankle, this vessel often does not provide adequate flow to heal a distal toe, or foot ulcer. An important anatomical concept, the angiosome, is discussed in a subsequent section of this chapter. It is extremely important that the clinician maps out the underlying blood supply that feeds the location of the ulcer prior to making therapeutic decisions.

Clinical Signs and Symptoms of Arterial Macrovascular Dysfunction

The clinical history should focus on the recent and remote functional status of an individual. The majority of patients with underlying atherosclerosis will be asymptomatic making the physical exam and Doppler study extremely important. In most reports, for every symptomatic patient, there is on average three to four patients who have asymptomatic peripheral arterial disease (PAD).[9] The prevalence of PAD increases from 3%–10% to upwards of 20% overall for patients over the age of 70.[10] The most common symptom of arterial disease is claudication. This term is taken from the Latin "Claudicos," which literally means to limp. However, the patients will give a description of heaviness, tired legs, a dull ache, cramping, or pain rather than a complaint of limping. The hallmark finding for this diagnosis is a history of a consistent amount of exertion that results in symptoms. For example, claudication is likely if a patient states that he develops pain in the calf while walking to the mailbox from the garage on a daily basis. The symptoms must arise each time the exertion occurs and should be completely relieved by standing still for a couple of minutes. If however on several days the patient can ambulate for a mile and the next day only 100 yards induces similar symptoms, the likely diagnosis is "pseudoclaudication." Pseudoclaudication relates to a similar set of clinical symptoms as with claudication; however, they are caused by neurocompression, usually in the lumbosacral spine. In addition to inconsistent distances resulting in symptoms, the patient with pseudoclaudication will often describe the need to sit or stretch in order to eliminate the discomfort compared to true claudication in which patients usually stand still for several minutes. Time should be taken to carefully separate these two clinical entities. The anatomic area where the patient describes symptoms can provide a clue as to the location of the underlying atherosclerotic stenotic region of the blood vessel. The affected muscle group will be one level below the arterial stenosis. For example, a patient with thigh claudication will have a blockage in the external iliac artery. Calf pain is usually secondary to a blockage in the adductor canal within the superficial femoral artery. The natural history for patients with claudication is usually benign with 75% of patients remaining stable over time.[11] Rest pain is discomfort in the foot (usually below the level of the malleoli) that occurs consistently when the legs are placed horizontal. Patients initially are awakened with pain and go to the bathroom to take medicine or "stretch" and the pain subsequently resolves. It is actually the upright position that allows for the increased flow and the resolution of ischemic pain. Over time, the patients will begin to hang their feet over the side of the bed and, as symptoms progress, sleep in a lounge chair with their head up and feet down. Interestingly, patients will not usually share these symptoms with the clinician without a probing in-depth history. The patients tend to believe they simply sleep better in a chair, do not want to bother spouses by frequently getting up, and are getting a better night's sleep in the chair without realizing that the symptoms are what lead to the alterations in body position and sleeping patterns. This can occur because often the progression of vascular disease is slow, and the patients simply lose track of time and how they have been changing their habits to accommodate the symptoms. Tissue loss is the end-stage manifestation for PAD.

RESEARCH WISDOM

Risk Factors for Arterial Dysfunction

Risk factors for atherosclerosis include advanced age, non-white race, diabetes, and smoking.[13–16] Symptoms can present with ulceration and limb-threatening infections as there is not always a linear progression from asymptomatic atherosclerotic disease through claudication, rest pain, and ulceration. Amputation however is still surprisingly unlikely outside of the diabetic population.

The ulcers are usually secondary to minor skin trauma that the patient rarely remembers. Small, punched out lesions appear, frequently on the top of the foot or toes that are extremely painful. There is little exudation and the symptoms seem out of proportion for the small wound that is seen on exam as shown in Figure 11.1.[12] Classification systems include the Rutherford and Fontaine and should be utilized in order to accurately report a patient's status and to communicate with other clinicians using the same language (see Table 11.1).

Management of Ulcers Caused by Arterial Macrovascular Dysfunction

The ischemic ulcer is usually a dry, punched out wound located on the toes, dorsal foot, ankle, or less frequently the anterior tibial region. The ulcers are characteristically painful and have scant drainage. The pain often appears out of proportion to the size of the wound. Providing a moist environment will help with the pain and potentially allow for some granulation tissue formation, but these positives must be balanced against the danger of creating a macerated wound with a local infection. Oftentimes, the use of cadexomer iodine or a silver product that maintains a dry environment is the most appropriate solution while awaiting the macrovascular tests and possible revascularization. The decision to debride should be thought through very carefully as it is very possible to create a new, expanded nonhealing wound. In addition, frequently after a local debridement of an ischemic wound, the wound bed becomes necrotic within a day and the clinician can be pulled into a cycle of frequent debridements that never achieve a healing wound environment.

CLINICAL WISDOM

Role of Microorganisms and Arterial Ulcers

Bioburden management takes on a more important role in a patient with an ischemic ulcer. Since there is limited perfusion, and delivery of white cells to the wound, bacteria can multiply without the host being able to respond. Systemic antibiotics are frequently prescribed; however, it should be remembered that the antibiotic is carried through the blood stream, and it is unlikely that an adequate tissue level will be achieved within ischemic tissue. This is why the use of concomitant topical agents becomes so important in this patient population.

TABLE	**11.1**	**Classification Scheme for Both Arterial and Venous Disease**

Arterial

Fontaine		Rutherford		
Stage	*Clinical*	*Grade*	*Category*	*Clinical*
1	Asymptomatic	0	0	Asymptomatic
2a	Mild claudication	1	1	Mild claudication
2b	Mod-severe	1	2	Moderate
3	Rest pain	1	3	Severe
4	Ulcer/gangrene	2	4	Rest pain
		3	5	Minor tissue loss
		3	6	Major tissue loss

Venous **CEAP**

Clinical		*Etiology*		*Pathophysiology*	
C0	No visible signs	Ec	Congenital	Pr	Reflux
C1	Telangiectasia or reticular vein	Ep	Primary	Po	Obstruction
C2	Varicose veins	Es	Secondary	Pr,o	Reflux and obstruction
C3	Edema	En	None identified	Pn	No path identified
C4a	Pigmentation and/or eczema				
C4b	Lipodermatosclerosis and/or atrophie blanche				
C5	Healed venous ulcer	*Anatomic*			
C6	Active venous ulcer	As	Superficial vein		
S	Symptoms are present	Ap	Perforator vein		
A	Asymptomatic	Ad	Deep vein		
		An	No location noted		

Diagnostic Tests for the Arterial Macrovascular System

The initial arterial evaluation focuses on the macrocirculation and begins with the palpation of peripheral pulses. Ankle pulses are however not sufficient to detect impaired arterial circulation, and additional testing is frequently required for the patient with leg ulcerations.[17] When interpreting an ankle brachial index (ABI), it must be remembered that in patients with diabetes, renal failure, and often in the elderly, medial calcification of the blood vessel leads to an incompressible blood vessel resulting in falsely elevated values.[18] Performing an ankle arm index is useful not only for wound healing prediction but also as an overall marker for cardiovascular health.[19,20] A useful option for the patient with heavily calcified vessels is the use of a toe/brachial index (TBI).[21–23] Using the TBI in combination with Doppler waveform analysis, the wound clinician can obtain a more accurate picture of the macrovascular status of their patients. Only about 10% of patients presenting to an outpatient wound clinic will have isolated arterial disease as an etiology for their leg ulcer.[24] Arterial duplex scans, segmental pressures including toe pressures, pulse volume recordings, magnetic resonance angiography (MRA), and rapid sequence CT scans are other noninvasive macrocirculation studies that may be ordered. An interventional angiogram is still considered the gold standard at this time although many facilities are utilizing MRA as an alternative. After a complete assessment of the macrocirculation, the clinician's attention must be turned to the status of the microcirculation. Adequacy of macrovascular flow does not ensure that healing will occur or that the microcirculation is functional.

ARTERIAL MICROVASCULAR SYSTEM

The circulation of the skin arises from cutaneous branches off subcutaneously located musculocutaneous arteries. A single artery pierces the dermis and divides into smaller arterioles.[25] A superficial and deep plexus of arterioles and venules is present within the dermis, connected by multiple communicating vessels.[26] The deep plexus is parallel to the skin surface and is located deep in the reticular dermis. The superficial plexus also lies parallel to the skin surface just below the papillary dermis (subpapillary plexus). The majority of microcirculatory flow occurs in the superficial plexus. The vessels located at the plexus level include end arterioles, capillaries, and postcapillary venules. The venules are more numerous and can be recognized histologically by their multilaminated basement membranes in contrast to the homogeneous membrane seen in the arteriole.[27] Many of the physiological events in the microcirculation, including changes in permeability, white blood cell (WBC) diapedesis, and vasculitis as a result of immune complex deposition on the vessel wall, occur at the venule.[28] It is the superficial plexus that gives rise to the "capillary loop." Projections of the dermis, along with accompanying blood vessels and nervous tissue into the epidermis, make up the papillary system. Each papilla usually contains one capillary loop, consisting of an intra- and extrapapillary segment.[27]

The red blood cells (RBC) move through the capillary with a velocity of 0.4 to 0.8 mm per second and remain in the capillary for several seconds allowing for exchange of gases and fluids. Cardiac pulsations, autoregulation, and intrinsic vasomotion are all factors in capillary flow.[29] Filtration is favored at the arteriolar limb of the capillary loop and absorption at the venular limb. Increases in pressure at either end of the capillary loop will lead to increased interstitial edema formation as capillary pressure exceeds plasma oncotic pressure. The body has a built-in protective mechanism for capillary hypertension known as the venoarteriolar reflex. As the increased pressure in the capillary is sensed, a reflex sympathetic response leads to a constriction on the arterial side, thereby decreasing overall flow to the capillary and indirectly lowering the pressure. This mechanism is defective in the patient with diabetes. This defect, along with microsclerosis, which can occur in the microcirculation of the patient with diabetes, leads to abnormal responses to inflammation, infection, and wound healing.[30]

Arterial Microvascular Pathophysiology

The microcirculation is initially compromised by arterial insufficiency at the macro level. Over time, however, a series of compensatory mechanisms can allow for adequate tissue perfusion. Hypoxic tissue induces a process known as angiogenesis (creation of new blood vessels from existing capillary networks).[31] More recently, it has been discovered that endothelial progenitor cells (EPCs) can come from the bone marrow to hypoxic tissues and help create blood vessels de novo in a process known as vasculogenesis.[32] Although these processes will not achieve the same level of tissue perfusion that is possible with a healthy macro flow, it can be enough to allow for wound healing to occur. Vascular endothelial growth factor (VEGF), platelet-derived growth factor (PDGF), and hypoxia-inducible factor (HIF1alpha) are all important in the process and are known to be deficient in diabetic patients.[33] If a patient has documented, compromised macrovascular flow and is not a candidate for revascularization, he or she should undergo testing of the microcirculation in order to determine the level of compensation that has occurred and if healing is likely at that baseline value. As discussed below, the microcirculation can improve, stay the same, or worsen after an attempt at restoring the macrovascular flow.

The process of atherosclerosis occurs at the cellular level and there have been three main theories proposed over the years. The initial lesion that can be seen even in children, is the fatty streak.[34] There is an increase in the number of intimal

RESEARCH WISDOM

Atherosclerosis and Response to Injury

Both shear and mechanical stress can induce biochemical changes through intracellular signal transduction pathways that lead to enhanced atherosclerosis through alterations in cell death, proliferation, and cytokine production.[40–42]

macrophages most of which are filled with lipid droplets. These fatty streaks are benign and may not lead to further problems but are thought to be the precursor lesions to advanced atherosclerotic plaques in the adult.[35] Lesions can advance, gain lipid content, and vascularize to form stable or nonstable atherosclerotic plaques. These lesions can either compromise the lumen or acutely dislodge and result in embolic phenomenon, respectively. The first theory of atherosclerosis focuses on the level of cholesterol in the blood. In particular, oxidized low-density lipoprotein (LDL) appears to be chemotactic for monocytes and T cells and is directly injurious to the endothelial lining.[36,37] This process continues over time with the ultimate development of a lipid-laden atherosclerotic lesion. Other researchers have focused on the response to injury model as the primary etiology for atherosclerosis. More recently, infection and inflammatory processes have been proposed as a mechanism for atherosclerosis. Infections with Chlamydia and the influences of heat shock proteins are gaining attention as potential targets for therapeutic interventions.[38,39]

Clinical Signs and Symptoms of Arterial Microvascular Dysfunction

The clinical signs of abnormal microcirculation are more subtle than those of the macrocirculation and require keen observation and routine follow-up of patients with nonhealing wounds. A wound that has recently been debrided due to the presence of necrotic tissue along the periphery of the wound margin may redevelop the same necrotic tissue within 24 hours of the procedure. The clinician thinks it is secondary to desiccation and applies a wound gel and occlusion. The next day the wound bed is dusky and the perimeter is macerated. Another attempt at debridement results in a healthy appearing wound and perimeter, but the necrotic tissue returns again. This is a classic picture of a wound in which the microcirculation is inadequate to support the blood flow needed for healing. If this is not recognized, the clinician may inappropriately debride multiple times resulting in a much larger nonhealing wound than the baseline measurements. This is a clinical example of microcirculatory pathology. The problem facing the clinician is an absence of quantitative, reproducible measurement tools to accurately diagnose the problem and, often, inadequate knowledge of therapeutic modalities that might enhance the microcirculatory flow.

Diagnostic Tests for the Arterial Microvascular System

Specialized arteriovenous shunts (glomus bodies) important in thermoregulation, allow blood to bypass the capillary bed. This parallel circulation provides much greater blood flow than is

CLINICAL WISDOM

Inadequate Microcirculation for Healing

A clinical example of when the microcirculation is inadequate to support blood flow needed for healing is when a negative pressure therapy system is applied at a high pressure on continuous mode to a freshly debrided wound in the operating room. The first dressing take down reveals a dusky, nongranular bed. The surgeon reports the wound looked very good with brisk bleeding in the operating room. A follow-up debridement with the reapplication of negative pressure therapy at a lower pressure, and intermittent suction, results in a red, moist, granular wound at the next dressing change.

metabolically required at rest. The distinction between nutritive and nonnutritive flow is difficult to assess with indirect techniques.[43] For example, an indirect measurement of a near normal perfusion may be the result of shunted (nonnutritive flow) perfusion and may not reflect "nutritive" (cutaneous) flow. It is therefore critical to assess not only flow (oxygen transport) but also cellular metabolism (oxygen utilization and energy production). Intravital capillaroscopy can help visualize nutritive capillary flow and quantify capillary density. The laser Doppler can tell us about the microcirculatory flow, but one would need to add a transcutaneous oxygen measurement to understand if the oxygen delivered to the tissue was utilized. As noted above, high levels of either shunted (nonnutritive flow) or dermal (nutritive) blood flow would be detected but not differentiated by laser Doppler. ^{31}P NMR spectroscopy data could reveal at a cellular level oxygen consumption by the cell. Near infrared spectroscopy and positron emission tomography (PET scan) are additional examples of measurement tools for the microcirculation.[44,45] Recently, clinicians are attempting to quantify the pressure in the skin by employing laser Doppler technology.[46] The "skin perfusion pressure" might allow the wound clinician to use this value in combination with an ankle brachial pressure to begin to comprehensively analyze the perfusion on both the macro and micro level.

Management of Ulcers Caused by Arterial Microvascular Dysfunction

Patients who present with tissue loss are treated with a goal of restoring pulsatile flow to the wound bed whenever possible. For patients who will require concomitant or subsequent infrainguinal revascularization, it is more likely that a surgical rather than endovascular aortoiliac reconstruction would be performed in order to ensure optimal inflow. Infrapopliteal occlusive disease is preferentially treated by saphenous vein bypass unless the distribution of disease is clearly focal and amenable to simple balloon angioplasty. If adequate saphenous vein conduit is not available and tibial disease is extensive, then the choice of alternative autologous vein or prosthetic conduit is weighed against endovascular intervention. If a suitable tibial target with axial runoff to the foot can be found, PTFE bypass with a distal vein segment adjunct, such as a Miller cuff or Linton patch, is performed.[47] Otherwise, patients may be considered for extensive endovascular-based interventions.

These general strategies are then tailored as the individual case dictates. Factors that may shift treatment strategy toward endovascular intervention instead of surgical bypass include patient age, prohibitive operative risks, limited expected lifespan, unsuitable autologous conduit for distal revascularization, lack of adequate target vessel, or hostile leg that prohibits surgical intervention. Examples of a "hostile" leg include marked edema, severe venous stasis changes, and open ulcers in the region of bypass target vessel. Factors that may shift treatment strategy toward surgical intervention include severe renal insufficiency that precludes contrast dye administration required for endovascular intervention. Additional considerations include the relationship between expected patency rates and likelihood of limb salvage. Patients in whom short-term patency following endovascular intervention are sufficient for limb salvage are more likely to be treated by endovascular means than patients who require long-term patency to maintain limb salvage. It is critical therefore that communication between the wound care and vascular surgery team identifies specific goals of therapy, so that the most appropriate treatment option is selected. Short-term goals of wound healing might be achieved through less invasive procedures allowing for more "definitive care" procedures to be reserved for possible future symptomatic vascular disease.

A patient may have compromised macro flow but due to compensatory mechanisms such as the development of collateral flow be able to heal a wound. In a study of 111 patients with nonreconstructable vascular disease, the microcirculatory assessment was predictive of ultimate limb salvage.[48] The clinician can treat the microcirculation through the use of various modalities that can increase angiogenesis and local blood flow to the wound bed.[49] A concept known as the push-pull theory has been presented by the authors as a working theoretical construct.[50] The push is achieved by the macrovascular-based arterial reconstruction. Other forms of "push" include increasing cardiac output, volume resuscitation, and the use of medications in the treatment of shock. The pull component is achieved through the use of mechanical energy–based modalities that lead to vasodilation and subsequent angiogenesis.[49,51] These therapies "pull" the blood flow toward the microcirculation in a bimodal pattern that can be demonstrated through the use of a scanning laser Doppler.[52] The "pull" is essentially created by decreasing peripheral resistance and increasing the quantity of available capillaries, a process known as capillary recruitment. After the initial increase in flow, mediated by nitric oxide release from the endothelium within the microcirculation, a second phase of increased microcirculatory flow is achieved through the process of angiogenesis. Local microcirculatory perfusion can also be influenced by both vasoconstriction and adequate volume status. Noxious stimuli such as hypothermia, stress, pain and depression can all lead to increased sympathetic tone and subsequent decreased tissue perfusion.[53] Smoking, through the action of nicotine, can also result in decreased microcirculatory flow.[54] Several medications including beta-blockers have been thought in the past to negatively impact the microcirculation, but with improved imaging techniques appear to be safe.[55,56] Other medications (pentoxifylline) can be used to augment microcirculation and tissue perfusion.[57]

Management Strategies for Arterial Ulcers with Macro- and Microvascular Dysfunction

If a patient has a nonhealing wound, abnormal macrovascular flow studies, and microvascular studies (i.e., transcutaneous oximetry) that are adequate for healing, a trial of aggressive local wound care could be warranted. This assumes the patient does not have an infected wound or confounding comorbidity that would warrant rapid surgical correction. If after a 4-week treatment course no significant improvement in either wound dimensions or quality of tissue is noted, then further invasive studies followed by revascularization or other surgical interventions might be necessary. Approaching a wound patient in this manner avoids unnecessary high-risk procedures, puts a limit on treatment times, and can minimize potential harmful outcomes. If the microcirculatory studies are abnormal, a trial of treatments aimed at enhancing the microcirculation (i.e., electrical stimulation, growth factors, bioengineered tissue, and therapeutic ultrasound) could be used along with aggressive wound care for a short course. Systemic therapy along with life style modifications should also be employed where indicated.

When treating patients with ischemic ulcers, it is important to monitor for signs of infection. Ischemic tissue is vulnerable to infection due to decreased tissue perfusion with a concomitant decreased number of polymorphonuclear cells to fight infection.[58] The use of topical agents that control bioburden can play an important role in ischemic ulcerations; however, systemic antibiotics are required for deep infections and when infection appears to be advancing beyond the wound margins.

In situations in which patients have no open or endovascular options for reconstruction, and microcirculatory therapies have been exhausted, palliative symptomatic treatment should be considered if appropriate clinically. Pain control can be achieved through sympathetic block procedures and the use of spinal cord stimulators.[59] Often a side benefit of these therapies in addition to pain relief is increased microcirculatory flow. Hyperbaric oxygen should be considered for patients who either cannot undergo revascularization or have incomplete revascularization as evidenced by the continued nonhealing of a wound despite a functional bypass. A transcutaneous oxygen test should be conducted on the periwound tissue with and without 100% oxygen via a nonrebreather to identify potentially reversible

hypoxic tissue. More recently, measurements taken inside the hyperbaric chamber at pressures above 2.0 atmospheres absolute have been shown to be more predictive of a potential healing response with hyperbaric oxygen therapy.[60] Several reports have demonstrated healing of ischemic ulcerations through the use of pneumatic counter-pulsation therapy.[61–63]

Finally, amputation can be the most appropriate solution for some patients with ischemia and tissue loss. As previously described, when both the macro and micro flow is severely compromised, significant time and expense can be wasted with a patient who ultimately ends up with an amputation at the end of a long, difficult treatment. During these treatments, patients can decondition and ultimately be unable to ambulate with a prosthetic after their amputation. Therefore, the decision concerning limb loss should be individualized, multidisciplinary, and patient focused.

VENOUS MACROVASCULAR SYSTEM

There is a misconception amongst wound care clinicians that venous ulcerations are essentially all the same and rarely is there an effort to separate them by underlying pathophysiology. Most wound care literature reports healing outcomes by wound etiology without any attempt to divide venous ulcerations into subcategories. Despite the evidence supporting compression as the mainstay of therapy for venous ulcerations, it is common to see a patient in the clinic with a history of venous disease who has never received any compression therapy. In addition, the term venous ulcer is applied to many patients without any diagnostic testing. Many leg ulcers that are secondary to vasculitis, malignancy, vasculopathy, and trauma get labeled as venous ulcers, further confounding the results from case observational series. Improvements in both diagnostic ultrasound and an agreed-upon classification system should make the future reporting of this disease state more accurate and will hopefully allow clinicians to tailor therapeutic options for specific conditions. Recently, surgical-based procedures have been shown to help reduce the recurrence rate of venous ulcerations, which has historically been very high.[64] The goal of this section is to review the anatomy, pathophysiology, clinical signs and symptoms, diagnostic testing, and treatment options.

Approximately 7 million people in the United States suffer from venous insufficiency.[65] It is thought that throughout the Western world the overall prevalence of venous ulcerations approaches 1%, but over the past 20 years, the prevalence and characteristics of chronic venous insufficiency (CVI) have changed.[66] Due to the high prevalence of the disease, variability in diagnosis, treatment, and patient conformance, there are high economic costs that include outpatient clinic visits, home healthcare, hospitalizations, and supplies.[67–69] It is important for the wound care clinician to approach the patient with a suspected venous leg ulcer with a consistent, algorithmic approach and to deliver the best evidence-based therapies based on the individual patient's needs.

The veins in the lower extremity are divided into superficial, deep, perforator, and communicating veins. Perforating veins function as conduits between the superficial and deep system. The communicating veins however connect veins that are within the same system. In the foot, there are two subcutaneous venous networks located on the dorsum and plantar surface of the foot. A dorsal vein arch runs across the dorsal foot at about

---

> ### CLINICAL WISDOM
>
> #### Overall Medical Management of the Patient with Arterial Macro- and Microvascular Dysfunction
>
> Another aspect of treatment for the vascular wound patient is the overall medical management of their underlying atherosclerosis. Frequently this is overlooked in PAD. With coronary disease, there is frequently an organized treatment regimen, but due to the myriad of clinicians who care for a patient with a lower extremity wound and PAD, often these important treatments fall through the cracks. Smoking cessation is paramount not only for graft patency and wound healing but also for overall health.[13,14] Aggressive lipid lowering, hypertension control, and tight diabetic control are all important issues that require attention.[15]

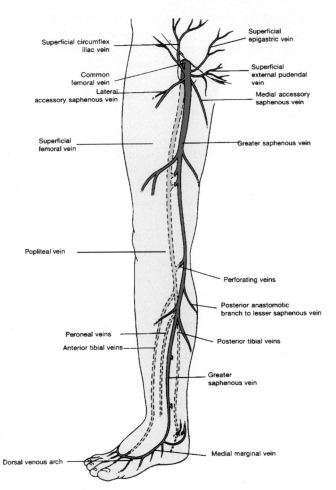

FIGURE 11.4 Normal venous anatomy. A schematic diagram demonstrates the veins of the lower extremity, which are divided into superficial, deep, and perforating veins.

the level of the metatarsal heads. The medial end of this arch continues anterior to the medial malleoli and up the medial side of the leg as the greater saphenous vein (GSV). Near the groin, the greater saphenous joins with multiple other veins at the confluence of the superficial inguinal veins, formally known as the saphenofemoral junction. The GSV is often duplicated in both the calf and thigh making accurate duplex examinations imperative (see Fig. 11.4).[70] The lateral end of the dorsal arch becomes the lateral marginal vein and ascends as the lesser saphenous

RESEARCH WISDOM

Role of Venous Sinuses

There are as many as 150 perforating veins in the lower extremity and over the years debate over their contribution to venous disease has not been definitively proven. Venous sinuses are large veins that reside within the calf muscles and have tremendous volume capacity. There are no valves within the sinuses and they act as holding chambers that empty with the rhythmic contraction of the calf muscles, leading investigators to call them the "peripheral heart."

vein. The lesser saphenous vein runs between the heads of the gastrocnemius muscle and approximately 5 cm proximal to the knee crease and empties into the popliteal vein (Fig. 11.4). In over two-thirds of patients with venous disease, an intersaphenous vein is located in the posteromedial thigh.[71] There is much duplication and anatomic variants within the venous system making the noninvasive assessment via duplex scanning difficult even for trained sonographers. There are bicuspid valves throughout the superficial venous system that ensure unidirectional flow toward the heart. There are more valves below the knee than above, and more on the medial side of the leg.

Deep veins of the lower extremity are paired with each corresponding artery. The proximal continuation of these paired veins is the popliteal vein, which continues as the femoral vein within the adductor canal in the lower thigh. Below the inguinal ligament the femoral vein joins the deep femoral (profunda vein) to become the common femoral. One of the important anatomic concepts for the wound clinician is to remember the continuation of the deep system into the external iliac vein, common iliac, and ultimately the inferior vena cava (Fig. 11.4). A patient presented to our hospital with a 3-day history of left lower leg swelling and erythema. She was admitted with cellulitis and, despite a normal white count and no fever, was started on antibiotics. Duplex scan of the leg was negative for deep vein thrombosis (DVT). After 4 days, there was no improvement in the swelling or redness and a second duplex was also read as negative. She then had a PICC line placed and was being considered for transfer to a subacute for long-term antibiotics. Her leg continued to swell and now she complained of numbness, and extreme pain, and there were areas of soft tissue breakdown along the medial lower leg. We were consulted and noticed engorged labial and perineal veins that led us to order a venogram to be performed through the groin. The patient had a 99% stenosis of the left common iliac vein secondary to a rare condition known as May Thurner syndrome.[72,73] After successful angioplasty and stent placement, the swelling and erythema resolved. Patients with frequent venous ulcerations and an inability to tolerate compression therapy need to be assessed for central venous stenosis as a number of reports cite an increasing frequency of iliac webs and stenotic lesions.[74]

Venous Macrovascular Pathophysiology

Overall, the purpose of the venous circulation is to return blood flow to the heart for reoxygenation. The overall movement of blood flow in the venous circulation is dependent on pressure differentials. Pressures in the right atrium average between 4 and 7 mm Hg and in the supine position the venous pressure at the ankle level is between 12 and 18 mm Hg.[75] Flow can proceed therefore from the ankle toward the heart in normal conditions in the recumbent position. When standing, the hydrostatic pressure at the ankle is 94 mm Hg. Venous return flows from the superficial system to the deep via the perforators, and then proximally toward the heart. The one-way valves act to ensure a directional flow pattern. The calf muscles act as a pump and eject over 60% of total venous volume with each contraction.[76] With repeated contractions, a residual venous volume is reached. This volume is known as the ambulatory venous pressure (AVP) and remains beneath 22 mm Hg in normal conditions. As AVP exceeds 30 mm Hg, the incidence of VLU increases.[77] Incompetent valves, poor muscle contractile function, or any outflow obstruction will result in elevated AVPs and increase the chances for VLUs.

Clinical Signs and Symptoms of Venous Macrovascular Dysfunction

The clinical signs and symptoms of venous disease can be readily recorded using the CEAP classification system (see Table 11.1). This system was initially created by the American Venous Forum in 1994.[78–80] A major revision of the CEAP classification was released in 2004.[81] The main components of the classification scheme describe the clinical, etiological, anatomical, and pathophysiological state of the venous system and the clinical consequences. Most papers in the vascular literature describe, at a minimum, the clinical scoring component of the CEAP when discussing venous leg ulcer patients. The revised CEAP added two subcategories of symptomatic and asymptomatic to the clinical score that ranges from C0 (no venous disease) to C6 (active venous ulcer). Chronic venous disorder refers to a term that refers to all clinical grades from C1 to C6 while CVI specifically refers to classes C3–C6. The nomenclature is important as many wound clinicians use the terms interchangeably. The E stands for etiology. The underlying cause for the venous pathology can be congenital, primary, secondary, or a category in which no venous pathology was identified. Congenital disorders such as Klippel-Trenauney refer to deformations of the venous system that are present at birth. Primary venous disease (PVI) refers to a degenerative condition of the vein walls and the valves and is more prevalent than secondary disease. This disorder is slowly progressive and can move from C1–C2 toward C4–C6 over time. Primary venous insufficiency should be separated from secondary due to important clinical and therapeutic reasons. Secondary venous insufficiency is what clinicians are classically taught about during their training. Some type of venous clot in the past leads to incomplete recanalization, increased venous pressures, and, over time, ulceration. Secondary venous insufficiency results in both reflux and obstructive noninvasive findings. Patients with secondary insufficiency often require anticoagulation and rarely benefit from saphenous vein ablation and might even be harmed by the procedure. The last two components of the CEAP, anatomical and pathophysiological classes, require a formal, comprehensive duplex scan in order to accurately classify.

Diagnostic Tests for the Venous Macrovascular System

The history and physical exam are performed prior to any noninvasive or invasive venous testing. Obvious questions include history of prior ulcerations, thrombotic episodes, venous surgery, medical conditions, and family history of varicose veins and/or vein clots. The patient needs to be examined in the standing position in order to evaluate the venous system. Sit down on a stool in a room with good lighting and look for dilated or tortuous veins. The distribution of varicose veins will commonly follow either the greater or the lesser saphenous vein distribution. Clinical signs of importance include the presence of a corona phlebectatica. This sign is diagnostic of elevated AVPs and appears as a flare of intradermal varices along the medial aspect of the foot. Lipodermatosclerosis (LDS) refers to the hardened subcutaneous tissue in the lower half of the leg that is so common in patients with venous disease. LDS has both an acute and a chronic presentation. The acute form is often misdiagnosed as cellulitis due to the presence of a demarcated, erythematous, inflammatory reaction that overlies an incompetent perforator.[82,83] The chronic variant demonstrates pigmented skin that is densely attached to the underlying inflamed subcutaneous tissue. The tissue is hard to palpate and "wood like." The location of chronic LDS coincides with the maximal sites of AVPs and is often the site of ulceration. White scar-like areas of the skin are referred to as atrophie blanche. Hyperpigmentation is secondary to macrophage uptake of local hemosiderin that has leaked from the microcirculation; however, a role for dermal melanocytes has been proposed.[84] The varices can be percussed to trace out the pattern of the vein (Tap test of Chevrier), and through a series of maneuvers, known as the Trendelenburg test, the clinician can identify the level and location of deep to superficial reflux.[85]

Although there are many diagnostic tests available for evaluating patients with venous disorders, the duplex scan has become the most important and should be considered a first-line assessment tool. Duplex scanning is a routine test to rule out acute DVT in the hospital setting. Duplex scanning is noninvasive, portable, and readily available. Accuracy is generally reported as over 90% for detecting femoral-popliteal thrombosis.[86] There are four important components of all duplex scans and these include visualization of the vein, compressibility of the vein wall, spontaneous venous flow, and the ability to augment flow with a compression force distal to the probe. There is a considerable drop in accuracy of DVT detection below the knee in most institutions. The majority of patients presenting to an outpatient wound care center however are ambulatory and not at high risk for DVT; yet, the vascular lab may only provide the clinician with a DVT rule out study when a "vein study" is ordered. A comprehensive venous system duplex scan is time consuming and requires additional expertise in performing.

Reflux is essentially a reversal of normal flow within the vein. There is always a small amount of physiological reversal of flow that is required to achieve vein valve wall apposition and closure. Reflux beyond this small quantity is pathological and should be measured for all vein segments. Duplex scanning is essential in order to accurately classify patients using the CEAP classification system.

In addition to duplex scanning, there are a number of other noninvasive tests available to the wound care clinician to assess venous function. Venous outflow can be measured with impedance and/or strain gauge plethysmography.[87,88] Air plethysmography can be used to analyze the overall calf muscle pump function and venous hemodynamics through a noninvasive test.[89]

RESEARCH WISDOM

Use of CEAP Classification

The use of the CEAP classification system is widespread in the vascular surgery field but is rarely discussed in the wound care community. Most healing outcomes related to venous leg ulcers fail to subclassify the VLU patients by CEAP criteria. Future subgroup analysis of these reports might help to identify responders from nonresponders for a wide variety of advanced wound care products.

Recent advances in radiological imaging have improved the accuracy with which a clinician can diagnose venous outflow obstruction. Classically, contrast ascending venography was the method of choice to evaluate the venous system, while descending venography was employed for detecting reflux. Computed tomography (CTV) or magnetic resonance imaging (MRV) can now help make the diagnosis of venous outflow obstruction.[90,91] The wound care clinician needs to keep this in mind when evaluating a recalcitrant venous leg ulcer patient. If the patient is complaining of extreme pain with the use of compression or the wound has failed to improve despite adequate compression, a consideration for central venous obstruction should be entertained.

VENOUS MICROVASCULAR SYSTEM PATHOPHYSIOLOGY

It is not the anatomy of the microcirculation that is unique in venous disease, but the pathophysiological alterations that are of most importance in the development of venous ulcerations. Historically, it was John Homans who published on the etiology of venous ulcers in 1917 that led investigators to follow a "stasis" model of venous insufficiency.[92] Additional theories describing potential etiologies for venous ulcer formation included arteriovenous fistula formation, diffusion block due to fibrin cuffs, and the activation and plugging of leukocytes.[93–95] The venous microcirculation was studied using quantitative morphometric analysis in 1997 by Pappas et al.[96] This study described the distribution of macrophages, mast cells, and the extracellular matrix in patients with and without venous disease. Current attention surrounds the role of fibroblast senescence, cytokine regulation of dermal fibrosis, and the role of matrix metalloproteinases.[97–99]

Clinical Signs and Symptoms of Venous Microvascular Dysfunction

The clinical signs of venous disease at the microcirculatory level include the visual appearance of the previously mentioned atrophie blanche. This area of white scar tissue essentially represents a dermal infarct and the skin immediately surrounding it can be painful. Despite conventional wisdom that venous ulcers are not painful, many of them actually are quite uncomfortable for patients. Many patients describe pain that is worse when lying down, which complicates the history and makes the clinician think of arterial causes. The microcirculatory impact of hypoxia can lead to dermal ischemic pain that is relieved with dependency and worsened with elevation. Paradoxically, these symptoms improve with compression as the elimination of microedema allows for increased microcirculatory perfusion. The skin immediately surrounding the venous ulcer can demonstrate lowered transcutaneous oxygen values and is at risk for ulceration with only minor trauma. The repetitive cycle of ulceration and healing leads to increased scar formation, which is poorly perfused and is at risk for recurrent ulceration. Even minor shifts of leg edema can lead to repeated ulcerations due to decreased elasticity of the subcutaneous tissue.

Diagnostic Tests for the Venous Microvascular System

Diagnostic testing for the microcirculatory component of venous disease is limited. Laser Doppler imaging, transcutaneous oxygen, and intravital video capillaroscopy were employed to analyze patients with venous disease at the microcirculatory level.[100] The findings included lowered transcutaneous oxygen levels, increased microcirculatory flow, a decrease in the number of capillaries and glomeruloid-like capillary architecture. This has led investigators to monitor the effects of topical agents before and after therapy at a microcirculatory level.[101,102] Others have tried to monitor the microcirculation in venous disease after a 4-week trial of a moist wound care product.[103]

Management Strategies for Venous Ulcers with Macro- and Microvascular Dysfunction

The most important aspect of treating patients with venous disease is the application of adequate compression therapy. The Cochrane review findings indicated that compression is always better than none, high compression is better than low compression, but failed to identify four layer as better than three layer.[104,105] Despite these findings, it is not uncommon for patients to present to the office without ever having received compression therapy. Lack of knowledge on the part of the clinicians and patient noncompliance are likely the two leading reasons for this outcome. The reader is referred to several references that describe the various forms of compression, that is, inelastic versus elastic, and to Chapter 19.[106]

Surgical interruption of the saphenous vein has been a well-described therapy for many years, but with the advent of radiofrequency and laser ablation techniques, most clinicians are considering the less invasive treatment. Initially, thought to augment venous leg ulcer healing, the ablation of the saphenous vein was shown to have a significant effect on reducing venous ulcer recurrence but not overall healing in a randomized controlled trial.[109–113] Patients should of course have documented reflux via duplex scan prior to undergoing any invasive therapy. Controversy still exists surrounding the treatment of perforator vein incompetence. The Linton procedure was an open surgical approach in which perforators were ligated at the subfascial level.[114] This surgery often resulted in wound complications that led to the development of the SEPS procedure

RESEARCH WISDOM

Medication Treatment

Medical therapy for venous ulcers plays a small role in the United States but is more prominent in the European community. Pentoxifylline has level one evidence to support its use in the comprehensive treatment of venous leg ulcers. The drug was studied at 400 mg three times a day in two studies while a third trial utilized 800 mg three times a day.[107] There are a myriad of other medication that have been studied, many of them with good supporting evidence.[108]

(subfascial endoscopic perforator surgery).[115] Surgeons have moved away from this procedure as it has proved time consuming and there are a fair number of cases in which the most distal perforators cannot be accessed endoscopically forcing the surgeon to use an incision in addition to the endoscopic procedure.

The local wound care is no different for venous ulcers than other types of chronic wounds. Most venous ulcers are highly exudative and require absorptive dressings. There has been little evidence to support the use of any one dressing over another.[116] It is more important to match the characteristics of the wound with the characteristics of the wound dressing. It is important to protect the periwound skin through the use of some protective barrier cream. This is especially important along the inferior margin of the wound because as the patient stands, the wound fluid moves down from the wound and can cause dermatitis and increasing skin loss due to the hostile nature of venous wound fluid. The compression therapy can be started at a low pressure and then gradually increased to try and increase patient acceptance of the treatment. Once the wound bed is stabilized, arterial disease ruled out, and compression initiated the patient should improve over 4 weeks with a decreasing wound area. Patients who fail to improve should be considered for biopsy to rule out alternative diagnosis and cultured and imaged to rule out central venous obstruction. Cultured skin substitutes have been shown to statistically increase the healing of venous leg ulcers and should be considered early if the patient fails the standard approach described.[117,118] In recalcitrant cases, consideration for tangential excision of the entire wound and subcutaneous tissue can be performed with subsequent implantation of dermal substitutes in an effort to completely remove the pathological tissue causing the recurrent ulcers. Other forms of skin grafting have insufficient evidence at this time.[119]

CASE STUDY

Venous Ulceration Case Study

JJ is a 65-year-old African American female with a history of type 2 diabetes, hypertension, and leg ulcers over the past 10 years. She has had numerous treatments and each time her wound would heal and then recur within 1 year of healing. The patient was wearing compression stockings during each recurrence and has been compliant with her prescribed therapies during each ulcer occurrence. During the most recent workup, a full duplex scan was ordered and the patient was found to have isolated severe saphenous reflux with a competent deep system. Her arterial Dopplers revealed biphasic waveforms and normal ankle pressures. A biopsy of the wound edge was negative for malignancy and the immunoflourescent stains were negative for the presence of vasculitis. The patient's sugars have been brought under good control, and after the wound failed to progress over 45 days, the decision was made to treat with a biological skin substitute. The patient was maintained in a multilayer compression wrap throughout the treatment and ultimately healed at 12 weeks. She was immediately placed in newly measured 30– to 40–mm Hg stockings and was referred to a vascular surgeon for saphenous venous ablation. The procedure was successful and postoperative duplex scanning revealed complete elimination of saphenous reflux. The patient maintained the use of her stockings and has remained ulcer free for 5 years.

Clinical Points

1. Always consider a wound biopsy for wounds greater than 1 year in duration or in those wounds that have an abnormal appearance.
2. Randomized controlled trial data support the use of compression therapy, biological skin substitutes, and pentoxifylline for venous ulcer healing and saphenous ablation for a decrease in recurrence rates.

Arterial Case Study

TI is a 44-year-old white male with a history of claudication since he was 15 years old. He is currently a stock clerk in a warehouse and is having a problem maintaining his position because of the limitations he experiences when trying to walk any distance greater than 400 ft. As well, he is currently suffering with a nonhealing wound located at the medial malleoli of the right leg. The wound is 1.8 cm^2, 0.1 cm deep, surrounded by a zone of hyperpigmentation, and completely filled with healthy-appearing granulation tissue. The wound has opened and closed several times over the past 5 years. The history is also positive for a prior interventional vascular procedure (balloon angioplasty) with concurrent use of urokinase (clot-dissolving medicine). A physical examination reveals a well-developed male with normal physical examination results. Pulses were present, with biphasic signals in both the dorsalis pedis and the posterior tibial vessels. When the pulses were examined after the patient exercised for 5 minutes, they were noted to be absent. A CAT scan performed on the legs revealed the presence of an abnormally located medial head of the gastrocnemius muscle. The muscle in effect "traps" the popliteal artery and vein during active motion. The condition is known as *popliteal entrapment syndrome*. This finding was confirmed with an angiogram. As the patient's foot was actively plantar flexed, one could see the cutoff of contrast flowing down the vessel. The treatment for this was the surgical removal of the medial head of the muscle, which freed up both the artery and the vein. The ulcer was then treated as a standard venous ulcer with local moist wound care and compression. The patient went on to heal and was able to resume normal activities again.

Clinical Points

1. The presence of a pulse does not preclude further investigation if the symptoms warrant. As well, we have demonstrated in this chapter that the presence of macrovascular flow does not always imply adequate microcirculation.
2. Consider evaluating both the ABI and the pulses after exercise in a patient with a history compatible with vascular disease and palpable pulses at rest.

CONCLUSIONS

Arterial disease is a growing problem in the United States and there is an increased awareness of PAD within the general population. Wound clinicians need to understand arterial anatomy and be able to identify which artery is most responsible for tissue perfusion within the region of the patient's wound. There are numerous treatment options, both surgical and endovascular, that may be appropriate to revascularize the patient with an arterial wound. The clinician needs to weigh many factors when deciding the best approach for a patient with an arterial wound. The durability of the procedure, the chance of distal embolization, the status of collateral flow, the health status and cardiac status of the patient, as well as the patient's underlying functional status. Without a multidisciplinary approach to these cases, there is a tendency to perform procedures that the clinician is comfortable with and a focus on "fixing the angiogram." With a renewed focus on cost-effectiveness and health-care reform, clinicians will need to be sure the procedure they select has the greatest outcome on both a clinical and an economic basis.

There are actually several evidence-based therapeutic options for treating venous ulcer patients. It is important to classify the venous ulcer patient using approved anatomical and clinical classification schemes that help the clinician identify possible treatment options. Untreated, venous disease leads to a myriad of skin changes that can place the patient at risk for frequent recurrences and bouts of cellulitis. The clinician needs to be mindful of the venous outflow anatomy proximal to the inferior vena cava when working up a patient with venous insufficiency and hypertension.

In both arterial and venous disorders, there is a strong potential for microcirculatory dysfunction and the clinician needs to consider testing methods and treatment options that address this circulatory network when organizing a treatment protocol.

REVIEW QUESTION

1. The following statements are true:
   A. HIF1alpha levels are normal or high in diabetic patients.
   B. Endothelial function is rarely impacted in diabetes.
   C. EPCs hone from the bone marrow and help revascularization through a process known as vasculogenesis.
   D. EPCs hone from the bone marrow and help revascularization through a process known as angiogenesis.
2. Atherosclerosis is thought to occur, in part, as a result of which of the following theories?
   A. Oxidized LDL cholesterol causing intimal damage
   B. A response to infectious agents, in particular Chlamydia
   C. An inflammatory process with heat shock proteins implicated
   D. An injury response phenomenon
   E. All of the above
3. The involved stenotic vein in May-Thurner syndrome is
   A. the inferior vena cava
   B. the external iliac vein
   C. the saphenous vein
   D. the left internal iliac vein
   E. the left common iliac vein
4. More accurate classification of venous disease can be achieved through the use of
   A. Fontaine classification system
   B. Wagner classification
   C. Rutherford classification
   D. CEAP classification
   E. Duke classification
5. The essential component of treatment for macro- and microvascular dysfunction of the venous system is:
   A. compression theraphy
   B. Pentoxifylene
   C. leg exercises
   D. leg elevation

REFERENCES

1. Ennis WJ, Meneses P. Technologies for Assessment of wound microcirculation. In: Krasner DL, Sibbald RG, Rodeheaver GT, eds. *Chronic Wound Care: A Clinical Source Book for Healthcare Professionals.* 4th ed. Malverne, PA: HMP Communications; 2007:417–426.
2. Weber K. In search of common ground. In: Weber K, ed. *Wound Healing in Cardiovascular Disease.* Armonk, NY: Futura; 1995:295–307.
3. Browse NL, Burnand KG. The cause of venous ulceration. *Lancet.* 1982;2(8292):243–245.
4. Ruckley CV. Socioeconomic impact of chronic venous insufficiency and leg ulcers. *Angiology.* 1997;48(1):67–69.
5. Van den Oever R, et al. Socio-economic impact of chronic venous insufficiency. An underestimated public health problem. *Int Angiol.* 1998;17(3):161–167.
6. Gillespie DL, et al. Venous ulcer diagnosis, treatment, and prevention of recurrences. *J Vasc Surg.* 2010;52(5 suppl):8S–14S.
7. Armstrong DG, et al. New opportunities to improve pressure ulcer prevention and treatment: implications of the CMS inpatient hospital care present on admission indicators/hospital-acquired conditions policy: a consensus paper from the International Expert Wound Care Advisory Panel. *Adv Skin Wound Care.* 2008;21(10):469–478.
8. Balakrishnan C, et al. Reconstruction of sacral defects following necrosis of buttocks due to embolization of internal iliac artery using a transverse lumbar flap. *Can J Plast Surg.* 2009;17(3):e8–e10.
9. Norgren L, et al. Inter-Society Consensus for the management of peripheral arterial disease (TASC II). *Eur J Vasc Endovasc Surg.* 2007;33(suppl 1):S1–S75.
10. Selvin E, Erlinger TP. Prevalence of and risk factors for peripheral arterial disease in the United States: results from the National Health and Nutrition Examination Survey, 1999–2000. *Circulation.* 2004;110(6):738–743.
11. Norgren L, et al. Inter-Society Consensus for the management of peripheral arterial disease (TASC II). *J Vasc Surg.* 2007;45(suppl S):S5–S67.

12. Sieggreen M. Lower extremity arterial and venous ulcers. *Nurs Clin North Am.* 2005;40(2):391–410.

13. Willigendael EM, et al. Smoking and the patency of lower extremity bypass grafts: a meta-analysis. *J Vasc Surg.* 2005;42(1):67–74.

14. Willigendael EM, et al. Influence of smoking on incidence and prevalence of peripheral arterial disease. *J Vasc Surg.* 2004;40(6):1158–1165.

15. MRC/BHF Heart Protection Study of cholesterol lowering with simvastatin in 20,536 high-risk individuals: a randomised placebo-controlled trial. *Lancet.* 2002;360(9326):7–22.

16. Management of peripheral arterial disease (PAD). TransAtlantic Inter-Society Consensus (TASC). *Int Angiol.* 2000;19(1 suppl 1): I–XXIV, 1–304.

17. Moffatt C, O'Hare L. Ankle pulses are not sufficient to detect impaired arterial circulation in patients with leg ulcers. *J Wound Care.* 1995;4(3):134–138.

18. Al-Qaisi M, et al. Ankle brachial pressure index (ABPI): an update for practitioners. *Vasc Health Risk Manag.* 2009;5:833–841.

19. Newman AB, et al. The Cardiovascular Health Study Group. Ankle-arm index as a predictor of cardiovascular disease and mortality in the Cardiovascular Health Study. *Arterioscler Thromb Vasc Biol.* 1999;19(3):538–545.

20. Wutschert R, Bounameaux H. Predicting healing of arterial leg ulcers by means of segmental systolic pressure measurements. *Vasa.* 1998;27(4):224–228.

21. Muro Y, et al. An evaluation of the efficacy of the toe brachial index measuring vascular involvement in systemic sclerosis and other connective tissue diseases. *Clin Exp Rheumatol.* 2009;27(3 suppl 54): 26–31.

22. Martin Borge V, et al. Peripheral arterial disease in diabetic patients: utility of the toe-brachial index. *Med Clin (Barc).* 2008; 130(16):611–612.

23. Fleck CA. Measuring toe brachial index. *Adv Skin Wound Care.* 2008;21(1):20–22.

24. Baker SR, et al. Aetiology of chronic leg ulcers. *Eur J Vasc Surg.* 1992;6(3):245–251.

25. Ryan T. Cutaneous circulation. In: Goldsmith LA, ed. *Physiology, Biochemistry, and Molecular Biology of the Skin.* Oxford, UK: Oxford University Press; 1991:1019–1064.

26. Jakubovic HR, Ackerman AB. Structure and function of skin: development, morphology, and physiology. In: Moschella H, ed. *Dermatology.* Philadelphia. PA: WB Saunders; 1992:3–79.

27. Braverman IM, Yen A. Ultrastructure of the human dermal microcirculation. II. The capillary loops of the dermal papillae. *J Invest Dermatol.* 1977;68(1):44–52.

28. Yen A, Braverman IM. Ultrastructure of the human dermal microcirculation: the horizontal plexus of the papillary dermis. *J Invest Dermatol.* 1976;66(3):131–142.

29. Braverman IM. The cutaneous microcirculation. *J Invest Dermatol Symp Proc.* 2000;5(1):3–9.

30. Korzon-Burakowska A, Edmonds M. Role of the microcirculation in diabetic foot ulceration. *Int J Low Extrem Wounds.* 2006;5(3):144–148.

31. Li WW, et al. The role of therapeutic angiogenesis in tissue repair and regeneration. *Adv Skin Wound Care.* 2005;18(9):491–500; quiz 501–502.

32. Velazquez OC. Angiogenesis and vasculogenesis: inducing the growth of new blood vessels and wound healing by stimulation of bone marrow-derived progenitor cell mobilization and homing. *J Vasc Surg.* 2007;45(suppl A):A39–A47.

33. Waltenberger J. VEGF resistance as a molecular basis to explain the angiogenesis paradox in diabetes mellitus. *Biochem Soc Trans.* 2009;37(pt 6):1167–1170.

34. Stary HC. Evolution and progression of atherosclerotic lesions in coronary arteries of children and young adults. *Arteriosclerosis.* 1989;9 (1 suppl):I19–I32.

35. Stary HC, et al. A definition of initial, fatty streak, and intermediate lesions of atherosclerosis. A report from the Committee on

36. Li H, et al. An atherogenic diet rapidly induces VCAM-1, a cytokine-regulatable mononuclear leukocyte adhesion molecule, in rabbit aortic endothelium. *Arterioscler Thromb.* 1993;13(2):197–204.

37. Quinn MT, et al. Oxidatively modified low density lipoproteins: a potential role in recruitment and retention of monocyte/macrophages during atherogenesis. *Proc Natl Acad Sci U S A.* 1987;84(9):2995–2998.

38. Saikku P, et al. Serological evidence of an association of a novel Chlamydia, TWAR, with chronic coronary heart disease and acute myocardial infarction. *Lancet.* 1988;2(8618):983–986.

39. Lu X, Kakkar V. The role of heat shock protein (HSP) in atherosclerosis: Pathophysiology and clinical opportunities. *Curr Med Chem.* 2010;17(10):957–973.

40. Shaw A, Xu Q. Biomechanical stress-induced signaling in smooth muscle cells: an update. *Curr Vasc Pharmacol.* 2003;1(1):41–58.

41. Mayr M, et al. Biomechanical stress-induced apoptosis in vein grafts involves p38 mitogen-activated protein kinases. *FASEB J.* 2000;14(2):261–270.

42. Davies PF. Endothelial mechanisms of flow-mediated atheroprotection and susceptibility. *Circ Res.* 2007;101(1):10–12.

43. Iabichella ML, Melillo E, Mosti G. A review of microvascular measurements in wound healing. *Int J Low Extrem Wounds.* 2006;5(3):181–199.

44. Nioka S, et al. A novel method to measure regional muscle blood flow continuously using NIRS kinetics information. *Dyn Med.* 2006;5:5.

45. Schrey AR, et al. Functional evaluation of microvascular free flaps with positron emission tomography. *J Plast Reconstr Aesthet Surg.* 2006;59(2):158–165.

46. Terashi H, et al. Dynamic skin perfusion pressure: a new measure of assessment for wound healing capacity and alternative angiosome in critical limb ischemia. *Plast Reconstr Surg.* 2010;126(4):215e–218e.

47. Trubel W, et al. Experimental comparison of four methods of end-to-side anastomosis with expanded polytetrafluoroethylene. *Br J Surg.* 2004;91(2):159–167.

48. Ubbink DT, et al. Prediction of imminent amputation in patients with non-reconstructible leg ischemia by means of microcirculatory investigations. *J Vasc Surg.* 1999;30(1):114–121.

49. Ennis WJ, Lee C, Meneses P. A biochemical approach to wound healing through the use of modalities. *Clin Dermatol.* 2007;25(1):63–72.

50. Ennis WJ. Microcirculation: the push-pull theory. In: Meneses P, ed. *Diabetic Limb Salvage Conference.* Washington, DC: Georgetown University; 2007.

51. Hightower CM, Intaglietta M. The use of diagnostic frequency continuous ultrasound to improve microcirculatory function after ischemia-reperfusion injury. *Microcirculation.* 2007;14(6):571–582.

52. Ennis WJ, et al. Evaluation of clinical effectiveness of MIST ultrasound therapy for the healing of chronic wounds. *Adv Skin Wound Care.* 2006;19(8):437–446.

53. Coulling S. Fundamentals of pain management in wound care. *Br J Nurs.* 2007;16(11):S4–S6, S8, S10 passim.

54. Arrick DM, Mayhan WG. Acute infusion of nicotine impairs nNOS-dependent reactivity of cerebral arterioles via an increase in oxidative stress. *J Appl Physiol.* 2007;103(6):2062–2067.

55. Pullar CE, et al. Beta-adrenergic receptor agonists delay while antagonists accelerate epithelial wound healing: evidence of an endogenous adrenergic network within the corneal epithelium. *J Cell Physiol.* 2007;211(1):261–272.

56. Ubbink DT, et al. Effect of beta-blockers on peripheral skin microcirculation in hypertension and peripheral vascular disease. *J Vasc Surg.* 2003;38(3):535–540.

57. Wollina U, Abdel-Naser MB, Mani R. A review of the microcirculation in skin in patients with chronic venous insufficiency: the problem and the evidence available for therapeutic options. *Int J Low Extrem Wounds.* 2006;5(3):169–180.

Vascular Lesions of the Council on Arteriosclerosis, American Heart Association. *Circulation.* 1994;89(5):2462–2478.

58. Schmidt K, et al. Bacterial population of chronic crural ulcers: is there a difference between the diabetic, the venous, and the arterial ulcer? *Vasa*. 2000;29(1):62–70.

59. Pedrini L, Magnoni F. Spinal cord stimulation for lower limb ischemic pain treatment. *Interact Cardiovasc Thorac Surg*. 2007;6(4):495–500.

60. Fife CE, et al. The predictive value of transcutaneous oxygen tension measurement in diabetic lower extremity ulcers treated with hyperbaric oxygen therapy: a retrospective analysis of 1,144 patients. *Wound Repair Regen*. 2002;10(4):198–207.

61. Kavros SJ, et al. Improving limb salvage in critical ischemia with intermittent pneumatic compression: a controlled study with 18-month follow-up. *J Vasc Surg*. 2008;47(3):543–549.

62. Delis KT, Knaggs AL. Duration and amplitude decay of acute arterial leg inflow enhancement with intermittent pneumatic leg compression: an insight into the implicated physiologic mechanisms. *J Vasc Surg*. 2005;42(4):717–725.

63. Delis KT. The case for intermittent pneumatic compression of the lower extremity as a novel treatment in arterial claudication. *Perspect Vasc Surg Endovasc Ther*. 2005;17(1):29–42.

64. Nelzen O, Bergqvist D, Lindhagen A. Venous and non-venous leg ulcers: clinical history and appearance in a population study. *Br J Surg*. 1994;81(2):182–187.

65. Weingarten MS. State-of-the-art treatment of chronic venous disease. *Clin Infect Dis*. 2001;32(6):949–954.

66. Bradbury AW. Epidemiology and aetiology of C4–6 disease. *Phlebology*. 2010;25(Suppl 1): 2–8.

67. Bickers DR, et al. The burden of skin diseases: 2004 a joint project of the American Academy of Dermatology Association and the Society for Investigative Dermatology. *J Am Acad Dermatol*. 2006;55(3):490–500.

68. Olin JW, et al. Medical costs of treating venous stasis ulcers: evidence from a retrospective cohort study. *Vasc Med*. 1999;4(1):1–7.

69. van Gent WB, et al. Conservative versus surgical treatment of venous leg ulcers: a prospective, randomized, multicenter trial. *J Vasc Surg*. 2006;44(3):563–571.

70. Cavezzi A, et al. Duplex ultrasound investigation of the veins in chronic venous disease of the lower limbs—UIP consensus document. Part II. Anatomy. *Eur J Vasc Endovasc Surg*. 2006;31(3):288–299.

71. Delis KT, Knaggs AL, Khodabakhsh P. Prevalence, anatomic patterns, valvular competence, and clinical significance of the Giacomini vein. *J Vasc Surg*. 2004;40(6):1174–1183.

72. Ziad EA, et al. May-Thurner syndrome: an uncommon cause for deep vein thrombosis. *Harefuah*. 2009;148(12):818–819, 855.

73. Moudgill N, et al. May-Thurner syndrome: case report and review of the literature involving modern endovascular therapy. *Vascular*. 2009;17(6):330–335.

74. Raju S, Darcey R, Neglen P. Unexpected major role for venous stenting in deep reflux disease. *J Vasc Surg*. 2010;51(2):401–408; discussion 408.

75. Meissner MH, et al. The hemodynamics and diagnosis of venous disease. *J Vasc Surg*. 2007;46(suppl S):4S–24S.

76. Christopoulos DG, et al. Air-plethysmography and the effect of elastic compression on venous hemodynamics of the leg. *J Vasc Surg*. 1987;5(1):148–159.

77. Nicolaides AN, et al. The relation of venous ulceration with ambulatory venous pressure measurements. *J Vasc Surg*. 1993;17(2):414–419.

78. Beebe HG, et al. Classification and grading of chronic venous disease in the lower limbs. A consensus statement. *Eur J Vasc Endovasc Surg*. 1996;12(4):487–491; discussion 491–492.

79. Beebe HG, et al. Classification and grading of chronic venous disease in the lower limbs. A consensus statement. *Int Angiol*. 1995;14(2):197–201.

80. Beebe HG, et al. Classification and grading of chronic venous disease in the lower limbs–a consensus statement. *Organized by Straub Foundation with the cooperation of the American Venous Forum at the 6th Annual Meeting*, February 22–25, 1994, Maui, Hawaii. *Vasa*. 1995;24(4):313–318.

81. Eklof B, et al. Revision of the CEAP classification for chronic venous disorders: consensus statement. *J Vasc Surg*. 2004;40(6):1248–1252.

82. Vesic S, et al. Acute lipodermatosclerosis: an open clinical trial of stanozolol in patients unable to sustain compression therapy. *Dermatol Online J*. 2008;14(2):1.

83. Greenberg AS, et al. Acute lipodermatosclerosis is associated with venous insufficiency. *J Am Acad Dermatol*. 1996;35(4):566–568.

84. Kim D, Kang WH. Role of dermal melanocytes in cutaneous pigmentation of stasis dermatitis: a histopathological study of 20 cases. *J Korean Med Sci*. 2002;17(5):648–654.

85. Bradbury A, Ruckley CV. Clinical presentation and assessment of patients with venous disease. In: Gloviczki P, ed. *Handbook of Venous Disorders*. London, UK: Edward Arnold; 2009:331–341.

86. Miller N, et al. A prospective study comparing duplex scan and venography for diagnosis of lower-extremity deep vein thrombosis. *Cardiovasc Surg*. 1996;4(4):505–508.

87. Hirai M, Yoshinaga M, Nakayama R. Assessment of venous insufficiency using photoplethysmography: a comparison to strain gauge plethysmography. *Angiology*. 1985;36(11):795–801.

88. Perhoniemi V, et al. Strain gauge plethysmography in the assessment of venous reflux after subfascial closure of perforating veins: a prospective study of twenty patients. *J Vasc Surg*. 1990;12(1):34–37.

89. Ting AC, et al. Air plethysmography in chronic venous insufficiency: clinical diagnosis and quantitative assessment. *Angiology*. 1999;50(10):831–836.

90. Carpenter JP, et al. Magnetic resonance venography for the detection of deep venous thrombosis: comparison with contrast venography and duplex Doppler ultrasonography. *J Vasc Surg*. 1993;18(5):734–741.

91. Chung JW, et al. Acute iliofemoral deep vein thrombosis: evaluation of underlying anatomic abnormalities by spiral CT venography. *J Vasc Interv Radiol*. 2004;15(3):249–256.

92. Homans J. The etiology and treatment of varicose ulcer of the leg. *Surg Gynecol Obstet*. 1917;24:300–311.

93. Pratt G. Arterial varices, a syndrome. *Am J Surg*. 1949;77:456–460.

94. Burnand KG, et al. Pericapillary fibrin in the ulcer-bearing skin of the leg: the cause of lipodermatosclerosis and venous ulceration. *Br Med J (Clin Res Ed)*. 1982;285(6348):1071–1072.

95. Coleridge Smith PD, et al. Causes of venous ulceration: a new hypothesis. *Br Med J (Clin Res Ed)*. 1988;296(6638):1726–1727.

96. Pappas PJ, et al. Morphometric assessment of the dermal microcirculation in patients with chronic venous insufficiency. *J Vasc Surg*. 1997;26(5):784–795.

97. Pappas PJ, et al. Dermal tissue fibrosis in patients with chronic venous insufficiency is associated with increased transforming growth factor-beta1 gene expression and protein production. *J Vasc Surg*. 1999;30(6):1129–1145.

98. Stanley AC, et al. Reduced growth of dermal fibroblasts from chronic venous ulcers can be stimulated with growth factors. *J Vasc Surg*. 1997;26(6):994–999; discussion 999–1001.

99. Weckroth M, et al. Matrix metalloproteinases, gelatinase and collagenase, in chronic leg ulcers. *J Invest Dermatol*. 1996;106(5):1119–1124.

100. Junger M, et al. Microcirculatory dysfunction in chronic venous insufficiency (CVI). *Microcirculation*. 2000;7(6 pt 2):S3–S12.

101. Cesarone MR, et al. Faster healing of venous ulcers with crystacide: a clinical and microcirculatory 8-week registry study. *Panminerva Med*. 2010;52(2 suppl 1):11–14.

102. Belcaro G, et al. Improvement of microcirculation and healing of venous hypertension and ulcers with Crystacide: evaluation with a microcirculatory model, including free radicals, laser Doppler flux, and PO2/PCO2 measurements. *Angiology*. 2007;58(3):323–328.

103. Andriessen A, Polignano R, Abel M. Monitoring the microcirculation to evaluate dressing performance in patients with venous leg ulcers. *J Wound Care*. 2009;18(4):145–150.

104. O'Meara S, Cullum NA, Nelson EA. Compression for venous leg ulcers. *Cochrane Database Syst Rev.* 2009(1):CD000265.

105. Iglesias C, et al. VenUS I: a randomised controlled trial of two types of bandage for treating venous leg ulcers. *Health Technol Assess.* 2004;8(29):iii, 1–105.

106. Partsch H. Compression therapy. *Int Angiol.* 2010;29(5):391.

107. Jull A, et al. Pentoxifylline for treating venous leg ulcers. *Cochrane Database Syst Rev.* 2007(3): CD001733.

108. Gohel MS, Davies AH. Pharmacological agents in the treatment of venous disease: an update of the available evidence. *Curr Vasc Pharmacol.* 2009;7(3):303–308.

109. Wright DD. The ESCHAR trial: should it change practice? *Perspect Vasc Surg Endovasc Ther.* 2009;21(2):69–72.

110. Gohel MS, et al. Long term results of compression therapy alone versus compression plus surgery in chronic venous ulceration (ESCHAR): randomised controlled trial. *BMJ.* 2007;335(7610):83.

111. Gloviczki P. Commentary. Comparison of surgery and compression with compression alone in chronic venous ulceration (ESCHAR study): randomised controlled trial. *Perspect Vasc Surg Endovasc Ther.* 2005;17(3):275–276.

112. Gohel MS, et al. Randomized clinical trial of compression plus surgery versus compression alone in chronic venous ulceration (ESCHAR study)—haemodynamic and anatomical changes. *Br J Surg.* 2005;92(3):291–297.

113. Barwell JR, et al. Comparison of surgery and compression with compression alone in chronic venous ulceration (ESCHAR study): randomised controlled trial. *Lancet.* 2004;363(9424):1854–1859.

114. Field P, Van Boxel P. The role of the Linton flap procedure in the management of stasis dermatitis and ulceration in the lower limb. *Surgery.* 1971;70(6):920–926.

115. O'Donnell TF. The role of perforators in chronic venous insufficiency. *Phlebology.* 2010;25(1):3–10.

116. Nelson EA. Compression therapy, dressings and topical agents for venous ulcer healing. *Phlebology.* 2010;25(suppl 1):28–34.

117. Zaulyanov L, Kirsner RS. A review of a bi-layered living cell treatment (Apligraf) in the treatment of venous leg ulcers and diabetic foot ulcers. *Clin Interv Aging.* 2007;2(1):93–98.

118. Fivenson D, Scherschun L. Clinical and economic impact of Apligraf for the treatment of nonhealing venous leg ulcers. *Int J Dermatol.* 2003;42(12):960–965.

119. Jones JE, Nelson EA. Skin grafting for venous leg ulcers. *Cochrane Database Syst Rev.* 2007(2):CD001737.

CHAPTER 12

Management of the Neuropathic Foot

Nancy Elftman and Joan E. Conlan

CHAPTER OBJECTIVES

At the completion of this chapter, the reader will be able to:

1. Discuss the pathogenesis of the neuropathic foot.
2. Identify patients at risk for foot ulceration due to lack of protective sensation.
3. Conduct a focused systems review and examination to determine co-impairments that can affect wound healing.
4. Assess the patient's footwear, wound, sensation, temperature, and foot pressure distribution, and examine for Charcot joint and osteomyelitis.
5. Discuss management with orthotics, special shoes, and other adaptive devices.
6. Discuss surgical management of the neuropathic foot.
7. Provide care of the skin and nails of the neuropathic foot.

As you know, advancements in medication and technology now extend the lives of patients with previously fatal diseases: the prognosis has changed from fatality to chronic complications.[1] The chronic disease complication addressed in this chapter is the neuropathic foot, a common complication of **peripheral neuropathy**, degeneration involving peripheral nerves. The objective of management of the problem is to control its progression and reduce amputations.

The patient with peripheral neuropathy often has dysvascular components that must be addressed by a medical team, rather than one specialty (see Chapter 11). With the team approach, the limb can be evaluated, treated, and monitored through follow-up to provide continued ambulation for the patient.[2] The team goal is the prevention or delay of amputation and/or limb salvage of lower extremities. Although the individual training programs of the healthcare professionals on the team typically include normal foot anatomy and biomechanics, few describe the neuropathic foot and associated complications.[3] This chapter aims to provide this information, which is critical to effective team care.

In the formation of clinical teams, there has been a trend to include practitioners of several disciplines, including the wound care, advanced practice, or wound ostomy continence nurse (CWOCN) (ET); diabetologist/endocrinologist; vascular surgeon; physical therapist; orthotist/pedorthist; orthopaedic surgeon/podiatrist; and dermatologist. The disciplines playing the most important roles are nurse educators, who encourage high-risk patients to modify their behavior; orthotists, for recommendation of suitable footwear, stockings, and orthotic devices (shoe inserts, pads, etc.); and primary-care providers, to remove calluses, treat minor trauma, and provide healthcare. Physical therapists will play a role in all of these aspects of care. Referrals should be available to vascular surgeons and other specialists when specified by a physician.[4]

PATHOGENESIS AND TYPICAL PROGRESSION

The neuropathic process is poorly understood, and there are many theories regarding its etiology. For example, many believe that all peripheral neuropathy is caused by hyperglycemia—high levels of glucose in the blood—and advocate tight blood glucose regulation.[5] But as we will see, hyperglycemia is not the only etiology. When attempting to understand the pathogenesis of peripheral neuropathy, you are likely to encounter the following obstacles:

- Lack of a clear definition of diabetic neuropathy (discussed shortly)
- Separation of diabetes from other potential etiologies of neuropathy
- Absence of single, repeatable tests of neuropathy that are not dependent on either expensive technology or subjective clinical judgment
- Varied manifestations of neuropathy: distal symmetric, mononeuropathies, autonomic neuropathies

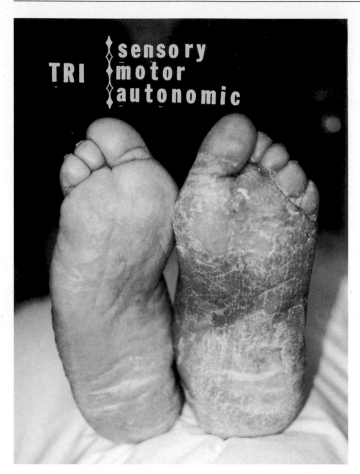

FIGURE 12.1 Feet of a patient with sensory, motor, and autonomic neuropathies. Manifestations of motor neuropathy (deformity, clawed toes, toe amputation, foot imbalance needing immediate intervention) and autonomic neuropathy (dry, cracked skin) are evident. Note the difference in trophic changes between the feet. (Reprinted with permission from N. Elftman, Clinical management of the neuropathic limb. *J Prosthet Orthot.* 1991;4(1):1–12. Copyright © American Academy of Orthotists and Prosthetists.)

Peripheral neuropathy can involve sensory, motor, and autonomic nerves. The neuropathic foot is typically affected by all three; that is, it is a *poly neuropathy*. The three types often occur simultaneously (Fig. 12.1):

- Sensory neuropathy—loss of sensation, leaving the patient incapable of sensing pain and pressure. The patient has no sense of identity with the feet.
- Motor neuropathy—loss of intrinsic muscles, resulting in clawed toes (Fig. 12.2) and eventual foot drop. The ankle jerk reflex is absent.[6]
- Autonomic neuropathy—loss of autonomic system function, resulting in the absence of sweat and oil production, leaving skin dry and nonelastic.

Onset and Typical Progression

Peripheral neuropathy can develop gradually or suddenly:

- Gradual onset. Neuropathies that develop gradually are usually painless. The exact cause is unknown but may be related to duration of diabetes and level of blood sugar control. Symptoms may include numbness, tingling, burning, and a pins-and-needles sensation.

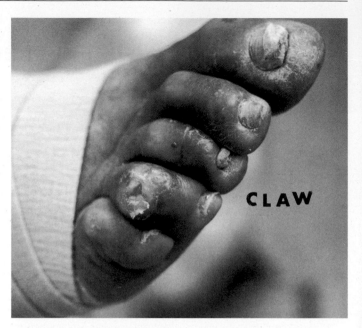

FIGURE 12.2 Clawed toes. Note the corn on the fourth toe, caused by rubbing from the top of the shoe.

- Sudden onset. Those that develop suddenly (or acutely) are almost always painful. Then, just as suddenly, the pain disappears, leaving sensory loss.

In the clinical setting, no initial problem is too small to address. The clinical team must treat minor trauma immediately to prevent deterioration of the condition. There is a destructive chain of trauma surrounding the typical progression of the neuropathic foot, as follows:

1. Trauma
2. Inflammation
3. Ulceration
4. Infection
5. Absorption
6. Deformity
7. Disability

This chain can be broken with effective care, including a thorough examination and objective measurement, immediate and focused treatment, and patient education.[2]

Conditions Associated with Peripheral Neuropathy

The medical history is a useful way to identify neuropathy that may accompany many chronic disease processes. The most common disease processes resulting in peripheral neuropathy are the following:

- Diabetes
- Spina bifida
- Hansen disease
- Systemic erythematosus lupus
- Acquired immunodeficiency syndrome (AIDS), human immunodeficiency virus (HIV) infection, AIDS-related complex
- Chemotheraphy
- Vitamin B deficiency
- Multiple sclerosis

- Uremia
- Vascular disease
- Charcot-Marie-Tooth muscle disease

Congenital sensory loss, as in spina bifida, is especially important to identify because the patient will never have experienced normal sensation and will be unable to evaluate his or her own sensory status.[7–9]

Toxins and toxic syndromes can also cause insensitivity in the limbs. These include abuse of or exposure to alcohol, arsenic, lead, steroids, the antituberculosis medication isoniazid, and pharmaceuticals containing gold.

Many other factors may also promote neuropathy; thus, all patients must be evaluated, regardless of reported history.

Diabetic Neuropathy

The most common disease process seen in peripheral neuropathy is diabetes. Statistics on diabetes are growing. It affects 194 million people worldwide. During their lifetimes, 15% to 25% of type 1 and type 2 diabetic patients face the risk of foot ulceration, a major complication. Within this population, some patients have recurrent ulceration. For 2% to 6% of patients with diabetes, these ulcers occur anually.[10] The medical costs related to diabetes in the United States is currently $14 billion per year. About 25% of all hospital visits among patients with diabetes are due to infected and/or ischemic diabetic foot ulcers.[10] Included in this cost are 88,000 lower extremity amputations per year, of which 50% to 70% could have been prevented by team management. It is estimated that 85% of the lower extremity amputations were preceded by a foot ulcer. Successful team management not only can reduce the cost of these ulcers but reduce the presence of comorbidities, thus improving the patient's quality of life.[10] More than 14 million Americans have diabetes (half are undiagnosed), with 700,000 cases diagnosed per year. In the general population, 1 in 20 has diabetes. Many diabetics are diagnosed when they present a nonhealing foot ulcer.[11–16] Of major concern is the mortality rate after amputation, which is 50% within 3 to 5 years. The rate of contralateral amputation is 50% within 4 years.[17] The World Health Organization has estimated that the number of diabetics will climb to 366 million by 2030.[18]

Although there are several different divisions of diabetes, the two main categories are insulin-dependent diabetes mellitus (IDDM), or type I, and non–insulin-dependent diabetes mellitus (NIDDM), or type II. In IDDM, the insulin deficiency is due to loss of pancreatic islet cells. Type 1 can develop at any age but often presents in childhood or adolescence. In type 2 diabetes, body cells develop resistance to the effects of insulin. Initially, the pancreatic islet cells produce more, but over time, insulin production fails and blood glucose levels rise dramatically. Type 2 used to be seen solely in adults but now occurs at any age. About 90% of patients with type 2 diabetes are overweight.[19]

Some dysvascular patients are also diabetic. These comorbidities significantly increase the risk of neuropathic foot, especially following infection. As discussed in Chapter 11, vascular disease impairs delivery of antibiotics to the infected limb, reducing the potential for healing. One limb may be severely insensitive while the other may be only mildly affected (see Fig. 12.1). Refer patients with loss of vascularity to a vascular surgeon for possible correction or improvement.

The Role of Pressure in Pathogenesis of the Neuropathic Foot

Pressure is a critical risk factor in development of most neuropathic foot ulcers. Of all amputations, 86% could have been prevented by patient education and appropriate footwear.[4] Various sources and levels of pressure produce characteristic types of stress that lead to ulceration and destruction of tissue in the neuropathic foot. These are as follows:

- Ischemic necrosis is usually seen on the lateral side of the fifth metatarsal head and is due to wearing a shoe that is too narrow. The ischemia is caused by a very low level of pressure (2–3 psi) over a long period of time, causing death of the tissue. As the progression of breakdown continues at the metatarsal heads, due to migration of fat pads, bone and skin are left to absorb shock.
- Mechanical disruption occurs when a direct injury caused by high pressure (600+ psi) inflicts immediate damage to tissue.
- Inflammatory destruction occurs with repetitive moderate pressures (40–60 psi). Inflammation develops and weakens the tissue, leading to callus formation and ulceration from thousands of repetitions per day.
- Osteomyelitis (and other sepsis) destruction is the result of a moderate force in the presence of infection. Infection is spread as forces are applied by intermittent pressure.[20]

Other pathways to ulceration include Exposure to heat or chemicals or stepping on a foreign object are common traumas that damage the skin, which occurs due to the loss of sensation, absence of the withdrawal reflex response, and loss of cortical signaling regarding danger and seeking help.

The incidence of ulceration is 71% on the forefoot, with the third metatarsal head most commonly affected, followed by the great toe and first and fifth metatarsal heads. Once breakdown has begun on the foot, 53% of the contralateral limbs follow the progression of breakdown within 4 years.[21] The highest incidence of ulceration occurs at sites of previous ulceration. Thus, you should review the patient's history carefully for previous ulcers.[22] Observation is also helpful in detecting breakdown of recently healed ulcers: a newly healed ulcer is covered by thin, fragile skin that requires time to mature and become strong. However, the potential for breakdown in this area always remains high. In completely healed ulcer areas, scar tissue may adhere to underlying structures. The healed areas are composed of tissues of different density and, therefore, compress uniquely, causing shear between opposing tissue durometers.[21,23]

SYSTEMS REVIEW AND EXAMINATION

A focused systems review and examination for the patient with neuropathy is required to determine the co-impairments that will affect wound healing and require management. Four systems to review for this patient population are the neuromuscular system, the vascular system, the musculoskeletal system, and the integumentary system.

Neuromuscular System

A foot with neuropathy has toes that are clawed (see Fig. 12.2). It is incapable of sensing trauma. The rigid anesthetic foot is more likely to break down than is a flexible anesthetic foot.[24] Evaluate the anesthetic foot carefully and bilaterally.

RESEARCH WISDOM

Interventions for Paresthesia

Paresthesia may be helped by use of a transcutaneous electronic nerve stimulator (TENS) unit, which generates small pulses of electricity similar to an electric massage. Another method of controlling the discomfort is with topical creams.[27,28] See Chapter 14 for more information.

Any form of peripheral neuropathy can produce the discomfort of paresthesia: prickling, burning, and jabbing sensations.[25,26] The length of this period of discomfort varies among patients. Neuromuscular system examinations to assess for neurologic changes are the focus of the foot screening process and are described in detail later.

Vascular System

Peripheral vascular disease (PVD) is a serious complication affecting millions of Americans. Of the 500,000 vascular-related ulcerations, 10% are arterial and 70% are venous ulcerations; some individuals have both venous and arterial diseases.[16] Many patients with neuropathy also have PVD. Therefore, it is critical to review the vascular history (to identify strategies that are being used to manage vascular problems) before planning any intervention. Some of the related circulatory system diseases that usually accompany neuropathy and management recommendations are described here. Chapter 11 describes the pathogenesis and management of vascular problems in more detail. Chapter 6 discusses noninvasive vascular testing for patients with diabetes.

Atherosclerosis is also known as hardening of the arteries. The interior wall of arteries is usually smooth but with atherosclerosis platelets, calcium, and connective tissue deposit on the walls. In early stages, the patient may experience intermittent claudication or cramping in the lower limb, which goes away with rest. As the disease progresses, symptoms appear when the patient is not walking (rest pain).[16] Arterial compromise can be noted by the loss of hair growth, shiny skin, atrophy, and cool skin over the toes.[29]

Atherosclerosis leads to impaired circulation in the legs and is one of the most important causes of gangrene, leading to amputation.[30] Arterial ischemic ulcers are located on tips of (or between) toes, on heels, on metatarsal heads, on sides or soles of the foot, and above the lateral malleoli. The ulcer will look punched out, with well-demarcated edges, and be nonbleeding (Fig. 12.3). The ulcer base may be deep and pale or black and necrotic. Treatment involves vascular reconstruction, bed rest, and immobilization. Arterial ulcers have a poor prognosis. Misdiagnosis of an arterial ulcer as a venous ulcer can lead to serious complications.

The venous stasis ulcer has a better prognosis for healing than does the arterial ischemic ulcer. Veins are less elastic than arteries. The valves within veins no longer function to return blood to the heart against gravity, leaving blood to pool in the lower limb. The pooling does not allow new oxygenated blood into the area, and the cell walls of the veins begin to break down. The waste blood products begin to weep through the lower limb. Venous stasis ulcerations are commonly located in the anteromedial malleolus and pretibial areas. The ulcerations are irregular in shape, surrounded by bluish brown skin. These ulcers are exudative and show evidence of bleeding.

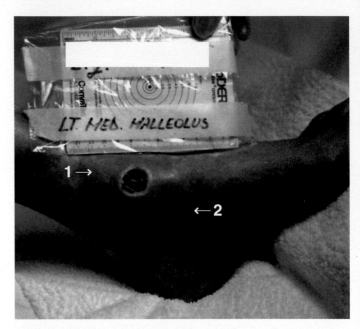

FIGURE 12.3 Ischemic ulcer in chronic proliferative phase and absence of epithelialization phase. Note: (1) punched-out ulcer appearance with rolled wound edges and (2) dependent rubor. (Copyright © C. Sussman.)

Treatment of venous stasis ulcerations begins with leg elevation.[31] The limb must be treated with compression bandages or an Unna boot. The Unna boot is a semirigid dressing of gelatin and zinc oxide (Fig. 12.4). Its application protects vulnerable

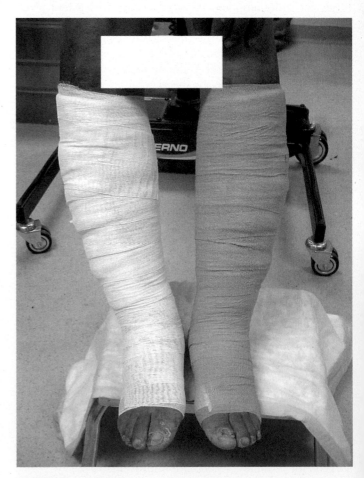

FIGURE 12.4 Unna boot.

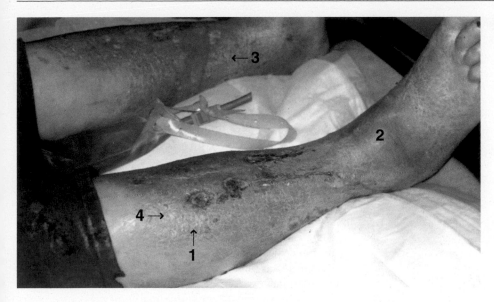

FIGURE 12.5 Stasis dermatitis. There is an absence of the epithelialization phase. Note evidence of (1) Brawny edema, (2) trophic skin changes, (3) hemosiderin staining (hyperpigmentation), and (4) multiple shallow ulcers. Precursors to venous ulceration (Copyright © B.M. Bates-Jensen.)

skin from the weeping exudate, especially below the ulcer site. The Unna boot is applied wet. When it dries, it forms a nonelastic, nonexpandable, nonshrinkable, porous mold that sticks to the skin. This treatment has been used on venous ulcers for 100 years. When applied across a joint, it is a means of controlling edema. The motion of the joint generates a pumping action.[1]

Chronic venous stasis of the lower limb without an open ulceration will typically show signs of edema. It may also have small water blisters or weeping. All these signs indicate that compression should begin (Figs. 12.5 and 12.6). In addition, when venous stasis ulceration occurs on one limb, you should begin compression therapy on the contralateral side. Treat the limb with pressure-gradiated stockings daily. Pressure-gradiated stockings exert a higher compression at the metatarsal heads and decreased pressure above the ankle to facilitate pumping action and assist the venous system in removing fluids from the lower limb (Fig. 12.7). Most patients do well with compression

in the range of 30 to 40 mm Hg at the foot and ankle. When applying these stockings, remember to avoid seams around bony prominences, and never place a zipper over the malleoli.

Antiembolism stockings are not designed for the ambulatory patient and do not supply the pumping action required. Antiembolism compression is for the recumbent hospitalized patient.

The prosthetic shrinker sock (Fig. 12.8A–C) should be used following a major limb amputation to reduce edema and shape the residual limb. The prosthetic shrinker applies both circumferential and vertical (distal to proximal) compression.[32] Chapter 18 describes procedures for management of edema.

Musculoskeletal System Examination

The musculoskeletal system examination includes examination of joint integrity, range of motion, skeletal deformity, and muscle strength. Motor neuropathy will distort skeletal

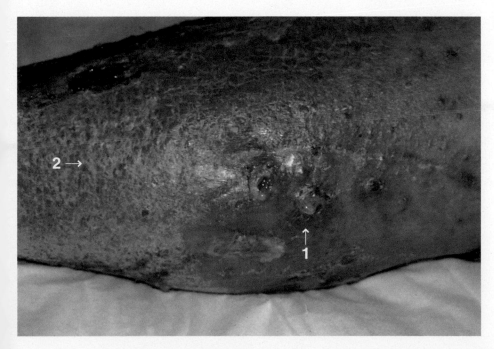

FIGURE 12.6 Close-up view of same leg as in Figure 12.5. Note evidence of (1) edema leakage through wounds, (2) scaling and crusting (trophic changes) due to lipodermatosclerosis. (Copyright © B.M. Bates-Jensen.)

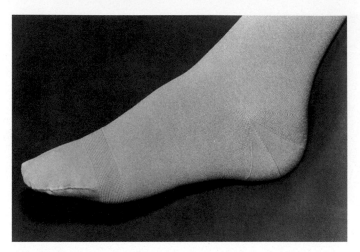

FIGURE 12.7 The full foot compression stocking begins compression at the metatarsal heads and decreases compression above the ankle to assist in the venous pumping mechanics. (Courtesy of Juzo-Julius Zorn, Inc., Cuyahoga Falls, Ohio.)

alignment, and Charcot joint will leave a foot deformed, as will be discussed later in this chapter. An analysis of abnormal gait should also be included. Beginning with the joint range of motion review, it is important that the foot has a dorsiflexion

range of at least 10 degrees to allow ambulation without harm to the great toe.[33] The forces on the plantar surface can peak to 275% of body weight when running and 80% when walking.[34] There is an absence of the ankle jerk reflex when neuropathy is advanced to glove-and-stocking distribution.[35]

Leg length discrepancy affects 70% to 80% of the population and often does not cause pain or deformity. A discrepancy can relate to chronic complications, such as hammertoes, hallux valgus, and referred joint disruption of the ankle, knee, hip, and lower back. A 2-cm discrepancy is sufficient to cause symptoms and requires shoe lifts with physical therapy. Any lift over 1/4 in. should be placed on the sole of the shoe. The full discrepancy should be reduced only gradually to allow the body to respond to changes as the pelvis levels.[36]

There is a constant concern with toe deformities that may result in ulceration. In the case of claw toe deformity, the toes are dorsiflexed at the metatarsal-phalangeal joints, with flexion at the interphalangeal joints.[37] The great toe should be examined for deformity. A fibrous proximal joint can cause ulceration that is especially difficult to relieve. Great toe extension can be seen when weight bearing, because the patient will thrust the toe into extension when ambulating, causing calluses and discoloration on the distal tip near the nail from contacting the shoe. Great toe pronation is seen on the medial/plantar surface of the great toe. Hallux rigidus refers to limited range of

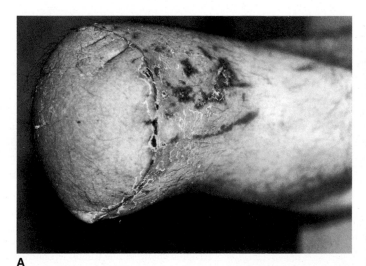

A

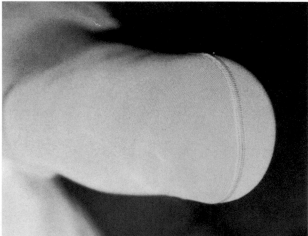

B

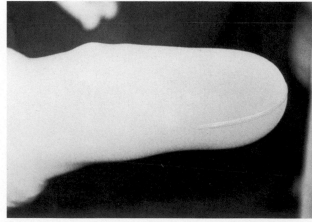

C

FIGURE 12.8 A: The prosthetic shrinker assists in shaping the limb following major amputation surgery. Postop bulbous residual limb of below knee (transtibial) amputee. **B:** The prosthetic shrinker assists in shaping the limb following major amputation surgery. Application of prosthetic shrinker. (Courtesy of Juzo-Julius Zorn, Inc., Cuyahoga Falls, Ohio.) **C:** The prosthetic shrinker assists in shaping the limb following major amputation surgery. Final residual limb shape for prosthetic application. (Courtesy of Juzo-Julius Zorn, Inc., Cuyahoga Falls, Ohio.)

motion in the proximal great toe metatarsal-phalangeal joint and requires a rigid rocker-bottom shoe to allow ambulation without excessive pressure on the great toe. Hallux valgus (bunion) is the increased valgus angle of the great toe in relation to the metatarsal, requiring a shoe that can be modified and molded to conform to the medial bunion formation.

Toe amputations may be required for single or multiple toes (see Fig. 12.1). The amputation may be a disarticulation or a resection (metatarsal shaft is removed). The distal end of the amputation site must be followed carefully and protected from trauma. Common complications must be addressed with the neuropathic limb. Bursa formation over the navicular prominence is due to the constant high forces and must be provided with an area of pressure relief before ulceration occurs. A sinus tract formation will result when previous areas of ulceration heal over a pocket of bacteria instead of healing from internal to external tissues. The small pocket of bacteria will be moved anteriorly through the tissues, causing infection to spread.

Motor neuropathy produces common abnormal gait characteristics in the neuropathic population. The shoes are worn on the lateral side of the sole because of a varus deformity (Fig. 12.9). This weakness often causes ankle injuries. After further deterioration, foot drop can occur. The stiffness in the complex joint structures leads to abnormal motion in the foot's function. Muscle atrophy, imbalances, and deformity lead to abnormal concentration of forces and shear forces that are precursors to wound formation.[38]

CLINICAL WISDOM

Modification of a Standard-Depth Shoe

To compensate for varus gait abnormalities, shoes need to be modified. The modifications required are (1) a full, lateral-flare sole, as shown in Figure 12.9, (2) a strong counter to support the heel, and (3) a high top to support the ankle. A standard-depth shoe can be modified by an orthotist, or a shoe repairperson may be able to do the job, if guided. Although not all orthotists will agree to modify an existing shoe, others will. This will save the patient money.

Integumentary System Examination

Toenail deformities are commonly seen in the neuropathic foot. Hypertrophic nails are caused by onychomycosis (nail fungus) infection (Fig. 12.10) and are common in the diabetic population. The nails tear the lining of the shoe, creating rough areas that abrade the toes. Nail care for fungus, ingrown toenails, and trimming must be performed by trained medical personnel to ensure that injury is not inflicted.

Soft corns are hyperkeratotic lesions between toes (usually between the fourth and fifth toes). They result from pressure of an opposing toe in a region that is moist.[39] Injury and maceration of the toes is commonly controlled by the use of lamb's wool between the toes or tube foam to space toes and prevent friction (Fig. 12.11A–C, Exhibit 12.1).

Dryness of the skin with small skin fissures is the result of autonomic neuropathy in which the sweat and oil production is decreased and moisture must be replaced. Loss of hair growth may be indicative of vascular impairment.

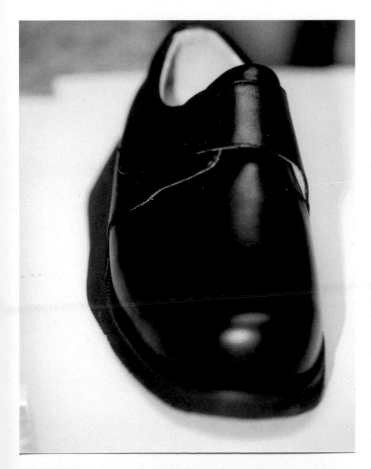

FIGURE 12.9 Lateral shoe flare to reduce varus deformity progression due to motor neuropathy. (Courtesy of Nancy Elftman.)

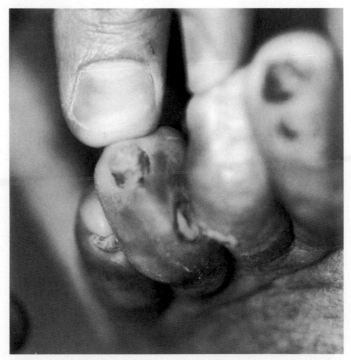

FIGURE 12.10 This foot has soft corns between toes, thickened toenails, and onychomycosis (fungal) infection.

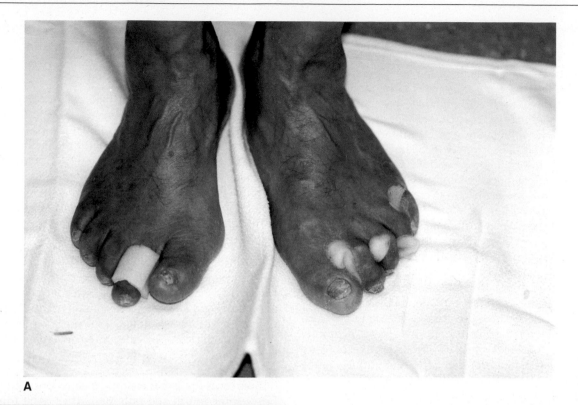

A

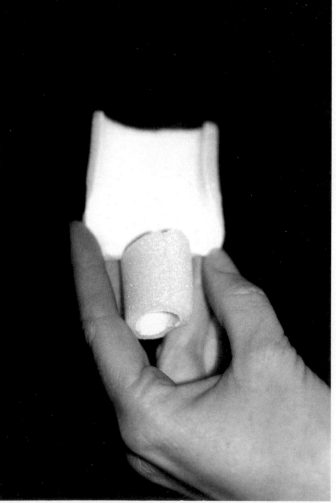

B

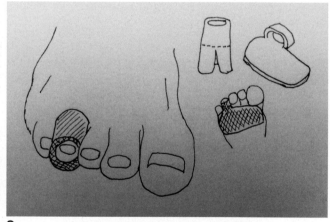

C

FIGURE 12.11 A: To keep the web space open and dry, use tube foam or lamb's wool. (Courtesy of Nancy Elftman.) **B:** The tube foam should be cut to allow a "tail" under the foot. This extension will deter migration of the pad. (Courtesy of Nancy Elftman.) **C:** Diagram of construction of a tube foam separator.

CLINICAL WISDOM

Tube Foam and Lamb's Wool for Quick Relief of Pressure on Toes

Claw toes, hammer toes, calluses, corns, and small ulcerations can be relieved of pressure by inserts and shoe modifications and spaced with tube foam or lamb's wool separators to allow air flow. Separators prevent maceration and skin breakdown; they should be removed before and replaced after bathing. In addition, the custom tube foam separator serves as a toe separator, reduces shear from the shoe, cushions metatarsal heads, and can be used as a positioner for overlapping toes. Figure 12.11A shows lamb's wool pieces placed between toes. Figure 12.11B shows a tube foam toe separator in place. Figure 12.11C and Exhibit 12.1 illustrate and describe the steps to create a tube foam separator. The tube foam is available from podiatric supply companies.

Another common occurrence is burns, which may be due to either heat or chemicals, such as over-the-counter foot remedies. Soaking the foot in hot water is a specific cause of burns. A common wisdom is that neuropathic patients should *never* soak their feet. The insensitive foot cannot produce the warning signals necessary to prevent severe burns.

Necrobiosis lipoidica diabeticorum is a dermatologic condition that may be seen on the shin (along the tibia) in diabetic patients (Fig. 12.12). The condition manifests as irregular patches of degenerated collagen with reduced numbers of fibrocytes. The dry, scaly areas have been infiltrated with chronic inflammatory cells.[40] The round, firm plaques of reddish brown to yellow are seen three times more often in women than in men.[41,42] Necrobiosis can be confused with venous stasis disease but does not require or respond to extensive treatment. Indeed, these ulcerations require only protective dressings.

A callus (or *tyloma*) is a yellowish gray lesion that may be flat or raised and spread over a large area (see Chapter 3). Calluses typically are caused by friction (shear), irritation, and/or pressure. There is hyperemia and thickening of the skin. The skin is compressed, and superficial layers of callus are laid down. Treatment requires that the friction, irritation, or pressure to the area be relieved. The callus may be reduced mechanically with sanding tools and callus reducers. The pumice stone is used as a wet tool on wet skin. The callus reducer debrides dry callus with a dry tool (Fig. 12.13).[43]

Keratoderma plantaris is a condition characterized by keratin cracks and ulcerations. It develops when autonomic neuropathy reduces sweat and oil gland production, reducing the moisture and elasticity of the skin. As keratin builds up, it creates small fissures that allow bacteria to enter, and infection to begin. The entire sole around the margin of the heel may undergo diffuse thickening and develop fissures, which will be painful if the foot is sensate or will go undetected if insensate (see Fig. 12.14). Prevention includes reduction of keratin buildup and retention of skin moisture.[39]

Many forms of rashes and infections must be evaluated and treated in the neuropathic foot. These are usually discovered by inspection, rather than patient discomfort. Typical rashes in the diabetic population include shin spots and diabetic bullae.[43] Infections include *Pseudomonas* infection, which is bacterial growth that occurs within a moist environment. Because

EXHIBIT 12.1

Instructions for Making a Foam Toe Separator

Make a custom foam toe separator (Fig. 19-8B,C) by the following steps:

1. Select a size of tube foam with a diameter that will not constrict the toe.

2. Cut a 21/2–3-in. piece of the foam.

3. To make the toe cuff:

   a. Measure back 1/2 to 3/4 in. from one end of the tube foam and mark.

   b. Cut across the diameter of the tube three fourths of the way through.

   c. Slit up the tube to the marking on the side that is cut to the diameter cut (see diagram).

   d. The foam will flatten out (see diagram).

   e. The tube will slip over the toe and the flat section will be located on the plantar surface of the foot.

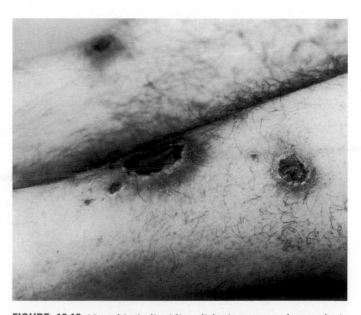

FIGURE 12.12 Necrobiosis lipoidica diabeticorum: a dermatologic condition often present in the diabetic, neuropathic limb.

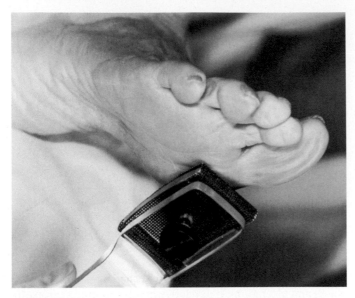

FIGURE 12.13 Callus reducer: a tool used dry on dry callus to remove buildup and reduce the superficial layers.

of the impaired circulation and immunosuppression seen in peripheral neuropathy, signs and symptoms of infection are usually absent in the neuropathic foot, even though the infection is present and virulent. See Chapter 17 for strategies to assess and treat infection.

Gangrene is another finding that may be discovered during the integumentary system review. There are two types of gangrene: wet and dry. Dry gangrene is due to loss of nourishment to a part, followed by mummification. The area is dry, black, and shriveled. When dry gangrene is present, there is a line of demarcation at which the body will autoamputate the affected

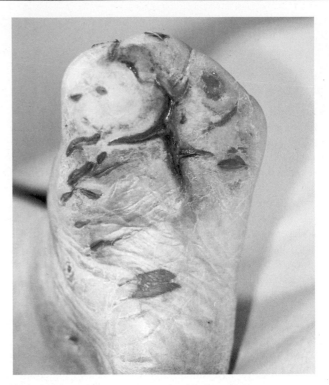

FIGURE 12.14 Typical neuropathic foot with keratoderma plantaris. Note the dry, cracked skin, dirt imbedded in the skin, open wounds, and the absence of dressing, due to lack of awareness of the condition.

area. This process of auto-amputation could take weeks to months.[37] It is nature's way of protecting the body from infection and should not be disturbed. Figure 12.15A shows a foot with dry gangrene.

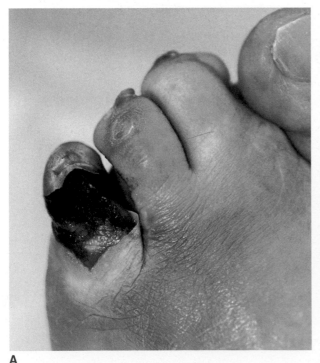

A

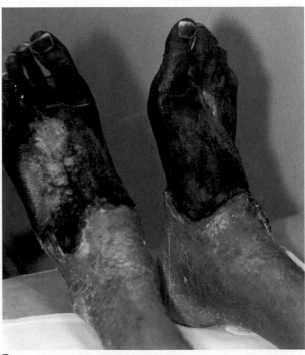

B

FIGURE 12.15 A: Wet gangrene and possible infection. **B:** Dry gangrene. In either condition urgent referral to a surgeon is indicated.

Wet gangrene is the necrosis of tissue, followed by destruction caused by excessive moisture. Bacterial gases accumulate in the tissue. The line of demarcation is ill defined, and the limb is painful, purple, and swollen. Wet gangrene is common when infection exists.[39,44] Figure 12.15B shows wet gangrene of the fifth toe. A patient with wet gangrene needs immediate referral to the surgeon.

FURTHER VISUAL AND PHYSICAL ASSESSMENTS

Examination of the neuropathic limb includes assessment of footwear, the wound itself, sensation, temperature, and pressure.

Footwear Assessment

Examine the patient's footwear for patterns of wear indicating excessive pressure. Shoes should show a normal wear pattern on the lateral heel of the sole, as contrasted with the pattern in Figure 12.9. Shoes should be resoled on a regular basis to keep sides from wearing down. Inserts are replaced as required when relief modifications are no longer sufficient and shock absorption is decreased.

Examine the ends of the patient's toes for injury caused by a short shoe. Notice in Figure 12.16 that the toe with a short-shoe injury extends to the end of the shoe insole. Alignment is required when fitting a shoe for proper weight distribution and length measurement. We discuss this later in the chapter. The interventions section of this chapter provides instructions in footwear management.

Wound Grading

The Wagner scale[45] for grading neuropathic ulcers and the stages are listed in a table just like Table 12.1. Ulcers with low grades are managed by conservative measures, whereas ulcers with higher grades are a direct threat to limb loss and require surgical

TABLE 12.1	Wagner Scale
Grade	**Description**
Grade 0	Skin intact (Fig. 12.13A)
Grade 1	Superficial ulcer (Fig. 12.13B)
Grade 2	Deeper ulcer to tendon or bone (Fig. 12.13C)
Grade 3	Ulcer has abscess or osteomyelitis (Fig. 12.13D)
Grade 4	Gangrene on forefoot (Fig. 12.13E)
Grade 5	Gangrene over major portion of foot

management. The neuropathic limb often suffers from dysvascularity as well; therefore, the system is often used for both populations. For continuity of documentation and communication, the team must understand the Wagner scale of ulcer grading and use it consistently. The preferred conservative method of treatment is also guided by the Wagner grade. Figure 12.17A–F

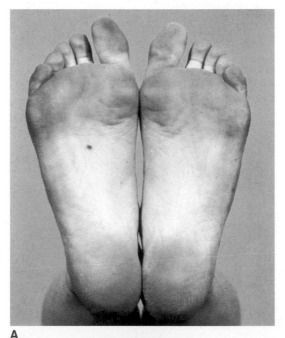

A

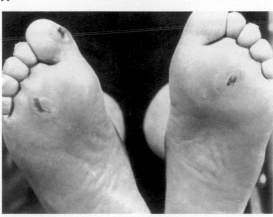

B

FIGURE 12.17 A: Skin intact, Wagner grade 0. **B:** Superficial ulcer, Wagner grade 1.

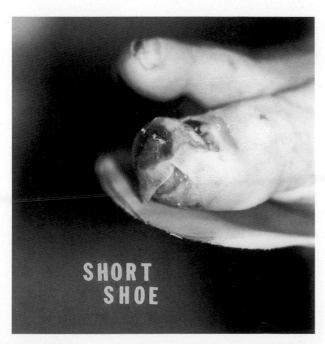

FIGURE 12.16 Short shoe. The toe extends to the end of the insole. (Reprinted with permission from N. Elftman, Clinical management of the neuropathic limb. *J Prosthet Orthot*. 1991;4(1):1–12. Copyright © American Academy of Orthotists and Prosthetists.)

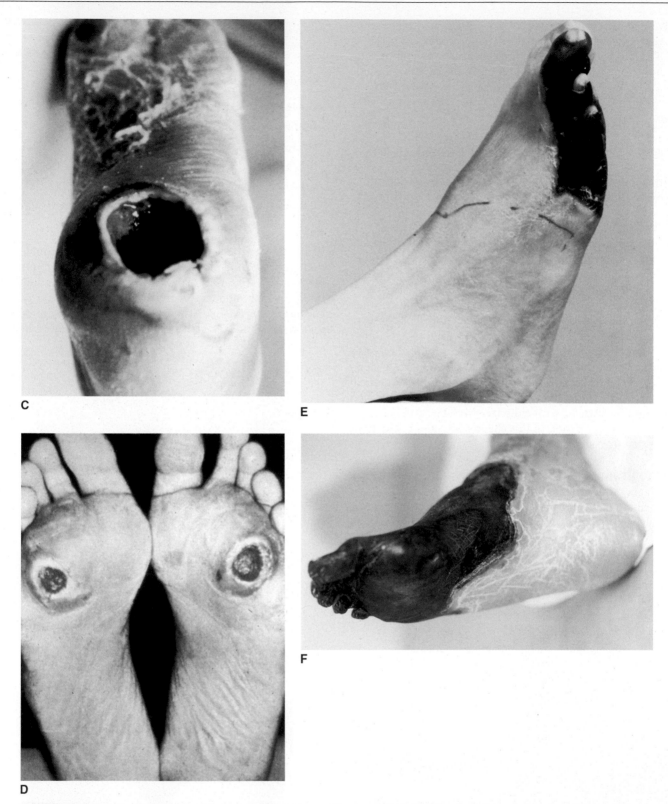

C

E

D

F

FIGURE 12.17 (*continued*) **C:** Deeper ulcer to tendon or bone, Wagner grade 2. **D:** Ulcer has abscess or osteomyelitis, Wagner grade 3. **E:** Gangrene on forefoot, Wagner grade 4. **F:** Gangrene over major portion of foot, Wagner grade 5.

EXHIBIT 12.2

Conservative Management by Wagner Ulcer Grade

Wagner Ulcer Grade and Treatment Protocol	
Grade 0	Depth shoes and shock-absorbing insert.
Grade 1	Cast, ODS splint, or wound care shoe to reduce weight at ulceration site; antibiotic intervention as required.
Grade 2	Debridement and cast, ODS splint or wound care shoe for weight distribution; antibiotics as required.
Grade 3	Remove infected tissue, cast and antibiotic intervention.

provides photos illustrating each of the six Wagner grades, from 0 to 5. Exhibit 12.2 shows how the different grades dictate different treatment strategies.[46]

Sensation Testing

Most clinicians evaluate sensation using reliability tested Semmes-Weinstein monofilaments, which can be obtained commercially in elaborate sets for precise measurement of protective sensation, but research has consolidated the testing to three sizes of monofilaments for grading the insensitive foot (Exhibit 12.3):[47]

- The 4.17 monofilament supplies 1 g of force. Patients who can feel this have normal sensation.
- The 5.07 monofilament supplies 10 g of force. If the patient cannot feel this, he or she does not have protective sensation and cannot sense trauma to the foot to cease weight bearing. Failure to sense the 10-g monofilament is used as the determining factor for use of protective footwear and accommodative orthotics.
- The 6.10 monofilament supplies 75 g of force. A large percentage of patients do not feel this largest monofilament. A loss of sensation at 75 g indicates an insensate foot that must be accommodated and followed closely.

The monofilament is a single-point perception test. The examiner places the monofilament on the skin, presses until the monofilament bends, and removes it from the skin surface. The patient is to respond when he or she feels the pressure sensation. To avoid errors in testing, the monofilament is never used in areas of scarring, calluses, or necrotic tissue. Figure 12.18 shows the proper method for the monofilament testing procedure. Note the bend of the monofilament. This must occur to measure correct pressure sensation. Monofilament testing is never used in areas of scarring, calluses, or necrotic tissue.

Notice that monofilament testing is not to be confused with the testing for sharp/dull sensation. The sharp/dull test stimulates multiple nerves, as opposed to a single-point perception test.

Bilateral monofilament testing is especially important for the unilateral and bilateral amputee to determine areas of insensitivity and progression of the neuropathy.

Loss of protective sensation, history of prior ulceration, and reduced circulatory perfusion are important factors in development of foot ulcers. A risk classification system based on these factors[48] is useful in identifying patients who would benefit from different levels of intervention. Risk is classified by four grades:

- 0, no loss of protective sensation
- 1, loss of protective sensation (no deformity or history of plantar ulceration)
- 2, loss of protective sensation and deformity or abnormal blood flow without history of plantar ulcer
- 3, history of plantar ulcer

Three interventions have proven effective in reducing risk of ulceration: protective footwear, patient education, and frequent clinic follow-up. For example, when a patient's ulcer is grade 0, preulceration, and the patient can sense the 10-g monofilament (has protective sensation), he or she will sense pain before damage occurs to the feet. Patients in this category usually do well with a standard shoe of correct sizing and a simple shock-absorbing pad.

In contrast, the patient without protective sensation will need very different interventions. These patients will not cease ambulating when damage begins to tissues. Patients with feet such as those in Figure 12.14 who walk into the clinic are insensate. They require extra-depth shoes with a total-contact accommodative insert to distribute pressure and reduce forces on areas of potential breakdown. Orthotics are discussed shortly.

Testing for vibratory sensation may be accomplished by using the bioesthesiometer. This instrument is essentially an electrical tuning fork that uses repetitive mechanical indentation of skin delivered at a prescribed frequency and amplitude.[49] The simple graduated tuning fork is a rapid means of sensory testing.[50,51] Bear in mind that the purpose of all sensory testing equipment is to identify those at risk.[52]

Upper and lower extremity peripheral neuropathy is present when sensation testing reveals that the level of sensation loss is symmetric and equidistant from the spine in both arms and legs. It is important to evaluate the hands of these patients carefully. Physical signs of upper extremity involvement include cheiroarthropathy (motor neuropathy in the upper extremity), a condition in which the patient cannot touch the palms together in the prayer position. The first sign of motor neuropathy in the hand is atrophy of the web space between the thumb and first finger. Consideration of the hand deficit must be taken into account for donning, doffing, and choice of closures for orthotics and footwear.[53] Little attention has been paid to the diabetic hand syndrome, or limited joint mobility (LJM), in which the joints of the fingers and wrists become limited. This condition occurs in 30% to 50% of people who have had type 1 diabetes for more than 15 years. To test for LJM, have the patient place the hands flat on a table. Patients with severe LJM will not be able to flatten the fingers onto the table. The skin will also be thick and can be tented on the back of the metacarpophalangeal (MCP) joint[54] (Fig. 12.19).

Surface Temperature Testing

Since the time of Hippocrates, physicians have known that body temperature variations offer important clues for diagnosing disease. The objectives and procedure for acquiring surface temperatures are discussed at the end of this section.

EXHIBIT 12.3

Screening Form for Diabetes Foot Disease

Name: _____ Date: _____ ID#: _____

I. Medical History *(Check all that apply.)*
___ Peripheral neuropathy
___ Retinopathy
___ Cardiovascular disease
___ Nephropathy
___ Peripheral vascular disease

(For Sections II & III, fill in the blanks with an "R," "L," or "B" for positive findings on the right, left, or both feet.)

II. Current History
1. Any change in the foot since the last evaluation? Y ____ N ____
2. Current ulcer or history of a foot ulcer? Y ____ N ____
3. Is there pain in the calf muscles when walking that is relieved by rest? Y ____ N ____

III. Foot Exam
1. Are the nails thick, too long, ingrown, infected with fungal disease? Y ____ N ____
2. Note foot deformities
____ Toe deformities
____ Bunions (hallus valgus)
____ Charcot foot
____ Foot drop
____ Prominent metatarsal heads

Amputation *(Specify date, side, and level.)*

3. Pedal Pulses *(Fill in the blanks with a "P" or an "A" to indicate present or absent.)*

Posterior tibial:
Left ____ Right____
Dorsalis pedis:
Left ____ Right ____

4. Skin Condition *(Measure, draw in, and label the patient's skin condition, using the key and the foot diagram below.)*

C = Callus
U = Ulcer
R = Redness
W = Warmth
M = Maceration
PU = Preulcerative lesion
F = Fissure
S = Swelling
D = Dryness

Dorsal

Right Foot   Left Foot

IV. Sensory Foot Exam *(Label sensory level with a "+" in the five circled areas of each foot if the patient can feel the 5.07 Semmes-Wienstein (10-g) nylon filament and "-" if the patient cannot feel the filament.)*

V. Risk Categorization *(Check appropriate box.)*
___ Low-Risk Patient

All of the following:
___ Intact protective sensation
___ Pedal pulses present
___ No severe deformity
___ No prior foot ulcer
___ No amputation
___ High-Risk Patient

One or more of the following:
___ Loss of protective sensation
___ Absent pedal pulses

___ Severe foot deformity
___ History of foot ulcer
___ Prior amputation

VI. Footwear Assessment *(Fill in the blanks.)*
Does the patient wear appropriate shoes? Y ____ N ____
Does the patient need inserts? Y ____ N ____
Should therapeutic footwear be prescribed? Y ____ N ____

VII. Education *(Fill in the blanks.)*
Has the patient had prior foot care education? Y ____ N ____
Can the patient demonstrate appropriate self-care?
Y ____ N ____

VIII. Management Plan
(Check all that apply.)
___ Provide patient education for preventive foot care.
Date: _____

Diagnostic studies:
___ Vascular laboratory
___ Other: _____
___ Schedule follow-up visit.

Footwear recommendations:
___ None
___ Athletic shoes

___ Accommodative inserts
___ Custom shoes
___ Depth shoes

Refer to:
___ Primary care provider
___ Diabetes educator
___ Orthopaedic foot surgeon

___ RN foot specialist
___ Orthotist
___ Podiatrist
___ Pedorthist
___ Endocrinologist
___ Rehab specialist
___ Vascular surgeon
___ Other: _____

Date: _____   _____
                            Provider Signature

NOTES:

Reprinted from *Feet Can Last a Lifetime: A Health Care Provider's Guide to Preventing Diabetic Foot Problems,* Institute of Diabetics and Digestive and Kidney Diseases, U.S. Department of Health and Human Services, National Institutes of Health, Bethesda, MD.

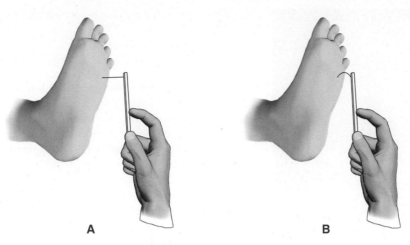

A   **B**

FIGURE 12.18 Sensory foot exam. The sensory testing device is a 10-g (5.07 Semmes-Weinstein) nylon filament mounted on a holder that has been standardized to deliver a 10-g force when properly applied. Research has shown that a person who can feel the 10-g filament in the selected sites is at reduced risk for developing ulcers. (1) The sensory exam should be done in a quiet and relaxed setting. The patient must not watch while the examiner applies the filament. (2) Test the monofilament on the patient's hand so he or she knows what to anticipate. (3) The five sites to be tested on each foot are indicated on the screening form. (4) Apply the monofilament perpendicular to the skin's surface (part A of figure). (Reprinted with permission from *Feet Can Last a Lifetime: A Health Care Provider's Guide to Preventing Diabetic Foot Problems*. Institute of Diabetes and Digestive and Kidney Diseases, U.S. Department of Health and Human Services, National Institute of Health, Bethesda, MD.)

Thermography is the measurement of temperature. Most thermographic tools used in wound care convert infrared radiation to a numerical measurement and display the reading on a monitor.[51] For example, thermocouples (or thermistors) are recording devices that, when touched to the skin for 10 seconds, give a numeric display of temperature.[55] In contrast, the infrared thermometers shown in Figure 12.20A,B allow accurate, immediate spot temperature reading, and the feature of scanning the foot quickly with or without skin contact.

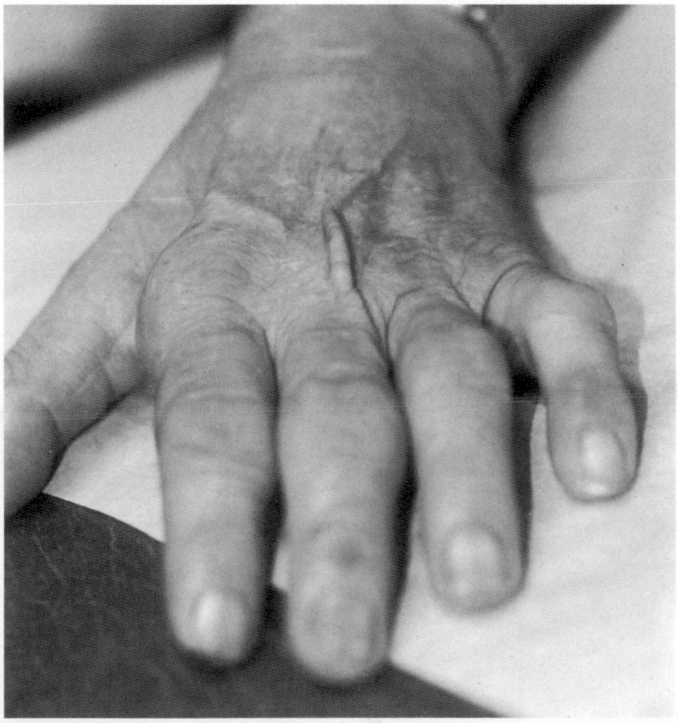

A high temperature reading provides objective evidence of tissue damage and inflammation produced by repeated mechanical (pressure) trauma or infection.[56,57] When evaluating the normal, healthy limb, the most distal aspects are cool. Muscular areas with good blood supply are warmer than bony regions. Arches are several degrees warmer than heels or toes.[55] Excessive heat in an area of the foot is a vascular response to trauma. The trauma may be due to external forces, infection, Charcot joint, or other internal complications. Certainly you could feel the increased heat manually, but without instrumentation to record actual numbers, you will not be able to provide the objective documentation needed for follow-up and comparison.

Implications of Temperature Testings

To perform temperature testing, use a surface-sensing temperature device (thermocouple or infrared). Record temperatures in predetermined areas, usually those related to common areas of breakdown. If you discover one definite area with a temperature 3°F higher than that of adjacent areas, you can assume that this is an area of high pressure or stress. Even if there is no current breakdown, you must relieve the pressure in this area and the redistribute it over the remaining weight-bearing surfaces. Upon follow-up of this same patient, you should notice a decrease in the temperature differentiation as healing of the tissue progresses.

In a comparison of contralateral limbs, suspect vascular impairment when one limb is significantly colder or distal portions of the foot show an extreme drop in temperature. A chronic hot spot points to the presence of a chronic stress or an underlying bone or joint problem. Bear in mind, however, that increased temperature tells that there is a problem and where it is—not what it is![23]

FIGURE 12.19 Neuropathic hand. Motor neuropathy testing reveals tenting on the back of the MCP joint, clawing of the fingers, and atrophy of the web space between the thumb and the first finger.

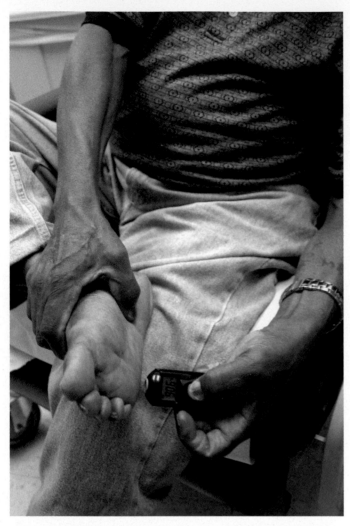

FIGURE 12.20 Tempgun infrared thermometer. Used with permission: James Birke, PT, PhD.

Objectives and Procedure for Taking Temperature

Objectives for taking temperature:

- To evaluate baseline temperature at sites of high incidence of ulceration
- To determine presence of inflammation
- To evaluate sites of baseline-elevated temperature for decrease in temperature after intervention to relieve pressure

Procedure for taking and recording temperature using a thermocouple

1. Expose the bare skin of the foot to the room temperature for 5 to 10 minutes before recording any temperature.
2. Take temperature at 10 locations on the sole of foot and toes (shown by circles on foot evaluation form Exhibit 12.3).
3. Follow steps for measuring temperature.
4. Record readings in degrees at each location on foot evaluation form and date.
5. Record readings at each location on successive evaluations below the initial reading and date.

Procedure for Use of an Infrared Scanner Thermometer

Follow these steps in measuring temperature with an infrared scanner thermometer:

1. Temperature testing may be done with or without contact of skin.
2. Read the first number seen.
3. Avoid pressure against the skin that causes ischemia.

Use of Temperature Testing for Self-Care

A recent study evaluated the effectiveness of at-home infrared temperature monitoring as a preventive tool in diabetics at high risk for lower extremity ulceration and amputation. The study group measured temperatures in the morning and evening and were instructed to reduce their activity and contact the study nurse when temperatures increased. This group had significantly fewer foot complications due to early warning of inflammation and tissue injury.[58]

Pressure Testing

A variety of devices have been used for many decades to determine pressure distribution while standing and walking. For example, force plates have given us valuable information regarding peak pressures during ambulation, but are limited in that they represent only a single step on the plate. Attempts to place sensors in the shoes have been unreliable because of the sensor structure and attachment within the shoe.[59] Another option is the Harris mat, which provides a grid analysis of pressure distribution, imprinting low foot pressures in large, light squares and heavier pressures in smaller, darker squares (Fig. 12.21).[2] The Harris mat can be used for static and dynamic assessment, can provide permanent records, and is relatively inexpensive.

Recent developments in computer-aided documentation have included devices, which provide full-color three-dimensional pressure recordings that can be used for static or dynamic documentation. Computer-aided devices are also being used to produce live scanning of the foot in order to provide a positive mold for orthotics, as well as for custom shoes.[60] Using three-dimensional, digital computer graphics, a plastic sock may be molded to the patient and converted to a shoe cast.[61]

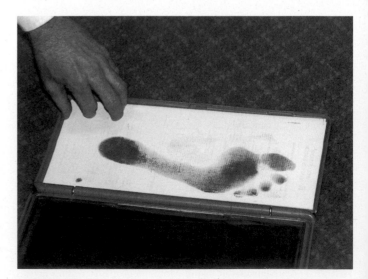

FIGURE 12.21 Harris mat pressure testing record. Darker areas represent higher pressure.

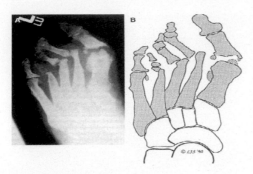

FIGURE 12.22 Charcot foot A. anteroposterior radiograph reveals osteolytic destruction of metatarsophalangeal joints, with pencil-like tapering of the metatarsal shafts resembling "sucked candy" or "licked peppermint stick". **B** Graphic represents the radiographic findings. (This article was published in Sanders LJ, Frykberg RG: Diabetic neuropathic osteoarthropathy: the Charcot foot in Fryberg RG, editor: The high risk foot in diabetes mellitus, New York, 1991, Churchill Livingstone, © Elsevier. Reprinted with permission.

Charcot Joint Examination

Charcot joint (Charcot arthropathy) is a relatively painless, progressive, and degenerative arthropathy of single or multiple joints, caused by underlying neuropathy. The neuropathy may be periosteal and not cutaneous. There are several theories behind the causes of Charcot joint, as follows:

- Multiple microtraumas to the joints cause microfractures. These fractures lead to relaxation of the ligaments and joint destruction.[62] (Fig. 12.22).
- There is increased blood flow and bone reabsorption (osteolysis). Patients with Charcot joints have bounding pulses.
- Changes in the spinal cord lead to trophic changes in bones and joints.
- Osteoporosis is accompanied by an abnormal brittleness of the bones, leading to spontaneous fracture.[63]

In clinical observations, the limb is usually painless, swollen, and red. Unhealed painless fractures are often visible with radiography. In advanced Charcot disease, there are multiple fractures, accompanied by extensive bone demineralization and reabsorption. Later stages reveal architectural distortion of the foot, with shortening and widening of the joint.[42] The foot joints most commonly affected are the following:

- tarsometatarsal (30%)
- metatarsophalangeal (30%)
- tarsus (24%)
- interphalangeal (4%)

Charcot joint is frequently misdiagnosed and mistreated, leaving the patient with deformities that require further medical intervention and/or expensive footwear (see Fig. 12.23). The acute stage will show a foot that is 5°F to 10°F hotter than the contralateral limb in the same area. The red, hot, swollen foot will usually not have a skin opening or ulceration. Laboratory tests, including radiographs, may not show changes in the acute stage to differentiate Charcot disease from other diagnoses.

The duration of the catastrophic destruction, dissociation, and eventual recalcification found with Charcot joint will vary with the individual, but the average healing time in a cast for

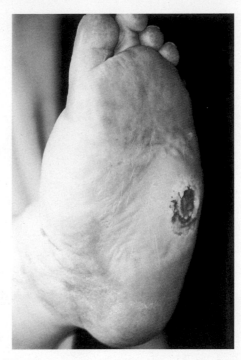

FIGURE 12.23 Classic Charcot rocker bottom foot deformity. Note ulceration over bony deformity surrounded by callus formation.

the hindfoot is 12 months; for the midfoot, 9 months; and for the forefoot, 6 months. By evaluating with comparative temperature measurements of the contralateral foot, the stages can usually be verified by radiograph. As the involved foot temperature increases, the destruction and dissociation are taking place. The temperature gradually decreases as recalcification is in progress. A radiograph shows that recalcification is complete when temperatures bilaterally are within 3°F.

The treatment plan for acute Charcot joint is total contact casting, discussed later in this chapter. The cast must be changed in 1 week to accommodate volume changes. Following the period of volume changes, the cast should be changed every 2 to 3 weeks. When the temperature is equal to that of the other limb, the patient may be weaned gradually from the cast to a splint, then to shoes. Follow-up should continue to ensure that there is no recurrence of an episode of Charcot joint.

Osteomyelitis Examination

The clinical manifestations, including laboratory data, of Charcot joint and osteomyelitis (bone infection) are very similar, and the patient should be monitored closely to verify the diagnosis. With osteomyelitis, you will often observe the presence of an opening in the skin to allow an entrance for bacteria to infect the bone (see Fig. 12.24A,B). Take the temperature over the best surrounding skin. Refer for immediate medical management. The recalcification would not occur radiographically as in Charcot disease. Verification may be made for osteomyelitis with a three-phase bone scan or biopsy (Fig. 12.24C).[22] The more common or familiar method of evaluating for osteomyelitis involves the use of radiographs as seen in Figure 12.25.

Diabetic patients with foot ulcers that expose bone should be treated for osteomyelitis, even if there is no evidence of inflammation.[64]

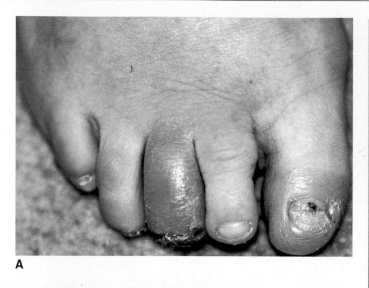

A

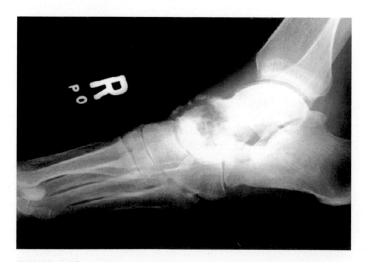

B

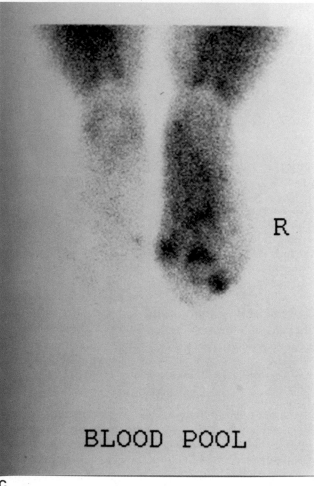

C

FIGURE 12.24 A: Red, hot, swollen toe: infection suspected. (Courtesy of Nancy Elftman.) **B:** Distal tip of inflamed toe. (Courtesy of Nancy Elftman.) **C:** Blood pooling of inflamed toe: infection confirmed. (Courtesy of Nancy Elftman.)

INTERVENTIONS

Interventions for the neuropathic foot include application of orthotics and other adaptive equipment, total-contact casting, and the use of splints and other devices. We discuss surgical management and skin care separately.

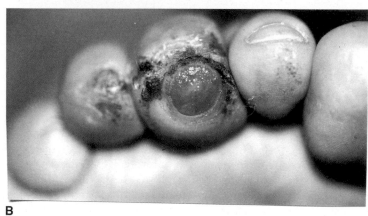

FIGURE 12.25 Radiograph showing osteomyelitis of talonavicular joint.

Orthotics and Adaptive Equipment

Treatment of the neuropathic foot requires accommodation, relief of pressure/shear forces, and shock absorption. This can be achieved with accommodative inserts, special shoes, socks, and blocks.

Accommodative Inserts

Accommodative inserts do not apply correction; they are used to fill the spaces between the flat shoe and the foot contours. All inserts are applied on the underlying surface in contact with the shoe, never in contact with the foot. The surface in contact with the foot is always a solid, uninterrupted surface that will not apply edges for the foot to receive shear forces. There are different types of inserts, as follows:

- Soft: cushioning/accommodation; improves shock absorption
- Semirigid: some cushion/accommodation; affords pressure relief
- Rigid: hard, single layer of plastic; controls abnormal foot and leg motion[65]

For example, metatarsal head (MTH) pads are soft cushioning inserts. They are placed proximal to the MTHs to redistribute the weight from the heads to the metatarsal shafts as well as to increase the transverse arch of the foot (Fig. 12.26).

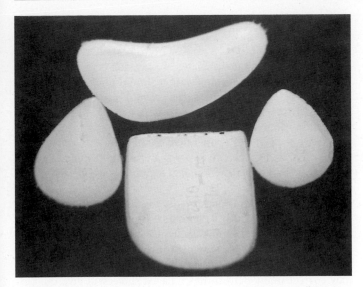

FIGURE 12.26 Metatarsal pads made of soft durometer to aid in pressure relief of metatarsal heads and increase transverse arch of foot. (Courtesy of UCO International, Inc., Wheeling, Illinois.)

A variety of materials are available for more sophisticated accommodative inserts, and it is important to understand the benefits and limitations of the material you will be using. Figure 12.27 shows the several different layers that make up an accommodative insert. Cellular polyethylene foams, such as Aliplast, Plastazote, and Pelite, are composed of a mass of bubbles in a plastic and gas phase. The bubbles are cells with lines of intersection called *ribs* or *strands*, and the walls are called *windows*. In closed-cell materials, the gases do not pass freely; open-cell material has no windows, leaving many cells interconnected, so that gas may pass between cells. Cell walls are not totally impermeable to the flow of gases. Under a sustained load (especially the heavy patient), gases are squeezed out; when the load is removed, gases are drawn back into the cells.[66] These materials will bottom out from compaction of the materials as cells fracture under repetitive stress. For example, Plastazote, when used alone, has a limited effective period of about 2 days. However, when Plastazote is combined with Poron to form a single unit, the combined attributes of both perform well for 6 to 9 months[67,68] The advantages of these foams are low-temperature molding, nontoxicity, water resistance, and washability without absorbency of fluid.[69]

The Aliplast/Plastazote ™ insert is an immediate preparation and can be provided within a clinic setting, but it has a relatively short life of compressibility (6–8 months). Plastazote is a closed-cell polyethylene foam that can be heated to 280°F and molded directly onto the patient's foot.[21] Care must be taken never to mold the toes or create ridges that the toes will ride over as the patient ambulates. By combining materials over a cast model of the foot, the composite type of insert can achieve all goals of the accommodative insert and provide a minimum life of 1 year.

An insert with a Plastazote surface in contact with the foot can be used as a diagnostic tool for future follow-up. The self-molding properties of Plastazote reveal deep sock prints in areas of high pressure. These high-pressure areas should be noted and relieved in future insert designs for the patient.

Temperature testing can help you evaluate the effectiveness of accommodative inserts. As noted earlier, areas of high trauma will have increased temperature. After the patient has worn accommodative inserts, the temperature differentiation

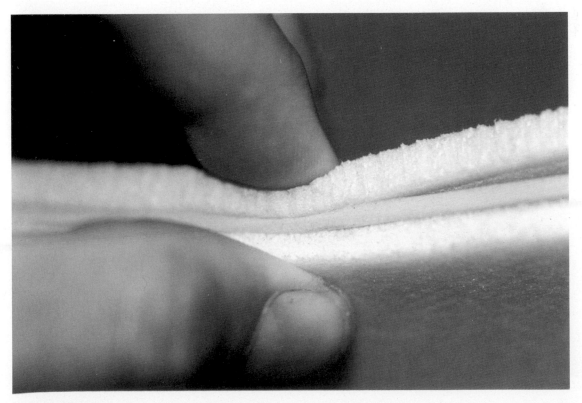

FIGURE 12.27 Accommodative inserts require multiple layers of varied durometer materials. Compression should reduce thickness by half. (Courtesy of Nancy Elftman.)

CLINICAL WISDOM

Choose Crepe Sole Shoes for Pressure Relief

Crepe soles, which are full of air cells, provide pressure relief to the plantar surface, whereas air or water "pillows," which are enclosed in an inflexible compartment, create pressure.

will decrease if the proper accommodation has been achieved. If the temperature has not decreased in the area, the relief may require enhancement, or there may be other underlying complications to be investigated.

Shoes

Shoes for the insensitive foot should be of soft leather that will conform to abnormalities on the dorsal surface and allow for the depth of an accommodative insert. Leather gradually adapts to the slope of the foot and will retain shape between wearings. The leather will breathe and absorb perspiration.[69]

The patient should not depend on the "feel" of a shoe for correct size. The shoe must be full width and girth and allow 1/2 to 3/4 in. of space beyond the longest toe to prevent distal shoe contact through the gait cycle. Figure 12.28A–D shows modifications of the shoe appropriate for the insensitive foot. Standard modifications of extra-depth shoes for the neuropathic patient include stretching of the soft toe box for clawed toes, flared

lateral soles to discourage varus instability, and shank/rocker bottom for a partial foot, hallux rigidus, or decreased motion at the metatarsal heads. A rocker bottom should be added to the shoe when metatarsophalangeal extension is to be avoided.[21] When properly fit, the instep leather should not be taut.

There are three tests to determine the proper fit of shoes (Fig. 12.29A,B):

Length: Allow 1/2 to 3/4 in. of space in front of longest toe.

Ball width: With the patient weight bearing, grasp the vamp of the shoe, and pinch the upper material; if leather cannot be pinched, it is too narrow. The ball should be in the widest part of the shoe.[70]

Heel to ball length: Measure the distance from the patient's heel to the first and fifth metatarsal heads. Bend the shoe to determine toe break, and repeat measurements on the shoe. They should be close to the same measurements.[71]

The simple addition of shoes instead of walking barefoot may correct many deformities.[72] Laced shoes will give the best control, but they must be broken in slowly, beginning with 2 hours per day and slowly adding time.[21] Cutout sandals are not recommended because they can cause irritation along the borders of the sandal and straps.[73]

To evaluate pressures within a shoe, there is a pressure-sensitive sock that is coated with dye-filled wax capsules. The capsules fracture when a certain pressure threshold is exceeded, leaving dye stains in areas of high pressure.[69]

To protect a healing area in which dressings will be applied, a healing shoe lined with Plastazote will allow greater circumference and volume adjustability.

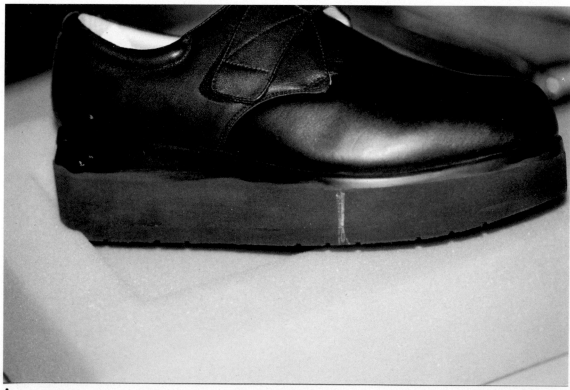

A

FIGURE 12.28 A: Common shoe modifications for the neuropathic foot. Rocker sole for limited great toe motion and forefoot complications. (Courtesy of Nancy Elftman.)

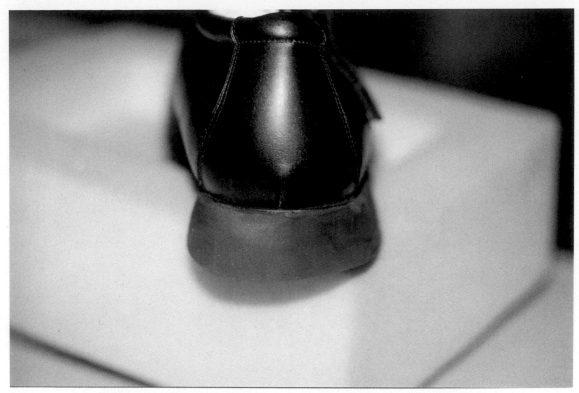

B

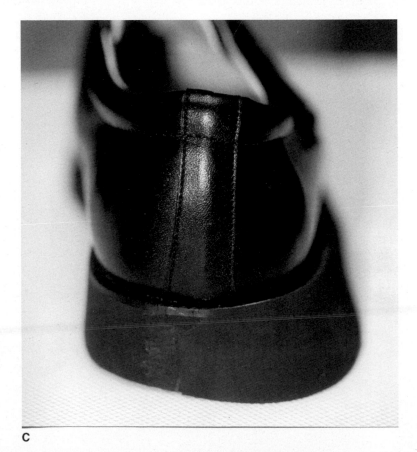

C

FIGURE 12.28 (*continued*) **B:** Common shoe modifications for the neuropathic foot. Heel wrap to widen heel contact surface and increase stability. (Courtesy of Nancy Elftman.) **C:** Common shoe modifications for the neuropathic foot. C. Lateral flare for varus deformity. (Courtesy of Nancy Elftman.)

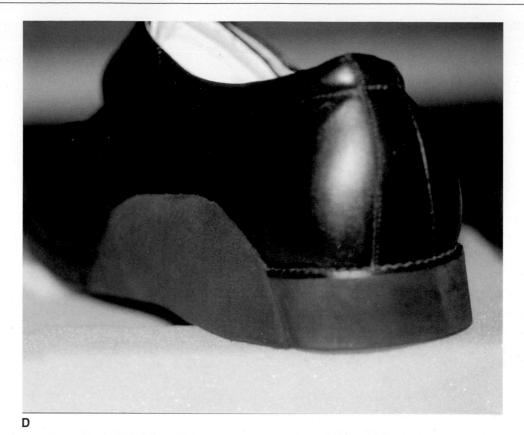

D

FIGURE 12.28 (*continued*) **D:** Common shoe modifications for the neuropathic foot. D. Bolster for midfoot medial support. (Courtesy of Nancy Elftman.)

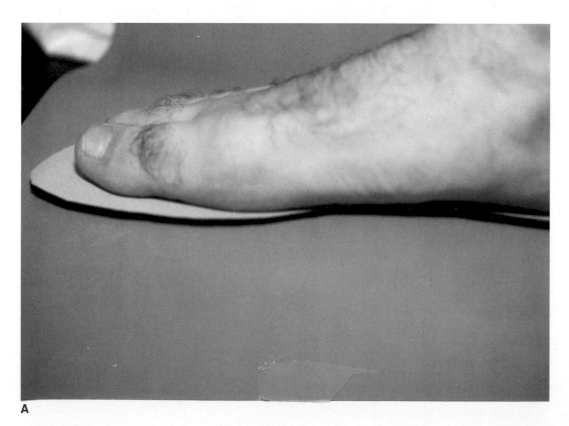

A

FIGURE 12.29 **A:** The neuropathic foot requires shoes that have a space of 1/2 to 3/4 in. of space beyond the longest toe. (Courtesy of Nancy Elftman.)

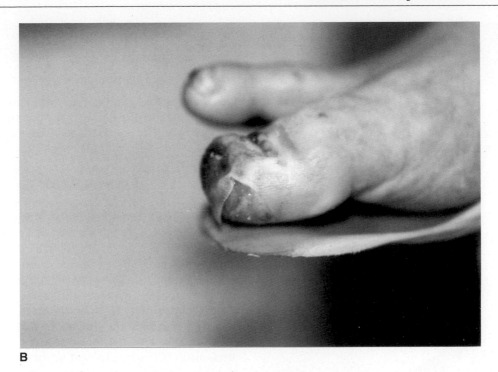

B

FIGURE 12.29 (*continued*) **B:** The wound on the distal end of the great toe due to a short shoe. (Courtesy Nancy Elftman.)

Socks

Socks for the neuropathic limb should have no mended areas or seams over bony prominences. A cotton/acrylic blend will assist in the wicking of perspiration away from the foot.[74] The sock should be fully cushioned and have a nonrestrictive top. The partial foot requires a sock that will conform to the shape without distal prominent seams or excess material at the distal end. For the active patient, socks can be obtained with silicone over high-stress areas to prevent shear for full or partial feet.

Blocks

The partial foot may require a block within the shoe for the area of amputation. The purpose of a block is to reduce migration of the partial foot and medial/lateral shear for the toe amputation. No block or "prosthetic toe" is used for a central digit amputation. The low pressures applied by a block to central digits cause ischemic ulcerations on opposing surfaces. Medial or lateral amputations (first and fifth toes) may require a block to hold the foot in the correct position within the shoe. The forefoot block holds the shoe leather away from the distal end of the foot and discourages distal migration of the foot. All forms of blocks must have space from the amputation site and be an integral part of the insert, not added to an existing orthotic. Forefoot blocks require a rigid rocker sole to prevent ulceration to distal end.

By utilizing state-of-the-art foams and room temperature vulcanized (RTV) silicone elastomers, shear can be reduced in areas of skin grafts, chronic ulcerations, and calcanectomies within more rigid orthotics. The viscoelastomer gel is a two-part gel that can be adjusted for durometer desired. The mixture can be used for shock absorption and shear reduction. Scar-adherent areas can benefit from a medium durometer mixture. The disadvantage is weight, so it should be used in small areas. Low-density foams can be designed into orthotics, such as toe breaks and forefoot blocks and reliefs. Reliefs for heel pain can be designed into the insert or shoe sole as a Sach heel. Sach heels use soft and medium durometer soling to simulate plantar flexion and provide shock absorption at heel strike.

Total-Contact Casting

The total-contact casting (TCC) method provides decreased plantar pressures by increasing weight bearing over the entire lower leg[75] (Fig. 12.30). Brand introduced the total-contact cast to the United States in the 1950s to redistribute walking pressures, prevent direct trauma to the wound, reduce edema, and provide immobilization to joints and soft tissue. The average healing time for ulcerations treated with TCC is 6 weeks.[73]

TCC provides decreased plantar pressures by increasing weight bearing over the entire lower leg, so that no part of the foot takes more than 5 psi. It has been successful as a treatment for plantar ulcerations but requires careful application, close follow-up, and patient compliance with scheduled appointments to minimize complications.[75] TCC has also been used for patients without as well as with evidence of severe peripheral vascular disease.[76]

Application methods vary by institution. Steps for application of the Carville-type TCC are given here solely for reference, as these casts are applied only by skilled technicians:

1. The ulcer is covered with a thin layer of gauze.
2. Cotton is placed between the toes to prevent maceration.
3. A stockinette is applied.
4. A 1/4-in. piece of felt is placed over the malleoli and anterior tibia.
5. Foam padding is placed around toes.
6. A total-contact plaster shell is molded.
7. The shell is reinforced with plaster splints.
8. A walking heel is attached.
9. A fiberglass roll is applied around the plaster.

A window is never cut into the cast or there may be localized swelling, shear stresses, and, eventually, a secondary wound.[21]

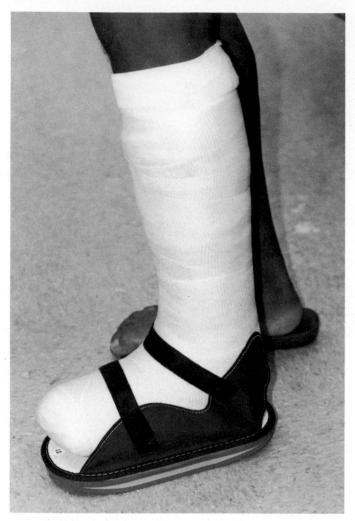

FIGURE 12.30 Total-contact cast.

CLINICAL WISDOM

Bathing While Wearing a TCC

A seal-tight cast and bandage protector is a heavyweight plastic vinyl bag that slips over the cast and forms a seal that is watertight. The product is convenient to use, durable, and has a sueded sole to minimize slippage in the shower.

The patient is instructed to ambulate only 33% of usual activity. The cast is removed in 5 to 7 days and reapplied. New casts are applied every 2 to 3 weeks.[75] To allow thorough drying, the patient should not stand or walk on the cast for 24 hours.[73]

A common complication of the neuropathic patient is severe foot deformity, including joint subluxation or dislocation, following neuropathic fractures or Charcot joint. The presence of severe foot deformity has been shown to be predictive of prolonged healing time for patients treated with TCC. Sinacore et al.[77] found that fixed foot deformity prolonged healing of ulcers with TCC when located in the midfoot and rear foot. Ulcers located in the midfoot healed in 73 ± 29 days, and rear foot ulcers healed in 90 ± 19 days. Individuals without fixed deformities with chronic diabetes mellitus and those with forefoot ulcers healed in 41 days. Therefore, early detection during the musculoskeletal examination of a fixed foot deformity in a patient with an ulcer located in the midfoot or rear foot can be used to determine a prognosis that healing time will be significantly longer when a TCC is used as the treatment intervention.

While not as effective as total contact, a posterior splint covers the posterior lower leg and plantar foot surface, and is held in place with elastic wrap. The splint acts to protect the plantar surface. This procedure may be chosen for the patient with

CASE STUDY

Charcot Arthropathy

The patient was a 44-year-old woman with a 15-year history of type 2 diabetes mellitus. She had neuropathic extremities to mid-calf bilaterally, loss of sensation, and motor function demonstrated by bilateral foot drop. She had a right foot Charcot arthropathy 4 years ago. The extremity was treated with a series of total-contact casts for 11 months and gradually weaned to ankle-foot orthotics with shoes. The contralateral side used ankle-foot orthosis to control foot drop.

The patient came to the clinic for an emergency check-up due to a weekend traumatic injury to the left foot. She recalls twisting the left ankle and slight discomfort. Within an hour, there was swelling so she went to a local emergency department. The patient was told that she had possibly torn a ligament and was put in a precautionary plaster cast with a rubber walking pad.

When the patient came to the clinic 2 days later, she was in a great deal of discomfort and the plaster cast seemed to

have absorbed exudate. The toes were left exposed in the cast and had swollen beyond the confines of the distal cast edge. When the cast was removed, it was observed that the walking pad had been forced through the plaster on the plantar surface and traumatized the entire plantar midfoot. The patient had Charcot arthropathy of the midfoot that was further destroyed by the nonreinforced walking pad. The edges of the plaster caused open abrasions to the exposed toes, leading to infection.

The patient was treated for abrasions and put into a total-contact cast. After 16 months, the Charcot episode was over but the foot was left with deformities that could not be accommodated in a standard shoe. A custom shoe was ordered for the left foot deformity.

Key Points

1. Immediate total-contact casting could have reduced the deformities and length of treatment.
2. A total-contact cast differs from a standard short leg cast and should be applied by a skilled technician.

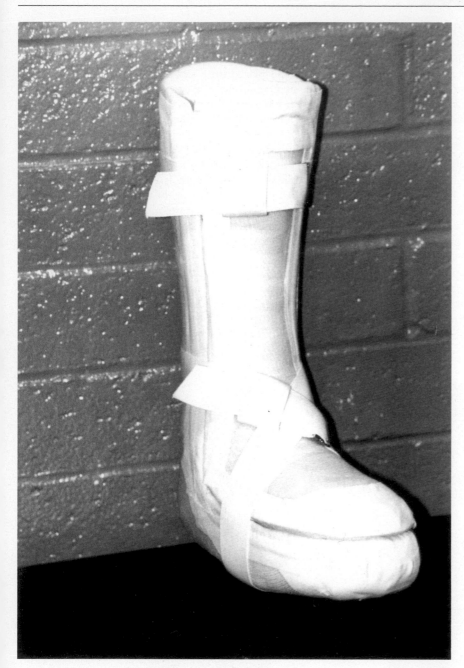

FIGURE 12.31 The ODS splint will be fit with a cast shoe for ambulation. (Courtesy of Nancy Elftman.)

a limb compromised by poor circulation or when the patient cannot tolerate the confinement of a cast.[78]

Healing Cast Shoe

There have also been attempts to heal ulcers by using a healing cast shoe molded of plaster. This healing cast shoe must be changed in 3 days, then reapplied every 10 days. Results have reported healing of plantar ulcers in 39 days.[79] Contraindications for the use of a healing cast shoe include infection (redness, swelling, warmth, fever) and hypotrophic skin (thin, shiny appearance, marked dependent edema).[73]

Orthotic Dynamic System Splint

The orthotic dynamic system (ODS) splint was developed to take advantage of the casting method of a TCC with the inclusion of a custom-molded insert that could be removed and

reliefs modified. With all of the advantages of the TCC, the advantages that were added with the ODS splint included the possibilities for daily inspection, regular cleaning/dressings/debridement, and adjustments to areas of excessive pressure and/or friction (Fig. 12.31).

The Plastazote/Aliplast insert is first molded to the patient's foot and trimmed to follow the plantar surface, with 1/4 in. of length added beyond toes. A stockinette is placed on the leg, the insert is positioned, and another stockinette is applied to hold the insert in place. A padded TCC is applied, using fiberglass only. The cast is bivalved; straps are added; edges are finished; and the insert is removed, relieved, and replaced to unweight the area of ulceration. After insert modification, it is replaced within the splint, and the patient may ambulate with a rocker-bottom cast shoe under the splint. The patient is instructed on volume control with sock thickness.

The disadvantage will lie with compliance of the patient. The splint design allows donning and doffing by the patient, therefore allowing him or her to remove the cast. The total contact of a healing cast cannot be compared in its superiority, but the clinical experience of the authors suggests that the advantages of being able to inspect the ODS daily and adjust it for patient comfort are a great asset in the treatment protocol.

Neuropathic Walker

The neuropathic walker is a combination of an ankle-foot orthosis (AFO) and a boot that is custom designed to be total contact for weight distribution (Fig. 12.32A,B). The ankle is locked to reduce force through the Lisfranc joint and/or ankle. The design is indicated for the patient with changes of Charcot joint in the tarsal and ankle joints, chronic recurrence of Charcot disease, and chronic ulcerations. The orthosis is easily donned and doffed, and is fabricated of a copolymer plastic with a closed-cell lining. The removable insert may be adjusted to reassign weight-bearing areas on the plantar surface. The insert may also be formed over chronic breakdown areas, such as the malleoli, posterior heel, and bunions, to reduce pressure.

The rocker sole allows for easy ambulation, but the contralateral shoe must be adjusted for height.

When casting for the neuropathic walker, the patient's limb is wrapped and placed on a soft foam block until the plaster is set. The plantar surface will accommodate without excessive pressures on bony prominences. Modifications of the positive model include smoothing the plantar surface but never removing plaster. Any area that has had plaster removed during modification will be an area of excess pressure in the finished orthosis. The distal end is built up at the medial and lateral metatarsal areas and the length is extended 1/2 in. to allow room for the toes and to decrease the chances of maceration.

Fabrication is completed on the modified positive cast. The insert is first fabricated, finished, and placed in position. The posterior Plastazote lining is pulled over the insert, followed by the copolymer (plastic) vacuum-formed shell. The entire posterior section is finished and trimmed. The anterior Plastazote is positioned, and the copolymer shell is applied over the entire posterior. There should be a 1/2- to 1-in. overlap of copolymer on the finished orthosis. The Velcro straps and rocker bottom are attached (apex of rocker proximal to MTH).

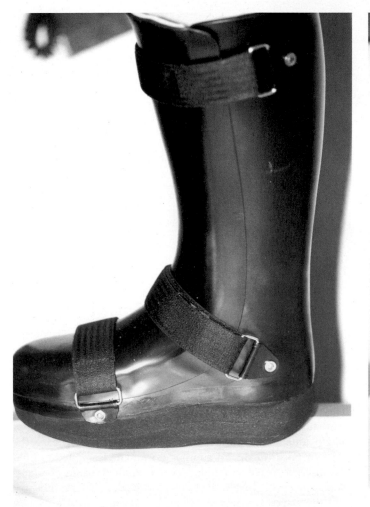

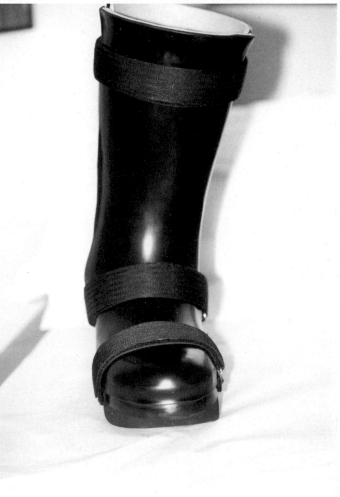

A **B**

FIGURE 12.32 A: The custom neuropathic walker has a rocker sole and provides total contact for the high-risk foot. (Courtesy of Nancy Elftman.) **B:** The orthosis fits the individual and supports deformity. (Courtesy of Nancy Elftman.)

Instruct the patient to check the skin daily for redness and possible breakdown. During follow-up, assess and record temperatures of the plantar surface. Your measurements may suggest that adjustments of insert pressures are needed. Sock management will be very important to continue a snug fit of the orthosis and volume control.

Total-Contact Ankle-Foot Orthosis

Like the neuropathic walker, the total-contact ankle-foot orthosis (AFO) is used for the patient who has an area of trauma in the mid-or hindfoot. The orthosis includes a custom, removable insert and is lined with Plastazote. This orthosis must be fit within a shoe, and this may be difficult in standard shoes. The casting procedure is the same as that for the neuropathic walker. The toes are open, and the anterior shell terminates at midfoot.

Other Devices

Short leg walkers and orthopaedic walkers have been used by some clinics, but they compromise the total-contact feature. The walkers have become popular as alternatives to cast immobilization but the indications for their use are for foot and ankle fractures, sprains, acute ligament/muscle, and postsurgical immobilization. Although prefabricated walkers (Fig. 12.33) are not custom-made to provide total contact, they do contain some features that may assist in reducing movement of the limb within the walker.[80] The walkers can be improved in function with the addition of a wide base, rocker sole, and custom insert.[81] The low-risk patient does well in the orthosis with a custom insert. In contrast, the high-risk patient with sensory neuropathy may be better served by a custom total-contact orthosis.[82]

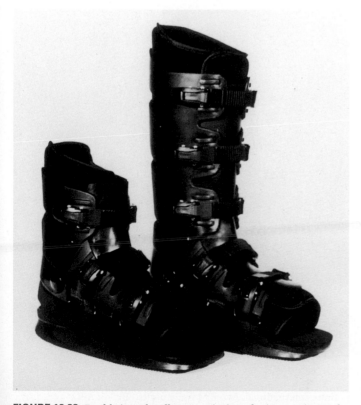

FIGURE 12.33 Prefabricated walker to assist in reducing motion at the ankle. (Courtesy of Darco International, Huntington, West Virginia.)

Patellar tendon-bearing (axial resist) AFO designs are intended to decrease forces on the plantar weight-bearing surface of the foot. The design is only minimally effective in reducing the load off the lower leg.[83] The patellar tendon-bearing design AFO has been used successfully for calcanectomy, plantar skin graft, and heel ulceration. This orthosis is contraindicated in the patient with vascular impairment because of the excess restriction in the popliteal area of arterial flow.

The prosthesis has been the orthotic replacement when the amputation case is complicated and the patient is not a candidate for prosthetic management. The prosthesis becomes a useful device for transfers and limb protection. This is always a creative design, with no two the same, unique to the individual and his or her needs.

As discussed in Chapter 10, the nonambulatory patient must be examined carefully for pressure ulceration due to positioning. Heel ulcers are particularly difficult to off-load in the recumbent position (Fig. 12.34A). For these patients, the prefabricated soft ankle-foot orthosis (soft AFO) can help. It is constructed of a soft foam over a semirigid posterior/plantar support. The device allows decreased pressure at the posterior, medial/lateral, and plantar areas of the heel (Fig. 12.34B). The soft outer construction decreases trauma to the contralateral leg.[80]

Off-Loading of Foot Ulcerations

In the treatment of foot ulcerations, the wound care protocol must include debridement/cleansing and simultaneous off-loading of the affected area; that is, pressure and shear affecting the area must be relieved. Many patients are given crutches, a walker, or a wheelchair, but they must have the upper body strength, cardiovascular reserves, and/or motivation to use assistive devices.[80] Bed rest eliminates the pressures on the foot but promotes deconditioning of the patient.[81] Thus, the wound care team should consider custom as well as prefabricated off-loading devices for each individual patient.

Custom Plastazote Healing Sandals

The custom Plastazote healing sandal contains a molded foot bed and has a rigid rocker sole (Fig. 12.35). The device is lightweight but requires considerable time and experience to fabricate.[80] The Carville sandal has been used as a successful off-loading shoe and interim device following the TCC and before definitive shoewear.[84]

Prefabricated Off-Loading Alternatives

Prefabricated devices are inexpensive alternatives for off-loading ulcerations. The following prefabricated products are improved in function by the addition of a customized accommodative insert. The area of off-loading can be designed using the patient's floor reaction imprint (Harris mat) as a pattern. Follow-up appointments should include temperature measurements to ensure proper off-loading. If temperature is increased, the off-loading area must be increased. Lower temperature indicates decreased inflammation and healing progression.[85]

Post Op/Med Surg/Cast Shoe

An inexpensive alternative for wound off-loading is a postoperative shoe (rigid sole) or cast shoe (roller sole) containing an off-loading insert (Fig. 12.36). These shoes adjust for bandage volume but do not offer an intimate fit to control foot motion.[82]

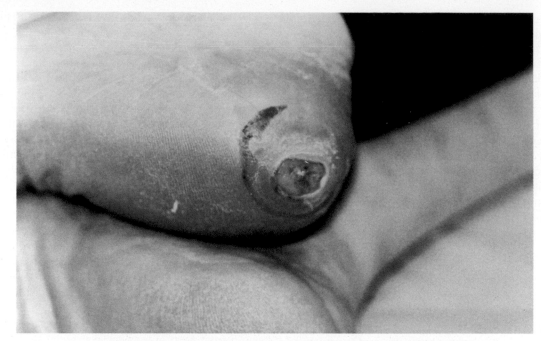

A

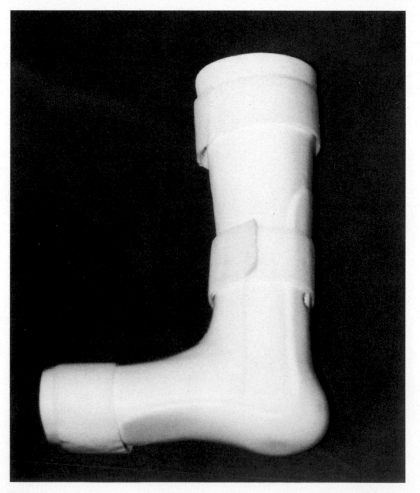

B

FIGURE 12.34 A: Common heel ulceration. (Courtesy of Boston Brace International, Avon, Massachusetts.) **B:** Soft AFO for the recumbent patient to off-load heel ulceration and prevent trauma to contralateral limb. (Courtesy of Boston Brace International, Avon, Massachusetts.)

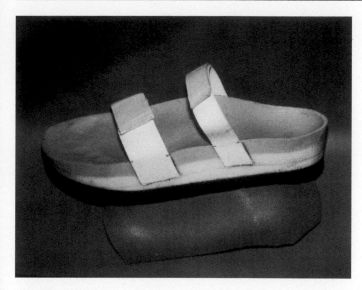

FIGURE 12.35 Plastazote Healing Sandal developed at Carville to provide a molded foot bed and rigid rocker sole. (Courtesy of the Department of Health and Human Services, Division of National Hansen's Disease Program.)

These shoes usually require extensions to Velcro straps and minor modifications. Use of the shoes as off-loading devices requires careful monitoring of the patient.

Wedged Shoe

The wedged shoe (Fig. 12.37) has full contact with the plantar surface of the foot but reduces load forces applied from the ground. The sole angle is designed to shift weight bearing away from the ulcerated area. The wedge shoe is contraindicated when the patient does not have the range of motion to accompany the shoe angle. A patient with poor proprioception, who is fitted with this shoe, may not be able to ambulate without assistive devices.

Half Shoes

Many clinics use the half shoe (Fig. 12.38) to suspend the ulcerated area, providing complete off-loading of the ulcerated

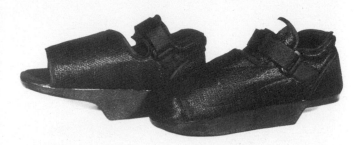

FIGURE 12.37 Wedged shoe reduces floor reaction forces to healing plantar surfaces. (Courtesy of Darco International, Huntington, West Virginia.)

area. The forefoot half shoe provides a pressure-free area for the forefoot, especially for the common ulcerations of the hallux. The heel relief shoe suspends the heel for noncontact. These devices may be contraindicated for the patient with limited ankle motion or balance problems associated with proprioception. Assistive devices may be required to reduce incidence of falls.[80,81]

Wound Healing Shoe Systems

Wound healing shoes are designed for the practitioner who does not have casting facilities or available support to off-load ulcerations by TCC or ODS splint. The basic wound shoe (Fig. 12.39) provides a base that allows relief of pressure for the dorsum, medial, lateral, and posterior ulceration. The plantar contact system (Fig. 12.40) enables the practitioner to off-load plantar ulcerations with four layers (multiple durometer) of material (Fig. 12.41A). The system is to be worn until the ulceration has healed. On final closure of the wound, a long-term material layer is added, and the wound shoe becomes the casual slipper to be worn at all times when definitive off-loading footwear is not being used (Fig. 12.41B). A previous ulceration site is susceptible to breakdown repeatedly, and the wound shoe used as a casual slipper ensures that pressure relief is achieved at all times. The patient must never walk barefooted.

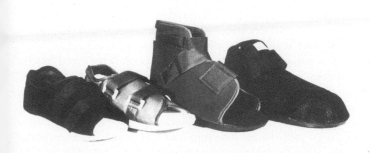

FIGURE 12.36 Post op/med surg/cast shoes: An inexpensive alternative to off-loading a wound on the plantar foot surface when plantar insert is supplied. (Courtesy of Darco International, Huntington, West Virginia.)

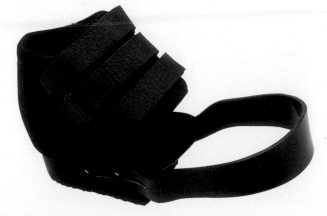

FIGURE 12.38 Half shoes suspend ulcerated area to eliminate external pressure. (Courtesy of Bauerfeind USA, Inc., Kennesaw, GA.)

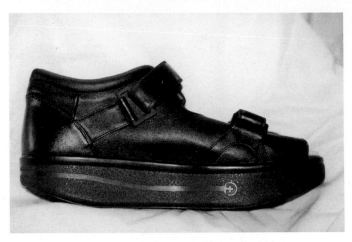

FIGURE 12.39 The wound healing system provides optimal environment for wound care protocol and simultaneous off-loading to encourage healing. (Courtesy of Darco International, Huntington, West Virginia.)

The floor reaction imprint (Harris mat, Fig. 12.42) is helpful to use as a pattern for the off-loading position, but is not necessary. The top layer to contact the foot is always a solid interface that will mold to the foot contours. There are two layers of higher durometer that will be relieved using available tools (scissors, scalpel, blade). With lower grade ulcers (Wagner 0 and 1), one off-loading layer is sufficient (Fig. 12.41C), whereas higher grade ulcers require two off-loading layers (Fig. 12.41D). On wound closure, a shock-absorbing layer is to be added to prolong use of the system as a slipper (Fig. 12.41E).

For ulcerations that are not weight bearing (not plantar surface), the double-layer upper construction can be trimmed to off-load pressure areas without allowing window edema to occur (Fig. 12.43A,B). The Velcro system is adjustable for bandage volume. The off-loading system allows for minimal dressings, which will usually add excess pressure areas when the patient is weight bearing.

The goal of the wound healing shoe system is to allow partial weight bearing while off-loading the high-risk foot with

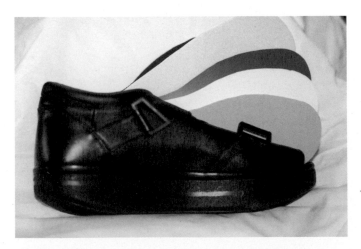

FIGURE 12.40 The wound shoe system allows off-loading of plantar, as well as dorsal wounds.

ulcerations. The combination of state-of-the-art wound care preparations and off-loading delivers optimal outcomes, as well as unlimited adjustments to forces applied.

SURGICAL MANAGEMENT

The most conservative treatment of foot infections is antibiotic therapy, but this is not always sufficient to treat aggressive, virulent cases.[86] Surgical intervention may be in the best interest of the patient if conservative therapy is not an option or has proven ineffective. Options should be discussed frankly with the patient and the family. Explain the necessity of surgical debridement of all osteomyelitis and nonviable tissue.[87] Reassure them that the surgeon will preserve as much length and width as possible to balance the motor function.[8] Finally, emphasize that the goal of amputation is reconstruction and ambulation.

Metatarsal osteotomies can eliminate the intrinsic stresses caused by elongated or plantarflexed metatarsal joints in neuropathic limbs and decrease the number of amputations.[88] Toe resections are the most distal amputation choices available. Expected outcomes of each toe resection are as follows:

- First toe—Interphalangeal disarticulation for an infected distal phalanx gives good balance. When possible, a wafer of the proximal phalanx should be left to maintain the position of the sesamoids beneath the first metatarsal head.
- Second toe—Disarticulation results in loss of lateral support of the first toe. A second ray resection is usually better to avoid secondary hallux valgus.
- Third or fourth toes—The remaining toes will tend to shift to close the gap.
- All five toes—A long forefoot lever is left with good weight-bearing properties.[8]

The advantages of the partial foot amputation are the following:

- It preserves end weight-bearing function.
- It preserves proprioception.
- It provides for limited disruption of body image.
- It requires only shoe modification/orthosis or limited prosthesis. Limitations of the partial foot amputation are the loss of normal foot function related to loss of forefoot lever length and associated muscles, and the challenges presented in selecting appropriate adaptive equipment.

The Chopart's amputation is selected when a patient retains sensation in the heel pad. Metatarsals and tarsals are removed, leaving a very short limb. It is difficult to suspend a shoe without the aid of an AFO or prosthesis.

The transmetatarsal/Lisfranc amputation is preferred for the resultant length of foot; amputation is through the metatarsals. The longest partial foot amputation is the distal metatarsal amputation, in which the toes are amputated. This level will require a short shoe or forefoot block to prevent forward motion.

In all partial feet, it is important to watch for an equinus deformity. The toes are no longer present, and visual inspection is more difficult without their reference.

Whether from trauma or chronic infection, the partial removal of the calcaneus is a follow-up challenge for the orthotist. Removing weight bearing from the heel is difficult, and the patient who has had a calcanectomy must be followed carefully.

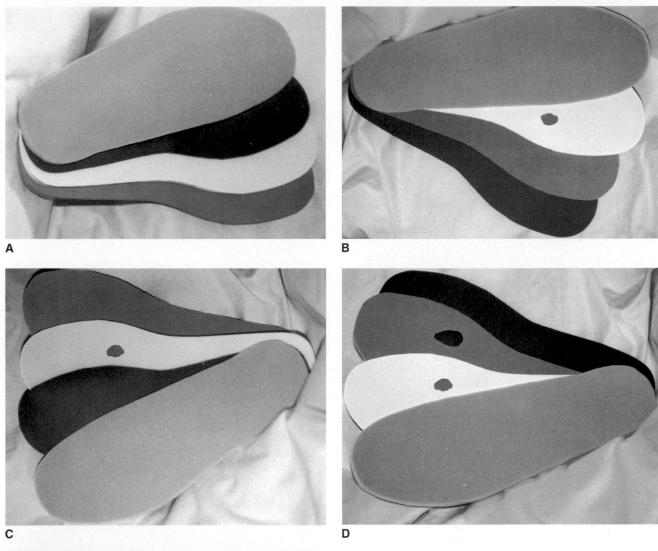

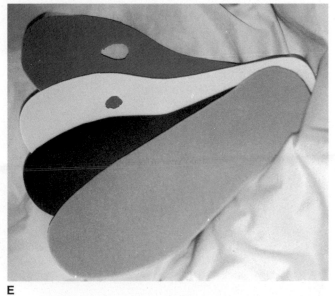

FIGURE 12.41 A: Plantar layers provide immediate in-clinic off-loading of wounds using four color-coded materials of varying durometers. **B:** Upon the healing of the ulceration, the material order is changed to utilize the shoe as an off-loading house shoe. **C:** Superficial wounds (Wagner grade 0 + 1) use one off-loading modified layer. **D:** Wagner grade 2+ ulcerations will require two off-loading layers. **E:** Upon healing of the superficial layer, the order of the materials is changed to provide an off-loading shoe for home ambulation.

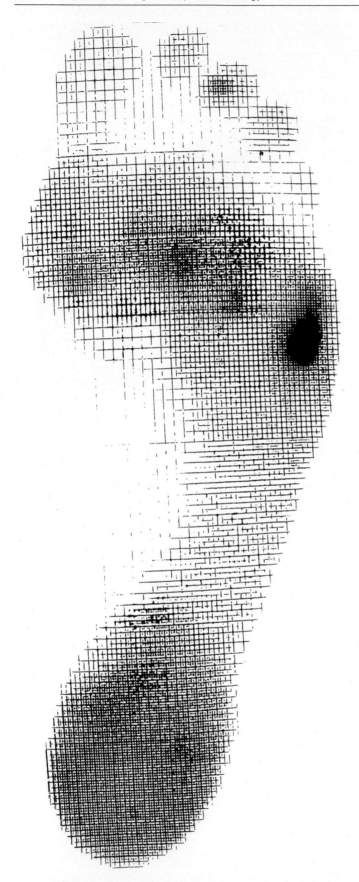

FIGURE 12.42 Floor reaction imprint (Harris mat) serves as pattern for plantar off-loading. (Courtesy of National Pedorthic Services Inc, Milwaukee, Wisconsin.)

The most successful methods of controlling future breakdown have involved the patellar tendon-bearing (axial resist) orthosis or the neuropathic walker. A soft RTV foam has been used to fill a void between the orthosis and the heel area. The same orthotic treatment is useful for chronic heel ulcers and plantar skin grafts that require reduction in weight-bearing and shear forces.

CARE OF THE SKIN AND NAILS OF THE NEUROPATHIC FOOT

Routine noninvasive skin and nail care is vital to promote foot health in patients with peripheral neuropathy. The medical community has long recognized the need for this skilled area of clinical expertise. You should also teach basic foot care to the patient and family, and encourage them to examine the patient's feet daily for early detection of complications.

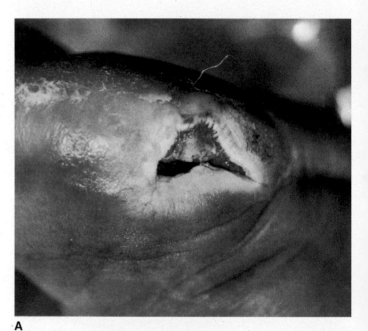

FIGURE 12.43 A: Lateral foot ulceration, not a weight-bearing surface. **B:** Upper construction allows relief of pressure for nonplantar ulcerations without window edema consequence.

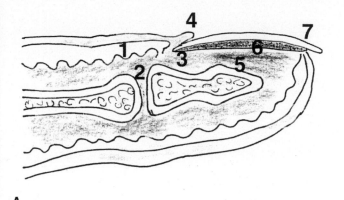

A

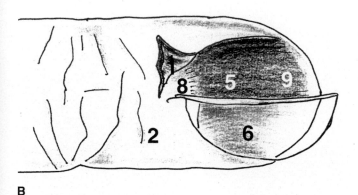

B

FIGURE 12.44 A: Anatomy of the nail. Cross section. **B:** Nail diagram. (1) nail matrix, (2) nail root, (3) nail fold, (4) eponychium, (5) nail bed, (6) nail body, (7) free edge, (8) lunula, (9) hyponychium.

This section includes the procedures, implements, and techniques for optimal results.

It is important to promote conditions as close as possible to normal skin for neuropathic patients because they already have compromised utility of the skin's attributes. With routine care, the performance of the skin as protection of the body can be improved.[89]

Nails are composed of hard keratin, a modification of the horny epidermal cells of the skin. The white crescent shape of the lunula at the proximal end of each nail is caused by air mixed in the keratin matrix. The nail plate originates from the proximal nail fold and attaches to the nail bed (Fig. 12.44A,B).

CLINICAL WISDOM

Facts About Nails

- Nails grow approximately 0.1 mm per day, or 3 mm per month.
- Nails grow faster in daytime and summer.
- Fever and serious illness slow growth rates.
- Pregnancy enhances growth.
- Nails grow more rapidly in men and young people than in women and the elderly.
- Toenails grow one-half to one-third the rate of finger nails.[90]

It grows about 1 mm per week unless inhibited by disease. Regeneration of a lost toenail occurs in 6 to 8 months.[89]

Noninvasive Skin and Nail Care

Before beginning skin and nail care, thoroughly inspect feet and ankles for breaks in the skin. Look for ulcers, heel fissures, maceration between the toes, or imbedded objects. When nails are neglected and overgrown, they can break the skin of the neighboring toe. Abnormal nails that are not given routine care can accumulate excess keratin and debris under the nails and in the nail folds, creating an ideal environment for bacteria to grow.[91] Poor hygiene necessitates routine foot care. The poorly managed foot will require professional treatment twice a month until the skin and nails are conditioned; routine care can be managed monthly. All tools should be cleaned and sterilized, or disposed of, to reduce cross-contamination. The procedure for basic skin and nail care for neuropathic feet is discussed here and illustrated in Figure 12.45A–H:

1. Wash hands and prepare sterilized tools (Fig. 12.45A).
2. Submerge feet into warm water (not to exceed 95°F, use thermometer). You can also use water, that is three parts water to one part vinegar. Vinegar softens the skin and nails.[92]
3. While wearing gloves, make a paste of baby shampoo (or any mild soap) and baking soda in the palm of your hand and gently massage over the entire foot.
4. Rinse and wrap feet individually in towels.
5. Expose toes and apply Blue Cross cuticle remover.
6. Using the curette, gently remove dead skin and loose cuticle from the toes (Fig. 12.45B).
7. Rinse.
8. Using the nail clippers, cut the nail straight across. Do not cut what you cannot see. Always have good lighting (Fig. 12.45C).
9. Thinner, more fragile nails can be cut using the smaller cuticle nippers (Fig. 12.45D).
10. Ingrown toenails are a puncture wound. To prevent them, use the ingrown nail file to smooth sharp corners that can dig into the skin (Fig. 12.45E).
11. Smooth rough edges of nails with an emery board. The patient may take the emery board home for self-care (Fig. 12.45F).
12. Massage emollient into feet but not between toes. Avoid lotions with fragrance, because they contain alcohol that will dry the skin. Vaseline, lanolin, or even Crisco may be used as a moisture barrier to contain the moisture within the skin. Remind the patient to use caution when using emollient to prevent slipping and falling. Removing excess and covering with socks will help to minimize the hazard.
13. Educate the patient regarding appropriate footwear.

There are nails that are difficult to trim. The safest way to trim the pincer nail is to file it straight across, rather than to risk cutting the skin (Fig. 12.45G). Some nails have grown into a "tent" shape. This tenting is usually caused by years of wearing pointed shoes. When trimming this type of nail, be aware of the skin under the nail at the dorsal apex. A condition called *onycholysis*, separation of the nail plate from the nail bed, can be caused by nail traumas and disorders. If onycholysis has been present for an extended period (6 months or more), the structure of

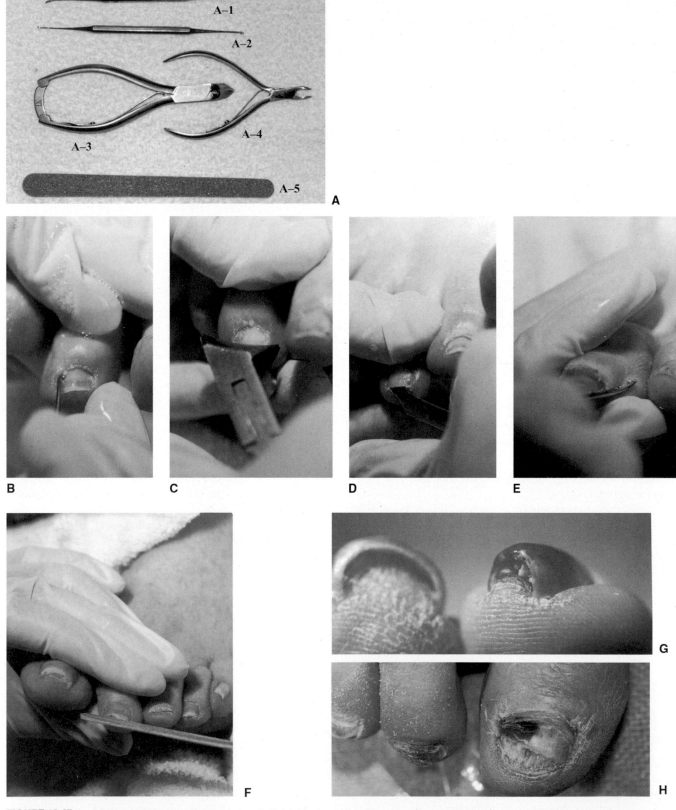

FIGURE 12.45 A: Tools for nail care: (1) ingrown nail file, (2) curette, (3) clippers, (4) cuticle nippers, (5) emery board. **B:** Use curette to loosen and remove debris. **C:** Clippers to cut nails. **D:** Cuticle nipper for fragile nails and small spaces. **E:** Ingrown nail file to round sharp corners. **F:** Emery board to smooth edges. **G:** Pincer nail. **H:** Nail with hematoma.

the nail bed can change, and the nail plate will no longer attach to the nail bed. At this point, the condition becomes permanent. Keep the patient's nails short to prevent them from catching on surroundings and tearing off.[93] Some patients will have nails that are atrophied, due to their illness. Figure 12.45H reveals an atrophied nail with a hematoma.

Care of Heel Fissures

Patients with autonomic neuropathy can have very dry, nonelastic skin, due to the lack of sweat and oil production. Deep heel fissures develop from the dry skin, creating an opportunity for bacteria and debris to invade the skin, causing ulcerations and infection (Fig. 12.46A).

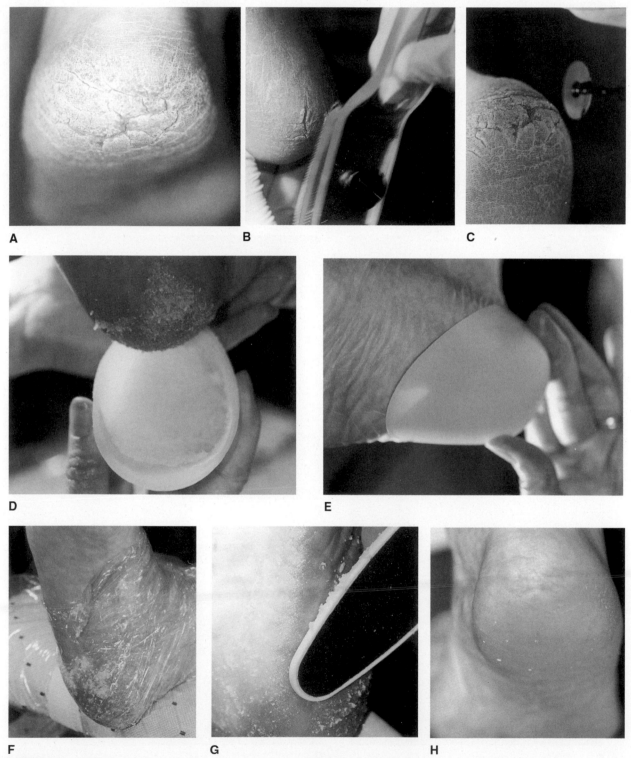

FIGURE 12.46 **A:** Heel fissures: dry, cracking hyperkeratotic heel. **B:** Callus reducer; used dry on dry skin. **C:** Dremel tool to reduce callus. **D:** Heel cup to concentrate basic callus paste. **E:** Heel cup on foot. **F:** Plastic wrap to apply and contain basic callus paste on large areas. **G:** Foot file to exfoliate heel callus. **H:** Heel fissures after first treatment.

EXHIBIT **12.4**

Back to Basics Paste

1 cup kosher salt
1/2 cup Epsom salts
8 tbsp baking soda
8 tbsp mineral oil

Care of heel fissures begins with the basic callus care procedure. Use a dry callus reducer on dry skin with one-directional strokes. A Dremel tool is a cordless, rotary tool with disposable abrasive disks. With proper training, you can use this tool in the same fashion as a callus reducer to remove very thick hyperkeratotic skin. It is important for you and the patient to wear coverings for your eyes, nose, mouth, and hair, because use of the Dremel tool generates airborne particles. Use of a HEPA air filter device would give added protection. Do not attempt to finish a difficult case in one session; several appointments will be required to reduce the build-up. The procedure for care of heel fissures is discussed here and shown in Figure 12.46B–H:

1. Wash hands and don gloves.
2. Use the callus reducer (Fig. 12.46B) or Dremel tool (Fig. 12.46C) to decrease the hyperkeratotic thickness.
3. Wrap the foot in a warm, moist towel for 5 minutes.
4. Remove towel, apply Vick's VapoRub™ to heel, followed by Back to Basics Callus Paste (Fig. 12.46D, Exhibit 12.4). The paste can be held in place with a plastic heel cup or plastic wrap, followed by a towel wrap, for 10 minutes (Fig. 12.46E,F).
5. Unwrap foot and remove paste from the heel with a wet foot file (Fig. 12.46G).
6. Rinse the foot and apply a moisture barrier emollient (Fig. 12.46H).
7. Wipe excess emollient off and don socks and shoes.

Once the patient's feet are conditioned, routine foot care can be maintained with 4- to 6-week follow-up appointments.

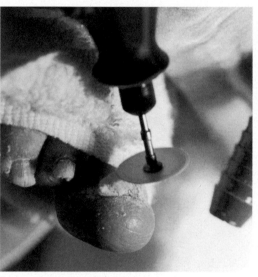

A

B

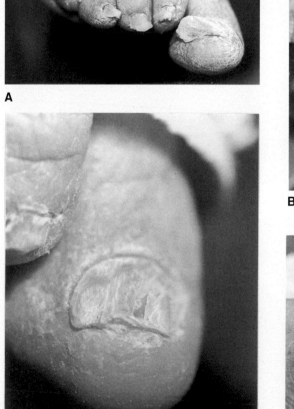

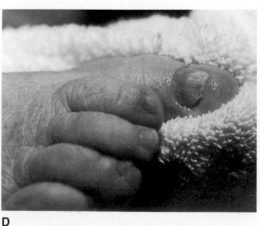

C

D

FIGURE 12.47 **A:** Reducing hypertrophic nails: hypertrophic nails. **B:** Dremel tool to reduce nail thickness. **C:** Reduced nail with raised nail bed. **D:** Completed nail procedure after conditioning.

Care of the Hypertrophic Nail (Onychauxis)

The hypertrophic nail may be caused by damage to the matrix, fungal infection, age, and/or vascular complications. Hypertrophic nails that have been neglected need to be thinned to make shoe fit possible and to prevent secondary infections due to traumatization of the prominent nail.

The most effective and expedient method for thinning the nail is to use the cordless rotary Dremel tool as described in the previous procedure. Follow these steps for reducing hypertrophic nails (Fig. 12.47A–D):

1. Wash hands, don gloves, mask, eye shield, and hair covering. Instruct patient to put on similar coverings.
2. Examine the skin around the nail for damage (Fig. 12.47A).
3. If there are no signs of broken skin or infection, secure toe with thumb and index fingers and move other toes away from the working area.
4. Turn Dremel on and move sanding disc in a proximal to distal direction, with slow, even strokes until nail is thinned (Fig. 12.47B). Take care when thinning the nail, as you may encounter a raised nail bed (Fig. 12.47C).
5. Wash and dry the thinned nail and apply a conditioning agent such as Tineacide. Use of this or comparable product will allow future nail care to be more effective by keeping the nail and surrounding skin conditioned (Fig. 12.47D).

Care of a Callus (Hyperkeratosis)

A callus typically forms in an area of high pressures and shear forces, typically on the plantar surface. It is the body's protective mechanism for an area of chronic irritation. To the neuropathic patient, the callus is indicative of chronic trauma (repetitive stress injury) that may lead to skin breakdown and serious complications.[94] Lack of sensation prevents the neuropathic patient from reacting to high pressures that can produce an ulceration.

Reduction of callus is required on an ongoing basis to prevent ulceration. The majority of plantar ulcerations in neuropathic patients are located in the forefoot, especially at the great toe and first, second, and fifth metatarsal heads.[91]

The procedure for callus reduction is as follows:

1. Wash hands.
2. Don gloves and hold foot securely with one hand. In the other hand, use the dry callus reducer in one direction over the dry callused area. When the screen fills with debris, tap on a hard surface, clear the screen, and continue the process. After the callus is reduced, give the screen to the patient with instructions on home use.

CLINICAL WISDOM

Callus Care

Avoid corn medications that can produce chemical burns; they contain salicylic acid. Vick's VapoRub™ will act quickly to soften the hardened skin. Petrolatum is the daily treatment to provide a moisture barrier after bathing.

CLINICAL WISDOM

Bathroom Surgery

Remind patients to never perform "bathroom surgery." Self-inflicted wounds due to razor blades and other sharp objects are common with patients who lack protective sensation.

3. When the callus is reduced, ulceration may be revealed under the callus (Fig. 12.49). Reduce the callus but do not open the skin. An off-loading insole will be necessary to reduce the pressure and shear to the area.
4. Once the callus is reduced, wrap the foot in a warm, moist towel for 5 minutes.
5. Remove the towel and apply Vick's VapoRub™, followed with Back to Basics Paste (see Exhibit 12.4). Cover with plastic wrap and towel for 10 minutes.
6. Gently remove paste with foot file, rinse, and pat dry.
7. The patient may need to be seen weekly to reduce the callus in stages.
8. Assess footwear to determine what is causing callus formation. Therapeutic depth shoes with accommodative inserts should be worn by all patients with neuropathic feet.[91]

You can also use a cordless Dremel rotary tool to reduce callus:

1. When learning to use the Dremel, begin with the less powerful Mini-Mite cordless model until skills are developed. Practicing on hoof trimmings purchased from a pet supply company will give similar experience to working on callus and hypertrophic nails. When proficient, the more powerful Multi-Pro model can be used.
2. When using a Dremel, thin the callus thickness by sanding in one direction (proximal to distal). Do not work in an area for a long period because the prolonged friction can cause overheating at the skin surface.
3. Continue with steps 2 through 7 in the procedure for callus reduction above.

SELF-CARE TEACHING GUIDELINES

The patient is the most important member of the clinical team caring for a neuropathic limb. Teach the patient that no complication is too small to bring to the team's attention.

Foot Inspection

Self-care begins with daily inspections of the feet, with the help of mirrors, magnifying glasses, and family members, when necessary. Examination includes footwear and orthotics for wear and foreign objects. The diabetic patient must understand that their own ability to perform this examination effectively may be complicated by other disease processes, including retinopathy, autonomic neuropathy (loss of smell and sensory signals), and decreased mobility of joints. They may therefore need to recruit family members to assist them. Overall, patients and family members require systematic instruction in the proper skills required for daily foot inspection and detection of impending trauma.

The neuropathic patient may neglect foot care. Figure 12.48A–D is a pictorial case study of a neuropathic patient who neglected regular foot and nail care. In spite of the overgrown, hypertrophic nails and callus formation, he continued to don his socks and shoes. Once foot and nail care were initiated, the skin and nails improved in appearance and there was reduced risk of injury to adjacent skin.

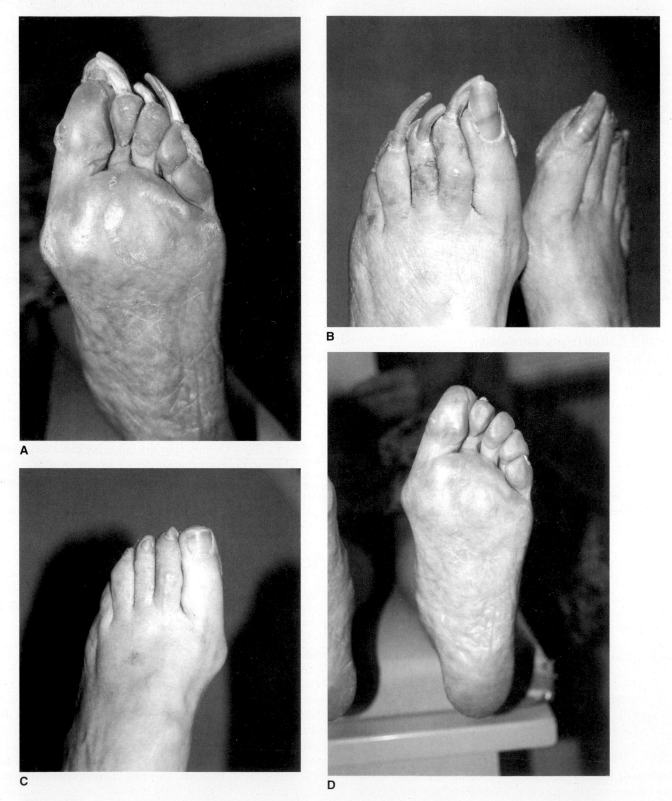

FIGURE 12.48 **A:** The neuropathic patient may neglect foot care. The patient continues to don shoes over excessive nail growth. **B:** The neuropathic patient may neglect foot care. The patient continues to don shoes over excessive nail growth. **C:** Condition of feet after an extensive foot care procedure. **D:** Condition of feet after an extensive foot care procedure.

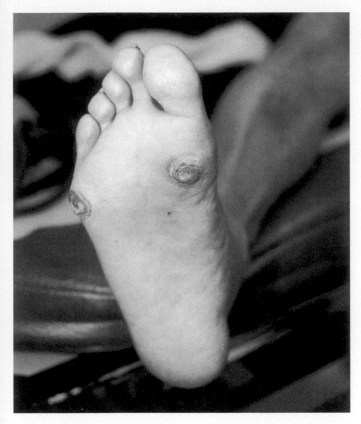

FIGURE 12.49 Foot requiring callus reduction and redistribution of weight-bearing forces at first and fifth metatarsal head.

Precautions and Risk Reduction Methods

There are several precautions for the patient with a neuropathic limb. The skin is very susceptible to damage and infection, and it must be treated carefully. It is advised that the patient not soak the feet in water because the chance of burns is always present, and the soaking will leave the skin moist and susceptible to fungal infection. Prolonged soaking can remove the natural protective barrier from the skin and lead to other infections. Feet should be washed with a nondrying soap, then towel-dried. After drying, petroleum jelly can be applied to retain natural moisture and the feet covered with socks. Care should be taken not to use creams with perfumes (alcohol), because they will further dehydrate the skin.

Dehydrated skin is especially susceptible to trauma. Adhesives of any form should never be applied directly to the skin of a neuropathic limb. On removal of the adhesive, there is a risk of loss of the outer layer of skin, leaving an area open to infection. The adhesives could be in the form of tape, a Band-Aid, or over-the-counter self-adhesive pads.

In selecting footwear, the patient should choose not only the correct size and width but also shoes with no stitching over the forefoot. The stitched areas will never mold to the foot; instead, they will cause breakdown of the skin, especially over bony areas. Socks should be seamless and without holes or repairs (Fig. 12.50). Tube socks do not contour to the foot without folds that can cause irritation, and therefore should not be used. The fabric of the socks should be a blend of fibers to wick perspiration, and should be non-constricting at the calf. The choice of white or light colors will enable the patient to

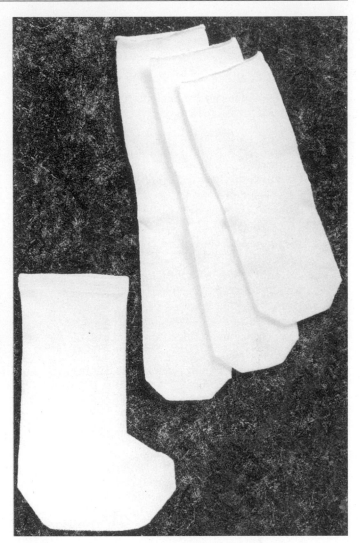

FIGURE 12.50 Specialty socks designed for the neuropathic partial and macerated foot. (Courtesy of Knit rite, Inc., Kansas City, Kansas.)

easily detect drainage due to trauma. When breaking in new shoes, the patient should wear two thin socks on each foot. The double socks will allow shear to occur between them and will decrease the probability of blistering from new leather.

Patients with a partial foot need special socks made of highly elastic fibers. The sock shape will conform to the partial foot length and shape. The single size fits a Chopart's amputation, as well as a long transmetatarsal amputation. There are no folds or seams to cause friction.

Toe socks decrease maceration between toes (see Fig. 12.50). The moist environment between the toes encourages fungal growth and may lead to ulceration and bacterial infection. The seamless construction helps to reduce overlapping of lesser toes but must be compensated for in shoe size. Advise patients to keep current on product recalls and warnings. For example, one hair removal system published a product alert on its device because of problems occurring with diabetic patients. Small areas were bleeding after hair was removed, leaving an entrance for bacteria and possible infection! Over 50% of the over-the-counter foot care products should never be used by a patient with a neuropathic limb or diabetes. There are occasionally warnings, but they are in very fine print.

EXHIBIT 12.5

Self-Care Guidelines for the Patient with Neuropathic Foot

Self-Care Guidelines for Patient with Neuropathic Foots	Instructions Given (Date/Initials)	Demonstration or Review of Material (Date/Initials)	Return Demonstration or States Understanding (Date/Initials)
1. Foot Inspection Methods a. Use mirror to check feet b. Use magnifying glass to check feet c. If blind, family member performs foot inspection			
2. Foot Inspection Item a. Toe nails: check for broken, cracked, or sharp nails b. Broken skin: check between toes, along sides of feet, tops and ends of toes, sole of foot c. Soft toe corns: check between toes d. Callus: check for cracks e. Drainage: check for any drainage from a sore f. Odor: check for odor from any source on the foot			
3. Patient Understands a. Significance of findings of foot inspection: break in nails, skin, or callus b. When to notify health-care provider if there is break in nails, skin, or callus c. To notify health-care provider immediately if there is any injury to the feet			
4. Foot Care Routine a. Wash feet with nondrying soap and towel dry b. Apply coating of petroleum jelly to all skin surfaces of feet c. Cover coated feet with clean white socks			
5. Foot Care Precautions a. Never walk barefoot b. Never use adhesive tape products on the skin c. Never put feet in hot water or apply a heating pad or hot pack d. Never soak feet e. Never apply over-the-counter foot care products to remove corns or callus, or to treat nails			
6. Shoe Wear Orthotic Inspection a. Choose shoes that are correct size and width b. Make sure there is no stitching over the forefoot of shoe c. Check for wear: heels, soles, tops, inside, bottom, edges, counter d. Always check shoes, socks, and orthotics for foreign objects; remove objects before donning			
7. Exercise Precautions a. Never jog b. Walk with short, slow steps			
8. Preferred Exercises a. Aerobic: low impact b. Swimming (wear soft bathing shoes in water to protect feet, dry feet thoroughly following) c. Cycling: protect feet and ankles from trauma d. Dancing e. Chair and mat exercises			
9. Importance of Follow-Up with Health-Care Provider			

Patients must also take care when choosing a form of exercise. Teach the patient that, when we walk, each step carries one and one-half times our body weight; jogging increases the force to three times the body weight.[95] The patient with a neuropathic limb would be advised to choose an exercise program that includes aerobics, swimming, cycling, dance, or chair exercises. Even walking should include slow, short steps only—no jogging.[96]

It is critical to teach the patient with a neuropathic limb never to walk barefoot. Even in the pool or on the beach, water shoes should be worn. Hot sand can cause burns, and undetected objects in the sand can cause injury. Burns can be caused by the floorboard of an automobile, as well as by any warmth-producing equipment.

Finally, patients should examine the interior of their shoes before every donning. Small objects can easily drop into a shoe.

Compliance/Acceptance Issues

Given these many instructions in self-care, it is not surprising that compliance/acceptance problems arise in patients with neuropathic limbs, especially diabetic patients. Bear in mind that they do not willfully neglect self-care activities, but simply are not aware of the possible dangers and may not have received adequate instruction or motivational messages.[2] Patients with peripheral neuropathy may also have other complications that reduce compliance. Many cannot see (retinopathy), feel (sensory neuropathy), or smell (autonomic neuropathy) that there is an infection or a potential problem. This is one reason that it is important to solicit help from a family member or caregiver in adhering to self-care guidelines.

Exhibit 12.5 is a checklist of instructional items with documentation to verify learning and understanding for the patient with neuropathic foot.

CONCLUSION

As the population ages, the medical community will be faced with the increasing demand for basic, noninvasive foot care with minimal risk of transmitted infections and skin conditions. Attention to foot care has become a recognized requirement for aging and, especially, neuropathic patients. Healthcare professionals are seeking information and specialized training relating to foot care in the clinical setting. Their efforts are being rewarded with fewer amputations, and patients are being educated in self-care. Self-care has allowed early detection and medical attention to conditions that would otherwise result in catastrophic events. Routine foot care is an integral part of comprehensive care for the neuropathic patient, and its presence will greatly improve the quality of life to those in the greatest need. See Chapter 13 for more information about foot and nail care in the nondiabetic foot.

REVIEW QUESTIONS

1. Motor neuropathy involves
   A. No sense of identity with the feet
   B. Loss of intrinsic muscles
   C. Absence of sweat production
   D. All of the above
2. Upper and lower peripheral neuropathy is present when
   A. Sensation loss in both legs is symmetrical
   B. Sensation loss in both arms and legs is asymmetric and equidistant from the spine
   C. Sensation loss in both arms and legs is symmetric and equidistant from the spine
   D. Sensation loss in both legs is asymmetrical
3. Objectives for taking temperatures are
   A. To evaluate baseline temperature at the site of high ulceration
   B. To determine the presence of inflammation
   C. To evaluate baseline temperatures after pressure has been relieved
   D. All of the above
4. Characteristics of a Charcot foot includes
   A. Microtraumas to joints leading to microfractures
   B. Decrease in blood flow
   C. Absence of trophic changes in joints
   D. Decrease in bone reabsorption
5. Expected outcomes of each toe resection are
   A. First toe: poor balance
   B. Second toe: loss of medial support
   C. Third or fourth toes: remaining toes will shift to close the gap
   D. All five toes: poor weight-bearing properties

RESOURCES

Acor Orthopedic
18530 South Miles Pkwy Cleveland, OH 44128 (800) 237-2267 fax (216) 662-4547 Materials/fabrication tools Prefab orthoses Custom and diabetic shoes

Alimed, Inc.
297 High Street Dedham, MA 02026 (800) 225-2610 fax (800) 437-2966 Materials/wound supplies Wheel chairs/positioning Specialty diabetic products

Apex Foot Health
170 Wesley St. South Hackensack, NJ 07606 (800) 526-2739 fax (800) 526-0073 Materials/tools Prefab orthoses Modifiable footwear

Boston Brace International
20 Ledin Dr. Avon, MA 02322 (800) 262-2235 fax (800) 634-5048 Soft ankle foot orthosis (AFO)

Brown Medical Industries
481 South 8th Ave. East Hartley, IA 51346 (800) 843-4395 fax (712) 336-2874 Cast and bandage protector

Comfort Products, Inc.
705 Linton Ave. Croydon, PA 19021 (800) 822-7500 fax (215) 785-5737 Diabetic socks

Darco International, Inc.
810 Memorial Blvd. Huntington, WV 25701 (800) 999-8866 fax (304) 522-0037 Wound healing shoe system P/O med/surg shoe/cast boot Neuropathic shoes/walker

Deltatrak, Inc.
5653 Stoneridge Dr. Pleasanton, CA 94588 (800) 962-6776 fax (925) 467-5949 Infrared thermometer

Ipos, North America, Inc.
2045 Niagara Falls Blvd. #8 Niagara Falls, NY 14304 (800) 626-2612 fax (716) 297-0153 Heel and forefoot relief shoes

Juzo-Julius Zorn, Inc.
P.O. Box 1088 Cuyahoga Falls, OH 44223 (800) 222-4999 fax (800) 645-2519 Neuropathic/compression stockings Sleeves/gloves/gauntlets Prosthetic shrinker/suspension

Knit-Rite, Inc.
120 Osage Ave. Kansas City, KA 66105 (800) 821-3094 fax (800) 462-4707 Diabetic/partial foot socks Prosthetic socks/shrinkers Prosthetic suspension

Measurements, Inc.
2946 Ponce de Leon New Orleans, LA 70119 (504) 949-1192 fax (504) 943-3489 Infrared thermometer

Moore Medical, Inc.
389 John Downey Dr. New Britain, CT 06050 (800) 234-1464 fax (800) 944-6667 Wound care supplies/material Tools/tube foam/crest pad support Medical supplies

North Coast Medical, Inc.
187 Stouffer Blvd. San Jose, CA 95125-1042 (800) 821-9319 fax (408) 277-6824 Monofilaments

Theradynamics
7283 W. Appleton Ave. (800) 803-7813 fax (414) 438-1051 Milwaukee, WI 53216 Floor reaction imprint (Harris) Material/fabrication equipment Prefabricated orthoses

UCO International, Inc.
16 E. Piper Ln. # 130 Prospect Heights, IL 60070 (800) 541-4030 fax (847) 541-4144 Material/specialty pads (MTH) Tools and equipment Prefabricated orthoses

Care of the Skin and Nail of the Neuropathic Foot Resources

Antoine de Paris
P.O. Box 1310 Solvang, CA 93464 (805) 688-0666 fax (805) 686-00330 (800) 222-3243 Pedicure tools Nail clipper #30 Cuticle nipper #14 Ingrown nail file #86

Moore Medical Products
389 John Downey Dr.
P.O. Box 2740 New Britain, CT 06060-2740 (800) 234-1464 http://www.mooremedical.com Tube foam Lamb's wool Curette Dremel tool

Sally's Beauty Supply (nationwide franchise)
Blue Cross cuticle remover Foot files Emery boards

Tineacide
(800) 307-8818

REFERENCES

1. Brenner M. *Management of the Diabetic Foot.* Baltimore, MD: Williams & Wilkins; 1987.
2. Shipley D. Clinical evaluation and care of the insensitive foot. *Phys Ther.* 1979;59:13–22.
3. Bowker J. Commentary. *Diabetes Spectr.* 1992;5:335.
4. Veves A, Boulton A. Commentary. *Diabetes Spectr.* 1992;5:336–337.
5. Green D, Waldhausl W. A forum on neuropathy. *Diabetes.* 1988;10.
6. Ellenberg M. Diabetic neuropathic ulcer. *J Mt Sinai Hosp.* 1968;35:585–594.
7. Bowker J. Neurological aspects of prosthetic/orthotic practice. *J Prosthet Orthot.* 1993;5(2):52–54.
8. Bowker J. Partial foot and Syme amputations: an overview. *Clin Prosthet Orthot.* 1987;12:10–13.
9. Letts M. The orthotics of myelomeningocele. In: *Atlas of Orthotics.* St. Louis, MO: CV Mosby; 1985;300–306.
10. Nouvong A, Hoogwerf B, Mohler E, et al. Evaluation of diabetic foot ulcer healing with hyperspectral imaging of oxyhemoglobin and deoxyhemoglobin. *Diabetes Care.* 2009;32(11):2056–2061.
11. Weingarten M. Commentary. *Diabetes Spectr.* 1992;5:342–343.
12. Pecoraro R, Reiber G, Burgess E. Pathways to diabetic limb amputation: basis for prevention. *Diabetes Care.* 1990;13:513–521.
13. Fylling C. Conclusions. *Diabetes Spectr.* 1992;5:358–359.
14. Bamberger D, Stark K. Severe diabetic foot problems: avoiding amputation. *Emerg Decis.* 1987;3(8):21–34.
15. Olin J. Peripheral arterial disease. *Diabetes Forecast.* October 1992;78–81.
16. Newman B. A diabetes camp for Native American adults. *Diabetes Spectr.* 1993;6:166–202.
17. Harkness L, Lavery L. Diabetes foot care: A team approach. *Diabetes Spectr.* 1992;5:136–137.
18. Jerrell M. Management of the diabetic foot. *O & P Bus News* August 2005;28–33.
19. Robbins D. Office guide to diagnosis and classification of diabetes mellitus and other categories of glucose tolerance. *Diabetes Care.* 1991;14(Suppl 2):3–4.
20. Brand P. Neuropathic ulceration. *The Star.* May/June 1983:1–4.
21. Brand P. Management of sensory loss in the extremities: management of peripheral nerve problems. *J Rehab.* 1980;862–872.
22. Ashbury A. Foot care in patients with diabetes mellitus. *Diabetes Care.* 1991;14(Suppl 2):18–19.
23. Brand P. *Insensitive Feet—A Practical Handout on Foot Problems in Leprosy.* London, UK: The Leprosy Mission; 1977.
24. Jahss M. Shoes and shoe modifications. In: *Atlas of Orthotics.* St. Louis, MO: CV Mosby; 1985:267–279.
25. Tsairis P. Differential diagnosis of peripheral neuropathies. In: *Management of Peripheral Nerve Problems.* Rancho los Amigos; 1980:712–725.
26. Thomas P. Clinical features and differential diagnosis. In: *Peripheral Neuropathy.* vol. 2. Philadelphia, PA: WB Saunders; 1984:1169–1185.
27. Wakelee-Lynch J. Relieving pain with peppers. *Diabetes Forecast.* June 1992;35–37.
28. Dailey G. Effect of treatment with capsaicin on daily activities of patients with painful diabetic neuropathy. *Diabetes Care.* 1992;15:159–165.
29. *Diabetes Mellitus: Management and Complications.* New York, NY: Churchill Livingstone; 1985:234–235, 277–293, 360–361.
30. Apelqvist J, Castenfors J, Larsson J. Prognostic value of systolic ankle and toe blood pressure levels in outcome of diabetic foot ulcer. *Diabetes Care.* 1989;12:373–378.
31. Cherry G, Ryan T, Cameron J. Blueprint for the treatment of leg ulcers and the prevention of recurrence. *Wounds.* 1992;3:1–15.
32. Field M. The use of garments to create compression. *Biomech Desk Ref.* 6:139–140.
33. Perry J. Normal and pathological gait. In: *Atlas of Orthotics.* St. Louis, MO: CV Mosby; 1985:83–96.

34. Mann R. Biomechanics of the foot. In: *Atlas of Orthotics*. St. Louis, MO: CV Mosby; 1985:112–125.

35. Thomas P, Eliasson S. Diabetic neuropathy. In: *Peripheral Neuropathy*. vol. 2. Philadelphia, PA: WB Saunders; 1984:1773–1801.

36. Boughton B. Experts debate long and short of limb length discrepancy. *Biomechanics*. 2000;7:139–140.

37. Oakley W, Catterall R, Martin M. Aetiology and management of lesions of the feet in diabetes. *Br Med J*. 1956;56:4999–5003.

38. Sussman C, Strauss M, Barry D, et al. Consideration of the motor neuropathy for managing the neuropathic foot. *J O & P Suppl*. 2005;17(2):s28–s31.

39. Cailliet R. *Foot and Ankle Pain*. Philadelphia, PA: F.A. Davis; 1983:181–189.

40. Yale J. *Yale's Podiatric Medicine*. 3rd ed. Baltimore, MD: Williams & Wilkins; 1980:135–136.

41. Wilson J, Foster D. *Textbook of Endocrinology*. Philadelphia, PA: WB Saunders; 1992:1294–1297.

42. Olefsky J, Sherman R. Diabetes. In: *Insensitive Feet—A Practical Handout on Foot Problems in Leprosy*. London, UK: The Leprosy Mission; 1977.

43. Yale J. *Yale's Podiatric Medicine*. 3rd ed. Baltimore, MD: Williams & Wilkins; 1980:159–160.

44. Yale J. *Yale's Podiatric Medicine*. 3rd ed. Baltimore, MD: Williams & Wilkins; 1980.

45. Wagner FEW. The dysvascular foot: a system for diagnosis and treatment. *Foot Ankle*. 1981;2:64–122.

46. Wagner F. A classification and treatment program for diabetic, neuropathic and dysvascular foot problems. *Foot Ankle*. 1983;1–47.

47. Birke J, Sims D. Plantar sensory threshold in the ulcerative foot. *Br Lepr Relief Assoc*. 1986;57:261–267.

48. Birke J. Management of the diabetic foot. *Wound Care Manage*. 1995.

49. Ashbury A. Diabetic neuropathy. *Diabetes Care*. 1991;14 (Suppl 2):63–68.

50. Thivolet C, Farkh J, Petiot A. Measuring vibration sensations with graduated tuning fork. *Diabetes Care*. 1990;13:1077–1080.

51. National Aeronautics and Space Administration. Mission accomplished (thermography aids in the detection of neuromuscular problems). *NASA Tech Brief*. January 1993:92.

52. Apelqvist J, Larsson J, Agardh C. The influence of external precipitating factors and peripheral neuropathy on the development and outcome of diabetic foot ulcers. *J Diabetic Complications*. 1990;4:21–25.

53. Barber E. Strength and range-of-motion examination skills for the clinical orthotist. *J Prosthet Orthot*. 1993;5(2):49–51.

54. Huntley A. Taking care of your hands. *Diabetes Forecast*. August 1991;11–12.

55. Bergtholdt H. Temperature assessment of the insensate. *Phys Ther*. 1979;59:18–22.

56. Chan A, MacFarlane I, Bowsher D. Contact thermography of painful neuropathic foot. *Diabetes Care*. 1991;14:918–922.

57. Fierheller M, Sibbald RG. A clinical investigation into the relationship between increased periwound skin temperature and local wound infection in patients with chronic leg ulcers. *Adv Skin Wound Care*. 2010;23:369–79.

58. Lavery L, Higgins K, Lanctot D, et al. Home monitoring of skin temperatures to prevent ulceration. *Diabetes Care*. 2004;27:2642–2647.

59. Zhu H, Maalej N, Webster J. An umbilical data acquisition system for measuring pressures between foot and shoe. *IEEE Trans Biomed Eng*. 1990;37:908–911.

60. Lord M. Clinical trial of a computer-aided system for orthopaedic shoe upper design. *Prosthet Orthot Int*. 1991;15:11–17.

61. McAllister D, Carver D, Devarajan R. An interactive computer graphics system for the design of molded and orthopedic shoe lasts. *J Rehabil Res Dev*. 1991;28:39–46.

62. Sims D, Cavanagh P, Ulbrecht J. Risk factors in the diabetic foot: recognition and management. *Phys Ther*. 1988;68:1887–1916.

63. DeJong R. *The Neurologic Examination*. New York, NY: Harper & Row; 1969:742–743.

64. Newman L, Palestro C, Schwartz M. Unsuspected osteomyelitis in diabetic foot ulcers: Diagnosis and monitoring by leukocyte scanning with indium in oxyquinoline. *Diabetes Spectr*. 1992;5:346–347.

65. Lockard M. Foot orthosis. *Phys Ther*. 1988;68:1866–1873.

66. Kuncir E, Wirta R, Golbranson F. Load-bearing characteristics of polyethylene foam: An examination of structural and compression properties. *J Rehabil Res Dev*. 1990;27:229–238.

67. Pratt D. Medium term comparison of shock attenuating insoles using a spectral analysis technique. *J Biomed Eng*. 1988;10:426–428.

68. Pratt D. Long term comparison of shock attenuating insoles. *Prosthet Orthot Int*. 1990;14:59–62.

69. Levin M, O'Neal L. *The Diabetic Foot*. St. Louis, MO: CV Mosby; 1988.

70. Hack M. Fitting shoes. *Diabetes Forecast*. January 1989.

71. McPoil T. Footwear. *Phys Ther*. 1988;68:1857–1865.

72. McPoil T, Adrian M, Pidcoe P. Effects of foot orthoses on center-of-pressure patterns in women. *Phys Ther*. 1989;69:66–71.

73. Coleman W, Brasseau D. Methods of treating plantar ulcers. *Phys Ther*. 1991;71:116–122.

74. Dwyer G, Rust M. Shoe business. *Diabetes Forecast*. June 1988;60–63.

75. Mueller M, Diamond J, Sinacore D. Total contact casting in treatment of diabetic plantar ulcers. *Diabetes Care*. 1989;12:384–388.

76. Sinacore D, Mueller M, Diamond J. Diabetic plantar ulcers treated by total contact casting. *Phys Ther*. 1987;67:1543–1549.

77. Sinacore OR, Elsner R, Rubenow C. *Healing Rates of Diabetic Foot Ulcers in Subjects with Fixed Charcot Deformity*. Platform Presentation, Physical Therapy 1997 APTA Scientific Meeting and Exposition; San Diego, CA: APTA, May 30–June 4, 1997.

78. Birke J, Novick A, Graham S, et al. Methods of treating plantar ulcers. *Phys Ther*. 1991;71:41–47.

79. Diamond J, Sinacore D, Mueller M. Molded double-rocker plaster shoe for healing a diabetic plantar ulcer. *Phys Ther*. 1987;67:1550–1552.

80. Armstrong DG, Lavery LA. Healing the diabetic wound with pressure off-loading. *Biomechanics*. 1997;4:67.

81. Fleischli JG, Laughlin TJ. TCC remains the gold standard for off-loading plantar ulcers. *Biomechanics*. 1998;5:51–52.

82. Giacolone VF. Diabetic footwear: pressure relief modalities. *Podiatr Today*. 1998;10:16–20.

83. Lauridsen K, Sorensen C, Christiansen P. Measurements of pressure on the sole of the foot in plaster of paris casts on the lower leg. *J Int Soc Prosthet Orthot*. 1989;13:42–45.

84. Nawoczenski DA, Birke JA. Management of the neuropathic foot in the elderly. *Top Geriatr Rehab*. 1992;7:36–48.

85. Armstrong DG, Lavery LA, et al. Infrared dermal thermometry for the high-risk diabetic foot. *Phys Ther*. 1997;77:169–171.

86. McIntyre K. Control of infection in the diabetic foot: The role of microbiology, immunopathology, antibiotics, and guillotine amputation. *J Vasc Surg*. 1987;5:787–802.

87. Lai C, Lin S, Yang C. Limb salvage of infected diabetic foot ulcers with microsurgical free-muscle transfer. *Diabetes Spectr*. 1992;5:356–357.

88. Tillow T, Habrshaw G, Chrzan J. Review of metatarsal osteotomies for the treatment of neuropathic ulcerations. *Diabetes Spectr*. 1992;5:357–358.

89. Stanley J. *Structure and Function in Man*. 3rd ed. Philadelphia, PA: WB Saunders; 1974:65–68.

90. Kechiijian P. How do nails grow? *Nails*. May 1993;78–79.

91. O'Neal LW. Surgical pathway of the foot and clinicopathologic conditions. In: Bowker JH, Pfeifer MA, eds. *The Diabetic Foot*. 6th ed. St. Louis, MO: CV Mosby; 2000:501–506.

92. Ruscin C, Cunningham G, Blaylock A. Foot care protocol for the older client. *Geriatr Nurs*. 1993;210–212.

93. Sher RK. The nail doctor. *Nails*. 1977;94–95.

94. Harkless LB, Satterfield VK, Dennis KJ. Role of the podiatrist. In: Bowker JH, Pfeifer MA, eds. *The Diabetic Foot*. 6th ed. St. Louis, MO: CV Mosby; 2000:690.

95. Furman A. Give your feet a sporting chance. *Diabetes Forecast*. April 1989;17–22.

96. Graham C. Neuropathy made you stop. *Diabetes Forecast*. December 1992;47–49.

Teresa J. Kelechi

CHAPTER OBJECTIVES

At the completion of this chapter, the reader will be able to:

1. Describe the clinical presentation and management of three foot problems: tinea pedis, plantar fasciitis, and onychomycosis.
2. Discuss miscellaneous conditions affecting the foot, including xerosis and anhidrosis, hyperhidrosis, cellulitis, maceration, hyperkeratotic lesions, fissures, and onychauxis.
3. Describe four patient education points related to the prevention of foot disorders.
4. List three referral criteria for foot complications.

Foot problems plague approximately 70% of individuals 65 years of age and older.[1] These conditions, which affect the nails, skin, and fascia, require skillful intervention to preserve the patient's functional ability and maintain quality of life. They can also lead to more serious complications, such as infections, wounds, and, in some cases, amputation.[2] Patients with diabetes and impaired circulation can be at greater risk for such complications.[3] Therefore, it is critical that you assess the patient's feet as part of your routine care. Inspect the patient's skin and toenails; investigate complaints of itching, pain, and temperature irregularities and other odd sensations; and provide interventions to ameliorate or prevent more serious foot problems.

In the previous chapter, we discussed foot care interventions, such as debriding toenails, paring hyperkeratotic lesions (corns and calluses), and other strategies for the prevention and management of foot complications in patients with peripheral neuropathy. This chapter focuses instead on common foot problems.

TINEA PEDIS

Tinea pedis ("athlete's foot") is the most common mycotic disorder of the feet. It results from infection by dermatophytes, a class of aerobic fungi that feed on keratin in dead layers of skin, hair, and nails.[4] *Trichophyton rubrum* is the species of dermatophyte most prevalent in the United States and the one most commonly associated with tinea pedis. Dermatophytes invade, infect, and persist in the stratum corneum and sometimes are successful in penetrating below the surface of the epidermis and its appendages. The skin responds to the superficial infection by increased proliferation, which leads to scaling and epidermal thickening.[5]

Dermatophytes can be acquired from the soil, animals, and other humans. The most common source in the United States is infected individuals and their belongings (towels, bath mats, etc.). Contributing factors include warmth and high humidity, with constant occlusion.

Ten percent of the population is estimated to be infected by a dermatophyte at any given time. This high incidence has been attributed to the increased use of broad-spectrum antibiotics, the expanding number of immunocompromised patients, such as those with HIV or AIDS, aging, and lifestyle changes. There is also an increased incidence of fungal infections among gardeners and farmers; individuals who regularly wear boots or sports shoes such as ice hockey skates; and individuals who frequent sports facilities, pools, and communal leisure facilities. Individuals with hepatic, renal, and endocrine diseases (e.g., diabetes mellitus) are at higher risk; as the incidence of diabetes increases, so does the risk of dermatophytoses. In fact, the prevalence of fungal foot infections in people with diabetes is often underestimated. Many health-care providers mistake marked mycoses on the soles of the feet for dry skin; therefore, people with diabetes require more diagnostic, therapeutic, and preventive care in terms of mycotic diseases than previously thought.[6]

Signs and Symptoms

Exhibit 13.1 identifies the clinical findings of tinea pedis. Symptoms include pruritus, scaling, redness, painful or uncomfortable breaks in the skin, weeping, odor, and disability.[1,4]

Diagnosis

Laboratory studies are generally indicated, because greater diagnostic accuracy occurs when the clinical diagnosis is verified by

EXHIBIT 13.1

Clinical Presentation of Tinea Pedis

1. Whitish, macerated interdigital spaces
2. Erythematous skin with vesicles, scales, or fissures
3. Malodor from bacterial superinfection, which can mask the underlying fungal infection
4. Thickened, scaly, dry patches on the soles and sides of feet
5. Lesions that are noninflammatory scaly, acute or subacute eczematous-like, chronically lichenified, nodular and granulomatous, bullous and pustular, or resembling pyoderma
6. Associated infections involving the hair follicle and nail, persistent hyperpigmentation and/or hypopigmentation, and secondary bacterial infection

laboratory data. This verification is especially important when the use of systemic therapy is anticipated. Aqueous potassium hydroxide preparation (KOH) and fungal cultures can be performed.

KOH specimens should be obtained from the active border or edge of a lesion or scale by scraping a skin sample from the site of infection. If a vesicle or bulla is present, the roof is an appropriate specimen. In pustular lesions, the purulent debris is acceptable. Place the material on a glass slide and add 10% to 20% KOH, with or without dimethyl sulfoxide (DMSO). If DMSO is added, heating is not necessary. A fungal stain, such as chlorazol black E or Parker blue-black ink, can be added to highlight the hyphae. A positive KOH specimen will show multiple septate hyphae.[5] A negative result does not necessarily exclude the possibility of dermatophyte infection; therefore, a culture of the sample helps identify the causative fungal organism.[4]

Fungal cultures are recommended for persistent and difficult conditions that require specific identification. Various methods of obtaining cultures have been described in the literature, such as using a sterile toothbrush or rubbing moistened sterile swabs or gauze pads over the affected area, and then pressing into the surface of the dermatophyte test medium to be cultured. The laboratory should be contacted for the acceptable method of obtaining the culture and which medium is to be used.

Differential diagnosis is indicated to rule out psoriasis, eczema, candidiasis, bacterial infection, and other dermatoses.

The diagnosis of tinea pedis is generally classified into three categories: interdigital toe web infections, plantar moccasin-type infection, and vesiculobullous tinea pedis.

Interdigital toe web infections usually start as dermatophyte infections with an interplay between various bacterial species and, although rare, *Candida* species. Scaling is the initial feature, and, when the bacteria proliferate, maceration occurs (Fig. 13.1). The terms *dermatophytosis simplex* and *dermatophytosis complex* have been proposed to address two forms of interdigital infection: *simplex* refers to the features of scaling and, at times, fissures, whereas *complex* includes a highly macerated, leukokeratotic symptomatic process in which dermatophytes can be recovered in only one-third of patients. This variety of interdigital infection is mainly caused by an overgrowth of a myriad of bacterial species.[7]

Plantar moccasin-type infection results in diffuse, hyperkeratotic scaling of the plantar surface and is often associated with toenail involvement. The skin can become red, with severe itching in some cases. The main feature is small scales that often appear as small, round areas of peeling skin.

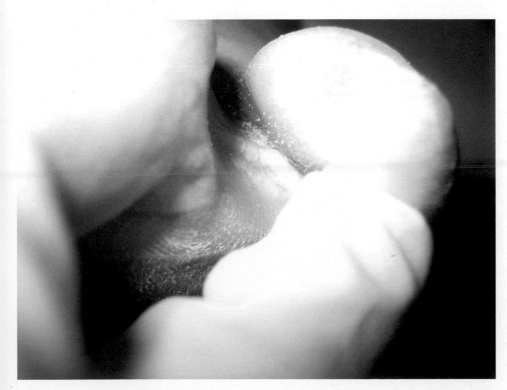

FIGURE 13.1 Tinea pedis interdigital toe web infection.

EXHIBIT   13.2

Common topical antifungal products

- Azoles: clotrimazole (Lotrimin®) applied for 4 weeks or per package directions (over the counter).
- Allylamines: terbinafine (Lamisil®) or naftifine (Naftin®) applied for 1 week or per package directions (over the counter).
- Azoles: clotrimazole (Lotrimin®) and econazole (Spectazole®) applied for 4 weeks (prescription).
- Allylamines: terbinafine (Lamisil®), naftifine (Naftin®), and butenafine (Mentax®) applied for 1 week (prescription).
- Ciclopirox 0.77% gel, applied once or twice daily for interdigit tinea.

Vesiculobullous tinea pedis presents as acute, highly inflammatory eruptions, particularly on the arch and side of the foot. The dermatophyte species *T. mentagrophytes* is primarily responsible. People with recurrent episodes tend to have low-grade scaling between exacerbations of acute inflammation. Differing environmental factors, such as seasonal temperature, sweating from physical activities, and types of shoe wear, influence the growth of the fungus. When sufficient proliferation and penetration of the stratum corneum occur, the epidermis comes into contact with fungal antigens, and a T cell–mediated immune contact allergic response occurs.[7]

Management

Treatment modalities for tinea pedis include general and specific interventions, which are often varied and include both topical and oral medications. General interventions involve the use of topical antifungal agents, which are indicated for simple interdigital and noninflammatory moccasin-type dermatophytoses. According to a recent systematic review of topical treatments for fungal infections of the skin and nails of the foot, there is good evidence that allylamines, azoles, butenafine, ciclopiroxolamine, tolciclate, and tolnaftate are effective compared to placebo for the treatment of fungal infections of the skin.[4] Allylamines are more effective than azoles. Exhibit 13.2 presents common topical products including allylamines and azoles.

CLINICAL WISDOM

Terbinafine hydrochloride cream (Lamisil Cream 1%, available over the counter) should be applied twice daily until clinical signs and symptoms of tinea pedis significantly improve, usually by day 7. Drug therapy should be provided for a minimum of 1 week, not to exceed 4 weeks. Interdigital tinea pedis may respond to ciclopirox 0.77% gel, applied twice daily for 4 weeks.[8]

RESEARCH WISDOM

For most dermatophytic infections of the foot, topical agents are usually effective and less expensive than oral agents. Recent advances in short-term therapies, such as the use of terbinafine emulsion gel for 5 days or simple film-forming solutions, have reduced the costs of treatment dramatically and enhanced adherence.[10]

Specific interventions for tinea pedis vary according to the type of infection. For dermatophytosis complex, a topical fungicidal agent, such as an allylamine (terbinafine), alternated with a double antibiotic ointment, such as Polysporin, or with broad-spectrum antibacterial agents, such as Castellani paint, aluminum chloride, and various tinctures of dye (gentian violet), can be used. If the toenails are infected, treat this reservoir of fungi as well. Topical therapy of the skin is often required for several weeks to eradicate residual fungus and prevent relapse. Monitor the patient's progress closely. As an adjunct to topical antifungals such as terbinafine, a 40% urea cream has been found beneficial in the treatment of the erythema, scaling, and pruritus. It has been especially useful when severe hyperkeratoses (very thickened skin) are present. Instruct patients to apply the 40% urea cream once daily and the ciclopirox cream twice daily for 2 to 3 weeks.[9]

Vesiculobullous tinea pedis with acute, highly inflammatory eruptions requires topical or systemic corticosteroids in conjunction with antifungal agents for acute attacks (Fig. 13.2). The choice of topical or systemic therapy depends on the extent and severity of the process. The use of combination topical corticosteroid-antifungal mixtures requires caution, however, as these medications contain fluorinated corticosteroids to reduce the inflammatory response. Moreover, steroid therapy should be withdrawn once the cell-mediated immune response is curtailed or there is evidence that symptoms are relieved, and it should never exceed 4 weeks. Contraindications for the use of combination products include application on occluded areas and use in children less than12 years of age and immunosuppressed patients.[11]

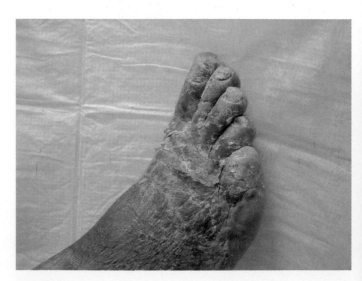

FIGURE 13.2 Severe inflammatory tinea pedis.

CLINICAL WISDOM

Tinea pedis can mimic dry skin. Dry skin tends to be flaky, whereas infected skin tends to produce small, round scales that give the appearance of the skin peeling.

The complications of both topical and systemic therapy should be discussed with each patient. The most common side effects of topical therapy include irritation, burning, itching, and dryness. Systemic therapy side effects can occur with terbinafine (Exhibit 13.3) and itraconazole (Exhibit 13.4). Patients who have known hypersensitivities to topical and systemic antifungal therapy should not take these drugs.

Surgical intervention is usually not indicated. However, some patients elect to have the infected toenail plate permanently removed, due to continuing nail deformity.

Outcome measures for successful treatment of tinea pedis include skin that is free of scaling, flakiness, and peeling, and relief of symptoms, such as itching or discomfort. Suspect treatment failure if the skin has not improved after 1 month of treatment. In such cases, it may be wise to obtain a skin culture. It is important to treat any proven foot dermatophytosis, as it is a significant risk factor for the development of acute bacterial cellulitis (discussed later in this chapter).[12]

Prevention

Prevention of tinea pedis is a lifelong goal. Many individuals experience several acute exacerbations during their lifetimes. Prevention goals are to minimize damp, moist skin caused by footwear and avoid environments that promote fungal growth, such as contaminated showers. The following self-care tips can help to prevent recurrences:

- Dry feet well after bathing and showering, making sure to dry between the toes.
- Use antifungal powders such as Zeasorb AF or sprays twice daily to minimize moisture on the feet and between the toes.
- Use skin sealant/antiseptic products such as Liquid Band-Aid, which act as moisture barriers between the toes. This helps repel moisture as well.
- Change socks frequently, especially when damp.
- Wear socks made of fabrics that are most conducive to wicking moisture away, including synthetic blends with nylon. While cotton is still advocated, it tends to absorb moisture and "hold" it next to the skin.
- Change shoes frequently and especially when they become wet.

CLINICAL WISDOM

Systemic antifungal agents can be hepatotoxic. It is important to rule out existing liver dysfunction because these agents could potentiate unknown liver disorders. Because of this, liver function studies are indicated prior to treatment with oral itraconazole and terbinafine, per package insert.

EXHIBIT 13.3

Side Effects of terbinafine (Lamisil)

- Gastrointestinal disorders, including diarrhea and dyspepsia
- Dermatologic disorders, including rash, pruritus, and urticaria
- Liver enzyme abnormalities
- Taste disturbance
- Visual disturbance

Members of households may choose to use separate tubs and showers from those who are affected to prevent the transmission from one person to another; the surface should be cleaned after each use with a solution that kills fungus such as bleach-containing products.

PLANTAR FASCIITIS

Plantar fasciitis is the most common form of heel pain. It is caused by inflammation, microruptures, hemorrhages, and collagen degeneration of the plantar fascia. The sequelae are fibrosis and possible ossification between the origin of the flexor digitorum brevis and the fascia.

The causes of plantar fasciitis are variable and multifactorial.[13] The major underlying factor is overuse injury to soft tissue, involving repetitive, excessive loading impact on heel strike over time. Anatomic, biomechanical, and environmental factors contribute to damage:

- Anatomic risk factors include pes planus, subtalar joint pronation, cavus foot, unequal leg length, tarsal coalition, and low or high foot arch.

EXHIBIT 13.4

Side Effects of Itraconazole (Sporanox)

- Gastrointestinal disorders
- Edema
- Fatigue
- Fever
- Malaise
- Skin disorders, including rash and pruritus
- Central and peripheral nervous system problems, including headache
- Psychiatric disorders, including decreased libido
- Hypertension
- Hypokalemia
- Albuminuria
- Abnormal hepatic function
- Impotence

- Biomechanical forces include tight Achilles tendon with inflexibility, weak plantar flexors, weak ankle flexors, weak intrinsic muscles, obesity, sudden weight gain, pregnancy, and sudden trauma.
- Environmental factors include changes in activity level; a rapid increase in training activities related to speed, intensity, and duration; running on steep hills, poor/hard surfaces, or barefoot on sand; running wearing worn-out athletic shoes; wearing shoes with poor support; inadequate stretching; excessive walking on the job; and excessive standing on hard, unyielding surfaces.

Athletic activities that have been linked to plantar fasciitis are running, distance running, tennis, gymnastics, and basketball.

Signs and Symptoms

The clinical features of plantar fasciitis include subjective symptoms of pain or discomfort. The pain can be described as a slow, dull ache; intense achiness; or burning sensation. The pain can be sharp, pinpoint, or knifelike. Patients often complain of pain in the heel when standing after periods of rest, especially during the first step in the morning.[14] This pain diminishes with each successive step, but can return late in the afternoon after prolonged weight bearing. It is usually described as nonradiating and well localized to the medial aspect of the heel pad. The symptoms are predominantly unilateral, but bilateral involvement occurs in 10% of cases.[13]

Diagnosis

Palpation over the medial calcaneal tuberosity produces a localized point tenderness. The pain can be reproduced during passive dorsiflexion of the ankle or toes and when standing on the toes to tighten the plantar fascia. If the condition is chronic, you will be able to palpate thickening, nodularity, and tautness along the fascia.

Diagnostic tests such as radiographs, bone scans, and blood studies are generally reserved for ambiguous presentations. A radiograph can be normal or reveal a horizontal bone spur projecting from the calcaneal tuberosity. The spur is not necessary in making the diagnosis, but its presence indicates chronic inflammation.[15]

Other related problems that can mimic plantar fasciitis include but are not limited to[16]

- Heel pad atrophy
- Tarsal tunnel syndrome
- Achilles tendonitis
- Calcaneal fracture
- Stress fracture
- Compartment syndrome

CLINICAL WISDOM

One of the most common complaints of heel pain associated with plantar fasciitis is the report that the pain is excruciating upon first rising in the morning, when the foot touches the floor. This is a hallmark symptom of fasciitis.

- Complete or partial plantar fascia rupture
- Systemic disorders, such as lupus erythematous, rheumatoid arthritis, ankylosing spondylitis, Reiter syndrome, gout, and vascular insufficiency

Patient assessment and diagnosis include a thorough history (e.g., reports of heel pain) and physical examination. The procedure for examining the patient is as follows:

1. Ask patient to stand. Assess for a rigid cavus foot (high arch) or pes planus (flat foot).
2. Ask patient to walk. The gait should be observed for any excessive pronation (ankles turning inward) on heel strike. Observe for a limp that might occur with weight bearing when the foot touches down on its lateral aspect.
3. Ask patient to dorsiflex (move foot upward toward leg) and plantar flex (push toes downward toward floor). Assess range of motion of the ankle for inversion and eversion to identify a tight heelcord.
4. Inspect the shoes for any abnormal wear and the quality of arch support within them. Shoes that do not fit properly or are in poor condition should be replaced. Athletic-type walking shoes with proper arch supports are indicated.

Management

Interventions include treating pain, restoring flexibility to the ankle and arch, strengthening the muscles in and around the foot, and gradually resuming activities. Conservative measures are described.[17]

General measures include rest, ice application, stretching, and muscle strengthening. A conservative rest program involves a decrease in activity for 6 weeks. Local ice application several times per day (conservative) includes ice massage for 6 to 7 minutes or application of an ice pack for 20 to 40 minutes four to six times a day. The patient should apply ice long enough to achieve a numbing affect, while avoiding frostbite injury.

Conservative stretching is considered by some to be the most important aspect of the treatment regimen, although evidence to support stretching as a best practice is limited. Demonstrate gastrocnemius and soleus stretches to the patient and have him or her repeat the demonstration. Gastrocnemius stretch is performed by having the patient lean forward into a wall and place the affected foot 12 to 18 in. from the wall, with the foot flat against the floor and the knee straight. The soleus stretch is performed in the same manner, but with the knee slightly bent. The stretch can be obtained in the seated position by placing a towel under the ball of the foot and gently pulling it upward. Proper

CLINICAL WISDOM

A bag of frozen vegetables, such as peas, can be placed in a plastic zipper bag and labeled *ice bag*. Or, the patient can place a foam cup filled with water in the freezer. When frozen, place the cup in a plastic zipper bag and massage the foot with the ice. Another method is to fill a 20-oz soda bottle with water and freeze. The frozen bottle can be placed on the floor, and the affected foot can be "rolled" over the bottle to ice the foot.

stretching involves a gentle pulling pressure in the muscle with the tendon being stretched, without causing an increase in pain.

Encourage the patient to apply ice prior to stretching. In addition, the patient may choose to take a nonsteroidal anti-inflammatory drug (NSAID) or other anti-inflammatory agent prior to stretching. Recommend that the patient stretches for 10 to 20 seconds on rising in the morning, with 15 repetitions, repeated at least two to five times per day.

You should also teach the patient conservative muscle strengthening exercises. For example, instruct the patient to pick up articles off the floor, using only the toes. The patient can also dorsiflex and plantar flex the foot several times during the day. Patients should observe you demonstrating the exercises and then perform these exercises several minutes each day for at least 6 weeks.

Specific interventions include the use of medications, support devices, strapping, shoe wear, and orthotics.[13] NSAIDs can be prescribed for pain management. In acute cases, NSAIDs are prescribed for a 7- to 10-day course up to 1 month, depending on the drug and degree of symptom management required. Patients should be encouraged to check with their health-care provider before starting a regimen of NSAIDs, because of the side effects.

Conservative support devices include use of heel cups, pads, lifts, and arch support inserts placed in both shoes. These devices relieve tension on the plantar fascia by reestablishing the arched shape of the foot. Cups and pads are especially beneficial to the elderly when there is atrophy of the plantar heel pad. If tenderness is localized, a cutout can be made into any of these three types of shoe inserts to relieve pressure over the tender area. Pedorthists, physical therapists, chiropractors, and podiatrists can recommend the proper inserts and orthotics when needed.

Strapping, splinting, and other methods of immobilizing the foot help to reestablish or maintain the arch of the foot, stabilize the first metatarsal head, decrease forefoot pronation, control heel valgus (turning outward), and change the foot strike position. Strapping is considered to be beneficial in the acute phase of plantar fasciitis. Night splints can be obtained from specialty shoe stores and pharmacies and worn at night to keep the foot in proper alignment (dorsiflexed), thus preventing relaxation of the fascia, which, when supported, is less painful. Sports medicine or physical therapy professionals can perform the strapping procedure and recommend splints. The splints can also be obtained from specialty footwear and online stores.

Good walking shoes and athletic-type footwear are also part of the treatment plan. Shoes with a firm heel, proper heel cushioning, and adequate longitudinal arch support are recommended. Orthotics within the shoes can relieve symptoms by providing adequate resistance to the mechanical forces applied to the foot. Patients can be referred to an orthotist, pedorthist, podiatrist, or other foot care–related specialist for orthotic devices. Evidence about which types of devices (customized or off-the-shelf) are most effective at reducing discomfort is lacking.

If no improvement is noted within 6 weeks, you can consider referring the patient to physical therapy, although there are conflicting data regarding the benefit of certain physical therapy modalities, such as pulsed ultrasound, phonophoresis, monochromatic near infrared light, and high-energy shock wave therapy.[18,19] Additionally, recommendations for contrast soaks can be made: warm and cold soaks for 15 minutes twice

---

CLINICAL WISDOM

When historical or physical findings of plantar heel pain are unusual or routine treatment proves ineffective, consider an atypical cause of heel pain, such as stress fracture of the calcaneus or heel spur syndrome.

---

a day, beginning with a warm soak for the first half and followed by a cold soak for the remaining time.

If improvement is only minimal after another 6 to 8 weeks, a steroid injection may be necessary. A corticosteroid injection into the calcaneal attachment can help control the inflammation of plantar fasciitis. The major risks are fascia rupture, associated with degeneration of the fascia, and fat-pad atrophy. Steroid injections tend to be very painful. Measures to reduce the pain include use of a local anesthetic and corticosteroid cryospray before the injection, and use of medial injection parallel to the fascia. Three injections may be given 2 to 4 weeks apart.[20] Evidence to support the long-term effectiveness of injections remains scant. If pain is recalcitrant to treatment, surgery may be an option. Candidates for surgery are limited to those with significant pain and disability in activities of daily living after conservative therapy has been exhausted.[21,22] Exhibit 13.5 presents complications related to plantar fasciitis treatment.

Outcome measures of successful treatment of plantar fasciitis include a reduction in pain after 4 to 6 weeks of conservative treatment and cessation of symptoms after 8 months to a year. Referral criteria include patients whose symptoms last longer than 6 months or who present with chronic symptoms of many months to years duration. Consultation with a foot care specialist in sports medicine, orthopedics, podiatry, pedorthy, or physical therapy depends on the patient's responsiveness to conservative treatment. Follow-up is generally appropriate within 6 weeks from onset of treatment.

Prevention

Self-care strategies for prevention of exacerbations include wearing proper footwear with adequate arch supports and

---

EXHIBIT 13.5

Complications of Plantar Fasciitis Treatment

A. Orthotics—Toe jamming, heel irritation, and slippage from an improper fit
B. Nonsteroidal anti-inflammatory drugs—Gastrointestinal upset most common (see package insert for comprehensive list of adverse reactions)
C. Strapping—Allergy to tape or prep adhesive, blistering, and irritation
D. Shoes—Ill-fitting footwear, leading to blisters, corns, calluses, and pain
E. Steroid injections—Fat-pad atrophy, pain and degeneration of the fascia, and plantar fascia rupture
F. Surgery—Decrease in strength and function

avoiding extreme dorsiflexion of the feet, such as bending down on the forefoot, which puts excessive pressure on the toes and metatarsal heads of the feet. This position causes extreme tension on the fascia and can induce microtears. The patient should also avoid excessive trauma from sports-related "pounding" of the feet during activities on hard surfaces, such as concrete.

ONYCHOMYCOSIS

Onychomycosis (tinea unguium) is an infection of the toenails in which fungal organisms invade the nail unit via the nail bed or nail plate. If left untreated, the infection can cause insidious, progressive destruction of the nail plate (Figs. 13.3 and 13.4).

Onychomycosis is precipitated by environmental factors, including repeated microtrauma to the nail and its structures. This can occur, for example, in athletic activities in which repeated trauma to the nail weakens the seal between the nail plate and nail bed, allowing fungal organisms to penetrate the nail unit.[23] Athletes are also at high risk because of profuse sweating, with runners particularly prone to onychomycosis. In addition, chronic exposure of nails to water, as with regular swimming activity, can double the risk of developing onychomycosis.[24] Exogenous heat and hyperhidrosis (excessive sweating), as seen in people who wear shoes or boots every day for prolonged periods of time, also increase the risk. Data suggest that people who wear sandals are less vulnerable to fungi because their feet are exposed to the air.

Onychomycosis is also more common in certain populations. The elderly are at increased risk because of the slower growth of the nail and decreased circulation that accompanies aging. Males are at greater risk than females, though postmenopausal women are affected because estrogen appears to exert a protective effect in younger women. Immunocompromised patients are also at risk: extensive use of chemotherapeutic, systemic antibiotic, and immunosuppressive therapies, and infection with the human immunodeficiency virus (HIV) predispose to the condition. Finally, a history of cancer, diabetes, circulatory impairment, psoriasis, tinea pedis interdigitalis, the moccasin form of tinea pedis, and other foot infections increases the risk.[25–27]

Three main classes of fungi cause onychomycosis. Dermatophyte fungi account for 90% of these infections. They include *T. rubrum, Epidermaophyton floccosum,* and *T. mentagrophytes.* Yeasts, including *Candida albicans,* account for 8%,

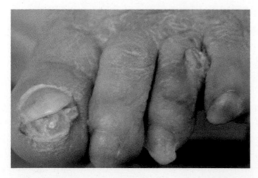

FIGURE 13.3 Onychomycosis demonstrating hyperkeratosis and hypertrophy of the nail plate with a deformed, thick, crumbly nail. The plate is thickened, deformed (misshapened), brittle, and crumbly.

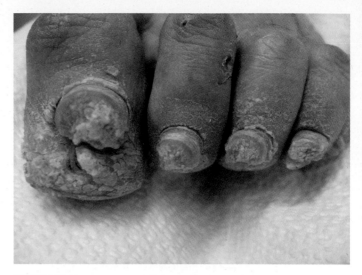

FIGURE 13.4 Onychomycosis involving multiple nail plates.

and nondermatophyte molds, including *Aspergillus* species, *Scopulariopsis brevicollis, Scytalidium dimidiatum, Scytalidium hyalinum, Fusarium* species, and *Acremonium* species, account for 2% of onychomycosis. Mixed infections involving two or more fungi can occur.

The initial pathophysiology involves a mild inflammatory response to the fungi once they have invaded the nail bed, causing hypertrophy of the bed. Hyperkeratosis and hypertrophy of the nail plate results in a discolored, deformed, thick, crumbly nail that can become loosened from the nail bed.[28]

Signs and Symptoms

Onychomycosis presents with three classic signs: discoloration, with white, brown, or yellow patches or streaks; subungual hyperkeratosis and debris; and onycholysis (loosening or separation of all or part of the nail plate from the bed). In addition, four patterns of onychomycosis are seen: distal subungual, proximal subungual, white superficial, and *Candida.* Each pattern is associated with a different entry point of the fungi into the nail unit and a different appearance of the infected nail.

Distal subungual onychomycosis is the most common type, and *T. rubrum* is the most common cause. The distal nail plate turns yellow or whitish brown, with hyperkeratotic debris accumulation under the nail. The plate often becomes thickened, deformed, brittle, and crumbly. These changes can make wearing shoes uncomfortable or painful.[23]

Proximal subungual onychomycosis, which is caused by a variety of dermatophytes, appears more frequently in immunocompromised patients. Fungi invade the proximal nail fold and cuticle, and then infect the deeper portion of the plate. The proximal nail plate develops a white color in patchy areas. The surface remains smooth and intact. Hyperkeratotic debris can accumulate under the plate.

White superficial onychomycosis (WSO) is most often caused by the dermatophyte *T. mentagrophytes* and a variety of other molds. Fungi directly invade the surface of the plate, producing a white, soft, dry, powdery, crumbly appearance. The plate does not thicken and continues to adhere to the nail bed. It can occur in patients with HIV infection.[29,30]

CLINICAL WISDOM

Many nail conditions can mimic onychomycosis. These include psoriasis, eczema, lichen planus, ischemic conditions, congenital nail disorders, yellow nail syndrome, and pseudomonas infections. In addition, dystrophic nails (nails that are abnormal in appearance, shape, and/or texture) can result from trauma.

Candida onychomycosis is mainly caused by *C. albicans*. It is a rare syndrome, limited to patients with chronic mucocutaneous candidiasis. The nail plate thickens and turns yellow-brown.[23]

The hallmark symptom of onychomycosis is nail discoloration, which commonly occurs as the nail plate thickens. Pain can result from pressure on the nail bed from ill-fitting footwear. The patient might also experience tenderness and trauma to adjacent soft skin folds from the thickened nails, and embarrassment from disfigured, discolored, and deformed nails.

Diagnosis

As a rule, laboratory studies are conducted when onychomycosis cannot be managed by standard mechanical or pharmacologic treatments. Histologic analysis via nail culture should be conducted in resistant clinical situations in which fungal infection is suspected. Because specimen processing can require special techniques, it can take several days to obtain results. Contact a local laboratory for requirements. If a diagnosis is still not possible using microscopic exam or histologic analysis, biopsy of the nail bed is indicated. Several diagnostic approaches are described in detail in the literature.[31–33]

Management

Treatment of onychomycosis includes general measures such as foot hygiene and mechanical manual debridement with nippers. More specific measures include use of topical preparations, systemic agents, and surgical nail removal. Monotherapy is often ineffective in the treatment of onychomycosis; thus, combination therapies are preferable.

You can promote topical nail reduction using urea compound (20%–40%) under a thin film dressing. You may also use manual debridement in conjunction with antifungal nail lacquers and creams.[34] Recent evidence shows that a common topical treatment delivered through a transungual drug delivery system (TDDS), or colorless nail lacquer, is a step forward from previous ineffective topical agents. Two common TDDS ciclopiroxolamine 8% (Penlac®) and amorolfine 5% (Loceryl®) are applied to the nail daily, layered over each other, and then every 7 days the layers are removed with nail polish remover or alcohol. This daily regimen is continued until the nail is clear of infection, which might take up to 6 to 9 months. There is general consensus that topical monotherapy (where only one agent is used) should be used where less than 50% of the nail surface is affected, without matrix involvement.[35] The overall cure rates of topical therapy and particularly monotherapy are relatively low, and relapse rates are relatively high.

Anecdotal data suggest that patients who use various herbal and over-the-counter topical preparations have experienced

EXHIBIT 13.6

Guidelines for systemic antifungal therapy for onychomycosis

Terbinafine, 250 mg every day for 12 weeks. Adverse reactions include headache; gastrointestinal symptoms, such as diarrhea, dyspepsia, abdominal pain, nausea, diarrhea, and flatulence; dermatologic symptoms, such as rash, pruritus, and urticaria; liver enzyme abnormalities; taste disturbance; and visual disturbance.

a reduction in symptoms associated with onychomycosis. Tea tree oil, Vick's VapoRub, and vinegar all have been reported to lessen the severity of symptoms but evidence is lacking to support their use.[36]

Systemic antifungal agents, such as terbinafine (Lamisil), are useful (Exhibit 13.6). Data from a plethora of studies of drug therapies yield inconsistent findings about the efficacy, best treatment regimens, and cost-effectiveness of these treatments.[37–45] Baseline liver function studies are obtained prior to initiation of oral therapy and during its course. Refer to package insert for prescribing information.[46] It is important to review the literature pertaining to the best practices for prescribing oral antifungal therapy, as open studies and randomized controlled trials are proliferative, and newer findings could change prescribing practices.

Most recent data suggest that the combination of topical and oral therapies is most effective when nail fungus is resistant to topical treatments of greater than 2 months duration.[46] Combination therapy can reduce the duration and cumulative dosage of oral therapy.[23] In the future, combined therapies with new oral antimycotics and antifungal lacquers, and treatments combined with surgical, laser, or chemical removal of the affected nail regions, may improve results. Novel treatment approaches are evolving, such as nail exposure to photo therapies, which exert an antifungal effect.[47]

The optimal clinical effect for systemic therapy is seen some months after cessation of treatment and is related to the period required for outgrowth of healthy nail. It can take up to 12 months for nail cure. The duration of treatment is based on prescribing recommendations, mycological cure, and outcome measures, including a nail free of discoloration, thickness, and crumbly texture.[35] It is important to remind patients that a "perfect" nail may not be an attainable goal. However, a nail plate that is much less thick is cosmetically more appealing and does reduce the risk of injury to the underlying nail bed.

Referral criteria include treatment failure with systemic agents (after 9–12 months of nail growth, even after systemic therapy has been completed) and patient dissatisfaction with mechanical debridement. Refer patients who are unable to take systemic therapy to foot care specialists for evaluation for more aggressive treatment, such as removal of the nail plate by surgical or chemical methods, particularly when severe toenail deformities exist. Patients who elect conservative measures, such as mechanical debridement, should see foot care professionals every 2 to 3 months.[2] Quality of life is important to consider during all aspects of treatment and should be included as part of the history.[48]

Prevention

Measures to prevent fungal infection or reinfection are critical.[49] Patients should be instructed on the following key points:

- Wear properly fitting shoes. Alternate between two pairs so you do not wear the same pair every day. Shoes with a high toe box of extra depth can accommodate thickened nails.
- Wear thin acrylic or acrylic-cotton blend socks, such as those worn by runners. These wick the moisture away from the skin, rather than absorbing it, keeping the skin drier. The socks should be changed frequently if they do become moist.
- Wash the feet daily and pay close attention to drying well between the toes.
- Trim toenails straight across, smoothing any rough or jagged edges and following the contour or shape of the toe.
- Alert health-care professionals of any changes in the nail or skin.

MISCELLANEOUS CONDITIONS

This section presents information on miscellaneous foot conditions. For each condition, the definition, pathophysiology, key points, and general guidelines for management are provided.

Xerosis and Anhidrosis

Xerosis and **anhidrosis** describe excessively dry, flaky skin that can be particularly severe on the heels and bottoms of the feet. Anhidrosis is often related to autonomic dysfunction caused by endocrine or neurologic disorders, which results in loss of moisture production in the skin and severe flaking (Figs. 13.5 and 13.6).

Management of xerosis and anhidrosis includes the following:

- Teach the patient to avoid prolonged soaking of feet in hot water because it can cause excessive drying by depleting moisture from the skin. Soaking should be eliminated or limited to 5 to 10 minutes.
- Apply topical hydrating products such as emollients and seal them with petrolatum-based products several times each day and at bedtime. The condition can require a prescription-strength product if symptoms do not resolve after 4 weeks.

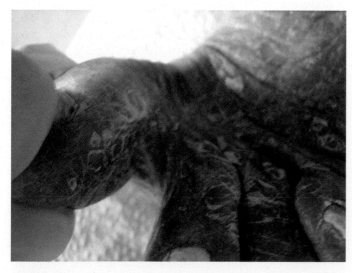

FIGURE 13.5 Anhidrosis of the foot.

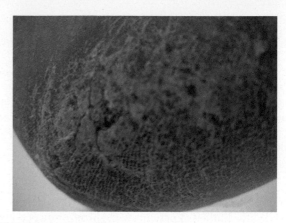

FIGURE 13.6 Dry skin on heel.

- Products containing humectants attract and retain moisture on the skin.
- Instruct the patient to wear proper footwear and socks, which are barriers between the skin and shoe, to reduce friction.

Hyperhidrosis

Hyperhidrosis is excessive moisture production related to endocrine/neurologic or sweat gland disorders. Management includes the following:

- Teach the patient to change acrylic or acrylic-blend socks several times each day.
- Suggest that the patient use spray antiperspirants on skin and absorptive powders daily or more frequently as needed. Prescription-strength antiperspirant (e.g., Drysol) may be needed to treat recalcitrant sweating.
- Footwear should be of leather or canvas/cloth material that is breathable.

Cellulitis

Cellulitis is inflammation and subsequent infection of the connective tissue between adjacent tissues and organs, and commonly results from bacterial infection. It gives the overlying skin a reddish appearance. Infection can be located in the toes, dorsum and plantar surface of the feet, and lower leg skin. The initial insult is often trauma. Risk factors include wounds and immunodeficiency syndromes.

Management of cellulitis includes the following:

- Order diagnostic testing, such as radiographs or magnetic resonance imaging, to rule out osteomyelitis.
- Initiate proper antibiotic therapy.
- Initiate wound care, if wound is present.
- Teach patient to dress the wound and prevent mechanical, thermal, and chemical injury to the area.
- Instruct patient to report worsening of symptoms, such as increased size, drainage, redness, pain, and fever.
- Instruct patient to take pain relievers.

Maceration

Macerated toe web spaces can result from rigid or fixed toe deformities or functional impairments, such as stiffness, which prevent the patient from bending over to dry the feet and areas between the toes. Excessive moisture gets trapped and can lead to fungal and bacterial infections.

Management of maceration includes the following:

- Implement moisture control practices, such as drying well between toes after bathing or showering and wiping toe web spaces with drying agents (e.g., alcohol) for up to 1 week. Spray antiseptics can be used, which also offer a drying effect.[50]
- Use absorptive material placed between toes to keep toes from rubbing together and to reduce moisture. This should be changed daily.
- Apply skin sealants to the toe web spaces as a moisture barrier. Liquid antiseptic products such as Liquid Band-Aid and New-Skin are available from drug stores and major discount chains and can be sprayed or "painted" between the toes.
- Apply absorptive powder between toes and in shoes to reduce moisture.
- Instruct the patient to wear thin acrylic or acrylic-blend socks when wearing shoes.
- Advise the patient to change shoes frequently.
- Once maceration is treated, skin moisture barrier/protectant wipes can be used between the toes as a moisture barrier.

If maceration persists for longer than 10 to 14 days, consider the presence of an interdigital tinea pedis and/or superimposed bacterial infection. Topical antifungal and antibacterial agents should be used for up to 1 month. Oral antifungal agents may be warranted if the fungal infection is recalcitrant to topical therapies.

Hyperkeratotic Lesions

Hyperkeratotic lesions, commonly referred to as corns and calluses, are circumscribed masses of a hornlike collection of epidermal cells that are thicker in the center and gradually taper, becoming thinner at the periphery. They form as a result of abnormal intermittent or chronic weight-bearing pressure and/or shear sliding stresses. Corns are technically known as helomas. Hard corns arise on top of or on the sides of the toes; soft corns arise between the toes (Fig. 13.7). Calluses, or tylomas, are found on the plantar surface of the feet under prominent weight-bearing areas and on the medial and lateral aspects of the sides of the feet and great toes (Fig. 13.8).

Management of hyperkeratotic lesions includes the following:

- Reduce amount of thickened keratoses by either mechanical debridement (buffing) or paring with sharp debridement. Instruct the patient to gently buff areas two to three times per week with a pumice stone and file board before taking a shower or bath. Alternatively, you can use a topical keratolytic agent containing urea, such as Carmol lotion, cream, or gel to "thin" the thickened epidermis and reduce hyperkeratoses, especially on the heels.

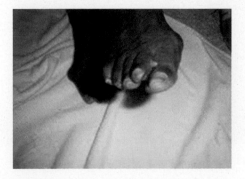

FIGURE 13.7 Example of a corn in the interdigital space.

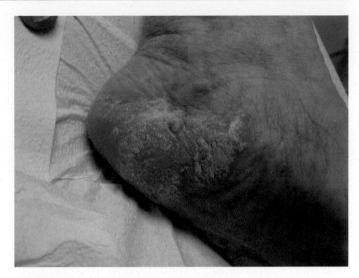

FIGURE 13.8 Callus formation.

- Teach the patient to pad the area with a proper over-the-counter pad, as directed. Choices include silicon-based products such as nonadhesive and reusable sleeves that fit over the toes.
- Recommend pressure relief shoes, such as those with a high toe box and padded cushion inserts. There are numerous commercially available inserts and orthotics that can further reduce the buildup of calluses by redistributing weight from bony prominences.

Fissures

Fissures are cracks in the dermis that cause a partial-thickness wound. They are common in the heel (Fig. 13.9). Management includes the following:

- Reduce keratotic tissue around fissure, if present, by mechanical or chemical debridement.
- Cleanse the area and apply a thin dressing, such as thin film, thin hydrocolloid, or sheet hydrogel, and dressing cloth tapes, to close the wound. A skin sealant or adhesive such as Dermabond can be used to fill and seal the fissure.
- Change the dressing weekly to allow for closure of wound. If the fissure is draining, red, inflamed, or extremely painful, consider an infection and treat accordingly.
- Instruct the patient on moisturizing protocol to prevent further fissures.
- Instruct the patient to wear shoes at all times and to avoid slippers or sandals that "flop" against the heel, causing excessive friction.

Onychauxis

Onychauxis describes hypertrophic toenails that result from trauma, aging, genetic predisposition, or other factors unrelated to onychomycosis. Management includes

- Mechanical debridement
- Teaching the patient to reduce the toenails at home if functionally able, using proper equipment such as nail files
- Instructing the patient to obtain extra-depth shoes or shoes with a high toe box to accommodate thickened toenails

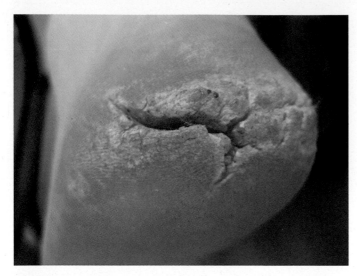

FIGURE 13.9 Fissure.

SELF-CARE TEACHING GUIDELINES

Specific self-care teaching guidelines were presented earlier for each specific foot problem discussed. The following are some general guidelines for self-care for all foot problems.

It is important to instruct patients to purchase shoes that accommodate structural deformities and swelling, offer support and cushioning, and are easy to put on and take off. Proper shoes are important for preventing a variety of complications. Those that are too narrow can cause blisters and corns, and shoes that are too short can cause toenail injury and hammertoes. Shoes that offer little support can lead to foot pain. Finally, shoes should be considered functional aids, rather than stylish accompaniments to clothing. Unfortunately, culture often dictates dress codes. Help your patients to understand that proper footwear can prevent serious foot complications, provide relief from excessive pressure and mechanical stress, and add to quality of life by reducing foot pain.

Teaching guidelines for general foot care should address the following:

- Proper self-care practices to include general information on bathing, drying well between toes, and avoiding excessive soaking. No bathroom surgery!
- The importance of daily self-inspection of feet and the areas between the toes. The patient can place a mirror on the floor, so that the patient can inspect the plantar surface of the foot for any cracks, discolorations, drainage, redness, and swelling. For individuals with limited vision, help from family members and caregivers can be required to inspect the feet.
- The need to wear shoes or slippers at all times, even when getting up at night to go to the bathroom.
- Information on purchasing proper shoes to accommodate structural deformities, diabetes, and other individuals needs.
- When to report problems to the health-care provider, such as abnormal sensations and pain in the legs at night or when ambulating.
- Reminding the health-care provider to inspect the feet routinely during each visit.

CONCLUSION

Foot problems continue to plague a disproportionately high percentage of older adults, affecting functional abilities and quality of life. In particular, problems affecting the toenails, skin, and plantar structures of the foot can have profound consequences such as severe infections or foot deformities. Help patients preserve their foot health by routinely including questions about the feet in the patient history, inspecting the skin and nails during the physical examination, and vigorously investigating complaints of heel and plantar foot pain. The evidence-based interventions discussed in this chapter can help guide you in ameliorating and/or preventing more serious foot problems and improving the patient's quality of life.

CASE STUDY

Mr. D. is a 72-year-old patient with a history of diabetes, CVA, hypertension, and high cholesterol. He also has chronic venous insufficiency. He lives alone in an apartment. He has some functional impairment due to right-sided weakness from his CVA. He has a long history of tinea pedis and onychomycosis. The major problem is his inability to bend over and care for his feet (see Fig. 13.10), and thus his toenails are extremely discolored, thickened, and now becoming so long that they are causing trauma to his skin. He also cannot put on compression stockings to manage edema. What is the most appropriate care approach for Mr. D?

a. Place him on a daily dose of an antifungal agent to decrease the nail thickness
b. Provide assistance with nail debridement and proper skin care
c. Tell his caregiver to apply topical urea agents to thin the nails and skin

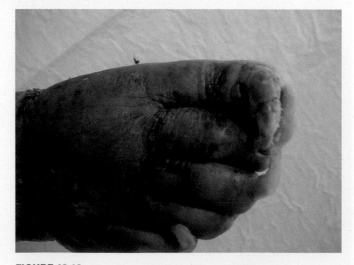

FIGURE 13.10 A patient with poor self-care abilities.

REVIEW QUESTIONS

1. How does the clinical presentation of tinea pedis differ from dry skin (xerosis)?
   A. Tinea pedis generally causes large blisters and drainage.
   B. The skin tends to have small areas that resemble peeling skin.
   C. Tinea pedis causes severe itching, whereas dry skin does not.

2. What is the hallmark symptom of plantar fasciitis?
   A. Foot cramps during the night
   B. Plantar foot bruising and discoloration
   C. Pain upon rising when foot touches floor

3. What are the best types of socks fabrics to wick away moisture from the skin?
   A. Acrylic blends
   B. 100% cotton
   C. Wool blends

4. Maceration is common between the toes. It generally is indicative of
   A. uncontrolled diabetes
   B. poor hygiene
   C. excessive moisture

5. A nail was recently removed due to onychauxis. The most important care consideration is to
   A. prevent trauma to the nail bed
   B. apply antifungal cream to the toe
   C. soak the foot in bleach water

REFERENCES

1. Havlickova B, Czaika VA, Friedrich M. Epidemiological trends in skin mycoses worldwide. *Mycoses.* 2008;51(suppl 4):2–15.
2. Standards of medical care in diabetes-2010. American Diabetes Association. *Diabetes Care.* 2010;33(suppl 1):S11–S61.
3. Frykberg RG, Zgonis T, Armstrong DG, et al. Diabetic foot disorders. A clinical practice guideline (2006 revision). American College of Foot and Ankle Surgeons. *J Foot Ankle Surg.* 2006;45 (5 suppl):S1–S66.
4. Crawford F, Hollis S. Topical treatments for fungal infection of the skin and nails of the foot. *Cochrane Database Syst Rev. Issue 3:*2009.
5. Korting HC, Kiencke P, Nelles S, et al. Comparable efficacy and safety of various topical formulations of Terbinafine in tinea pedis irrespective of treatment regimen. *Am J Clin Dermatol.* 2007;8:357–361.
6. Kikuchi I, Tanuma H, Morimoto K, et al. Usefulness and pharmacokinetic study of oral terbinafine for hyperkeratotic-type tinea pedis. *Mycoses* 2008;51:523–531.
7. Gupta AK, Skinner AR, Cooper EA. Intergidital tinea pedis (dermatophytosis simplex and complex) and treatment with ciclopirox 0.77% gel. *Int J Dermatol.* 2005;42(suppl 1):23–27.
8. de Chauvin MF, Viguie-Vallanet C, Kienzler JL, et al. Novel, single-dose, topical treatment of tinea pedis using terbinafine: results of a dose-finding clinical trial. *Mycoses* 2008;51:1–6.
9. Fungal nail infections: diagnosis and management. *Prescrire Int.* 2009;18:26–30.
10. James IG, Loria-Kanza Y, Jones TC. Short-duration topical treatment of tinea pedis using terbinafine emulsion gel: results of a dose-ranging clinical trial. *J Dermatol Treat.* 2007;8:163–168.
11. Olkhovskaya KB, Perlamutrov Y. Step-wise treatment of athlete's foot (tinea pedis) using isoconazole combined with a corticosteroid followed by isoconazole alone. *Mycoses* 2008;51(suppl 4):50–51.
12. Bristow IR, Spruce MC. Fungal foot infection, cellulitis and diabetes: a review. *Diabet Med.* 2009;26:548–551.
13. Lee SY, McKeon P, Hertel J. Does the use of orthoses improve self-reported pain and function measures in patients with plantar fasciitis? A meta-analysis. *Phys Ther Sport.* 2009;10:12–18.
14. Neufeld SK, Cerrato R. Plantar fasciitis: evaluation and treatment. *J Am Acad Orthop Surg.* 2008;16:338–346.
15. Jeswani T, Morlese J, McNally EG. Getting to the heel of the problem: plantar fascia lesions. *Clin Radiol.* 2009;64:931–939.
16. Stapleton JJ, Kolodenker G, Zgonis T. Internal and external fixation approaches to the surgical management of calcaneal fractures. *Clin Podiatr Med Surg.* 2010;27:381–392.
17. Crawford F, Thomson CE. WITHDRAWN. Interventions for treating plantar heel pain. *Cochrane Database Syst Rev.* 2010;20(1): CD000416.
18. Marks W, Jackiewicz A, Witkowski Z, et al. Extracorporeal shock-wave therapy (ESWT) with a new-generation pneumatic device in the treatment of heel pain. A double blind randomised controlled trial. *Acta Orthop Belg.* 2008;74:98–101.
19. Dogramaci Y, Kalaci A, Emir A, et al. Intracorporeal pneumatic shock application for the treatment of chronic plantar fasciitis: a randomized, double blind prospective clinical trial. *Arch Orthop Trauma Surg.* 2010;130:541–546.
20. Kalaci A, Cakici H, Hapa O, et al. Treatment of plantar fasciitis using four different local injection modalities: a randomized prospective clinical trial. *J Am Podiatr Med Assoc.* 2009;99:108–113.
21. Bazaz R, Ferkel RD. Results of endoscopic plantar fascia release. *Foot Ankle Int.* 2007;28:549–556.
22. McMillan AM, Landorf KB, Barrett JT, et al. Diagnostic imaging for chronic plantar heel pain: a systematic review and meta-analysis. *J Foot Ankle Res.* 2009;13(2):32.
23. Finch JJ, Warshaw EM. Toenail onychomycosis: current and future treatment options. *Dermatol Ther.* 2007;20:31–46.
24. Welsh O, Vera-Cabrera L, Welsh E. Onychomycosis. *Clin Dermatol.* 2010;28:151–159.
25. Helfand AE. Primary considerations in managing the older patient with foot problems. In: Halter JB, Ouslander JG, Tinetti ME, et al., eds. *Hazzard's Geriatric Medicine and Gerontology.* 6th ed. New York, NY: McGraw-Hill; 2009.
26. Kockaert M, Neumann M. Systemic and topical drugs for aging skin. *J Drugs Dermatol.* 2003;2(4):435–441.
27. Nazarko L. Caring for older skin: preventing and treating dryness. *Nurs Residential Care.* 2009;11(7):333–336.
28. Trivedi NA, Shah PC. A meta-analysis comparing efficacy of continuous terbinafine with intermittent itraconazole for toenail onychomycosis. *Indian J Dermatol.* 2010;55:198–199.

29. Aman S, Nadeem M, Haroon TS. Successful treatment of proximal white subungual onychomycosis with oral terbinafine therapy. *J Coll Physicians Surg Pak*. 2008;18:728–729.

30. Moreno-Coutiño G, Toussaint-Caire S, Arenas R. Clinical, mycological and histological aspects of white onychomycosis. *Mycoses*. 2010;53:144–147.

31. Garcia-Doval I, Cabo F, Monteagudo B, et al. Clinical diagnosis of toenail onychomycosis is possible in some patients: cross sectional diagnostic study and development of a diagnostic rule. *Br J Dermatol*. 2010;163:743–751.

32. Wilsmann-Theis D, Sareika F, Bieber T, et al. New reasons for histopathological nail-clipping examination in the diagnosis of onychomycosis. *J Eur Acad Dermatol Venereol*. 2010. [Epub ahead of print]

33. Shenoy MM, Teerthanath S, Karnaker VK, et al. Comparison of potassium hydroxide mount and mycological culture with histopathologic examination using periodic acid-Schiff staining of the nail clippings in the diagnosis of onychomycosis.. *Indian J Dermatol Venereol Leprol*. 2008;74:226–229.

34. Malay DS, Yi S, Borowsky P, et al. Efficacy of debridement alone versus debridement combined with topical antifungal nail lacquer for the treatment of pedal onychomycosis: a randomized, controlled trial. *J Foot Ankle Surg*. 2009;48:294–308.

35. Shemer A, Nathansohn N, Trau H, et al. Ciclopirox nail lacquer for the treatment of onychomycosis: an open non-comparative study. *J Dermatol*. 2010;37:137–139.

36. Proksch, E. (2008). The role of emollients in the management of disease with chronic dry skin. *Skin Pharmacol Physiol*. 2008;25:75–80.

37. Sigurgeirsson B. Prognostic factors for cure following treatment of onychomycosis. *J Eur Acad Dermatol Venereol*. 2010;24:679–684.

38. de Berker D. Clinical practice. Fungal nail disease. *N Engl J Med*. 2009;360:2108–2116.

39. Baron R, Hay RJ, Garduno JI. Review of antifungal therapy, Part II. Treatment rationale, including specific patient populations. *J Dermatol Treat*. 2008;19(3):168–175.

40. Kumar S, Kimball AB. New antifungal therapies for the treatment of onychomycosis. *Expert Opin Investig Drugs*. 2009;18:727–734.

41. Trivedi NA, Shah PC. A meta-analysis comparing efficacy of continuous terbinafine with intermittent itraconazole for toenail onychomycosis. *Indian J Dermatol*. 2010;55:198–199.

42. Lecha M, Effendy I, deChauvin MF, et al. Treatment options- development of consensus guidelines. *Eur Acad Dermatol Venererol*. 2005;19(suppl 1):25–33.

43. Takahata Y, Hiruma M, Shiraki Y, et al. Treatment of dermatophyte onychomycosis with three pulses of terbinafine (500 mg day for a week). *Mycoses*. 2009;52:72–76.

44. Baron R, Hay RJ, Garduno JI. Review of antifungal therapy and the severity index for assessing onychomycosis: Part I. *J Dermatol Treat*. 2008;19(2):72–81.

45. Nakano N, Hiruma M, Shiraki Y, et al. Combination of pulse therapy with terbinafine tablets and topical terbinafine cream for the treatment of dermatophyte onychomycosis: a pilot study. *J Dermatol*. 2006;33:753–758.

46. Jacobson A, Zajac L. Nail disorders every clinician should know. *Clin Advis*. 2008;11:24–30.

47. Qiao J, Li R, Ding Y, et al. Photodynamic therapy in the treatment of superficial mycoses: an evidence-based evaluation. *Mycopathologia*. 2010;170:339–343.

48. Warshaw EM, Foster JK, Cham PM, et al. NailQoL: a quality-of-life instrument for onychomycosis. *Int J Dermatol*. 2007;46:1279–1286.

49. Nail fungal infections—topic overview. Retrieved August 20, 2010 at http://www.webmd.com/skin-problems-and-treatments/tc/fungal-nail-infections-topic-overview

50. Stroud S, Kelechi TJ. Itching and sores between the toes; maceration or fungal infection. *Adv Nurs Pract*. 2008;16:26.

CHAPTER 14

Management of Malignant Cutaneous Wounds and Fistulas

Barbara M. Bates-Jensen and Susie Seaman

CHAPTER OBJECTIVES

At the completion of this chapter, the reader will be able to:

1. Explain the significance, pathophysiology, and assessment of malignant cutaneous wounds.
2. Describe methods of managing bleeding, exudate, and odor in malignant cutaneous wounds.
3. Describe interventions for management of pain related to malignant cutaneous wounds.
4. Explain the significance and pathophysiology of fistulas.
5. Identify the factors to be considered when assessing the client with a fistula.
6. Examine management methods for the client with a fistula.
7. Design a pouching procedure for a fistula.

This chapter explores your role when caring for a patient with a malignant cutaneous wound that has little or no healing potential. In these cases, symptom reduction is a primary goal and typically focuses on pain management, odor control, management of bleeding, and pouching for fistula output. Malignant wounds and fistulas are often complex and difficult to manage, and both creativity and sensitivity are required.

MALIGNANT CUTANEOUS WOUNDS

Malignant cutaneous wounds are skin wounds that develop secondary to cancer. They can occur from a primary skin cancer, from local spread of soft tissue tumors, or via lymphatic or blood vessels (metastatic spread). They are also known in the literature as *malignant fungating wounds* when they exhibit nodular, fungal-like growth that protrudes above the skin surface and *malignant ulcerating wounds* when there are deep erosions or craters. These wounds present both a physical and an emotional challenge for patients and even experienced clinicians. Often unsightly, malodorous, and painful, these wounds are a blow to self-esteem and may cause social isolation at the very time when the patient needs more time with family and friends (see Figs. 14.1–14.5). In caring for patients with malignant cutaneous wounds, your primary goal should be to improve the patient's quality of life through symptom palliation. Develop a treatment plan aimed at minimizing pain and infection, managing exudate and odor, and controlling bleeding.

Significance of Malignant Cutaneous Wounds

Malignant cutaneous lesions may occur in up to 5% of patients with cancer and 10% of patients with metastatic disease. In the largest US study done at a single site to date, Lookingbill et al.[1] retrospectively reviewed data accumulated over a 10-year period from the tumor registry at Hershey Medical Center in Pennsylvania. Of 7,316 patients, 367 (5.0%) had cutaneous malignancies. Of these, 38 patients had lesions as a result of direct local invasion, 337 had metastatic lesions, and 8 had both. A secondary analysis from the same registry found that 420 patients (10.4%) out of 4,020 with metastatic disease had cutaneous involvement.[2] Krathen et al.[3] performed a meta-analysis of nine studies examining the incidence of cutaneous metastasis from data collected from patient registries and autopsy reports. Excluding patients with melanoma, leukemia, and lymphoma, cutaneous metastasis was found in 1,080 out of 20,380 cancer patients for an incidence rate of 5.3%. The most common origins of metastasis are cancers of the breast, skin (melanoma), lung, head and neck, colon, rectum, and ovary.[1-6] Although these types of cancer account for the majority of skin involvement, it is important to note that metastatic cutaneous lesions may arise from any type of malignant tumor.[7-10] In some cases, the tumor of origin may not be identified.[11]

Cutaneous metastasis of internal cancer may predict survival time. In a retrospective study of 200 patients who developed cutaneous metastasis over a 46-year period, the median survival time after cutaneous involvement was 6.5 months.[12] Survival time varied by primary diagnosis. Median survival after cutaneous metastasis of the three most commonly observed cancers were 2.9 months for bronchopulmonary cancer, 13.8 months for breast cancer, and 15.5 months for melanoma.

Pathophysiology of Malignant Cutaneous Wounds

Malignant cutaneous lesions may develop secondary to local invasion of a primary tumor, or to metastasis from a distant site.[7,8]

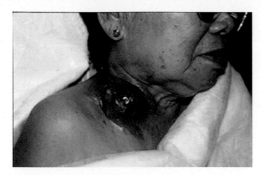

Figure 14.1 Fungating tumor secondary to metastasis of head and neck cancer. Note extreme friability of tissue. Requires extreme care to reduce bleeding with wound care. Reprinted with permission, © Gwen Thomas.

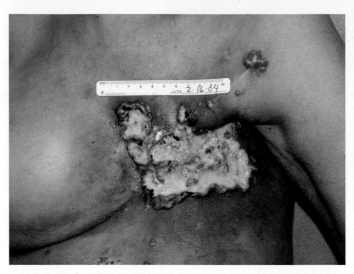

Figure 14.3 Eight years post mastectomy with ulcerative malignant lesion. Note necrotic center and friable edges. Note new metastatic nodule forming above ulcer. Reprinted with permission, © Susie Seaman.

Local invasion may initially manifest as inflammation with induration, redness, heat, and/or tenderness. The skin may have a *peau d'orange* appearance, and the area may be fixed to the underlying tissue. As the tumor infiltrates the skin, one or more ulcerating and/or fungating wounds develop.

In metastatic disease, tumor cells detach from the primary site and travel via blood and/or lymphatic vessels or tissue planes to distant organs, including the skin.[7,8] The resulting cutaneous lesions commonly present as well-demarcated nodules, ranging in size from a few millimeters to several centimeters.[7] Their consistency may vary from firm to rubbery. There may be pigmentation changes noted over and around the lesions, from deep red to brown-black. In general, these nodules are painless and may initially be misdiagnosed as epidermal cysts, lipomas, or other benign dermatoses. Cutaneous metastasis may also present as inflamed erythematous patches or plaques,[13] violaceous papules and vesicles, or alopecia. Over time, any of these lesions may ulcerate, drain, and become very painful. When patients with a history of cancer present with nodules, rashes, or inflamed skin, cutaneous metastasis must be a differential diagnosis.

Tumor cells secrete growth factors that promote metastasis, angiogenesis, extracellular matrix deposition, and, thus, tumor growth and extension.[14,15] Abnormalities in capillary development and lymphatic flow cause changes in local tissue perfusion that lead to increased tumor growth with simultaneous tissue death and alterations in local edema and exudate. As the tumor grows larger, it is unable to sustain sufficient vascular growth to support the entire mass. This results in fragile capillaries, poor perfusion, altered collagen synthesis, and resultant tissue ischemia and necrosis.

As noted earlier, the resulting lesion may be fungating, with the tumor mass extending above the skin surface with a fungus or cauliflower-like appearance, or it may be erosive and ulcerative.[7] The wound bed may be pale pink to red with very *friable* tissue, tissue that is fragile and bleeds easily, or completely necrotic, or a combination of both. Bleeding may be a challenge to control. In addition, the presence of necrotic tissue provides an ideal environment for overgrowth of anaerobic organisms, which may result in significant malodor.[16,17] The surrounding skin may be erythematous, edematous, fragile, and exceedingly tender to touch. Maceration may occur in the presence of excessive wound exudate.

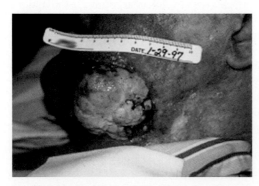

Figure 14.2 Fungating tumor from local invasion of oral cancer. Significant drainage and odor. Later developed an oral-cutaneous fistula. Reprinted with permission, © Gwen Thomas.

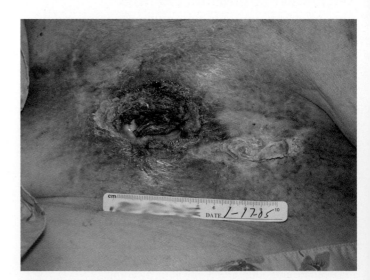

Figure 14.4 Cutaneous metastasis of breast cancer, four years post mastectomy and radiation therapy. Note thick dry eschar with dried exudate covering moist underlying wound. Significant odor. Reprinted with permission, © Susie Seaman.

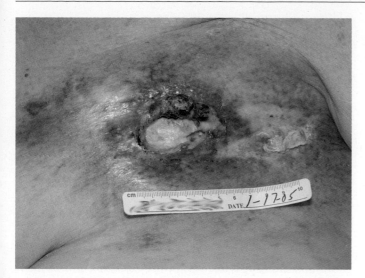

Figure 14.5 Same wound as shown in Figure 14-1, immediately following sharp debridement of eschar and thorough cleansing with skin cleanser. Note fungating area at superior edge of wound with friable tissue. Note slough and exposed rib in wound bed. Fragile surrounding skin secondary to radiation therapy. Surrounding redness from high vascularity of area. Reprinted with permission, © Susie Seaman.

Assessment of Malignant Cutaneous Wounds

A comprehensive evaluation of the patient and the malignant wound is necessary to create an individualized treatment plan. Assessment of malignant cutaneous wounds includes all parameters of wound assessment (see Chapter 3). Thorough assessment is important not only to determine treatment needs but also to document wound improvement or deterioration and to evaluate treatment effectiveness.

Expect malignant cutaneous wounds to change in size and appearance over time depending on the aggressiveness of the tumor and any treatment provided, including surgery, chemotherapy, and/or radiation.

Assess the following wound characteristics:

• *Location.* Depending on its location, the wound may impair the patient's mobility and functional level. This finding may demonstrate the need for occupational therapy, which can help in facilitating activities of daily living and functional ability. Wound location will also influence the dressing selection and dressing fixation because malignant cutaneous wounds may be located in wrinkled skin or highly uneven anatomic sites. The location of the wound also has significant psychological impact. If the wound is located in an area where it is easily covered from public view, the patient will respond differently than if the wound is located such that hiding it is not possible.

• *Wound appearance.* Assessment of the appearance of a malignant cutaneous wound is not very different from assessment of any other wound type. However, there are some special considerations.[18] Wound appearance should be evaluated for size, specifically looking for undermining and deep structure exposure. The wound should be assessed as fungating or ulcerative, with objective assessment of the percentage of viable versus necrotic tissue. Tissue should be assessed for friability and bleeding. Odor and exudate amount should be monitored and the presence of a fistula documented.

• *Wound colonization versus infection.* Identification of heavy bacterial colonization provides information on the deterioration or response of the wound to palliative care and impacts decisions regarding topical therapy and dressing selection. Malignant wounds that are heavily colonized require special attention to cleansing, odor-reducing antibacterial agents and dressings, and exudate management. Clinically infected malignant wounds with increased erythema, induration, pain, and fever require systemic antibiotic therapy. It can be challenging, however, to differentiate between the signs of infection and the signs of tumor extension, which are similar. Rapid onset of cellulitis and fever can point toward infection.

• *Surrounding skin.* Evaluate the skin surrounding the wound for color, integrity, and the presence of nodules or other signs of malignant progression. Typically, the skin surrounding malignant cutaneous wounds is erythematous. The skin may be fragile, macerated, or denuded as a result of excess exudate. You will often be able to predict the extension of the wound by observing the presence of nodules or eruptions in the skin surrounding the wound site. Surrounding skin may also exhibit signs of radiation damage, with erythema and other evidence of poor tissue perfusion. Tumor extension or metastasis will influence which dressing type and fixation method you select. For instance, you may need to use nonadherent dressings or methods other than tape for affixing the dressing. Significant deterioration in the surrounding skin presents challenges in selecting the appropriate dressing because applying larger and larger dressings may become necessary, and successfully securing the dressing may become problematic.

• *Symptom assessment.* The degree of symptoms experienced by the patient will depend on wound location, depth of tissue invasion and damage, nerve involvement, and the patient's previous experience with pain and use of analgesia.[19,20] Pain assessment is critical, because these wounds are often very painful, and adequate analgesia can control the pain and improve quality of life. Pain may include deep pain that is characterized by continuous aching or stabbing and superficial pain such as burning and stinging that may be associated only with dressing changes. If pain symptoms are the result of dressing changes, use of a short-acting topical analgesic with a rapid onset will make dressing changes more bearable for the patient. Pruritis is also commonly associated with these wounds. If the pruritic symptoms are related to dressings, the remedy may be as simple as trying a different dressing. More typically, pruritus may be a side effect of systemic analgesia and, if significant to the patient, may warrant change in pain medication or new systemic medications.

• *Complications.* It is essential to assess the potential for serious complications.[18] Evaluation should include potential for hemorrhage or vessel compression and obstruction, especially when the malignant wound is located close to major blood vessels. Wounds in the neck and chest area pose the threat of airway obstruction. Less serious complications include minor local bleeding, which is common secondary to capillary fragility. If you observe local bleeding, consider the use of nonadherent dressings, use extreme care in dressing removal, and be prepared to implement interventions to control it.

• *Psychosocial adaptation.* Assess how the patient and family are coping with the malignant wound and cancer diagnosis.[21,22] Question patients on how the wound affects their daily life,

CLINICAL WISDOM

If the lesion is not very friable, the patient may be able to get in the shower. This not only provides for local cleansing but also gives the added psychological benefit of helping the patient to feel clean. The patient should be instructed to allow the shower water to hit the skin above the wound and then allow it to gently run over the wound.

activities, and relationships. Assess the availability of social support networks in the community and question patients regarding their use.

- *Treatment effectiveness.* Assess treatment effectiveness at each dressing change. If the wound appears to be degenerating, you may need to change the treatment. These wounds may require more frequent treatment adjustments than other wound types.

Management of Malignant Cutaneous Wounds

Control of bacterial colonization, exudate, odor, bleeding, and pain are the cornerstones of management for malignant cutaneous wounds.[17–20,23–25] In determining the appropriate treatment regimen, the abilities of the caregiver must also be considered. The limited information on treatment effectiveness reflects the absence of evidence-based care in this area and the extreme need for further research and dissemination of findings.[26]

Infection Control: Wound Cleansing and Debridement

Infection control is facilitated by wound cleansing and debridement to remove necrotic debris, decrease bacterial counts, and thereby reduce odor. Judicious use of appropriate topical antimicrobials may also help control bacterial counts in the wound.[18]

If there is friable tissue or the patient is not able to shower, irrigate the wound gently with normal saline or a wound cleanser. For wounds without tissue friability that have increased necrosis and/or odor requiring more aggressive cleansing, low-pressure irrigation with normal saline can be performed using a 35-mL syringe and a 19-gauge needle or angiocatheter held a few inches away from the wound. Saline has the advantage of not disturbing any tissue that might be healthy, but a disadvantage is the lack of odor-reducing ingredients.

Skin cleansers, used to give patients bedbaths or to cleanse the perineal area with diaper changes, are highly efficacious at controlling odor in cutaneous tumors that have significant tissue necrosis and a high bacterial burden. Because they contain antiseptics, the use of skin cleansers alone will frequently be sufficient to control odor without the need for further products. They are also useful to gently cleanse the surrounding skin. However, the patient may experience burning from skin cleansers, especially if the wound has a large amount of viable tissue, and in that case, they should be avoided in favor of saline or wound cleansers.

Short-term use of antimicrobial solutions, such as povidone-iodine, sodium hypochlorite solution, or hydrogen peroxide are recommended by some authors in the palliative care of wounds, especially wounds that have dry gangrene or offensive odor.[20] The rationale for choosing an antimicrobial solution is the decrease of bacterial burden on the surface of the wound, with resultant decrease in odor. However, these chemicals can have their own odor that may be offensive to the patient. Significant burning, wound desiccation resulting in dressing adherence, and skin irritation are also associated with these products. If they are utilized, limit the time of use to no more than 2 weeks. An alternative to these antimicrobials is a polyhexamethylene biguanide (PHMB)-based solution. PHMB has been used as an antimicrobial for many years in products like PHMB-impregnated dressings and contact lens solutions.[27] A retrospective analysis comparing PHMB-soaked gauze to Ringer's lactate–soaked gauze in the treatment of venous ulcers demonstrated faster healing and lower infection rates in patients treated with PHMB.[28] To use on malignant wounds, PHMB-soaked gauze should be applied to the wound for 15 minutes and then removed. An appropriate dressing should then be applied.

Wound cleansing is followed by necrotic tissue debridement, if necessary. Necrotic tissue in malignant cutaneous wounds is typically moist yellow slough. Black eschar may be present in the absence of exudate, but this is less common. Necrotic tissue in these wounds may be extremely malodorous. Conservative debridement strategies are the basis for odor control. Autolysis, enzymatic, gentle mechanical, and/or conservative sharp debridement are the preferred options. Autolytic debridement is best achieved by using dressings that maintain a moist wound bed[29]; however, this should be weighed against the potential for increased odor that may occur in that occlusive environment. Topical enzymatic debriding agents can be applied to the wound and have the advantage of keeping the wound moist. Using care to prevent pain, gentle scrubbing of the necrotic tissue with saline-moistened gauze may facilitate removal of loose necrotic tissue. Cautious sharp debridement of necrotic tissue by clinicians trained in this procedure can be performed, taking special care to avoid bleeding, which may be difficult to control. If compatible with the palliative care goals of the patient, surgical debridement may be indicated in malignant wounds with a large amount of necrotic tissue. This procedure can significantly decrease odor, exudate, and will assist in decreasing the risk of infection.

Clinical wound infection may be effectively treated with topical antibiotic preparations or topical antimicrobial dressings (such as silver-impregnated products, PHMB-based dressings or gels), in conjunction with systemic antibiotics. A topical preparation may be necessary in infected malignant wounds treated with systemic antibiotics. The decreased perfusion and vasculature throughout the tumor may impede systemic antibiotic dissemination, making the combination approach more successful.

Management of Exudate

There tends to be significant exudate in malignant wounds due to local inflammation and edema that are commonly present. The goal in the management of exudate is to provide a moist wound environment to prevent trauma from dressing adherence that can occur if the wound dries out.[29] Keep the wound moist, but not wet. Choose dressings that will both conceal and collect exudate *and* odor. It is crucial to use dressings that absorb and contain exudate because a patient who experiences unexpected drainage on clothing or bedding may experience significant feelings of distress and loss of control. Specialty

CLINICAL WISDOM

Debridement of malignant cutaneous wounds is best done by enzymatic, autolytic, or conservative sharp methods and gentle mechanical methods (such as low-pressure irrigation), as opposed to wet-to-dry dressings, which are traumatic and painful and can cause significant bleeding upon removal.

dressings, such as foams, alginates, or starch copolymers, are notably more expensive than gauze pads or cotton-based absorbent pads. However, if the use of these dressings reduces cost by reducing the need for frequent dressing changes (improving quality of life for the patient), they are cost-effective, both in terms of dollars spent and quality of care.

In wounds with low exudate, the goal is to maintain a moist environment and to prevent dressing adherence and bleeding. Dressing choices for wounds in this category include nonadherent contact layers, such as Adaptic (Systagenix), Dermanet (DeRoyal), Mepitel (Mölnlycke), petrolatum gauze (numerous manufacturers), and Tegapore (3M Health Care). Amorphous hydrogels, sheet hydrogels, and hydrocolloids may also be helpful for low exudate wounds. Hydrocolloids are contraindicated with fragile surrounding skin and may increase odor. Semipermeable film dressings are also contraindicated with fragile surrounding skin. Nonadherent dressings are best for the primary contact layer because they minimize the trauma to the wound associated with dressing changes.

Wounds with high exudate require attention to absorbing and containing exudate. Dressings such as alginates, foams, starch copolymers, gauze, and soft cotton pads are all possible selections. Seaman[30] suggests nonadherent contact layers (such as petrolatum gauze) for the primary dressing on the wound bed, covered with soft, absorbent dressings (such as gauze and abdominal binder dressings) for secondary dressings to contain drainage. The dressing should be changed one to two times daily, depending on the amount of exudate. When drainage increases, the use of calcium alginate dressings to decrease the frequency of dressing changes may be considered.

Protection of the surrounding skin is an important aspect of exudate management. Using ostomy skin barriers on the skin surrounding the wound and then taping dressings to the skin barriers (changing the barriers every 5–7 days) are one method

CLINICAL WISDOM

Use of menstrual pads as secondary dressings may be helpful for wounds with heavy exudate. These pads have the added benefit of clothing protection because of the outer plastic lining. Instruct patients to leave the paper backing over the adhesive so the pad will not adhere to clothing. Also, recommend unscented pads, as the scented pads can have a very strong smell, especially if the wound is close to the nose.

CLINICAL WISDOM

When using ostomy barriers on the surrounding skin, determine the correct location by applying the absorbent cover dressing first. Once that is on, then apply the ostomy barrier along the edge of the cover dressing; this will ensure that the barrier is in the correct spot when tape is applied. Another trick to avoid pulling the barrier off prematurely when removing the dressing is to cover the barrier with a layer of adhesive tape first. Then when taping the dressing in place, the tape used to secure the bandage contacts the tape on the barrier (tape-to-tape contact instead of tape-to-barrier contact), and pulls off easier upon removal.

of protecting surrounding skin from both excess drainage and tape, and the resultant skin stripping with dressing changes. Another method of protecting the surrounding skin is use of a barrier ointment to the skin surrounding the ulcer. The barrier protects fragile tissue from maceration and the caustic effects of the drainage on the skin. Do not use barrier ointments if the skin is already macerated; the ointment will make this worse. Consider use of a liquid skin sealant instead. Dressings can be held in place with Montgomery straps or tape affixed to a skin barrier placed on healthy skin, flexible netting, tube dressings, sports bras, panties, and the like.[18]

Odor Control

Odor control is by far the most challenging management aspect of malignant cutaneous wounds and one of the most distressing to cancer patients.[22,31] Approaches to odor control include use of topical medications, dressings, systemic medications, and environmental manipulation.

One treatment available for topical use in several formulations and well supported in the literature for odor control is the antibiotic metronidazole (Flagyl, Helidac, MetroCream, MetroGel, Noritate Cream).[17,18,20,30,32–38] Application of MetroGel (Galderma Laboratories), 0.75% metronidazole in a hydrogel carrier, to wounds results in a decrease in wound odor in 2 to 3 days, even in the presence of resistant odor.[34–37] Typically, metronidazole gel is applied to the wound in a thin layer, then covered with nonadherent contact layer and absorbent bandage, and dressings are changed once to twice daily, depending on the amount of exudate. An irrigant solution can be made by either crushing metronidazole tablets or using metronidazole powder in sterile water and creating either a 0.5% solution (5 mg/mL) or a 1% solution (10 mg/mL).[39,40] This solution may be used to moisten gauze for packing into a wound and may be very effective for filling malodorous undermined or tunneled areas. Care must be used with this method to prevent adherence of the gauze to the wound and subsequent bleeding and pain. Topical treatment may be sufficient for controlling odor. If odor persists, odor is severe, or clinical infection is suspected, systemic metronidazole 500 mg taken orally three to four times a day may also be administered, but caution should be used because of the adverse gastrointestinal (GI) effects that may occur.[17,20]

Another topical treatment is the antimicrobial agent Iodosorb gel, an iodine complex in a starch copolymer

RESEARCH WISDOM

A disadvantage of metronidazole gel is that both brand names and generic equivalents are expensive. Kalinski et al.[33] studied the use of a compounded topical formulation of metronidazole in the odor control of 16 patients with malignant wounds. Metronidazole gel 0.75% was formulated by blending 3.6 g of metronidazole powder with 10 mL of propylene glycol to make a gelatinous base. Once this was well mixed, 480 mL of hydroxypropyl methylcellulose was added and blended until the metronidazole was completely dissolved. This was made by a compounding pharmacist and packaged in 2- or 4-oz jars. The metronidazole formulation was applied to malignant wounds once a day in a 1- to 1.5-mm-thick layer and covered with a nonadherent contact layer and gauze. Odor was completely eliminated in 10 patients within 24 hours, and significantly reduced in the other 6 patients. The formulation was safe without adverse side effects. The per gram cost was 3% of that of commercial metronidazole.

CLINICAL WISDOM

Use of peppermint oil or other aromatherapy products in the environment around the patient may help in masking wound odor. A container of charcoal or kitty litter under the bed may also absorb and decrease odor in the patient's room. If room sprays are used, educate patients to use odor eliminator sprays, not deodorant sprays. Deodorant sprays add a sweet smell to the room that may be disturbing to the patient. Caregivers may apply mentholatum under their nostrils when changing wound dressings if the odor is troubling to them.

(cadexomer iodine). This product contains slow-release iodine and has been shown to decrease bacterial counts in wounds without cytotoxicity.[41,42] Seaman has had clinical experience with this product in reducing odor associated with venous ulcers. Cadexomer iodine is available in a 40-g tube and is applied to the wound in a 1/8-inch layer. An advantage of this product is exudate absorption, in that each gram absorbs 6 mL of fluid. Disadvantages include cost (comparable with metronidazole 0.75% gel) and possible burning on application.

A PHMB-based gel is now available for odor control. Prontosan gel contains PHMB, which decreases bacterial counts, and Betaine, which is a surfactant that softens and loosens necrotic debris. It should be applied to wounds in a 3- to 5-mm layer, covered with a nonadherent contact layer and absorbent pad. The gel can also be applied to gauze packing for deeper wounds.

An additional topical treatment for managing odor is the use of charcoal-based dressings. Charcoal will absorb and decrease odor. There are many different versions of these dressings; some can be placed directly next to the wound, while others are secondary dressings. Many charcoal dressings are inactivated if they become moist. Their use can be costly, so the benefit of using charcoal dressings should be weighed against less expensive and possibly more effective options.

Controlling Bleeding

Bleeding, which can vary from capillary oozing to frank hemorrhage, is common in malignant wounds due to the friability of the tissue. These patients may also have coagulation defects that increase their risk of bleeding.[43,44] It must be controlled since bleeding is not only distressing to the patient and caregiver, but it also prolongs the dressing change procedure, causes the bandages to adhere to the wound, and can worsen the chronic anemia that many of these patients experience.

Prevention is the best strategy and involves the use of a gentle hand in dressing removal and thoughtful attention to the use of nonadherent dressings or moist wound dressings. On wounds with low exudate, the use of hydrogel sheets, or amorphous hydrogels under a nonadherent contact layer, may keep the wound moist and prevent dressing adherence. Even highly exudating wounds may require a nonadherent contact layer to allow for nontraumatic dressing removal. When dressings do adhere to the wound during removal, they should be soaked off with normal saline or water to lessen trauma to the wound bed.[23]

If bleeding does occur, the first intervention should be the application of direct pressure over the wound for 10 to 15 minutes.[18,23] Hold saline-moistened gauze against the wound; this will help prevent the gauze from adhering and causing a new episode of bleeding upon removal. Adding an ice pack may help control bleeding and also contribute to local comfort. If pressure and/or ice are ineffective, several other options exist.

The local application of hemostatic dressings such as purified gelatin (Gelfoam), oxidized regenerated cellulose (Surgicel), collagen (available as sheets, powders, or sponges), combination collagen/oxidized regenerated cellulose (Promogran), fibrin sealants, or calcium alginates may be of use to control mild bleeding.[44] Gauze soaked in 1:1,000 epinephrine or topical cocaine can be applied to the wound to control bleeding but also may result in systemic side effects.[44] Topical formalin, applied to the wound by soaking gauze, is an effective chemical hemostat.[43,44] Sucralfate paste, made by crushing a 1-g sucralfate tablet in 5 mL of water-soluble hydrogel, can be applied directly to bleeding areas and left in place.[23,43] Two fibrinolytic inhibitors, tranexamic acid and aminocaproic acid, have been used either orally or topically (crushed tablets in solution) to control bleeding in cancer patients.[45,46] These drugs prevent the breakdown of fibrin clots and have also been used topically to control wound bleeding in patients with hemophilia.[47] You can also treat small bleeding points with silver nitrate sticks.

If bleeding continues or is severe, more aggressive palliation may be necessary. Radiation therapy may be useful in achieving hemostasis.[44,48] Additionally, super-selective angiography with transcatheter embolization of the arteries supplying the tumor can be very effective in controlling bleeding and may lead to shrinkage of the lesion.[49–51]

For patients receiving palliative or hospice care, caregivers should be educated on measures to take for catastrophic hemorrhage.[18] This includes notifying hospice staff (do not call 911), having dark towels ready to cover the bleeding area, and elevating the area of bleeding if comfortable for the patient. A rapid acting sedative, such as midazolam 2.5 to 5.0 mg IV or SQ, can be administered to calm the patient. The caregiver should be encouraged to sit with the patient and speak in a comforting tone.

Minimizing Pain

Several types of pain are associated with malignant cutaneous wounds: deep aching, sharp pain, burning or stinging sensations, and superficial pain related to procedures. Deep pain should be managed by regularly scheduled oral, subcutaneous, or parenteral analgesics, with extra premedication prior to dressing changes. Opioids may be needed preprocedurally, and rapid-onset, short-acting formulations may be especially useful for those already receiving other opioid medication. Use of nonsteroidal anti-inflammatory drugs may be beneficial for mild pain.[20] Ice packs may also provide local control of mild pain.

For management of superficial pain related to procedures, topical lidocaine, lidocaine-prilocaine, tetracaine, or benzocaine may be useful.[20,30] Different formulations are available in sprays, gels, creams, and ointments. Although eutectic mixture of local anesthetics (EMLA) cream, a combination of lidocaine and prilocaine, is FDA-approved in the United States for use only on intact skin, it is approved and used in many countries on leg ulcers prior to sharp debridement. EMLA has demonstrated adequate local anesthesia in leg ulcer debridement.[52,53] Its use on malignant wounds has not been studied and would be considered off-label but would be an acceptable practice if in the best interest of the patient. Dosage is 1 to 2 g/10 cm², up to a maximum of 10 g. It should be applied to wounds under occlusion for 45 to 60 minutes prior to procedures such as wound cleansing or debridement. Excessive dosing of EMLA can lead to methemoglobinemia and should be avoided.[54] Liposomal lidocaine (LMX-4%, LMX-5%) is formulated for rapid penetration into the skin. It is FDA-approved for pain relief of minor cuts, abrasions, burns, and skin irritations. Use in malignant wounds would be considered off-label. Liposomal lidocaine absorbs rapidly, requires only a 30-minute application time without occlusion, and has been found be as efficacious as EMLA prior to dermal procedures.[55] The maximum recommended dose is a thick layer applied to an area no greater than 100 cm².

Another option for topical analgesia is the use of topical opioids, which bind to peripheral opioid receptors.[56,57] Back and Finlay[58] reported the use of diamorphine 10 mg added to an amorphous hydrogel and applied to the wounds of three patients on a daily basis. Two of the patients had painful pressure ulcers, and the third had a painful malignant wound. All three patients were on systemic opioids. The patients noted improved pain control on the first day of treatment. Krajnik and Zbigniew[59] reported the case of a 76-year-old woman with metastatic lesions on her scalp that caused severe tension pain. Ibuprofen 400 mg three times a day was ineffective, and because the pain was in a limited area, the authors applied morphine 0.08% gel (3.2 mg morphine in 4 g of amorphous hydrogel). The patient's pain decreased from 7 on a 10-point visual analogue scale (VAS) to 1 within 2 hours of gel application. Pain increased back to 6 on the VAS at 25.5 hours postapplication. Therefore, the gel was reapplied daily and maintained pain control with no side effects. Zeppetella et al.[60] demonstrated the efficacy of topically applied morphine sulfate 10 mg/mL in 8 g Intrasite gel in the treatment of five hospice patients with painful pressure ulcers. The results of this pilot study were later validated in a larger randomized controlled study by the same authors.[61] Sixteen hospice inpatients with painful pressure or malignant wounds were randomized to receive topical morphine as described above or placebo (water for injection 1 mL in 8 g Intrasite gel) to their wounds. After 2 days of treatment, patients entered a 2-day washout period and then were crossed over to the opposite group for 2 more days. Patients assigned a numerical rating score to the analgesia that they obtained in each 2-day period, the lower score indicating better pain relief. Topically applied morphine provided significantly lower scores compared to pretreatment and placebo ($p < 0.001$). The treatment was well tolerated. Wound care clinicians should consider this option for topical pain relief in the care of patients with localized pain from a cutaneous tumor. Because wound care is performed frequently in these patients, the addition of topical opioids, applied with dressing changes, may be an excellent adjunct to the pain management plan.

Other Management Options

Many patients in the early stages of cutaneous metastasis or local invasion may be candidates for more aggressive care aimed at tumor shrinkage and the resulting decrease in pain, exudate, bleeding, and odor. These treatments may include surgical removal of problematic nodules or debulking of fungating masses,[18] transcatheter embolization,[44,48–50,62] local radiation therapy,[63,64] topical or intra-arterial chemotherapy,[65,66] and/or radiofrequency ablation.[67] Bufill et al. reported the case of a 59-year-old woman with an extensive fungating chest wall tumor secondary to breast cancer whose tumor completely resolved following local intra-arterial chemotherapy.[68] She died 10 months later with only a palpable breast mass but no open wound.

Despite the fact that patients may eventually succumb to the underlying cancer and that there may no longer be a curative treatment available, individual patients may benefit from temporary improvement in the lesion through more aggressive palliative treatments. Consult with the patient's primary provider about the feasibility of these treatments for individual patients.

Outcome Measures for Malignant Cutaneous Wounds

The expected outcome for most malignant cutaneous wounds is that the wound will deteriorate and increase in size. Outcome measures are, therefore, related to palliation of symptoms, not wound healing. The major goals of therapy are to control infection, manage exudate, reduce odor, control bleeding, and minimize pain. Outcomes of therapy relate to the success of the treatment in meeting these goals.

Outcomes related to infection control include the lack of signs/symptoms of infection, including increased erythema, exudate, odor, and pain. There may be no reports of the need for prescribed systemic antibiotics, indicating prevention of infection.

Outcomes related to effective management of exudate include the amount and type of exudate and possibly the number of dressing changes per day to manage exudate. Other

---

CLINICAL WISDOM

Alvarez et al.[20] describe the use of a mixture of lidocaine ointment and zinc oxide cream (Balmex) compounded at their hospital pharmacy to render a 2.75% lidocaine topical formulation for use on painful wounds. They suggest application twice a day, covered by a nonadherent primary dressing with or without a secondary absorbent dressing.

options for outcome measures related to exudate are the number of accidental leaks of exudate through to clothing or maceration of surrounding skin because of excessive moisture.

Patient or caregiver reports of wound odor or even of the amount of time family members spend with the patient on a daily basis are good measures of outcomes related to achieving effective odor control. Reports regarding increased or decreased use of topical antimicrobials will indicate whether or not odor is controlled.

Outcome measures for controlling bleeding may include monitoring of hemoglobin and hematocrit status and prevention of excessive trauma to the wound by the wound dressing, as well as frequency of bleeding events.

Pain outcome measures must include patient self-report with an evidence-based tool for assessment of pain. Additional outcomes related to pain and discomfort may be related to the patient's perception of the wound dressing itself. The dressing should be perceived as comfortable, accessible, user-friendly, and as staying in place for the desired time period. The amount of analgesia required by the patient is not a good outcome measure for pain because the implication is that as the analgesia amount decreases the outcome improves, and this is generally not the case with palliative care. In fact, in many instances, the amount of analgesia will increase over the course of therapy.

In general, with malignant cutaneous wounds, outcomes are focused on alleviation of suffering related to the wound. Achievement of comfort, general psychological well-being, and a satisfactory level of physical functioning can all be measures of patient outcomes.

Patient and Caregiver Education Related to Malignant Cutaneous Wounds

Your patients with malignant cutaneous wounds, and their caregivers, require the same education you would provide to patients and caregivers about basic wound care. Discuss the frequency of and procedures for dressing changes, including when to premedicate to manage pain. Identify and reinforce the variety of alternatives for odor control. Also make sure to educate patients and caregivers about reportable conditions. Teach them to report the following conditions to their health-care provider:

- Excessive or malodorous exudates
- Pruritus or cellulites
- Severe emotional distress
- Increased or change in pain
- Bleeding
- Fever
- Unusual or major change in the wound appearance

- Inability of the caregiver to manage wound care
- Inability to obtain needed wound care supplies

Dealing with a cancer diagnosis is traumatic enough without the added physical and psychological burden of a malignant wound.[69] Lo et al.[70] interviewed 10 patients with malignant fungating wounds to examine how this condition affected their lives. Central issues that negatively affected quality of life were pain, social isolation secondary to exudate and odor, and ignorance of both patients and health care providers regarding appropriate wound care. It was concluded that the key to improving quality of life for these patients was access to a wound care team or specialist who educated them on how to care for the wound with appropriate dressings, and how to control exudate and odor. Education must also focus on the psychosocial aspects of having a malignant wound. Patients may report feelings of fear, grief, disgust, loss of control and self-esteem, and anxiety.[71,72] They may feel embarrassed and stigmatized, and may withdraw from loved ones. Caregivers may experience feelings of helplessness and fear about caring for the patient and wound. Both patients and caregivers may feel repulsed by the malignant wound. The clinician can facilitate a trusting relationship with the patient and caregivers by reviewing the goals of care and by openly discussing issues that the patient may not have talked about with other providers. For example, it is helpful to acknowledge odor openly and then discuss how the odor will be managed. Attention to the cosmetic appearance of the wound with the dressing in place can assist the patient in dealing with body image disturbances. Use of soft flexible dressings that can fill a defect and protect clothing may help to restore symmetry and provide security for the patient. Lastly, the clinician can model calm and competent care of the wound to the patient and caregiver and give them the sense that they can handle this difficult situation.

Assisting the patient and the caregiver to cope with the distressing symptoms of the malignant wound such that odor and bleeding are managed, exudate is contained, and pain is alleviated, will improve the quality of life for these patients and contribute to the goal of satisfactory psychological well-being. Education must include realistic goals for the wound. In these patients, the goal of complete wound healing is seldom achievable; however, quality of life and satisfying relationships can be maintained and nurtured, even as the wound degenerates. Continual education and reevaluation of the effectiveness of the treatment plan are essential to maintaining quality of life for those suffering from a malignant wound.

The following case illustrates the positive effect that the wound care clinician can have on patients with malignant cutaneous wounds.

CASE STUDY

An anxious 82-year-old woman with breast cancer with cutaneous metastasis to the left chest wall was referred to the Wound Healing Center. She was accompanied by her daughter, who was also very anxious and worried. The patient had undergone a mastectomy and radiation therapy 4 years prior and had developed chest wall metastasis 8 months before referral. Current wound care included no cleansing, and she

kept the wound covered with dry gauze, which would adhere to the wound. Her main complaint was of severe pain, which she rated an "8" on a scale of 0 to 10 and described as a constant ache with intermittent sharp pains in the area of the tumor metastasis. Current pain management consisted of oral hydrocodone with acetaminophen, one tablet four times a day. She felt that pain was something that could not be controlled and that she would have to live with it. Her second complaint was of severe malodor associated with the wound, and she stated that her main goal in coming to the Wound Healing Center was to learn how to care for the wound and decrease the odor.

Assessment revealed a 5 × 5 cm moderately dry necrotic wound on the left chest wall (see Fig. 14.1) with severe malodor, scant tan exudate from the lower edge, and very thin, fragile surrounding skin.

The necrotic tissue was sharp debrided without damaging viable tissue or causing pain or bleeding. The wound was then thoroughly cleaned and rinsed with a skin cleanser, resulting in almost total elimination of odor. It was noted that the superior edge of the wound was fungating and mildly friable and there was rib exposure at the base of the wound (see Fig. 14.2). The daughter was instructed on the following daily wound care:

1. Cleanse the wound and skin with skin cleanser and pat dry.
2. Apply a thin coat of metronidazole gel 0.75% across the wound.
3. Cover with one to three layers of petrolatum gauze (one layer to start and add more layers if the wound dries out and the dressing adheres to the tissue).
4. Cover the wound and surrounding skin with an absorbent ABD pad and secure with chest stockinette.

A long discussion was undertaken with the patient and daughter regarding pain management. The oncologist was contacted, and started the patient on Duragesic patch 25 µg to be changed every 72 hours. The patient was continued on the hydrocodone for breakthrough pain.

The patient returned to the clinic 2 weeks later. She was in much better spirits and reported complete control of the odor. She was now on Duragesic patch 50 µg, with use of two to four hydrocodone per day and reported pain at a 2 to 3 on a numerical rating scale of 0 to 10, which was acceptable to her. She felt very encouraged by her progress, and her daughter reported that she was much more interactive with the family. The patient and her daughter were extremely appreciative of the simple interventions that had been undertaken to improve the patient's quality of life.

The patient continued with monthly reassessments in the Wound Healing Center and, 3 months later, reported problems with bleeding from the tumor. She had been hospitalized for one significant episode of bleeding and had undergone angiography and catheter embolization of the artery feeding the tumor. This had stopped any major bleeding but she reported continued seepage from the friable areas of the tumor and was quite scared by this. Assessment revealed an area of friable tissue with no large vessels visible. Bleeding was easily controlled in the clinic with pressure and silver nitrate application. She was reassured that bleeding was normal and that she and her daughter could handle all but the most severe of bleeding episodes with the following steps, advancing to each subsequent step if bleeding was not controlled:

1. Rest in reclined position with chest and head elevated.
2. Apply local pressure with water-moistened gauze for 15 minutes.
3. Apply oxidized regenerated cellulose and collagen (Promogran) to any bleeding areas and continue pressure for 15 minutes.
4. Apply ice packs to the area for 15 to 20 minutes.
5. Gently apply silver nitrate with the use of silver nitrate sticks (the daughter was instructed in this and the patient was given a prescription for same).
6. Contact physician or Wound Healing Center if bleeding continues. As the patient was not on hospice care, she was instructed to go to the emergency room for any significant, high-volume bleeding.

When the patient was assessed the next month, she reported mild episodes of bleeding that were controlled with pressure alone. She stated that once she had been taught that bleeding was normal from these types of wounds, she had not worried about it and it had not been a problem. Pain and odor remained under good control, despite the fact that the wound was obviously larger, with increased rib exposure.

This patient lived 11 months with quality of life, free of odor and significant pain, and died peacefully at home. With support and education, she and her family learned to live quite comfortably, despite the enlarging malignant wound.

FISTULAS

A **fistula** is an abnormal passage or opening between two or more body organs or spaces. Fistulas with openings from one internal body organ to another (such as from small bowel to bladder or from bladder to vagina) are *internal* fistulas, whereas those with cutaneous involvement (such as small bowel to skin) are termed *external* fistulas. Exhibit 14.1 presents common fistula terminology related to internal and external fistula types.

The most commonly seen fistulas involve the skin and GI tract, and are called *enterocutaneous fistulas*. However, fistulas can occur between many other body organs and spaces. The organs involved and the precise location of the fistula can significantly complicate care; for example, fistulas between the

small bowel and the vaginal vault, as well as those involving the esophagus and skin, present extreme challenges in wound care. Fistulas involving the pancreas are also typically problematic, as are enterocutaneous fistulas. This chapter predominantly addresses enterocutaneous fistulas although we briefly discuss vaginal fistula management techniques later in the chapter.

Significance of Fistulas

In most cases, the goal of care is fistula closure (spontaneous or surgical). Interventions to promote spontaneous closure include attention to fluid and electrolyte balance, prevention of sepsis and infection control, maintenance of adequate nutrition, and protection of surrounding tissues.[73] Spontaneous closure of enterocutaneous fistulas with adequate medical management can occur in 60% to 85% of cases.[74–77] Adequate medical management includes nutrition supplementation and support, for example, enteral or parenteral with or without somatostatin infusion. The time required to achieve closure ranges from 5 to 26 days, thus requiring long-term treatment plans for all patients with fistulas. Of the enterocutaneous fistulas that will close spontaneously, 90% will do so within a 4- to 7-week time frame.[73,76,78,79] Therefore, if the fistula has not spontaneously closed with adequate medical treatment (e.g., management of sepsis and parenteral or enteral nutrition with or without somatostatin infusion) within 7 weeks, the goal of care may change from fistula closure to management of the fistula for quality of life.

Palliative care is particularly needed when the chances of fistula closure are limited by other nonmodifiable factors. Factors that inhibit fistula closure include complete disruption of bowel continuity, distal obstruction, presence of a foreign body in the fistula tract, an epithelium-lined tract contiguous with the skin, presence of cancer, previous radiation, and Crohn's disease.[73] Goals of care for palliative fistula management involve containment of effluent, management of odor, increased comfort, and protection of the surrounding skin and tissues.

Pathophysiology of Fistula Development

Among all cancer patients, those with GI cancers and/or those who have received irradiation to pelvic organs are at highest risk of fistula development. Fistula development occurs in 1% of patients with advanced malignancy, typically in relation to either obstruction from the malignancy or from irradiation side effects.[80] Radiation therapy damages vasculature and underlying structures. In cancer-related fistula development, management is almost always palliative.

Fistula development is not limited to patients with cancer. Postsurgical complications can also increase a patient's risk for fistula development. Many clinicians have reported the majority of fistula cases as arising from anastomotic breakdown immediately following surgical procedures.[78,81] In addition, postsurgical adhesions (scar tissues) can promote fistula development by obstructing the normal intestinal passageway. Moreover, by reducing tissue perfusion, an inadequate blood supply during surgery, tension on a suture line, improper suturing technique, and an aggressive surgical procedure can promote vulnerability to fistula formation in surgical patients. Patients with inflammatory bowel disease, Crohn's disease in particular, are prone to fistula development because of the effects of the disease process on the bowel itself. Because Crohn's disease is a transmural disease, involving all layers of the bowel wall, patients with Crohn's are prone to fistula development. Crohn's disease can occur anywhere along the entire GI tract; however, it often involves the perianal area, with fissures and fistulas as common findings. Initially, the disease is managed medically with steroids, immunotherapy, and metronidazole for perianal disease. There is no cure for Crohn's disease; thus, if medical management fails, the patient may elect surgical removal of the area of bowel affected with the disease, and creation of an ostomy. In later stages of disease, if medical and surgical management has failed, multiple fistulas may present clinically, and the goal for care becomes palliative, with symptom control as the primary objective.

Other factors contributing to fistula development include the presence of a foreign body next to a suture line, distal obstruction, hematoma/abscess formation, tumor or additional disease in the bowel anastomotic site, and inadequate blood supply.[82] Each of these can contribute to fistula formation by promoting an abnormal passage between two body organs. Typically, the contributing factor provides a path of least resistance for evacuation of stool or urine along the tract, rather than through the normal route. Such is the case with hematoma or abscess formation. In some cases, the normal passageway is blocked, as with tumor growth or obstructive processes.

Assessment of Fistulas

Assessment of the fistula involves assessment of the source, output, location, and fluid and electrolyte status.

- *Source.* Evaluation of the fistula source may involve use of diagnostic tests, such as radiographs, to determine exact structures involved in the fistula tract. Computed tomography and magnetic resonance imaging may be required to rule out abscess or complicated fistula tracts.[73] Assessment of the fistula source also involves evaluation of fistula output for odor, color, consistency, pH, and amount.[83] These all provide clues to the fistula origin.
- *Output.* Fistulas with highly odorous output likely originate in the colon or may be related to cancerous lesions. Fistula output with minimal odor may be from the small bowel. Color also provides clues to the source. Clear or white output is typical of esophageal fistulas. Green output usually indicates a fistula originating from the gastric area. Light brown or tan output may indicate a small bowel fistula. The consistency of small bowel output varies from thin and watery to thick and pasty, whereas output from colonic fistulas has a pasty to a soft consistency. The volume of output may suggest the source of the fistula. For small bowel fistulas, output volume may range from 500 to 3,000 mL over 24 hours. Esophageal fistula output may be as high as 1,000 mL over 24 hours.
- *Location.* Assessment of the orifice location, the proximity of the orifice to bony prominences, the regularity and stability of the surrounding skin, the number of fistula openings, and the level the fistula orifice exits onto the skin all influence treatment options. *Fluid and electrolyte balance.* Fistulas of GI origins are more likely to prompt fluid and electrolyte disruptions. Patients with ECFs are at high risk for fluid volume deficit or dehydration, and assessment of hydration is essential. These patients are also at risk for metabolic acidosis, because of the loss of large volumes of alkaline small bowel contents. Significant losses of sodium and potassium are also common with small bowel fistulas. Monitor laboratory values frequently.

Exhibit 14.2 identifies the typical composition of output from a variety of GI organs involved in fistulas.

CLINICAL WISDOM

The location of the fistula often impedes containment of fistula output. Skin integrity should be assessed for erythema, ulceration, maceration, or denudement from fistula output. Typically, the more caustic the fistula output, the more impaired the surrounding skin integrity. Multiple fistula tracts may also hamper containment efforts.

Management of Fistulas

The mortality rate among patients with an enterocutaneous fistula is 5% to 21%, even with appropriate management. Thus, a variety of interventions are critical.

Nutrition Management

One of the cornerstones of fistula management is attention to nutrition. Most fistula patients with enterocutaneous fistulas are malnourished and become more so as the duration of time with the fistula increases. Fluid and nutritional requirements may be greatly increased, while simultaneously the functioning of the GI system may be greatly impaired. Lack of adequate intake of protein and calories, inadequate digestion and absorption of nutrients, extreme losses of nutrient-rich output, and increased metabolic demands from infection also contribute to nutritional deficits. Consultation with a nutritionist or dietician is highly encouraged early in the management of the fistula patient.

Protein and calorie needs vary, based on the type of fistula, amount of output, status of the patient prior to fistula development, and infection status. The route for nutritional supplementation depends on the anatomic location of the fistula and on the patient's ability to take in adequate nutrition orally. As a general guideline, the GI system should be used whenever possible for nutritional support. Using the GI tract allows the intestines to continue performing usual functions, thus maintaining normal physiology of the tract. When the GI tract is not used, the villi can atrophy and lose their absorptive capabilities. If nutrition can bypass the fistula site, absorption and tolerance are better with use of the intestinal tract. Enteral nutrition is preferred when the fistula is located in the *most* proximal or distal portions of the GI tract.

For enterocutaneous fistulas, bypassing the fistula orifice is not always feasible. If the small bowel fistula is located distally, there may be enough of the intestinal tract available to absorb nutrients adequately prior to the fistula orifice. If the fistula is located more proximally, there may not be enough intestinal tract available for adequate nutrient absorption. Specific solutions or feeding regimens should be ordered in consultation with the dietician because he or she can recommend the most appropriate supplement. Many of these patients must be managed with intravenous hyperalimentation (TPN) during the early stages of fistula management.

Include the patient and family in discussions of nutrition management. Explain that patients with enterocutaneous fistulas should see a reduction in fistula output within 7 days of TPN therapy. Encourage the patient and caregivers to inform the primary care provider if after 7 days there is no change in fistula output. In such cases, adding somatostatin infusion has demonstrated improvements and spontaneous closure in some patients.[73,75,76]

Management of Output

Gauze dressings with or without charcoal filters may be used when the output from the fistula is less than 250 mL over 24 hours and is not severely offensive in odor. However, in the majority of cases, the fistula should be managed with an ostomy pouching technique. Pouching the fistula allows for odor control, containment of output, and protection of the surrounding skin from damage. When the enterocutaneous fistula occurs in a wound, use of negative pressure wound therapy (NPWT) has demonstrated effectiveness.

Pouching Procedure: General Instructions

The pouching procedure involves three basic steps: cleansing the surrounding skin with warm water, without soap or antiseptics; applying a skin barrier paste to fill uneven skin surfaces and create a flat surface on which to apply the pouch; and applying the pouch. Variations on this basic procedure are discussed shortly.

Choose the type of pouch according to the location and fistula output. Pediatric pouches are often smaller and may be useful for hard-to-pouch areas where flexibility is needed, such as the neck for esophageal fistulas. If the fistula output is watery and thin, choose a pouch with a narrow spigot or tube for closure. In contrast, a fistula with a thick, pasty output would be better managed with a pouch with an open end and a clamp for closure.

Pouches must be emptied frequently, at least when one-third to one-half full. There are several wound drainage pouching systems that will allow for visualization and direct access to the fistula through a valve or door. This allows you to open the pouch for drainage and then reclose it. These wound management pouches are available in large sizes and often work well for abdominal fistulas.[84–86] Colostomy caps (small, closed-end pouches) may be very useful for low-output fistulas.

Specific pouching techniques that are useful in complex fistula management include troughing, bridging, and saddlebagging.[82] Alternatively, use of NPWT may be used. These techniques are particularly helpful when dealing with fistulas that occur in wounds, most commonly the small bowel fistula that develops in the open abdominal wound.

Troughing

Troughing is useful for fistulas that occur in the posterior aspect of large abdominal wounds (Fig. 14.6).[87] Line the skin surrounding the wound and fistula with a skin barrier wafer and seal the edge of the nearest wound with skin barrier paste. Then apply thin film dressings over the top or anterior aspect of the wound, down to the fistula orifice and the posterior aspect of the wound. Last, use a cut-to-fit ostomy pouch to pouch the opening in the thin film dressing at the fistula orifice. Wound exudate drains from the anterior portion of the wound (under the thin film dressing) to the posterior portion of the wound and out into the ostomy pouch, along with fistula output. The trough technique does not prevent fistula output from contaminating the wound site.

Bridging

The bridging technique prevents fistula output from contaminating the wound site and allows for a unique wound dressing to be applied to the wound site (Fig. 14.7). Bridging is appropriate for fistulas that occur in the posterior aspect of large abdominal wounds, where it is important to contain fistula output away from the wound site. Using small pieces of skin barrier wafers, build a bridge by consecutively layering the skin barriers together until the skin barrier has the appearance of a wedge or bridge and it is the same height as the depth of the wound.[82] Using skin barrier paste, adhere the skin barrier wedge to the wound bed (it will not harm the healthy tissues of the wound bed) next to the fistula opening. Then cut an ostomy pouch to fit the fistula opening, using the wedge or bridge as a portion of intact surrounding skin to adhere the pouch.[82] Finally, dress the anterior aspect of the wound with the dressing of choice.

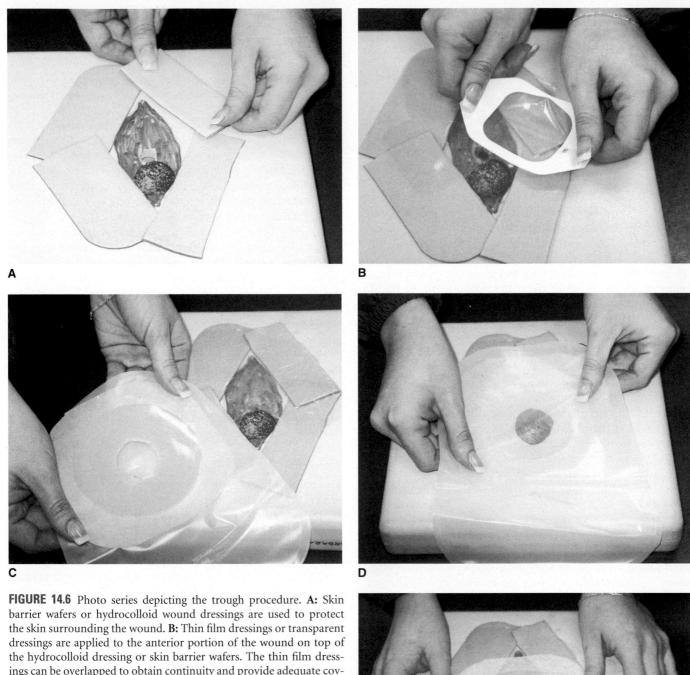

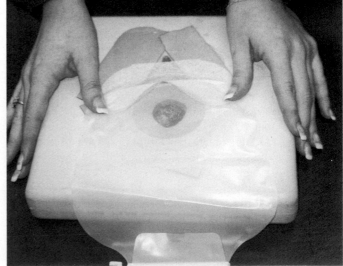

FIGURE 14.6 Photo series depicting the trough procedure. **A:** Skin barrier wafers or hydrocolloid wound dressings are used to protect the skin surrounding the wound. **B:** Thin film dressings or transparent dressings are applied to the anterior portion of the wound on top of the hydrocolloid dressing or skin barrier wafers. The thin film dressings can be overlapped to obtain continuity and provide adequate coverage. The fistula area is left open and not covered by the thin film dressings. **C:** An ostomy pouch is sized for the fistula opening and prepared appropriately. **D:** The ostomy pouch is applied over the open fistula site. **E:** The ostomy pouch is applied over and on top of the thin film dressing covering the anterior portion of the wound. (Courtesy of Barbara Bates-Jensen.)

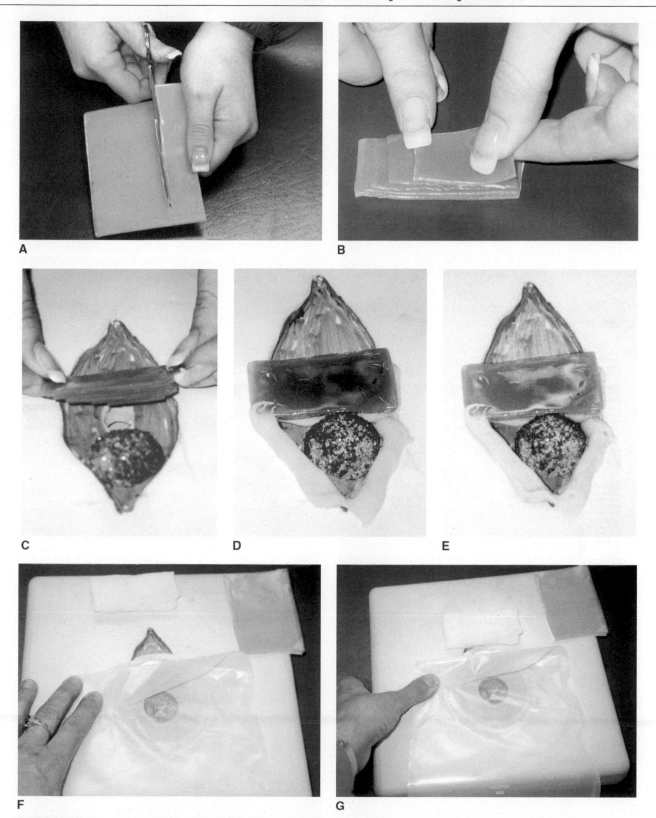

FIGURE 14.7 Photo series depicting the bridging procedure. **A:** A skin barrier wafer is cut into strips. **B:** The strips of skin barrier wafer are applied on top of each other to create a "bridge." **C:** The skin barrier "bridge" is applied to the wound. **D:** The skin barrier "bridge" is secured in the wound bed using skin barrier paste. The paste is also used around the fistula site as necessary to create an even surface. **E:** The skin barrier "bridge" is in place and the anterior portion of the wound can be seen to be clear of the fistula area. **F:** An ostomy pouch is sized and cut to fit the fistula area. The ostomy pouch is applied over the fistula, using the skin barrier "bridge" as part of the adhesive surface area for pouch application. **G:** A wound dressing can be applied to the anterior portion of the wound that is now protected from fistula output by the ostomy pouch.

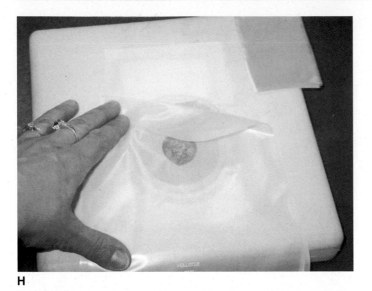

H

FIGURE 14.7 (*continued*) **H:** The wound dressing can be changed more frequently than the fistula pouch system if necessary. This system allows the wound to be treated with a different approach than the fistula area. (Courtesy of Barbara Bates-Jensen.)

Saddlebagging

Saddlebagging is used for multiple fistulas, where the fistula orifices are close together and it is important to keep the output from each fistula separated (Fig. 14.8). Using two (or more for multiple fistulas) cut-to-fit ostomy pouches, cut fistula openings on the back of the pouch, off-center or as far to the side as possible. Cut the second pouch to fit the next fistula and off-center as far to the other side as possible. Cleanse the skin with warm water, and apply skin barrier paste around the fistulas orifices. Apply the ostomy pouches. Where they contact each other (down the middle), they are affixed/adhered to each other in a "saddlebag" fashion. Figure 14.9 shows the saddlebag procedure in use.

Multiple fistulas can also be managed with one ostomy pouching system accommodating the multiple openings. This method is appropriate when fistula openings are close together and there is no need to separate drainage.[88] Figure 14.10 demonstrates multiple fistulas managed with one large pouching system.

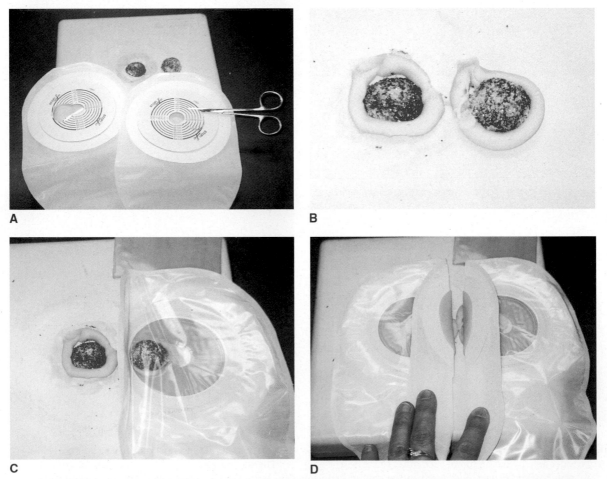

A

B

C

D

FIGURE 14.8 Photo series depicting the saddlebagging procedure. **A:** Two ostomy pouches are used to pouch each of the fistulas present separately. This will allow for unique containment of fistula output for each site. Ostomy pouches are sized and cut to fit the fistula openings. The fistula openings are cut off-center, as far to one edge of the pouch skin barrier backing as possible. **B:** Skin barrier paste is used around the fistula openings to provide for a smooth adhesive area and fill in any dips or crevices around the fistula openings. **C:** Each ostomy pouch is applied to the fistula site. **D:** The adhesive area of the pouch closest to the second fistula site is not firmly adhered to the skin; rather, it is left (or bent up) in a nonadhered manner.

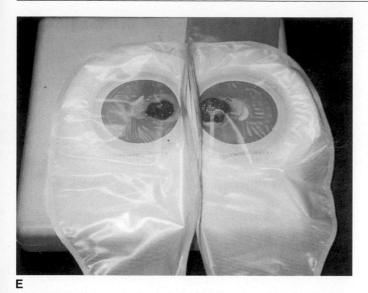

E

FIGURE 14.8 (*continued*) **E:** The nonadhered middle sections of the two pouches are adhered to each other to create the "saddle." Both pouches will require simultaneous changing as it is nearly impossible to change one without changing the other because of the adherence of one pouch to the other in the middle section. (Courtesy of Barbara Bates-Jensen.)

Closed suction drainage system and Negative Pressure Wound Therapy

A similar method of managing fistulas is by a closed suction drainage system. Jeter et al.[89] describe the use of a Jackson-Pratt drain and a continuous, low suction in fistula management. After cleansing the wound with normal saline, the fenestrated drain of the Jackson-Pratt is placed in the wound on top of a moistened gauze opened up to line the wound bed (primary contact layer); a second fluffed wet gauze is placed over the drain, and the surrounding skin is prepared with a skin sealant.

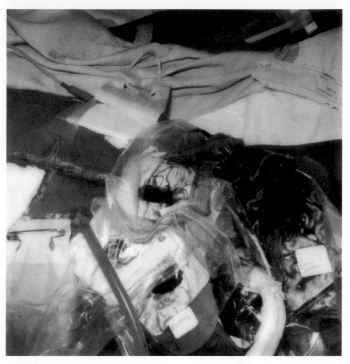

FIGURE 14.9 Saddlebagging procedure in use. Photo demonstrates an abdomen with multiple fistula sites and draining wound sites. Each site was pouched separately with the saddlebagging technique used for most because of the close proximity of many of the sites. The midline abdominal wound shows a posterior fistula that was pouched using the bridging technique. (Courtesy of Copyright © Barbara Bates-Jensen.)

Next, the entire site is covered with a thin film dressing, crimping the dressing around the tube of the drain where it exits the wound. The tube exit site is filled with skin barrier paste, and the Jackson-Pratt is connected to the low, continuous wall

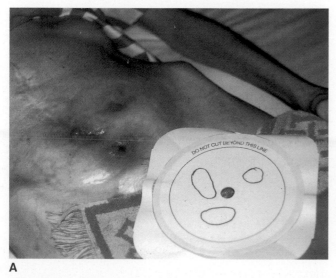

A

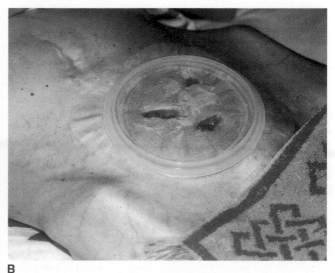

B

FIGURE 14.10 Photo series depicting the use of one pouch for multiple fistulas. **A:** Three major fistula sites evident on abdomen (from long-standing Crohn's disease). A two-piece pouch is used and the skin barrier wafer portion is cut to fit the fistula openings. Pouch with large opening has been cut to fit the three fistula sites. Caution must be used to cut the pouch barrier so that the fistula openings are cut with attention to how the skin barrier will be applied on the skin (it is common to accidentally reverse the images if not aware). **B:** Skin barrier portion of two-piece pouch applied. Skin barrier paste has been used around the fistula openings to help apply the pouch.

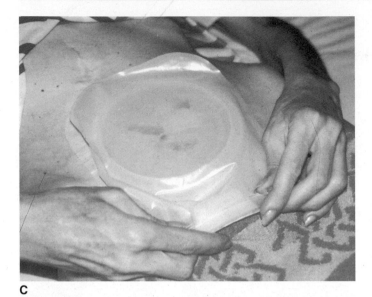

C

FIGURE 14.10 (*continued*) **C:** Pouch attached to skin barrier and closure clamp applied. (Courtesy of Barbara Bates-Jensen.)

suction. The connection site may have to be adjusted or may require the use of a small "Christmas tree" connector or device and secured with tape. Jeter et al. advise changing the system every 3 to 5 days.[89]

The suction catheter technique is most effective when fistula output is liquid and watery. Fistula output that is pasty, thick, or chunky will clog the suction catheter, making the system ineffective. Insertion of the suction catheter into the fistula opening will prevent fistula closure because the body responds to the catheter as a foreign object. However, laying the catheter in the wound around the fistula opening will not prevent fistula closure. A soft catheter should be used to prevent undue trauma to the wound bed.

Commercially available NPWT devices are also available from a variety of companies and provide similar therapy and may assist in promoting healing of enterocutaneous fistulas. NPWT is suggested for two goals: obtaining complete pressure-related closure of acute fistulas as an aid to enterocutaneous fistula closure and segregating the fistula from the abdominal wound to obtain sufficient healing and stabilization of the patient to allow for surgical repair of a chronic fistula (Figs 14.11 and 14.12). In both cases, the device is not intended as a method of containing or managing enterocutaneous fistula output. Patients must be on TPN therapy with nothing by mouth and the fistula must be assessed prior to initiation of therapy. Pressure is usually continuous at 150 to 175 mm Hg for acute enterocutaneous fistulas and may be lower for chronic enterocutaneous fistulas.[90]

Vaginal Fistulas

Vaginal fistulas present complex management problems. Whether the fistula involves the bladder or intestine, manifestations are continual leakage of stool or urine (depending on fistula origins) through the vaginal vault, with erosion and denudation of the sensitive vaginal epithelium, as well as the perineal skin. Containment of the fistula output is extremely

difficult because of the anatomic constraints of the perineal area. Female urinary containment pouches can be tried, as can soft, cuplike devices inserted into the vaginal vault to direct output flow into a tube and drainage bag system. Use of commercially available fecal incontinent systems in which the bowel catheter is inserted in the vaginal vault may also be useful. Use of skin protector ointments, attention to odor control, and some form of fistula output containment are essential for these patients. Consultation with the enterostomal therapy (ET) nurse or ostomy nurse is extremely advantageous in any of these cases because clinical experience plays a major role in successful of the complex fistula.

Management of Odor

Pouching to contain the fistula output will usually contain odor as well. If odor continues to be problematic with an intact pouching system, oral medications that decrease stool odor may be helpful, such as bismuth subgallate and charcoal compositions.[91] Taking care to change the pouch in a well-ventilated room will also help with odor. If odor is caused by anaerobic bacteria, some clinicians suggest the use of 400 mg metronidazole orally three times a day.[80]

Reduction of Output Volume

Management of high-output fistulas may be improved with administration of octreotide acetate 300 µg subcutaneously

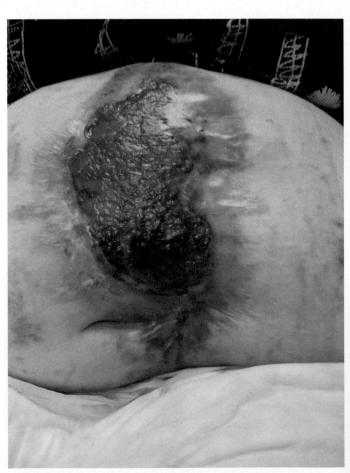

Figure 14.11 Open abdominal wound with fistula located at base of wound, lateral to umbilicus with erythema and ulceration surrounding fistula opening. (Copyright © T.E. Serena.)

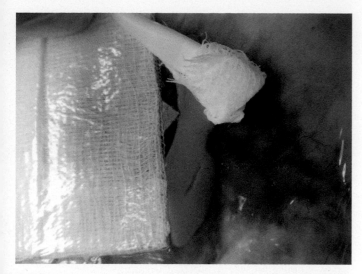

FIGURE 14.12 Same patient as shown in Figure 14-11 with wound and fistula ready for application of negative presssure wound therapy. (Copyright © T.E. Serena.)

over 24 hours.[80,92] Octreotide is an analog of Somatostatin with fewer side effects and a longer half life. Somatostatin has a half life of <3 minutes and therefore must be administered as a continuous intravenous infusion for the duration of the therapy. Octreotide and lanreotide are two synthetic analogues of somatostatin and may be administered subcutaneously over a period of hours or days. Octreotide may be given for the prevention of enterocutaneous fistulas with pancreatic involvement following pancreatic surgery in high-risk patients.[92] Typically, octreotide is given subcutaneously as 100 μg every 8 hours for a period of at least 7 days. Evidence supporting use of octreotide or somatostatin for treatment of existing enterocutaneous fistulas is mixed.[73,92] The current suggested approach is to treat the enterocutaneous fistula initially with nutrition support (e.g., enteral or TPN) and, if no response in fistula output within a week, to add therapy with somatostatin or octreotide to reduce volume of fistula output.[73]

Surgical Management

Surgical management may be indicated for fistula closure and for palliative care. However, fistula recurrence has been reported in 20% of persons within 3 months following surgery.[93] Optimizing the patient with adequate nutrition and hydration prior to surgical procedures is desired, and the exact timing of the intervention is highly individualized.

Options for surgical management include surgical resection, bypass, diversion, or endoscopic use of fibrin tissue glue.

- Surgical resection involves removal of the diseased area of the intestine, including the fistula site, with end-to-end anastomosis and temporary diversion to protect the healing site.
- Surgical bypass involves using end-to-end anastomosis of the intestinal tract, bypassing or going around the fistula site. The intestinal tract just before and just after the fistula opening are anastomosed together, effectively isolating and separating the area of the intestine containing the fistula opening.

- Surgical diversion involves creation of an ostomy located proximal to the fistula site, thus diverting the fecal stream before it reaches the fistula site.
- Endoscopic procedures using fibrin tissue glue have been reported to seal low-output fistulas and anal fistulas, with no adverse effects and early healing.[94–96]

Outcome Measures for Fistulas

Outcome measures for fistula care relate to the potential for fistula closure, maintenance of nutrition and fluid and electrolyte balance, and management of the fistula output. For a newly developed fistula, the goals of care are fistula closure, and the major outcome measure is slowing of fistula output, with eventual closure of the fistula site.

When fistula closure is not likely to occur spontaneously and the patient is not a surgical candidate, focus the outcomes of care on preserving the patient's quality of life with the fistula. These outcome measures may include decrease in fistula output; management of fistula odor, as measured by patient/caregiver self-report; and maintenance of nutrition and fluid and electrolyte balance, as monitored by frequent laboratory values.

Patient and Caregiver Education for Fistulas

Prior to patient and caregiver teaching, you need to assess the patient's self-care ability and the caregiver's ability. Consider their level of education, manual dexterity, and willingness to learn. The patient and caregiver must be taught the management method for the fistula, including pouching techniques, how to empty the pouch, odor control methods, and strategies for increasing fluid and nutritional intake. As you have learned, many of the pouching techniques used to manage fistulas are complicated; thus, continual surveillance by an expert, such as an ET nurse or ostomy nurse, may be wise.

CONCLUSION

Patients with malignant cutaneous wounds and fistulas require basic wound care, creativity in specific management strategies, and thoughtful attention to the psychosocial implications of the wound's cutaneous manifestations. Both conditions are common in palliative care, and cure is not a goal. Instead, the goals of palliative intervention are to control infection, manage drainage and odor, reduce discomfort, ensure nutrition and hydration, and provide for optimal functional capacity. At all times, direct your care toward alleviating the distressing symptoms and improving the patient's quality of life.

Involvement of the caregiver and family in the plan of care is important. To meet the needs of the patient and family, access to the multidisciplinary care team is crucial, and consultation by an ET or certified wound, ostomy, or continence nurse is highly desirable.[97–99]

REVIEW QUESTIONS

1. Malignant cutaneous lesions may occur
   - **A.** in up to 5% of patients with cancer and 10% of patients with metastatic disease
   - **B.** in up to 25% of all cancer patients
   - **C.** very rarely, no studies have documented the occurrence
   - **D.** in up to 10% of all cancer patients and 50% of patients with metastatic disease
2. Malignant cutaneous wounds occur secondary to
   - **A.** local invasion of a tumor
   - **B.** spread via lymphatics and blood vessels
   - **C.** surgical removal of primary tumor
   - **D.** A. and b
3. Enterocutaneous fistulas are usually managed initially by
   - **A.** surgically closing the fistula opening
   - **B.** medical management consisting of bowel rest and nutritional support
   - **C.** high-dose antibiotics and steroids to reduce infection and inflammation
   - **D.** surgical resection and end-to-end anastomosis
4. Which of the following best exemplifies conditions and treatments that predispose to fistula development?
   - **A.** Intra-abdominal sepsis, surgery, chronic diverticulitis
   - **B.** Surgery, anal malformation, chronic diverticulitis
   - **C.** Chronic's diverticulitis, intra-abdominal sepsis, surgery, Crohn disease
   - **D.** Radiation therapy, intra-abdominal sepsis, surgery, Crohn's disease
5. If bleeding occurs from a malignant cutaneous wound the first intervention should be:
   - **A.** Application of a hemostatic dressing
   - **B.** Direct pressure for 10–15 minutes
   - **C.** An ice pack applied to the area
   - **D.** Application of gauze soaked in 1:1,000 epinephrine

REFERENCES

1. Lookingbill DP, Spangler N, Sexton FM. Skin involvement as the presenting sign of internal carcinoma. *J Am Acad Dermatol.* 1990;22:19–26.
2. Lookingbill DP, Spangler N, Helm KF. Cutaneous metastases in patients with metastatic carcinoma: a retrospective study of 4020 patients. *J Am Acad Dermatol.* 1993;29:228–236.
3. Krathen RA, Orengo IF, Rosen T. Cutaneous metastasis: a meta-analysis of data. *South Med J.* 2003;96:164–167.
4. Marcoval J, Moreno A, Peyrí J. Cutaneous infiltration by cancer. *J Am Acad Dermatol.* 2007;57:577–580.
5. Saeed S, Keehn CA, Morgan MB. Cutaneous metastasis: a clinical, pathological, and immunohistochemical appraisal. *J Cutan Pathol.* 2004;31:419–430.
6. Chopra R, Chhabra S, Samra SG, et al. Cutaneous metastases of internal malignancies: a clinicopathologic study. *Indian J Dermatol Venereol Leprol.* 2010;76:125–131.
7. Nashan D, Müller ML, Braun-Falco M, et al. Cutaneous metastasis of visceral tumors: a review. *J Cancer Res Clin Oncol.* 2009;135:1–14.
8. Hu SC, Chen GS, Lu YW, et al. Cutaneous metastases from different internal malignancies: a clinical and prognostic appraisal. *J Eur Acad Dermatol Venereol.* 2008;22:735–740.
9. Mueller TJ, Wu H, Greenberg RE, et al. Cutaneous metastasis from genitourinary malignancies. *Urology.* 2004;63:1021–1026.
10. Serrano ML. Cutaneous metastases of hepatocellular carcinoma. *Clin Exp Dermatol.* 2009;34:e567–e569.
11. Carroll MC, Fleming M, Chitambar CR, et al. Diagnosis, workup, and prognosis of cutaneous metastases of unknown primary origin. *Dermatol Surg.* 2002;28:533–535.
12. Schoenlaub P, Sarraux A, Grosshans E, et al. Survival after the occurrence of cutaneous metastasis: a study of 200 cases. *Ann Dermatol Venereol.* 2001;128:1310–1315.
13. Bottoni U, Innocenzi D, Mannooranparampil TJ, et al. Inflammatory cutaneous metastasis from laryngeal carcinoma. *Eur J Dermatol.* 2001;11:124–126.
14. Tortora G, Ciardiello F, Gasparini G. Combined targeting of EGFR-dependent and VEGF-dependent pathways: rationale, preclinical studies and clinical applications. *Nat Clin Pract Oncol.* 2008;5:521–530.
15. Nguyen A, Hoang V, Laquer V, et al. Angiogenesis in cutaneous disease: part I. *J Am Acad Dermatol.* 2009;61:921–942.
16. Bowler PG, Davies BJ, Jones SA. Microbial involvement in chronic wound malodour. *J Wound Care.* 1999;8:216–218.
17. Alexander S. Malignant fungating wounds: managing malodour and exudate. *J Wound Care.* 2009;18:374–382.
18. Seaman S. Management of malignant fungating wounds in advanced cancer. *Semin Oncol Nurs.* 2006;22:185–193.
19. Naylor W. Assessment and management of pain in fungating wounds. *Br J Nurs.* 2001;10(suppl 22):S33–S36.
20. Alvarez OM, Kalinski C, Nusbaum J, et al. Incorporating wound healing strategies to improve palliation in patients with chronic wounds. *J Palliat Med.* 2007;10:1161–1189.
21. Alexander S. Malignant fungating wounds: epidemiology, aetiology, presentation and assessment. *J Wound Care.* 2009;18:273–280.
22. Piggin C, Jones V. Malignant fungating wounds: an analysis of the lived experience. *Int J Palliat Nurs.* 2007;13:384–391.
23. Alexander S. Malignant fungating wounds: managing pain, bleeding and psychosocial issues. *J Wound Care.* 2009;18:418–425.
24. McDonald A, Lesage P. Palliative management of pressure ulcers and malignant wounds in patients with advanced illness. *J Palliat Med.* 2006;9:285–295.
25. Hawthorn M. Caring for a patient with a fungating malignant lesion in a hospice setting: reflecting on practice. *Int J Palliat Nurs.* 2010;16:70–76.
26. Adderly U, Smith R. Topical agents and dressings for fungating wounds. *Cochrane Database Syst Rev.* 2007;2:CD003948.
27. Mulder GD, Cavorsi JP, Lee DK. Polyhexamethylene biguanide (PHMB): an addendum to current topical antimicrobials. *Wounds.* 2007;19:173–182.
28. Andriessen AE, Eberlein T. Assessment of a wound cleansing solution in the treatment of problem wounds. *Wounds.* 2008;20:171–175.
29. Seaman S. Dressing selection in chronic wound management. *J Am Podiatr Med Assoc.* 2002;92:24–33.
30. Seaman S. Home care for pain, odor, and drainage in tumor-associated wounds. *Oncol Nurs Forum.* 1995;22:987.
31. Young CV. The effects of malodorous fungating malignant wounds on body image and quality of life. *J Wound Care.* 2005;14:359–362.

32. Bale S, Tebble N, Price P. A topical metronidazole gel used to treat malodorous wounds. *Br J Nurs*. 2004;13(suppl):S4–S11.

33. Kalinski C, Schnepf M, Laboy D, et al. Effectiveness of a topical formulation containing metronidazole for wound odor and exudate control. *Wounds*. 2005;17:84–90.

34. Newman V, Allwood M, Oakes RA. The use of metronidazole gel to control the smell of malodorous lesions. *Palliative Med*. 1989;3:303–305.

35. Bower M, Stein R, Evans TRJ, et al. A double-blind study of the efficacy of metronidazole gel in the treatment of malodorous fungating tumours. *Eur J Cancer*. 1992;28A:888–889.

36. Poteete V. Case Study: eliminating odors from wounds. *Decubitus*. 1993;6(4):43–46.

37. Finlay IG, Bowszyc J, Ramlau C, et al. The effect of topical 0.75% metronidazole gel on malodorous cutaneous ulcers. *J Pain Symptom Manage*. 1996;11:158–162.

38. Clark J. Metronidazole gel in managing malodorous fungating wounds. *Br J Nurs*. 2002;11(6 suppl):S54–S60.

39. Whedon MA. Practice corner: what methods do you use to manage tumor-associated wounds? *Oncol Nurs Forum*. 1995;22:987–990.

40. McMullen D. Topical metronidazole. Part II. *Ostomy/Wound Manage*. 1992;38(3):42–46.

41. Holloway GA, Johansen KH, Barnes RW, et al. Multicenter trial of cadexomer iodine to treat venous stasis ulcer. *West J Med*. 1989;151:35–38.

42. Danielsen L, Cherry GW, Harding K, et al. Cadexomer iodine in ulcers colonised by *Pseudomonas aeruginosa*. *J Wound Care*. 1997;6:169–172.

43. Prommer E. Management of bleeding in the terminally ill patient. *Hematology*. 2005;10:167–175.

44. Pereira J, Phan T. Management of bleeding in patients with advanced cancer. *Oncologist*. 2004;9:561–570.

45. Dean A, Tuffin P. Fibrinolytic inhibitors for cancer-associated bleeding problems. *J Pain Symptom Manage*. 1997;13:20–24.

46. Grocott P. Care of patients with fungating malignant wounds. *Nurs Stand*. 2006;21:57–66.

47. Coetzee MJ. The use of crushed tranexamic acid tablets to control bleeding after dental surgery and from skin ulcers in haemophilia. *Haemophilia*. 2007;13:443–444.

48. Huang SF, Wu RC, Chang JTC, et al. Intractable bleeding from solitary mandibular metastasis of hepatocellular carcinoma. *World J Gastroenterol*. 2007;13:4526–4528.

49. Broadley KE, Kurowska A, Dick R, et al. The role of embolization in palliative care. *Palliat Med*. 1995;9:331–335.

50. Morrissey DD, Andersen PE, Nesbit GM, et al. Endovascular management of hemorrhage in patients with head and neck cancer. *Arch Otolaryngol Head Neck Surg*. 1997;123:15–19.

51. Coldwell DM, Sewell PE. The expanding role of interventional radiology in the supportive care of the oncology patient: from diagnosis to therapy. *Semin Oncol*. 2005;32:169–173.

52. Blanke W, Hallern B. Sharp wound debridement in local anaesthesia using EMLA cream: 6 years' experience in 1084 patients. *Eur J Emerg Med*. 2003;10:229–231.

53. Rosenthal D, Murphy F, Gottschalk R, et al. Using a topical anaesthetic cream to reduce pain during sharp debridement of chronic leg ulcers. *J Wound Care*. 2001;10:503–505.

54. Hahn IH, Hoffman RS, Nelson LS. EMLA-induced methemoglobinemia and systemic topical anesthetic toxicity. *J Emerg Med*. 2004;26:85–88.

55. Eidelman A, Weiss JM, Lau J, et al. Topical anesthetics for dermal instrumentation: a systematic review of randomized, controlled trials. *Ann Emerg Med*. 2005;46:343–351.

56. Sawynok J. Topical and peripherally acting analgesics. *Pharmacol Rev*. 2003;55:1–20.

57. Zeppetella G, Porzio G, Aielli F. Opioids applied topically to painful cutaneous malignant ulcers in a palliative care setting. *J Opioid Manage*. 2007;3:161–166.

58. Back IN, Finlay I. Analgesic effect of topical opioids on painful skin ulcers. *J Pain Symptom Manage*. 1995;10:493.

59. Krajnik M, Zbigniew Z. Topical morphine for cutaneous cancer pain. *Palliative Med*. 1997;11:325.

60. Zeppetella G, Paul J, Ribeiro MD. Analgesic efficacy of morphine applied topically to painful ulcers. *J Pain Symptom Manage*. 2003;25:555–558.

61. Zeppetella G, Ribeiro MD. Morphine in intrasite gel applied topically to painful ulcers. *J Pain Symptom Manage*. 2005;29:188–119.

62. Tokunaga Y, Hosogi H, Nakagami M, et al. A case of chest wall recurrence of breast cancer treated with paclitaxel weekly, 5′-deoxy-5-fluorouridine, arterial embolization and chest wall resection. *Breast Cancer*. 2003;10:366–370.

63. Fritz P, Hensley FW, Berns C, et al. Long-term results of pulsed irradiation of skin metastases from breast cancer. *Strahlenther Onkol*. 2000;176:368–376.

64. Veness MJ. The important role of radiotherapy in patients with non-melanoma skin cancer and other cutaneous entities. *J Med Imaging Radiat Oncol*. 2008;52:278–286.

65. Leonard R, Hardy J, van Tienhoven G, et al. Randomized, double-blind, placebo-controlled, multicenter trial of 6% miltefosine solution, a topical chemotherapy in cutaneous metastases from breast cancer. *J Clin Oncol*. 2001;19:4150–4159.

66. Pacetti P, Mambrini A, Paolucci R, et al. Intra-arterial chemotherapy: a safe treatment for elderly patients with locally advanced breast cancer. *In Vivo*. 2006;20:761–764.

67. vanSonnenberg E, Shankar S, Parker L, et al. Palliative radiofrequency ablation of a fungating symptomatic breast lesion. *Am J Roentgenol*. 2005;184(3 suppl):S126–S128.

68. Bufill JA, Grace WR, Neff R. Intra-arterial chemotherapy for palliation of fungating breast cancer. *Am J Clin Oncol*. 1994;17(2):118–124.

69. Goode ML. Psychological needs of patients when dressing a fungating wound: a literature review. *J Wound Care* 2004;13:380–382.

70. Lo S, Hu W, Hayter M, et al. Experiences of living with a malignant fungating wound: a qualitative study. *J Clin Nurs*. 2008;17:2699–2708.

71. Piggin C. Malodorous fungating wounds: uncertain concepts underlying the management of social isolation. *Int J Palliat Nurs*. 2003;9:216–221.

72. Lund-Nielsen B, Müller K, Adamsen L. Malignant wounds in women with breast cancer: feminine and sexual perspectives. *J Clin Nurs*. 2004;14:56–64.

73. Makhdoom ZA, Komar MJ. Nutrition and enterocutaneous fistulas. *J Clin Gastroenterol*. 2000;31(3):195–204.

74. Berry SM, Fischer JE. Classification and pathophysiology of enterocutaneous fistulas. *Surg Clin North Am*. 1996;76(5):1009.

75. Ryan JA, Adye BA, Weinstein AJ. Enteric fistulas. In: Rombeau, JL, Caldwell, MD, eds. *Clinical Nutrition, Volume II. Parenteral Nutrition*. Philadelphia, PA: WB Saunders; 1986:419–436.

76. Rose D, et al. One hundred and fourteen fistulas of the gastrointestinal tract treated with total parenteral nutrition. *Surg Gynecol Obstet*. 1986;163(4):345.

77. Rombeau J, Rolandelli R. Enteral and parenteral nutrition in patients with enteric fistulas and short bowel syndrome. *Surg Clin North Am*. 1987;67(3):551.

78. Fischer JE. Enterocutaneous fistulas. In: Najarian JS, Delaney JP, eds. *Progress in Gastrointestinal Surgery*. St. Louis, MO: CV Mosby; 1989.

79. Kurtz R, Heimann T, Aufses A. The management of intestinal fistulas. *Am J Gastroenterol*. 1981;76:377.

80. Waller A, Caroline NL. Stomas and fistulas. In: Waller A, Caroline NL, eds. *Handbook of Palliative Care in Cancer*. Boston, MA: Butterworth-Heinemann; 1996:81–86.

81. Chamberlain RS, Kaufman HL, Danforth DN. Enterocutaneous fistula in cancer patients: etiology, management, outcome and impact on further treatment. *Am Surg*. 1998;64(12):1204.

82. Rolstad BS, Bryant RA. Management of drain sites and fistulas. In: Bryant RA, ed. *Acute and Chronic Wounds: Nursing Management.* 2nd ed. St. Louis, MO: CV Mosby; 2000:317–341.

83. Hess CT. Assessing a fistula, part 1. *Nursing.* 2002;32(8):22.

84. Schaffner A, Hocevar BJ, Erwin-Toth P. Small bowel fistulas complicating midline surgical wounds. *J Wound/Ostomy Continence Nurs.* 1994;21(4):161–165.

85. O'Brien B, Landis-Erdman J, Erwin-Toth P. Nursing management of multiple enterocutaneous fistulae located in the center of a large open abdominal wound: a case study. *Ostomy/Wound Manage.* 1998;44(1):20.

86. Benbow M. The use of wound drainage bags for complex wounds. *Br J Nurs.* 2001;10(19):1298–301.

87. Wiltshire BL. Challenging enterocutaneous fistula: a case presentation. *J Wound/Ostomy Continence Nurs.* 1996;23(6):297–301.

88. Wessel LC. Application of a wound pouch over an enterocutaneous fistula: a step-by-step approach. *Ostomy Wound Manage.* 2002;48(9):26–28,30.

89. Jeter KF, Tintle TE, Chariker M. Managing draining wounds and fistula: new and established methods. In: Krasner D, ed. *Chronic Wound Care.* King of Prussia, PA: Health Management Publications; 1990:240–246.

90. V.A.C. (r) *Therapy Clinical Guidelines. A Reference Source for Clinicians.* San Antonio, TX: KCI, January 2005.

91. McKenzie J, Gallacher M. A sweet smelling success. *Nurs Times.* 1989;85(27):48–49.

92. Gray M, Jacobson T. Are somatostatin analogues (octreotide and lanreotide) effective in promoting healing of enterocutaneous fistulas? *J WOCN.* 2002;29(5):228–233.

93. Lynch AC, Delaney CP, Senagore AJ, et al. Clinical outcome and factors predictive of recurrence after enterocutaneous fistula surgery. *Ann Surg.* 2004;240(5):825–831.

94. Hwang TL, Chen MF. Short note: randomized trial of fibrin tissue glue for low-output enterocutaneous fistula. *Br J Surg.* 1996;83(1):112.

95. Hammond TM, Grahn MF, Lunniss PJ. Fibrin glue in the management of anal fistula. *Colorectal Dis.* 2004;6:308–319.

96. Singer M, Cintron J, Nelson R, et al. Treatment of fistulas-in-ano with fibrin sealant in combination with intra-adhesive antibiotics and/or surgical closure of the internal fistula. *Dis Colon Rectum.* 2005;48(4):799–808.

97. Harris A, Komray RR. Cost-effective management of pharyngocutaneous fistulas following laryngectomy. *Ostomy/Wound Manage.* 1993;39(8):36–44.

98. Beitz JM, Caldwell D. Abdominal wound with enterocutaneous fistula: a case study. *J Wound/Ostomy Continence Nurs.* 1998;25(2):102.

99. Lange MP, et al. Management of multiple enterocutaneous fistulas. *Heart Lung.* 1989;18:386.

R. Scott Ward

CHAPTER OBJECTIVES

At the completion of this chapter, the reader will be able to:

1. Identify five etiologies of burn injuries.
2. Compare and contrast four different burn depths.
3. Identify two tools for estimating the size of a burn.
4. Discuss a range of pathophysiologic effects of different burn injuries.
5. Describe three common surgical interventions for burn injury.
6. Discuss the nonsurgical management of burn wounds.
7. Educate patients and their caregivers about pain, self-care measures, and what to expect during wound healing.

A burn injury is damage to the skin and sometimes underlying tissues caused by heat, chemicals, radiation, friction, or electricity. The American Burn Association reports that, in the United States, about 500,000 patients per year seek some kind of medical care for burn injury.[1] Although researchers had noted a general trend toward decreased emergency department visits for burn injures over many decades, the incidence of visits for burns has remained reasonably consistent since the year 2000.[2] In 2008, 79 US hospitals with primary burn centers reported over 127,000 admissions for burn injuries.[1] Seventy-one percent of reported burn patients were males and seventeen percent of patients were children under 5 years of age. Scalding is the most common cause of burns in children younger than 5 years of age,[1,3,4] whereas fire and flame are the leading cause of burns in other age groups.[5] In general, hospital stays for survivors of burn injury arc about 1 day per percent of total body surface area (TBSA) burned, plus additional days of outpatient care and rehabilitation. Those patients who do not survive are hospitalized for an average of 3 weeks. As these data suggest, burn injury is costly in terms of human suffering and mortality and places a tremendous financial burden on the health-care industry.

BURN CLASSIFICATION

Burn injury is generally described or classified by the *etiology* (cause) of burn, the *depth* of the burn, and the *size* of the burn.

Etiology of the Burn

The damage sustained in a burn injury depends on the properties of the injurious agent and the intensity and duration of the exposure. Causes of burn injury include heat, chemicals, radiation, friction, and electricity.

Thermal Injury

Heat-related burn injury may also be referred to as thermal injury. Thermal injury can result from contact with flame, hot liquids, or a hot object.

Flame Burns

Direct contact with a flame can result in a flame burn. This can happen, for example, when clothing catches on fire. A burn that results from a flash of intense heat caused by a sudden explosion or ignition of gases (sometimes referred to as a flash burn) is also considered a flame burn. Flame burns are the most common cause of burn injury in adults[1] (Fig. 15.1).

Scald Burns

Contact with hot liquid can result in a scald burn. Scald burns may occur with immersion in a liquid or when a liquid is poured, spilled, or splashed. Scald burns also include burns caused by steam. Patterns of the scald should match the parent's or caregiver's description of the scalding incident. A lack of correspondence suggests the possibility of abuse. Adults can sustain a full-thickness burn if exposed to hot liquids at the following temperatures and durations:

- 150°F for 2 seconds
- 140°F for 5 to 10 seconds
- 130°F for 30 seconds
- 120°F for 5 minutes

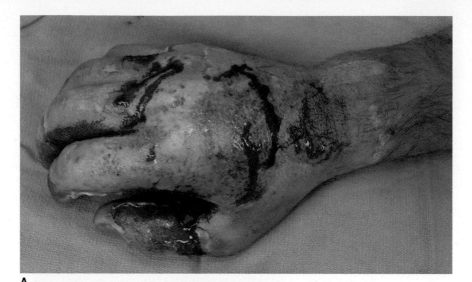

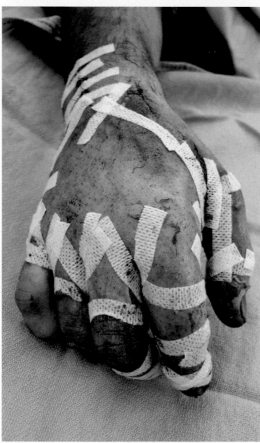

FIGURE 15.1 Deep flame/grease burn to hand. **A.** Before graft. **B.** After sheet graft placed.

It takes even less time for an infant, toddler, or elder to suffer a full-thickness scald burn at the same temperatures. Scald burns are the most common cause of burn in children younger than 5 years old[1] (Fig. 15.2). Hot water heaters in homes and businesses should be set at 110°F since, at this temperature, several hours of immersion would be necessary to produce a full-thickness burn. Nevertheless, children should be supervised when in contact with hot water at this "safe" temperature.

Contact Burns

These burns occur when a hot object comes in contact with the skin. Cigarette burns and stove and oven injuries are examples of contact burns. Other objects that commonly lead to contact burns include radiant heaters, hot dishes, clothing irons, hair curling irons, hot automobile parts such as radiators or exhaust pipes, hot industrial equipment such as soldering guns, and light bulbs. The marks left on the skin may resemble the pattern of the surface contacted.

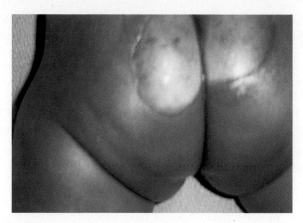

FIGURE 15.2 Partial-thickness scald burn. The buttocks of this infant show a second-degree burn as a result of being intentionally immersed in scalding water.

Chemical Burns

Chemical burns can be caused by direct contact with the skin with either acidic or basic caustic agents.[6]

- Acids cause a precipitation or denaturing of proteins that produce a coagulative effect in tissue. The resultant burns are often dry and clearly demarcated, and the tissue is firm or hard. One known exception to the acid reaction is hydrofluoric acid, which produces a liquefaction necrosis.
- Bases tend not only to denature proteins but also to cause saponification of fats. Thus, alkali burns create a liquefactive necrosis that can lead to deep burns, with variable demarcation and marked edema.

Chemicals such as elemental metals, phosphorus, and hydrocarbons can cause injury to the skin as well.[7] Besides the duration of contact, the strength and concentration and nature of the agent affect the extent of the tissue damage.

Radiation Burns

Radiation burns occur when cells of the skin are damaged by exposure to ionizing radiation. Radiation can also contribute to cellular changes that promote the initiation of various forms of cancer. For example, exposure to UV radiation from the sun is the most common cause of both radiation burn and skin cancer.[8] Some radioactive isotopes, and some radiology tests and therapies, can also be a source of burn injury, but these are rare. The ionizing radiation damages tissue cells that are exposed to the radiation source and also have profound systemic effects as well as difficulty with healing.[9]

Friction Burns

Friction from skin rubbing against a surface creates both abrasion and heat that can damage tissue. A common example of friction burns are "carpet burns." Athletes such as basketball, soccer, or volleyball players commonly experience "court burns," and rock climbers "rope burns" (Fig. 15.3). The example of a rock climber who uses ropes to ascend and descend in the climbing can experience "rope burns" when the friction from the rope rubs skin off. This does not always happen but it often does. These were all simply provided to

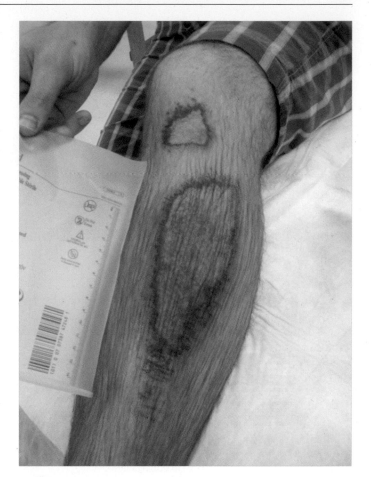

FIGURE 15.3 Friction burn. (Used with permission. Copyright © Teresa Conner Kerr.)

try to allow the reader to get an idea of the various types of potential causes of friction burns. Serious friction burn injuries also have been reported in association with treadmill use.[9] In the literature, it is reported that this most commonly occurs when a child who is in the area reached for the moving treadmill track and the track creates a friction burn on the hand.

Electrical Burns

Electrical burns are complex injuries that occur when an electrical current passes through the body. They are created by tissue resistance to the passage of the current or by direct electrical current damage to tissue.[10,11] Skin is resistant to electrical current, but when a strong enough current enters and eventually exits the body, wounds in the skin and associated tissue are created. The wound created at the site of contact with the current is referred to as the *entrance wound*. Depending on the path the electrical current takes through the body, one or more wounds can be created at the exit sites. These wounds are referred to as *exit wounds* (Fig. 15.4). Flame burns may also occur as a result of the flash of heat or from sparks igniting clothing.[12]

An entrance wound (sometimes referred to as the contact site) is generally a focal injury that is dry, often has an appearance similar to a full-thickness burn, is often depressed, and is commonly smaller in size than the exit wound. In contrast, an

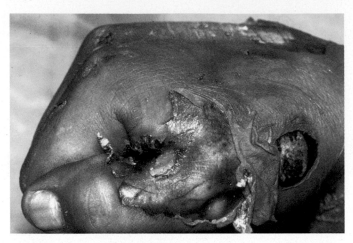

FIGURE 15.4 Electrical hand burn.

exit wound (also referred to as the ground site) may be very untidy. This is because energy builds up at the site of the current ground and then "explodes" through the skin. These exit wounds are commonly dry. The dryness of the wounds is likely a result of heat-related cauterization of vascular tissue by the electrical current.

As the electrical current passes through the body, it follows no predictable pathway, but its direction is likely influenced by the resistance of the tissues it encounters.[10] The range of resistance of internal tissues from low to high is nerve, blood vessels, muscle, skin, tendon, fat, and then bone. Obviously, if the current affects the heart, it can cause arrhythmias. Patients should be monitored for other potential consequences of electrical current passage, such as neuropathy.

Depth of the Burn

Burns can range in depth from superficial injuries that only damage the epidermis to very deep burns that affect tissue below the subcutaneous fat. A burn injury becomes progressively more severe the deeper the burn is and the larger the surface area of injury. Therapy and healing are also related to the depth of the injury: deeper burn injures commonly require surgical intervention to progress to healing.

Burn injuries have historically been classified as first-, second-, third-, or fourth-degree burns. Today, they are more universally classified as superficial-thickness (first degree), partial-thickness (second degree), full-thickness (third degree), or subdermal (fourth degree) (Fig. 15.5) More than one depth of burn often can be found on any individual patient.[13]

FIGURE 15.5 Depth of injury is commonly classified by depth of tissue injury (which corresponds to classic burn degree designations) as superficial-thickness (first degree), partial-thickness (second degree), full-thickness (third degree), or subdermal (fourth degree).

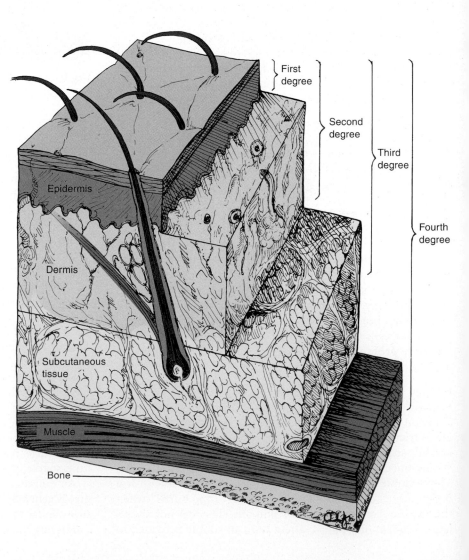

TABLE 15.1	Common Characteristics of Burn Wounds Related to Depth of Injury				
Depth of Burn	Appearance	Pain	Edema	Time to Healing	Scarring
Superficial	Pink, red, erythematous; dry surface; no blisters	Resting inflammatory pain and tender to touch	Minimal tissue edema	2–5 d	No scarring
Superficial partial-thickness	Blisters; moist, bright red surface; blanches with normal capillary refill	Very painful, sensitive to touch, pressure, temperature change	Minimal to moderate tissue edema	7–4 d	Minimal or no scarring
Deep partial-thickness	May have broken blisters; red, pale or white; moist; blanching with delayed capillary refill	Painful; sensitive to touch and pressure	Moderate to marked tissue edema	21–35 d	Scarring
Full-thickness	Dry, firm, leathery eschar; white or pale yellow to a dark red or black; no blanch or refill	Insensate to touch; pain associated with inflammation of associate viable tissue	Marked tissue edema	Weeks; requires skin grafting	Scarring
Subdermal	Relevant tissue exposure	Damaged tissue is generally insensate; inflammatory pain of associated viable tissue	Moderate to marked tissue edema	Weeks; requires surgical intervention	Scarring; potential for tissue defects

As shown in Table 15.1, each type of burn has a distinct clinical presentation, time to healing, potential for scarring, and other characteristics. Despite the availability of a variety of assessment technologies, for practical purposes, most health-care providers use the clinical presentation to assess burn depth.[14]

Superficial-Thickness Burns

Superficial-thickness burns affect only the epidermal layer of the skin. These wounds are dry, erythematous, and painful (Fig. 15.6A,B). They commonly heal within 2 to 5 days, without scarring, and do not generally require medical intervention. Dehydration and pain control may require some broader medical care in the case of a superficial burn over a large surface area. A sunburn without blistering is a very good example of a superficial burn.

Partial-Thickness Burns

Burn injuries that destroy the epidermis and some of the dermis are referred to as **partial-thickness burns**. The appearance, pain, healing time, and potential for scarring that is associated with a partial-thickness burn wound depends on the extent of damage the dermis incurs. The depths of partial-thickness burns are commonly divided into two categories: superficial partial-thickness and deep partial-thickness.

Superficial partial-thickness burns destroy the epidermis and involve damage to the papillary layer of the dermis (Fig. 15.6B). A common indication of this depth of wound is the presence of blisters on the wound surface. Once blisters are denuded, the wound will appear moist, red, and very painful, with the potential for some edema. A burn wound of this depth will also blanch and refill with pressure. These wounds

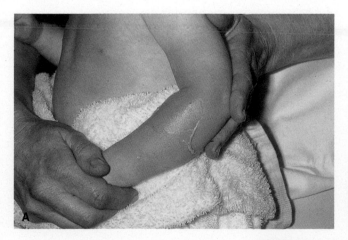
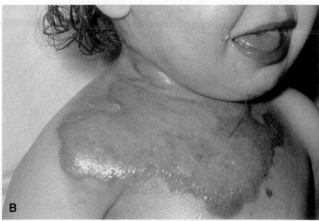

FIGURE 15.6 A,B. Superficial burns.

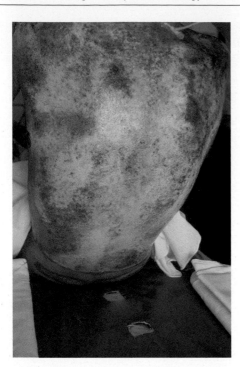

FIGURE 15.7 Example of a deep partial-thickness (second-degree) burn.

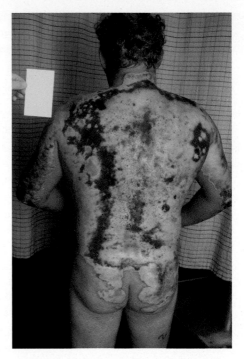

FIGURE 15.8 Example of a full-thickness (third-degree) burn.

may take 7 to 14 days to heal. Some wounds that are classified as partial-thickness may take up to 21 days to heal (Table 15.1). The longer time to healing is an indication that the injury was deeper in the dermis. A true superficial partial-thickness wound should heal well with appropriate wound management that encourages migration of epithelium from wound boundaries and from existing basal cells associated with skin appendages. These wounds should heal without scarring.

Deep partial-thickness burns destroy the epidermis and the papillary layer of the dermis, and damage the reticular layer of the dermis (Fig. 15.7). These wounds are typically moist, painful, edematous, and red; however, the deeper the wound is in the dermis, the more likely it is to take on a pale or white appearance. These wounds generally take at least 21 to 35 days to heal, and often require more time (Table 15.1). As with superficial

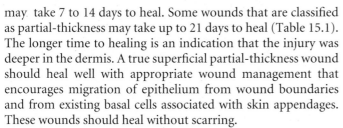

CLINICAL WISDOM

Patients may have wounds at depths that are hard to differentiate. This occurs most often for wounds that are partial-thickness and deep partial-thickness. It can be challenging at times, despite clinical indicators, to be sure of the actual depth of burns as they reach the deeper reaches of the dermis. It is often simply a matter of time and the best indicator of depth is the time it takes for a wound to heal or differentiate. If you are unsure about the real depth of a partial-thickness wound, it is common practice to allow the wound time to progress to healing. Two weeks is a good discriminating target. If the wound is healed or close to healing by 2 weeks, it was likely a true partial-thickness wound. The longer it takes beyond 2 weeks indicates a deep partial-thickness wound or even a full-thickness wound.

partial-thickness burns, the length of time to healing provides an indicator of the depth of injury. With very deep burns, few basal cells remain to epithelialize the wound; therefore, the epidermis is thin and susceptible to shear. There is also increased capillary damage and this leads to more swelling. Because of the depth of injury and delay in healing, there is an increased likelihood of scarring with these wounds.

Full-Thickness Burns

Full-thickness burns obliterate the entirety of the epidermis and dermis (Figs. 15.8 and 15.9). These burns may damage the subcutaneous fat but do not damage the muscle fascia. These wounds are characterized by a dry, firm, leathery eschar that lacks pliability. The color of the eschar may range from white or pale yellow to a dark red or black. Because of the damage to the vascular tissue, the wounds do not blanch or refill, and because of the loss of normal skin-related nerve tissue, they are insensate to touch and

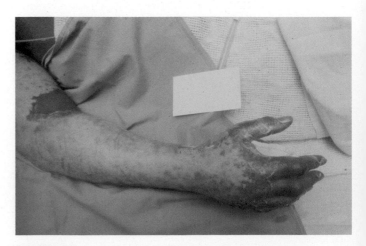

FIGURE 15.9 Example of a full-thickness (third-degree) burn.

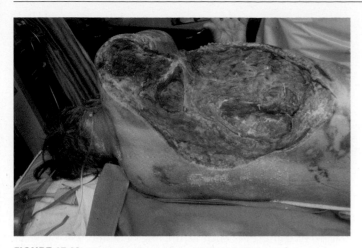

FIGURE 15.10 Example of a subdermal (fourth-degree) burn.

temperature. Although the patient will not feel pain if the wound itself is touched, he or she will experience ongoing inflammatory pain in viable tissue adjacent to the wound. There can also be significant swelling associated with these wounds. These wounds can take several weeks to heal, and the preferred intervention to achieve wound closure is skin grafting (Table 15.1). Scarring is expected with the healing of these wounds.

Subdermal Burns

Subdermal burns are a result of tissue damage that penetrates through the fascial layer of muscle and destroys deep tissues (Fig. 15.10). These wounds may result in damage to muscle, nerve, bone, and related structures like capsules and bursae. Indeed, subdermal burns are characterized by exposure of related tissue.

The appearance of the wound is generally related to the cause of the burn. For example, if the wound was caused by flame, the tissue might appear charred. If a chemical, there might be the presence of eschar secondary to the coagulation necrosis associated with the causative chemical. The denatured tissue caused by the chemical burn is often gray or brown. The damaged tissue is commonly anesthetic, while there is evident inflammatory pain in the adjacent viable tissue. There will be edema associated with these wounds. The healing times for subdermal burns can be several weeks, and these wounds typically require surgical intervention to achieve wound closure. These wounds will also exhibit associated scarring.

Size of the Burn

The size of a burn injury is reported as an estimated percent of the TBSA that is injured. Two methods are commonly used to determine this estimated percentage. In either method, the TBSA of the burn is diagrammed and the percentage of the burn is calculated based on the diagram of the area burned.

- The Lund and Browder chart, shown in Figure 15.11, provides a methodology of documenting percentages of TBSA area that allows for age and development.[15]
- The Rule of Nines, shown in Figure 15.12, was developed by Tennison and Pulaski. This method for estimating surface area divides the body into 11 different areas equal to 9% each with the final 1% for the genitalia, allowing for a 100% sum.[16]

The Rule of Nines allows for a quick estimate of body surface area and is often used in triage situations, while the Lund and Browder chart allows a more accurate representation of the body surface estimate. Note that, in general, burns that involve the hands, feet, face, genitalia, perineum, or major joints are considered serious because of the potential effect of the injury on function.

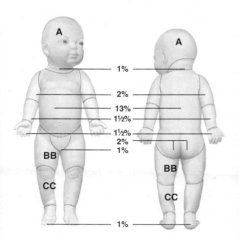

Area of Body	Relative percentage of body surface (varies by age)					Estimated percentage of body area with:	
	0-1 years	1-4 years	5-9 years	10-15 years	Adult	2nd degree burns	3rd and 4th degree burns
Head	19	17	13	10	7		
Neck	2	2	2	2	2		
Anterior Trunk	13	13	13	13	13		
Posterior Trunk	13	13	13	13	13		
Right buttock	2	2	2	2	2		
Left buttock	2	2	2	2	2		
Genitalia	1	1	1	1	1		
Right upper arm	4	4	4	4	4		
Left upper arm	4	4	4	4	4		
Right lower arm	3	3	3	3	3		
Left lower arm	3	3	3	3	3		
Right hand	2	2	2	2	2		
Left hand	2	2	2	2	2		
Right thigh	5	6	8	8	9		
Left thigh	5	6	8	8	9		
Right lower leg	5	5	5	6	7		
Left lower leg	5	5	5	6	7		
Right foot	3	3	3	3	3		
Left foot	3	3	3	3	3		

Totals: [   ] + [   ] = [   ]

FIGURE 15.11 Adaptation of the Lund and Browder chart to estimate TBSA of a burn injury.

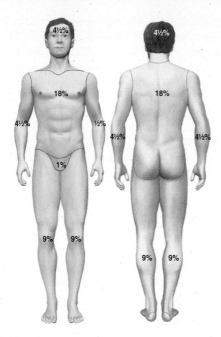

FIGURE 15.12 Adaptation of the Figure of Nines chart to estimate TBSA of a burn injury.

BURN PATHOPHYSIOLOGY

A number of physiologic changes occur as a result of a burn injury and subsequent biological actions to fight infection and heal the wounds.[17] Essentially all body systems are affected by a burn injury. Exhibit 15.1 shows a schematic overview of the physiologic changes associated with a severe burn. This section goes into details on specific changes for most burns including pain, cardiovascular effects, increased metabolism, risk for infection, and pulmonary complications. For information about psychophysiologic stress see Chapter 2.

Pain

Local pain results from the tissue damage, damaged nerves, and stimulation of nociceptors by inflammatory mediators. Adjacent and regional pain will occur as a result of swelling and locally released and circulating inflammatory pain mediators. Heightened anxiety associated with a burn injury will also increase the perception of pain.[18,19] Pain is treated using pharmaceuticals and psychological interventions.[20] See Chapter 22 for more on pain and interventions.

Cardiovascular Effects

The major vascular response to a burn injury is a fluid shift from the vascular system to the interstitium.[21,22] The fluid shift occurs when burn injury induces local, short-term systemic changes in capillary dynamics. These include an increase in capillary permeability with an associated increase in both capillary hydrostatic pressure and interstitial osmotic pressure. Together, these mechanisms prompt a movement of fluid from the vascular system to the interstitium. Significant edema can develop. Historically, this fluid shift was a common cause of mortality in patients with deep burn injuries, because the resulting decreased perfusion of core organs led to organ failure.

This fluid shift is particularly remarkable within the first 24 hours post burn. During this time, patients are provided intravenous fluid to counteract the hypovolemia.[22,23] After about 24 hours, capillary permeability begins to return to normal.

Fluid-replacement therapy is life-saving, but it does have the adverse effect of adding to the amount of tissue swelling. This can increase the risk of constriction in cases where circumferential burns are present. If a full-thickness burn is circumferential, the swelling associated with the trauma can lead to compression injury of deeper tissue such as blood vessels and nerves. If the circumferential injury is on a limb, a tourniquet effect might result that could lead to ischemia-related damage to structures distal to the site of the constriction.[22,24] The extremities should be monitored for tightness, cyanosis, loss of pulses, and peripheral nerve complaints such as tingling or numbness. Surgical treatment to relieve the compression is discussed shortly.

One of the initial cardiac responses to loss of vascular fluid volume is decreased cardiac output.[25] This in turn leads to a hypermetabolic state that results in increased heart rate.[26]

Increased Metabolism

Burns lead to an increase in resting metabolic rate as the system responds to the injury and fights bacterial load. Normal metabolic rates can increase at least as much as 50% in a 25% burn, and that rate can double in a burn of larger than 40%.[27–29] Even with increased nutritional supplements, this increase in metabolism also can lead to a loss of lean body mass as skeletal muscle proteins are catabolized to provide energy. There are several formulas for determining the caloric needs of patients with burns. The most commonly used formula is the Curreri formula, which allows for calculation requirements for adults and children.[30,31] The Galveston formula is used for children.[32] The Harris-Benedict equation is designed to calculate the calorie needs of adults.[33] These formulas apply to the phase of recovery that includes wound healing. Most clinicians consider these formulas helpful but note that the formulas tend to overestimate the calorie needs of patients.[34,35] Protein requirements increase because of increased energy requirements leading to protein breakdown for an energy source, structural loss due to the wound, and protein requirements in wound healing. Muscle breakdown is the major source for use in energy production. Providing an increased load of protein will not stop the breakdown of muscle, but it will provide protein that will allow for replacement of the catabolized tissue. Fat is required for energy and to provide essential fatty acids needs. It is often recommended that at least 30% of replacement calories consist of fat. Carbohydrates are necessary to provide an energy source and as a protein-sparing mechanism. Increased vitamin and mineral replacement is also a part of diets for patients. See Chapter 7 for comprehensive nutrition information.

Increased Risk for Infection

Burns break the skin barrier, and microbial colonization of burn wounds typically occurs rapidly. The surface of the burn wound is an avascular, warm, protein-laden environment that is ideal for microbial propagation. These factors, along with a decrease in immune responses, put patients with burns, especially large burns, at high risk for infectious complications.

Surface infections can delay wound healing and increase scarring.[36] Microbial incursion beyond the skin can lead to sepsis.[37,38] The microorganisms that initially occupy burn

EXHIBIT **15.1**

Overview of Physiological Changes Associated with a Severe Burn

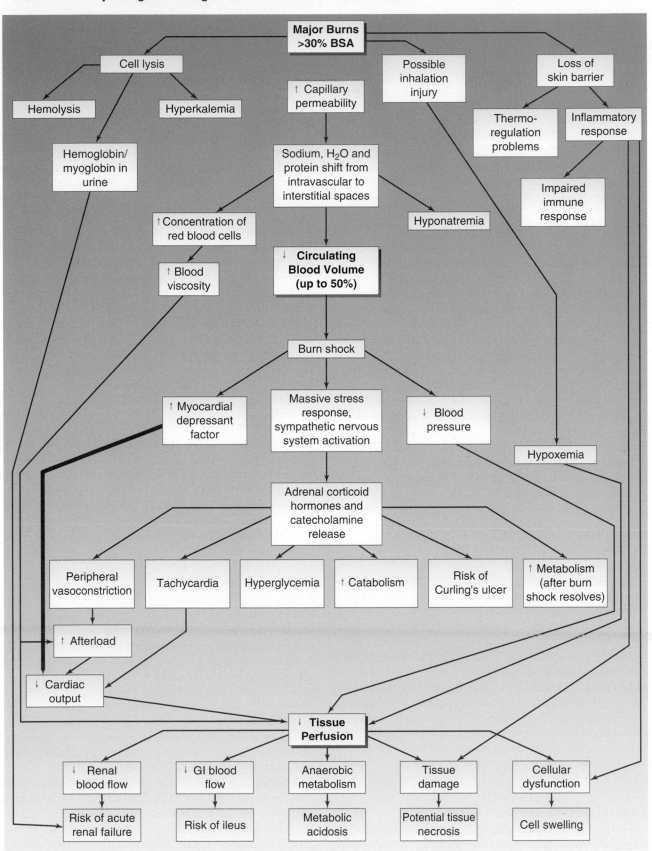

wounds are flora from the patient's skin (gram-positive). These bacteria migrate onto the wound surface within the first few days after the burn.[39] Within the next few days through the first week, the wound will likely become colonized with additional microbes including additional gram-positive and gram-negative bacteria, and yeasts from patient's gastrointestinal and upper respiratory systems.[39] Additional flora can be spread from health-care workers and the hospital environment.[40]

Environmental control measures include hand washing and the use of personal protective equipment, especially gloves, gowns, and masks.[40] Excellent wound care, including the use of antimicrobial topical agents, sterile dressings, sterile debridement tools, and clean linens (towels, blankets, wash clothes, drapes, etc.) will also aid in fighting infection. Monitor both the wounds and the patient for signs of current or impending infection. Finally, the excision and closure of burn wounds as early as possible following the injury will decrease the likelihood of infectious complications. Chapter 18 discusses management of infection.

Pulmonary Complications

The pulmonary system may be affected in two ways following a burn injury. The first problem is pulmonary edema, which can result from the fluid shift previously discussed. Although this edema will affect lung function, if the fluid shift is appropriately managed and oxygenation status is maintained (oxygen saturation of >90%), then this is often an acute problem.

The second problem is inhalation injury. Inhalation injury may consist of a chemical injury to the airways caused by inhalation of toxic products of combustion that damage cells. Inhalation injury can include the compromise of gas transport secondary to inhaling gases such as carbon monoxide or cyanide. Inhalation injury can also occur as a result of direct trauma to the upper airways from inhaling hot gases.[41] An inhalation injury might be suspected if the patient has facial burns, singed nasal hair, a harsh cough, changes in breath sounds, carbonaceous sputum, and a history of a closed-space fire or the presence of chemical irritants in the air.[41]

BURN WOUND TREATMENT

The seriousness of the condition of any patient with a burn increases if any of the following are also present: an inhalation injury, a preexisting medical condition that may complicate treatment, and concomitant trauma when the burn injury occurred.[42] Electrical injury is one of the variables that increases the seriousness of a burn injury, along with the others listed. Age, both very young and very old, also can increase the complexity of burn wound treatment.[43,44]

Treatment of burn wounds is directed at managing infection and directing the wounds toward closure. Surgical intervention, most commonly consisting of skin grafts, is common with deep partial-thickness and full-thickness burns. Nonsurgical wound care procedures are sufficient to manage superficial and partial-thickness wounds. They are also used to help control the microbial load of burn wounds prior to skin-grafting procedures.

Surgical Intervention in Burn Care

Types of surgical interventions commonly used in burn treatment include *escharotomy, excision, and skin grafting*.

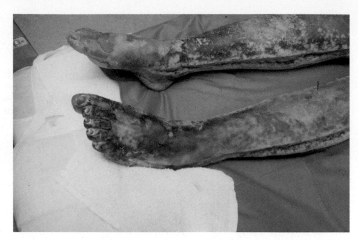

FIGURE 15.13 Bilateral escharotomies. There is a lateral escharotomy on the left leg and a medial escharotomy on the right leg.

Escharotomy

The combination of edema and a lack of pliability of the eschar associated with a circumferential full-thickness burn can compress structures such as blood vessels and nerves. **Escharotomy** is a medial and lateral surgical incision through the depth of the eschar with a scalpel (Fig. 15.13). The goal is to allow expansion of the subdermal space, decompress the subdermal tissue, and decrease constriction on vascular and nerve structures.[24] The edges of the incision will immediately part because of the tissue pressure. Signs of success of this intervention include a decrease in tightness, return of normal pulses, vascular perfusion, and improvement of the tingling or numbness.

Excision of the Burn Wound

The surgical procedure of removing the burn eschar is called **excision**. Excision must be carefully completed to prepare a wound bed that will be amenable to subsequent skin grafting. Excision typically consists of tangential removal of consecutive layers of burn eschar until viable tissue is exposed.[45] It is important that the tissue exposed at the end of the excision of the eschar be vascularized and capable of supporting a skin graft.

Skin Grafts

Harvesting and Placing Skin Grafts

A **skin graft** is a section of skin that is surgically removed from one area of the body (*donor site*) and transferred to another area to cover an area of damaged or missing skin such as a burn. One or more donor sites may be utilized for harvesting the skin graft, depending on the size of the excised burn wound. Donor sites are ideally located in areas where skin is healthy and not associated with an existing burn wound. The donor skin is harvested using a surgical instrument known as a dermatome. The skin that is harvested is generally at a superficial partial-thickness depth, and a graft at that depth is referred to as a split-thickness graft.

After placing the skin graft on the excised burn wound, the surgeon secures the graft to the wound bed with sutures, surgical staples, synthetic adhesives, or fibrin glue. In patients with large TBSA wounds or limited donor site availability, the skin graft is expanded through meshing of the harvested skin; that is,

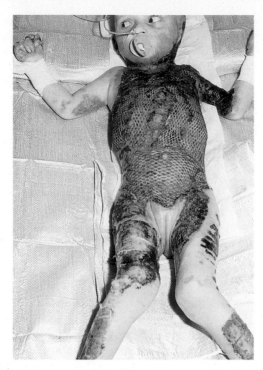

FIGURE 15.14 Mesh grafting is necessary to cover large areas of the body such as in this young child with third-degree burns. (Reprinted with permission from CC studio\photo Researchers, Inc.)

the harvested skin has many small incisions made into it using a small machine (called a mesher). The graft is then referred to as a *meshed graft* (see Fig. 15.14). The cuts or incision in the harvested skin let the graft be expanded for coverage of a larger surface area. The meshed graft may also help with acceptance of the graft by preventing hematomas or seromas because fluids can more readily escape through the cuts in the meshed graft. If the graft is not meshed, it is referred to as a *sheet graft*. Dressings and splints are placed on the graft to protect it from shear. (Fig. 15.2A,B)

Types of Grafts

To minimize the risk of tissue rejection and promote permanent acceptance of the graft, skin grafts should be harvested from the patient. These types of grafts are known as *autografts* or *homografts*. Skin harvested from another species such as a pig (*heterografts* or *xenografts*) or from cadavers (*allografts*) can provide a temporary biologic covering for an excised wound, but are not used for permanent coverage. Such temporary grafts might be used if the size of the excised wound is large and there is insufficient donor skin available.[46]

Other options for wound coverage include cultured epidermal autografts and synthetic skin coverings.[47] *Cultured epidermal autografts* are grown from a patient's own epidermis in culture, and eventually transferred to the patient. They can be helpful for patients with large wounds, although they often prove to be quite fragile at the graft site and can lead to scarring. Synthetic skin substitutes are collagen-based replacements for the dermis. Once accepted, they are often followed by an epidermal skin graft.[48]

Skin grafts may differ in thickness.

- A *split-thickness skin graft*, the most common type, includes the entire epidermis and part of the dermis. The depth, which

is 12/1,000 inch or less, allows the donor site to heal as a superficial partial-thickness wound does, and also will allow for reharvesting if necessary.
- A *full-thickness skin graft* includes all elements of the skin. When a full-thickness skin graft is taken, the deficit left requires coverage with another graft. Because of this, full-thickness skin grafts are generally only used to cover very small areas.[46]

Excision and grafting may be completed during the same operative time, or in two stages. Often, two-stage procedures involve excision of the burn wound on 1 day and harvesting and placement of the skin graft on the following day. Considerations regarding the decision for a single-stage or a two-stage procedure include: the size of the area requiring excision, potential and intraoperative blood loss (can be related to area and depth of planned excision), patient tolerance of the procedure, patient age, and patient comorbidities. The success of two-stage procedures is considered better than single-stage procedures.[49]

Nonsurgical Management of Burn Wounds
Management of Infection
Nonsurgical care of a burn wound varies according to the depth of the wound; however, most wound types require cleansing to decrease the bacterial load on the wound. The common practice in most burn care centers is to bathe or shower off the wounds using tap water.[50] Some centers use a variety of antiseptic additives to bath water; although there are no data to suggest this is necessary, it may be a useful preventive measure against cross-contamination (see Chapter 27).

Debridement of burn wounds is also common. Techniques include mechanical, sharp, or surgical debridement (see Chapter 17). Enzymatic or biological debridement is rarely, if ever, used. Debridement of partial-thickness wounds can be particularly painful. Always provide analgesic medication 30 to 60 minutes prior to the procedure. In general, cleansing and debridement should be gentle but efficient, minimizing the time required to complete the procedure. Chapter 22 describes methods to mitigate painful debridement and other burn/wound pain.

Management by Depth of Burn
Burn management varies by depth of burn severity. In this section, goals as well as treatment options are provided to guide the plan of care.

Superficial-Thickness Burns

The care of a superficial-thickness burn is simple, often requiring only the application of a moisturizer on the wound. The goal is to provide an environment that encourages reepithelialization of the wound.

Partial-Thickness Burns

The goal of wound management of partial-thickness burns is to prepare them for primary healing. First, they should be cleansed. There is some controversy about whether it is most effective to debride blisters or to leave them intact, with no clear evidence supporting either technique conclusively.[51] It is generally felt that small, sturdy blisters can be left intact, but large or fragile blisters should be debrided. If there is a concern about infection, then an antibacterial agent may also be applied to the wound surface.[52] The most common antimicrobial agents used on partial-thickness wounds are ointments or creams.

Cover the wound with mesh gauze impregnated with petroleum gel, with a secondary dressing of plain gauze, held in place with elastic netting.[53] Partial-thickness wounds are exudative, so choose a dressing unlikely to adhere to the wound surface. In general, any dressing that will encourage the maintenance of a moist wound surface, decrease trauma to the healing tissue, and thus encourage wound closure, is acceptable.[54] Again, partial-thickness wounds can be particularly painful, so keep cleansing and debridement gentle and brief. Once partial-thickness wounds have healed, moisturizers should be used to help the new epithelium remain moist and pliable.

Full-Thickness Burns

Debridement of full-thickness burn wounds is accomplished in the operating room as part of surgical excision and skin grafting. The clinician's goal is therefore to prepare the wound for surgical management by controlling infection, rather than to promote primary healing.[52] First, the wounds are cleansed and treated with antimicrobial topical agents to help diminish the bacterial load on the wound surface. The most common topical agent used is a silver sulfadiazine cream. This cream is then covered with a gauze dressing held in place with elastic netting. Dressings should be applied in a way that will allow movement. This is especially important for any dressing applied to the area of a joint; moreover, encourage patients who are medically stable to use the burned extremity.[55]

Subdermal Burns

Subdermal burns are treated with moist wound healing procedures as described until surgical coverage of the wound is completed.

Burn Dressings, Ointments, and Creams

Of the variety of dressings available for burns, many can be helpful in achieving the goals of wound management.[56] For example, depending on the depth and size of the burn wounds, moisture-retentive hydrogels can be used. Patients generally consider these comfortable. Silver-impregnated gauze dressings (see Chapter 20) have also become more common in burn care.[57,58]

As noted earlier, topical agents are commonly used in burn care to decrease the microbial load at the site of the burn wound.

CLINICAL WISDOM

Maintaining Mobility and Functional Movement

It is critical that the patient maintain mobility and function. Therefore, pliable dressings must be chosen and applied in a manner that tolerates movement of burned extremities. If a gauze wrap or elastic wrap is incorporated into the dressing, a figure of eight wrap around joints is a good way of completing that wrap. It is recommended that the intersection of the figure of eight wraps occur on the flexor surface of the joint. DO NOT restrict joints. It should also be noted that no matter how secure a dressing might seem, movement will loosen and possibly disrupt the dressing. Movement is a good thing. Be willing to encourage and allow for movement and replace dressings as necessary.

They are most commonly used in association with an ointment or a cream base for ease of application.[59] Antimicrobial agents can also be mixed in solution and are sometimes used as a part of a wet dressing.

Ointments are oleaginous-based topical agents with antibacterial agents added. When used on wounds, ointments are typically applied one to three times daily. Toxicity of ointments is rare and is more likely when ointments are applied to large surface areas for an extended period of time. Ointments should not be used in the eyes. Some commonly used products include the following:

- Bacitracin is an ointment that is effective against gram-positive organisms through the inhibition of cell-wall synthesis. The development of bacitracin-resistant organisms appears to be rare, and there is also a low risk of hypersensitivity reactions. It is safe for application on children and adults.
- Polymyxin B sulfate is useful against gram-positive organisms, possibly because it causes alteration of the membrane permeability of bacteria.
- Neomycin is an ointment that is helpful against gram-positive organisms, likely because it inhibits protein synthesis. Cutaneous sensitivity reactions occur more frequently with neomycin, however, and there is a risk of ototoxicity with prolonged use of this ointment.

Antibacterial agents are also available in cream (water-soluble preparation) bases. Most creams are typically applied one to two times daily. Toxicity of creams varies with different products, but in general may be increased with extended use of the agent. Some commonly used products include the following:

- Silver sulfadiazine is effective against gram-negative bacteria, gram-positive bacteria, and *Pseudomonas* and is currently the most extensively used topical agent for burn wounds in the United States. The bactericidal mechanism of silver sulfadiazine is likely directed at the cell membrane or cell wall. There is no pain associated with application of the cream, and many patients report that it is comfortable and soothing upon application. The formation of resistant organisms is rare. Cutaneous sensitivity is rare. Although a transient leukopenia has been reported after the first few days of use, the leukopenia is typically not severe, remits even with continued use of the drug, and is not correlated with septic episodes. Because of the possibility of kernicterus (associated with sulfonamide therapy), silver sulfadiazine should not be used at term pregnancy, on premature infants, or on infants younger than 2 months of age.
- Mafenide acetate 0.5% cream (Sulfamylon) is active against gram-negative and gram-positive pathogens, including *Pseudomonas*. Sulfamylon is readily absorbed into the eschar and therefore can be a powerful alternative to silver sulfadiazine. However, the chance of developing a sulfa allergy is higher with mafenide acetate than it is with silver sulfadiazine. Secondary hyperventilation may result as a consequence of a drug-induced metabolic acidosis secondary to inhibition of carbonic anhydrase. Therefore, a patient's respiratory status and acid-base balance should be monitored while the drug is being used. The drug can also cause pain *after* application. It is recommended that this topical agent be used primarily on small wounds, or for as short a time as possible on large wounds.

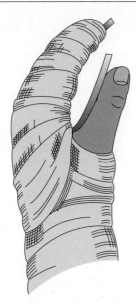

FIGURE 15.15 Splinted hand.

Management of the Skin-Grafted Burn Wound

The skin graft is dressed after placement on the excised burn wound. The goals of the dressings associated with a skin graft are to protect the graft from shearing or displacement, to minimize the likelihood of hematoma or seroma formation under the graft, and to decrease the possibility of infection.

Skin grafts are commonly dressed with soaked gauze that is irrigated frequently to keep the wound bed moist. A splint is incorporated as a part of the dressing over the gauze for mechanical protection of the site; that is, it shields the site from disruption of the developing connections between the graft and the wound bed (Fig 15.15). Figure 15.16 shows a good functional outcome of a hand that was properly splinted during the healing process.

The dressing is often finished off with some form of compression wrap to prevent formation of a hematoma or seroma. These dressings are changed every 1 to 2 days, and the grafts are inspected to assess the adherence of the graft to the wound bed. If upon inspection a subgraft hematoma or seroma

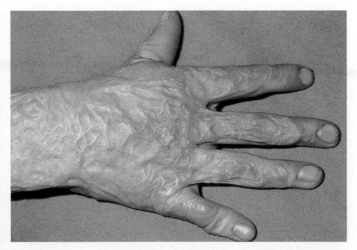

FIGURE 15.16 Functional outcome of a hand properly splinted during healing. (Reprinted with permission from Dr. P. Maraggi Images and Text Copyright © 2011 Photo Researchers, Inc. All Rights Reserved.)

is noted, it can be removed by needle aspiration or by carefully incising the graft to express the blood or fluid. Elevation of grafted extremities is generally recommended to decrease the risk of hematoma or seroma formation due to increased vascular pressure at the graft site. This adherence is sometimes referred to as "graft take."

These initial dressings are used until the graft has adhered. The initial adherence of the graft is through surface tension created by the serum at the wound site. This is quickly followed by establishment of a fibrin matrix that allows a progressively firmer adherence. Within a few days, the graft should begin to vascularize. Anastomosis of the vascular structures between the wound bed and the skin graft not only nourish the transplanted skin, but also help secure the graft. This can be noted by the graft turning pink or red. Once the graft has adhered, or "taken," a different type of dressing is often used. A common choice is an ointment-based dressing covered with petroleum gauze and covered in a light gauze wrap.

The destruction of sebaceous and sweat glands with a deep burn decrease the ability of the skin to self-moisturize. This can lead to dry and flaking, or cracked skin. Thus, once the graft has fully healed, moisturizer should be applied to the skin frequently. Note that most sites of skin grafts can be expected to scar.

Management of the Donor Site

The surgical donor site is managed with interventions similar to those used for partial-thickness burn wounds.[52] The goal is to maintain a moist tissue bed that will encourage primary healing, decrease pain, and control infection.

Donor-site wounds are painful and often have a serosanguineous or sanguineous exudate. The wounds need to be kept moist so that the dressing does not adhere to drying or coagulating exudates and damage the healing tissue upon removal. Dressings that are commonly applied to donor sites include the following:

- Petroleum-impregnated gauze is generally placed over an ointment base and then covered with a light gauze wrap

---

CLINICAL WISDOM

Vascular Support for Extremity Grafts

It is necessary to provide some vascular support for an extremity graft if upper or lower extremities will be dependently positioned or if a patient will be ambulating. A useful way of accomplishing this is to apply a double layer of elastic wrap over a burn dressing prior to the dependency. This pressure to support the peripheral vascular tree is likely to be more effective if the elastic wraps are not placed over a bulky dressing. Once the patient has resumed a position of elevation of the limb, it is important to remove the dressing to inspect the grafts for signs of hematoma formation. If hematomas are present, they should be evacuated. Some clinics have also applied dressings such as Unna boots to grafted sites to allow for early ambulation of patients post skin grafting.

covered with elastic netting. These mesh gauze dressings often have to be changed twice daily.

- Polyurethane semipermeable transparent films are generally self-adhesive and vapor-permeable. These dressings require less frequent dressing changes, every 3 to 5 days in the absence of infection, and therefore pose less potential trauma to the healing donor site. They are recommended for wounds with light to moderate exudates.
- Hydrocolloid dressings help maintain the moist wound surface and can provide a useful barrier to infection. These dressings require changing every 2 to 4 days in the absence of infection. They are recommended for wounds with moderate exudates and often are applied to small donor sites.
- Calcium alginate dressings are highly absorptive and eventually turn to a gel that can be washed off the healed wound surface. They can be left in place for up to 7 days in the absence of infection. Alginate dressings are indicated for donor sites with a high amount of exudates.

Once the donor site is healed, apply moisturizers to maintain the moisture and pliability of the new epithelium. Detailed imformation about dressings is found in chapter 20.

CONCLUSION

The etiology, depth, location, and size of a burn injury are important in understanding the treatment plan for patients with burns. As with any wound, the seriousness of the injury is increased the deeper the injury is and the larger the surface area it covers. Superficial-thickness and many partial-thickness burns can be expected to heal spontaneously with proper care. Deep partial-thickness and full-thickness burns most commonly require escharotomy, excision, and skin grafting procedures to minimize the risk of major infection and to allow progression to healing. Subdermal burns are categorized by exposed deep tissues and are typically caused by flame (charred appearance) or chemical (eschar necrosis) or electrical injury (entrance and exit wounds). Surgical management is usually a part of care for deep partial-thickness, full-thickness, and subdermal burn wounds and includes surgical debridement, escharotomy, and skin grafting of different types. Key nonsurgical management for burn wounds incorporates debridement, cleansing, infection control, appropriate dressings and topical agents, therapeutic use of assistive devices, exercise, and activities of daily living rehabilitation.

SELF-CARE TEACHING GUIDELINES

Prior to discharge, the planned home care of the wounds must be determined. An essential next step in burn management is to teach the patient and/or caregivers how to manage the burn wounds at home. This chapter focuses on treating the burn wound as it heals. Chapter 16 has information about management of the scar at home.

Goals of home care
- Perform a needs assessment of the patient for home care.
  a. Advise the patient and/or caregiver about the elements of care they are expected to provide

  b. Determine the patient's and/or caregiver's willingness and ability
  c. Determine the psychosocial implications of the burn and burn home care. Refer to social services or psychological practitioner.
- Determine how the learner's abilities will be assessed.
  a. Determine if there are concomitant medical and social conditions that influence the learner's ability to learn.
  b. Demonstrate and receive return demonstration of the patient's and/or caregiver's ability to use care products, perform procedures and explain the reasons for what they are doing correctly.
- Educate the patient on topics such as are listed in next section.
- See that the recommended supplies and appliances are available for home use.
- Provide the patient or caregiver a number to call with questions or concerns.
- Provide a directive to contact the health-care provider immediately if the wound changes for the worse. This would be indicated by any one or combination of the following:
  ✓ Increase or change in pain
  ✓ Increase in swelling
  ✓ Increase in redness or a change in color in the unburned skin around the wound
  ✓ Previous red granulation tissue may become pale
  ✓ Malodor
  ✓ General sickness (nausea, fever, achiness, weakness, etc.)
- Date and time of scheduled follow-up appointment with the health-care provider.
- Remember that at each follow-up visit, it is vital to assess the way care is being provided and to add new material as readiness to incorporate is demonstrated.

Education Topics
A checklist of appropriate teaching topics might include the following:

- Depth of burn(s) and what that means for care and prognosis
- Common characteristics of the depth of burn(s) that are present and what to expect over time as the wound heals (e.g., contractures, reduction in edema, improved range of motion, pain, purities, improved activities of daily living)
- Wound care including irrigation, bandaging, positioning, and skin care,
- Importance of good nutrition, including the need for plenty of fluids, high-quality protein, etc. (see Chapter 7)
- Importance and methods for proper pain management at all times and especially before cleansing, dressing changes, or other treatments (see Chapter 22)
- Importance of proper washing and dressing of the burn wound(s), including the schedule of the care and methods for applying dressings
- The when, where, why, and how of appliance use (e.g., dynamic, static, or serial static splints)
- Skin check for pressure points, maceration, secondary trauma, sensory deficits, hyperalgesia, dryness
- Importance of following all directions and risks of nonadherence to the regimen of care

CASE STUDY

C.K. is a 44-year-old male who was injured in a house fire. The patient was napping, was awakened by the smell of smoke, and his shirt caught on fire while he was escaping the house. He ran outside and dropped and rolled and put the flames on his shirt out. He sustained a TBSA burn of 35%. Partial-thickness burns (20.5%TBSA) were located on the upper anterior trunk, the posterior trunk, the anterior head and neck, the upper left arm, and part of the right arm and dorsal right hand. Full-thickness burns (14.5% TBSA) were located on the anterior trunk, the dorsal left arm, and the dorsum of the left hand. There were no associated injuries and no inhalation injury, and the patient was fully oriented and had no significant past medical history.

For the first 7 days of treatment of the wounds, the patient was cleansed using a gentle shower over a hydrotherapy tub. Initially, some blisters related to the partial-thickness wounds were debrided, and additional necrotic skin was removed. The full-thickness burns were cleansed. Following cleansing and gentle drying of the wounds, bacitracin ointment was applied to the partial-thickness wounds and they were covered with petroleum-impregnated gauze that was held in place with a gauze roll wrap and elastic netting. The full-thickness burns were cleansed, and silver sulfadiazine cream was applied to the eschar, which was then covered with a gauze wrap and elastic netting. These dressing changes were completed twice each day.

The partial-thickness wounds responded well to the wound care and healed spontaneously and completely by postburn day 15. On postburn day 7, the patient was scheduled for excision of the full-thickness burns. The excision was completed on postburn day 7 and the excised wounds were grafted on postburn day 8. Skin graft donor sites for the skin grafts were harvested from both lower extremities. The graft sites were dressed with wet bulky dressings, splinted, and covered with a compressive wrap. Irrigation catheters were incorporated into the dressings to allow staff to add solution to the dressings to keep them moist. These initial surgical dressings were removed on post-graft day 2, and the grafts were adherent and showed signs of vascularization, and no hematoma or seroma formation was noted. Wet bulky dressings were applied for 2 additional days at which time the grafts were well adhered and looked to be well vascularized because of their rich pink appearance. At this time, the grafts were dressed with bacitracin ointment and then covered in petroleum-impregnated gauze that was held in place with a gauze roll wrap and elastic netting.

On post graft day 6, the grafts had healed, and moisturizer was applied to the graft skin. Following harvesting of the skin, the donor sites were dressed with polyurethane semipermeable transparent film dressings that were left in place for 5 days. The majority of the donor site wounds were healed by day 5, and the few remaining open wounds were dressed with bacitracin and gauze as previously described. The donor sites were fully healed by day 8 postgraft.

CASE STUDY

V. R. is a 26-year-old female who was cooking a pot of pasta in a restaurant kitchen when a coworker knocked the pot off the stove. The liquid splashed down her left side. She immediately began to run cool water over the burns, after which the restaurant manager transported her to a local emergency room. There were no associated injuries, the patient was fully oriented, was not pregnant, reported smoking occasionally, and had no significant past medical history. The scald burn was calculated to be a TBSA burn of 10%. Partial-thickness burns (4.0%TBSA) were located on the left lower lateral and anterior thigh and the upper part of the anterior lower leg. Full-thickness burns (6.0% TBSA) were located on the left lower leg and the dorsum of the left foot.

For the first 5 days of treatment of the wounds, the patient was cleansed using a gentle shower over a hydrotherapy tub. Initially, necrotic skin related to the partial-thickness wounds was removed. Following cleansing and gentle drying of the wounds, bacitracin ointment was applied to the partial-thickness wounds, and they were covered with petroleum-impregnated gauze that was held in place with a gauze roll wrap and elastic netting. The full-thickness burns were cleansed and were clearly demarcated as deep burns within the 5 days post burn. The full-thickness burns were cleansed, and silver sulfadiazine cream was applied to the eschar, which was then covered with a gauze wrap and elastic netting. These dressing changes for both wound depths were completed twice each day.

The partial-thickness wounds responded well to the wound care and healed spontaneously and completely by postburn day 9. On postburn day 5, the patient was scheduled for excision of the full-thickness burns. The excised wounds were grafted on postburn day 6. Skin graft donor sites for the skin grafts were harvested from the right thigh. The graft sites were dressed with wet bulky dressings, splinted, and covered with a compressive wrap. Irrigation catheters were incorporated into the dressings to allow staff to add solution to the dressings to keep them moist. These initial surgical dressings were removed on postgraft day 2, and the grafts were adherent and showed signs of vascularization, and no hematoma or seroma formation was noted. Wet bulky dressings were applied for 2 additional days at which time the grafts were well adhered and looked to be well vascularized because of their rich pink appearance. At this time (postgraft day 4) the grafts were dressed with bacitracin ointment, covered in petroleum-impregnated gauze and then wrapped in two layers of compression wrap to provide pressure support for the vascular tissue in the leg. This additional compression was important to allow the leg to be placed in a dependent position to allow

CASE STUDY *(continued)*

the patient to sit and begin supervised ambulation (ambulation began post graft day 6). The dressings were removed from the leg to allow graft inspection. The grafts tolerated the dependent positioning and eventual ambulation, showing continuing vascularization and no signs of blistering or seroma formation. The dressings, including the two layers of compression wrap, were continued until the grafts had fully healed on day 10 post graft.

On day 10 post graft, moisturizer was applied to the graft skin. The donor sites were dressed with polyurethane semipermeable transparent film dressings that were left in place for 2 days when they became dislodged. New polyurethane semipermeable transparent film dressings were applied and remained in place through day 6 post graft when the donor site wounds were healed. The donor sites were fully healed by day 6 post graft, and then moisturizer was applied to these healed wounds.

REVIEW QUESTIONS

1. A full-thickness burn may be characterized by
   A. broken blisters, moist wound surface, pain, and minimal to moderate edema
   B. dry and leathery wound surface, no pain to touch, marked tissue edema
   C. moist wound surface, no blisters, pain, minimal tissue edema
   D. pink and erythematous wound surface, no pain, marked edema

2. Which of the following statements is true about the healing of burn wounds (without surgical intervention)?
   A. Superficial-thickness burns will heal in 5 to 10 days with no scarring.
   B. Superficial partial-thickness burns will heal in 3 to 5 days with no scarring.
   C. Deep partial-thickness burns will heal in 14 to 21 days and will predictably scar.
   D. Full-thickness burns will take many weeks to heal and will predictably scar.

3. How is the size of a burn injury described and what methods are available to describe the extent of the injury?
   A. Percent total body surface area burned calculated with the Lund and Browder chart or using the Rule of 10s
   B. Actual total body surface area burned calculated with the Lund and Browder chart or using the Rule of 10s

C. Percent total body surface area burned calculated with the Lund and Browder chart or using the Rule of 9s
D. Actual total body surface area burned calculated with the Lund and Browder chart or using the Rule of 9s

4. The Lund and Browder chart helps with estimated of burn size by
   A. allowing the burn to be estimated by % of body part, age, and development
   B. dividing the body into 11 areas of 9% each with a final 1% for the genitalia
   C. dividing the body into 10 equal areas of 10% each
   D. dividing the body into areas that are burned and areas that might be burned

5. Some factors that affect the severity of burn injury include
   A. depth of burn, size of burn, anatomical location of burn, preexisting medical conditions, and concomitant trauma
   B. depth of burn, time of day the burn occurred, size of burn, concomitant trauma
   C. depth of burn, anatomical location of burn, whether the burn occurred at home or at work
   D. depth of burn, size of burn, preexisting medical conditions, date of the burn

REFERENCES

1. http://www.ameriburn/org/2009NBRAnnual Report.pdf
2. Taira B, Singer AJ, Thode HC, et al. Burns in the emergency department: a national perspective. *J Emerg Med*. 2010;39(1):1–5.
3. Dissanaike S, Rahimi M. Epidemiology of burn injuries: highlighting cultural and socio-demographic aspects. *Int Rev Psychiatry*. 2009;21:505–511.
4. Guzel A, Aksu B, Aylanc H, et al. Scalds in pediatric emergency department: a 5-year experience. *J Burn Care Res* 2009;30:450–456.
5. Renz BM, Sherman, R. The burn unit experince at Grady Memorial Hospital: 844 cases. *J Burn Care Rehabil*. 1992;13:426–436.
6. Palao R, Monge I, Ruiz M, et al. Chemical burns: pathophysiology and treatment. *Burns* 2010;36:295–304.
7. Edlich RF, Farinholt HM, Winters KL, et al. Modern concepts of treatment and prevention of chemical injuries. *J Long Term Eff Med Implants*. 2005;15:303–318.

8. Lucas RM, McMichael AJ, Armstrong BK, et al. Estimating the global disease burden due to ultraviolet radiation exposure. *Int J Epidemiol*. 2008;37:654–667.
9. Varghese BV, Thomas S, Balakrishnan NB, et al. Accidental radioistope burns management of late sequelac. *Indian J Plast Surg*. 2010 September, 43(suppl): S88–S91.
10. Fish RM, Geddes LA. Conduction of electrical current to and through the human body: a review. *Eplasty*. 2009;12:e44.
11. Luz DP, Millan LS, Alessi MS, et al. Electrical burns: a retrospective analysis across a 5-year period. *Burns*. 2009;35:1015–1019.
12. Esses SI, Peters WJ. Electrical burns: pathophysiology and complications. *Can J Surg* 1981;24:11–14.
13. Hettiaratchy S, Papini R. Initial management of a major burn: II assessment and resuscitation. *BMJ*. 2004;329:101–103.
14. Jaskille AD, Shupp JW, Jordan MH, et al. Critical review of burn depth assessment techniques: part I. Historical review. *J Burn Care Res*. 2009;30:937–947.

15. Lund CC, Browder NC. The estimate of areas of burn. *Surg Gynecol Obstet.* 1944;79(4):352–358.

16. Artz C, Saroff HS. Modern concepts in the treatment of burns. *JAMA.* 1955;159:411–417.

17. Hettiaratchy S, Papini R. Initial management of a major burn: I overview. *BMJ.* 2004;328:1555–1557.

18. Choiniere M, Melzack R, Rondeau J, et al. The pain of burns: characteristics and correlates. *J Trauma.* 1989;29:1531–1539.

19. Colloca L, Benedetti F. Nocebo hyperalgesia: how anxiety is turned into pain. *Curr Opin Anaesthesiol.* 2007, 20:435–439.

20. Wiechman AS, Patterson DR, Sharar SR, et al. Pain management in patients with burn injuries. *Int Rev Psychiatry.* 2009;21:522–530.

21. Lund T, Onarheim H, Reed RK. Pathogenesis of edema formation in burn patients. *World J Surg.* 1992;16:2–9.

22. Latenser BA. Critical care of the burn patient: the first 48 hours. *Crit Care Med.* 2009;37:2819–2826.

23. Alvarado R, Chung KK, Cancio LC, et al. Burn resuscitation. *Burns.* 2009;35:4–14.

24. Orgill DP, Piccolo N. Escharotomy and decompressive therapies in burns. *J Burn Care Res.* 2009;30:759–768.

25. Porter JM, Shakespeare PG. Cardiac output after burn injury. *Ann R Coll Surg Engl.* 1984;66:33–35.

26. Giantin V, Ceccon A, Enzi G, et al. Heart rate and metabolic response to burn injury in humans. *J Parenter Enteral Nutr.* 1995;19(1):55–62.

27. Dickerson RN, Gervasio JM, Riley ML, et al. Accuracy of predictive methods to estimate resting energy expenditure of thermally-injured patients. *J Parenter Enteral Nutr.* 2002;26:17–29.

28. Deitch EA. Nutritional support of the burn patient. *Crit Care Clin.* 1995;11:735–750.

29. Demling RH, Seigne P. Metabolic management of patients with severe burns. *World J Surg.* 2000;24:673–380.

30. Curreri P, Richmond D, Marvin J, et al. Dietary requirements of patients with major burns. *J Am Diet Assoc.* 1974;65:415–417.

31. Curreri P. Assessing nutritional needs for the burned patient. *J Trauma.* 1990;30(12 suppl):S20–S23.

32. Hildreth M, Carvajal HF. A simple formula to estimate daily caloric requirements in burned children. *J Burn Care Rehabil.* 1982;3:78–80.

33. Harris JA, Benedict FG. *A Biometric Study on Basal Metabolism in Men.* Carnegie Institute of Washington, Washington, DC; 1919.

34. Hildreth M, Herndon DN, Desai MH, et al. Reassessing caloric requirements in pediatric burn patients. *J Burn Care Rehabil.* 1988;9:616–618.

35. Turner WJ, Ireton CS, Hunt JL, et al. Predicting energy expenditures in burned patients. *J Trauma.* 1985;24:11–16.

36. Singer AJ, McClain SA. Persistent wound infection delays epidermal wound maturation and increases scarring in thermal burns. *Wound Repair Regen.* 2002;10:372–377.

37. Pruitt BAJ, McManus AT, Kim SH, et al. Burn wound infections: current status. *World J Surg.* 1998;22:135–145.

38. Robson MC. Burn sepsis. *Crit Care Clin.* 1988;4:281–298.

39. Altoparlak U, Erol S, Akcay MN, et al. The time-related changes of antimicrobial resistance patterns and predominant bacterial profiles of burn wounds and body flora of burned patients. *Burns.* 2004;30:660–664.

40. Weber J, McManus A. Infection control in burn patients. *Burns.* 2004;30:A16–A24.

41. McCall JE, Cahill TJ. Respiratory care of the burn patient. *J Burn Care Res.* 2005;26:200–206.

42. Burn Center Referral Criteria. In: American Burn Association; 2006. http://www.ameriburn.org/BurnCenterReferralCriteria.pdf

43. Ryan MR, Schoenfeld DA, Thorpe WP, et al. Objective estimates of the probability of death from burn injuries. *N Engl J Med.* 1998;338:362–366.

44. http://www.ameriburn.org/BurnCenterReferralCriteria.pdf

45. Mosier MJ, Gibran, N.S. Surgical excision of the burn wound. *Clin Plast Surg.* 2009;36:617–625.

46. Sheridan R. Closure of the excised burn wound: autografts, semipermanet skin substitutes, and permanent skin substitutes. *Clin Plast Surg.* 2009;36:643–651.

47. Chern PL, Baum CL, Arpey CJ. Biologic dressings: current applications and limitations in dermatologic surgery. *Dermatol Surg.* 2009;35:891–906.

48. Fohn M, Bannasch H. Artificial skin. *Methods Mol Med.* 2007;140:167–182.

49. Gore DC, Chinkes D, Heggers J, et al. Association of hyperglycemia with increased mortality after severe burn injury. *J Trauma.* 2001;51:540–544.

50. Pankhurst S, Pochkhanawala T. *Wound Care.* 2nd ed. London, UK: Whurr Publishers; 2002.

51. Flannagan M, Graham J. Should burn blisters be left intact or debrided? *J Wound Care.* 2001;10:41–45.

52. Hermans MH. Results of an internet survey on the treatment of partial-thickness burns, full-thickness burns, and donor sites. *J Burn Care Res.* 2007;28:835–847.

53. Hudspith J, Rayatt, S. First aid and treatment of minor burns. *BMJ.* 2004;328:1487–1489.

54. Saba SC, Tsai R, Glat P. Clinical evaluation comparing the efficacy of aquacel ag hydrofiber dressing versus petrolatum gauze with antibiotic ointment in partial-thickness burns in a pediatric burn center. *J Burn Care Res.* 2009;30:380–385.

55. Quinn KJ, Courtney JM, Evans JH, et al. Principles of burn dressings. *Biomaterials.* 1985;6:269–377.

56. Wasiak J, Cleland H, Campbell F. Dressings for superficial and partial thickness burns. *Cochrane Database Syst Rev.* 2010;10:18–48.

57. Elliott C. The effects of silver dressings on chronic and burns wound healing. *Br J Nurs.* 2010;19:S32–S36.

58. Silver dressings—do they work? *Drug Ther Bull.* 2010;48:38–42.

59. Palmieri TL, Greenhalgh DG. Topical treatment of pediatric patients with burns: a practical guide. *Am J Clin Dermatol.* 2002;3:529–234.

CHAPTER 16

Management of Scar

R. Scott Ward

CHAPTER OBJECTIVES

At the completion of this chapter, the reader will be able to:

1. Explain the process of scar formation.
2. Identify complications caused by scar formation.
3. Describe common examination techniques used to assess and document scar tissue.
4. Describe intervention strategies used to treat impairments related to scar formation.

The formation of scar tissue during wound healing can lead to both cosmetic and functional complications. The hypertrophy associated with scar formation can be disfiguring and is particularly distressing when located at body sites commonly exposed to the public (i.e., face, hands, arms, etc.). Contraction of the forming scar often leads to further disfigurement. Functional deficits occur principally when the scar is situated over joint surfaces, particularly over joints of the extremities. Scarring of the face may also compromise functions such as feeding or speech. Moreover, pruritis, some pain, or other annoying paresthesias may accompany scar formation.

More than 2000 years ago, the ancient Greek physician Hippocrates acknowledged the problems of scar formation as a torsion resulting from healed burns.[1] Early documentation of surgical correction of scar contractures is included in the writings of the 16th century surgeons Camillo Ferrara and Wilhelm Fabry of Hilden.[1] Fabry of Hilden also described the use of splinting apparatuses to help correct joint deformities secondary to scar contraction. Modern versions of these devices are still used today to control the problems created by active scar formation.

In contemporary health-care settings, scar tissue is managed operatively, pharmaceutically, or with conservative measures, including pressure therapy, massage, silicone, exercise, splinting, positioning, and warming. Each of these treatments corrects some problem related to the progression of scarring and has demonstrated effectiveness in clinical studies, or has been accepted as effective because of anecdotal evidence of success. Further, the use of combinations of some of these treatments has resulted in increased improvement in function and appearance. Nevertheless, it is essential to bear in mind that none of these interventions can cure or stop the process of scarring. Current scientific investigation is uncovering more information

about the cause of scarring and may lead to new therapies, such as the use of growth factors that would be aimed more directly at the actual development of scars. Before we turn to contemporary therapies, we discuss the pathophysiology of scar tissue formation, and methods of testing and measurement.

SCAR TISSUE: FORMATION AND COMPLICATIONS

Scars are classified as *normotrophic*, *hypertrophic*, or *keloid*. A normotrophic scar is a visible scar that is not raised above the height of the normal skin (Fig. 16.1). A hypertrophic scar is raised but does not grow beyond the original wound boundaries (Fig. 16.2)[2–5] A keloid scar is raised and does extend past the original boundaries of the wound (Figs. 16.2–16.4).[2–5]

Formation of any scar begins with the proliferation and stimulation of fibroblasts during the inflammatory phase of wound healing. We discuss the process here, identify markers that allow for prediction of scar formation, and consider the most common complications.

Pathophysiology of Scar Tissue Formation

As you learned in Chapter 2, inflammation follows any tissue trauma. Several cell lines are recruited during the inflammatory response to control local infection, debride damaged tissue, nourish surviving and regenerating cells, and release factors that stimulate repair. One cell line that is stimulated to proliferate is fibroblasts. These are the cells of origin for scar tissue.

Fibroblasts produce elastin and collagen; however, the ratio of elastic fibers to collagen is less in scar than in normal skin. The secreted elastin becomes elastic fibers that provide normal dermis, or scar, with elasticity and flexibility. The secreted collagen develops into collagen fibers that mainly provide tensile

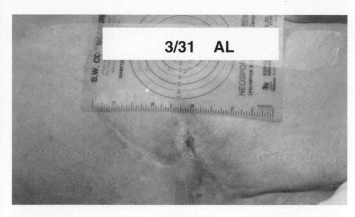

FIGURE 16.1 The wound is completely resurfaced and is in the remodeling phase. (Copyright © C. Sussman.)

strength but also afford some flexibility within the normal dermis. The collagen secreted by fibroblasts in scar tissue is laid down in an unorganized, whorl-like pattern. Again, collagen in scars is produced at a much greater rate than in normal skin.

Like all connective tissue, normal dermis and scars contain ground substance, or extracellular matrix, which provides some cushion, and allows for the diffusion of oxygen and nutrients in the vicinity. Scar tissue is well vascularized and highly metabolic.

Although scar formation begins with the proliferation and stimulation of fibroblasts during inflammation, the process of scarring continues for weeks, if not months, in most individuals. This is in part because the fibroblast-promoting growth factors continue to be released through the proliferative and remodeling phases of wound healing. Examples of some of these growth factors include platelet-derived growth factor (PDGF), tumor necrosis growth factor-ß (TGF-ß), and insulinlike growth factor (IGF). The interaction of these growth factors with other substances in scar tissue formation is not well understood.

We do know, however, that in all healing wounds, collagen deposition strengthens the wound site, and collagen degradation remodels the wound. When wounds demonstrate an imbalance between the rate of collagen deposition and degradation such that the rate of collagen production exceeds the rate of degradation, a scar that is raised and thick—that is, either a hypertrophic or a keloid scar—forms.[6,7] As a scar actively forms, it lacks suppleness and is red and raised. During this "phase" of scarring, the scar is commonly referred to as *immature scar*. As the scar matures in due course, the redness fades, the scar levels out to some degree, and the scar tissue softens (Fig. 16.5). It commonly takes 6 to 18 months for a scar to mature.[8]

Predictors of Scar Formation

Several clinically observed and documented markers allow for some prediction of scar formation. These include wound depth, skin pigmentation, and other factors.

The deeper the wound, the more likely it is that the wound will scar. This increased risk of scarring is likely due to extended healing time and the associated formation of granulation tissue.[9–11] In this same light, the length of time it takes for a wound to heal, thereby also implicating the chronicity of inflammation, will also influence scar formation.

Highly pigmented skin has been described as being more susceptible to scarring.[10,11] The reason for this increased risk is not entirely clear.

Skin tension appears to be a contributor to scarring.[10,11] Tension can lead to microdamage, which in turn may lead to inflammation that stimulates fibroblasts to create collagen.

Young people tend to scar more than elderly people do.[10,11] This might be due to the "tighter" skin and generally more active lifestyle (causing frequent skin tension) of younger individuals, compared with the "loose" skin and decreased elasticity of the skin in elderly people.

Although scars can form on any part of the body, it is generally agreed that the location of a wound may contribute to the amount of eventual scarring.[10,11] Hypertrophic scarring is more likely at the shoulder, upper arm, upper back, dorsal feet, and buttocks.[11] Keloids most commonly appear somewhere between the ears and the waist or from the elbow to the shoulder.[12]

Finally, there is probably some genetic predisposition to scar formation.[13]

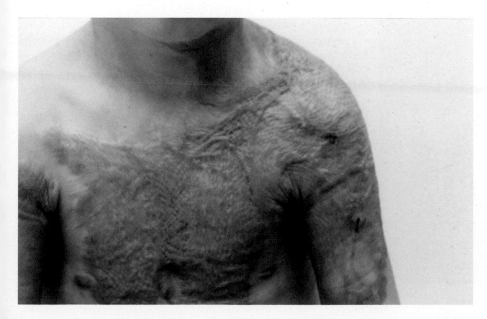

FIGURE 16.2 Hypertrophic scar. (Copyright © 2001, R. Scott Ward.)

FIGURE 16.3 Immature keloid scar. (Copyright © 2001, R. Scott Ward.)

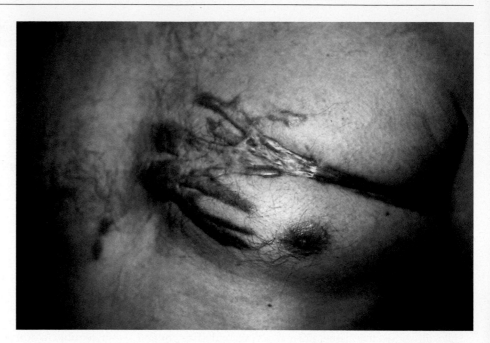

Complications of Scar Formation

Cosmetic changes are a possible complication of scarring. The location of the scar might be thought to influence cosmesis initially. For example, a facial scar is likely to be more a consistent challenge than a scar that is commonly hidden on the body. However, this does not hold true if the person swims or lives in a warm climate that necessitates shorts or other light clothing. Generally, interactions with people beyond health-care providers, family, and friends may be difficult and, therefore, a person may confine himself or herself socially.

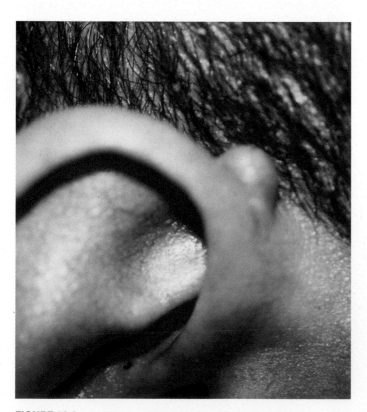

FIGURE 16.4 Keloid scar. (Copyright © 2001, R. Scott Ward.)

Social isolation reduces quality of life and can lead to lowered self-esteem. Particularly following a trauma such as a burn, patients may hesitate to participate in their normal relationships and activities, thereby losing some of their sense of worth or contribution. Disfigurement can result in a deceased self-esteem for women and men,[14] adolescents,[15] and children.[16] Low self-esteem and quality of life can also be affected by other complications of scarring, such as contraction, changes in sensation, itching, and color variability in the scar.

Hypertrophic scar contracts while it is maturing.[17–22] Contraction of scar may intensify a cosmetic deformity and can also restrict mobility. When a scar is forming over a joint or on a particular side of an extremity, the contraction will affect the related motion. For example, a scar located on the anterior surface of the elbow (the antecubital fossa) will be expected to contract the arm into flexion and could lead to limits of extension of the elbow. Scars on the dorsal surface of the toes will "pull" the toes into extension and limit toe flexion.

If intervention is not provided and the scar contraction is allowed to progress, it can become a fixed scar contracture. Prevention of fixed contracture is one of the primary reasons for long-term follow-up care of patients with scars.

The process of contracture formation can also result in the shortening of associated soft tissue, such as muscle, ligament, and joint capsule. The combination of all of these shortened structures makes it extremely challenging to recover any functional mobility without invasive surgical revision. The regrettable part of surgical revision is the possibility of the very same outcome because of the scarring that results from the surgical wound.

Scar is typically less densely innervated than is normal skin; thus, sensory loss is common. Patients may experience a "dulled" ability to recognize any of the protective sensations normally present in the skin, such as touch, pain, and temperature.[23] Because of these elevated sensory thresholds, a patient may be at risk for trauma to the scar and should be taught to inspect the scar regularly for scrapes, cuts, small burns, or other damage. Interestingly, even though there is a loss of cutaneous temperature sensation, some patients complain of their scar

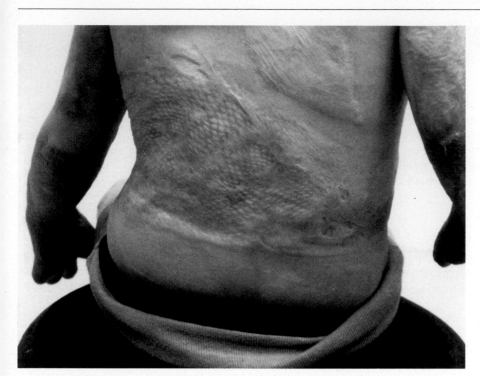

FIGURE 16.5 Maturing keloid scar. (Copyright © 2001, R. Scott Ward.)

being very sensitive to cold. Patients may describe numbness, tingling, or shooting pain in the scar during cold weather.

Pruritis is also common, both in maturing scar tissue and as a chronic problem in some scars. The itching is probably a result of several contributing factors. A low level of inflammation may be present in forming scar, and substances released during inflammation, such as histamine and substance P, can contribute to itch. The scar also lacks oil-producing glands. The deficiency of skin oils results in a dry surface that may cause itching. It should also be noted that the dry scar is less supple and, therefore, more prone to cracking, which may lead to the development of sores. Patients should avoid scratching the scar because of the risk of blistering or skin breakdown. Instead, encourage the patient to apply lotion to the scar frequently. Lotion may help to decrease itchiness and prevent the scar from cracking. Advise patients to avoid perfumed lotions because they might cause a rash or skin irritation.

Additional ingredients, such as vitamin E or aloe, are often included in lotions because they are purported to decrease or cure scars. Although neither of these additives will aggravate or worsen a scar, there is also no current evidence that they will improve the appearance of a scar or cure the scar.[24-26]

Patients may also report that their scar changes color from time to time, between varying shades of red, purple, brown, and gray. Position often affects the color changes. Generally, the color intensifies if a limb is in a dependent position. Elevation of the body part should help diminish the amount of color. Extreme ambient environmental temperatures, either hot or cold, might also increase the color of a scar. Color changes associated with position or temperatures are not permanent. However, if a maturing scar is exposed to sunlight, there is a risk that the scar will become permanently hyperpigmented. The mechanism for this hyperpigmentation in scar is not understood at this time, although it may be related to a potential increase in melanocytes and melanin in the scar tissue.[27] A maturing scar *must* be kept protected from sunlight.

ASSESSMENT OF SCARS

Assessment of a scar's characteristics and sequelae is essential to determining appropriate intervention strategies. Begin by assessing the scar tissue itself to determine whether the scar is immature or mature. Then assess the patient for complications of scar formation.

CLINICAL WISDOM

If a patient is experiencing a rash or skin irritation, discontinue the soap currently being used for hygiene and body washing and try a mild, nonperfumed lotion. If you are not sure whether it is the soap or lotion that is causing the irritation, have the patient change the soap first for a few days. If the rash has not gone away, try a nonperfumed lotion. If both the soap and lotion are changed to nonperfumed brands and the rash does not go away, consult a physician.

CLINICAL WISDOM

Sun Protection

The patient should apply a waterproof sun block or a sunscreen that is at least a sun protection factor (SPF) 30 before engaging in any outdoor activity. It is also wise to wear light, sun-protective clothing and hats to guard against the rays of the sun. The extra clothing is recommended even when the patient is wearing compression garments. Remember, too, that ultraviolet rays are also present on cloudy days.

CLINICAL WISDOM

Cosmetics

Patients with permanent discoloration of scars might benefit from the use of cosmetics. Cosmetics are most useful over areas of visible scarring, such as the hands and face. There are hypoallergenic forms of makeup that can be used to provide a covering for discoloration and minor deformity. Cosmetics with a sunscreen should be selected to protect the scar tissue from the sun.

Assessing Scar Maturity

A scar that is immature is more likely to respond to treatment. To determine maturity, assess color, pliability, height, and texture.

Color

The color of a scar reflects both vascularity and pigmentation. Generally, immature scars appear hypervascular and, therefore, may be red or violescent. The same scar may turn a deep purple if it is on a body part that is held in a dependent position or is exposed to cold for a period of time. This coloration begins to fade and should generally return to near-normal skin tone through the process of scar maturation. After the scar has matured, it may be either hypopigmented or hyperpigmented. Patients should understand that variations of the pigment of the scar are probably permanent if they are present following scar maturation.

Pliability

Mature scars are generally more pliable than immature scars. To assess the pliability of a scar, simply pinch it: a scar that is not pliable will be difficult to pinch up between your fingers because of the stiffness of the tissue. Also, a scar that is not pliable will typically move as a unit when manipulated.

Height

The height of a scar provides information about the level of hypertrophy of the scar. Height may be difficult to quantify; however, a scar that is raised above the plane of the normal adjacent skin demonstrates hypertrophy. The scar will not necessarily flatten as it matures, without some intervention.

Texture

The texture of the scar may also indicate hypertrophy. As scar tissue is being actively deposited, if it becomes hypertrophied to any degree, the texture of the scar will deviate from that of the normal surrounding skin. Describe a scar's texture as objectively as possible. Adjectives such as *rough*, *uneven*, or *bumpy*, although not necessarily scientific and certainly not quantitative, communicate the presence of an atypical texture, compared with normal smooth skin.

Scar Rating Scales

Scar measurement tools allow some objectification of observed scar traits; however, each of these scales involves observation and some judgment regarding the scar. In 1990, Sullivan et al.[28] published the Vancouver Scar Scale as a method for assessing burn-related scars (Table 16.1). This scale uses the variables of pigmentation, vascularity, pliability, and height of the scar to describe the current status of the tissue. Scores are assigned based on variances of these variables from normal, with normal being zero. A higher score represents a worse scar.

Another scar rating scale uses photographs (Exhibit 16.1).

In this scale, qualities of the scar, including smoothness of scar surface, border height, scar thickness, and color differences, are rated by evaluating color photographs of the scar.[29] The quality of the photographs and the experience of the evaluator may affect the reliability of this tool; however, if it is

TABLE 16.1 Ratings Used in the Vancouver Scar Scale to Measure Scar Formation

Pigmentation	Vascularity	Pliability	Height	Score
Normal—color that closely resembles the color over the rest of the body	Normal—color that closely resembles the color over the rest of the body	Normal	Normal—flat	0
Hypopigmentation	Pink	Supple: flexible with minimal resistance	Raised < 2 mm	1
Hyperpigmentation	Red	Yielding: giving way to pressure	Raised < 5 mm	2
	Purple	Firm: inflexible, not easily moved, resistant to manual pressure	Raised > 5 mm	3
		Banding: ropelike tissue that blanches with extension of the scar		4
		Contracture: permanent shortening of scar, producing deformity or distortion		5

NOTE: The higher the score reported, the worse the scar.
Reprinted from Sullivan T, Kermode J, McIver E, et al. Rating the burn scar. *J Burn Care Rehabil.* 1990;11:256–260, with permission.

EXHIBIT 16.1						
Ratings Used in a Photographic Scar Scale to Measure Scar Formation						
1. Scar Surface	−1 Smooth	0 Normal	1 Rough	2 Rough	3 Rough	4 Rough
2. Scar Border Height	−1 Depressed	0 Normal	1 Raised	2 Raised	3 Raised	4 Raised
3. Scar Thickness	−1 Thinner	0 Normal	1 Thicker	2 Thicker	3 Thicker	4 Thicker
4. Color Differences (between scar and adjacent normal skin)	−1 Hypopigment	0 Normal	1 Hyperpigment	2 Hyperpigment	3 Hyperpigment	4 Hyperpigment

NOTE: The scale ranges from −1 to 4 for each characteristic. Generally, the higher the score reported, the worse the scar. Reprinted from Yeong EK, Engrav LH, et al. Improved burn scar assessment with use of new scar-rating scale. *J Burn Care Rehabil.* 1997;18:353–355, with permission.

used within a particular setting, it may prove useful not only for measuring scar formation but for documenting the scar by photograph as well.

Assessing Complications of Scar Formation

A decrease in range of motion and associated joint mobility is a major impairment caused by scar contraction. Assessment procedures for examining range of motion include standard goniometry. Also assess functional limitation secondary to contraction, including activities of daily living and instrumental activities of daily living.

As already noted, disfigurement is a common problem associated with contraction. Two methods that can be used to portray the disfigurement are written description and photography. For example, describe scarring that occurs on the dorsum of the hand, involving the web spaces of the fingers, as "development of web space syndactyly."

Sensation is another impairment that follows scarring.[23] Perform sensation testing to identify the degree of sensory ability over a scar. Document any decreased sensation. Make sure to include self-care for skin protection in your patient education.

INTERVENTIONS FOR THE TREATMENT OF SCAR

As noted earlier, a variety of interventions are available for the treatment of scar formation. These include surgery, medications, and conservative measures.

Surgical Interventions

Surgery is considered in cases where conservative measures of scar control have not completely corrected or controlled scarring. It is indicated to improve specific cosmetic or functional deformities. A patient's particular needs, goals, and medical history are important matters for deliberation when finalizing any judgment regarding surgery. The success of surgery in correcting or controlling a scar depends on the location of the scar, timing of the surgery, extent of the deformity, and surgical technique.

- *Location*. At most anatomic locations, scar tissue can be revised; however, areas such as the head and face, neck, and axillae respond more poorly to surgical modification than do other areas.[30]

- *Timing*. Most scar revisions are performed after the scar tissue has matured. However, individual considerations and the extent of any deformity must be considered when decisions about reconstructive surgery for correction of scar are made.
- *Extent*. The larger the deformity or scar, the more extensive the surgery will be.
- *Technique*. Surgical techniques vary, and the type used for any scar revision will be influenced by the factors previously discussed. Small scars can simply be excised and the excision site can then be primarily closed. Larger scars may be excised and a graft placed to cover the wound.

The selection of graft type is important, as grafting may lead to further scar formation. Generally, split-thickness meshed skin grafts will scar to some degree, whereas full-thickness skin grafts, skin flaps, or split-thickness sheet grafts are less likely to scar. Of course, there is a risk that a donor site for a skin graft might scar. There is clearly a risk of scarring at the donor site of a full-thickness skin graft or a skin flap. Such donor sites will require further skin coverage, either with another split-thickness skin graft or, if the donor site is small enough, primary closure.

Another technique used in revising larger scars is *serial excision*, or *segmental scar reduction*. This is achieved by excising a central portion of the scar and primarily closing the wound. This procedure is then replicated over a period of several months until the entire scar has been removed.

Surgical realignment of scar tissue may be considered when scar formation causes abnormally high skin tension lines. This contributes to contracture formation. Z-plasty, Y-V plasty, and local advancement or rotational flaps are surgical techniques used to realign or replace scar and break up tension lines.[31] Tension lines are the direction of pull on the skin at any surface region created by the natural elasticity of the skin and the underlying muscle.

Tissue expanders, which are silicone balloons surgically implanted in the subcutaneous fat or under the muscle, are injected with saline and are used to increase the surface area of normal skin adjacent to the scar. This expanded area of skin eventually can be transferred as a flap to cover an excised area of scar. Tissue expansion allows for better matches of skin color, thickness, and texture than do techniques such as grafting.

Inform any patient considering scar revision that the scar may form again. This would then require continuing treatment to control the new scar.

Pharmaceutical Interventions

Some scar tissue responds to injection of cortisone-related medications. Such medications likely are effective because of their capability to increase activity of collagenase in breaking down the scar.

Conservative Measures

Conservative measures for scar formation include pressure therapy, massage, silicone, exercise, splinting, positioning, and warming.

Pressure Therapy

As noted earlier, the longer the healing time, the more likely it is that a wound will form scar tissue. Thus, pressure therapy is typically recommended when a wound takes longer than 14 days to heal. Most clinicians advise that pressure garments or devices be worn for an average of 23 hours a day while the scar is maturing. Regularly check the fit of the supports because pressure garments do stretch and wear out. Alter or replace existing garments as often as necessary to promote desired outcomes. Figures 16.6 and 16.7 show pressure garments.

Companies manufacture pressure garments in a variety of colors to match a variety of skin tones. Manufacturers offer garments that fit the face, neck, upper extremity, torso, hand, and lower extremity. They also are generally willing to fabricate atypical garments for special circumstances, such as a hand with an amputated finger. Although the different manufacturers may have slightly different methods for measuring each body part for a pressure garment, generally, limb circumferences every 1 inch to 1–1/2 inches are required. Assuring a proper fit of the face, torso, and hands is a bit more complex, and manufacturers' methods for taking measurements of these parts vary to some extent. Specific directions for measurement techniques can be obtained by contacting the manufacturer directly. A list of custom pressure garment suppliers is provided at the end of the chapter.

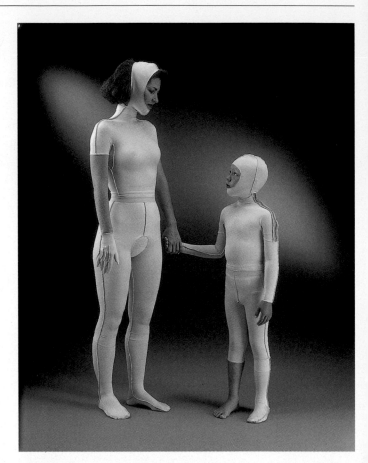

FIGURE 16.7 Examples of styles of pressure garments than can be used on different areas of the body. Styles available in adult and child sizes. They also may be custom made.

Patients need complete instructions in putting on and wearing pressure garments. After a bath or shower, the patient should apply some lotion to the scar and put on a clean pressure garment. Meanwhile, the garment previously worn should be washed and dried. The pressure garment can be washed either by hand or on a delicate cycle in a washing machine with mild detergent and warm (not hot) water. If the garment is washed by hand, it should be rinsed thoroughly after washing. The pressure garment should be dried in the air (do not dry in the dryer or by placing the garment on a heater). The garment will dry faster if it is first rolled up in a towel and gently wrung to remove extra water. Pressure garments will not tolerate dry cleaning and should not be ironed. Recommend that the patient have at least two of each type of garment worn so that a clean one is always available.

Some patients find the experience of wearing pressure garments challenging. Commonly expressed concerns about the garments include the appearance, the discomfort (tightness), getting the garment on and off, and how hot they make the patient. Compliance will increase if patients understand the consequences of scar formation, are given a color choice, and are educated about the benefits and care of the garments. As patients wear a pressure garment over time, they typically feel more accepting of the treatment.[32,33]

Patients commonly have difficulty in donning a pressure garment on a limb where a dressing is in place. Attempting to pull the pressure garment over the dressing is difficult and commonly dislodges it. This problem generally can be overcome by

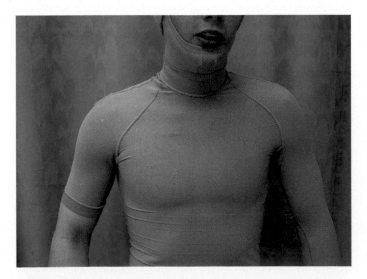

FIGURE 16.6 Patient wearing pressure garments that cover the trunk, full left arm, upper right arm, axillae, shoulders, neck and chin.

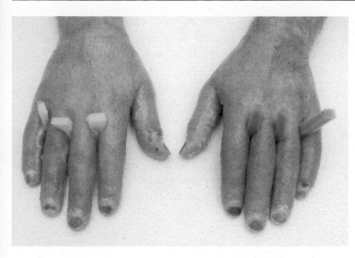

FIGURE 16.8 Self-adherent wrap and cotton elasticized pressure supports may be used to control edema and scarring. Coban™ self-adherent wrap was applied to the fingers in this figure. Tubigrip™ was used to cover the arm and hand in this figure. (Copyright © 2001, R. Scott Ward, PT, PhD.)

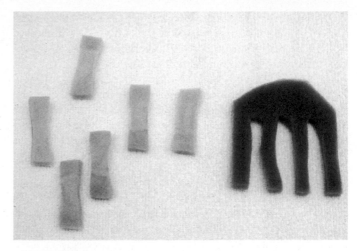

FIGURE 16.9 Examples of how foam was cut for placement in the web spaces of the fingers under a pressure support glove. (Copyright © 2001, R. Scott Ward, PT, PhD.)

pulling on nylon hosiery over the dressed limb and then donning the pressure garment over the nylon hosiery.

Pressure to a scar can also be applied through the use of elastic wraps, self-adherent stretch wraps, or elasticized cotton tubular bandages as shown in Figure 16.8. Manufacturers of custom pressure garments also produce noncustom, general fit supports. These less expensive, noncustom options can also be advantageous in treating lymphedema or postwound edema. Early pressure can decrease edema formation and facilitate wound healing. This may also have some effect on eventual scarring because, as mentioned previously, delayed wound healing has been linked to increased scar formation.

It can be difficult to fit certain areas of the body appropriately with a fabric pressure garment, because the fabric will generally form a bridge between bony prominences or over anatomic arches. Difficult-to-fit areas include the central portion of the face, palm of the hand, interscapular region, and sternal region. Foam, thermoplastic splinting material, and rubberized compounds can be placed under a pressure garment to conform better to these areas (Fig. 16.9). These "inserts" can also be used to augment pressure provided by a well-fitting pressure garment in areas such as the web spaces of the hand (Fig. 16.10). Custom-fitted, rigid, transparent, plastic material

has also been used successfully to control scarring of the face and could certainly be considered for other areas.[34,35]

Massage

Evidence for the effectiveness of massage in controlling scar formation is scarce. Massage should be useful in mobilizing superficial tissues by loosening the adhesions of scar to the tissue; however, massage does not appear to decrease scarring or to improve variables of scar formation, such as vascularity, pliability, and height.[36] Although massage does not appear to improve the scar itself, supplementary benefits of massage may include lubrication of the scar to prevent drying and cracking of the skin, a decrease in reported pruritis, and the psychologic benefits of touch. Aggressive massage of early forming scar tissue should be avoided because it may cause blisters or skin breakdown.

Silicone

A silicone polymer gel (the viscosity of silicone used for scar treatment) is produced in sheets or pads that are applied directly over a maturing scar. These manufactured gel pads are commonly offered in several shapes and sizes for application to scars on different areas of the body. They are most commonly used over small areas and in areas where sufficient pressure cannot be applied to a scar. Although silicone gel has been used in treating scar hypertrophy, the mechanism of action for its effect is not known.[26,37,38]

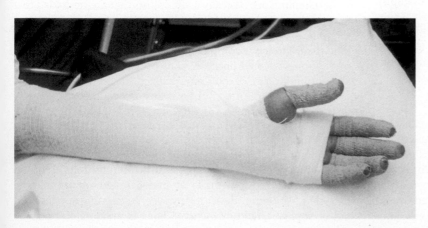

FIGURE 16.10 Application of the foam inserts placed in the web spaces of hands. A pressure support glove is then applied over these inserts. The foam inserts increase the pressure applied to web spaces of fingers and toes and can be used over other areas that may require additional pressure. (Copyright © 2001, R. Scott Ward, PT, PhD.)

Reported complications associated with silicone gel application include local rash, skin breakdown, and a lack of durability of some brands of silicone. If a rash develops, the use of the gel product should be suspended temporarily. In general, the rash clears up readily, and, because the rash does not predictably reoccur at the same location, the gel may be reapplied, once the site is clear of the rash. Skin breakdown appears to occur almost exclusively in cases where a rash develops and the use of the gel sheet is not interrupted. No systemic complications related to the use of silicone have been reported.

Exercise

Exercise is vital in counteracting the contraction associated with active hypertrophic scar. Directed exercise to prevent deconditioning, functional limitation, and disability is also extremely important. When determining an exercise prescription for a patient with a scar, consider the following factors: location, size (surface area of the scar), and status (phase of wound healing). For example, in some acute situations immediately following a grafting procedure or following tendon repair associated with a skin wound, any type of exercise may be delayed to allow for appropriate healing. Patient variables that also must be considered in the preparation of an exercise prescription include medical history and current medical status, age, level of cognition, perceived or real level of cooperation, and goals for recovery.

Encourage the patient to put as much stretch on the scar as is safely indicated to prevent as much scar contraction as possible. Blanching of the scar is a reasonable clinical indication that the scar is being sufficiently stretched, and the stretch should not exceed the patient's pain tolerance. Stretching of a scar should be done with a slow, sustained elongation of the tissue. Stretching and exercise will also help to prevent other associated soft tissues from shortening. Any of several types of exercise may be appropriate for patients with scars.

Active Exercise

Active exercise is the preferred method of exercise in treating scar. This type of exercise allows a patient to control the extent and amount of stretch placed on a scar. Active exercise will also help to overcome any loss of strength or endurance associated with varying levels of muscle disuse sometimes associated with injuries that lead to scar formation. An active exercise program should be prescribed and monitored by a physical therapist.

Active-Assisted Exercise

Active-assisted exercise allows patients who cannot quite achieve full range of motion to be assisted by the therapist. Encourage patients to complete as much of the motion as they can by themselves; then apply additional stretch to maximize tissue elongation. Weights may be used to enhance a stretch. The patient may also provide the assistance to active motion by using equipment such as reciprocal pulleys.

Passive Exercise

Passive exercise is effective but does not encourage patient independence. This form of stretching may be necessary if a patient is otherwise unable to stretch a scar because of such problems as weakness or paralysis, or when the patient is otherwise cognitively unable to participate in a prescribed active exercise program. Passive exercise may also be indicated when a wound is acute enough that a well-intentioned but overzealous patient might compromise healing. During passive exercise, avoid overstretching the scar or exceeding a patient's pain tolerance. Be aware that overly aggressive stretching might lead to heterotopic ossification.[39] Passive exercise should progress to active-assisted or active exercise as soon as possible.

Strengthening Exercise

A decrease in normal use of a muscle (or muscle group) can lead to a decrease in strength of that muscle. Strength testing should be a part of any physical examination associated with scarring. If strength deficits are found, prescribe a series of resistance exercises to help the patient regain lost strength. Strengthening exercises will also assist with any decreases in endurance or conditioning.

Directed Functional Exercise

Scar contraction can also lead to an inability to strengthen a muscle through its normal range of motion. These scar contraction-related impairments of strength or range of motion can lead to functional limitations. Institute age-appropriate functional exercises to improve motor skills, enhance confidence in daily activities, and allow the patient to resume his or her expected daily role in society.

Splinting

Splints are generally indicated for the positioning of a scar to avoid deformation or to maintain or increase the stretch on a scar.[40] A variety of effective prefabricated splints are available, but you can also fabricate a *conforming splint* using thermoplastic material. A conforming splint is custom-fit to a patient and matches the patient's anatomic shape. Since a poorly fitted prefabricated splint might apply some pressure to the scar, a conforming splint is preferred for controlling scar formation.

Clinicians also classify splints as static, dynamic, or serial splints. A *static splint* has a fixed shape and maintains a position through immobilization of the splinted part. Static splints are commonly used in the early phases of scar formation. They are generally molded and applied following an exercise treatment to maintain the elongation of the scar achieved during the session. They may be left on for an extended period of time to preserve range of motion gains.

Dynamic splints apply a force, or a stretch, to a body part or allow resistance to movement for exercise. This type of splint can be used to continue a gentle force to scar, thus providing an extended period of stretching.

Serial splints are basically static splints that are remolded to a newly achieved position of a body part. Serial splints (or casts) might be used if a scar is particularly difficult to stretch. A maximal tissue stretch is completed, and then the splint is reformed to the new stretched position. This procedure is followed serially until full range of motion is realized.

Discontinue splinting if there is any associated pain, sensory disturbance (numbness, tingling, etc.), or skin breakdown.

Positioning

Positioning may be used to sustain tissue elongation to counter scar contraction.[41] Preferred anticontracture positions are listed in Table 16.2. Custom-made or prefabricated splints may be used as "positioning" devices. However, positioning devices need not be sophisticated or expensive. For example, pillows may be

TABLE 16.2	Preferred Anticontracture Positions for Major Joints
Joint/Joint Complex	**Preferred Position**
Neck	Hyperextension, no rotation
Shoulder	Abduction (90 degree), slight horizontal flexion
Elbow	Extension, supination
Wrist/hand	Slight wrist extension, slight MCP flexion, PIP/DIP extension, thumb abduction
Trunk	Straight postural alignment
Hip	Extension, abduction (20 degree), no rotation
Knee	Full extension
Ankle/foot	Neutral ankle (no plantar flexion), neutral toes

used to position the hips or shoulders, and high-top tennis shoes make a reasonable positioning device for the foot and ankle.

Warming

Thermal agents are commonly used to treat scar or the sequelae of scarring. Warming the scar, in particular, may have the most effect on the tissue because of the high concentration of collagen in scar. Gersten and others demonstrated that collagen tissue is most effectively stretched when a blend of heat and gentle stretch are provided.[42,43] Superficial forms of heat may also provide the most effective method of heating surface scar and allowing enhanced elongation of the tissue; however, very little research exists to support the efficacy of superficial heat on integumentary scarring.

Because scars are also normally hypesthetic, use caution when applying thermal agents to the scar tissue. Complete a sensory examination first, and inspect the tissue frequently to ensure that no tissue damage is occurring secondary to the heat or coupling media.

SELF-CARE TEACHING GUIDELINES

Patients and their caregivers should be trained to apply and assess scar control techniques. This includes care of the scar, pressure supports, silicon gel, exercise, splints, and positioning. Allow patients and caregivers sufficient time to observe the proper techniques, and follow this with plenty of opportunities to practice the techniques while supervised. These steps will enhance the confidence of the patients/caregivers in their

abilities. Also provide written and illustrated supplemental materials. Having a patient/caregiver demonstrate the appropriate interventions is a logical discharge goal for patients with actively forming scars.

Educate patients and caregivers about the reasons for treatments being used and the goals of the interventions. An increased understanding will lead to greater acceptance of the treatment. Patients are more likely to take some personal responsibility regarding their care if they truly buy in to the plan.[44,45] Reassurance that you will be willing to provide further assistance and advice, should it be needed, will also quell some concerns they might have about forgetting a component of the intervention or asking questions that arise concerning the progression of the scar. The supplemental material provided might be sufficient for some, but a contact phone number with an invitation to call can also be reassuring.

CONCLUSION

When considering treatment for a scar, consider all aspects of the scarring process. This includes not only the location and appearance of the scar, but also the limitations that result from the contraction of the scar. It is important to remember that scarring is a process and that it commonly takes several months for a scar to mature. Therefore, much of what is done to treat scar cannot be employed on a short-term basis only. Scar management requires high-quality patient education and follow-up to monitor the progression of the scarring properly for the best possible clinical outcome.

CASE STUDY

B.G. is a 34-year-old Caucasian female with healed full-thickness burns to the dorsum of her left hand and the dorsal surface of all left fingers. She is 3 weeks post–split-thickness autografting to the hand wound. Her burn injury included partial-thickness burns to her left arm that have fully healed. She is otherwise healthy, with no significant past medical history.

On examination, there is no evidence of scarring on the left arm over the site of the partial-thickness burns. The skin-grafted areas of the left hand are showing signs of scarring. The tissue is red, has a mildly decreased pliability, and is slightly raised and uneven. Range of motion measurements demonstrated the following limitations: the left wrist is

0- to 80-degree extension, 0- to 65-degree flexion; an average loss of 20 degrees of motion in the left MCPs of the fingers; an average loss of 25 degrees in the motion. Tissue stretches will be taught to the patient and should be performed six or more times daily. Interventions will also include

- Active range of motion exercises, including encouraging full use of the hand in normal daily functional activities. The active motion exercises should be performed following each session of passive stretches. The hand should be used actively for all normal activities.
- Measurement and application of a custom-fit, antiscar support glove. The patient will be educated on the application and care of the pressure garment. One to two additional gloves will be ordered.

- Application of moisturizer to the scar, as needed, for itching and discomfort. The patient will be educated in the indication for application of moisturizer, including itching, discomfort, and "scaliness."

All of these interventions will continue through to maturation of the scar, which may be 6 to 18 months. The frequency of the stretching and range of motion exercises may be decreased, depending on the level of ongoing limitation and impairment.

The discharge outcome for this patient would be a scar that closely matches normal skin pigment, is relatively pliable, is smooth, and does not limit mobility and function of the hand.

REVIEW QUESTIONS

1. Predictors of scar formation can include:
   A. Depth and duration of healing.
   B. Skin pigmentation and tension
   C. Age and location.
   D. All of the above.
2. To determine a scar's maturity assess:
   A. Color, range of motion, disfigurement, and pliability.
   B. Color, pliability, height, and texture.
   C. Pliability, mobility, contraction, and texture.
   D. Mobility, range of motion, contraction, and color.
3. The Vancouver Scar Scale measures the scar's:
   A. Pigmentation, vascularity, pliability and height.
   B. Color differences, thickness, surface, and vascularity.

C. Height, surface, pliability and pigmentation.
D. Surface, height, thickness and color differences.
4. Which statement regarding grafting is incorrect?
   A. Grafting may lead to further scar formation.
   B. Split-thickness sheet grafts are less likely to scar.
   C. Full-thickness skin grafts are more likely to scar.
   D. Donor sites are at risk for scarring.
5. Methods to counter scar contraction include all of the following except:
   A. Massage and active exercise.
   B. Active-assistive exercise and splinting.
   C. Positioning and passive exercise
   D. Splinting and strengthening exercise

RESOURCES

Custom Pressure Garment Manufacturers

Barton-Carey Medical Products
26963 Eckel Road, Suite 303
Perrysburg, OH 43551
(800) 421-0444

Bio-Concepts, Inc.
2424 East University Drive
Phoenix, AZ 85034-6911
(800) 421-5647
www.bio-con.com

Gottfried Medical, Inc
4105 West Alexis Road
Toledo, OH 43623
(800) 537-1968
www.gottfriedmedical.com

Juzo
P.O. Box 1088
Cuyahoga Falls, OH 44223
(216) 923-4999
www.juzousa.com

Torbot Group, Inc.
Jobskin Division
653 Miami Street
Toledo, OH 43605
(800) 207-1074
www.torbotgarments.com

Medical Z
6800 Alamo Downs Parkway
San Antonio, TX 78238
Phone: (800) 368-7478
www.gottfriedmedical.com

REFERENCES

1. Thomsen M. It all began with Aristotle—the history of the treatment of burns. *Burns Incl Therm Inj.* 1988;14(suppl):S1–S8.
2. Burd A, Huang L. Hypertrophic response and keloid diathesis: two very different forms of scar. *Plast Reconstr Surg.* 2005;116(7):150e–157e.
3. Slemp AE, Kirschner RE. Keloids and scars: a review of keloids and scars, their pathogenesis, risk factors, and management. *Curr Opin Pediatr.* 2006;18(4):396–402.
4. Tuan TL, Nichter LS. The molecular basis of keloid and hypertrophic scar formation. *Mol Med Today* 1998;4(1):19–24.
5. Kose O, Waseem A. Keloids and hypertrophic scars: are they two different sides of the same coin?" *Dermatol Surg.* 2008;34(3):336–346.
6. Ladin DA, Garner WL, et al. Excessive scarring as a consequence of healing. *Wound Repair Regen.* 1995;3(1):6–14.
7. Armour A, Scott PG, et al. Cellular and molecular pathology of HTS: basis for treatment. *Wound Repair Regen.* 2007;15(suppl 1):S6–S17.
8. Hunt T. Disorders of wound healing. *World J Surg.* 1980;4:289–295.
9. van der Veer WM, Bloemen MC, et al. Potential cellular and molecular causes of hypertrophic scar formation. *Burns* 2009;35(1):15–29.
10. Davies DM. Plastic and reconstructive surgery. Scars, hypertrophic scars, and keloids. *Br Med J (Clin Res Ed).* 1985;290(6474):1056–1058.
11. Deitch EA, Wheelahan TM, et al. Hypertrophic burn scars: analysis of variables. *J Trauma* 1983;23(10):895–898.
12. Cohen IK, McCoy BJ. The biology and control of surface overhealing. *World J Surg.* 1980;4:289–295.
13. Lewis WHP, Sun KKY. Hypertrophic scar: a genetic hypothesis. *Burns* 1990;16:176–178.
14. Lawrence JW, Fauerbach JA, et al. Visible vs hidden scars and their relation to body esteem. *J Burn Care Rehabil.* 2004;25(1):25–32.
15. Robert R, Meyer W, Bishop S, et al. Disfiguring burn scars and adolescent self-esteem. *Burns* 1999;25:581–585.
16. Abdullah A, Blakeney P, Hunt R, et al. Visible scars and self-esteem in pediatric patients with burns. *J Burn Care Rehabil.* 1994;15:164–168.
17. Clark JA, Cheng JCY, Leung KS, et al. Mechanical characterization of human postburn skin during compression therapy. *J Biomech.* 1987;20:397–406.
18. McHugh AA, Fowlkes BJ, et al. Biomechanical alterations in normal skin and hypertrophic scar after thermal injury. *J Burn Care Rehabil.* 1997;18(2):104–108.
19. Nedelec B, Ghahary A, et al. Control of wound contraction. Basic and clinical features. *Hand Clin.* 2000;16(2):289–302.
20. Steed DL. Wound-healing trajectories. *Surg. Clin. North Am.* 2003;83:547.
21. Shin D, Minn KW. The effect of myofibroblast on contracture of hypertrophic scar. *Plast Reconstr Surg.* 2004;113(2):633–640.
22. Li B, Wang JH. Fibroblasts and myofibroblasts in wound healing: force generation and measurement. *J Tissue Viability* 2009.
23. Ward RS, Tuckett RP. Quantitative threshold changes in cutaneous sensation of patients with burns. *J Burn Care Rehabil.* 1991;12(6):569–575.
24. Cuttle L, Kempf M, et al. The efficacy of Aloe vera, tea tree oil and saliva as first aid treatment for partial thickness burn injuries. *Burns* 2008;34(8):1176–1182.
25. Juckett G, Hartman-Adams H. Management of keloids and hypertrophic scars. *Am Fam Physician.* 2009;80(3):253–260.
26. Morganroth P, Wilmot AC, et al. JAAD online. Over-the-counter scar products for postsurgical patients: disparities between online advertised benefits and evidence regarding efficacy. *J Am Acad Dermatol.* 2009;61(6):e31–e47.
27. Sowemimo GO, Naim J, Harrison HN, et al. Repigmentation after burn injury in the guinea-pig. *Burns Incl Thermal Inj.* 1982;8:345–357.
28. Sullivan T, Smith J, et al. Rating the burn scar. *J Burn Care Rehabil.* 1990;11(3):256–260.
29. Yeong EK, Mann R, et al. Improved burn scar assessment with use of a new scar-rating scale. *J Burn Care Rehabil.* 1997;18(4):353–355; discussion 352.
30. Kraemer MD, Jones T, Deitch EA. Burn contractures: incidence, predisposing factors, and results of surgical therapy. *J Burn Care Rehabil.* 1988;9:261–265.
31. Viera MH, Amini S, et al. Do postsurgical interventions optimize ultimate scar cosmesis. *G Ital Dermatol Venereol.* 2009;144(3):243–257.
32. Rosser P. Adherence to pressure garment therapy of posttraumatic burn injury. *J Burn Care Rehabil.* 2000;21(pt 2):S178.
33. Ripper S, Renneberg B, et al. Adherence to pressure garment therapy in adult burn patients. *Burns* 2009;35(5):657–664.
34. Shons AR, Rivers EA, et al. A rigid transparent face mask for control of scar hypertrophy. *Ann Plast Surg.* 1981;6(3):245–248.
35. Powell BW, Haylock C, et al. A semi-rigid transparent face mask in the treatment of postburn hypertrophic scars. *Br J Plast Surg.* 1985;38(4):561–566.
36. Patino O, Novick C, et al. Massage in hypertrophic scars. *J Burn Care Rehabil.* 1999;20(3):268–271; discussion 267.
37. O'Brien L, Pandit A. Silicon gel sheeting for preventing and treating hypertrophic and keloid scars. *Cochrane Database Syst Rev.* 2006;(1):CD003826.
38. Berman B, Perez OA, et al. A review of the biologic effects, clinical efficacy, and safety of silicone elastomer sheeting for hypertrophic and keloid scar treatment and management. *Dermatol Surg.* 2007;33(11):1291–1302; discussion 1302–1303.
39. Nassabi H, Raff T, et al. Manifestation of multifocal heterotopic ossifications with unusual locations as a complication after severe burn injury. *Burns* 1996;22(6):500–503.
40. Richard R, Ward RS. Splinting strategies and controversies. *J Burn Care Rehabil.* 2005;26(5):392–396.
41. Rudolf R. Construction and the control of contraction. *World J Surg.* 1980;4:279–287.
42. Gersten JW. Effect of ultrasound on tendon extensibility. *Am J Phys Med.* 1995;34(2):362–369.
43. Warren CG, Lehmann JF, et al. Heat and stretch procedures: an evaluation using rat tail tendon. *Arch Phys Med Rehabil.* 1976;57(3):122–126.
44. So K, Umraw N, et al. Effects of enhanced patient education on compliance with silicone gel sheeting and burn scar outcome: a randomized prospective study. *J Burn Care Rehabil.* 2003;24(6):411–417; discussion 410.
45. Robinson JH, Callister LC, et al. Patient-centered care and adherence: definitions and applications to improve outcomes. *J Am Acad Nurse Pract.* 2008;20(12):600–607.

Management by Wound Characteristics

Barbara M. Bates-Jensen

The Bates-Jensen rules for wound therapy are based on wound characteristics:

- If the wound is dirty, clean it.
- If there is leakage, manage it.
- If there's a hole, fill it.
- If it's flat, protect it.
- If it's healed, prevent it from recurring.

While simplistic and only addressing wound characteristics, these rules do provide general guidance for wound management.

Understanding the impact of wound characteristics on treatment options provides a template for intervention. Often, the physical appearance of the wound is the driving force behind treatment options. Part III presents management of wound healing by examination of physical characteristics commonly observed in wounds. Specific interventions by the clinician are required by the presence of necrotic tissue; exudate, infection, and biofilms; and edema. Clean, proliferating wounds; use of advanced wound therapy; and scar tissue present additional opportunities and obstacles for optimal therapy.

Part III begins with a chapter on management of necrotic tissue. A description of the significance and pathophysiology of necrotic debris in the wound bed opens the discussion. Five methods of debridement are presented: mechanical, enzymatic, sharp, autolysis, and biosurgical. Chapter 17 presents each debridement method with indications for use, contraindications, advantages, disadvantages, and procedures for implementation. Importance of initial and serial or maintenance debridement is discussed. Outcome measures and self-care teaching guidelines for other health-care workers, family caregivers, and patients conclude the chapter.

Chapter 18 reviews management of exudate, infection, and biofilms. The significance of infection and biofilm development in inhibiting wound healing are presented. This chapter provides information on diagnosis of infection with attention to differentiation of infection versus inflammation and colonization, as well as information on biofilm development. Wound culture is one of the primary methods of diagnosing infection, and this chapter includes procedures for tissue biopsy, needle aspiration, and quantitative swab techniques. Methods of wound cleansing and irrigation, proper use of antimicrobials, and management of exudate with topical dressings are presented to finish out the chapter.

Chapter 19 focuses on the management of edema. Procedures for managing edema and quantitative and qualitative parameters to measure to determine intervention outcomes are presented. Elimination and control of edema may be accomplished through leg elevation, exercise, and the use of compression therapy. Included in the chapter are expected outcomes and helpful hints for using a variety of compression methods. The next two chapters in Part III examine wound management of the clean wound and use of advanced wound therapy. Chapter 20 provides discussion on wound management of the clean wound with topical wound care products for moist wound healing. Discussion includes inert and passive products such as gauze, lint, and fiber products and modern moist wound dressings. The features of an "ideal" wound dressing are presented. Generic wound product categories of film dressings, foams, hydrocolloids, hydrogels, alginates, hydroactive dressings, and combination/miscellaneous dressings are presented. Chapter 21 follows with information on advanced wound therapies. Background, indications, and contraindications for use of growth factors and biological skin substitutes are presented. The section on growth factors is extensive and covers a wide variety of growth factors. This chapter provides the clinician with a quick reference for determining appropriate use of advanced therapy for wound care.

The final chapter in this section, Chapter 22: Management of Wound Pain provides a comprehensive discussion of wound pain physiology, as well as practical tools for assessing and treating wound pain. Management of wound pain is covered for a variety of different wounds in conjunction with generic management principles. An extensive section on self-care teaching guidelines completes this chapter.

The chapters on wound management by wound characteristics in Part III all include tools, such as procedures for specific interventions, self-care teaching guidelines, and guidelines for measuring outcomes. The procedures and guidelines included in these chapters provide the clinician with a "toolbox" for daily practice in wound management. Each chapter focuses on simplifying the often-complex task of determining which interventions are appropriate for patients with wounds. Each follows the simple rules for therapy stated at the beginning of Part III. If the wound is dirty or if necrotic debris and infection are present, clean the wound. Debride the devitalized tissue and identify and treat infection. If the wound is leaking excess exudate or if edema is present, manage the drainage. Control the edema and contain excess exudate. Provide for a moist wound environment, not a wet wound environment. If there is a hole or if significant tissue has been lost at the wound site, provide for tissue replacement with a wound dressing, or fill the hole. If the wound is flat, in the process of reepithelialization, or scarring, protect it from external trauma and complications related to scarring. Finally, if the wound is healed, prevention of future wounds is critical.

Management of Necrotic and Nonviable Tissue

Barbara M. Bates-Jensen and Thomas E. Serena

CHAPTER OBJECTIVES

At the completion of this chapter, the reader will be able to:

1. Define the terms *eschar* and *slough*.
2. Explain the importance of debridement in wound healing.
3. Differentiate between initial and maintenance debridement.
4. Identify indications for mechanical, enzymatic, sharp, autolytic, and biosurgical debridement.
5. Describe advantages and disadvantages for mechanical, enzymatic, sharp, autolytic, and biosurgical debridement.
6. Identify three characteristics for evaluating the effectiveness of debridement.

The word *necrosis* comes from the Greek word *nekros* meaning a corpse. It refers to the process by which living tissues die. The presence of necrotic tissue in the wound bed inhibits healing: necrotic tissue is a medium for bacterial growth and infection, and a physical barrier to epidermal resurfacing, wound contraction, and the formation of granulation tissue.[1-4] Healing cannot proceed until the wound is free of necrotic and *nonviable tissue*, tissue that is devitalized or burdened with dead and senescent cells. *Debridement*, the removal of nonviable or necrotic tissue, has become an essential principle in the treatment of acute and chronic wounds. In chronic wounds, debridement is key to wound bed preparation. Wound bed preparation, a concept based on a synthesis of research and clinical experience in the management of chronic wounds, is attention to total wound management aimed at accelerating endogenous healing and incorporates four factors that must be addressed by the clinician when developing a care plan for chronic wounds.[5,6] The four components are referred to in total with the acronym TIME, where "T" refers to nonviable or deficient tissue, "I" refers to infection or inflammation, "M" indicates moisture imbalance, and "E" refers to a nonadvancing or undermined wound edge.[6] Debridement plays a role in three of these areas: removal of nonviable or deficient tissue, removal of infection or contamination, and treatment of a nonadvancing or undermined edge. As such, debridement is an integral part of wound bed preparation. This chapter focuses on the importance of debridement in treating wounds: frequency of debridement, what tissue should be removed and how to identify it, methods for debridement, and debridement technique.

It is important to properly identify necrotic tissue. The three distinct characteristics that permit identification are presented. There are several methods for wound debridement. The indications, advantages, and disadvantages for each of the techniques are reviewed. Finally, clinicians must be able to evaluate the effectiveness of debridement.

SIGNIFICANCE OF DEBRIDEMENT

Debridement has become the cornerstone in the comprehensive management of patients with nonhealing wounds. Removal of necrotic tissue, foreign debris, and bacteria from the surface of the wound is necessary for healing. Debridement is thought to further support wound healing by

- Stimulating a response to prevent infection
- Reducing inflammatory cytokines, fibronectin, and metalloproteinases produced from chronic inflammation due to the presence of necrotic tissue
- Promoting DNA synthesis and keratinocyte growth, both of which are inhibited by products of the inflammatory response
- Converting the chronic nonhealing wound physiology to that of an acute wound[7,8]

The classic example of the importance of debridement was published by Steed and the Diabetic Ulcer Study Group in 1996.[8] The authors analyzed the data from a pivotal trial looking at the safety and efficacy of becaplermin (platelet-derived growth factor [PDGF]-BB) in the treatment of diabetic foot ulcerations. They established for the first time that regular aggressive sharp wound debridement resulted in superior healing. Two studies provide additional support for initial sharp debridement as important in wound healing: one in diabetic foot ulcers and the second in venous leg ulcers. In a retrospective analysis of a study on the effect of bioengineered tissue for treating diabetic foot ulcers, Saap and Falanga found that ulcers that were debrided more aggressively (determined by comparison of wound images after debridement to those from initial study entry and summarized as a debridement performance index) were twice as likely to heal by study completion compared to those with less aggressive debridement.[11] In venous leg ulcers, Williams et al. also showed initial debridement to be essential. In a prospective controlled trial examining the effect of a single sharp debridement episode using a curette with nonhealing venous leg ulcers, those ulcers that were debrided averaged higher surface area reductions than those ulcers that were not debrided.[10] Thus, the support for at least initial debridement of chronic wounds is strong. Debridement has become the standard of care and is recommended for all chronic wounds in national treatment guidelines, such as those published by the Wound Healing Society.[11–13] Health-care providers can choose from multiple debridement methods: sharp, mechanical, enzymatic, autolytic, and biosurgical. The type of debridement chosen will depend on the status and nature of the wound (e.g., type and volume of necrotic tissue, presence of underlying infection or bacterial bioburden, wound size, pain, vascularity of the wound and adjacent tissue), the condition of the patient (e.g., comorbid conditions such as sepsis), the skill and licensure of the practitioner, access to providers, patient preference, cost and reimbursement, and the care setting.

DEBRIDEMENT FREQUENCY

One of the current issues in debridement is when to debride and how often. Clinical practice guidelines recommend initial debridement to remove the obvious necrotic tissue and maintenance debridement to maintain readiness of the chronic wound bed for healing.[11–13] *Maintenance debridement*, also called *serial debridement*, is debridement that occurs multiple times during the course of managing the chronic wound. Although maintenance debridement is recommended, as with initial debridement, there are limited guidelines on what type of debridement should be used for maintenance debridement. The value of maintenance debridement has been questioned, and there is controversy related to potential overuse of serial surgical debridement, which is complicated by reimbursement regulations.

There is growing opinion that an initial aggressive surgical debridement may obviate the need for future multiple debridements. At present, most experts recommend an excisional debridement at the time of presentation. This entails removal of all nonviable tissue and a margin of normal skin. This may be critical as the edge (e.g., the 2–3-mm rim of the wound) of chronic wounds has been shown to exhibit distinct pathogenic changes (e.g., hyperproliferative/hyperkeratotic epidermis, dermal fibrosis, increased procollagen synthesis), and fibroblasts exhibit senescence and impaired migration.[14,15] Thereafter, maintenance debridement involves removing unhealthy tissue, slough, and bacterial biofilm that builds up on the wound. In the author's clinic, the initial sharp debridement is performed with a scalpel (see Fig. 17.1). Subsequent debridement can be performed using a curette (see Fig. 17.2). This aggressive approach may not be appropriate for all practitioners or for all patient care settings. The effectiveness of this treatment plan is

FIGURE 17.1 Sharp debridement using a scalpel. (Copyright T.E. Serena).

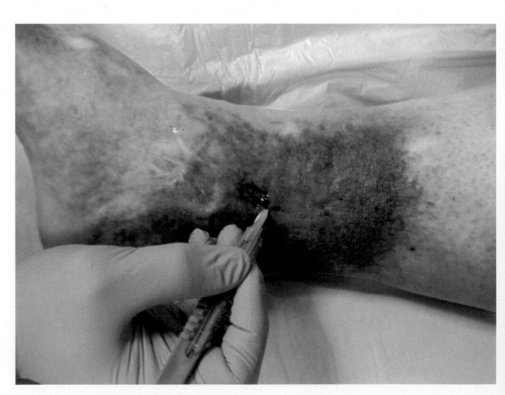

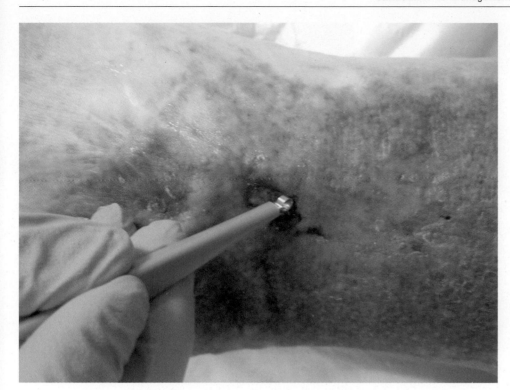

FIGURE 17.2 Sharp debridement using a curette. (Copyright T.E. Serena.)

currently under study. Others have also examined serial surgical debridement. Cardinal and colleagues evaluated serial surgical debridement of diabetic foot ulcers and venous leg ulcers by retrospectively examining the results of two large controlled prospective randomized trials of topical wound treatments and found that for both diabetic foot ulcers and venous leg ulcers, centers where patients were debrided more frequently were associated with higher rates of wound healing and wound closure.[16]

Continuous debridement is a form of maintenance debridement that uses topical therapy to provide debridement on an ongoing basis. Continuous debridement may be the treatment of choice for patients with nonhealing chronic wounds who are not candidates for maintenance debridement using sharp debridement methods.[17] Once continuous debridement (or even maintenance debridement) is initiated, it should not be discontinued just because the wound bed appears healthy on visual assessment. A wound that appears healthy may not be capable of adequate healing at a microbial, biochemical, or cellular level.[17] Since only 25% to 50% of chronic wounds (especially diabetic foot ulcers and venous leg ulcers) have been shown to heal with up to 20 weeks of treatment, continuous debridement may provide an additional boost to the proportion of chronic wounds that achieve complete healing.[18–20] Provision of continuous debridement may be effected with use of polyacrylate or medical-grade honey dressings (both discussed below).[20]

RECOGNITION OF TISSUE FOR DEBRIDEMENT

Nonviable tissue includes necrotic tissue, cellular debris, senescent nonfunctional cells, and bacterial biofilms, and all are tissues appropriate for debridement. Recognition of tissue appropriate for debridement requires knowledge of the appearance of normal healthy tissues and experience. Necrotic tissue and cellular debris are easiest to identify and are discussed next. Senescent nonfunctional cells and bacterial biofilms are more difficult to identify and are discussed at the end of this section.

Characteristics of Necrotic Tissue

As tissue dies, it changes in color, consistency, and adherence to the wound bed. Understanding these characteristics permits the clinician to recognize and remove necrotic tissue from the wound (see Figs. 17.3 and 17.4).

Color and Consistency of Necrotic Tissue

Initially, necrotic tissue appears white or gray. Prolonged ischemia may lead to necrosis of underlying tissues producing areas of gray or blue skin, or white devitalized tissue.[21,22] As necrosis increases in severity, the color progresses to tan or yellow, and finally, to brown or black.

Consistency refers to the cohesiveness of debris. It can be described as thin and stringy or thick with clumps of nonviable material. Consistency of the necrotic tissue changes depending on the hydration of the tissue, which is typically related to the length of time the tissue has been ischemic. Initially, the consistency of ischemic tissue may be mucoid with a high water or moisture content. Later, the material becomes stringy in nature as the tissue desiccates. Eventually, as the wound is exposed to air, the necrotic debris dehydrates, becoming leathery, dry, and hard. The tissue type affected also influences the consistency of the necrotic tissue. For example, as subcutaneous fat dies, it takes on a stringy consistency. In contrast, degenerating muscle or tendon will tend to become thick and tenacious.

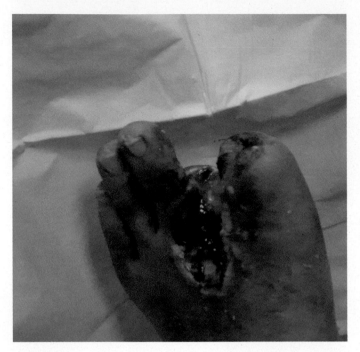

FIGURE 17.3 Loosely adherent slough in a diabetic wound. (Copyright T.E. Serena.)

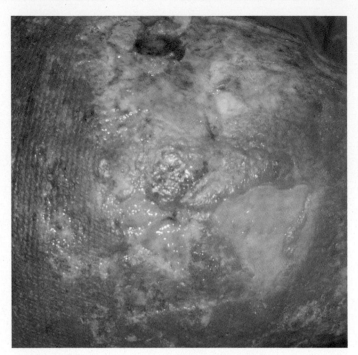

FIGURE 17.5 Loosely adherent slough frequently seen on venous leg ulcers. (Copyright T.E. Serena.)

The terms *slough* and *eschar* refer to different levels of necrosis and are described according to color and consistency.[21–23]

- *Slough* is yellow (or tan) fibrin debris and has a moderate to high water content. It frequently lies on top of the wound with minimal to moderate adherence to the wound bed.
- *Eschar* is brown or black necrotic tissue. It may be soft or hard and represents full-thickness tissue destruction.[21–23]

Necrosis of dermal and fat tissue may be compounded by infection following contamination by normal skin flora.[21,23] The debris may appear as yellow fibrinous slough.

Adherence of Necrotic Tissue

Adherence refers to the adhesiveness of the debris to the wound bed and the ease with which the two are separated. In general, the more the water content present in the necrotic debris, the less the debris adheres to the wound bed. Figure 17.5 depicts several large venous leg ulcers with loosely adherent slough. This loosely adherent material is seen frequently in this ulcer type. Necrotic tissue tends to become more adherent to the wound bed as the level of damage increases and as moisture in the wound decreases. Clinically, eschar is more firmly adherent than yellow slough. Figure 17.6 shows necrotic material tightly adhered to the margin of a heel ulcer in a diabetic patient.

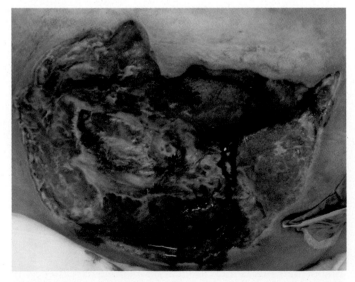

FIGURE 17.4 A sacral ulcer with necrotic tissue in the base of the wound. (Copyright T.E. Serena.)

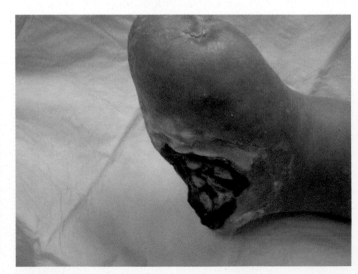

FIGURE 17.6 Eschar firmly adherent to the margins of a complex diabetic heel ulcer. (Copyright T.E. Serena.)

TABLE 17.1	**Debridement Time Frames**			
Necrotic Tissue Type	Debridement Choice	Expected Outcomes	Time Frame Guide	Notes
Eschar	Autolysis	1. Eschar nonadherent to wound edges 2. Necrotic tissue lifting from wound edges 3. Necrotic tissue soft and soggy 4. Color change from black/brown to yellow/tan	14 d	Depending on type of dressing used for autolysis, may proceed at more rapid rate.
Eschar	Enzymatic preparations	1. Eschar nonadherent to wound edges 2. Necrotic tissue lifting from wound edges 3. Necrotic tissue soft and soggy 4. Color change from black/brown to yellow/tan 5. Change from eschar to slough	14 d	Requires compliance on dressing changes in order to be effective.
Eschar	Sharp	1. Removal/elimination of eschar, if done one time or significant change in amount and adherence, if sequential	Immediate if one time, 7 d if sequential	If sequential sharp debridement used in conjunction with enzymatic preparation or autolysis, may expect clean wound base in 7 d.
Slough or fibrin	Autolysis or enzymatic preparations	1. Necrotic tissue lifting from wound base 2. Necrotic tissue stringy or mucinous 3. Tissue color yellow or white 4. Change in amount of wound covered—gradual decrease to wound predominantly clean	14 d	Will require moderate amount of exudate absorption and protection of surrounding tissues from maceration.
Slough or fibrin	Sharp	1. Removal/elimination of necrotic slough if done one time or significant change in amount and adherence, if sequential	Immediate if one time, 7 d if sequential	If sequential sharp debridement used in conjunction with enzymatic preparation or autolysis, may expect clean wound base in 7 d.

Table 17.1 classifies necrotic tissue types according to the characteristics of color, consistency, and adherence. Exhibit 17.1 identifies guidelines for assessing necrotic tissue.

Location of Necrotic Tissue

Necrotic tissue may be observed in chronic wounds with various etiologic factors.

Arterial/Ischemic Wounds

Necrotic debris in the ischemic wound usually appears as dry gangrene. It may have a thick, dry, or desiccated black/gray appearance. It is usually firmly adherent to the wound bed. Dry gangrene is often surrounded by an erythematous halo (see Figs. 17.7 and 17.8). Arterial wounds as a rule should not be debrided until revascularization as the surrounding tissue does not have adequate perfusion to support the procedure, resulting in worsening of the wound. In the presence of active infection, the wound should be debrided immediately regardless of the need for revascularization. However, the standard of care for dry gangrene or an arterial wound without clinical signs of infection is revascularization to optimize blood supply to the wound before debridement to

EXHIBIT 17.1

Necrotic Tissue Assessment Guideline

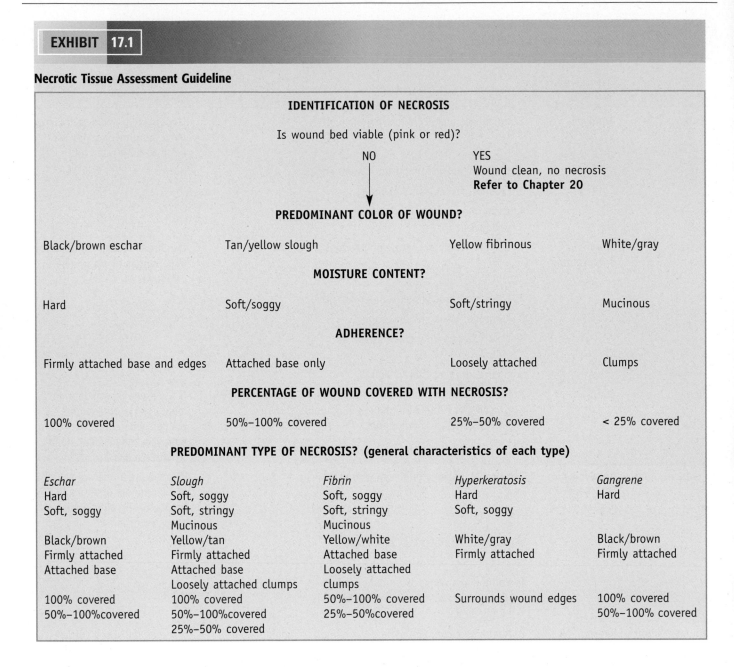

ensure potentially viable tissue is not removed unnecessarily. Once blood flow has been reestablished, the wound may be debrided. This can be accomplished by waiting 4 to 8 days after an open bypass or 3 to 4 weeks following endovascular surgery before performing any definitive debridement on a noninfected wound.[24]

Diabetic Neuropathic Ulcers

Neuropathic or neurotrophic wounds usually present with hyperkeratosis surrounding the wound in addition to necrotic tissue. These wounds are most common on the plantar aspect of the foot. This hyperkeratosis appears as callus formation at the wound edge, which should be shaved down to normal-appearing or bleeding skin (see Fig. 17.9). It is standard practice in debriding diabetic neuropathic wounds to excise the wound completely on initial presentation, removing a margin of 1 to 2 mm of intact skin. The edges of the wound should be beveled at a 44-degree angle (see Fig. 17.10).

Venous Leg Ulcers

Venous leg ulcers can present with blisters, slough or, less commonly, eschar. The wound bed in a majority of chronic venous ulcers becomes covered with a yellow fibrinous material, slough. Eschar may be attributed to desiccation of the wound and necrotic debris. It is not typically seen when the patient is receiving compression therapy.

Pressure Ulcers

Necrotic debris that occurs in pressure ulcers is directly related to the degree of tissue destruction. In the early stage of pressure sore formation, the tissue may appear firm and hard (indurated), with a purple or black discoloration on intact skin. This is indicative of the death of tissues between the skin and an underlying bony prominence. The overlying skin appears purple in color, called *deep tissue injury*. In time, the skin may die and an eschar appears, a phenomenon referred to as *demarcation*. In most cases, it takes 3 to 7 days for the wound to fully demarcate.

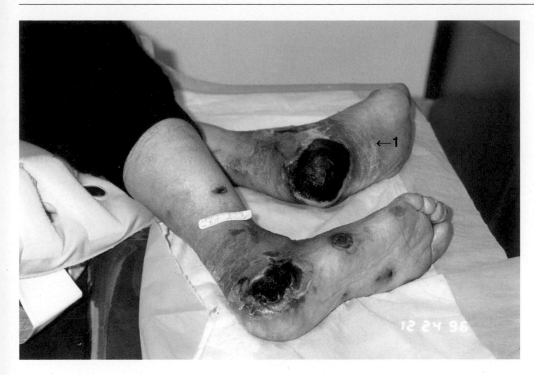

This sequence of events has been confirmed histologically.[21–23] The firm, black eschar represents full-thickness destruction of the skin and often the subcutaneous tissues. Figure 17.4 is a large sacral pressure ulcer prior to debridement. The central portion of the wound is covered with necrotic material.

Characteristics of Senescent Nonfunctional Cells and Bacterial Biofilms

Senescent nonfunctional cells generally occur on the periphery of the wound, at the rim or wound edge. Typically they extend 2 to 3 mm from the edge of the wound. In diabetic foot ulcers, the 1 to 2 mm at the edge of the wound contains senescent nonfunctional cells and contributes to the hyperkeratotic tissue observed in these wounds.

Biofilms develop on the base of chronic wounds. A *bacterial biofilm* is a polymicrobial sessile community of microorganisms that develop on the surface of chronic wounds, not reaching critical colonization levels and thus, not causing classic wound infection.[25] The biofilm is an effective barrier to topical dressings and antimicrobial therapy and as such inhibits healing. Bacterial biofilms have been shown to be present

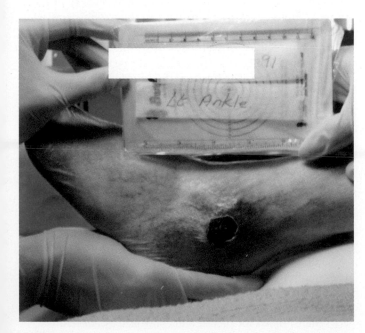

FIGURE 17.8 Classic ischemic ulcer with chronic inflammation noted surrounding the ulcer, covered with dry black eschar. (Copyright C. Sussman.)

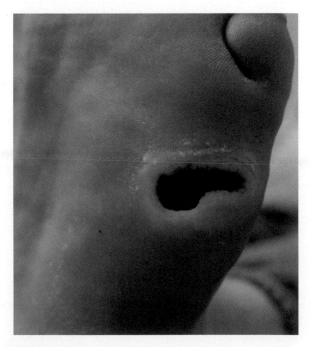

FIGURE 17.9 Diabetic neuropathic ulcer with callus around the margins of the wound. (Copyright T.E. Serena.)

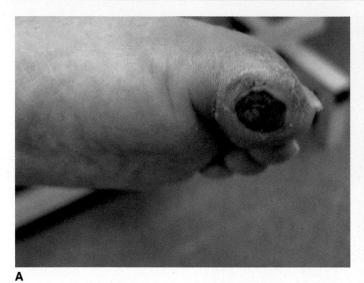

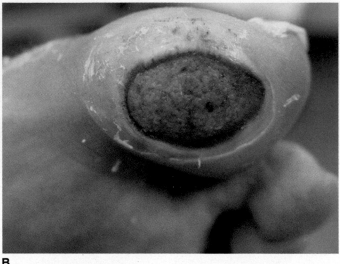

A   B

FIGURE 17.10 Diabetic ulcer on the great toe (**A**) before and (**B**) after initial debridement. (Copyright T.E. Serena.)

in greater than 60% of chronic wounds[26] and are an invisible layer that is formed by an extracellular matrix that binds to the wound base.[24] Chronic wounds with biofilms may present with healthy-appearing wound tissue on visual inspection and signs of inflammation surrounding the wound. The erythematous halo surrounding the wound is not associated with other signs of local infection (e.g., swelling, induration, tenderness, or malodor). Remember that while all infections are associated with inflammation, not all inflammation is associated with infection. In the case of the nonhealing wound, the issue is chronic inflammation due to arrested wound healing in the inflammatory phase. Suggestions for biofilm removal include wound base debridement using sharp debridement with blades, scalpel, curettes or hydrosurgical debridement.[24]

DEBRIDEMENT OF NECROTIC TISSUE

As previously noted, debridement is the therapeutic intervention of choice for necrotic tissue.

A variety of debridement methods are available to the wound care practitioner: mechanical, enzymatic (or chemical), sharp, autolytic, and biosurgical. The methods are not mutually exclusive: more than one type can be used on the same wound. The choice of method is largely based on preference of the health-care professional. Health-care professionals make the decision on debridement type based on appearance of the wound bed, wound type, amount and type of necrotic tissue, practitioner skill and experience, access to the practitioner, patient condition, and care setting. See Appendix 17A for general guidelines in choosing the method of debridement for chronic wounds. Reimbursement for debridement is available under several CPT (current procedural technology) codes and ICD-10 diagnostic codes. Coding varies according to the health-care professional's status. The debridement codes are updated frequently by Centers for Medicare and Medicaid Services (CMS). Clinicians need to stay abreast of these changes. Practitioners should only use the debridement codes specific to their specialty. In addition, clinicians should check with their certifying boards to ensure that certain types of debridement, particularly sharp

debridement, are within their scope of practice. This may vary by region.

Mechanical Debridement

Mechanical debridement is the application of a physical force to remove necrotic tissue. Historically, the most common form of mechanical debridement was the wet-to-dry gauze dressings. These dressings have fallen from favor because of the need for frequent dressing changes and pain associated with their use. Hydrodebridement consists of the application of water, saline, or similar solution to the wound bed. This may be as simple as irrigating the wound using a syringe and needle or angiocatheter or more complex with commercially available products such as pulsed lavage or hydrosurgery devices, which use high-speed jets of fluid. The commercially available hydrosurgery products are used almost exclusively in the operating room, and while discussed under mechanical debridement, they perform sharp debridement. Surgeons will often rely on these mechanical debridement techniques for patients requiring extensive intraoperative debridement. The Versajet® (Smith and Nephew) employs a high-speed water jet to remove nonviable tissue and is one example of these devices. In these systems, a high-pressure jet stream of sterile normal saline is pumped to a disposable handheld cutting/aspirating tool. The high-velocity saline jet crosses an open chamber and cuts the tissue, which is drawn up into the chamber due to the partial vacuum created by the saline jet (termed the Venturi effect). Caputo and colleagues compared hydrosurgical debridement with conventional surgical debridement in lower extremity ulcers on 41 patients in a prospective randomized controlled clinical trial. Hydrosurgery use was associated with significantly shorter average debridement time in the operating room (10.8 minutes) compared to standard surgical debridement time (17.7 minutes).[27] Although this did not translate into shorter time to complete wound healing, the shorter operating room time represents cost savings. The quality of debridement using hydrosurgery systems allows for precise and controlled eschar removal.[28,29] Further, hydrosurgery also reduces bacterial burden in wounds.[30]

Another mechanical debridement technique involves the use of ultrasound (see Chapter 26 for more information on use of ultrasound for debridement). There are several of these units available commercially (SonicOne®, Misonix, Farmingdale NY; Sonoca®, Soring, North Richland Hills, TX.; M.I.S.T® Celleration, Eden Prairie MN; and Qoustic® Arobella Medical, Minnetonka, MN). The ultrasound employed in these devices is low frequency (20–100 kHz) as opposed to diagnostic and therapeutic ultrasound which is high frequency in nature. Ultrasound works by streaming ultrasonic waves via saline through the tissue resulting in cellular stimulation, bacterial killing, and a process called cavitation.[28] *Cavitation* is debridement caused by microbubbles in the tissues. Cavitational effects from the ultrasonic energy form gas bubbles within the saline dripped from the probe; it is visible to the patient and the clinician as a fine mist. Depending on the frequency and intensity of the sound waves, the gas bubbles may rapidly expand and implode (a cavitational effect), resulting in fibrin destruction and debridement.[31,32] The process loosens nonviable tissue and kills bacteria, decreasing bioburden and resultant biofilm development, without damaging healthy tissue.[34] Ultrasound debridement can be complementary to traditional antimicrobial agents and enables the destruction of antibiotic-resistant pathogens.[34] This can be an excellent technique in wounds that are painful or in areas in which traditional debridement is not feasible. Noncontact, low-frequency ultrasound promotes wound healing when used in conjunction with standard wound care[33,34] and has demonstrated some debridement effects in a controlled, randomized clinical trial and clinical series.[33–35] Case Study: pediatric wound—Hemangioma in this chapter illustrates a case in which noncontact nonthermal ultrasound debridement was employed for a wound associated with a segmental hemangioma in an infant. Sharp or enzymatic debridement was not possible.

Advantages of Mechanical Debridement

The advantages of mechanical debridement include the following:

- Mechanical debridement methods can be used in a variety of health-care settings and for a variety of nonviable tissues.
- Hydrosurgical debridement is effective in operative surgical debridement at lower cost.
- Noncontact nonthermal ultrasound may decrease the bacterial burden on the wound, when done correctly, and it can be used in conjunction with other treatment options. It may also offer an alternative to sharp debridement methods in patients who are not candidates for other sharp debridement methods.

CLINICAL WISDOM

Procedures and Contraindications for Use of Ultrasound

Noncontact nonthermal low-frequency ultrasound is typically delivered as a 4- to 5-minute treatment three times a week for 12 weeks. Contraindications to ultrasound debridement therapy include malignant wounds, radiation wounds or tissue previously treated with radiation, thrombophlebitis, and bleeding disorders.[34] The health-care professional should wear protective gear such as fluid proof gown, goggles and mask or face shield, and gloves.[34] If the patient experiences discomfort or pain with the therapy, topical analgesics such as 4% lidocaine may be used.[32]

CLINICAL WISDOM

Rationale for Avoiding Use of Wet-to-Dry Gauze Dressings

Wet-to-dry gauze dressings should be avoided for the following reasons:

- Wet-to-dry gauze dressings as a form of mechanical debridement are nonselective, removing healthy tissue in addition to dead tissue.
- Wet-to-dry gauze dressings are difficult to apply correctly.
- Wet-to-dry gauze dressings cause pain on removal.
- Wet-to-dry gauze dressings may be more costly in terms of labor and supplies.
- Wet-to-dry gauze dressings may cause maceration of the skin surrounding the wound.
- Wet-to-dry gauze dressings may release airborne organisms and cause cross-contamination.[36]

Considerations for Use of Irrigation

Wound irrigation removes necrotic debris from the wound bed by using pressurized fluids. The two most common techniques are pulsatile lavage and high-pressure irrigation. Pulsatile lavage is described in Chapter 28.

High-pressure irrigation involves the use of devices that deliver the irrigant solution to the wound at pressures between 8 and 12 pounds per square inch (psi). Use of a 35-mL syringe with a 19-gauge angiocatheter attached delivers fluids to the wound with high-pressure irrigation. This provides enough force to separate and remove necrotic tissue from viable tissue, yet not so much as to drive bacteria deeper into the wound tissues. The clinician performing high-pressure irrigation must use protective equipment against potential bacterial contamination. In addition, the use of this type of debridement may lead to the aerosolization of bacteria.

Procedure for Wound Irrigation

Equipment needed:

- Sterile normal saline
- Goggles
- Clean gloves (one pair)
- 35-mL syringe and 19-gauge needle or angiographic catheter
- Irrigation tray
- Trash bag
- Gauze sponges (4 × 4 inch^2 or Kerlix super sponges) *or* cover/topper sponges

Frequency: Apply with each dressing change.
Indications: All wounds.
Contraindications: Use "gentle" irrigation on clean wounds and more vigorous irrigation on necrotic wounds.

Procedure:

1. Explain procedure to the patient and caregiver.
2. Wash hands.
3. Prepare supplies.
   a. Open gauze or cover sponges.
   b. Fill syringe with an irrigant.

- Use normal saline or a nonionic surfactant wound cleanser.
- Antimicrobial solutions, such as povidone-iodine, may destroy healthy wound tissues and should be used cautiously—*for short-term treatment on wounds with necrotic tissue present.*

4. Apply goggles and clean gloves (to protect from splashing and cross-contamination).
5. Remove dirty dressing and dispose in a trash bag.
6. Remove gloves, dispose in a trash bag, and apply clean gloves (to protect from cross-contamination).
7. Evaluate the wound.
8. Flush the wound with an irrigant. Hold the needle/catheter 1 to 2 inches from the wound bed.
   a. Irrigate forcefully to debride loose, necrotic tissue mechanically.
   b. May attach a 14-French straight catheter to irrigate tunnels and large undermined areas.
   c. Irrigate gently if wound is clean or free of necrotic debris.
9. Dry surrounding skin with gauze or cover sponges.
10. Apply prescribed dressing, according to procedure for dressing.
11. Remove gloves and dispose in a trash bag, dispose of the trash bag, and wash hands.
12. Review procedure with patient and caregiver.

Enzymatic Debridement

Enzymatic (also called *chemical*) *debridement* involves applying a concentrated, commercially prepared chemical (enzyme) to the surface of the nonviable, necrotic tissue, in the expectation that it will digest the devitalized tissue or loosen the bonds between the nonviable tissue and healthy tissue. A physician's order is required, and manufacturer's guidelines should be followed. At present in the United States there is only one commercially available enzymatic agent, a collagenase marketed under the name Santyl® (Health Point, Dallas, TX). Collagenases selectively degrade nonviable collagen with minimal toxicity to normal tissue. Enzymatic debridement can be used alone or in combination with other modalities such as sharp debridement.[36]

Advantages and Disadvantages of Enzymatic Debridement

Enzymatic preparations have yielded consistently positive results in wound debridement.[37] The advantages of enzymatic debridement include the following:

- It is selective, working only on necrotic tissue.
- It is effective in combination with other debridement techniques, such as sequential sharp debridement and autolytic debridement.

The disadvantages include the following:

- Enzyme preparations can be more costly than sharp debridement.
- Often, enzymatic use is prolonged more than necessary, further increasing costs.
- Enzymatic debridement can be slow to achieve a clean wound bed.

Considerations for Enzymatic Debridement

Enzymatic debridement can be used on patients with infected wounds and with patients on anticoagulant therapy when surgical debridement is contraindicated.[38] Enzymatic preparations are not active in dry environments, and most are not intended for use on a dry eschar without proper preparation. The eschar must be cross-hatched with a No. 10 scalpel blade to allow the enzyme to penetrate the necrotic debris and the wound surface kept moist for the preparations to be successful. As an alternative, the enzyme may be applied at the edge of the eschar or at the periphery of the wound to encourage separation of the eschar from the healthy tissue. A common error with the use of enzymatic debriding agents is their use on thick necrotic tissue or eschar. These tissues are best removed surgically to expedite the healing process.

Enzymes also require a specific pH range for best results, and many are inactivated by heavy metals (such as those often found in wound cleansers, topical dressings, and antimicrobial solutions). The wound should be cleansed with normal saline or a pH-neutral cleanser. Antimicrobial cleansers such as povidone-iodine and those containing heavy metals should be avoided as they inactivate the enzymes. Additionally, topical dressings with antimicrobial agents such as silver dressings also inactivate enzymatic agents, causing up to a 50% loss in activity.[39]

Enzymatic agents are applied once or twice daily. The enzymatic agent is applied directly to the wound and may cause a brief, transient stinging or burning sensation. Different enzymatic agents should not be used in combination. Use of a secondary dressing is required, and most manufacturer guidelines recommend moist gauze dressings. Use of other moisture-retentive dressings may facilitate enzymatic debridement, but the choice of the dressing should match the expected dressing change frequency for the enzyme preparation. The surrounding skin must be monitored for potential maceration and the wound observed for potential infection.

As stated previously, there is only one enzymatic debriding agent available in the United States: collagenase. Collagenase has been shown to be effective in animal models[40] and in several randomized controlled clinical trials on patients with pressure ulcers and venous leg ulcers.[41–44] Boxer and colleagues compared collagenase to a placebo in 47 patients with pressure ulcers treated from one to 14 weeks and found significantly more wounds treated with collagenase achieved complete debridement compared to those treated with placebo.[41] Lee and Ambrus found similar results when they investigated collagenase versus a placebo in 11 patients with 28 pressure ulcers treated for 4 weeks. They reported more improvement (defined on a global scale that included amount of necrotic tissue, purulent drainage, and inflammation) in those treated with collagenase compared to the placebo.[42] Palmieri and colleagues examined collagenase use in 30 patients with leg ulcers treated for 14 days. They reported significantly less necrotic tissue in those wounds treated with collagenase at day 6 and 14 compared to the placebo.[43] Konig compared collagenase and autolytic debridement with a polyacrylate dressing in 42 patients with leg ulcers and did not find a significant difference between the two approaches to debridement over 21 days.[44] The evidence shows collagenase is more effective than a placebo ointment at debridement of necrotic tissue from pressure ulcers and leg ulcers but there is insufficient data to determine whether collagenase is faster at debridement of necrotic tissue than autolytic dressings with a polyacrylate dressing.[38]

Enzymatic debridement is effective as an alternative to sharp debridement and can be very effectively used in combination debridement approaches. Combined enzymatic debridement usually entails initial sharp debridement followed by debridement with enzyme preparations and subsequent maintenance of sharp debridement at dressing changes. Use of moisture-retentive dressings with enzymatic preparations provides for autolytic debridement in conjunction with the enzymatic debridement process.

Procedure for Enzymatic Debridement

Equipment needed:

- Sterile normal saline
- Enzymatic preparation
- Gauze (rolled or 4 × 4 inch²) or cover/topper sponges
- Cleansing solution
- Clean gloves (two pairs)
- Paper tape, trash bag

Frequency: Follow manufacturer's guidelines.

Indications: All necrotic wounds; moist necrotic wounds are best. If the wound has dry eschar, remove or *cross-hatch* the eschar with a No. 10 scalpel blade to improve effectiveness.

Contraindications: Do not use on clean wounds, dry gangrene, or dry ischemic wounds, unless vascular consultation or ankle-brachial index has been obtained and circulatory status determined.

Procedure:

1. Explain dressing and procedure to the patient and caregiver. Inform the patient that there may be a slight, transient burning or stinging sensation when the enzyme preparation is applied to the wound.
2. Wash hands.
3. Prepare dressing supplies.
   a. Open gauze or cover/topper sponges and moisten with normal saline (most of the enzymatic ointments require a moist dressing for maximum effectiveness) or prepare topical cover dressing.
   b. Tear tape.
4. Apply clean gloves (to protect from cross-contamination).
5. Remove dirty dressing and dispose in a trash bag.
6. Remove gloves and dispose in a trash bag (gloves have been contaminated with the dirty dressing).
7. Apply clean gloves (to protect from cross-contamination).
8. Evaluate the wound.
9. Clean the wound; use normal saline or pH-neutral wound cleanser. *Avoid* antimicrobial solutions, such as povidone-iodine, which destroy enzymatic activity in the enzyme preparations.
10. Apply the enzymatic ointment with a tongue blade or cotton-tipped applicator to wound bed the thickness of a nickel. As an alternative, the enzymatic ointment may be applied directly to the gauze dressing to be applied to the wound surface.
11. Cover the wound with the cover or topper sponges. A dressing other than gauze or cover/topper sponges may be used for appropriate topical therapy as the secondary dressing for the wound.
12. Secure the dressing with paper tape, if applicable. Write the date and time, and initial the tape.
13. Remove gloves and dispose in a trash bag, dispose of the trash bag, and wash hands.
14. Review the procedure with the patient and caregiver.

Sharp Debridement

Sharp debridement is also called *instrumental debridement* because it involves the use of a scalpel, forceps, curette, scissors, or other sharp instrument to remove nonviable tissue. Being the most rapid form of debridement, it can be highly effective and is the preferred method of debridement of necrotic tissue. As mentioned above, there is growing opinion that initial sharp debridement should remove all nonviable tissue as well as one to two millimeters of normal tissue surrounding the ulcer. Subsequent sharp debridement can be more conservative, removing slough and any new areas of dead tissue. Subsequent debridement can also be achieved using enzymatic agents as mentioned in the previous section. In contrast, there may be situations in which *sequential conservative instrumental debridement* (SCID), a procedure in which sterile instruments are used to remove loose avascular tissue, may be appropriate. One such instance would be debridement performed in a skilled nursing facility. Sequential conservative instrumental debridement can speed the removal of necrotic debris when used in combination with other modalities, such as enzymatic agents.

Advantages and Disadvantages of Sharp and Sequential Conservative Instrumental Debridement

Of course, the main advantage of sharp and sequential conservative instrumental debridement is the speed of converting a necrotic wound to a clean wound. Another advantage is that, in most states, SCID can be performed by registered nurses or physical therapists in any health-care setting and does not require transfer to an acute facility. Check individual state practice acts before proceeding.

The disadvantages of SCID and sharp debridement include the following:

- Debridement requires a level of experience or skill and specific education. Health-care professionals who use SCID and sharp debridement must demonstrate their competence in sharp wound debridement skills and meet licensing requirements.[45]
- Reimbursement may be denied if sharp debridement is performed by a nonphysician (such as a nurse). Reimbursement depends on individual state practice acts for nurses.
- Sharp debridement may be painful for the patient, and therefore, analgesia (topical or systemic) may be needed.
- There is a potential for complications such as blood loss, infection, and injury to underlying structures.

Considerations for Sharp Debridement

Sharp debridement and SCID are indicated over other methods for removing thick, adherent, and/or large amounts of nonviable tissue particularly when signs and symptoms of cellulitis and sepsis are present. As noted previously, one multicenter, randomized, controlled trial found that centers that used sharp debridement frequently experienced better healing rates than did those that used sharp debridement less frequently.[8] The highest degree of healing (83%) occurred in the center that used sharp debridement most frequently. Subsequent studies have confirmed higher levels of healing in diabetic foot ulcers and venous leg ulcers when

CLINICAL WISDOM

Licensing Issues

Registered nurses and physical therapists may perform SCID and sharp debridement. Nurses are required to (and PTs should) complete an educational course on wound debridement with competence validation of wound debridement skills. A qualified mentor validates the student's skill performing debridement on a wound model, such as a pig's foot, and on patients. Not all states allow nurses or PTs to perform sharp debridement. Individuals should check with their state board of registered nursing, the state nursing practice act, and the PT licensing agency for validation of practice requirements for performing wound debridement.

debridement was used more frequently.[12,13,16] There is a strong relationship between sharp debridement and wound healing, particularly in diabetic foot ulcers and venous leg ulcers.[16]

There are special indications for debridement in relationship to pressure ulcers. Sharp debridement should be performed when gross necrotic tissue, sepsis, or advancing cellulitis is present and should be done with physician collaboration and probable systemic antibiotic coverage. Pressure ulcers on heels that present with black, hard eschar may be left intact, provided that they are inspected daily and are stable, nonerythematous, and nontender; if signs and symptoms of pathology develop (redness, sogginess, or mushy feel to the area or frank purulent drainage), debridement should be considered.

Use of atraumatic surgical techniques should be used when performing debridement on chronic wounds to avoid damaging healthy tissues. In general, sterile surgical instruments are recommended over the use of disposable suture removal kits. Tools included in disposable suture removal kits may be dull, causing damage to the skin edge and underlying tissue.[24] Basic debridement tools include scalpel blades, forceps, scissors, and curettes. Grasp only the tissue that is to be excised (prevents damage to viable tissue), and use No. 10 or No. 20 scalpel blades to sequentially slice off thin layers of tissue. The blades should be changed frequently as they can become dull quickly. Use of curettes is helpful in removing the gelatinous material that accumulates on the top of granulation tissue in the wound base. The wound should be debrided until there is no visible grey or black tissue or substances present and only red (muscle), healthy yellow (subcutaneous fat), and white (fascia, tendon) tissues remain. One method for determining what tissue is nonviable and how much tissue to remove is to paint the entire wound surface with methylene blue prior to debridement. The blue staining binds irreversibly to nonviable tissue and can ensure that no contaminated tissue is inadvertently left in the wound.[24]

In wounds that appear healthy, it may be necessary to debride 2 to 3 mm of the wound edge to adequately remove senescent nonfunctional cells. Debridement of the wound base with blades or curettes or hydrosurgical debridement can remove biofilm.[46]

Sharp debridement should be repeated whenever necrotic tissue reappears. It is unlikely that one initial sharp debridement episode will successfully remove the necrotic tissue that continually accumulates in chronic wounds. As noted earlier, sharp debridement may be used as maintenance debridement to eliminate biofilm and senescent cells to support healing.

CLINICAL WISDOM

Safe Sharp Debridement

A key to successful, safe sharp debridement is knowledge of anatomy. Debridement training is available online and at wound care meetings and seminars. For example, most educational wound conferences offer preconference workshops in wound techniques. These conferences combine on-site didactic knowledge with expert instruction and skill attainment using animal models.

Serial debridement is typically less aggressive than the initial debridement procedure.

Procedure for SCID Debridement

Equipment needed:

- Silver nitrate sticks, Gelfoam, or hemostatic dressing (optional). If extensive debridement is anticipated, sutures should be available to control excessive bleeding.
- Sterile normal saline
- Gauze or cover/topper sponges
- Instrument set
- No. 10, No. 15, or No. 20 scalpel blades or curettes
- Wound dressing of choice
- Clamp (Kelly or mosquito)
- Suture removal set
- Sterile gloves (one pair)
- Clean gloves (one pair)
- Paper tape, trash bag
- Cotton-tipped applicators
- Scissors (small, fine, serrated; and large, with or without serrations)
- Forceps (Adson—with or without teeth—or Adson-Brown—multiple teeth)

Frequency: Perform according to clinical judgment and physician's orders.

Indications: All necrotic wounds. If the wound has dry eschar, autolytic or enzymatic debridement may be used first to soften necrosis and facilitate sharp removal of debris.

Contraindications: Do not perform if you feel uncomfortable or cannot identify what you are removing. Do not perform on clean wounds, dry gangrene, or dry ischemic wounds unless vascular consultation has been obtained and circulatory status determined.

Procedure:

1. Verify physician orders.
2. Explain the procedure to the patient and caregiver.
3. Premedicate the patient for pain and relaxation.
   a. Topical: lidocaine (Xylocaine) spray or solution or benzocaine (Hurricaine) spray. Lidocaine spray can be used as a gauze compress directly to the wound site for 10 minutes for effective topical anesthesia or may be locally injected.
   b. Systemic: oral, intramuscular, or intravenous as a preoperative/predebridement regimen. Administer approximately 30 minutes prior to therapy to increase patient tolerance and compliance with procedure.

4. Assemble equipment.
5. Arrange for an assistant if applicable.
6. Provide adequate lighting.
7. Position the patient.
8. Wash hands.
9. Prepare clean field and equipment.
10. Apply clean gloves (to protect from cross-contamination).
11. Remove dirty dressing and dispose in a trash bag.
12. Clean the wound (follow manufacturer's guidelines on use of cleaning solutions). Warm the solution to 96°F to 100°F for patient comfort, if applicable. Use normal saline or a nonionic surfactant wound cleanser.
13. Evaluate the wound.
14. Remove gloves and dispose in a trash bag (gloves have been contaminated with the dirty dressing). Open the suture removal kit and/or scalpel.
15. Apply sterile gloves (to prevent introduction of new bacteria into the wound). (When wound care is being carried out in the home or long-term care setting, the procedure may be performed using only clean gloves.)
16. Removal of the eschar: Using forceps (e.g. from the suture removal kit), lift the dead tissue or eschar and cut it with scalpel or scissors. Grasp dead tissue and hold it taut so that the line of demarcation between viable and nonviable tissue can be clearly seen. Creating tension between the viable and nonviable tissue assists in debridement. Cut the dead tissue with care, layer by layer if necessary, to prevent injuring large amounts of healthy tissue. The removal of a margin of healthy tissue is acceptable as long as the patient has received adequate analgesia. If indicated, use clamp to fold over the necrotic debris allowing visualization of the line of demarcation between healthy and dead tissue. Bleeding is indicative of healthy tissue.
17. Remove as much nonviable tissue as possible. Try to keep the procedure time down to 15 to 30 minutes. Longer procedures should be reserved for the operating theater.
    a. Consider reevaluation or consultation when any of the following are present:
      • Elevated temperature and/or signs and symptoms of systemic infection
      • Failure of the wound to progress after 4 weeks. Consider biopsy of the wound edge to confirm the clinical diagnosis.
      • Cellulitis *or* gross purulence/infection
      • Impending exposed bone or tendon
      • Abscessed area
      • Extensively undermined area
    b. Aggressiveness of debridement should be guided by the following:
      • The amount of necrotic tissue present
      • Patient pain and discomfort
      • The skill of the practitioner performing the procedure
      • Time schedule and limits to avoid patient and provider fatigue (15–30 minute) Stop debriding when the following occurs:
      a. There is bone or tendon exposed or exposure is imminent.
      b. You are close to a fascial plane.
      c. You are close to a vessel or nerve that may be injured.
      d. You get nervous.
18. Provide postdebridement care:
    a. Cleanse the wound with normal saline.
    b. Apply wound therapy of choice.
    c. Document procedure with a complete procedure note. The following should be included:
      • Preoperative and postoperative diagnosis (e.g. pressure ulcer)
      • Procedure performed including the level of debridement (partial or full-thickness debridement, debridement of subcutaneous tissue)
      • Anesthesia used
      • Indication for the debridement
      • Document that the patient consented
      • Document that a "time-out" was taken before beginning the procedure
      • A complete description of the procedure including the method of hemostasis (e.g. direct pressure, suture ligature)
      • How the patient tolerated the procedure
      • List any complications.
19. Secure the wound therapy with paper tape if necessary, write the date and time, and initial the tape.
20. Remove gloves and dispose in a trash bag, dispose of the trash bag, and wash hands.
21. Review the procedure with the patient and caregiver.

Autolytic Debridement

Autolytic debridement is the process of using the body's intrinsic debriding mechanisms to remove nonviable tissue; it is a method that supports endogenous healing. It begins with adequate wound cleansing washing out the partially degraded nonviable tissue followed by the application of a moisture-retentive dressing. Maintaining a moist wound environment allows collection of fluid at the wound site; this in turn promotes rehydration of the dead tissue and allows enzymes within the wound to digest necrotic tissue. Autolysis is facilitated by cross-hatching if the wound is covered with dry eschar. This method along with enzymatic debridement approaches may be appropriate for patients in long-term care or home care settings and for those who cannot tolerate other methods.

Two types of moisture-retentive dressings, medical-grade honey and polyacrylate moist dressings, have been suggested as methods to provide for continuous autolytic debridement.[20] Medical-grade honey dressings cause movement of fluid from the wound bed into the open wound because of high osmotic pressure created by the concentrated honey and the wound fluid. The osmotic pull of the honey draws lymph from the deeper tissues.[47] Lymph fluid contains proteases that could contribute to the debriding activity of honey. Another possible action is the ability of honey to convert inactive plasminogen to plasmin which breaks down fibrin and the resultant bond of slough and eschar to the wound bed.[20] In the laboratory, honey has been shown to prevent biofilm formation.[20] Polyacrylate moist dressings use Ringer solution, which is physiologically complete, and provide continuous rinsing and cleansing of the wound. The dressing has a mean debridement rate of 38% and has been shown more effective than moist gauze dressings and equal to enzymatic preparations.[44,47–49]

Advantages and Disadvantages of Autolytic Debridement

The advantages of autolysis:

• Improvement can occur rapidly (there should be observed progress within 7 days).

- Autolysis is selective, working only on necrotic tissue and thereby preserving healthy tissues.
- It is effective in combination with other debridement techniques.
- Specific types have been suggested as possible methods for continuous debridement.

Disadvantages include the caregiver education required for treatment compliance. The patient and caregiver must be informed and aware of the wound appearance, odor, and exudate under the dressing during autolysis since this can be disturbing. Also, autolysis is typically slower than sharp debridement to achieve a clean wound bed. There may also be an increased incidence of infection.

Choice of Dressings for Autolytic Debridement

Autolysis is performed using one of the following dressing choices (but any moisture-retentive dressing can achieve autolysis):

- Transparent film dressings. They function best over dry eschar. They are nonabsorptive, rapidly creating a fluid environment.
- Hydrocolloids. These dressings work best over moist wounds with necrosis. They provide minimal absorptive capacity while maintaining a moist wound environment.
- Hydrogels promote autolysis by maintaining a moist wound environment. In a randomized, controlled trial comparing a hypertonic hydrogel versus wet-to-dry gauze, Mulder and colleagues[50] found that the hydrogel safely removed dry adherent eschar from wounds. Other investigators have also found hydrogels to be effective in digesting and removing necrotic debris from wounds.[51-56]

The choice of dressing depends on the appearance of the wound. For instance, a wound that is covered with a dry eschar might be autolytically debrided using a thin film dressing, whereas a deep wound with moderate exudate would benefit from an alginate dressing or one with more absorptive capacity.

Procedure for Autolytic Debridement: Application of a Moisture-Retentive Dressing

Equipment needed:

- Sterile normal saline
- Skin sealant
- Moisture-retentive dressing (e.g., transparent film, hydrocolloid, hydrogel dressing)
- Clean gloves (two pairs)
- Paper tape, trash bag

Frequency: Apply every 3 to 5 days. Always change the dressing when fluid leaks occur.

Indications: All necrotic wounds, for dry eschar, may cross-hatch eschar to facilitate autolysis.

Contraindications: Do not use for dry gangrene or dry ischemic wounds unless vascular consultation has been obtained and adequate circulatory status determined.

Procedure:

1. Explain dressing and procedure to the patient and caregiver.
2. Wash hands.
3. Prepare dressing supplies.
   a. Open dressing.
   b. Be sure that dressing size is at least 2 inches larger than wound area to be covered.
4. Position the patient.
5. Apply clean gloves (to protect from cross-contamination).
6. Remove dirty dressing and dispose in a trash bag. (There is likely to be an odor, and the wound drainage may appear disturbing.)
7. Remove gloves and dispose in a trash bag (gloves have been contaminated with the dirty dressing).
8. Apply clean gloves (to protect from cross-contamination).
9. Evaluate the wound.
10. Clean the wound. Use normal saline or a nonionic surfactant wound cleanser.
11. Apply the dressing according to manufacturer's guidelines.
12. Secure the dressing, write the date and time, and initial the dressing.
13. Remove gloves and dispose in a trash bag, dispose of the trash bag, and wash hands.
14. Review the procedure with the patient and caregiver.

Biosurgical Debridement

Biosurgery, or *maggot debridement therapy (MDT)*, is the application of uninfected maggots to the wound to remove the nonviable tissue. Fly larvae, either *Lucilia sericata* or *Phaenicia sericata*, are applied to the wound.[57] Generally, they are left in the wound from 1 to 4 days.[58-60] The maggots secrete proteolytic enzymes that break down necrotic tissue and then ingest the liquefied tissue.[57,58] The secretions also have antimicrobial properties that are helpful in preventing bacterial growth and proliferation, including methicillin-resistant *Staphylococcus aureus*. In vitro studies have shown that the secretions also promote the growth of human fibroblasts.[58] This effect contributes to improved granulation in wounds debrided by maggots.[59] In addition to the secretion of proteolytic digestive enzymes that dissolve the necrotic tissue, maggots secrete various cytokines and tissue growth factors that can increase local tissue oxygenation.[60] MDT is also effective in the presence of resistant strains of bacteria.

Biosurgery has not been widely used in the past 50 years. In the past, it was used as a last resort for serious wounds that failed multiple alternative therapies.[61] However, maggots are making a comeback particularly since several enzyme debriding agents have been removed from the market. MDT has been compared to other wound management treatments and compares favorably. It decreases time to debridement, performs a more precise debridement as viable tissue is protected, and does so at a lower cost.[62] MDT has demonstrated superiority over other conventional methods of treatment and is appropriate for ulcers of various etiology.[63]

Advantages and Disadvantages of Biosurgery

Advantages of biosurgery include the following:

- Since only nonviable matter is liquefied and digested, biosurgery is considered a selective debridement method.
- Biosurgery reduces bacterial burden.
- The technique has possible growth-stimulating effects.

Some disadvantages of biosurgery are

- Availability
- Slower rate of debridement when compared to sharp debridement
- Removal and disposal of larvae
- Client and family preference and/or approval for larval treatment

Patients and caregivers may be uncomfortable with larval therapy. Education is important when using this modality.

Considerations for Biosurgery

Several studies have examined the effect of MDT on healing rates in specific wound types. Sherman[60] studied the effects of MDT on lower extremity ulcers in 18 diabetic patients that failed to respond to conventional wound therapy. After 5 weeks, the conventionally treated wounds still had 33% of their surface covered with necrotic tissue, whereas the wounds treated with MDT were completely debrided in 4 weeks. One randomized controlled trial of 12 subjects evaluated the cost effectiveness of biosurgical debridement on venous ulcers, and concluded that this method of debridement, when compared with hydrogel therapy, was cost-effective and efficacious.[62]

Biosurgical debridement is not suitable for all wounds. Maggots are effective in environments where fluid and oxygen are readily available and where wound pH is relatively stable. The ideal dressing for wounds treated with MDT allows oxygen exchange for the maggots, prevents maggots from escaping, and is appropriate for wound characteristics.[61]

OUTCOME MEASURES

There are three characteristics for evaluating the effectiveness of debridement: the type of necrotic tissue, the amount of necrotic tissue, and the adherence of necrotic tissue to the wound bed. These outcome measures are specific to the type of debridement used. For example, outcome measures for sharp debridement are typically achieved faster than the same outcomes when other, less aggressive debridement techniques are used. Outcomes for debridement include the time to the development of granulation tissue, the time to removal of all nonviable tissue, and time to complete healing.

Necrotic Tissue Levels

The quantity of necrotic tissue in the wound bed should diminish progressively with appropriate therapy. The amount of necrotic tissue can be measured in several ways: by linear measurements (measuring the length and width of the necrotic debris), visual assessment of the percentage of the wound bed covered with nonviable tissue, digital planimetry (measuring the area of the wound using photographic analysis), and photography.

A linear measurement entails measuring the length and width (in centimeters) of the visible necrotic debris; multiplying length by width determines surface area of the necrosis. The percentage of the wound bed covered by necrotic tissue can be quantified by viewing the wound bed in four quadrants, like a pie cut into four pieces, with each equal to 25% of the wound. Judge the percentage of the wound covered with nonviable tissue. A rating scale similar to the following may be used:

1 = None visible
2 = <25% of wound bed covered
3 = 25%–50% of wound covered
4 = >50% and <75% of wound covered
5 = 75%–100% of wound covered

Planimetry involves tracing the wound necrotic tissue and then retracing on a digital tablet (computerized planimetry), tracing the necrotic tissue from a photograph on a computer, or on graph paper. Using a digital tablet calculates the surface area automatically after the image is retraced using the digital pen attached to the digital tablet. Computerized planimetry involves capturing a photograph of the wound, uploading the image onto a compatible computer, and using the cursor of the mouse to manually delimit the necrotic tissue. The computer software then calculates the surface area based on the manual outline from the photograph. Use of noncomputerized planimetry involves retracing the outline of the necrotic tissue on graph paper and then counting the number of graph blocks contained in the tracing. Laplaud and colleagues examined reliability and reproducibility of three of these methods, visual assessment, use of a digital tablet for planimetry, and use of photographs and computerized planimetry for determining the amount of necrotic tissue in chronic wounds.[64] Use of computerized planimetry was better than the digital tablet method of determining percent of necrotic tissue with improved reproducibility and reliability. Of interest, visual assessments were close to the computerized planimetry calculations.[64] For clinical practice, visual assessment of percent of necrotic tissue present was reliable and reproducible, and thus it is recommended for daily clinical practice.

Type of Necrotic Tissue

When conservative methods of debridement are used, including mechanical, autolytic, and enzymatic techniques, the type of necrotic tissue should change as the wound improves. As the necrotic tissue is rehydrated, the appearance will change from a dry, desiccated eschar to soft slough and, finally, to a loose tissue that does not adhere to the wound bed. The color usually changes as well, the black/brown eschar giving way to yellow or tan slough. Rate the type of necrotic tissue by using a scale similar to the following:

1 = None visible
2 = White/gray nonviable tissue and/or nonadherent yellow slough
3 = Loosely adherent yellow slough
4 = Adherent, soft black eschar
5 = Firmly adherent, hard black eschar

Adherence of Necrotic Tissue

Adherence of the necrotic tissue should decrease as debridement progresses. Initially, the necrotic tissue may be firmly attached to the wound base as well as the wound edges. As conservative debridement methods proceed, the necrosis begins lifting, loosens from the edges of the wound, and eventually disengages from the base of the wound. Evaluate adherence using a rating scale similar to that for types of necrotic tissue. General guidelines for debridement times are presented in Table 17.1.

REFERRAL CRITERIA

Debridement in arterial/ischemic ulcers is contraindicated. Arterial testing (e.g. Ankle/Brachial Index, vascular studies) to evaluate circulatory status should be performed prior to debridement. If the patient has significant arterial disease (ABI < 0.7), referral to a vascular specialist is indicated. In addition, if you do not feel comfortable or have limited or no experience in debridement, you may want to refer to a health-care provider with more experience.

Debridement of vasculitic wounds can lead to deterioration of the ulcer. If there is any question as to the etiology of the ulcer, a biopsy should be performed. The following patients may warrant a referral to a physician or an advanced practice nurse:

- Patients with dry gangrene or dry ischemic wounds (for vascular consult)
- Patients with elevated temperature or those with signs and symptoms of systemic disease (e.g. sepsis)
- Consultation should be considered if the wound fails to progress over a period of time. Four weeks is the generally accepted time frame for the wound to improve (consider consultation with other health-care practitioners: PTs, dietitians, wound care nurse, and physicians)
- Patients with evidence of cellulitis *or* gross purulence/infection
- Patients with bone, tendon, prosthetic devices or vital structures visible in the wound or impending exposure are a concern
- Patients showing evidence of an abscessed area or patients with extensively undermined areas present in the wound

SELF-CARE TEACHING GUIDELINES

Individualize patient and caregiver instruction in self-care to the topical therapy care routine, the patient's wound, the patient's learning style and coping mechanisms, and the ability of the patient/caregiver to perform procedures. Exhibit 17.2 presents self-care teaching guidelines related to necrotic tissue management.

CASE STUDIES

Two case studies demonstrating the importance of debridement as the management technique for necrotic and nonviable tissue are presented.

CONCLUSION

Debridement is a critical component of good wound care. Prompt removal of nonviable tissue both eliminates a physical impediment to healing and reduces the bacterial burden within the wound bed. A variety of debridement methods exist: mechanical, enzymatic, sharp, autolytic, and biotherapy.

EXHIBIT 17.2

Self-Care Teaching Guidelines

Self-Care Guidelines Specific to Necrotic Tissue	Instructions Given (Date/Initials)	Demonstration or Review of Material (Date/Initials)	Return Demonstration or Verbalizes Understanding (Date/Initials)
1. Type of wound and reason for necrotic tissue			
2. Significance of necrosis			
3. Topical therapy care routine:			
a. Clean wound.			
b. Apply enzymatic preparation (if appropriate).			
c. Apply autolytic dressing—transparent film, hydrocolloid, or hydrogel.			
d. Apply polyacrylate or medical-grade honey dressing.			
4. Frequency of dressing changes			
5. Expected change in wound appearance during debridement			
6. When to notify the health-care provider:			
a. Signs and symptoms of infection			
b. Failure to improve			
c. Evidence of undermining			
d. Impending bone or joint involvement			
7. Importance of follow-up with health-care provider			

Pediatric Wound—Hemangioma

A 5-month-old infant presented to the wound clinic with a segmental hemangioma. Although most of these lesions are benign and resolve spontaneously, this particular hemangioma was growing rapidly, endangering the vision in her left eye. The hemangioma had not responded to corticosteroids. Therefore, laser therapy was attempted. However, the laser therapy was complicated by the development of a complex wound over the hemangioma (see Fig. 17.11). The challenge faced by the wound care specialist at this point was how to debride the dead tissue from the surface of the ulcerated hemangioma. Sharp debridement was far too risky due to the vascular nature of the lesion. Similarly, enzymatic debridement, biosurgery, and occlusive debridement techniques were not practical given the location of the wound on the face and the proximity to the eye. The surgeon chose noncontact nonthermal ultrasound applied daily. More information on ultrasound use in debridement specific to this case can be found in Chapter 26. Anterior and lateral views of the wound 1 week later reveal a healthy-appearing granulating base (see Fig. 17.12A,B). After 6 weeks of therapy, the wound was closed and the hemangioma had begun to involute (see Fig. 17.13). The final figure is 2 years after treatment and plastic surgery (see Fig. 17.14).

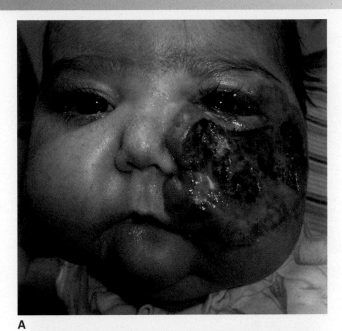

A

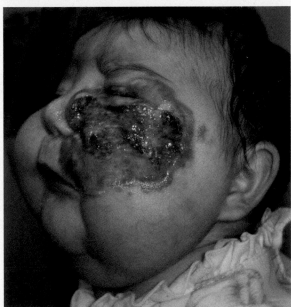

B

FIGURE 17.12 A,B: Anterior and lateral views after 1 week of ultrasound debridement. (Copyright T.E. Serena.)

Source: Serena TE. Wound closure and gradual involution of an infantile hemangioma using a noncontact, low-frequency ultrasound therapy. *Ostomy and Wound Management* 2008; 54(2):68–71.

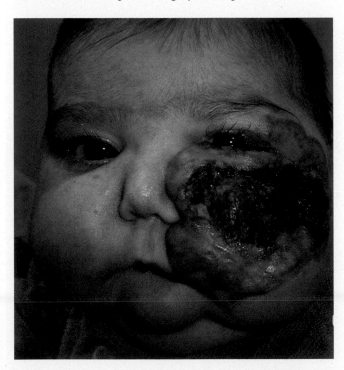

FIGURE 17.11 Segmental hemangioma in a 5-month-old infant, Presentation. (Copyright T.E. Serena.)

CASE STUDY

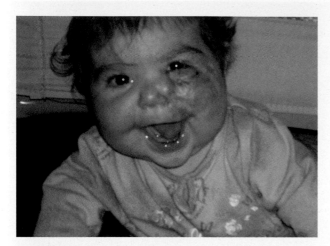

FIGURE 17.13 Healed ulceration and early involution of the hemangioma at 6 weeks. (Copyright T.E. Serena.)

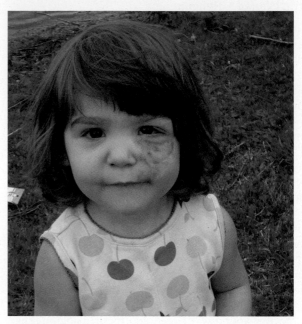

FIGURE 17.14 Two years after treatment and plastic and reconstructive surgery. (Copyright T.E. Serena.)

CASE STUDY

Diabetic Foot Ulcer

A 72-year-old diabetic presents with a plantar neuropathic foot ulceration of 6 weeks duration (see Fig. 17.15). The wound is treated aggressively with excisional debridement (see Fig. 17.16). A topical antimicrobial ointment is applied daily with a dry dressing. A fixed ankle walker is used for off-loading. On the subsequent visits, debridement consisted only of removal of callus surrounding the ulcer or any loose slough in the base of the wound. Figure 17.17A–E demonstrates the progression of healing over a 5-week time period.

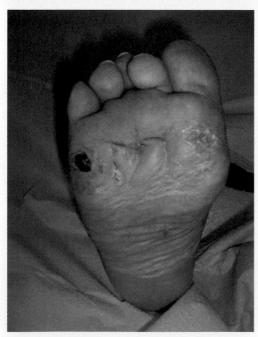

FIGURE 17.15 Diabetic neuropathic plantar ulcer in a 72-year-old gentleman. (Copyright T.E. Serena.)

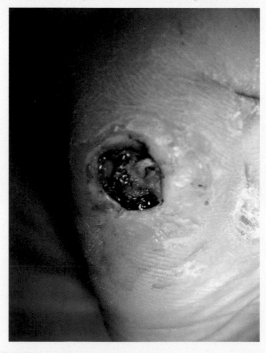

FIGURE 17.16 Aggressive initial debridement. (Copyright T.E. Serena.)

CASE STUDY

A

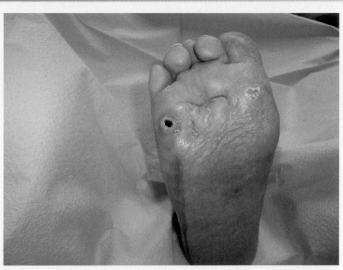

B

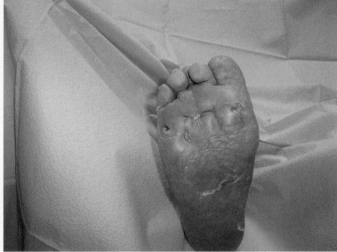

D

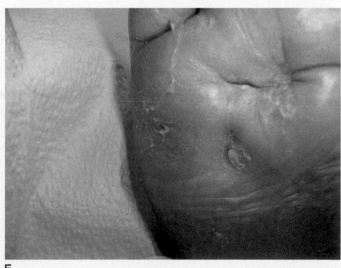

E

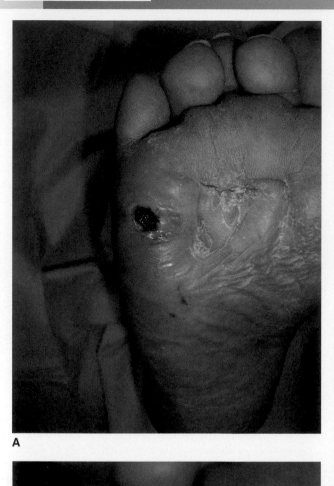

C

FIGURE 17.17 A–E: Progression to healing. (Copyright T.E. Serena.)

Sharp debridement and SCID are the method of choice for the rapid removal of necrotic material. It is favored in wounds with extensive and adherent necrosis. It is also the method of choice if signs of cellulitis are present. Other debridement methods may be used in conjunction with SCID and sharp debridement, particularly if the debridement does not result in a completely clean granulated base. The more rapidly a clean wound bed is achieved, the faster wound closure can be expected.

REVIEW QUESTIONS

1. Debridement is essential to achieving healing in acute and chronic wounds.
   True
   False

2. Which of the following wounds should not be debrided?
   A. Pressure and venous ulcers
   B. Vasculitic and arterial ulcers
   C. Diabetic and arterial ulcers
   D. Vasculitic and pressure ulcers

3. A patient presents with a sacral wound that is 100% covered with thick, adherent black eschar. Which of the following debridement techniques is the best choice at this time?
   A. Mechanical
   B. Enzymatic
   C. Autolytic
   D. Sharp

4. Which of the following techniques would be considered mechanical debridement?
   A. Maggot therapy
   B. An occlusive dressing
   C. Pulsatile lavage
   D. Scalpel debridement

5. Maintenance debridement is recommended because it assists with which of the following:
   A. Removes buildup of additional necrotic tissue in the wound bed.
   B. Removes bacterial biofilm development on the base of the wound.
   C. Removes initial load of necrotic tissue from base of wound.
   D. Removes 1 to 2 mm of healthy granulation tissue throughout the wound bed.
   E. Both a and b are correct.
   F. Options a, b, and c are correct.

RESOURCES

Wound Healing Society Guidelines for the treatment of diabetic, venous, pressure and arterial. www.woundheal.org

Falanga V, Brem H, Ennis WJ, et al. Maintenance debridement in the treatment of difficult-to-heal chronic wounds. Recommendations of an expert panel. *Ostomy Wound Manage.* 2008;(Suppl):2–13.

REFERENCES

1. Loo WT, Sasano H, Chow LW. Pro-inflammatory cytokine, matrix metalloproteinases and TIMP-1 are involved in wound healing after mastectomy in invasive breast cancer patients. *Biomed Pharmacother.* 2007;61(9):548–552.

2. Bucalo B, Eaglstein W, Falanga V. Inhibition of cell proliferation by chronic wound fluid. *Wound Repair Regen.* 1993;1:181–186.

3. Rogers AA, Burnett S, Moore JC, et al. Involvement of proteolytic enzymes, plasminogen activators, and matrix metalloproteinases levels in the pathology of pressure ulcers. *Wound Repair Regen.* 1995;3:273–283.

4. Armstrong DG, Lavery LA, Nixon BP, et al. Is is not what you put on, but what you take off: techniques for debriding and offloading the diabetic foot wound. *Clin Infect Dis.* 2004;39:S92–S99.

5. Schultz G, Mozingo D, Romanelli M, et al. Wound healing and TIME: new concepts and scientific applications. *Wound Repair Regen.* 2005;13(4)(suppl):S1–S11.

6. Schultz GS, Sibbald RG, Falanga V, et al. Wound bed preparation: a systematic approach to wound management. *Wound Repair Regen.* 2003;11(suppl):S1–S28.

7. Attinger CE, Bulan E, Blume PA. Surgical debridement: the key to successful wound healing and reconstruction. *Clin Podiatr Med Surg.* 2000;17:599–630.

8. Steed DL, Donohoe D, Webster MW, et al. Diabetic Ulcer Study Group. Effect of extensive debridement and treatment on the healing of diabetic foot ulcers. *J Am Coll Surg.* 1996;183:61–64.

9. Saap LJ, Falanga V. Debridement performance index and its correlation with complete closure of diabetic foot ulcers. *Wound Repair Regen.* 2002;10:354–359.

10. Robson MC, Cooper DM, Aslam R, et al. Guidelines for the treatment of venous ulcers. *Wound Repair Regen.* 2006;14:649–662.

11. Whitney J, Phillips L, Aslam R, et al. Guidelines for the treatment of pressure ulcers. *Wound Repair Regen.* 2006;14:663–679.

12. Williams D, Enoch S, Miller D, et al. Effect of sharp debridement using curette on recalcitrant nonhealing venous leg ulcers: a concurrently controlled, prospective cohort study. *Wound Repair Regen.* 2005;13:131–137.

13. Steed DL, Attinger C, Colaizzi T, et al. Guidelines for the treatment of diabetic foot ulcers. *Wound Repair Regen.* 2006;14:680–692.

14. Brem H, Stojadinovic O, Diegelmann RF, et al. Molecular markers in patients with chronic wounds to guide surgical debridement. *Mol Med.* 2007;13(1–2):30–39.

15. Brem, H, Golink MS, Stojadinovic O, et al. Primary cultured fibroblasts derived from patient with chronic wounds: a methodology to produce human cells and test putative growth factor therapy such as GMC SF. *J Transl Med.* 2008;6:75.

16. Cardinal M, Eisenbud DE, Armstrong DG, et al. Serial surgical debridement: a retrospective study on clinical outcomes in chronic lower extremity wounds. *Wound Repair Regen.* 2009;17:306–311.

17. Falanga V, Brem H, Ennis WJ, et al. Maintenance debridement in the treatment of difficult-to-heal chronic wounds. Recommendations of an expert panel. *Ostomy Wound Manage.* 2008;(suppl):2–13.

18. Margolis DJ, Allen-Taylor L, Hoffstad O, et al. Healing diabetic neuropathic foot ulcers: are we getting better? *Diabet Med.* 2005;22:172–176.

19. Thomas DR, Diebold MR, Eggemeyer LM. A controlled, randomized, comparative study of a radiant heat bandage on the healing of stage 3–4 pressure ulcers: a pilot study. *J Am Med Dir Assoc.* 2005;6:46–49.

20. Fleck, CA. Chakravarthy D. Newer debridement methods for wound bed preparation. *Adv Skin Wound Care.* 2010;23(7):313–315.

21. Shea D. Pressure sores: classification and management. *Clin Orthop.* 1975;112:89–100.

22. Witkowski JA, Parish LC. Histopathology of the decubitus ulcer. *J Am Acad Dermatol.* 1982;6:1014–1021.

23. Enis JG, Sarmiento A. The pathophysiology and management of pressure sores. *Orthop Rev.* 1973;2:25–34.

24. Cornell RS, Meyr AJ, Steinberg JS, et al. Debridement of the noninfected wound. *J Vasc Surg.* 2010;52:31S–6S.

25. Martin JM, Zenilman JM, Lazarus GS. Molecular microbiology: new dimensions for cutaneous biology and wound healing. *J Invest Dermatol.* 2010;130:38–48.

26. James GA, Swogger E, Wolcott R, et al. Biofilms in chronic wounds. *Wound Repair Regen.* 2008;16:37–44.

27. Caputo WJ, Beggs DJ, DeFede JL, et al. A prospective randomized controlled clinical trial comparing hydrosurgical debridement with conventional surgical debridement in lower extremity ulcers. *Int Wound J.* 2008;5:288–294.

28. Mosti G, Mattaliano V. The debridement of chronic leg ulcers by means of a new fluidjet-based device. *Wounds.* 2006;18:227–237.

29. Mosti G, Iabichella ML, Picerni P, et al. The debridement of hard to heal leg ulcers by means of a new device based on Fluidjet technology. *Int Wound J.* 2005;2:307–314.

30. Granick MS, Posnett J, Jacoby M, et al. Efficacy and cost-effectiveness of a high-powered parallel waterjet for wound debridement. *Wound Repair Regen.* 2006;14:394–397.

31. Serena TE, Lee SK, Lam K, et al. The impact of noncontact non-thermal low-frequency ultrasound on bacterial counts in experimental and chronic wounds. *Ostomy Wound Manage.* 2009;55(1):22–30.

32. Stanisic MC, Provo BJ, Larson DL, et al. Wound debridement with 25 kHz ultrasound. *Adv Skin Wound Care.* 2005;18(9):484–490.

33. Kavros SJ, Miller JL, Hanna SW. Treatment of ischemic wounds with noncontact low-frequency ultrasound: the Mayo Clinic experience 2004–2006. *Adv Skin Wound Care.* 2007;20(4):221–226.

34. Ramundo J, Gray M. Is ultrasonic mist therapy effective for debriding chronic wounds? *J Wound Ostomy Continence Nurs.* 2008;35(6):579–583.

35. Ennis WJ, Formann P, Mozen N, et al. Ultrasound therapy for recalcitrant diabetic foot ulcers: results of a randomized, double-blind, controlled multicenter study. *Ostomy Wound Manage.* 2005;51(8):24–39.

36. Lawrence JC, Lilly HA, Kidson A. Wound dressings and airborne dispersal of bacteria. *Lancet.* 1992;339(8796):807.

37. Falanga V. Wound bed preparation and the role of enzymes: a case for multiple actions of therapeutic agents. *Wounds.* 2002;14:47–57.

38. Ramundo J, Gray M. Enzymatic wound debridement. *J Wound Ostomy Continence Nurs.* 2008;35(3):273–280.

39. Shi L, Ermis R, Kiedaisch B, et al. The effect of various wound dressings on the activity of debriding enzymes. *Adv Skin Wound Care.* 2010;23(10):456–462.

40. Mekkes J, Zeegelaar J, Westerhof W. Quantitative and objective evaluation of wound debriding properties of collagenase and fibrinolysin/deoxyribonuclease in a necrotic ulcer animal model. *Arch Dermatol Res.* 1998;290:152.

41. Boxer MN, Gottesman N, Bernstein H, et al. Debridement of dermal ulcers and decubiti with collagenase. *Geriatrics.* 1969;24:75–86.

42. Lee LK, Ambrus JL. Collagenase therapy for decubitus ulcers. *Geriatrics.* 1975;30(5):91–93, 97–98.

43. Palmieri B, Magri M. A new formulation of collagenase ointment (Iruxol Mono) in the treatment of ulcers of the lower extremities: a randomized, placebo-controlled, double-blind study. *Clinical Drug Investigation.* 1998;15(5):381–387.

44. Konig M, Vanscheidt W, Augustin M, et al. Enzymatic versus autolytic debridement of chronic leg ulcers: a prospective randomized trial. *J Wound Care.* 2005;14(7):320–323.

45. Wound, Ostomy, and Continence Nurses Society. *Guideline for Prevention and Management of Pressure Ulcers: WOCN Clinical Practice Guideline Series.* Glenview: IL: Wound, Ostomy, and Continence Nurses Society; 2003.

46. Bowling FL, Strickings DS, Edwards-Jones V, et al. Hydrodebridement of wounds: effectiveness in reducing wound bacterial contamination and potential for air bacterial contamination. *J Foot Ankle Res.* 2009; 2:13.

47. Cutting KF. Honey and contemporary wound care: an overview. *Ostomy Wound Manage.* 2008;53(11):49–54.

48. Bruggisser R. Bacterial and fungal absorption properties of a hydrogel dressing with a superabsorbent polymer core. *J Wound Care.* 2005;14:438–442.

49. Paustian C, Stegman MR. Preparing the wound for healing: the effect of activated polyacrylate dressing on debridement. *Ostomy Wound Manage.* 2003;49(9):34–42.

50. Mulder GD, Romanko KP, Sealey J, et al. Controlled randomized study of a hypertonic gel for the debridement of dry eschar in chronic wounds. *Wounds.* 1993;5(3):112–115.

51. Flanagan M. The efficacy of a hydrogel in the treatment of wounds with non-viable tissue. *J Wound Care.* 1995;4(6):264–267.

52. Bale S, Banks V, Haglestein S, et al. A comparison of two amorphous hydrogels in the debridement of pressure sores. *J Wound Care.* 1998;7(2):65–68.

53. Mulder GD, Romanko KP, Sealey J, et al. Controlled randomized study of a hypertonic gel for the debridement of dry eschar in chronic wounds. *Wounds.* 1993;5(3):112–115.

54. Flanagan M. The efficacy of a hydrogel in the treatment of wounds with non-viable tissue. *J Wound Care.* 1995;4(6):264–267.

55. Bale S, Banks V, Haglestein S, et al. A comparison of two amorphous hydrogels in the debridement of pressure sores. *J Wound Care.* 1998;7(2):65–68.

56. Colin D, Kurring PA, Quinlan D, et al. Managing sloughy pressure ulcers. *J Wound Care.* 1996;5(10):444–446.

57. Prete PE. Growth effects of *Phaenicia sericata* larval extracts on fibroblasts: Mechanism for wound healing by maggot therapy. *Life Sci.* 1997;60(8):505–510.

58. Mumcuoglu KY. Clinical applications for maggots in wound care. *Am J Clin Dermatol.* 2001;2(4):219–227.

59. Wollina U, Liebold K, Schmidt WD, et al. Biosurgery supports granulation and debridement in chronic wounds—clinical data and remittance spectroscopy measurement. *Int J Dermatol.* 2002;41(10):635–639.

60. Sherman RA. Maggot therapy for treating diabetic foot ulcers unresponsive to conventional therapy. *Diabetes Care.* 2003;26(2):446–451.

61. Sherman RA, Hall MJR, Thomas S. Medicinal maggots: an ancient remedy for some contemporary afflictions. *Annu Rev Entomol.* 2000;45(1):55–81.

62. Wayman J, Nirojogi V, Walker A, et al. The cost effectiveness of larval therapy in venous ulcers. *J Tissue Viability.* 2000;10(3):91–94.

63. Gupta A. A review of the use of maggots in wound therapy. *Ann Plast Surg.* 2008;60(2):224–227.

64. Laplaud AL, Blaizot X, Gaillard C, et al. Wound debridement: comparative reliability of three methods for measuring fibrin percentage in chronic wounds. *Wound Repair Regen.* 2010;18:13–20.

Debridement Choices for Chronic Wounds

Wound Type	Tissue Type	Consistency	Adherence	Amount of Debris	Debridement Choices	Rationale and Notes
Pressure sores	Black/brown eschar	Hard	Firmly adherent, attached to all edges and base of wound	75%–100% wound covered	1. *Autolytic*—best choice is transparent film dressing. May use hydrocolloid or hydrogel; score eschar with scalpel for more rapid results. 2. *Enzymatic ointment with secondary dressing*—must score eschar with scalpel.	1. Transparent film dressings trap fluid at the wound surface with no absorptive capabilities, providing for more rapid hydration of the eschar and facilitating autolysis. Hydrocolloid/hydrogel dressings have an absorptive capacity and may require more time for autolysis. 2. Enzymatic ointments effective against collagen and protein may be most effective.
	Black/brown eschar or Yellow/tan slough	Soft, soggy Soft, stringy	Adherent, attached to wound base, may or may not be attached to wound edges	50%–100% wound covered	1. *Autolytic*—best choices are hydrocolloids and hydrogels; composite dressings may also be beneficial. 2. *Enzymatic ointment with secondary dressing.* 3. *Sharp, serial, or one time*—may be used alone or in conjunction with any of the above methods	1. Hydrocolloids and hydrogels provide for absorption of mild to moderate amounts of exudate while maintaining a moist wound environment to facilitate autolysis. 2. Enzymatic ointments effective against collagen and protein may be most effective. May need to protect intact skin from enzyme and excess exudate.
	Yellow/tan slough	Soft, stringy	Adherent, attached to wound base; may or may not be attached to wound edges or loosely adherent to wound base	Less than 50% wound covered	1. *Autolytic*—best choices are hydrocolloids and hydrogels. 2. *Enzymatic ointment with secondary dressing.* 3. *Sharp, serial, or one time*—may be used alone or in conjunction with any of the above methods.	1. Hydrocolloids and hydrogels provide for absorption of mild to moderate amounts of exudate while maintaining a moist wound environment to facilitate autolysis. 2. Enzymatic ointments effective against collagen and protein may be most effective. May need to protect intact skin from enzyme and excess exudate.

	Tissue type	Consistency	Adherence	Amount	Debridement method	Rationale/Notes
	Yellow slough	Mucinous	Loosely adherent to wound base, clumps scattered throughout wound	50%–100% wound covered	1. *Autolytic*—best choices are hydrocolloids and hydrogels. 2. *Enzymatic ointment with secondary dressing.*	1. Hydrocolloids and hydrogels provide for absorption of mild to moderate amounts of exudate while maintaining a moist wound environment to facilitate autolysis. 2. Enzymatic ointments effective against collagen and protein may be most effective. May need to protect intact skin from enzyme and excess exudate. Should be discontinued when wound is predominantly clean.
Venous disease ulcers	Black/brown eschar	Hard	Firmly adherent, attached to all edges and base of wound	50%–100% wound covered	1. *Autolytic*—best choices are hydrocolloids and hydrogels. 2. *Enzymatic ointment with secondary dressing.*	1. Hydrocolloids and hydrogel dressings have absorptive capacity, which helps to prevent maceration of surrounding tissues and promotes autolysis. 2. Enzymatic ointments effective against fibrin may be most effective.
	Yellow slough	Soft, soggy, or fibrinous	Firmly adherent, attached to all edges and base of wound	50%–100% wound covered	1. *Autolytic*—best choices are hydrocolloids and hydrogels. 2. *Enzymatic ointment with secondary dressing.* 3. *Sharp, serial, or one time*—may be used alone or in conjunction with any of the above methods.	1. Hydrocolloids and hydrogel dressings have absorptive capacity, which helps to prevent maceration of surrounding tissues and promotes autolysis. 2. Enzymatic ointments effective against fibrin may be most effective. May need to protect intact skin from enzyme and excess exudate. Should be discontinued when wound is predominantly clean.
	Yellow slough	Fibrinous or Mucinous	Loosely adherent clumps scattered throughout wound	Any amount of wound covered	1. *Autolytic*—best choices are hydrocolloids and hydrogels. 2. *Enzymatic ointment with secondary dressing.*	1. Hydrocolloids and hydrogel dressings have absorptive capacity, which helps to prevent maceration of surrounding tissues and promotes autolysis. 2. Enzymatic ointments effective against fibrin may be most effective. May need to protect intact skin from enzyme and excess exudate. Should be discontinued when wound is predominantly clean.

(continued)

Debridement Choices for Chronic Wounds (*continued*)

Wound Type	Tissue Type	Consistency	Adherence	Amount of Debris	Debridement Choices	Rationale and Notes
Arterial ischemic ulcers	Black/brown eschar	Hard	Firmly adherent, attached to all edges and base of wound	50%–100% wound covered	1. *Autolytic*—best choices are hydrogels. 2. *Enzymatic ointment with secondary dressing.*	Must be certain of circulatory status prior to initiating debridement. 1. Hydrogel dressings have absorptive capacity, which helps to prevent maceration of surrounding tissues and promotes autolysis. The amorphous hydrogels are nonadherent and require a secondary dressing. 2. Enzymatic ointments: may need to protect intact skin from enzyme and excess exudate. Should be discontinued when wound is predominantly clean.
		Soft, soggy	Adherent, attached to wound base; may or may not be attached to wound edges	50%–100% wound covered	1. *Autolytic*—best choices are hydrogels. 2. *Enzymatic ointment with secondary dressing.* 3. *Sharp, serial, or one time.*	1. Hydrogel dressings have absorptive capacity, which helps to prevent maceration of surrounding tissues and promotes autolysis. The amorphous hydrogels are nonadherent and require a secondary dressing. 2. Enzymatic ointments effective against protein and collagen may be most effective. May need to protect intact skin from enzyme aw nd excess exudate. Should be discontinued when wound is predominantly clean.
Diabetic neuropathic ulcers	White/gray	Hard	Hyperkeratosis, callus formation at wound edges	Involves all/partial wound edges	1. *Sharp, serial, or one time*—saucerization or callus removal. 2. *Autolytic*—best choices are hydrocolloids and hydrogels.	1. Saucerization may be required at each dressingv change. 2. Hydrocolloids and hydrogels soften the callus formation, and th's may facilitate removal as the dressing is removed.

CHAPTER 18

Management of Exudate, Biofilms, and Infection

Barbara M. Bates-Jensen, Gregory Schultz, and Liza G. Ovington

CHAPTER OBJECTIVES

At the end of this chapter, the reader will be able to:

1. Discuss the clinical significance of wound exudate.
2. Describe wound exudate characteristics, including color, consistency, adherence, distribution, odor, and amount.
3. Compare and contrast wound contamination, colonization, and infection.
4. Identify the local and systemic signs of wound infection.
5. Describe the development and management of wound biofilms.
6. Describe procedures for obtaining wound cultures.
7. Describe wound cleansing procedures.
8. Discuss the appropriate use of topical antimicrobials in treating wound infection.
9. Describe methods of managing exudate.

In providing wound care, an ability to assess wound exudate is critical. You must be able to distinguish between normal exudate, which confirms the body's brief inflammatory response to tissue injury, and exudate that signals wound infection, which retards wound healing and must be treated. An ability to interpret the characteristics of wound exudate (also known as *wound fluid* and *wound drainage*) will also help you evaluate the effectiveness of topical therapy and monitor wound healing. This chapter explains how to assess wound exudate, how to identify and treat infection, how to manage wound biofilms, as well as how to cleanse and dress wounds to promote healing.

SIGNIFICANCE OF EXUDATE

The healthy wound normally has some evidence of moisture on its surface. Healthy wound fluid contains optimal ratios of endogenous chemicals, including enzymes such as proteases, and cytokines or growth factors, which play a role in promoting the efficient deposition of granulation tissue, regrowth of blood vessels, and reepithelialization of the wound.[1] The moist environment produced by wound exudate allows efficient migration of epidermal cells and prevents wound desiccation and further injury.[2]

In acute wounds that are healing by primary intention, exudate on the incision line is normal during the first 48 to 72 hours. After that time, the continued presence of exudate is a sign of impaired healing. Infection and *seroma*, a pocket of clear serous fluid that sometimes develops in the body, often after surgery, are the two most likely causes. Both infection and seroma impair healing.

In chronic wounds, increased exudate is a response to the inflammatory process or infection. As discussed in Chapter 2, increased capillary permeability causes leakage of fluids and substrates into the injured tissue. Wound exudate in chronic wounds has noticeable differences from exudate derived from acute wounds: higher levels of proteases, imbalance between tissue inhibitors of metalloproteinases and matrix metalloproteinases (MMPs), missing growth factors and cytokines, and a sustained presence of neutrophils and macrophages.[3–7] Further, chronic wound fluid contributes to the hostile environment in chronic wounds. The cellular environment in chronic wounds is one of prolonged inflammation and cellular dysfunction, both maintained and initiated by components present in chronic wound exudate. For example, keratinocytes at wound edges are hyperproliferative but this is not functional proliferation.[5] High levels of MMPs in chronic wound fluid can potentially be inhibited by wound dressings that incorporate protease inhibitors or other substances targeted at specific MMPs.[6,8] Research in this area is in its infancy but holds promise for more targeted management of chronic wound exudate that can directly affect wound healing.

General Assessment of Wound Exudate

Characteristics of exudate that can be evaluated in the clinical setting are color, consistency, adherence, distribution in the wound, presence of odor, and the amount present. Table 18.1

TABLE 18.1 **Wound Exudate Characteristics**			
Exudate Type	**Color**	**Consistency**	**Significance**
Sanguineous/bloody	Red	Thin, watery	Indicates new blood vessel growth or disruption of blood vessels, normal during proliferative phase of healing. If drainage is moderate in amount or occurs with minimal wound bed disturbance (friable granulation tissue), the wound should be evaluated for other signs of chronic wound infection.
Serosanguineous	Light red to pink	Thin, watery	Normal during inflammatory and proliferative phases of healing
Serous	Clear, light straw color	Thin, watery	Normal during inflammatory and proliferative phases of healing
Seropurulent	Cloudy, yellow to tan	Thin, watery	May be first signal of impending wound infection
Purulent/pus	Yellow, tan, or green	Thick, opaque	Signals wound infection; may be associated with odor

presents various types of wound exudate and associated characteristics. Figures 18.1 through 18.4 provide some examples of wound exudate.

Amount of Exudate

Estimating the amount of exudate in a wound can be difficult because of wound size variability. What might be considered a significant amount of drainage for a smaller wound may be considered a minor amount of drainage for a larger wound. This difficulty can be compounded by the type of topical dressing in use. Certain dressing types interact with or trap wound fluid, which can then mimic certain characteristics of exudate. For example, dressing residue from both hydrocolloid and alginate dressings can mimic purulent drainage upon removal of the dressing.

To achieve an accurate assessment of exudate amount, prepare the wound site by removing the wound dressing. Then cleanse the wound to remove dressing debris or residue from the wound bed. Then evaluate the wound for true exudate. When wound exudate character is more serous in nature, clinical observation of the wound alone is insufficient to quantify the amount of drainage. For thinner wound exudate, estimate the amount of drainage by noting the number of dressings saturated during a period of time. Clinical judgment of the amount of wound drainage requires some experience with expected wound exudate output in relation to the type of wound and current phase of wound healing, as well as knowledge of the absorptive capacity and normal wear time of different topical dressings.

When estimating the percentage of the dressing involved with the wound exudate, you are required to put a number to your visual assessment of the dressing. For example, you might determine that 50% of a hydrocolloid dressing was involved with wound drainage over a 4-day wearing period. Based on this information related to type of dressing, length of dressing wear time, and wound etiology, you might conclude that a "minimal" amount of exudate was present. Some have attempted to quantify wound exudate more objectively. For example, weighing wound dressings before application to the wound bed and upon removal provides an objective measure of wound exudate. This approach is time-consuming and not always practical in

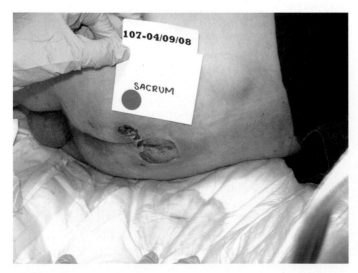

FIGURE 18.1 Serous exudate.

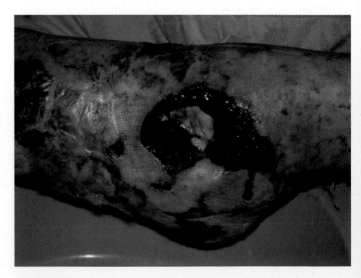

FIGURE 18.2 Sanguineous exudate. Evidence of infection present: erythema, edema, friable granulation tissue, nonviable tissue at base of the wound.

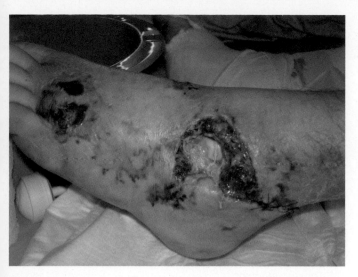

FIGURE 18.3 Same wound as in Figure 18.2. Purulent exudate scattered throughout wound bed.

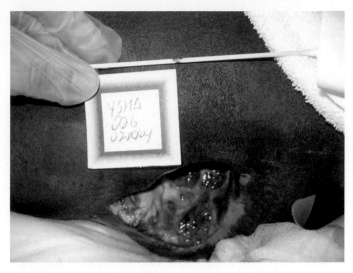

FIGURE 18.4 Serosanguineous exudate, see pink-tinged drainage on gauze dressing at base of the wound.

the clinical setting.[9] For wounds treated with negative pressure wound therapy, measuring the output in the negative pressure wound therapy device canister at regular intervals provides an objective measure of exudate amount.[9]

Type of Exudate

The color and consistency of wound exudate vary according to the type of wound, degree of moisture in the wound, wound healing phase, and presence of microorganisms in the wound. As indicated in Table 18.1, the color and consistency of exudate suggest the type, which in turn can indicate wound degeneration and infection. If an infection such as cellulitis is present (see Figs. 18.2 and 18.3), the exudate may be seropurulent or purulent in character. With further wound degeneration, the amount of exudate will remain high or increase, and its character may change to frank purulence. Always assume wound infection when the exudate is purulent. Infection may also be indicated by sanguineous exudate as occurs when granulation tissue is friable.

In an infected wound, microorganisms promote several characteristic changes: the exudate typically thickens, becomes purulent and malodorous, and remains moderate to copious. An example of these changes is seen with wound infection by *Pseudomonas* organisms, which produce a thick, malodorous, green drainage. *Proteus* infection, in contrast, may produce an ammonia odor. You can generally assume that wounds with foul-smelling drainage are either infected or filled with necrotic debris. True wound exudate can be differentiated from necrotic tissue with adequate debridement. Often, the removal of

the necrotic tissue dramatically reduces the amount of exudate and changes its character.

New biomolecular and genetic diagnostic methods can help identify specific enzymes, cytokines, and bacteria present in chronic wound exudate, which can be used to better target wound therapy. For example, use of mass spectrometric (MS) methods such as multidimensional protein identification technology (MudPIT) allows evaluation of the wound fluid proteome (the highly complex collection of high-abundant and low-abundant proteins in wound fluid). Use of MudPIT in conjunction with an immunodepletion approach that depletes high-abundant proteins has been shown to allow the identification of the more difficult to analyze low-abundant proteins.[10] This approach may allow further analysis of the dynamic range of proteins present in chronic wound fluid and provide more specific directions for advanced wound treatment that targets the low-abundant proteins, some of which have been identified as proinflammatory proteins.[10]

SIGNIFICANCE OF INFECTION

Bacteria are present in all chronic wounds and do not in themselves constitute an infection. The presence of bacteria in wounds is often described as meeting one of four conditions: contamination, colonization, critical colonization, or infection (see Fig. 18.5). These four conditions vary with respect to the behavior and location of the bacteria in the wound, as well as the effect on and response from the host.

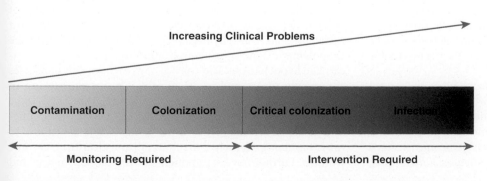

FIGURE 18.5 Relationship between wound contamination, colonization, and infection. As microorganisms increase in the wound and interact with the host, the need for clinical intervention increases as clinical evidence of problems with healing increase. Biofilms develop during critical colonization.

Bacterial *contamination* refers to the presence of nonproliferating bacteria on the wound surface with no injury to or visible signs of immune response from the host (e.g., erythema, edema, pain, heat, and purulent exudate). Bacterial *colonization* refers to the presence of proliferating bacteria on the surface of the wound, again with no injury to or immune response from the host. *Critical colonization* refers to the presence of bacteria in stalled wounds in the absence of classical signs and symptoms of inflammation—pain, heat, swelling, redness, and loss of function. This condition is also sometimes referred to as localized infection or occult or covert infection. As described below, recent data suggest that many chronic wounds that are "critically colonized" also have bacterial biofilms that generate chronic inflammation, which leads to elevated levels of proteases that degrade growth factors, receptors, and extracellular matrix proteins that are essential for healing. Bacterial *infection* refers specifically to the presence of proliferating bacteria within viable tissues—that is, they are no longer only on the superficial tissue but have invaded living tissues—to such an extent that injury to tissues occurs and a host immune response is evoked and visible. Most clinicians agree that greater than 10^5 organisms per gram of tissue indicate wound infection, but laboratories use different references, so what may be considered colonization in one facility might be considered true infection in another facility. Systemic signs of true infection include elevated temperature and white blood cell count, as well as confusion in the older adult.

Whenever host and wound conditions are favorable, infection can occur. Basically, infection represents an imbalance between bacterial numbers and/or virulence and the host's ability to defend itself. Wound infection delays healing in several ways. It extends the inflammatory response, delays collagen synthesis, slows epithelialization, and causes more injury to the tissues. Bacteria not only compete with fibroblasts and other cells for limited amounts of oxygen and other nutrients but also produce and release a variety of deleterious chemicals into the wound environment, such as toxins and proteases.[11]

Incidentally, if bacterial numbers are high, the combination of bacterial species is right, or the host immune response is depressed, then even in the absence of clinically observable signs of infection, wound healing can be delayed. Microbiologic research has shown that the presence of four or more bacterial groups in a wound is associated with delayed healing.[11]

Effects of Bacteria in Acute versus Chronic Wounds

Large, acute wounds generally react to bacterial burden differently than do small, chronic, ulcerative wounds. Acute wounds, in particular those with prolonged inflammatory responses, are more susceptible to bacterial invasion by skin flora. Sufficient numbers of skin flora organisms will cause acute wounds such as grafts and flaps to fail and, if untreated, lead to sepsis. Wounds involving the loss of large amounts of body surface area (15% of surface area or greater) are also at a greater risk for bacterial invasion.

In contrast, a small, chronic leg ulcer may remain unchanged for months or years, showing no signs of infection or sepsis, with the same organisms and a larger number of organisms present.[12] Indeed, the small chronic wound may go on to heal despite the presence of these organisms. Chronic wounds are often contaminated with skin flora, such as *Enterococcus*, *Staphylococcus*, *Bacillus*, or, occasionally, gram-negative organisms.[12] The number of microorganisms related to chronic wound infections is expanding and includes aerobes:[13]

- *Acinetobacter baumannii*
- Coliforms
- *Enterococcus faecalis*
- MRSA
- *Pseudomonas aeruginosa*
- *Staphylococcus aureus*
- *Staphylococcus epidermidis*
- *Streptococcus pyogenes*

and anaerobes:[13]

- *Bacteroides* spp.
- *Fusobacterium* spp.
- *Peptostreptococcus* spp.
- *Porphyromonas* spp.
- *Prevotella* spp.
- *Veillonella* spp.

These bacteria (especially staphylococci) are most often found in synergistic relationships with other bacteria. It is not unusual to identify anywhere from 1 to 8 different aerobic bacteria (average 2.7 organisms) from chronic wound cultures.[13] High levels of aerobic and anaerobic bacteria are commonly found in chronic wounds presenting with necrotic debris and in those with undermining. Deep chronic wounds and those with undermining have poor perfusion and support anaerobic bacteria because of the hypoxic wound environment.[13] The presence of a foul odor is usually associated with anaerobic organisms (such as *Bacteroides*, *Streptococcus*, *Enterobacter*, and *Escherichia coli*). Sharp debridement of necrotic tissue initially virtually eliminates these anaerobic organisms and decreases the number of aerobic organisms (such as *Staphylococcus aureus*) present in the wound as well.

Bacterial Biofilms in Chronic Wounds

Bacterial biofilms are well known in other medical specialities to cause a variety of chronic pathologies including periodontal disease, cystic fibrosis, chronic otitis media, and osteomyelitis.[14] Biofilms are characterized by an exopolymeric matrix of polysaccharides, proteins, and DNA synthesized by the multiple bacterial species (polymicrobial) comprising the biofilm community. Bacteria (and fungi) contained within the biofilm matrix are highly tolerant to killing phagocytic inflammatory cells (neutrophils and macrophages), antibodies, and exogenous antibiotics, antiseptics, and disinfectants. Several factors contribute to the increased tolerance of bacteria in biofilms to these agents, including reduced penetration of large proteins (antibodies) into the dense exopolymeric matrix, binding of oppositely charged molecules like antibiotics or cationic heavy metal ions (silver ion) by negatively charged components of the exopolymeric matrix, or neutralization of high reactive chemicals like hypochlorous acid (bleach) by reaction with molecules comprising the exopolymeric matrix. Also, some bacteria in mature biofilms become metabolically quiescent, and these "persister cells" are therefore highly resistant to antibiotics that disrupt bacterial metabolism. These factors contribute to make biofilms extremely difficult to kill and clear from chronic wounds. Furthermore, components of the biofilm matrix and products produced by bacteria in the biofilm stimulate chronic inflammation, which leads to persistently elevated levels of molecules like proteases and reactive oxygen species that kill wound cells and damage proteins that are essential for healing.

Assessment of the "bioburden" of wounds has traditionally relied upon relatively simple microbiology laboratory techniques that typically provide information on major bacterial or fungal species in swabs or biopsies that can grow under the nutritional and environmental conditions provided in the lab. These assessments of bacteria and fungi in wound samples have unquestionably generated important data that have been used for decades to help select therapeutic regimens for patients and their wounds. However, multiple publications have pointed out that, in many patients, measurements of total bacterial bioburden (expressed as colony-forming units per gram of tissue biopsy or 0–4+ levels of bacterial growth) alone do not correlate well with the failure of wounds to heal. This led to the concept of "critical colonization" or "occult infection" to explain the discrepancy, because there was an apparent link between microbial bioburden in these wounds and the impaired healing in the wounds. However, it was not clear what aspect of the relatively low total bioburden was 'critical' to impairing healing. More thorough evaluation of these 'standard' clinical microbiology assays led to the realization that these assays are inherently limited by the rather poor ability to culture or identify all (or even a high percentage) of the bacterial and fungal species that are actually present in an individual chronic wound. In other words, standard clinical microbiology assays only culture planktonic bacterial and fungal species that are able (capable) of growing on agar media plates supplemented with general nutrients in air at 37°C. Thus, it is reasonable to assume that a more complete picture of different bacterial species (aerobes, facultative anaerobes, and obligate anaerobes) and fungal species in a particular wound should improve the ability to assess the microbial bioburden on individual wounds and to indicate what therapeutic strategies would be optimal for each wound. Fortunately, in the last few years, sophisticated laboratory research techniques have been developed that allowed more complete assessment of bacterial bioburden. Advanced technology uses molecular methods that allow for identification of viable but nonculturable (VBNC) bacteria that remain undetected by traditional culture methods.[13] Specifically, these techniques demonstrated that a high percentage (60%) of chronic skin wounds have extensive bacterial biofilms that are highly tolerant to killing by endogenous phagocytic inflammatory cells and antibodies, as well as to exogenous antibiotics, antiseptics, and disinfectants.[15] The fact that standard clinical microbiology assays only measure planktonic bacteria, and do not measure bacteria in biofilms, suggested that the presence of "occult" bacteria protected in biofilms may be a major factor contributing to the "critical colonization" of wounds. In other words, the "critically colonized" state of wounds may actually be a euphemism for the presence of polymicrobial biofilms that are not detected by standard clinical microbiology assays, but stimulate chronic inflammation that leads to elevated levels of proteases and reactive oxygen species that degrade proteins in the wound that are essential for healing.

To address the problem of incomplete identification of bacterial and fungal species in wounds by traditional laboratory culturing techniques, researchers and clinicians turned to identifying bacterial and fungal species in wound samples based on their unique DNA sequences. The only reason this approach is feasible is because of the tremendous advances that have been made in rapid polymerase chain reaction (PCR) assays combined with the genomic nucleotide sequencing of thousands of bacteria and fungi in the last decade. Using open-access DNA databases and advanced pyrosequencing techniques, a pivotal paper published by Dowd et al.[16] reported that the bacterial and fungal complexity of chronic wound samples was much greater than previously thought. In fact, they found that, on average, approximately 60% of the bacterial species present in chronic pressure ulcers and approximately 30% present in diabetic ulcers were strict anaerobic bacteria, and many bacterial species were present that had never been reported in cultures of chronic wounds. These data suggest that many of the bacteria present in biofilms in a chronic wound may never be successfully cultured in the standard clinical microbiology laboratory due to obligate cooperation with other bacteria that create unique environmental conditions in a polymicrobial community of bacteria in biofilms. Most studies describing bacteriology of chronic wounds have agreed on the nearly universal presence of *Staphylococcus aureus* as well as *Pseudomonas aeruginosa* present in approximately half of chronic wounds along with a large population of anaerobic species.[15–19]

A second major concept recently reported by Wolcott et al.[20] showed that mature biofilms are rapidly reestablished in chronic wounds following surgical debridement, on the time frame of 24 to 72 hours. This indicates that sharp debridement opens a time-dependent therapeutic window to prevent the reestablishment of mature biofilms that are highly tolerant to host inflammatory response or to exogenous antimicrobial treatments.

Methicillin-Resistant *Staphylococcus aureus*

Methicillin-resistant *Staphylococcus aureus* (MRSA) is of special concern for patients with wounds. *S. aureus*, which is part of normal skin flora, is on the skin of approximately 20% to 50% of healthy adults and can persist in wounds.[21] Patients at the highest risk for developing MRSA colonization and infection are those with a chronic disease or history of intravenous drug abuse, frequent antimicrobial therapy, previous hospitalization, admission to an intensive care unit, or a prolonged stay in a health-care institution. All forms of *S. aureus*, including MRSA, can quickly invade and infect breaks in skin integrity, making wounds one of the most common sites of *S. aureus* and MRSA colonization and infection.

In the early 1940s, penicillin was found to be effective against *S. aureus*. Soon after its initial use, however, some strains of *S. aureus* began to produce the enzyme penicillinase, which inactivates antimicrobials, such as ampicillin, other penicillins, and cephalosporins. Methicillin was the first penicillinase-resistant semisynthetic penicillin; it continues to be used to treat *S. aureus* infections. The late 1960s and early 1970s saw the emergence of MRSA, with the first reports of outbreaks in both acute and long-term care facilities.[21]

MRSA infections are of concern because resistance to methicillin is associated with resistance to other antibiotics. A gene on the chromosome of resistant bacteria codes for abnormal penicillin-binding protein (PBP). The abnormal PBP confers resistance to methicillin by impairing methicillin binding.[21]

This abnormal PBP has a lower affinity for all penicillins; therefore, all penicillin-type antibiotics, which must bind to the PBP site in order to kill the bacteria, are ineffective in treating MRSA. Some strains of MRSA are also resistant to nonpenicillin antibiotics as well.

A recent study examined the occurrence of *Staphylococcus aureus* isolates as well as the resistance rates of the isolates to methicillin and to non–β-lactam antimicrobials from 1996 to 2008, using data from The Surveillance Network (TSN) Database-USA.[22] The TSN is a repository of antibiotic resistance data taken from culture results from more than 300 hospitals laboratories in the United States. These laboratories are nationally representative based on hospital bed size, patient population, and geographic region as determined by the U.S. Bureau of the Census. Several important trends emerged from analysis of the data. The total number of *S. aureus* isolates in the TSN database increased almost linearly from 1996 to 2005 (from 35,553 isolates to 236,849 isolates, a ~6.7-fold increase) then decreased progressively to approximately 80% of highest level in 2008 (190,654 isolates). MRSA isolates (9,115) accounted for approximately 26% of the total *S. aureus* isolates in 1996, and the percentage increased progressively to approximately 55% in 2005 (129,958) and then remained stable at approximately 53% of total isolates in years 2006 to 2008. The relative percentages of MRSA isolates were similar between general inpatients and inpatient-intensive care unit patients. Importantly, the largest increase of MRSA rate from 1996 to 2004 was for wound specimens (32%) compared to blood (24%) or respiratory specimens (22%) and in outpatients and young individuals. Interestingly, the TSN database showed consistent decreasing rates of resistance of among all *S. aureus* isolates for the non–β-lactam antimicrobial agents gentamicin, tetracycline, and trimethoprim-sulfamethoxazole (TMP-SMX) from approximately 10% in 1996 to approximately 5% in 2008. In contrast, resistance rates among all *S. aureus* isolates progressively increased from 1996 to 2002 for the non–β-lactam antimicrobial agents clindamycin, ciprofloxacin, erythromycin, and oxacillin, from approximately 20%–35% to 30%–50%; then resistance rates diverged for these four agents in 2005 to 2008, increasing for gentamicin and oxacillin to 55% to 65% while slightly decreasing for clindamycin and ciprofloxacin to 25% to 40%. More importantly, resistance of MRSA isolates to non–β-lactam antibiotics decreased for all except erythromycin, with less than 5% of MRSA isolates having resistance to tetracycline, gentamicin, or TMP-SMX.

Of particular concern is the discovery of the potential for MRSA to become resistant to vancomycin hydrochloride (Vancocin HCl) by acquiring a gene from vancomycin-resistant enterococci (VRE), leading to vancomycin-resistant *S. aureus*.[21] Because vancomycin is the drug of choice for treating MRSA, resistance to vancomycin presents critical problems.

Treatment of an MRSA wound infection involves antimicrobial therapy and prevention of cross-contamination, as discussed in detail shortly. Topical antimicrobial therapy specifically designed for MRSA-infected or MRSA-colonized wounds must be used cautiously for routine wound infections so that the antimicrobial will be available if the patient develops MRSA. Mupirocin (Bactroban) is specific for MRSA and can be used topically for wounds infected with the organism.

Prevention of cross-contamination between patients requires significant patient and caregiver education at all levels in the use of universal standard precautions and good hand washing procedures. Care must be taken to prevent contamination of not only multiple patients with the organisms but also multiple body systems within the same patient. An alternative method of preventing MRSA cross-contamination is by the use of ultraviolet light (see Chapter 25).

Distinguishing between Wound Colonization and Infection in Chronic Wounds

The classic local signs of infection—erythema, edema, pain, heat, and purulence—are usually reliable in acute wounds, but may be of less value in assessing chronic wounds such as pressure sores, diabetic foot ulcers, and venous ulcers. In these cases, the patient's overall condition may include the presence of a disease or medication that impairs the immune response. These chronic wounds may, however, still exhibit more subtle indicators of an imbalance of bacteria relative to the host's ability to defend against them. Gardner et al.[23] validated signs and symptoms of infection in chronic wounds. Increasing pain, friable granulation tissue, foul odor, and wound breakdown were found to be more valid indicators of local infection in chronic wounds than were the classic signs. Additionally, increasing pain and wound breakdown were found to be sufficient indicators, with a specificity of 100%.

Always evaluate wounds with continuing moderate to large amounts of seropurulent or purulent exudate for signs and symptoms of infection. Local signs of wound infection include erythema or skin discoloration, edema, warmth, induration, increased pain, and purulent drainage, with or without a foul odor. Table 18.2 gives local and systemic characteristics of wound infection.

Assessment of Wound Infection

Assessment of wound infection involves the following three components:

- Assessment of the patient's overall condition
- Observation of the wound and surrounding tissues to differentiate wound inflammation versus wound infection
- Wound cultures to determine colony count

Clinical signs of inflammation are often mistaken for infection. Table 18.3 presents clinical manifestations of both inflammation and infection. Advancing cellulitis indicates that the offending organism has invaded tissue surrounding the ulcer and is no longer localized. Advancing cellulitis begins as a small red or discolored area that is indurated, edematous, and warm to touch and progresses to involve other tissues. Left uncontrolled and untreated, cellulitis can result in sepsis.

Immunocompromised patients can fail to demonstrate any signs of infection, or the signs may be significantly diminished or very different. For example, in older adults, confusion or agitation may be the first indicator of infection, with elevated temperature occurring much later in the course of the illness. In some cases, a wound simply fails to progress, without obvious signs of infection. Immunocompromised patients may also exhibit signs of infection when the bacterial burden is less than that required for producing infection in immunocompetent patients. In immunocompromised patients, identification of the organism may be critical to effective treatment because the responsible organism may be opportunistic in nature and not the typical culprit.[24]

TABLE 18.2   Characteristics of Wound Infection

Local Signs of Infection (Acute and Chronic Wounds)	Systemic Signs of Infection (Acute and Chronic Wounds)
Erythema or skin discoloration	Elevated temperature
Edema	Elevated white blood cell count
Warmth	Confusion or agitation in older adults
Induration	Red streaks from wound
Increased pain	
Purulent wound exudate	
Local signs specific to chronic wounds:	
Friable granulation tissue	
Wound breakdown	
Foul odor	

Diagnosis of Wound Infection

For inpatients diagnosed with infection, antibiotic therapy is generally initiated immediately, and the culture reports are used to adjust or modify the antibiotic regimen.

The common method of confirming clinical infection is by colony count. As noted earlier, colony counts higher than 100,000 (10^5) organisms per gram of tissue or per mL of tissue fluid are considered confirmation of clinical infection.

A heavy bioburden (bacterial colonization in the wound) or compromised host resistance (e.g., immunocompromised or diabetic patients) can both result in bacterial colony counts higher than 100,000 organisms. Chronic wounds do not have to be sterile in order to heal. Also, some wounds heal uneventfully in the presence of bacterial colony counts greater than 100,000. However, when the bacterial burden in a wound is greater than this level, wound healing is typically impaired or

TABLE 18.3   Comparison of Wound Characteristics in Inflamed and Infected Wounds

Wound Characteristic	Inflammation	Infection
Erythema	Usually presents with well-defined borders. Not as intense in color. May be seen as skin discoloration in dark-skinned persons, such as a purple or gray hue to the skin, or a deepening of normal ethnic skin color.	Edges of erythema or skin discoloration may be diffuse and indistinct. May present as very intense erythema or discoloration with well-demarcated and distinct borders. Red stripes or streaking up or down from the area indicates infection.
Elevated temperature	Usually noted as palpable increase in temperature at wound site and surrounding tissues.	Systemic fever (may not be present in older adult populations). Look for acute confusion in older adults, as usually occurs prior to fever.
Exudate: odor	Any odor present may be due to necrotic tissue in the wound, liquefaction of necrotic tissue, and the type of wound therapy in use, not necessarily infection.	Specific odors are related to some bacterial organisms, such as the sweet smell of *Pseudomonas* or the ammonia odor associated with *Proteus*.
Exudate: amount	Usually minimal; if injury is recent, should see gradual decrease in exudate amount over 3–5 d.	Usually moderate to large amounts; if injury is recent, will not see decrease in exudate amount—amount remains high or increases.
Exudate: character	Bleeding and serosanguineous to serous.	Serous and seropurulent to purulent.
Pain	Variable. In acute stages, may be very tender and painful.	Pain is persistent and continues for an unusual amount of time. Must take wound etiology and subjective nature of pain into account when assessment is performed.
Edema and induration	May be slight swelling, firmness at wound edge.	May indicate infection if edema and induration are localized and accompanied by warmth.

delayed.[12] Moreover, wounds colonized with β-hemolytic streptococcus can exhibit impaired healing with colony counts less than 100,000.[12] In summary, diagnosis of infection requires critical evaluation of the wound, the patient, and the pathogen. Documentation of infection is based on the amount and type of the bacteria present in the wound tissue.

Methods of Quantitative Wound Culture

Quantitative wound culture is recommended to confirm the presence of infection. The technique for obtaining the culture specimen must capture bacteria in the wound tissue, not simply bacteria on the wound surface. Tissue biopsy, needle aspiration, curettage, and the quantitative swab technique are the most frequently used methods of quantitative wound culture. They are used to examine tissue for both aerobic and anaerobic organisms. Data show that biopsy, aspiration, and swab techniques are comparable in terms of sensitivity, specificity, and accuracy.[25] Curettage is suggested as a method that has improved accuracy and potential ability to destroy biofilm as well as identify microorganisms.[26] Each method is used in clinical practice.

Tissue Biopsy

Tissue biopsy is the removal of a piece of tissue with a scalpel or by punch biopsy. Before performing a tissue biopsy for wound culture, cleanse the area with sterile solution that does not contain antiseptic. To manage the patient's pain, treat the area with topical anesthetic or inject a local anesthetic. The biopsy is performed and pressure applied to the area to control bleeding. The biopsy tissue is promptly transported to the laboratory, where it is weighed, flamed to kill surface contaminants, ground and homogenized, and plated in various media in varying dilutions. Findings are expressed in number of organisms per gram of tissue.[27,28]

Needle Aspiration

Needle aspiration involves insertion of a needle into the tissue to aspirate fluid that contains microorganisms.[29,30] Intact skin next to the wound is disinfected with a substance such as povidone-iodine and allowed to dry. A 10-mL disposable syringe with 0.5 mL of air in it and a 22-gauge needle are used. The needle is inserted through intact skin; suction is achieved by briskly withdrawing the plunger to the 10-mL mark. The needle is moved backward and forward at different angles for two to four explorations. The plunger is gently returned to the 0.5-mL mark, the needle is withdrawn and capped, and the specimen is transported to the laboratory. In the laboratory, the aspirated fluid is diluted in broth and plated. Data are expressed in colony-forming units (CFU) per volume of fluid. If tissue is extracted by this technique, the weighing and grinding described for tissue biopsy processing also need to be done and, in this case, the data generated are in number of organisms per gram of tissue.

Curettage

Curettage has a stronger relationship with deep tissue wound biopsy than swab or needle aspiration.[26] Curettage is relatively noninvasive and is more sensitive and specific than swab culture. The technique has the advantage of reliably isolating anaerobic bacteria as well as disrupting biofilm in the area

CLINICAL WISDOM

Performing Tissue Biopsy and Needle Aspiration

By physical therapy practice acts, physical therapists are not allowed to perform tissue biopsy, needle aspiration, or curettage procedures. Physical therapists must work collaboratively with nursing and medicine to obtain these samples as required.

where it is performed. The procedure is conducted using a 3-mm curette with a single brisk harvest from the edge or just under the undermined area of the wound. This collects approximately 20 mg of tissue, which is sufficient for testing.[26] Further, the same organisms have been cultured with this technique from various locations in the wound.[26,27] (This procedure has also been used for maintenance debridement as a method of managing wound biofilm.)

Quantitative Swab Technique

As traditionally performed, swab cultures detect only surface contaminants and may not reveal the organism causing the tissue infection.[25] One of the problems with the routine swab technique for culturing a wound is that it has been performed in a variety of ways and, therefore, cannot be relied on to address the issue of bioburden in the tissues. Some recommend culturing the exudate in the wound prior to wound cleansing.[31,32] Others recommend that, after cleansing of the wound is complete, the culture be obtained using a Z technique (side to side across the wound from one edge to the other).[33,34] Others suggest irrigation of the wound with sterile water or saline and pressing of the swab against the wound margin or ulcer base to elicit fresh exudate.[35]

The recommended method of quantitative swab culture involves cleansing the wound with a solution that contains no antiseptic. The end of a sterile, cotton-tipped applicator stick is rotated in a 1-cm^2 area of the open wound for 5 seconds.[35] Pressure is applied to the swab to cause tissue fluid to be absorbed in its cotton tip. The swab tip is inserted into a sterile tube containing transport medium and sent to the laboratory. The end of the applicator that is not sterile is not inserted into the tube for culture.

At the lab, serial dilutions of the organisms are made on agar plates. A swab moistened with normal saline without preservative provides more precise data than does the use of a dry swab.[36] Results are expressed as organisms per swab, CFU per swab, or in a semiquantitative manner, such as scant, small, moderate, or large (1+ to 4+) bacterial growths.

Use of Quantitative Wound Culture for a Gram Stain

Tissue biopsy, needle aspiration, and the quantitative swab technique also can be used to obtain a specimen for Gram stain, a method recognized as a rapid diagnostic technique of infection.[36,37] For a Gram stain, the tissue fluid is placed on a slide, treated with various stains, and viewed under the microscope. In wounds in which swabs yielded less than 10^5 organisms, the Gram stain is considered to show no bacteria.

Procedures for Quantitative Wound Culture

Equipment needed:

- Gloves (clean and sterile)
- Sterile saline (nonbacteriostatic)
- Container to transport specimen
- Lab requisition
- Appropriate dressing materials

Culture technique-specific equipment needed:

- Punch biopsy/scalpel/3-mm curette
- Wound culture swab
- Anaerobic medium
- 10-mL syringe with 22-gauge needle
- Cork

Procedure preparation—for all methods

1. Wash hands. (Reduces transmission of microorganisms.)
2. Don clean gloves (and gown, if necessary). (Maintains universal precautions.)
3. Remove soiled dressings and discard in a plastic bag. Then remove and discard gloves. (Prevents contamination and spread of microorganisms.)
4. Clean the wound and surrounding skin with normal saline. (Removes contaminated debris.)

Procedure: swab method

1. Don sterile gloves and remove swab from culturette tube, taking care not to touch the swab or inside of the tube. (Maintains universal precautions and aseptic technique.)
2. Swab the wound area 1 cm² with sufficient pressure to obtain wound fluid. (Ensures collection of a good specimen.)
3. Use separate swabs if taking more than one specimen. Swab only a 1-cm² area of wound with each swab. (This ensures good culture specimen and prevents cross-contamination. Make sure to swab the wound instead of the wound edges to prevent contamination by skin flora and contaminated debris.)
4. Carefully place the swab into culturette tube without touching the swab or the inside, outside, or top of the container. (Prevents contamination and keeps those areas free of pathogens that could be spread to others who handle the tube.)
5. Crush ampule of medium in culturette and close securely, making sure the swab is surrounded by medium. (Keeps specimen from drying out and provides supporting medium.)

Procedure: anaerobic swab culture method

If collecting a specimen for anaerobic culture, take care to keep the anaerobic transport culture tube in an upright position to prevent carbon monoxide from escaping. Close container securely after swab is placed in tube. (Maintains anaerobic environment.)

Procedure: syringe method

1. Disinfect intact skin with antiseptic and allow skin to dry for 1 minute. (Anaerobic specimens are obtained from deep inside wounds.)
2. Place 0.5 mL of air in 10-mL disposable syringe with 22-gauge needle. Insert the needle into intact skin adjacent to the wound. Withdraw plunger to achieve suction and move the needle back and forth at different angles. (Prevents contamination at needle withdrawal site.)
3. Return the plunger gently to the 0.5-mL mark; do not insert drainage into the tissues. (This ensures a good specimen and prevents contamination from skin flora. Syringe method is used when large amounts of pus or drainage are present or for collecting tissue.)
4. Cork needle to send syringe/needle to laboratory as one unit. Do not recap or attempt to disconnect needle from syringe. (This maintains universal precautions and prevents injury from needle stick and spread of microorganisms.)

Procedure: tissue biopsy

1. Don sterile gloves. Obtain a biopsy specimen using a 3- to 4-mm dermal punch or a scalpel. (This allows for determination of the tissue level of microorganism contamination. Biopsy is usually performed by a physician or advanced practitioner.)
2. Place specimen in sterile container. (Prevents spread of microorganisms.)

Procedure: curettage

1. Don sterile gloves. Obtain approximately 20 mg of tissue using a brisk sweeping motion with the curette (3 mm) just under the edge of the wound or from the undermined margin of the wound. (This allows for determination of the tissue level of microorganism contamination. Curettage is usually performed by a physician, advanced practice nurse, or wound nurse.)
2. Place specimen in sterile container. (Prevents spread of microorganisms.)

Procedure: final steps—all methods

1. Remove and discard gloves in plastic bag. (Reduces transmission of microorganisms.)
2. Wash hands.
3. Don sterile gloves and apply sterile dressing to the wound. (Dressing absorbs drainage and immobilizes and protects the wound.)
4. Label specimen container(s) with the patient name, room number, date, time, and exact source of specimen. (This ensures proper identification of specimen. Proper source of specimen is important for laboratory to rule out normal flora from location.)
5. Place the container in a clean plastic bag, and have the specimen transported to the laboratory as soon as possible. (Plastic bag prevents spread of microorganisms. Immediate transport prevents overgrowth of microorganisms that can occur if the specimen is left at room temperature for an extended length of time.)
6. Dispose of soiled equipment into appropriate receptacle. (Maintains universal precautions.)
7. Wash hands. (Reduces transmission of microorganisms.)

MANAGEMENT OF EXUDATE AND INFECTION

Management of exudate and infection begins with wound cleansing. This is followed by the application of topical antimicrobials and antiseptic-containing dressings. In some cases,

EXHIBIT 18.1

Definitions of Antimicrobial Terms

Term	Definition
Antimicrobial	An agent that inhibits or kills microorganisms
Antiseptic	An agent that stops microorganism growth by either preventing microorganism multiplication—*bacteriostatic*, or by inhibiting microorganism action with resultant destruction—*bactericidal*. Agents are applied to living tissues.
Antibiotic	An organic chemical substance produced by a microorganism that when diluted in solution, has the ability to kill or prevent growth of other microorganisms. (e.g., penicillin)
Antibacterial	An agent that destroys or stops bacterial growth (e.g., bacitracin)
Antifungal	Agents that inhibit or kill fungi (e.g., nystatin)

systemic antimicrobials may also be prescribed. Management of exudate is also achieved with topical dressings.

Note that the terms *antimicrobial*, *antibiotic*, *antibacterial*, and *antiseptic*, although often used interchangeably, have slightly different definitions, according to the Food and Drug Administration (FDA). Exhibit 18.1 presents definitions of these terms for your reference.

Before we describe the various methods of wound cleansing, we explore some general methods of infection control.

General Measures for Infection Prevention and Management

In approaching the patient with a wound, one of your primary and ongoing concerns should be to prevent infection, or to control infection already present. General infection-control measures include the use of aseptic technique, hand washing, and adherence to universal precautions.

Aseptic Technique

One of the continuing debates in wound care is what type of aseptic technique is necessary in various health-care settings. *Asepsis* is a general term indicating activities that prevent infection or break the chain of infection. It is generally divided into two types: surgical asepsis and medical asepsis. *Surgical asepsis*, or *sterile technique*, is the method used in surgery in which all instruments and materials used are sterile, and all health-care providers involved wear sterile gloves, caps, masks, and gowns. In surgical asepsis, the nurse prepares a sterile field, dons sterile gloves, and follows surgical aseptic techniques in caring for the wound. *Medical asepsis*, or *clean technique*, involves procedures to reduce the number of pathogens and decrease the transfer of pathogens.

There are various viewpoints on which approach is most suitable for wound care patients; however, some general guidelines may help. Sterile technique is most appropriate in acute-care hospital settings, for patients at high risk for infection (e.g., advanced age, immunocompromised, diabetic) and for certain interventions, such as sharp wound debridement. Clean technique is most appropriate for patients in long-term care settings, home care, and some clinic settings, and for patients who are not at high risk for infection and are receiving routine wound care, such as dressing changes. Further research is needed to determine outcomes with the use of clean technique. Table 18.4 compares general guidelines for clean versus sterile technique for wound care patients.

TABLE 18.4   Clean versus Sterile Technique General Guidelines

Factor	Sterile Technique	Clean Technique
Settings	Acute care hospitals	Home care
	Clinics in acute care facilities	Long-term care facilities
		Community clinics
		Physicians' offices
Procedures	Invasive procedures	Routine procedures
	Sharp debridement	Dressing changes
Patients	Immunocompromised	Patients NOT at high risk for infection
	Advanced age or very young age	
	Diabetic	

Hand Washing and Universal Precautions

One thing about infection management that is not under debate is the importance of hand washing by all health-care professionals. Hand washing is the single most important means for preventing the spread of infection both in health-care facilities and in home settings.

Along with hand washing, make sure to follow universal precautions. In clinics, hospitals, and long-term care facilities, follow institutional procedures for disposal of contaminated materials in bags clearly identified as infectious waste (e.g., double-bagging out of isolation rooms, and use of red biohazard trash bags). In the home-care setting, disposal of contaminated waste is more problematic. Address disposal by identifying local waste collection procedures, and following agency protocols.

Appropriate hand washing and universal precautions together promote health maintenance for patients and caregivers and, as such, are critically important to include when instructing others in wound care. For example, in the home-care setting, instruct caregivers in hand washing technique as well as appropriate disposal of infectious waste products, such as used wound dressings, gauze used for wound cleansing, and other supplies used in wound care.

Wound Cleansing

Effective wound cleansing removes debris that supports bacterial growth and delays wound healing. Wound cleansing delivers cleansing solution to the wound by mechanical force, aids with separation of necrotic tissue from healthy wound tissues, and removes bacteria and dressing residue from the wound surface. The process of wound cleansing involves selecting a cleansing solution and a method of delivering the solution to the wound.

Choose a cleansing solution according to its efficacy and safety for use in the particular type of wound. Isotonic normal saline is generally preferred because it is physiologic, nontoxic, and inexpensive. Saline does not contain preservatives and must be discarded 24 to 48 hours after opening. Commercial solutions are available for wounds requiring more cleansing capacity to remove adherent debris from the wound surface. These wound cleansers contain surfactants that act to lower surface tension and to loosen matter from the wound surface. Nonionic surfactant wound cleansers are recommended as generally safe for use on healing wounds.

CLINICAL WISDOM

Normal Saline for Wound Cleansing

Two useful strategies for obtaining normal saline for wound care in the home setting:

1. Saline can be made at home by adding two teaspoons of table salt to 1 L of boiling water. Cool. Be sure to discard after 24 hours.
2. Pressurized saline sold for contact lens care may also be used. This preserved saline may be used for a longer duration, and the pressure from the canister is not sufficient to cause wound trauma.

For healthy, clean wounds, cleanse with normal saline, and do not use antimicrobial solutions or skin cleansers. Clean wounds do not need to be cleansed with antimicrobial solutions, because the goal of care is to clear low levels of contaminants from the wound. In fact, some studies suggest that antimicrobial solutions such as povidone-iodine, acetic acid, hydrogen peroxide, and sodium hypochlorite (Dakin solution) are toxic to fibroblasts *in vitro*.[38–41] On the other hand, *in vivo* studies have shown that these solutions can be used safely in wounds for short periods (4–7 days) to control bacterial levels, without compromising the healing process.[42] These seemingly contradictory research findings suggest that the effects of antimicrobial agents *in vivo* may differ from their effects *in vitro*, where cells are exposed to an environment vastly different from that of the wound tissue. Nevertheless, these solutions are cytotoxic to all types of cells (bacterial and host cells), and decisions regarding the duration of their use in open wounds should take into account the bacterial status of the wound (e.g., clean versus infected) and the desired outcome.

Most skin cleansers are not appropriate wound cleansers because they have been developed for external rather than internal use. What is appropriate for cleansing the skin is not appropriate for open wounds, because an open wound lacks the protection of intact epidermis and provides direct access to internal body structures. For healthy, clean wounds, cleanse with normal saline and avoid antimicrobial solutions and skin cleansers.

For infected wounds or those with necrotic debris, cleanse with normal saline or use a 10- to 14-day cleansing regimen with an antimicrobial solution. Do not use skin cleansers. Antimicrobial agents may play a minor role in wound cleansing for infected wounds, wounds with large amounts of necrotic debris, or those with large amounts of exudate; however, they should be employed in a manner similar to antibiotics, for 10 to 14 days only, and rinsed thoroughly from the wound with saline. Rinsing decreases the antimicrobial's cytotoxic effects in the wound. Antimicrobial cleansers should be discontinued when the wound is clean and free of debris.

It is very important to realize that new data with laboratory models, animal models, and patients show that planktonic bacteria can rapidly reform biofilm communities after wound cleansing and/or debridement, typically within 48 hours, and can reach the original resistance levels by 72 hours.[20] The clinical principle that should guide "biofilm-based wound care" is to reduce planktonic and biofilm bacterial burdens by any effective means (surgical debridement, curettage, irrigation, etc.) and then follow the debridement by covering the wound with an effective bacterial barrier dressing, of which there are many types including dressings with microbicidal metal ions (silver), quaternary amines, or occlusive films.[43]

Cleansing Methods

Methods for cleansing a wound include soaking, whirlpool therapy, scrubbing, and irrigation. Soaking is a form of hydrotherapy that includes a variety of methods, from the use of a bucket to a Hubbard tank, and may be useful for removing gross contaminants and loosening necrotic tissue. The softening that occurs with soaking helps to ease the separation of necrotic debris from healthy wound tissues. Wound soaking is appropriate only for wounds with large amounts of necrotic debris. Once a wound is clean and proliferating, wound soaking impedes healing and is therefore generally not appropriate.

RESEARCH WISDOM

Use of battery-powered, disposable pulsatile lavage irrigating devices—which irrigate with solutions and simultaneously use suction to remove the irrigation fluid and loosened wound debris—is more effective than whirlpool therapy in increasing the rate of granulation tissue formation.[44] Ulcers cleansed with pulsatile lavage had a rate of granulation tissue formation of 12.2% per week, compared with 4.8% per week for the whirlpool-treated group. However, caution is required. Use of pulsed lavage has been associated with outbreaks of multidrug-resistant (MDR) Acinetobacter baumannii infection due to the aerosolization of the organism during pulsatile lavage debridement of infected wounds.[45,46] This points to the need for infection-control procedures when using pulsed lavage therapy.

Whirlpool therapy may be useful for more than simply soaking and cleansing, as is the case when using whirlpool therapy to increase perfusion to an area. (See Chapters 27 and 28 for information on pulsatile lavage and hydrotherapy.) Antimicrobial agents should not be used in either a whirlpool or wound-soaking solution because of wound tissue toxicity. As with soaking, whirlpool therapy is not recommended for wounds that are clean and proliferating.

Scrubbing involves applying gauze or sponges with mechanical force in direct contact with a wound in order to enhance removal of debris and the efficacy of cleansing solutions. Scrubbing causes microabrasions in the wound, thus possibly delaying healing. Use of a nonionic surfactant cleansing solution limits the damage inflicted with scrubbing, and use of nonabrasive sponges also helps to decrease the damage to the healing wound tissues. The more porous the sponge, the less the damage inflicted on the wound surface. Nevertheless, even the use of nonionic surfactant cleansing solutions and nonabrasive porous sponges can injure the fragile wound tissue.

Wound irrigation can be performed using a variety of instruments and equipment. Wound irrigation is particularly appropriate for cleansing deep wounds with undermining or tunneling. Use a catch basin and towels to absorb and accumulate waste materials and irrigant runoff. Repeat the irrigation procedure at each dressing change. Protect your eyes, face, and clothing by using universal precautions. Some newer irrigation devices include a protective splashguard. Determine the amount of

CLINICAL WISDOM

Shallow Wound Cleansing Procedure

Cleanse from the center of the wound in a circular motion, working toward the edge of the wound and the surrounding tissues. Do not return to the center of the wound after cleansing at the edge of the wound or the surrounding tissues, because this will recontaminate the clean wound center.

CLINICAL WISDOM

Deep Wound Cleansing Procedure

Use of a catheter or a syringe to irrigate wounds with undermining and tunneling will not injure the tissues, and can effectively cleanse involved tissues under the skin surface. Flush with copious amounts of irrigant solution, and then gently massage the tissues above the tunneling to express the exudate accumulated in the tunnel. Repeat two or three times until the solution and fluids returned are clear. After the wound cleansing, the undermined spaces are usually packed loosely with packing materials, such as roller gauze or alginate rope products, to prevent infection from traveling up the tunnel.

pressure to apply during irrigation by balancing the goal of preserving healing wound tissues with the need to cleanse the wound effectively. Pressure force is described in pounds per square inch (psi). Pressure force under 4 psi is commonly referred to as low pressure, and can be obtained by use of bulb syringes or just by pouring solution over the wound bed. Pressure force between 4 and 15 psi is considered high pressure, and can be achieved by using commercial devices, a 35-mL syringe attached to a 19-gauge needle or angiocatheter, pulsatile lavage, or hydrotherapy.

High-pressure irrigation using any of these forms is a method of debridement—loosening and softening necrotic tissue for easy separation from healthy tissue. Pressurized irrigation removes bacteria and debris more effectively than do gravity or bulb syringe irrigation. As such, high-pressure irrigation is most effective for wounds with an inflammatory process. Use of high-pressure irrigation is not the method of choice for the healthy, proliferating wound, because fragile blood vessels and new tissue growth can be damaged.

Some available irrigation devices deliver solutions with too much pressure, thus driving bacteria and irrigant solution deeper into wound tissues. Pressures higher than 15 psi can cause trauma to the wound bed, forcing bacteria deeper into wound tissues. For example, use of a Water Pik at the middle and high settings provides 42 psi and more than 50 psi, respectively, both of which are too high and will drive bacteria farther into the wound tissues. Irrigation pressures between 4 and 15 psi are recommended.

Outcomes of Wound Cleansing

The clinical outcomes of wound cleansing are evaluated by taking account of the original intent of the cleansing and the wound assessment. For predominantly clean wounds with new tissue growth, cleansing is used only to remove dressing residue, prevent biofilm development, and if any additional cleansing is needed, a low-pressure irrigation system should be used. The goals of therapy with low-pressure irrigation are to dislodge wound dressing residue, reduce wound surface contaminants, and protect fragile new tissue growth. For wounds with necrotic tissue or debris, a high-pressure irrigation system should be used. Hydrotherapy and pulsatile lavage are not always available or appropriate for all patients, and

CLINICAL WISDOM

Wound Irrigation

Use of a 35-mL syringe with a 19-gauge angiocatheter or needle attached delivers saline at 8 psi and provides more effective removal of bacteria and debris than does use of a bulb syringe.

other devices, such as the 35-mL syringe and 19-gauge needle or angiocatheter, may be the best choice. The goals of therapy are to loosen and soften the necrotic debris for easier separation from healthy tissues, reduce the bacterial burden, remove dressing remnants, and prevent undue wound trauma.

Use of Topical Antimicrobials

The use of topical antimicrobials can be an area of confusion for clinicians. Systemic antimicrobial drugs are often superior to topical agents in treating invasive tissue infection because of the better penetration of systemic agents into the tissues via the blood supply. However, topical antimicrobials are often effective in limiting surface colonization, so that tissue defenses can clean up without continual reinfection from superficial bacteria. Some superficial infections respond better to topical agents and, in some cases, it is wise to use topical agents to avoid sensitizing the patient or creating resistant microorganisms. Some topical antimicrobials can damage healthy tissues, exacerbating tissue destruction or damaging tissue defenses.

Understanding how antimicrobials are prescribed is helpful for wound care clinicians. The proper selection requires determination of clinical infection in the wound, correct identification of the invading organism by culture and Gram stain, and consideration of pharmacology and toxicology. If an agent must be chosen prior to receiving laboratory results, the decision should be based on Gram stain smears (either positive or negative), the most likely pathogens involved in the disease process (for example, *E. coli* for a fecally incontinent patient with a sacral pressure sore), and the efficacy of the agent in similar situations.

Multiple factors influence the transcutaneous penetration of topical antimicrobial agents, including the physiochemical properties of the drug (polarity, stability, and solubility in base and lipids), nature of the pharmaceutical preparation (drug concentration, composition and properties of the base, and incompatible mixtures), method of application (inert delivery

CLINICAL WISDOM

Bacterial Overburden

The clinician should suspect a high bioburden of bacteria or biofilm development in the clean wound if healing or improvement does not occur within a 2-week time frame when the patient is receiving appropriate topical therapy. In these patients, treatment with topical antimicrobials and maintenance debridement strategies may be appropriate.

CLINICAL WISDOM

Factors Altering Response to Topical Antibacterials and Antiseptics

Patient response to antibacterial and antiseptic agents can be altered by age, disease processes (such as diabetes), malignancy, neurologic disorders, immune dysfunction, pregnancy, allergy, concomitant drug therapy, and biofilm development in the wound.

systems, time-released delivery systems, application in conjunction with occlusion, polar compounds to increase absorption, and substances that damage the stratum corneum to improve penetration), and nature of the skin (integrity of the epidermis, variability in skin thickness, and age).

Problems associated with topical antimicrobial use in wound care are related to the absorption of chemicals into the body tissues through the wound bed. There are cases in which absorption of certain chemicals contained in an antiseptic through the wound bed has caused systemic health problems. For example, iodine toxicity has occurred as a result of the use of povidone-iodine in open wounds with a large surface area.

The three main classes of topical antimicrobials used for wounds are antibacterials, antiseptics, and antifungals. Each is discussed separately.

Antibacterials

Antibacterial agents are chemicals that eliminate living bacteria that are pathogenic to the host or patient. Some examples of topical antibacterials are bacitracin (Betadine, Cortisporin, Neosporin, and Polysporin), gentamicin (Garamycin), metronidazole gel and cream (MetroGel, MetroCream, Noritate), mupirocin, and silver sulfadiazine (Silvadene, SSD). Topical antibacterials are sometimes used alone, sometimes in combination with systemic antibacterials, and sometimes in conjunction with other topical antibacterials. Because of their direct contact with the affected area, topical antibacterials can be administered in smaller doses than systemic antibacterials. They can achieve the same or better results than systemic agents, without the risk of toxicity. Moreover, problems of absorption, distribution, and availability to the infected site are reduced. Frequently, topical agents are used in conjunction with one another to give broader coverage, thereby increasing the rate of bactericidal action against a large spectrum of bacteria.

In addition, topical antibacterials may be used prophylactically. When used properly, they can be effective chemical barriers that impede the entrance of pathogenic organisms and diminish the local or systemic morbidity associated with infected wounds. When using topical antibacterials prophylactically, there is a risk of overgrowth of resistant organisms; therefore, use good clinical judgment.

Topical antibacterials are indicated when the patient has a diagnosed or suspected significant bacterial infection, as well as an indication for prophylactic use, such as underlying disease, increased risk of infection resulting from surgical procedures, viral or metabolic diseases, chemotherapy or radiation therapy, and/or prolonged corticosteroid administration. Contraindications

CLINICAL WISDOM

Routine Use of Topical Antibacterials

Routine use of topical antibacterials is strongly discouraged because it frequently leads to the development of resistant organisms. This is particularly true of mupirocin, which is effective against MRSA. If used inappropriately, it will not be effective when most needed.

include the excessive use of antibacterials for minor infections and nonbacterial pathogens. Inappropriate use of antibacterials subjects the patient to risk of drug toxicity, allergy, superinfection with resistant organisms, and unnecessary costs.[47]

The base, or vehicle, is the form in which the antibacterial agent is made available. In general, it is best to use a lotion or a paste for application to wet or weeping skin and wounds, as well as for areas that rub against each other, for example, groin areas and in between the toes. This is because lotions are usually less occlusive than ointments.

Reserve ointments for application to dry, cracked skin. Many ointments contain lanolin or wood alcohols, and patients can readily develop contact sensitivity to these substances.

Creams are convenient because, to some extent, they can be used for wet or dry surfaces and are easier than ointments to apply. Creams also do not typically contain lanolin, though they usually do contain a preservative or stabilizer, such as parabens or ethylenediamine dihydrochloride, both of which are known to occasionally cause sensitivity reactions. Some topical antibacterials are prepared with a synthetic base that may give them the properties of both creams and ointments.

Antiseptics

Antiseptics are a group of widely differing chemical compounds able to destroy or inhibit the growth of microorganisms, yet whose strength has been diluted enough to render them safe to use on living tissues. They can be inorganic or organic chemicals. Some examples of antiseptics are povidone-iodine, acetic acid, hydrogen peroxide, and hypochlorite. Povidone-iodine is effective against a wide range of microbial pathogens, from bacteria to viruses and fungi. Acetic acid is commonly used against infections caused by *Pseudomonas aeruginosa*. Hydrogen peroxide is an example of an oxidizing antiseptic: these liberate oxygen when in contact with pus, blood, or other organic substances.

Antiseptic agents are applied directly to tissue to destroy microorganisms or inhibit their reproduction or metabolic activity. By reducing organisms, antiseptics potentially hasten

CLINICAL WISDOM

Wound Healing and Antimicrobials

No antibacterial agent, whether bactericidal or bacteriostatic, is curative when used in isolation. Attention to nutritional factors, management of underlying pathology, and relief of causative factors are also required.

wound healing and diminish the local wound infection.[7] They are also employed clinically to disinfect instruments and infected material.

Antiseptics are available as hand scrubs, cleansers, irrigants, and protective dressings. It is important to remember, however, that the skin cannot be sterilized (made entirely free of microorganisms). Approximately 20% of the skin's normal resident flora is beyond the reach of antiseptics.[48] Excessive antiseptic use places patients at risk of allergy, drug toxicity, superinfection, and unnecessary costs. Further, excess antiseptic use poses significant public health concerns because this presents an environment that favors growth of bacteria that are resistance to antiseptics.

Use of topical antiseptics can interact with commonly used wound dressings and in doing so, lose their antimicrobial properties. In a study to examine the interaction, five clinically used antiseptics (Prontosan, Lavasept, Braunol, Octenisept, and Betaisodona) were tested in the presence or absence of 42 wound dressings against *Staphylococcus aureus*.[49] Povidone-iodine–based products showed sufficient antimicrobial activity in 64% to 78% of the combinations assessed. The octenidine derivate Octenisept showed sufficient antimicrobial activity in 54% of combinations. Polyhexamethylene biguanide (PHMB) derivatives demonstrated sufficient antimicrobial activity in 32% of the combinations. Thus, commonly used wound dressings dramatically reduce antibacterial activity of clinically used antiseptics and wound irrigating agents in vitro.[49]

Antiseptic-Containing Dressings

Some dressings contain and release antiseptic agents at the wound surface. The objective of these dressings is to provide long-lasting antimicrobial action in combination with the maintenance of a physiologically moist environment for healing. Iodine has been complexed with a polymeric cadexomer starch vehicle to form a topical gel or paste. The cadexomer moiety provides exudate absorption from the wound, which results in the concomitantly slow release of low concentrations of free iodine from the vehicle.[47] Cadexomer iodine is effective at reducing bacterial counts in chronic wounds, and also positively affects the healing process when compared with standard treatments (usually gauze and saline) and the cadexomer starch vehicle alone.[50–52] A 2010 Cochrane systematic review of antibiotics and antiseptics for venous leg ulcers concluded that some evidence supports use of cadexomer iodine. When cadexomer iodine was compared with standard care with all patients receiving compression, the pooled estimate from two trials for frequency of complete healing at 4 to 6 weeks indicated significantly higher healing rates for cadexomer iodine (RR 6.72, 95% CI 1.56 to 28.95). Surrogate healing endpoints such as change in ulcer surface area and daily or weekly healing rate also showed favorable results for cadexomer iodine.[53]

Silver (metallic, nanocrystalline, and ionic) has been incorporated into a wide variety of semiocclusive dressing formats, such as foams, hydrocolloids, alginates, and hydrofibers. All of these products release silver cations into the wound as they absorb or come in contact with wound exudate. Silver ions kill bacteria by several mechanisms including damaging cell walls, membranes, respiratory enzymes, and ribonucleoproteins[54,55]. Silver has proven efficacy against MRSA, vancomycin-resistant enterococci (VRE), and extended-spectrum β-lactamase producers.[54,55] Silver is also effective against biofilm.[54]

Honey works as an antimicrobial by the osmotic effect produced by the high sugar content and the presence of an enzyme that produces hydrogen peroxide.[54] Honey has an inhibitory effect on more than 50 different species of bacteria (broad-spectrum effectiveness) including MRSA and VRE.[56] Honey does not have any reported microbial resistance and has demonstrated effectiveness for a variety of wound infections as well as colonization and biofilms.[56] Clinicians should avoid using non–medical-grade honey as it can have viable spores and have unpredictable antibacterial activity.

Polyhexanide is an antimicrobial compound that is effective in infected or critically colonized acute and chronic wounds. It is also effective against biofilms. Like iodine, silver, and honey, it has a broad spectrum of effectiveness, no resistance, and minimal contact sensitization.[54] Polyhexanide is available as antiseptic wound irrigation solution (Prontosan® Wound irrigation solution, Lavanid® solution), hydrogels (Prontosan® Wound gel, Lavanid® wound gel), and wound dressings (Telfa® A.M.D., Kerlix® A.M.D., Kendall® A.M.D., XCell).[54] The duration of therapy is usually 2 to 5 days and generally should not exceed 14 to 21 days.[57] Polyhexanide is most effective when used at the critical colonization period to prevent wound infection.[54]

Superoxidized water (Microcyn) is a recently approved antiseptic.[54] It is pH-neutral with reactive species of chlorine and oxygen in a stable form. Superoxidized water is bactericidal with broad spectrum coverage. It is potentially active in the presence of biofilm with no contact sensitivity.[58] It can be applied directly to the wound or combined with other dressings or wound care products. Antimicrobial peptides are a new approach to topical therapy for wound infection. Antimicrobial peptides are small, cationic amphipathic compounds that are stored in granules of polymorphonuclear leukocytes and epithelial cells in most eukaryotes.[54] They are bactericidal against a broad spectrum of microorganisms and synergistic with other antimicrobials. Pexiganan, a peptide awaiting U.S. FDA approval, is applied in a 1% cream and is effective against most aerobic and anaerobic, gram-positive and gram-negative organisms.[59]

Topical antimicrobial therapy using iodine, silver, honey, polyhexanide or superoxidized water plays a role in eradicating bacteria prior to skin grafting, or to reduce odor associated with nonhealing necrotic ulcers (in persons for whom debridement and/or revascularization procedures are not an option), for wounds that are failing to heal (possible critical colonization), and removal of biofilm.[54] Iodine, silver, and honey specifically show inhibition or disruption of biofilm.[54]

Antifungals

About 50 species of fungi are pathogenic to humans. Antifungal agents include nystatin (Mycostatin), ketoconazole (Nizoral), and miconazole nitrate (Monistat-Derm). Not all antifungal agents are fungicidal; many are only fungistatic, and certain of them may owe their efficacy to a keratolytic action.

Fungi are eukaryotes, like the cells of plants and animals, including humans. Thus, designing drugs that can target fungi selectively is challenging. Broad-spectrum antifungal agents are in general nonselective and therefore, when taken systemically, are toxic. However, many antifungals have limited absorption through the epidermis, and therefore can be used in dermatologic preparations.

An antifungal agent is indicated when a patient has a diagnosed or strongly suspected significant fungal infection,

RESEARCH WISDOM

Treatment of Malodorous Wounds

Topical metronidazole has been shown to be effective in resolving odor in foul-smelling wounds. Use of a 1% solution or 0.75% gel applied twice daily reduced or eliminated odor in 80% to 90% of wounds in 4 to 7 days. Odor was significantly decreased in 2 days.[60–62]

as well as an indication for prophylactic antifungal use, such as underlying disease or an increased risk of fungal infection resulting from invasive procedures or environmental exposure (e.g., diarrhea, diaphoresis, poor hygiene, diabetes). The major contraindication for antifungal use is a known allergy to its ingredients. Antifungals must be used for the entire time prescribed to completely eliminate the infection.

Some areas are more difficult to treat, and some fungi are more difficult to eliminate because of a patient's underlying disease process. External factors that affect the antifungal agent's ability to penetrate the skin include temperature, ambient water vapor pressure, and drying agents such as powders, which reduce the excess moisture in the skin folds and may aid in the efficacy of antifungals.

Nonsporing anaerobes are a significant pathogen in ulcers with a foul smell and exposure to fecal contamination.[60] Metronidazole topical gel (MetroGel) has been shown to be effective in eliminating or decreasing the odor associated with these wounds.[60–62]

Topical Dressings for Management of Exudate

Effective management of exudate requires knowledge of the absorptive capacity of dressing materials and attention to fragile wound margins. Excess exudate on the wound edges can lead to maceration and destruction of the critical wound edge. Use of petrolatum products or other hydrophobic ointments around the wound can provide some protection for the wound edges. Use of a topical dressing that adequately absorbs the wound fluid will also protect the wound edges.

The choice of a dressing for a wound is, in many cases, dependent on the amount of drainage present in the wound and the expected drainage from the wound. For example, a wound that has been recently debrided of yellow necrotic tissue may have a history of moderate to large amounts of drainage; however, the amount of drainage postdebridement is expected to decrease. The topical dressing may also become not only

CLINICAL WISDOM

Caution About Petrolatum Around Wound Edges

If petrolatum products are being used for wound care and the patient is receiving physical therapy, the physical therapist must be notified. Petrolatum products can interfere with physical therapy technologies and are difficult to remove from the patient's skin prior to physical therapy interventions.

TABLE 18.5 Topical Treatment—Wound Dressings				
Wound Dressings: Generic Categories	**Not Absorbent**	**Low to Minimal Absorption**	**Minimal to Moderate Absorption**	**Moderate to Large Absorption**
Skin sealants	X			
Composite or combination dressings		X	X	
Transparent film dressings	X			
Gauze—woven		X		
Gauze—nonwoven			X	
Gauze—impregnated	X			
Calcium alginates			X	X
Collagen dressings		X	X	
Exudate absorbers—beads, pastes, powders, flakes			X	X
Hydrocolloids—regular, thin, pastes, granules		X	X	
Hydrogels—sheets, wafers, amorphous		X	X	
Foams		X	X	X
Hydrocolloid-hydrogel combinations		X	X	

the treatment but also the method of determining the efficacy of treatment. For example, by evaluating the dressing upon removal from the wound, you can judge what percentage of the dressing material has interacted with wound drainage. This can help you determine whether to continue treatment with the same dressing or to apply a new dressing. Table 18.5 identifies the generic product categories with notes about the absorptive capability of each dressing type. This information may be useful in choosing dressings for the exudative wound. Monitor closely any patient who has a wound with large amounts of exudate. The skin surrounding the wound can become macerated and, in some cases, a candidiasis or yeast infection can develop around the wound. The continual loss of proteins, fluids, and electrolytes in wound exudate can cause fluid and electrolyte disturbances in severe cases; at a minimum, the loss of proteins and wound healing substrates can slow or impede the wound healing progress. Finally, the presence of a wound with large amounts of draining exudate takes a toll on the patient's daily quality of life, disrupting normal function.

OUTCOME MEASURES

Appropriate characteristics to assess in evaluating the results of exudate management are the amount of exudate in the wound, type of exudate in the wound, and involvement of the wound dressing with the exudate present in the wound. Measurement of exudate is an intermediate outcome measure, and healing is the final outcome.

Amount of Exudate

The amount of exudate should diminish progressively in the wound if therapy is appropriate. The amount of exudate can be

measured by using clinical judgment to evaluate the distribution of moisture in the wound and the interaction of exudate with the wound dressing. A rating scale similar to the following may be used to quantify the amount of exudate:

1 = None = wound tissues dry
2 = Scant = wound tissues moist, no measurable exudates
3 = Small = wound tissues wet, moisture evenly distributed in wound, drainage involved 25% of wound dressing
4 = Moderate = wound tissues saturated, drainage may or may not be evenly distributed in wound, drainage involved >25% to <75% of wound dressing
5 = Large = wound tissues bathed in fluid, drainage freely expressed, may or may not be evenly distributed in wound, drainage involved >75% of wound dressing

Type of Exudate

The type of exudate should change as the wound improves and heals. As the wound passes through the inflammatory phase of wound healing, serous drainage should become more serosanguineous and then sanguineous in nature. As infection or necrosis is resolved, improvement should be reflected in the exudate type. Foul, purulent drainage should become merely purulent, then seropurulent, and finally serous and serosanguineous in character. Measurement of the type of exudate is best accomplished by the use of a rating scale, such as:

1 = Bloody = thin, bright red
2 = Serosanguineous = thin, watery, pale red to pink
3 = Serous = thin, watery, clear
4 = Purulent = thin or thick, opaque tan to yellow
5 = Foul purulent = thick, opaque yellow to green with offensive odor

REFERRAL CRITERIA

The determination of whether a patient is a candidate for wound management requires adequate assessment of the patient, with attention to evaluation for possible referral. For example, the following patients would warrant referral to a physician and/or an advanced practice nurse for medical evaluation, immediate intervention, or referral to another health-care professional for consultation:

1. Patients with wound exudate that is copious, malodorous, and prolonged should be evaluated further for infection, cellulitis, abscess, or progressive degeneration. In this case, the advanced practice nurse may choose to manage the patient initially. If the condition worsens or the patient fails to improve over a 2-week time frame, the physician should be consulted.
2. Patients with an elevated temperature or those on a downhill course should be evaluated further. Intervene as in No. 1.
3. Patients with no wound improvement over several weeks should be evaluated further. In this case, the advanced practice nurse may want to consult other health-care practitioners (e.g., physical therapists, dietitians, wound care nurses, and physicians).
4. Patients with evidence of cellulitis or gross purulence/ infection should be evaluated further. Intervene as in No. 1.
5. Patients with impending exposed bone or tendon present in the wound should be evaluated further. Intervene as in No. 3.
6. Patients with evidence of an abscessed area should be evaluated further. Intervene as in No. 3.
7. Patients with extensively undermined areas present in the wound should be evaluated further. Intervene as in No. 3.

SELF-CARE TEACHING GUIDELINES

Patient and caregiver instruction in self-care must be individualized to the topical therapy care routine, individual patient's wound, individual patient's and caregiver's learning styles and coping mechanisms, and ability of the patient/caregiver to perform procedures. The general self-care teaching guidelines in Exhibit 18.2 provide a model of information to teach, and should be individualized for each patient and caregiver.

CONCLUSION

Management of exudate and infection is part of preparing the wound for healing. Differentiation of infection from colonization can be difficult, since clinical signs and symptoms of each are similar. Colonization does not usually impair wound healing or invade wound tissues. In contrast, infection invades wound tissues with resultant cellulitis, inflammation, drainage and odor, and impaired wound healing. Knowledge of wound biofilm and the complexity of bacteria present in chronic wounds have increased our understanding of failure to heal in chronic wounds and is improving our diagnostic abilities.

Correct antimicrobial therapy can assist in bacterial contamination, prevention of biofilm, and infection. Use of antimicrobials should be undertaken with a thoughtful approach in wounds with signs of infection and cautiously used in wounds that are clean. Advancements in our understanding of wound cleansing, biofilms, antimicrobial use, and dressings to absorb wound exudate have made obtaining an infection-free, moist but not wet, wound ready for healing more attainable.

EXHIBIT 18.2			
Self-Care Teaching Guidelines			
Self-Care Guidelines Specific to Exudate and Infection Management	**Instructions Given (Date/Initials)**	**Demonstration or Review of Material (Date/Initials)**	**Return Demonstration or Verbalizes Understanding (Date/Initials)**
1. Type of wound and reasons for exudate			
2. Significance of exudate and infection			

3. Topical therapy care routine
  a. Clean wound.
  b. Apply absorptive dressing (note appearance of dressing when it interacts with wound drainage and on removal).
  c. Manage wound edges to prevent maceration.
  d. Apply secondary or topper dressing, as appropriate.			

4. Frequency of dressing changes			
5. Expected change in wound drainage during healing			

(continued)

EXHIBIT	18.2 (*continued*)

Self-Care Teaching Guidelines

Self-Care Guidelines Specific to Exudate and Infection Management	Instructions Given (Date/Initials)	Demonstration *or* Review of Material (Date/Initials)	Return Demonstration *or* Verbalizes Understanding (Date/Initials)

6. When to notify the health-care provider
  a. Signs and symptoms of infection
  b. Failure to improve
  c. Presence of odor
  d. Pus or purulent drainage
  e. Copious amounts of drainage
  f. Elevated temperature or signs of confusion in the older patient			

7. Universal precautions
  a. Hand washing
  b. Use of gloves during care procedures
  c. Disposal of contaminated materials			

8. Antibiotic regimen
  a. Oral medication use
  b. Topical medication use
  c. Antimicrobial cleanser use			

9. Importance of follow-up with health-care provider			

REVIEW QUESTIONS

1. Which of the following statements best describes wound colonization?
   A. The presence of proliferating microorganisms in viable wound tissues without a host response
   B. The presence of proliferating microorganisms in viable wound tissues with a host response
   C. The presence of proliferating microorganisms on the wound surface without a host response
   D. The presence of proliferating organisms on the wound surface with a host response

2. A client presents with a clean full-thickness wound. Which of the following solutions would be the best for use in cleansing?
   A. Povidone-iodine
   B. Normal saline
   C. Sodium hypochlorite solution
   D. Hydrogen peroxide

3. Cultures are indicated for which of the following pressure ulcers?
   A. All pressure ulcers involving loss of epidermis and dermis
   B. All full-thickness pressure ulcers
   C. Pressure ulcers with signs and symptoms of localized/systemic infection or bone involvement
   D. Pressure ulcers with necrotic tissue present and surrounding erythema

4. Which of the following reports typically indicates wound infection?
   A. Colony count of more than 1,000 organisms/mL
   B. Colony count of more than 5,000 organisms/mL
   C. Colony count of more than 10,000 organisms/mL
   D. Colony count of more than 100,000 organisms/mL

5. Which of the following agents can be used to prevent biofilm development after debridement?
   A. Hydrocolloid dressings
   B. Polyhexanide or medical grade honey dressings
   C. Saline moist gauze dressings
   D. Calcium alginate dressings

REFERENCES

1. Trengove NJ, Bielefeldt-Ohmann H, Stacey MC. Mitogenic activity and cytokine levels in non-healing and healing chronic leg ulcers. *Wound Repair Regen.* 2000;8(1):13–25.
2. Winter GD. Formation of the scab and the rate of reepithelialization of superficial wounds in the skin of the young domestic pig. *Nature.* 1965;193:293–294.
3. Rayment EA, Upton Z, Shooter GK. Increased matrix metalloproteinase-9 (MMP-9) activity observed in chronic wound fluid is related to the clinical severity of the ulcer. *Br J Dermatol.* 2008;158(5):951–961.
4. Bucalo B, Eaglstein WH, Falanga V. Inhibition of cell proliferation by chronic wound fluid. *Wound Repair Regen.* 1993;1(3):181–186.
5. Eubank TD, Marsh CB. Cytokines and growth factors in the regulation of wound inflammation. In: Sen C, ed. *Advances in Wound Care, Vol. 1: Translational Medicine: From Benchtop to Bedside to Community and Back.* New Rochelle, NY: Mary Ann Liebert, Inc.; 2010:211–216.
6. Wiegand C, Schonfelder U, Abel M, et al. Protease and pro-inflammatory cytokine concentrations are elevated in chronic compared to acute wounds and can be modulated by collagen type I in vitro. *Arch Dermatol Res.* 2010;302(6):419–428.
7. Moor AN, Vachon DJ, Gould LJ. Proteolytic activity in wound fluids and tissues derived from chronic venous leg ulcers. *Wound Repair Regen.* 2009;17(6):832–839.
8. Motzkau M, Tautenhahn J, Lehnert H, et al. Expression of matrix-metalloproteases in the fluid of chronic diabetic foot wounds treated with a protease absorbent dressing. *Exp Clin Endocrinol Diabetes.* 2010;PMID:21031342.
9. Dealey C, Cameron J, Arrowsmith M. A study comparing two objective methods of quantifying the production of wound exudate. *J Wound Care.* 2006;15(4):149–153.
10. Steinstraber L, Jacobsen F, Hirsch T, et al. Immunodepletion of high-abundant proteins from acute and chronic wound fluids to elucidate low-abundant regulators in wound healing. *BMC Res Notes.* 2010;3(1):355.
11. Bowler PG. The 10^5 bacterial growth guideline: reassessing its clinical relevance in wound healing. *Ostomy/Wound Manage.* 2003;49(1):44–53.
12. Thomson PD, Smith DJ. What is infection? *Am J Surg.* 1994;167(suppl 1A):7–11.
13. Association for the Advancement of Wound Care (AAWC). *Advancing your Practice: Understanding Wound Infection and the Role of Biofilms.* Malvern, PA: AAWC; 2008.
14. Phillips PL, Wolcott RD, Fletcher J, et al. Biofilms made easy. *Wounds Int.* 2010;1(3):1–6.
15. James GA, Swogger E, Wolcott R, et al. Biofilms in chronic wounds. *Wound Repair Regen.* 2008;16:37–44.
16. Dowd SE, Sun Y, Secor PR, et al. Survey of bacterial diversity in chronic wounds using pyrosequencing, DGGE, and full ribosome shotgun sequencing. *BMC Microbiol.* 2008;8:1–43.
17. Bjarnsholt T, Givskov M. Ecology of biofilms in chronic wounds. In: Sen C, ed. *Advances in Wound Care, Vol. 1: Translational medicine: From Benchtop to Bedside to Community and Back.* New Rochelle, NY; Mary Ann Liebert, Inc.; 2010:287–292.
18. Gjodsbol K, Christensen JJ, Karlsmark T, et al. Multiple bacterial species reside in chronic wounds: a longitudinal study. *Int Wound J.* 2006;3:225.
19. Valencia IC, Kirsner RS, Kerdel FA. Microbiologic evaluation of skin wounds: alarming trend toward antibiotic resistance in an inpatient dermatology service during a 10-year period. *J Am Acad Dermatol.* 2004;50:845.
20. Wolcott RD, Rumbargh KP, James G, et al. Biofilm maturity studies indicate sharp debridement opens a time-dependent therapeutic window. *J Wound Care.* 2010;19:320–328.
21. Boyce JM. Methicillin-resistant *Staphylococcus aureus*: detection, epidemiology, and control measures. *Infect Dis Clin North Am.* 1989;3:901–913.
22. Bordon J, Master RN, Clark RB, et al. Methicillin-resistant *Staphylococcus aureus* to non-β-lactam antimicrobials in the United States from 1996 to 2008. *Diagn Microbiol Infect Dis.* 2010;67:395–398.
23. Gardner SE, Frantz RA, Doebbling BN. The validity of the clinical signs and symptoms used to identify localized chronic wound infection. *Wound Repair Regen.* 2001;9:178–186.
24. Mosiello GC, Tufaro A, Kerstein MD. Wound healing and complications in the immunosuppressed patient. *Wounds.* 1994;6(3):83–87.
25. Stotts NA. Determination of bacterial burden in wounds. *Adv Wound Care.* 1995;8:28–52.
26. Kandula S, Zenilman JM, Melendez JH, et al. New frontiers of molecular microbiology in wound healing. In: Sen C, ed. *Advances in Wound Care, Vol. 1: Translational Medicine: From Benchtop to Bedside to Community and Back.* New Rochelle, NY: Mary Ann Liebert, Inc.; 2010:281–286.
27. Frankel YM, Melendez JH, Wang NY, et al. Defining wound microbial flora: molecular microbiology opening new horizons. *Arch Dermatol.* 2009;10:1193.
28. Robson MC, Heggars JP. Bacterial quantification of open wounds. *Milit Med.* 1969;134:19–24.
29. Wood GL, Gutierrez Y. *Diagnostic Pathology of Infectious Diseases.* Philadelphia, PA: Lea & Febiger; 1993.
30. Lee P, Turnidge J, McDonald PJ. Fine-needle aspiration biopsy in diagnosis of soft tissue infections. *J Clin Mibrobiol.* 1985;22:80–83.
31. Morrison MJ. *A Colour Guide to the Nursing Management of Wounds.* Oxford, UK: Blackwell Scientific Publications; 1992.
32. Pagana KD, Pagana TJ. *Mosby's Diagnostic and Laboratory Test Reference.* St. Louis, MO: Mosby-Year Book; 1992.
33. Cuzzell JZ. The right way to culture a wound. *Am Nurs.* 1993;93:48–50.
34. Alvarez O, Rozint J, Meehan M. Principles of moist wound healing: indications for chronic wounds. In: Krasner D, Rodeheaver GT, Sibbald RG, eds. *Chronic Wound Care: A Clinical Source Book for Healthcare Professionals.* 3rd ed. Wayne, PA: HMP Communications; 2001.
35. Levine NS, Lindberg RB, Mason AD, et al. The quantitative swab culture and smear: a quick simple method for determining the number of viable aerobic bacteria on open wounds. *J Trauma.* 1976;16(2):89–94.
36. Georgiade NG, Lucas MC, O'Fallon WM, et al. A comparison of methods for the quantification of bacteria in burn wounds. *Am J Clin Pathol.* 1970;53:35–39.
37. Duke WF, Robson MC, Krizek TJ. Civilian wounds: their bacterial flora and rate of infection. *Surg Forum.* 1972;23:518–520.
38. Lineaweaver W. Cellular and bacterial toxicities of topical antimicrobials. *Plast Reconstr Surg.* 1985;75:394–396.
39. Rodeheaver G. Topical wound management. *Ostomy/Wound Manage.* 1988;20:59–68.
40. Foresman PA, Payne DS, Becker D, et al. A relative toxicity index for wound cleansers. *Wounds.* 1993;5(5):226–231.
41. Hellewell TB, Major DA, Foresman PA, et al. A cytotoxicity evaluation of antimicrobial and non-antimicrobial wound cleansers. *Wounds.* 1997;9(1):15–20.
42. Bennett LL, Rosenblum RS, Perlov C, et al. An in vivo comparison of topical agents on wound repair. *Plast Reconstr Surg.* 2001;108(3):675–687.
43. Rhoads DD, Wolcott RD, Percival SL. Biofilms in wounds: management strategies. *J Wound Care.* 2008;17:502–508.
44. Haynes LJ, Brown MH, Handley BC, et al. Comparison of Pulsavac and sterile whirlpool regarding the promotion of tissue granulation. *Arch Phys Med Rehabil.* 1994;74(suppl 5):54.
45. Young LS, Sabel AL, Price CS. Epidemiologic, clinical, and economic evaluation of an outbreak of clonal multidrug-resistant *Acinetobacter baumannii* infection in a surgical intensive care unit. *Infect Control Hosp Epidemiol.* 2007;28(11):1247–1254.

46. Maragakis LL, Cosgrove SE, Song X, et al. An outbreak of multidrug-resistant Acinetobacter baumannii associated with pulsatile lavage wound treatment. *JAMA*. 2004;292(24):3006–3011.

47. Leaper DJ. Prophylactic and therapeutic role of antibiotics in wound care. *Am J Surg*. 1994;167(Suppl 1A):158S–159S.

48. Gilman G, ed. *Topical Agents for Open Wounds: Antibacterials, Antiseptics, Antifungals*. Reviewed by Rodeheaver G, Cooper JW, Nelson DR, Meehan M. Charleston, SC: Hill-Rom International; 1991.

49. Hirsch T, Limoochi-Deli S, Lahmer A, et al. Antimicrobial activity of clinically used antiseptics and wound irrigating agents in combination with wound dressings. *Plast Reconstr Surg*. 2010. [Epub ahead of print]

50. Harcup JW, Saul PA. A study of the effect of cadexomer iodine in the treatment of venous leg ulcers. *Br J Clin Pract*. 1986;40(9):360–364.

51. Ormiston MC, Seymour MT, Venn GE, et al. Controlled trial of Iodosorb in chronic venous ulcers. *Br Med J (Clin Res Ed)*. 1985;291(6491):308–310.

52. Skog E, Arnesio B, Troeng T, et al. A randomized trial comparing cadexomer iodine and standard treatment in the outpatient management of chronic venous ulcers. *Br J Dermatol*. 1983;109(1):77–83.

53. O'Meara S, Al-Kurdi D, Ologun Y, et al. Antibiotics and antiseptics for venous leg ulcers. *Cochrane Database Syst Rev*. 2010;(1):CD003557.

54. Lipsky BA, Hoey C. Topical antimicrobial therapy for treating chronic wounds. *Clin. Pract*. 2009;49(15):1541–1549.

55. Fonder MA, Lazarus GS, Cowan DA, et al. Treating the chronic wound: A practical approach to the care of nonhealing wounds and wound care dressings. *J Am Acad Dermatol*. 2008;58:185–206.

56. Kwakman PH, Van der Akker, JP, Guclu, A, et al. Medical-grade honey kills antibiotic-resistant bacteria in vitro and eradicates skin colonization. *Clin Infect Dis*. 2008;46:1677–1682.

57. Dissemond J, Gerber V, Kramer A, et al. A practice-orientated recommendation for treatment of critically colonized and locally infected wounds using polihexanide. *J Wound Tech*. 2010;7:27–33.

58. Gonzalez-Espinosa D, Perez-Romano L, Guzman-Soriano B, et al. Effects of pH-neutral, super-oxidised solution on human dermal fibroblasts in vitro. *Int Wound J*. 2007;4:241–250.

59. Ge Y, MacDonald D, Hait H, et al. Microbiological profile of infected diabetic foot ulcers. *Diabet Med*. 2002;19:1032–1034.

60. McMullen D. Topical metronidazole, part II. *Ostomy/Wound Manage*. 1992;38(3):42–48.

61. Jones P, Willis A, Ferguson I. Treatment of anaerobically infected pressure sores with topical metronidazole. *Lancet*. 1978;1:214.

62. Gomolin I, Brandt J. Topical therapy for pressure sores in geriatric patients. *J Am Geriatr Soc*. 1983;31:710–712.

CHAPTER 19

Management of Edema

Terry Treadwell, Evonne Fowler, and Barbara M. Bates-Jensen

CHAPTER OBJECTIVES

At the completion of this chapter, the reader will be able to:

1. Explain the various causes of edema.
2. Discuss assessment of the patient with edema.
3. Describe the general guidelines for compression therapy.
4. Discuss effective management strategies for various types of edema.

Edema is defined as "the presence of abnormally large amounts of fluid in the intercellular tissue spaces of the body, usually applied to demonstrable accumulation of excessive fluid in the subcutaneous tissues."[1] This abnormal collection of fluid has been a problem for patients and health-care providers for centuries. In early times, it was called "dropsy." This accumulation of fluid can be a recent occurrence (<72 hours), called acute edema, or it may have been present for a longer period of time, in that case called chronic edema. *Peripheral edema* involves the extremities, most commonly the lower legs, ankles, and feet. Without skillful assessment and timely intervention, peripheral edema can progress, leading to further tissue damage and functional impairment. There are two types of leg edema: venous edema and lymphedema. *Venous edema* consists of excess protein-poor interstitial fluid resulting from increased capillary permeability that cannot be accommodated by the normal lymphatic system.[2] This edema is a high-output failure of the vascular and lymph circulation, which occurs because the normal transport capacity of the intact lymphatics is overwhelmed by excessive flow of filtrate or fluid.[3] Common examples include heart failure, chronic venous insufficiency, hepatic cirrhosis, nephritic syndrome, and edema secondary to the inflammatory wound healing response. *Lymphedema* is protein-rich fluid within the skin and subcutaneous tissue that results from lymphatic system dysfunction.[4] Lymphedema is the result of low-output failure of the lymphatic system. The dysfunction of the lymphatic system can be due to a primary disorder (congenital dysplasia) or a secondary disorder (anatomical disruption such as seen with surgical dissection or recurrent infections).[3] The edema associated with wounds is often mixed, with initial features of venous edema (e.g., low-protein edema) as a result of the prolonged inflammation phase of wound healing coupled with damage to the lymphatic system (from the open wound), which leads to true lymphedema.

Lipedema is often misdiagnosed as lymphedema. Lipedema is abnormal adipose tissue accumulation in the lower extremities. Usually the dorsum of the foot is spared from edema. Massage and compression techniques used to treat edema and lymphedema are not useful for the management of this condition (Fig. 19.1).

Given the importance of edema management in wound care, we provide in this chapter a thorough exploration of the subject. The chapter begins with a discussion of the etiology and pathophysiology of edema and then explores assessment and management, including compression therapy and skin care.

SIGNIFICANCE

Many health-care providers fail to realize that "edema" is not a diagnosis unto itself but is a symptom. A symptom is defined as "any functional evidence of disease."[5] Excess fluid in the tissues is a symptom of an underlying condition and when detected by physical examination is called a "finding." Something is causing an excess accumulation of fluid in the tissues, and the disease causing the fluid accumulation is the diagnosis.

Because edema is a symptom and can be associated with a variety of diseases and conditions, determining the significance of the problem is difficult. Worldwide, the two most common causes of chronic and clinically significant edema are venous insufficiency and lymphedema (lymphatic obstruction). These are followed by an arteriovenous (AV) fistula and fluid overload, which in turn may indicate underlying cardiac or renal disease or malnutrition. Table 19.1 identifies the general characteristics of lower extremity edema from a variety of causes. The most likely cause of lower extremity edema in persons over age 50 is venous insufficiency with estimates that up to 30% of the U.S. population is affected.[6,7] Globally, secondary lymphedema caused by filariasis (infection with larvae transmitted

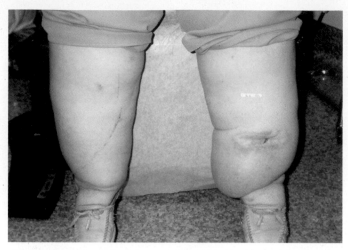

FIGURE 19.1 Lipedema. (Copyright © Evonne Fowler, RN, CNS, CWOCN.)

to humans from mosquitoes) is much more common, affecting 90 to 125 million persons worldwide.[3,8] Lymphedema, following axillary node dissection or radiation therapy for cancer, is most common in the United States,[9] affecting up to 80% of patients after surgery.[8] These figures do not include persons with chronic wounds and periwound edema.

Treatment of edema helps improve patient comfort and mobility, which in turn can lead to improved patient participation in the plan of care. Successful management of the edematous limb is also closely associated with successful wound healing and a decreased frequency of focal infections.[10–13] The importance of controlling edema in patients with wounds cannot be overemphasized. Indeed, studies showing the effectiveness of wound healing in venous ulcers without edema-control measures are almost nonexistent.[14] Poor epithelialization, decreased oxygenation[11] and nutrient diffusion, and decreased immune defense appear to be factors for problems in edematous limbs.[12,15,16] In many instances, treatment of edema itself may assist in wound healing and prevention.[16–18]

TABLE 19.1	Common Causes of Edema

Bilateral	Unilateral
1. Cardiac disease	1. Venous disease
2. Renal disease	2. Arterial disease usually AV fistulae
3. Hepatic disease	3. Lymphatic disease
4. GI disease	4. Operations
5. Immune disease and allergy	5. Trauma
6. Nutritional disease	
7. Endocrine disease	
8. Pregnancy	
9. Circulatory problems usually vena caval obstruction	
10. Drugs and medications	

ETIOLOGY OF EDEMA

If you are to choose effective treatment of edema, you must first understand the underlying etiology. A first step is to classify peripheral edema as *unilateral* or *bilateral* (Fig. 19.2A,B).

- *Unilateral lower extremity edema.* Causes include venous and arterial abnormalities, lymphedema, infection, trauma, and neoplasms.
- *Bilateral lower extremity edema.* Causes include congestive heart failure, systemic and metabolic abnormalities, endocrine dysfunction, inferior vena cava obstruction by tumor or inflammatory mass, *lipedema* (a condition involving excessive deposition and expansion of adipose cells), and pregnancy. In addition, malnutrition as a cause of edema is not widely appreciated in the United States, but when providing healthcare in underserved countries around the world, it can be a major problem. Another underappreciated cause of bilateral edema is drug-induced edema. Exhibit 19.1 shows a number of commonly used medications that can cause swelling of the extremities.

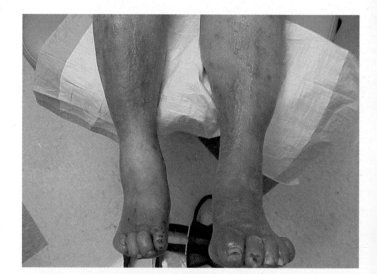

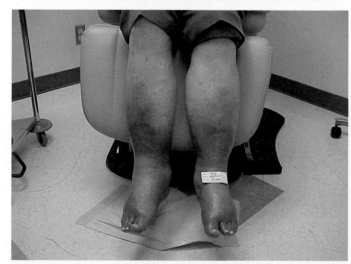

FIGURE 19.2 A,B: Determine whether the edema is unilateral (**A**) or bilateral (**B**) as shown. (Copyright © Evonne Fowler, RN, CNS, CWOCN.)

EXHIBIT   19.1

Drugs Causing Edema

- Calcium channel blockers (for example: amlodipine, diltiazem, felodipine, isradipine, nifedipine, verapamil)
- Antihypertensives
  - Hydralazine
  - Clonidine
  - Reserpine
- Minoxidil
- Beta-blockers (e.g., acebutolol, atenolol, betaxolol, bisoprolol, metoprolol, nadolol, penbutolol, propranolol)
- Cilostazol
- Gabapentin
- Hormones
  - Corticosteriods
  - Estrogen
  - Progesterone
  - Tamoxifen
  - Testosterone
- Monoamine oxidase inhibitors
- Anti-inflammatory drugs
  - Nonsteroidal anti-inflammatory drugs
  - Cox-2 inhibitors

Although the majority of lower extremity problems are due to venous disease, either insufficiency or occlusion, the underlying cause of the edema must be accurately identified if appropriate therapy is to be provided.

Unfortunately, edema may be the result of more than one etiology. For example, arterial ischemia may coexist with venous disease and the resultant edema and venous disease may also be associated with lymphedema. For this reason, all etiologies of edema must be considered and eliminated if the patient is to have successful therapy. Many times patients and providers are frustrated when therapeutic measures are less than successful in the treatment of edema. Many times the failure of therapy is because the underlying cause of edema has not been identified and appropriately treated.

PATHOPHYSIOLOGY OF EDEMA

As previously noted, edema occurs when excess fluid is present in the *interstitial space*, the area between cells and the capillaries. Exchange of nutrients, wastes, fluid, gases, electrolytes, and proteins from the vascular system, lymphatic system, and tissue cells occurs through this space. Fluid normally moves from the capillaries to the interstitial space and back again taking nutrients, oxygen, electrolytes, proteins, and other products to the cells and surrounding tissues and removing waste products. Pressure in this area may be low and attract fluid into the tissue or be high and force fluid into lymphatics and capillaries.[19] Up to 30 L of fluid each day pass from the capillaries into the interstitial spaces, and normally, an equal amount of fluid is returned to the circulatory system through the capillaries and removed by the lymphatics.[20] Edema occurs when this carefully regulated balance of fluid movement into and out of the tissues is upset.

Role of the Vascular System

As you know, hydrostatic pressure in the arteries, arterioles, and the arterial side of the capillaries comes largely from cardiac contraction. Hydrostatic pressure is exerted on blood in the veins, venules, and venous side of the capillaries by gravity and tissue pressures on the venous side of the circulation. By far, the greatest volume of blood at all times is in the veins (about two-thirds) while about one-fifth is in the arteries, arterioles, and capillaries.[21]

In the lower leg, the venous system is composed of a superficial system, a connecting perforating system, and a deep system. Blood normally flows from the superficial to the deep system through perforating veins and, at certain areas, at the groin and knee; the superficial system connects directly to the deep system. One-way valves in the veins prevent reflux. During muscle contraction, the muscles exert high pressures on the deep veins and pump blood toward the heart.

The Venous Muscular Pump

Venous pressure at the ankle is about 90 mm Hg, which is higher than venous pressure taken in a recumbent person whose ankle veins are at about the same level as the right atrium. However, when the leg and abdominal muscles are active, they compress the adjacent veins, emptying the blood and reducing venous pressure (until they fill up again when the muscles are relaxed). This compression, in combination with the function of the one-way valves in allowing blood to flow only toward the heart, is known as the *venous muscular pump*. The most important pump is the calf pump, but the quadriceps in the thigh and the foot pump also play roles in moving venous blood. Clearly the pump does not work without motion, an open unobstructed vein, and intact valves. When one, two, or all three of these fail, venous pressure can rise dramatically. When this happens in the superficial and deep systems or the deep system alone, edema, prominent varicose veins, and (eventually) venous skin ulcers may occur.[19–22]

Role of the Microcirculation

The flow of fluid to and from capillaries and lymphatics is governed by mechanisms defined by Dr. Starling over 100 years ago.[23] The controlling factors have to do with pressures inside and outside the capillary. When blood enters the arterial end of the capillary, the blood pressure is 30 to 35 mm Hg. Because of resistance to blood flow in the small vessels, the blood pressure drops further and is only 10 to 15 mm Hg at the venous end of the capillary. This makes the average pressure forcing fluid out of the vessels about 20 mm Hg.

Opposing this outward force of fluid from the capillary would be the pressure the tissues make pressing on the capillary wall to prevent fluid from leaking out of the capillary. Interestingly this opposing tissue pressure is 0 mm Hg. Since there is no opposing force to fluid leaking out of the vessels, the tendency is for fluid to leave the vessels and go into the interstitial space.

Unfortunately, it is not that simple. There are other forces involved called osmotic pressures which are generated by the proteins and other large molecules or solutes in the blood and interstitial space. When large molecules are concentrated in a fluid and on the other side of a permeable membrane is a fluid with fewer molecules, the fluid tries to move from an area of low concentration to one of high concentration so that the concentrations will be equal. This motion of fluid in relation to molecules results in pressure being generated, the oncotic pressure. The oncotic pressure in the plasma, because of the large number of protein molecules, is about 28 mm Hg pressure. The oncotic pressure of the interstitial fluid is approximately 8 mm Hg. This means that the net oncotic pressure (28–8 mm Hg) is 20 mm Hg, forcing fluid to stay in the capillary or flow into the capillary from the interstitial fluid.

When this is all combined, we see some interesting concepts. When blood enters the arterial end of the capillary, the force encouraging fluid to leave the capillary and go into the interstitial space is arterial pressure (30 mm Hg) minus the net oncotic pressure (20 mm Hg) holding the fluid in the capillary equals 10 mm Hg pressure forcing fluid into the interstitial space. About 30 L of fluid per day goes into the interstitial space in this manner.[3,10]

The entire equation changes when the blood reaches the venous end of the capillary. The pressure of the blood is only about 10 mm Hg. Now we have 10 mm Hg blood pressure forcing fluid out of the capillary minus the net oncotic pressure (20 mm Hg) holding the fluid in the capillary equals a *negative* 10 mm Hg pressure or 10 mm Hg pressure pulling fluid INTO the capillary from the interstitial space. This results in fluid being transferred back into the vascular system to be carried back to the heart. Each day, approximately 27 L of fluid from the interstitial space returns to the vascular system.

What happens to the other 3 L of fluid per day? It is removed along with 80 to 200 g of protein molecules, bacteria, cell residue, unwanted proteases, and cytokines by the lymphatics, the *other* circulatory system in the body.[3,10] The lymphatic system picks up this extra fluid (now called lymph) and returns it to the general circulation.

The lymphatic system consists of lymph vessels and lymph nodes. The lymphatics include valved capillaries and lymph collectors. The initial lymphatics reabsorb liquid and the lymph collectors act as transport vessels. Lymph collectors have muscular walls and valves. The contraction of the vessel walls acts as a pump to move the lymph along to the lymphatic ducts and then to the thoracic duct.[3] Lymphatic ducts do not have reabsorbing function. Extremities have both a superficial and deep lymphatic system. Lymph transport occurs from proximal to distal and from superficial to deep. Lymphatic drainage mostly follows the blood vessels and leads to regional lymph nodes. Nearly all of the lymph from the lower extremities and lower body flows to the thoracic duct. Lymph from the left side of the head, left arm, and some of the chest also drains into the thoracic duct and then rejoins the venous circulation. Lymph from the right side of the head and neck, right arm, and the thorax empties into the right thoracic duct. The right thoracic duct empties into the right subclavian and internal jugular vein. Thus, the upper venous system receives the large volume of lymph.[3] The body including the skin is divided into lymphatic drainage regions termed lymphotomes.[3] These lymphotomes are generally found in the dermis, and flow from lymphatic vessels varies around these lymphotomes (e.g.,drainage around the lymphotomes is in different, often opposite directions). Excess lymph can be directed along these drainage paths into functioning lymph vessels and back

into circulation. For example, when lymph nodes are removed after breast cancer, collateral lymphatic circulation can take over lymph transport.[3] The ability of the lymphatic system to circumvent or compensate for lost or damaged lymph nodes enables manual lymphatic drainage techniques to be successful in lymphedema management.[3] This approach is not successful with venous edema. Lymphedema may be primary or secondary. Primary lymphedema is classified according to age of onset:

- Congenital (onset before 1 year old)
- Praecox (onset at 1–35 years old)
- Tarda (onset after 35 years old)

Secondary lymphedema is caused by direct damage to the lymphatic system. As noted earlier, the most common cause of secondary lymphedema globally is filariasis, while the most common cause of secondary lymphedema in the United States is lymph node excision or damage from cancer therapy. Tumor invasion, infection, and direct trauma to lymph system can also cause secondary lymphedema.

As you can see, there are many potential causes for excess fluid to accumulate in an extremity. If the pressure in the arterial end of the capillary is increased (as seen in patients with fluid overload from congestive heart failure, renal failure, postoperative fluid overload, drugs, and others), more fluid will pass into the interstitial tissues. If the pressure at the venous end of the capillary is increased (as seen when one stands and in venous insufficiency and venous occlusion), less fluid is going to be reabsorbed. If the oncotic pressure is changed by a reduced amount of protein in the blood (as seen in nutritional problems, renal disease, liver disease, and some gastrointestinal problems) or an increased amount of protein in the tissues (as seen in conditions with damaged lymphatics), the balance of fluid into and out of the capillary will be altered. If the capillary is damaged and leaks more than it should (as seen in trauma, burns, inflammatory processes including infection, edema-causing drugs, and others), more fluid will pass into the interstitial space than can be handled. Damage to the lymphatics by either congenital problems or disease will result in more fluid and damaging products remaining in the tissues. The control of fluid in the tissues is a very precise process and is easily disrupted either temporarily or permanently by our actions or disease. Any disease or condition that could disrupt any portion of this carefully orchestrated physiologic process must be considered when evaluating the patient with edema.

Edema can be a problem in maintaining normal skin integrity and in the healing of wounds. The fluid impedes diffusion of oxygen and nutrients to the tissues, making maintaining healthy skin and healing wounds more difficult. Edema fluid is a good culture medium and, more importantly, inactivates the normal antistreptococcal properties of skin predisposing the patient with the swollen limb to infection. Edema fluid is known to delay wound healing by inhibiting mitogenic activity and DNA synthesis in cells, by having higher levels of proinflammatory cytokines which keep the microenvironment more inflammatory, and by having higher levels of proteases that destroy newly forming tissue matrix and growth factors. Edema fluid also induces a state of senescence in cells.[24] This puts cells into a state where they do not respond to growth factors and do not contribute to healing. Significant swelling of tissues can compress smaller blood vessels in the tissues, resulting in ischemia. Edema can be a sign of serious disease and can significantly contribute to other problems.

ASSESSMENT

Evaluation of the patient with edema is important because edema is more than just a cosmetic issue. Chronically swollen legs can cause a feeling of heaviness in the legs, be painful, and reduce ambulation and quality of life. Edema can be the first sign of a serious disease. For example, new onset of edema in a lower extremity may reflect pelvic tumors.

The etiology of the edema can be accurately determined by knowledgeable health-care providers in about 90% of cases on the basis of a good history and physical examination.[25] Unfortunately, many health-care providers do not conduct a good history and physical examination, a malady known as "hyposkillia."[26] Only about 10% of patients with swollen extremities should need laboratory evaluation and radiographic studies to determine the cause of the edema.

Patient History

A good patient history is necessary in the evaluation of the patient with the swollen limb. As has previously been mentioned, there are numerous diseases that can cause and contribute to edema. An adequate history entails pursuing information about these medical conditions that might cause edema. A family history is important when considering the patient with a swollen extremity. The incidence of varicose veins in someone with a family history can be up to three times higher than in someone who does not have a family history of the problem.[27,28] Genetic factors have been noted to increase the susceptibility of some patients to develop thrombophlebitis and venous ulcers.[29–31] A nutritional history should be included. Inadequate nutrition could be due to inadequate intake of food or many diseases. On the other hand, an excess of dietary intake could lead to increased intra-abdominal pressure, pressure on the veins, and subsequent lower extremity swelling. Does the patient have a history of malignancy or gastrointestinal disease? Does the patient have abdominal complaints of any kind? For example, swollen legs may be due to a previously undetermined pregnancy. There are other intra-abdominal causes of edematous extremities which must not be overlooked.

The patient's age and medication history are essential, because, as previously mentioned, a number of common medications can cause edema. Calcium channel blockers, prednisone, and anti-inflammatory drugs are common causes of edema.[6] Does the patient have a history of injury or operative procedures? These procedures may be overlooked as not important to report by patients. Yet they are important since the association between total knee replacements and chronic venous disease has been noted.[32] As an example, one of the authors saw a patient in their clinic with a massively swollen leg who, just in passing, mentioned that she had undergone a cardiac catheterization the week prior to the onset of the edema. Evaluation of the patient showed that the femoral vein had been damaged during the procedure resulting in an acute arteriovenous fistula between the femoral artery and femoral vein, causing her edema. After operative closure of the fistula, the edema resolved. The patient did not connect the procedure with the onset of the swelling. Is there a history of systemic disease? Heart, liver, and kidney disease are associated with edema. A history of HIV is important in the evaluation of the patient with lower extremity swelling especially if it is associated with an ulceration or other signs of chronic venous disease.[33] A history of pelvic or abdominal cancer or radiation therapy may also contribute to edema. Does the patient have a history of sleep apnea? Sleep apnea can cause pulmonary hypertension that can lead to leg edema.[6]

It is important to determine the occupation of the patient. Does the patient stand all day while working? Lower extremity edema may fail to respond to any therapy until the person can retire or change positions such that he or she is off his or her feet most of the day. Does the edema only occur at certain times? In women, edema of the lower extremities may be associated with their hormonal cycle (premenstrual edema).

The duration of the edema is important. Is the swelling a recent occurrence or has it been present for a length of time, perhaps even since shortly after birth? If the onset is acute (i.e., less than 72 hours), deep vein thrombosis should be strongly considered. Is there pain with the swelling? Pain needs to be documented and is generally done with a pain scale. It is important to qualify the pain. Does the pain occur when walking or just when standing or sitting? There is a little-remembered syndrome originally described by German physicians[34] of venous claudication which consists of tiredness, mild pain, and muscle weakness with activity of any extremity in which there is venous occlusion (upper or lower extremity). Since the patient may have associated arterial insufficiency, it is important to determine if the symptoms are due to arterial disease or venous disease. Similar to the intermittent claudication of arterial disease, the symptoms resolve with rest and recur with exercise. Important differences are that arterial pulses are present and evidence of venous obstruction is noted.[35]

Another important question relates to the response of the swelling to elevation. Asking if the swelling goes down overnight usually obtains the needed information. If the edema improves overnight, it is more likely venous edema as lymphedema generally does not improve overnight. Determine if there is a history of thrombophlebitis or pulmonary embolus; be sure to use terms understood by the patient (e.g., blood clots in the legs or lungs).

Physical Examination

Some elements of the physical examination include body mass index, distribution of edema, evaluation of pain, and assessment for pitting, varicosities, and skin changes and signs of systemic diseases.[6] Examination for evidence of the previously mentioned medical problems is essential. Examination of the patient for evidence of previous operative procedures and trauma is beneficial in case the patient's memory is deficient. Specific attention to the following areas is essential:

- Body mass index. Obesity is associated with sleep apnea and venous insufficiency.

- Abdominal exam. Numerous intra-abdominal problems can result in edema. Ascites from liver disease, metastatic cancer, prior radiation therapy, and tumors can all cause edema.
- Signs of systemic disease. Findings of heart failure, such as jugular vein distension and lung crackles, or liver disease such as spider hemangiomas and jaundice may be helpful in detecting a systemic cause of the edema.
- Distribution of edema. Unilateral edema is typically due to a local cause such as deep vein thrombosis, venous insufficiency, or lymphedema. Bilateral edema may be due to a local or systemic cause such as heart failure or kidney disease. Generalized edema is due to systemic disease. Examination of the extremities, trunk, and neck provide information on the extent of lymphedematous changes.[3]
- Pain or tenderness. Pain is usually associated with deep vein thrombosis or lipedema. Lymphedema is usually nontender.
- Pitting. Deep vein thrombosis, venous insufficiency, and early lymphedema usually present with pitting. Chronic lymphedema generally does not pit.
- Varicosities. If present, they may indicate venous insufficiency. Evaluation of the venous system entails direct and indirect venous evaluation. Looking at the extremity will reveal the presence or absence of varicose veins. Techniques for evaluation of the venous system for incompetent venous valves and venous insufficiency exist but are beyond the scope of this discussion (refer to Chapter 7).
- Kaposi-Stemmer sign. An inability to pinch a fold of skin on the dorsum of the foot at the base of the second toe is a sign of lymphedema.[36] Palpation may reveal thickened skin and fibrous changes in the subcutaneous tissues.[3]
- Skin changes. Hyperkeratosis with brawny induration is a characteristic of chronic lymphedema. *Hyperkeratosis* is a warty-like texture to the skin. Hemosiderin or brown staining of the lower legs and ankles is associated with venous disease.

The vascular examination is essential because arterial insufficiency is often mild and minimally symptomatic, yet significant when considering patients with edema and venous disease. Numerous studies have shown that up to 40% of patients with venous disease and ulceration will have significant peripheral vascular disease.[37] Even though the examiner may not be familiar with the techniques of the arterial examination, this is a skill that every person taking care of patients with lower extremity wounds *must* master. Inspection of all extremities for pulses should be done and signs of ischemia noted. If questions about the adequacy of the circulation arise, additional evaluation with Doppler studies and even invasive arterial imaging studies should be considered.

Palpation of the arterial system is important in the evaluation of the patient with edema because arterial problems such as abdominal aortic aneurysms, femoral artery aneurysms, and popliteal artery aneurysms can be large enough to compress the adjacent vein, resulting in venous hypertension and lower extremity edema. Examination of the popliteal fossa may also reveal the presence of a Baker cyst, a cystic mass coming out of the knee joint into the tissues behind the knee. These cysts commonly compress the vascular structures in the popliteal fossa, causing swelling of the leg below the knee.

Evaluation of the appropriate areas for enlarged lymph nodes is important and part of the examination for an edematous extremity. Enlarged lymph nodes due to infectious, inflammatory, or malignant diseases can obstruct veins and lymphatics, contributing to swollen extremities. This is especially true of the upper extremity where many diseases of the chest and lungs can result in edema.

Color, texture, and temperature of the skin should be evaluated. It should be noted that all "red legs" are not infected. In patients with ischemia or peripheral neuropathy, loss of control of the microcirculation occurs. When the leg is in the dependent position for any length of time, it turns red (*dependent rubor*). This can be differentiated from cellulitis by elevating the limb. If the limb becomes pale on elevation, it is not infected (pallor on elevation). If the color remains red when elevated, cellulitis may be present. *Hyperkeratosis*, a warty-like texture to the skin, and brawny induration are characteristic of lymphedema. Some of these characteristics can be seen in Figures 19.3 and 19.4. Venous edema is often associated with brown *hemosiderin* (a by-product of red blood cell breakdown) skin deposits on the ankles and lower legs.[6] When checking for the temperature of the skin, use the back side (dorsal surface) of your hand and fingers. The back

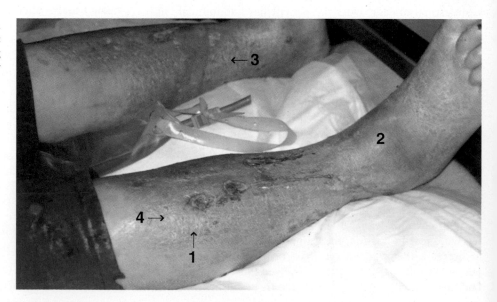

FIGURE 19.3 Chronic bilateral edema with evidence of (1) Brawny edema, (2) Trophic skin changes, (3) Hemosiderin staining (Hyperpigmentation), (4) Multiple shallow ulcers (Copyright © B.M. Bates-Jensen.)

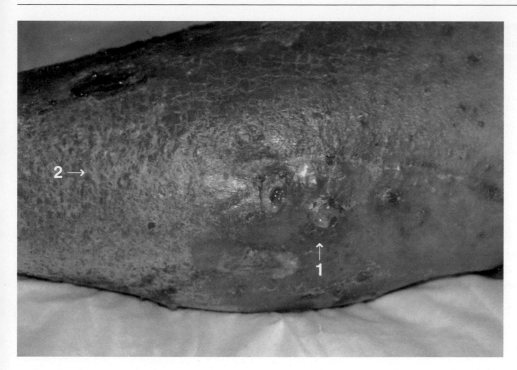

FIGURE 19.4 Close-up view of same leg as in Figure 19.3. Note evidence of (1) Edema leakage through wounds, (2) Scaling and crusting due to lipodermatosclerosis (Copyright © B.M. Bates-Jensen.)

of the hand is the most sensitive portion and can detect difference of temperature as small as one to two degrees.[38]

Extremities with long-standing venous disease will show evidence of chronic venous insufficiency and increased venous pressure. The skin may be thickened. Discoloration of the skin usually starting around the ankle and extending proximally is common. As the disease progresses, the chronic inflammatory condition in the subcutaneous tissues continues to do damage resulting in the classic "upside-down champagne bottle" leg. This is due to fibrosis of the tissues in the lower half of the leg and clinically is known as *lipodermatosclerosis* (see Figs. 19.3 and 19.4). The presence of this finding indicates chronic nature of the venous insufficiency. Interestingly, when this condition is severe, there may be little swelling of the lower portion of the leg. The subcutaneous tissues are so sclerotic and the skin so tight, swelling is not possible except in the upper portion of the leg where the tissues are less damaged.

Further visualization of the extremity will reveal the presence of swelling and the degree that is present. It is important to know how much of the extremity is involved by the swelling. Does the swelling just occur distally? Does it involve the entire extremity or just a portion of it? Are the toes or fingers involved? All of this information is important and will help in the determination of the diagnosis of the edema. How severe is the edema? The amount of pitting of the edema is the customary way to judge the severity of the edema with 1+ being the least amount to 4+ being the most severe. Table 19.2 shows the scale for evaluating the amount of edema. The diagnosis of the cause of the edema can be initiated once the extent and pattern of the edema are known. There are certain characteristics of the location and degree of edema that will point toward the correct diagnosis (see Table 19.3).

Evaluation of the swollen or edematous extremity would not be complete without the evaluation for the presence of an ulceration and drainage. If the leg is draining, the color, consistency, volume, and odor of the drainage should be noted. Is the drainage thin like serous fluid or thick like purulent fluid?

Is the drainage minimal or massive? All are important questions that will aid in the diagnosis of the cause of the drainage and determine the subsequent treatment. Evaluation and documentation of an ulcer and the surrounding tissue are important. The location of the ulcer or ulcers needs to be detailed. Ulcers need to be measured with a measuring, tracing, or laser device. If the ulcer is to be measured with a measuring tape, the measurement should be of the longest length, the perpendicular widest width, and the deepest depth. The condition of the periwound skin is important. Is it red, irritated, indurated, moist, or macerated? The status of the wound bed should be recorded. Is granulation tissue present? If so, how much of the wound bed is covered with granulation tissue? Is the granulation tissue healthy or discolored? All of this information is important in the evaluation of the patient with an edematous limb.

For patients with lymphedema, the severity can be classified according to clinical severity although there is not complete agreement among experts[3,39].

- Stage I: spontaneous, reversible tissue swelling leaving indentations, negative or borderline Stemmer sign, no palpable fibrous tissue.
- Stage II: spontaneous, irreversible tissue swelling with moderate or pronounced fibrosis; indentations are difficult to

TABLE 19.2	Edema Severity Scale	
Depth of Pitting	**Scale of Pitting**	**Severity**
0 to ¼ inch	1+	Mild
¼ to ½ inch	2+	Moderate
½ to 1 inch	3+	Severe
>1 inch	4+	Very severe

TABLE 19.3 Examination of the Swollen Lower Extremity				
	Lymphedema	Venous Edema	Medical Conditions: Cardiac-Renal-Hepatic Insufficiency	Medications
Symptoms and Pain	Heaviness; aching	Heaviness; aching	Usually none	Usually none
Bilateral	Yes/No	Yes/No	Yes	Yes
Pitting	No	Early: Yes Late: +/–	Yes	Yes
Skin Changes	Yes; Eventually thickening can be severe, Ulceration rare	Yes; Atrophic, Pigmentation, Possible ulcers	Shiny, no trophic changes	None
Location	Diffuse, more distal than proximal (from lymph drainage areas)	Ankles and legs; Occasionally foot	Bilateral, greatest distally May appear over back (sacral) in recumbent patient	Leg; Occasionally foot
Benefit with Elevation	Minimal: over several days	Yes: Almost complete in several hours up to one day	Yes: Almost complete in several hours up to 1 d	Yes

produce. Stemmer sign positive, lymphostatic dermatosis (firm, indurated tissues).

- Stage III: lymphatic elephantiasis (extreme swelling), usually with pronounced skin alterations and gross shape changes due to overgrowth of epidermal, dermal, and subcutaneous tissue. Severity based on differences in limb volume is assessed as minimal (<20% increase), moderate (20% increase), or severe (>40% increase).

Adjunctive Tests

It should be remembered that with an astute history and physical examination, only a small percent of patients will need adjunctive tests to make the diagnosis of the edematous extremity. Laboratory tests should include studies that would define any medical condition that might be responsible for the edema, including liver function tests, renal function tests, nutritional evaluation, cardiac evaluation, and other indicated tests. For example, if the cause of the edema is thought to be associated with nephrotic syndrome, serum lipids should be evaluated in addition to basic laboratory studies. Special coagulation studies may be indicated in the patient with recurrent or a strong family history of thrombophlebitis. The use of Doppler flow studies, lower extremity pressure measurements and ankle-brachial index, and contrast studies to evaluate for arterial disease have already been discussed (refer to Chapter 7).

The test of choice for evaluation of the venous system is the duplex ultrasound scan.[40] It provides a fast, cost-effective, reliable, noninvasive method of evaluating the venous system of any extremity. It can detect diseases of the venous system such as obstruction from clots or extrinsic masses and reflux in the deep or superficial venous systems due to damaged or nonfunctioning venous valves. Conditions with increased venous flow such as arteriovenous fistula can be detected. It helps outline the anatomy of the venous system in the event operative intervention is indicated.

Contrast venography is still an option for evaluation of the venous system. It outlines the venous anatomy and shows areas of venous obstruction and other abnormalities. It is indispensable in defining problems within the veins such as iliac vein web formation and certain venous compression syndromes. It is not to be done without significant reason because contrast phlebography has been associated with damage to venous valves.[41]

Other evaluations such as abdominal ultrasound may be indicated if intra-abdominal pathology is suspected. Special x-rays and scans may be indicated if malignancy is being considered as a cause of the edema. Rarely, plain film x-rays, nuclear medicine scans, and magnetic resonance imaging can be done to evaluate the soft tissues and bones of the extremities if this is deemed necessary. If there is need to evaluate the lymphatic system, lymphangiography and lymphatic scanning can be considered. These tests require significant skill in accomplishing them to get dependable results. A new, simpler technique for imaging lymphatics using near-infrared fluorescence is currently being evaluated.[42] This noninvasive technique detects the presence of lymphatics and can determine the physiology of lymphatic flow in the vessels.

MANAGEMENT OF EDEMA

Treatment of the edematous extremity depends on the diagnosis of the problem. With treatment, one may be able to make the swollen extremity smaller, but without addressing the underlying cause, the edema will quickly return. Because many of the causes of edema are chronic medical conditions, there is rarely a "quick fix" to the swollen extremity. Commitment and persistence on the part of the health-care provider, the patient, and the family are essential for good outcomes to be attained. Unfortunately, many get frustrated, give up, and just settle for the status quo with the swollen extremity. Interest in treating the swollen extremity often occurs only when acute problems arise.[43] The commitment to the treatment must include the patient for without the patient's involvement the chance of successful therapy is minimal. Compliance by the patient is the cornerstone of care for the swollen extremity, but many times, it is lacking.[44] Successful management depends on the patient's ability to cooperate; however, multiple pathologies—such as arthritis, obesity, limited mobility, or weakness—often complicate management. Lack of caregiver support may also hamper management. For positive outcomes, control of edema requires a commitment of the patient and/or caregiver in time, energy, as well as financial investment. Many times, a change in lifestyle is necessary.

The treatment of the swollen extremity involves removal of the edema fluid. All therapies involve assisting the body in mobilizing the fluid and removing it through the kidneys. From the very beginning, the task will be difficult if the patient has renal failure or renal insufficiency. In situations such as this, the nephrologist must be consulted to assist in the diuresis. In some cases, dialysis may be needed, at least on a temporary basis.

Treatment of extremity edema with diuretics is to be done judiciously. If the patient has symptoms of fluid overload and bilateral lower extremity swelling, diuretics will be of benefit. Unilateral extremity edema or edema without the presence of fluid overload will rarely be improved by diuretic therapy, and in these cases, diuretic use is not recommended. In the patient with lymphedema, the edema fluid has high protein levels, and diuretics will make the patient worse. Diuretics will mobilize the fluid, leaving the protein molecules behind and even more concentrated. This results in more damage to the subcutaneous tissues and makes removal of the highly concentrated protein-containing fluid even more difficult. In these cases, compression therapy and other specialized maneuvers are indicated but not diuretics.

Leg Elevation and Exercise

Another way to attempt to mobilize fluid out of an extremity is through elevation. There is no question that elevation of the swollen extremity will facilitate the mobilization of the fluid.[45,46] The theory of leg elevation is good, but the practice is more difficult. It is virtually impossible for a relatively active person to remain with an extremity elevated long enough to make a significant contribution to reduction of the edema.

CLINICAL WISDOM

Complete bed rest is discouraged. However, frequent 20- to 30-minute episodes of elevation throughout the day are recommended. People with cardiovascular conditions may have difficulty breathing when reclining with legs elevated. Those who are obese may have positioning problems with leg elevation. People at risk or who have edematous legs should not sit with legs dependent for long periods of time nor sit with legs crossed at the knees. These positions can slow the circulation and cause pooling of fluids at the ankles and lower legs. For those who sit in wheelchairs for extended times, elevation of foot risers is helpful.

When a person is up and down most of the time, the benefit of elevation is minimized. With that being said, it is always good to encourage the patient to elevate the swollen extremity as much as possible.

Another issue with extremity elevation has been the degree of the elevation. Many health-care practitioners encourage patients to elevate the legs "higher than the heart." That may be physiologically sound advice, but the position is difficult for persons to maintain due to discomfort. Having one's heart and head below the level of the feet is not a comfortable position in the first place and, in the second place, can result in cardiac and respiratory problems for many patients. Elevating the feet above the level of the hip joint, adequate fluid mobilization will occur. This is a position most people can manage, causes no physiologically untoward effects, and is easily accomplished by elevation of the foot of the bed.

Difficulties arise for patients who are unable to elevate their extremities such as those in wheelchairs for prolonged periods and those with neurologic impairments. In these cases, special efforts must be made to elevate the limbs to any degree possible. Extending the foot and leg rests on the wheelchair to manage some elevation is better than prolonged periods of dependency. Even patients with desk jobs requiring prolonged periods of sitting can be affected. We recommend that these patients put a small foot stool under the desk to get, at least, some elevation. An upside-down trash can placed under the desk can take the place of a foot stool if necessary.

Exercise is always recommended for the swollen extremity. The "calf muscle pump" is an important mechanism in managing fluid accumulation in everyone's lower extremities. This "pump" consists of five basic components: the superficial veins, the perforating veins (the connecting veins between the superficial and deep veins), the deep veins, the one-way valves in the veins, and the calf muscles. The calf muscles are confined by the fascia of the leg. When the muscles contract and enlarge, every structure in the leg which is surrounded by the fascia is compressed. This includes the arteries, veins, lymphatics, and soft tissues. When the veins and lymphatics are compressed, the fluid is forced out of them much like squeezing a tube of toothpaste. Because there are valves in these structures that only allow fluid to go in one direction, the pressure on these vessels forces blood and lymph toward the heart. This is an active process that helps overcome the pressures generated by sitting or standing. Unfortunately, this muscle pump does not function in patients who are unable to contract their muscles due to neurological disorders (stroke, spinal cord injury, spina bifida, coma, multiple sclerosis). Calf muscle pump function is also impaired in patients with chronic venous disease.[47–49] It, also, significantly malfunctions in patients with venous valve insufficiency. Since the valves are no longer directing the blood only toward the heart, each contraction of the muscle pump can force blood toward the foot or into the superficial veins of the leg in addition to the direction of the heart. When considering the toothpaste tube analogy, it is much like squeezing a tube of toothpaste that has no cap and has multiple holes in the sides and bottom of the tube.

When the calf muscle pump is not functioning, exercise either actively through walking, running, dancing, riding a bicycle, or similar activity or passively by way of ankle range of motion movements is recommended to increase the blood return to the heart.[50] The calf muscle pump can be activated by simply going from standing flat-footed to standing on one's toes and then returning to the flat-footed position. It has been recommended that this exercise should be repeated thirty times each hour to maximize calf muscle pump function.[51] Passive movements of the ankle in those unable to do it for themselves will also improve blood flow to the heart. Although increasing the calf muscle function and blood return to the heart will improve the swollen extremity, it has not been efficacious in improving healing of venous ulcers. The efficiency of the calf muscle pump with exercise can be greatly improved with the addition of compression bandages, especially in patients with venous valve failure and ambulatory venous hypertension (increased pressure in the lower extremity veins with standing or walking).

Compression Therapy

Compression therapy involves applying external pressure to a swollen extremity. It is designed to help mobilize the fluid in the tissues and overcome the ambulatory venous hypertension due to the damage to the venous system. Without any compression device, the skin is the only resistance to muscle contraction, and being elastic to some degree, it provides no significant compression to the extremity. Numerous techniques and bandages can be used, but they all have one thing in common—providing external compression to the swollen extremity. Compression therapy will improve swelling from both edema and lymphedema (high-protein fluid accumulation). Unfortunately, compression therapy alone is not a "magic bullet" for the swollen limb. When combined with treatment for the underlying condition, it can be effective. Because significant cooperation from the patient is required, successful treatment will involve persistence and understanding from both the patient and health-care provider.[43,44]

Preliminary Steps

There are several assessments that should occur prior to using compression therapy, including evaluation of the arterial circulation, underlying systemic conditions, and baseline leg

---

CLINICAL WISDOM

Preliminary Steps

One is always concerned about whether or not the patient can tolerate and be helped by compression therapy. Prior to instituting compression therapy, the health-care provider should be sure the patient is agreeable to its being used. Patients must be willing to tolerate the slight discomfort and inconvenience of wearing a compression garment or bandage for prolonged periods of time. Patients who insist that they must be able to take a shower and wash their legs each day will require a different approach than ones who can tolerate having a bandage on an extremity for as long as a week at a time. If the health-care provider tries to force the patient into a therapy he or she is not willing to do, both will be unhappy, and the patient will quickly become labeled as being noncompliant and difficult.[52]

---

characteristics. The patient considered for compression therapy should have previously been evaluated for the presence of arterial insufficiency, and lower extremity circulation should be assessed. The pulse exam includes locating and grading bilateral femoral, popliteal, dorsalis pedis, and posterior tibial artery pulses. A diminished or absent pulse indicates partial or complete arterial occlusion. If you are unable to palpate the dorsalis pedis or posterior tibial pulse, perform a Doppler assessment and ankle-brachial index (ABI). The results of the ABI allow determination of the amount of compression therapy that can be safely applied to reduce lower extremity edema. The ABI can be misleading in cases where the arteries are poorly compressible, such as in some cases of diabetes and severe atherosclerosis. In these situations, the ABI may be higher than would otherwise be expected.

Despite what is commonly thought, almost every patient with edema is a candidate for some type of compression therapy. Table 19.4 provides a basic guide to compression therapy for patients with peripheral arterial disease based on the ABI (measuring the systolic blood pressure at the ankle and the arm with a Doppler flow meter then dividing the ankle pressure by the arm pressure). If the patient has an ABI of 0.8 or higher, any compression system will be reasonable to use. If the ABI is between 0.5 and 0.8, the compression should be limited to no more than a three-layer bandage. If the ABI is below 0.5, many will say compression therapy should be used cautiously and under direction of an expert in edema management. Patients with edema must have a "reasonable" amount of circulation in order to develop edema. Patients with profoundly ischemic extremities rarely have edema. For this reason, essentially every patient with edema should have the benefit of carefully chosen compression therapy. If there is great concern about the circulation, the health-care practitioner should start with a mild, single-layer compression device such as an ace wrap or tube grip. The patient should be instructed to remove the bandage if the toes should turn blue or the leg becomes extremely painful. Surprisingly to many, this rarely occurs. The patient should be seen in two to three days to check the leg. The provider will be surprised that the swelling is better, and the patient's extremity has suffered no untoward effects. The patient will tell you how much better the extremity feels since the swelling is improved. This approach is supported by two clinical studies.[53,54]

In the first study, 24 patients from 63 to 92 years of age with lower extremity ulcers were evaluated. The mean ABI was 0.62 with a range from 0.3 to 0.78. All were treated with short-stretch compression bandages (bandages that have minimal stretch when the muscle contracts [see below]) with a mean treatment duration of 1.8 years. In these patients, digital blood pressure measurements were done before and after applying the short stretch compression. The mean toe pressure without compression was 47.6, and the mean toe pressure with compression was 47.9.[53] Using short-stretch compression did not affect the patient's already tenuous circulation.

The second study of short-stretch bandages in patients with arterial insufficiency (ABI between 0.5 and 0.8) showed similar results. Five patients had an ABI of 0.5 to 0.6, 4 patients had an ABI or 0.6 to 0.7, and 6 patients had an ABI of 0.7 to 0.8. All received a short-stretch compression bandage (Coban 2 Lite®, 3M) for up to 14 days with the bandages being changed every 4 days. The average pressure at the ankle under the bandage

| TABLE 19.4 | Compression Therapy, Circulation and Recommendations for Use |

Ankle-brachial Index	Bandage	Subbandage Pressure (mm Hg)	Classification of Compression	Recommendations for Use
≥0.8	• Custom stocking (Jobst™, Sigvaris™, or equivalent) • Four-layer bandage	40–50	High compression	Lymphedema
	• Custom stocking (Jobst™, Sigvaris™, or equivalent) • Four-layer bandage	30–40	Moderate compression	Edema with/without ulceration Edema that persists in spite of lower level compression options Ulcer failing to heal (may be venous or other)
	• Jobst™, Sigvaris™, or equivalent • Custom Fit • Double reverse elastic wrap • Four-layer bandage • Some three-layer bandages	25–35	Low to moderate compression	Edema secondary to venous insufficiency Edema in patient able to participate in exercise rehabilitation
0.7—0.5	• Jobst™, Sigvaris™, or equivalent • Two- or three-layer bandages • Elastic wraps • Paste bandage	17–25	Low compression	Nonambulatory with edema failing 16–19 mm Hg stockings Dependent edema Arterial disease with edema
	Jobst™, Sigvaris™, or equivalent TED stockings, prophylaxis only	16–18	Antiembolism stockings	Nonambulatory with edema Deep vein thrombosis prophylaxis
<0.5	Only with medical supervision	-		

was 28 mm Hg. At the end of the 14-day study, no patient had any pressure related skin damage, and no patient reported pain related to tissue hypoxia. Laser Doppler examination of the extremities showed that there was an increase in arterial perfusion of the tissues and a reduction of the edema.[54] This study confirms the utility of using selected compression therapy with patients with arterial insufficiency and edema of the extremity.

Another issue that comes up is whether or not to compress patients with systemic conditions causing edema, specifically heart failure, cellulitis, and deep vein thrombosis. In times past, patients with acute pulmonary edema from heart failure were treated with "rotating tourniquets" to impede venous return to the heart and prevent mobilization of the edema fluid. A tourniquet was placed on any two extremities tight enough to impede venous return. These were rotated to the other two extremities every 10 to 15 minutes in the hope that the digitalis (the only cardiac stimulatory agent available at the time) would take effect, making the heart pump strong enough to manage the fluid load. This obviously occurred before the time of diuretics. Today, most patients with heart failure are quickly placed on a number of medications to allow the heart to pump better and diuretics to eliminate the excess fluid from the body. If a patient is in heart failure, is fluid overloaded, and has pulmonary edema, compression therapy is not indicated. If the patient is being treated for heart failure and does not have pulmonary edema, compression therapy for lower extremity edema may be effective without untoward systemic circulatory effects. Many times, it is the only therapy that helps remove the excess fluid from the extremities and is essential if there is drainage from the legs.

RESEARCH WISDOM

Improving Arterial Flow with Compression

When the limb is swollen and the interstitial tissues are filled with fluid, the pressure compresses all the vessels in the tissues. This compression restricts blood flow in the vessels. With compression therapy and removal of the fluid, the pressure on the vessels decreases, allowing more flow through them. No matter how much flow is going into and out of the tissues before compression, the flow will be increased when the edema is reduced. One study has shown a 60% increase in arterial blood flow as measured by nuclear magnetic resonance flow studies following compression therapy.[55] Use of intermittent compression therapy in patients with critical limb ischemia and nonhealing wounds can produce complete wound healing and limb preservation; use of compression therapy can make even an ischemic extremity better.[56]

Controversy exists as to the role of compression therapy in the treatment of cellulitis. The swollen limb is more prone to develop streptococcal infection, the edema fluid in the limb is a good culture media for bacteria, and edema in the tissue slows diffusion of antibiotics from the vascular system to the tissues where the bacteria reside. The concern in compressing a leg with cellulitis is that bacteria-containing fluid will be pushed out of the leg into the circulation, making the patient septic. Fortunately, this is a very rare occurrence if at all. Compression therapy in conjunction with antibiotic therapy will speed the patient's recovery.

Another controversial issue is compressing the limb of a patient with thrombophlebitis. No one wants to "squeeze" a blood clot out of a leg resulting in a pulmonary embolus. However, health-care practitioners would have no hesitation about recommending leg elevation in a patient with thrombophlebitis. By facilitating blood flow out of the leg, would this make a pulmonary embolus more likely? Should a patient with thrombophlebitis be encouraged to ambulate? Would that activity predispose to more pulmonary emboli? The answer to all above questions is "no." Leg elevation does not predispose to pulmonary emboli nor does patient ambulation. After anticoagulation is begun, the incidence of pulmonary embolism is the same in patients who ambulate as in those who do not and is the same in patients who elevate their legs as in those who do not.[57] This is also true for compression therapy. Compression of the limb with thrombophlebitis results in increased venous flow preventing further clotting, occludes superficial veins that could clot, and does not cause an increase in pulmonary embolism.[58] For the treatment of the swollen extremity in the patient with thrombophlebitis, begin the patient's anticoagulation and compress the extremity. The only contraindication to compression therapy is pain in the leg so severe that compression cannot be tolerated. In that case, compression is begun as soon as symptoms will allow.

It is also essential to gather baseline data on lower extremity edema and any existing ulcers as this data will allow for evaluation of meaningful outcomes. There are a variety of methods to measure lower extremity edema including leg circumference measurements, subjective clinical assessment of pitting edema, patient self-report, volumetry, and high-frequency ultrasound measurement.

Lower leg circumference measurements can be obtained for multiple sites on the extremity or just for the ankle. Obtain a baseline measurement of the circumference in centimeters of both lower legs during the initial assessment prior to compression therapy, and at regular intervals throughout therapy. Comparing baseline measurements to follow-along measurements allows determination of the success of therapy to reduce edema. Use a measuring tape on the leg circumference at the largest portion of the calf (10 cm below the inferior rim of the patella) and the smallest portion of the ankle (5 cm above the superior rim of the lateral malleolus) as demonstrated in Figure 19.5. Use of a tension-controlled measuring tape can help minimize measurement error.[59] For consistent measurements, the ankle and leg sites can be marked with a semipermanent marker. Ankle measurements are associated with subjective clinical ratings of pitting edema, reliable, practical, and feasible in the clinical setting.[59]

Also assess for pitting edema using subjective clinical ratings. If the edema is pitting, grade the severity on a four-point scale from mild to very severe using the guide presented in Table 19.2. Figure 19.6 shows 4+ very severe pitting edema.

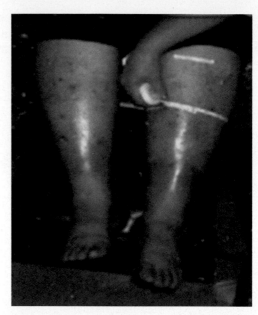

FIGURE 19.5 Correct measurement of an edematous leg. (Copyright © Evonne Fowler, RN, CNS, CWOCN.)

Patient self-report of edema presence, frequency, and severity over the previous week should be obtained at baseline as well as each follow-up visit. Patient self-report of edema characteristics is correlated with health-care provider assessments.[59] Questions to ask patients for self-report include but are not limited to the following[59]:

- Over the past week, how often did you have swelling of your ankles (from not at all to every day)?
- What level of swelling did you experience (from extreme to very little)?
- How much were you bothered by swelling in your ankles (from not all to extremely)?
- During what times of day did you have swelling in your ankles (from morning only to morning, afternoon, and evening)?
- Did swelling in your ankles limit your normal activity?

Volumetry involves use of commercially available equipment to determine the leg volume by capturing water displacement as a method of calculating the leg volume. A volumeter is

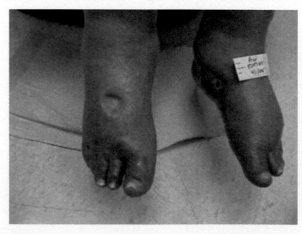

FIGURE 19.6 Severe 4+ pitting edema. (Copyright © Evonne Fowler, RN, CNS, CWOCN.)

a clear rectangular box or another container with a spout at the top of one side. The volumeter is filled with water until water rushes out the spout. The water is allowed to stabilize, and then the patient's foot and ankle are placed in the volumeter and the displaced water collected and measured. The amount of water displaced in milliliters equals the volume of the foot and ankle.[59] The difficulty with volumetry lies in the time required to set up equipment and conduct the measurements and problems with reproducibility of measures.[60]

Use of high-frequency ultrasound (HFU) measurement of dermal thickness has also been used to quantify edema.[61] Edema produces an increase in dermal thickness and HFU produces high-resolution images of the dermis that allows accurate measurements.[62] This process has been used to quantify edema in venous leg ulceration.[61,63] As with circumference measurements, a standard location is chosen for obtaining an ultrasound image. The patient is placed in a side-lying position, and images are obtained at 7.5 cm above the medial malleolus. The dermis is measured on the image from the epidermis to the interface of the dermis with the subcutaneous fat layer. HFU dermal measurements of edema are responsive to change and can be useful in monitoring edema reduction with compression therapy.[63]

The next item to be considered before compression therapy is instituted is which of the multiple compression systems will be best for the patient. One must be aware that there are different indications for each of the systems although many may be used for any cause of edema. All compression devices should provide a graded compression with the highest compression at the ankle gradually decreasing to the knee. Compression bandages that provide 35 to 45 mm Hg pressure at the ankle are considered "ideal" for treatment of edema and venous ulcers.[58] There are other classes of compression bandages that can be used successfully for the appropriate patient. Bandages providing <20 mm Hg pressure are considered to provide mild compression, 20 < 40 mm Hg medium compression, 40 < 60 mm Hg strong compression, and >60 mm Hg very strong compression.[64] Multilayer compression bandages have been considered the standard, but recent studies have shown that short-stretch bandages are at least as effective.[65,66]

Another approach to extremity compression involves the use of bandage systems that neither apply compression nor expand when the muscles of the leg contract. These bandage systems are called inelastic or short-stretch. In elastic compression bandage systems, a certain amount of pressure is applied to the leg, ideally 35 to 45 mm Hg,[64] to provide pressure to the extremity when the patient is sitting or walking. These systems are generally considered to be "long-stretch" bandages. Inelastic or short-stretch bandages conform to the leg and have minimal

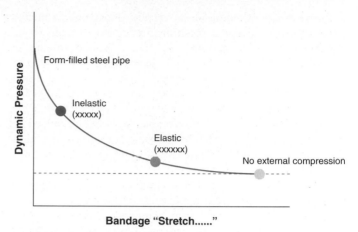

FIGURE 19.7 Dynamic pressure depends on bandage material. As shown in the graph, as the bandage material increases in inelasticity, the pressures on the leg muscles increase with walking activity. (From Mayrovitz HN, Larsen PB. Effects of compression bandaging on leg pulsatile blood flow. *Clin Physiol.* 1997;17(1):105–117.)

stretch. They are applied loosely with a pressure at the ankle when the patient is sitting of around 28 mm Hg pressure,[54] but when the patient is walking and the muscle is contracting and relaxing, there is no stretch. This allows high pressure to be generated on the leg. The pressure on the leg is directly related to the bandage materials—the more elastic, the less pressure generated on walking; the less elastic, the more pressure generated on walking as seen in Figure 19.7.[57] The short-stretch bandages generate significantly more pressure on the extremity when the patient is walking, yet when at rest, they provide minimal pressure. This implies that short-stretch bandages are ideal for patients who are mobile because of the high pressures generated on ambulation. It, also, implies that this type of bandage is best for the patient with arterial insufficiency (see above discussion) because the pressure when the patient is at rest is minimal. On the other hand, when patients are not very active and walk little, the long-stretch, more elastic bandage system may be the ideal choice since it provides significant pressure at rest even though it supplies less pressure when the patient is walking (see Fig. 19.8).

In today's environment, there is a great push to have patients take care of themselves, i.e. self-care. While self-care is the ideal,

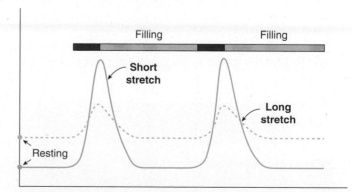

FIGURE 19.8 Working versus resting pressures—the role of compression material. As shown, the pressures achieved with short stretch bandages are higher during activity. (From Mayrovitz HN, Larsen PB. Effects of compression bandaging on leg pulsatile blood flow. *Clin Physiol.* 1997;17(1):105–117.)

CLINICAL WISDOM

What is the Best Compression Pressure for the Individual Patient?

The answer is that the best compression pressure for each patient is the one the patient will tolerate. It may not be what is best for the problem, but if the patient refuses to wear the compression device or takes it off as soon as he or she leaves the office, it is worthless. Remember, some compression is better than none.

in the treatment of venous ulcer over 50% of patients are unable to bandage their own legs, resulting in a decreased quality of life and a decreased healing rate.[67] As a result, before you choose the type of compression therapy for your patient with edema or an ulcer, find out about the patient's support system at home and their ability to return for follow-up. If a patient is unable to return to the wound center on a regular basis, arrangements must be made for the compression bandages to be changed by home health nurses. If this is not possible, types of compression that can be managed by the patient must be selected even if it is not the first choice of therapy.[68]

Frequency of bandage change should be considered before choosing the compression bandage system for the patient. As noted above, the majority of the compression devices are not "user friendly" and require a trained health-care provider to apply them. Most of the compression bandages can be worn for about seven days. The time for bandage change is mainly dependent on the amount of drainage from the leg. If there is no drainage and the compression is for edema or lymphedema only, once per week is adequate. Patients with draining wounds will need bandage changes when the bandage gets wet. This may be only one or two days initially, but as the drainage and edema resolve, bandage changes may be spaced further apart. Many patients with open wounds with or without drainage may begin to complain of a bad odor from the bandage. This is also an indication to change the bandage.

Compression Stockings

Compression stockings or compression hose provide a graded compression from the ankle to below the knee to assist with mobilizing the edema fluid. There are four classes of compression stockings based on the amount of compression they provide, ranging from 14 to 18 mm Hg compression to 40 to 50 mm Hg compression. (Exhibit 19.2). There is debate about which is the most effective compression stocking, but, without any doubt, the most effective stockings are the ones that are worn. The literature supports the use of the 30 to 40 mm Hg compression because this is a good compromise between compression, comfort, and ease of use. The majority of compression stockings are ready-made and are reasonably priced. Many patients with large or unusually shaped legs may require custom-made compression stockings. These are more effective than the ones that do not fit the patient. Unfortunately, they are significantly more expensive. Compression stockings come in a variety of colors and styles to accommodate as many patient preferences as possible.

The compression stockings can cover the leg to the knee, to the middle of the thigh, or to the groin and lower abdomen in the form of panty hose. Compression stockings to the knee are adequate for most swollen extremities. Compression stockings that are the "thigh-high" variety tend to make too much pressure around the knee and compress the midthigh too much if they are to stay in place. If upper leg compression is needed from stockings, we recommend the panty hose variety.

The difficulty of getting the support stockings on the foot and leg is the main problem with their use. Because they fit snugly, they are difficult to stretch and to slide over the foot and heel. Many patients are unable to reach their feet, many do not have the arm and hand strength to apply the stockings, and many feel it is just too uncomfortable and too much trouble to wear them. There are devices such as the stocking butler shown in Figures 19.9A,B to assist in getting the stockings on the leg, but these have their own difficulties in terms of setup and ease of use. Another method is to have patients first place a thin sock or lady's knee-high stocking on the leg and pull the compression stocking over that. This allows the compression stocking to slide over the foot and ankle easier as shown in Fig. 19.10A–D. There is a company (Carolon®) who makes a two-layer support stocking. The thin inner layer provides 16 to 18 mm Hg compression. The outer layer easily slides over the inner layer with the combination of layers providing 30 to 40 mm Hg compression. This product has been much easier for the patient to get on than a snug, single-layer product of the same compression.

When compression stockings are used to treat edema associated with a venous ulcer or other open wound, additional problems are noted. When an open wound or ulcer is present, a dressing must be used to cover, treat, and protect it. It is very difficult to get compression stockings over a wound dressing without displacing it. If the wound is draining, the drainage may soil the stocking. The stockings then have to be washed more frequently, thus shortening their life span. The purchase of additional pairs of stockings is not cheap. For this reason, patients with open wounds and edema may be treated with the appropriate dressing followed by compression bandages until the wounds are healed. At that point in the patient's treatment, compression stockings can be recommended.

Elastic Compression Bandages

Compression bandages come in various types and degrees of compression. The variety allows the health-care provider to choose the compression bandage system most appropriate for the patient.

Single-Layer Elastic Compression Bandages

Single-layer compression bandages include the familiar ace wrap. Prior to the invention of rubber and elastic, compression could only be applied by tight wraps or garments that laced up around the leg. The use of rubberized compression devices are reported as early as 1877. In a report in 1878, rubber compression bandages promised to "effect a revolution in the treatment of eczema and ulceration of the leg."[69] The author reported 27 cases of various types of wounds and edema, all of whom did so well that the "claims are so extraordinary as to possibly give rise to a doubt as to their truth in the minds of those who were not assured of the writer's veracity." (p. 14)[69] Thus began the treatment of edema and venous ulcers with compression bandages that could stretch.

Currently, the most frequently used single-layer compression bandage is the ace wrap. It is readily available, inexpensive, and easy to use. It is useful when only mild compression

EXHIBIT 19.2	
Classes of Compression Stockings	
Class 1	14–19 mm Hg
Class 2	19–24 mm Hg
Class 3	25–35 mm Hg
Class 4	40–50 mm Hg

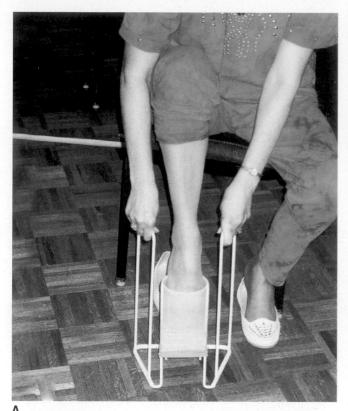
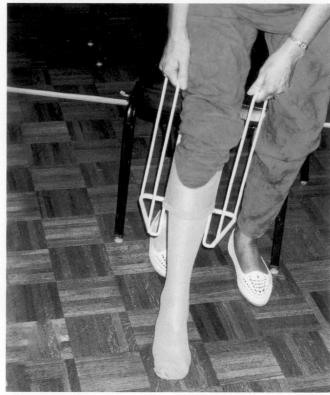

A   B

FIGURE 19.9 **A,B:** Using a stocking butler to apply compression stockings. (Copyright © Evonne Fowler, RN, CNS, CWOCN.)

of the extremity is needed. It can be removed by the patient and reapplied as desired. That is also one of the disadvantages of the dressing. Since it is easily applied, many untrained people feel they can adequately apply it. This leads to inappropriate application and inadequate pressure gradients from distal to proximal. The ace wrap is prone to slip, which requires frequent reapplication at best and can cause significant limb constriction at worst. Attempts to help these problems led to the development of the Coban® elastic wrap, which is similar to an ace wrap but adheres to itself minimizing slippage. Because the bandage sticks to itself, removal and reapplication is essentially impossible.

In an effort to combine convenience with single-layer compression, several elastic tubular bandages have been developed. These generally provide mild, consistent compression and are easy to slide on and keep on the extremity. When they no longer maintain their compression, they are discarded and replaced since the cost is very reasonable.

Multilayer Elastic (Long-stretch) Compression Bandages

Multilayer compression is just what the name implies—external compression of the extremity supplied by multiple layers of bandage. Multilayer compression can be supplied by two-layer, three-layer, and/or four-layer bandages systems—each layer adding additional compression. Because of this, multilayer bandages are considered to provide moderate to high compression. Obviously, this depends on the person applying the bandages. A recent study of skilled, experienced wound care nurses showed that 34.9% of the compression bandages they applied had insufficient pressure to be effective (<20 mm Hg

pressure). None were applied too tightly (>60 mm Hg pressure). Interestingly, 56.7% of the bandages with <20 mm Hg pressure were applied by wound care nurses with more than 10 years' experience. After institution of a training program that allowed the nurses to wrap extremities and have immediate feedback as to the subbandage pressure, only 4.8% of the bandages had insufficient pressure (<20 mm Hg pressure), but now 12.7% of bandages had >60 mm Hg pressure.[58] It appears that application of compression bandages is a skill that must be learned and practiced with accurate feedback to ensure that the bandage is being applied properly. Since multilayer compression systems provide significant pressure at rest, the patient must be educated as to potential problems. If the patient feels the bandage is too tight, we recommend sitting or lying with the feet elevated to see if the symptom will abate. Many times the patient is on his/her feet too much, the leg swells, and the bandage is perceived as too tight. If the tightness does not resolve after about two hours of elevation of the extremity or the leg is frankly painful, the patient is instructed to remove the bandage and call the health-care provider. The patient should be instructed about the possibility of the toes becoming numb or blue (cyanotic). These are indications for the patient to remove the bandage and call the health-care provider.

As health-care providers, we must ensure that everyone applying compression bandages is adequately trained. The inadvertent application of a multilayer compression bandage that is too tight is not all that uncommon. Keep track of how many complaints are forthcoming about tight bandages to see if more staff training may be needed. Fortunately or unfortunately, as the study above showed, the majority of bandages are

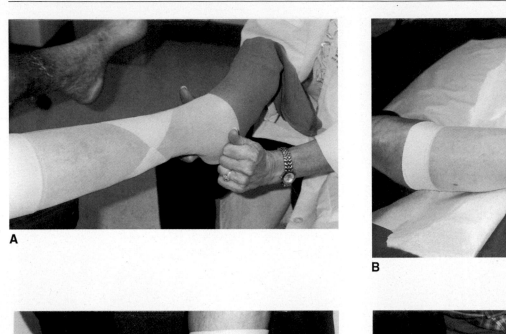

A

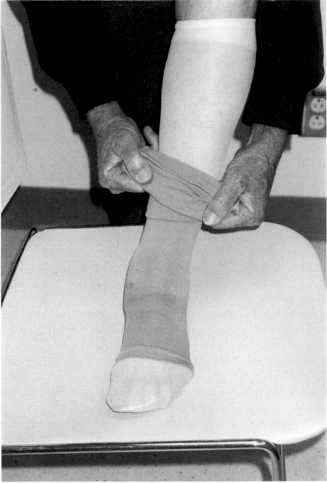

C

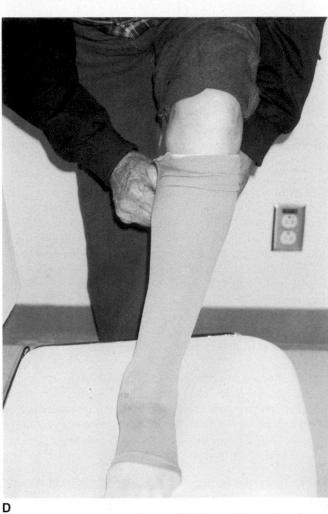

D

FIGURE 19.10 Applying compression stocking. **A.** Turn stocking inside out. A liner makes pulling on stocking easier. (Note dressing under the lining. The liner keeps the dressing positioned correctly.) **B.** Work stocking gradually up leg, smoothing out all wrinkles. (Stockings are available with or without toes.) **C.** Knee-high stockings halfway up showing zipper rear closure. **D.** Stocking extended to below the bend on the knee. Patient is positioning stocking. (Copyright © Evonne Fowler, RN, CNS, CWOCN.)

applied too loosely as providers try not to make the compression bandages too tight.

Many patients seem to be very "sensitive" to compression bandages and will tolerate minimal pressure on the extremity. This can be a source of frustration for the health-care provider, but remember the adage "some compression is better than no compression." Explain to the patient that less compression may not be as effective, but it is important to have some compression to help with the edema in the extremity. It is interesting that many times, over time, compression can be gradually increased until the original compression level is attained.

Inelastic (Short-stretch) Compression Bandages

Inelastic or short-stretch compression bandages do not stretch, but generate compression when the muscle of the extremity contracts. Since they do not stretch, they are applied loosely with minimal subbandage pressure. The classical short-stretch bandage is the Unna Boot developed in 1887 by Dr. Paul Gerson Unna, a young 37-year-old German physician. The original Unna boot was a gauze roll impregnated with zinc oxide. The bandage was applied directly over the skin and ulcer, if present. The bandage was covered with another gauze wrap to minimize getting the paste everywhere until it solidified. Since this bandage provided no compression unless the patient was walking, Dr. Duke at Duke University added a single-layer elastic bandage (ace wrap or Coban® wrap) over the paste bandage. This is the "Unna boot" bandage as used today, technically a "Duke boot." The bandage functions as described previously to decrease the edema in an extremity and is typically worn for about seven days before being changed. The paste bandages of today do contain zinc oxide, but may also contain calamine lotion, glycerin, aloe vera, and other moisturizing agents. One little-considered fact about the paste bandage is that it is well tolerated by patients with upper extremity edema and lymphedema.

Many patients who have chronic swelling of an extremity especially if it is due to lymphedema or chronic venous disease may develop dry, scaly skin. This can result in itching and cracking of the skin (see Fig. 19.11). The moisture in the paste bandage of the Unna (Duke) boot helps treat the dryness and relieves symptoms while providing compression. Figure 19.12A,B show an example of the Unna boot's effect on dry, scaly skin. Moisturizers with layer wraps can also improve skin irritation, dryness, and cracking (see Fig. 19.13A,B).

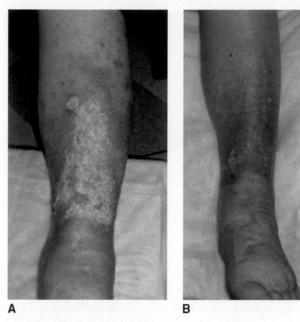

A   B

FIGURE 19.12 A,B. Effect of Unna boot on venous dermatitis and skin irritation. **A.** Edematous leg due to venous insufficiency with dermatitis. (Copyright © Terry A. Treadwell, MD.) **B.** The same leg as in Figure 19.12A after 5½ months of therapy with compression therapy using Unna Boot. (Copyright © Terry A. Treadwell, MD.)

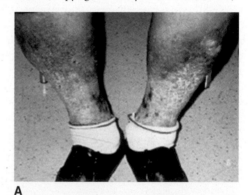

A

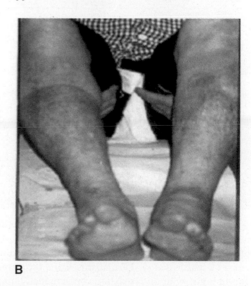

B

FIGURE 19.13 Effect of moisturizers on dry cracks and fissures. **A.** Edematous legs with dry skin and wounds present. **B.** Same legs as in Figure 19.13A, 1 week after using a moisturizing cream and multilayer wraps. (Copyright © Evonne Fowler, RN, CNS, CWOCN.)

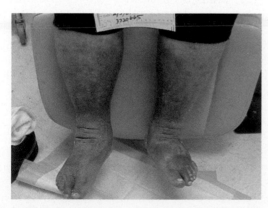

FIGURE 19.11 Bilateral edematous legs with dry cracks and fissures present. (Copyright © Evonne Fowler, RN, CNS, CWOCN.)

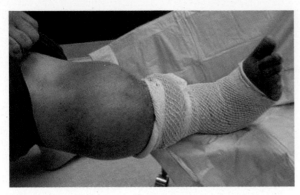

FIGURE 19.14 Example of compression bandage slippage from inappropriate application. (Copyright © Terry A Treadwell, MD.)

A new type of short-stretch compression bandage has recently been introduced, the Coban 2® and Coban 2 Lite® compression bandages (3M, Minneapolis, MN). The inner layer is foam fused to a layer of nonstretching Coban®. After this layer is wrapped over the extremity, it is covered with a special short-stretch Coban®. The Coban® layers stick together, providing stability for the bandage. The foam against the skin provides comfort and minimizes slippage of the bandage. With this short-stretch compression system, a primary dressing on the wound is needed if one is present. In evaluations of both short-stretch compression bandages and long-stretch elastic compression bandages, the Coban 2® and Coban 2 Lite® bandages were deemed more comfortable and had less slippage than other bandages tested.[66] (Figs. 19.14 and 19.15).

Since Coban 2® and Coban 2 Lite® are short-stretch bandages, they are useful for patients who are ambulatory and patients who have arterial insufficiency.[54] It is comfortably worn

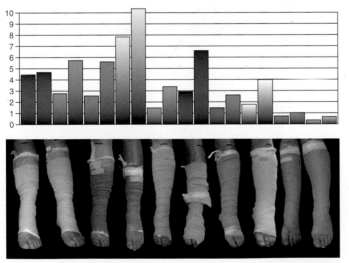

FIGURE 19.15 This graph presents data from a 48-hour wear test of 10 different compression bandage systems. All bandages were applied by experts for each system on one leg of 5 to 6 healthy volunteer participants ($n = 72$ participants). Participants wore the compression bandages for 48 hours with no restrictions on activities. Slippage was measured in centimetres at 24 and 48 hours. Photographs were taken at the same times to document slippage. The graph shows slippage in centimeters after 24 (first bar) and 48 (second bar) hours for each of the 10 compression bandage systems. (Copyright © Terry A Treadwell, MD.)

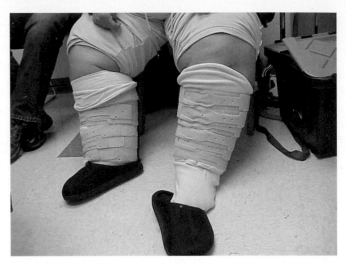

FIGURE 19.16 CircAid™ in place.

on the upper extremity when upper extremity compression bandaging is needed.

Other inelastic systems that provide short-stretch compression are removable for the patient to wash the leg and care for any wound or ulcer that might be present. These are beneficial for patients who may have difficulty returning for routine bandage changes. The CircAid Compression Bandage System® (Coloplast, Marietta, GA) is a nonelastic, adjustable system consisting of a legging with interlocking, nonelastic bands fastened with Velcro (Fig. 19.16). The garment can be removed for wound care and cleaning of the leg. It adjusts to the size of the leg as the edema resolves.

A second, similar device is the ReidSleeve® that is a custom-made device for the extremity, which can also be taken on and off and adjusted as needed.

The convenience of these devices should be apparent, but they do require training to apply them correctly. The cost of the devices also limits their use.

Compression Pump Therapy

The use of compression pumps for the treatment of edema, lymphedema, and venous ulcers is an additional therapeutic device for use in these patients but is generally considered an adjunctive therapy used with other compression systems. This device includes a sleeve with multiple air chambers (from three to ten) which fits over the entire leg from the foot to the groin. Once in place on the patient's extremity, the air pump is activated, and the chambers are inflated in sequence from the foot to the groin. After the sequence is completed, the chambers deflate only to reinflate and repeat the sequence. The pressure generated by the device is about 45 to 60 mm Hg at the ankle and progressively decreases in each chamber to the groin. The treatment may last one to two hours several times per day.

The therapy is effective in reducing edema but is inconvenient to use since the patient is confined to the bed or chair during the treatment periods. Following the treatment session, compression bandaging or compression stockings are needed to prevent a rapid recurrence of the edema. Unfortunately, this therapy is not covered by most insurance plans, making it difficult for the individual patient to obtain this expensive equipment.

Skin Care

Compression bandages and the diseases that result in their use can be very hard on the skin. Rashes, dryness, cracking, and other skin problems are not uncommon. Even healthy skin develops a dry, scaly appearance after many weeks under a compression bandage changed only once a week. Chronic venous disease can provide its own special problems with the skin of the lower extremities. Dryness and cracking of the skin is a frequently seen in patients with autonomic peripheral neuropathy with or without diabetes. Many times medications put on ulcers or wounds will result in skin problems, especially Neosporin® ointment. Wounds with significant drainage can cause skin breakdown from the retention of the protease-containing fluid on the skin (maceration). All of these issues need to be addressed when the patient has a bandage changed. Wash the extremity with soap and water followed by applying a moisturizing cream to the skin of the entire leg before reapplying the bandage. If the skin is too moist from wound fluid drainage, skin protection is also applied.

Consideration must be given to the development of an allergy to some portion of the compression bandage system. Patients may develop an allergy to Unna paste boots, cotton-containing bandages, ace wraps, and Coban® wraps as seen in Figures 19.17 and 19.18. Allergic reactions can occur with almost any product put on the skin. When this occurs, the

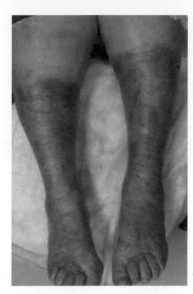

FIGURE 19.18 Allergy to ace wraps. (Copyright © Terry A Treadwell, MD.)

allergy is treated, and a different compression system is used to treat the edema or lymphedema.

Lower leg edema can cause skin problems such as pruritus, dryness, scaling, cracks, fissures, oozing of fluid from under the skin, and open wounds as shown in Figures 19.3, 19.4, and 19.19. Healthy skin is clean, dry, and supple. To keep the skin on the legs and feet soft, wash daily with a mild soap and water, dry, and apply a moisturizing cream. After washing the feet, while the skin is still damp and soft, use a coarse emery board to reduce callus formation on the feet. A foot file or emery board can also be used to smooth the nail edges and reduce the nail thickness. Keeping the legs and feet warm can improve circulation. Appropriate shoes or supportive slippers should be worn to avoid injury to the feet.

Encourage patients to treat dry, itching, and scaly skin by applying a warm oil treatment to the feet and legs daily for 1 week. Before reclining for the night, bath or shower. After drying off, rub warm mineral oil thoroughly into the feet and legs. Cover the feet and legs with a plastic wrap (i. e., Saran Wrap) to seal in the oil. Put on a pair of cotton socks. Remove the plastic wrap in the morning, wash and dry the feet well, and apply a

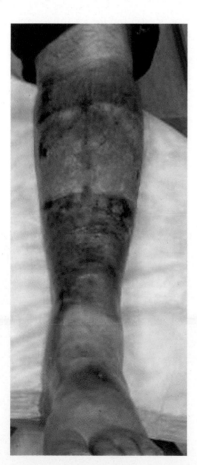

FIGURE 19.17 Allergy to cotton wrap from compression bandage system. Reprinted from Braden, B. (1987), a conceptual schema for the study of the etiology of pressure sores. Rehabilitation Nursing, 12(1), 9, with permission of the Association of Rehabilitation Nurses. Copyright © 1987 by the Association of Rehabilitation Nurses.

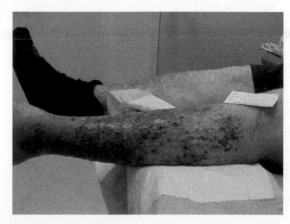

FIGURE 19.19 Venous dermatitis with weeping and oozing. (Copyright © Evonne Fowler, RN, CNS, CWOCN.)

thick moisturizing cream on the skin. Figure 19.13A,B shows the same legs after this treatment. If skin maceration occurs, discontinue the plastic wrap.

If a fungal infection is present, an antifungal cream may be necessary. In severe cases of fungal infection and infection of the nails, an oral antifungal agent may also be employed.

Figures 19.3 and 19.4 show severe cases of venous *dermatitis*, a condition that occurs due to the inflammation of the skin of the lower legs caused by chronic venous insufficiency and edema. Symptoms include itching, scaling, hyperpigmentation, and sometimes ulceration. Symptoms can be exacerbated when skin in the edematous extremity is subject to soaps, chemicals, or adhesives. Venous dermatitis may be extremely painful, with blistering and weeping skin. Using compression to control swelling can promote healing: either a paste bandage or multilayer wrap may be applied. The paste bandage has a calamine or zinc oxide base that aids in the healing of the irritated skin by its soothing and drying effect. It can also decrease the itching of the skin. Place a compression wrap (Coban) or a short-stretch bandage over the paste wrap to provide sustained compression. The multilayer wrap absorbs more fluid and provides sustained compression over a longer period of time. Apply a cream or advanced wound care product to the irritated skin prior to applying the multilayer wrap.

Venous dermatitis can also be treated with a 1-week course of Domeboro Soaks. Domeboro is an astringent agent made of aluminum acetate and used as a drying agent to decrease weeping, irritated, and itchy skin. Encourage patients to soak the legs and feet for 15 minutes twice a day (i.e., morning and evening). A soft foam, cloth, or brush can be used to cleanse the irritated skin. Dry the skin and apply an ointment to the irritated skin and cover with a petroleum-type dressing and a compression wrap. Apply a topical antibiotic ointment (Bactroban™) in the morning. Bactroban™ has documented effectiveness against resistant staph and strep and other common organisms found on the skin. Avoid Neosporin and bacitracin ointment, as they are known skin sensitizers. After the ointment, apply a petroleum-based dressing to keep the ointment in contact with the skin. Cover with a roller gauze and apply a compression wrap. In the evening, repeat the same procedure but use a corticosteroid ointment (fluocinonide, triamcinolone, or over-the-counter 0.1% hydrocortisone) in place of the antibiotic ointment. Do not apply the corticosteroid to open wounds. A course of oral antibiotics and/or prednisone may also be necessary.[70]

Special Concerns in Lymphedema

The swollen leg due to lymphedema needs special considerations. Lymphedema fluid is edema fluid containing high levels of protein. Lymphedema can be due to the lack or deficiency of normal lymphatic channels in the extremity from birth. Secondary causes of lymphedema result from damage to normal lymphatic channels. The causes of lymphedema are listed in Table 19.5. The treatment for lymphedema involves removal of the fluid and protein from the tissues. Lymphedema cannot be cured, and requires lifelong treatment to control symptoms that, if left untreated, will progress. One of the main problems is that, by the time patients with lymphedema are seen, their condition is usually pronounced. The aim of treatment is to stabilize the edema and empower the patient with the necessary skills to undertake self-care. Four components of treatment are used to achieve this goal: care of the skin, compression and support, exercise and elevation, and lymphatic massage.

Good skin care is essential for lymphedema patients, whose skin shows several characteristic qualities.

- The skin becomes brown in color.
- The texture of the skin has a woody hardness, with superficial hyperkeratosis, as shown in Figures 19.20 and 19.21. It may be fissured or folded. Mushroom-like papules of tissue can be present.
- Edema is usually nonpitting and involves the feet as well as the legs. The diameter from the ankle to the knee is almost uniform rather the inverted champagne bottle–like fibrosis seen in long-standing venous disease.

TABLE 19.5	Classification of Lymphedema Based on Causes	
Primary Lymphedema	**Secondary Lymphedema**	

Congenital (onset before 1 year old)
   Nonfamilial
   Familial (Milroy Disease)
	Filariasis	

Praecox (onset 1–35 years old)
   Nonfamilial
   Familial
	Lymph node excision +/– irradiation	

Tarda (onset after 35 years old)	Tumor invasion	
	Infection	
	Trauma	

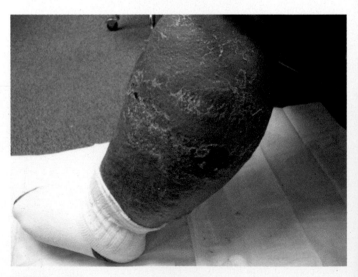

FIGURE 19.20 Lymphedema with woody hardness and superficial hyperkeratosis present. (Copyright © Evonne Fowler, RN, CNS, CWOCN.)

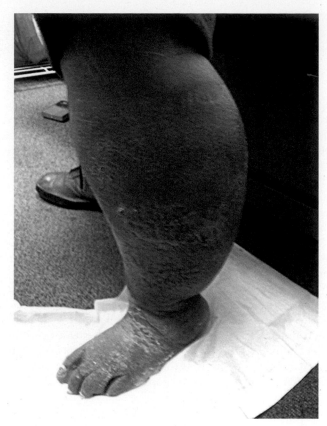

FIGURE 19.21 Lymphedema, notice the mushroom-like papules on the lower leg. (Copyright © Evonne Fowler, RN, CNS, CWOCN.)

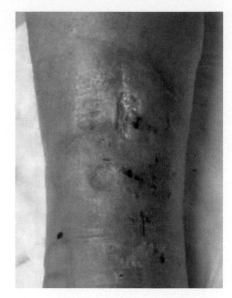

FIGURE 19.22 Acute postoperative wound following open reduction internal fixation of a leg fracture. Characteristics of edema and lymphedema can be seen. (Copyright © Terry A Treadwell, MD.)

- Infections may be present: Swelling of the feet with close apposition of the toes provides an ideal environment for fungal growth. Fissures can act as portals of entry for bacterial infection that can progress to cellulitis.[71]

Use of some or all of the skin care techniques just described has not been shown to provide significant benefits for patients with lymphedema unless other interventions are also implemented. These other measures include compression and support, as discussed earlier, exercise and elevation, also discussed earlier, and lymphatic massage.

Lymphatic massage, also referred to as *complex decongestive physiotherapy*, is a particular type of therapeutic massage and requires a skilled and certified therapist to instruct and administer.[3] It is now the standard of care for lymphedema in this country and has been the standard in other countries for some time.[3,72] Usually, a patient with lymphedema will be started on a course of complex decongestive physiotherapy along with temporary short-stretch compression bandages. This is combined with exercise and meticulous skin care to prevent infection that will further compromise the lymphatics. After the course is finished, the patient will be graduated to a compression garment, exercise, and elevation. Impressive results can be obtained by a dedicated, meticulous lymphedema therapist and a dedicated patient. Massage may be reinstituted for an acute exacerbation.

Although generally not appreciated, lymphedema is a problem with each wound we treat. When the tissues are damaged in any way by trauma, operation, or ulceration, the surrounding lymphatics are damaged. Thus, the periwound edema that is seen is mostly lymphedema and if optimum wound healing is to be realized, then compression therapy may be indicated (see Fig. 19.22).

OUTCOME MEASURES

Determining the effectiveness of therapy for edema involves comparison of baseline edema measurements with follow-along measurements and evaluation of patient self-report data. It is recommended to use more than one measure of edema and to include a process measure to evaluate outcomes of edema care. Outcome measures may include the following:

- Decrease in leg or ankle circumference
- Percent decrease in leg volume
- Decrease in subjective clinical pitting edema assessment rating
- Improvement in patient self-report edema measures
- Improvement in venous skin dermatitis

Process measures may also be helpful, especially for patients and caregivers for whom the treatment is challenging. For example, appropriate process measures might include

- Increased leg elevation time duration
- Increased frequency of leg elevation periods
- Increase in compression pressure tolerance
- Increase in length of time compression used/worn

Because edema management is often a lifelong process, setting realistic mutual goals for treatment with the patient and caregiver is prudent and may result in more positive outcomes.

SELF-CARE TEACHING GUIDELINES

Individualize patient and caregiver instructions in self-care to the cause of edema, exercise, elevation, compression, and skin care routine, signs and symptoms requiring health-care

CASE STUDY

Case Study #1:

A 47-year-old lady was seen with progressively increasing swelling of the left leg for 6 months. The patient denies any pain in the leg but does have a feeling of "heaviness" in the leg. She has noted an 11-pound weight gain in the past 6 months. She denied swelling of either lower extremity prior to the onset of the current symptoms. Her only abdominal complaint was that of mild constipation that had been a problem since the birth of her two children. The patient does work but has a desk job with minimal standing or walking. She has no history of recent operation or injury. She has no history of thrombophlebitis or "blood clots." There is no family history of clotting disorders. She has no history of cardiac, renal, or liver disease. She takes no medication except for birth control pills. She has no known allergies.

Examination:

The patient appears to be her stated age and shows no visible sign of chronic disease. Examination of the heart and lungs reveals no significant problems. Abdominal examination detected some mild lower abdominal tenderness, but no masses were felt. Examination of the extremities detected a normal right leg with no swelling. The left leg was swollen from the groin to the ankle with 3+ pitting edema. There was neither discoloration nor ulceration of the extremity. There was mild tenderness over the femoral triangle in the groin and the entire lower extremity. The patient had no detectable varicose veins. All arterial pulses in both legs were normal. Semmes-Weinstein exam of both lower extremities showed normal sensation.

The patient admitted that her family physician had ordered a venous ultrasound examination of the left leg, which had been reported as "normal." She had been treated with diuretics and thigh-length support stockings with no improvement in the edema.

In view of the negative ultrasound and swelling of the entire leg, a pelvic ultrasound was ordered. A 7-cm, solid left ovarian mass overlying and compressing the left iliac artery and vein was detected. The patient underwent operative removal of the mass that proved to be a benign ovarian teratoma on pathological exam. Postoperatively the edema of the left leg resolved and has not returned in the 8-month follow-up period.

CASE STUDY

Case Study #2:

A 68-year-old lady was referred to the wound center for treatment of what was called "bilateral venous ulcers." The patient had massively swollen legs with splitting of the skin and large volumes of drainage from each leg. She was wearing towels around the legs in an attempt to keep the fluid from draining on her floor. This condition developed over a one-month period of time and had been ongoing for 4 months. Despite all attempts, her physician and cardiologist had been unable to control the problem. The patient walked with difficulty because of the size and heaviness of the legs and the drainage. The patient had a history of congestive heart failure but was controlled with diuretics and cardiac medications. She had no recent episodes of pulmonary edema, shortness of breath, or other symptoms of cardiac decompensation. The patient had no history of renal disease, diabetes mellitus, or operative procedures. The patient is retired from a job with the state government. She has no history of thrombophlebitis, "blood clots," or pulmonary embolus. She is taking multiple medications including a calcium channel blocking agent and diuretics.

Examination:

The patient appears not to be feeling well and has a puddle of wound fluid on the floor around each leg. She has no neck vein distention. Examination of the lungs reveals decreased breath sounds but no rales or rhonchi. Cardiac exam does not reveal any arrhythmias or gallops. Examination of the abdomen is negative. Both lower extremities are swollen from the toes to the knees with 4+ pitting edema. There are multiple areas of drainage on each leg from sites of skin disruption. The patient has normal arterial pulses in each lower extremity. Both legs are tender from the swelling, but no redness is noted.

Despite the previous physician's suggestion, it was felt the patient was in mild, decompensated congestive heart failure. Electrocardiogram was negative, but her chest x-ray showed signs of early congestive heart failure.

The patient was treated with additional diuretics and cardiostimulatory agents to help remove the additional fluid from the body. The legs were treated with a dressing that absorbs large amounts of fluid (Sorbion®) and four-layer compression bandages changed every three days for the first week and then weekly thereafter. With this regimen, the excess drainage was controlled and the edema improved. After 4 weeks of this therapy, the legs stopped draining and mild edema (2+ bilaterally) was present. Continued compression bandaging for an additional 2 weeks reduced the edema even further. The patient was then changed to compression stockings (to-the-knee) without recurrence of the edema. The new cardiac medications were continued.

TABLE 19.6	Self-Care Teaching Guidelines for Edema Management

Self-Care Guidelines Specific to Edema Management	Instructions Given (Date/Initials)	Demonstration or Review of Material (Date/Initials)	Return Demonstration or Verbalizes Understanding (Date/Initials)
1. Cause and Type of edema			
2. Significance of edema			
3. Exercise plan—graduated walking program			
4. Lower extremity elevation procedures			
5. Compression			
a. Type of compression—stockings, wraps, Unna boots			
b. Application of compression			
c. Frequency of compression dressing changes			
6. When to remove compression and notify the health-care provider:			
a. Signs and symptoms of poor circulation in toes (purple/black toes, loss of sensation in toes)			
b. Pain not relieved by leg elevation			
c. Compression dressing odor, evidence of wound drainage on dressing, dressing slippage to ankle			
7. Importance of follow-up with health-care provider			
8. Compression therapy-ongoing			
a. Pumps			
b. Stockings			
c. Other devices			
9. Skin care regimen			
a. avoidance of chemicals and harsh soaps/detergents and solutions on edematous extremity			
b. Use of mineral oil and moisturizers or Domoboro soaks or other recommended strategies for skin breakdown.			

provider attention, the patient's wound if appropriate, the patient's learning style and coping mechanisms, and the ability of the patient/caregiver to perform procedures. Table 19.6 presents self-care teaching guidelines related to edema management.

CONCLUSION

Edema is not a disease but a symptom of an underlying condition. Before appropriate therapy can be instituted, the correct cause of the edema must be identified. Most diagnoses of edema can be made by a careful, thorough history and physical examination. Adjunctive tests are available to aid in the diagnosis when uncertainty exists. If the appropriate diagnosis is not identified, therapy is unlikely to result in a lasting improvement and will cause frustration on the part of the patient and the health-care provider. The mainstay of therapy for the swollen extremity is compression therapy in addition to treatment of the underlying cause. Multiple types of compression therapy are available today, each with its own good points and bad points. The health-care provider must determine which is the one most suited for the patient and will give the best result. Without patient compliance, no therapy will be successful. Experience, patience, and flexibility are most important for the health-care provider attempting to treat the patient with edema.

ADDITIONAL RESOURCES

- Moffatt C. World Wide Wounds [serial online]. http://www.worldwidewounds.com/2006/june/Moffatt/Four-Layer-Bandage-System-Part3.html
- Macdonald, JM & Geyer, MJ (Eds.) Wound and Lymphoedema Management, 2010 World Health Organization.

REVIEW QUESTIONS

1. Which of the following statements about edema is correct?
   A. Edema is a diagnosis.
   B. Edema is always caused by medication side effects.
   C. The majority of edema is caused by venous disease.
   D. The major treatment for edema is diuretic therapy.

2. The Kaposi-Stemmer sign is
   A. an inability to pinch a fold of skin on the dorsum of the foot at the base of the second toe which is a diagnostic tool for differentiating edema from lymphedema
   B. a sign of venous valvular disease
   C. a diagnostic test for determining arterial circulation status
   D. pinching the fold of skin on the dorsum of the foot at the base of the second toe to assess for pain

3. Treatment of venous edema includes which of the following?
   A. Diuretics and topical dressings
   B. Compression and a low sodium diet
   C. Exercise, compression, and elevation
   D. Diuretics, compression and diet

4. Unilateral edema is typically due to which of the following causes?
   A. A local cause such as deep vein thrombosis, venous insufficiency, or lymphedema
   B. A systemic cause such as heart failure, kidney or liver disease
   C. Drugs or medications
   D. Nutritional deficits

5. Which of the following does NOT provide adequate compression for edema?
   A. Short-stretch bandages like the Unna boot and the Coban 2® bandage
   B. Custom fit stockings
   C. Three- or four-layer bandages
   D. Antiembolic stockings

REFERENCES

1. *Dorland' Illustrated Medical Dictionary*. 24th ed. Philadelphia, PA: W.B. Saunders Co.; 1965:467.
2. Gorman WP, Davis KR, Donnelly R. ABC of arterial and venous disease. Swollen lower limb—1: General assessment and deep vein thrombosis. *BMJ*. 2000;320:1453–1456.
3. Macdonald JM, Ryan TJ. Lymphoedema and the chronic wound: The role of compression and other interventions. In: Macdonald JM, Geyer MJ, eds. *Wound and Lymphoedema Management*, Geneva, Switzerland: World Health Organization; 2010:63–83.
4. Mortimer PS. Swollen lower limb—2: Lymphoedema. *BMJ*. 2000; 320:1527–1529.
5. *Dorland' Illustrated Medical Dictionary*. 24th ed. Philadelphia, PA: W.B. Saunders Co.; 1965:1482.
6. Ely JW, Osheroff JA, Chambliss ML, et al. Approach to leg edema of unclear etiology. *J Am Board Fam Med*. 2006;19:148–160.
7. Alguire PC, Mathes BM. Chronic venous insufficiency and venous ulceration. *J Gen Intern Med*. 1997;12:374–383.
8. Rockson SG. Lymphedema. *Am J Med*. 2001;110:288–295.
9. Segerstrom K, Bjerle P, Graffman S, et al. Factors that influence the incidence of brachial oedema after treatment of breast cancer. *Scand J Plast Reconstr Surg Hand Surg*. 1992;26:223–227.
10. Macdonald JM. Wound healing and lymphedema: a new look at an old problem. *Ostomy/Wound Management*. 2001;47:52–57.
11. Kolari PH, Pekanmaki K, Pohiolo RT. Transcutaneous oxygen tension in patients with post-traumatic ulcers: treatment with intermittent pneumatic compression. *Cardiovasc Res*. 1988;22: 138–141.
12. Bucalo B, Eaglstein WH, Falanga V. Inhibition of cell proliferation by chronic wound fluid. *Wound Rep Reg*. 1993;1:181–186.
13. Argenta L, Morykwas M. Vacuum-assisted closure: a new method for wound control and treatment: clinical experience. *Ann Plastic Surg*. 1997;38:553–562.
14. Marston WA, Carlin WE, Passman MA, et al. Healing rates and cost efficacy of outpatient compression treatment for leg ulcers associated with venous insufficiency. *J Vasc Surg*. 1999;30(3):491–498.
15. Stadelmann WK, Digenis AG, Tobin G. Impediments to wound healing. *Am J Surg*. 1998;176 (suppl 2A):407.
16. Kawahara A, Yasuoka Y, Kawada H. Regulation of the interstitial fluid volume. *Nippon Rinsho*. 2005;63(1):31–36.
17. Kirstner RL. Diagnosis of chronic venous insufficiency. *J Vasc Surg*. 1986;3(1):185–188.
18. Browse NL. The diagnosis and management of primary lymphedema. *J Vasc Surg*. 1986:3(1):181–184.
19. McCance KL, Huether SE, Brashers VL, et al. *Pathophysiology: The Biologic Basis for Disease in Adults and Children*. 6th ed. Maryland Heights, MO: Mosby Elsevier Inc.; 2010:1091–1140.
20. Patient evaluation: the vascular consultation. In: Rutherford RB, ed. *Vascular Surgery*. 5th ed. Philadelphia, PA: W.B. Saunders Co.; 2000:9–11.
21. Guyton AC, Hall JE. *Textbook of Medical Physiology*. Philadelphia, PA: W.B. Saunders Co.; 1996:161–181, 183–197, 308–313, 178, 270.
22. Zierler RE, Strandness DE. Hemodynamics for the vascular surgeon. In: Moore WS. *Vascular Surgery*. 4th ed. Philadelphia, PA: Saunders; 1993:179–203.
23. Starling EH. Physiologic forces involved in the causation of dropsy. *Lancet*. 1896;1:1267–1270.
24. Mendez MV, Raffetto JD, Phillips T, et al. The proliferative capacity of neonatal skin fibroblasts is reduced after exposure to venous ulcer wound fluid: a potential mechanism for senescence in venous ulcers. *J Vasc Surg*. 1999;30:734–743.
25. Rutherford RB. Initial patient evaluation: the vascular consultation. In: Rutherford RB, ed. *Vascular Surgery*. 5th ed. Philadelphia, PA: W.B. Saunders Co.; 2000:9–11.
26. Fred HL. Hyposkillia: deficiency of clinical skills. *Tex Heart Inst J*. 2005;32(3):255–257.
27. Hirai M, Kaiki K, Nakayama R. Prevalence and risk factors of varicose veins in Japanese women. *Angiology*. 1990;41:228–232.
28. Carpentier PH. Epidemiology and physiology of chronic venous leg disease. *Rev Prat*. 2000;50:1176–1181.
29. Nagy N, Szolnoky G, Szabad G, et al. Tumor necrosis factor-alpha -308 polymorphism and leg ulceration–possible association with obesity. *J Invest Dermatol*. 2007;127(7):1768–1769; author reply 1770–1771.

30. Wallace HJ, Vandongen YK, Stacey MC. Tumor necrosis factor-alpha gene polymorphism associated with increased susceptibility to venaous leg ulceration. *J Invest Dermatol*. 2006;126(4):921–925.

31. Kim BC, Kim HT, Park SH, et al. Fibroblasts from chronic wounds show altered TGF-beta-signaling and decreased TGF-beta Type II receptor expression. *J Cell Physiol*. 2003;195(3):331–336.

32. Taylor RJ, Taylor AD, Smyth JV. *J Wound Care*. 2002;11:101–105.

33. Pieper B, Templin T, Ebright JR. *Adv Skin Wound Care*. 2006; 19(1):37–42.

34. Harms, E. Beitrage zur Traumatischen Achselvenenthrombose Bzw. Claudicato Venosa Intermittens. *Zentralbl F Chir*. 1938;65:946–951.

35. Allen EV, Barker NW, Hines EA. An approach to the diagnosis of vascular diseases of the extremities. In: Allen EV, Barker NW, Hines EA, eds. *Peripheral Vascular Diseases*. Philadelphia, PA: W.B. Saunders Co.; 1946:38.

36. Tiwari A, Cheng KS, Button M, et al. Differential diagnosis, investigation, and current treatment of lower limb lymphedema. *Arch Surg*. 2003;138:152–161.

37. Nelzen O, Bergqvis D, Lindhagen A. Leg ulcer etiology—a cross sectional population study. *J Vasc Surg*. 1991;14:557–564.

38. Lee B, Trainor F, Thoden W, et al. *Handbook of Noninvasive Diagnostic Techniques in Vascular Surgery*. New York, NY: Appleton-Century-Crofts; 1981:41.

39. Honnor A. Staging of lymphoedema and accompanying symptoms. *Br J Commun Nurs*. 2006; The Lymphoedema Supplement:6S–8S.

40. Tsintzilonis SK, Labropoulos N. Lower extremity ultrasound evaluation and mapping for evaluation of chronic venous disease. In: Bergan JJ, Shortell CK, eds. *Venous Ulcers*. Boston, MA: Elsevier; 2007:43–54.

41. Hermans MHE, Treadwell TA. An introduction to wounds. In: Percival S, Cutting K. eds. *Microbiology of Wounds*. Boca Raton, FL: CRC Press; 2010:108.

42. Rasmussen JC, Tan IC, Marshall MV, et al. Lymphatic imaging in humans with near-infrared fluorescence. *Curr Opin Biotech*. 2009;20:74–82.

43. Cullen GH, Phillips TJ. Clinician's perspectives on the treatment of venous leg ulceration. *Int Wound J*. 2009;6:367–378.

44. Edwards L. Views of patients deemed non-compliant. *Leg Ulcer Forum*. 2001;14:11.

45. Clement DL. Management of venous edema: insights from an international task force. *Angiology*. 2000;51(1):13–17.

46. Xia ZD, Hu D, Wilson JM, et al. How echographic image analysis of venous oedema reveals the benefits of leg elevation. *J Wound Care (England)*. 2004;13(4):25–28.

47. Araki CT, Back TL, Padberg Ft, et al. The significance of calf muscle pump function in venous ulceration. *J Vasc Surg*. 1994;7(4):872–879.

48. Back TL, Padberg FT, Araki CT, et al. Limited range of motion is a significant factor in venous ulceration. *J Vasc Surg*. 1995;22(5):519–523.

49. Yang D, Vandongen YK, Stacey MC. Changes in calf muscle function in chronic venous disease. *Cardiovasc Surg*. 1999;7(4):451–456.

50. Kan YM, Delis KT. Hemodynamic effects of supervised calf muscle exercise in patients with venous leg ulceration: a Prospective Controlled Study. *Arch Surg*. 2001;136(12):1364–1369.

51. Jull A, Parag V, Walker N, et al. The PREPARE Pilot RCT of Home-based Progressive Resistance Exercises for Venous Leg Ulcers. *J Wound Care*. 2009;18(12):497–503.

52. Treadwell TA. Effectively managing the patient not just the problem. *Wounds*. 2007;19(4):A8.

53. Top S, Arveschoug AK, Fogh K. Do short-stretch bandages affect distal blood pressure in patients with mixed aetiology leg ulcers? *J Wound Care*. 2009;18(10):439–442.

54. Sakurai T, et al. *Am J Physiol Heart Circ Physiol*. 2006;291(4):H176–H1767. ClinicalTrials.gov. Open label clinical study to assess the clinical safety of a new compression device in subjects with peripheral arterial vascular disease. http://clinicaltrials.gov/ct2/show/NCT00854516?term=ABPI+of+0.5).8&rank=1. Accessed May 7, 2010.

55. Mayrovitz HN, Larsen PB. Effects of compression bandaging on leg pulsatile blood flow. *Clin Physiol*. 1997;17(1):105–117.

56. Montori VM, Kavros SJ, Walsh EE, et al. Intermittent compression pump for nonhealing wounds in patients with limb ischemia The Mayo Clinic Experience (1998–2000). *Int Angiol*. 2002;21(4):360–366.

57. Mayrovitz HN, Macdonald JM. Medical compression: effects on pulsatile leg blood flow. *Int Angiol*. 2010;29(5):436–441.

58. Keller A, Muller ML, Calow T, et al. Bandage pressure measurement and training: simple interventions to improve efficacy in compression bandaging. *Int Wound J*. 2009;6:324–330.

59. Brodovicz KG, McNaughton K, Uemura N, et al. Reliability and feasibility of methods to quantitatively assess peripheral edema. *Clin Med & Res*. 2009;7(1/2):21–31.

60. Rabe E, Stucker M, Ottillinger B. Water displacement leg volumetry in clinical studies—A discussion of error sources. *BMC Med Res Methodology*. 2010;10:5 http://www.biomedcentral.com/1471-2288/10/5

61. Volikova AI, Edwards J, Stacey MC, et al. High-frequency ultrasound measurement for assessing post-thrombotic syndrome and monitoring compression therapy in chronic venous disease. *J Vasc Surg*. 2009;50:820–825.

62. Kong L, Caspall J, Duckworth M, et al. Assessment of an ultrasonic dermal scanner for skin thickness measurements. *Med Eng Phys*. 2008;30:804–807.

63. Hu D, Phan TT, Cherry GW, et al. Dermal oedema assessed by high frequency ultrasound in venous leg ulcers. *Br J Dermatol*. 1998;138:815–820.

64. Partsch H, Clark M, Mosti G, et al. Classification of compression bandages: practical aspects. *Dermatol Surg*. 2008;34:600–609.

65. Junger M, Partsch H, Ramelet A, et al. Efficacy of ready-made tubular compression device versus short-stretch compression bandages in the treatment of venous leg ulcers. *Wounds*. 2004;16:313–320.

66. Moffatt CJ, Edwards L, Collier M, et al. Randomized controlled 8-week crossover clinical evaluation of the 3m coban 2 layer compression system versus profore to evaluate the product performance in patients with venous leg ulcers. *Int Wound J*. 2008;5:267–279.

67. Fife C, Walker D, Thomson B, et al. Limitations of daily living in patients with venous stasis ulcers undergoing compression bandaging: problems with the concept of self-bandaging. *Wounds*. 2007;19(10):255–257.

68. Treadwell TA. Self-care. *Wounds*. 2009;21(8):A7.

69. Bulkley LD. On the use of the solid rubber bandage in the treatment of eczema and ulcers of the leg. *Arch Dermatology*. 1878, July. Reprinted by G.P. Putnam's Sons, New York, NY, 1878:4–14.

70. Cheville AL, McGarvey CL, Petrek JA, et al. Lymphedema management. *Semin Radiat Oncol*. 2003;13(3):290–301.

71. Casley-Smith JR. Changes in the microcirculation at the superficial and deeper levels in lymphoedema: the effects and results of massage, compression, exercise and benzopyrenes on these levels during treatment. *Clin Hemorheol Microcirc (Netherlands)*. 2000; 23(2–4):335–343.

72. Ukat A, Konig M, Vanscheidt W, et al. Short-stretch versus multilayer compression for venous leg ulcers: a comparison of healing rates. *J Wound Care*. 2003;12(4):139–143.

Management of the Wound Environment with Dressings and Topical Agents

Geoffrey Sussman

CHAPTER OBJECTIVES

At the completion of this chapter, the reader will be able to:

1. Describe the properties of ideal dressings.
2. Identify the limitations and appropriate use of inert dressings and interactive dressings.
3. List the classifications and uses of the six modern interactive dressing product groups.
4. Describe miscellaneous dressings that do not fit into any of the standard six groups, including new products on the market.
5. Explain the role of topical antimicrobials in wound management.

The aim of wound care is to provide the appropriate environment for healing by both direct and indirect methods, together with the prevention of skin breakdown. Dressings and topical agents are important aspects of the healing environment. They play a role in providing a moist environment absorbing excess exudates, lowering or removing wound bacteria, assisting in the removal of slough, and protecting the wound from contamination.

INTRODUCTION TO MOIST WOUND HEALING

Until about 50 years ago, traditional wound care theory indicated that

- Wounds should be kept clean and dry so that a scab can form over the wound.
- Wounds should be exposed to the air and sunlight as much as possible.
- When tissue loss is present, the wound should be packed to prevent surface closure before the cavity is filled.
- Wounds should be covered with dry dressings.

The problem with the first of these principles is that the scab, which is made up of the dehydrated exudate and dead tissue, is a barrier to healing. Scabs delay healing by hindering the movement of epidermal cells; this can lead to poor cosmetic results and scarring. The second principle recommends exposure to air; however, this reduces the surface temperature of the wound, further delaying healing. Reduced surface temperature can also result in peripheral vasoconstriction, affecting the flow of blood, oxygen, nutrients, and other factors to the wound. Exposure to air will also increase fluid loss and dry the

wound surface. When a wound with tissue loss is packed with dry gauze, as recommended in the third principle, the quality of healing is impaired by the adhesion of the gauze to the surface of the wound. This causes the wound to dry out and increases the risk of trauma on removal of the packing (the limitations and appropriate use of gauze and other inert dressings are discussed shortly). Finally, in opposition to traditional beliefs, wounds should not be covered with dry dressings: doing so does not provide a moist environment essential for wound healing; this is explained in the following section.

Benefits of Moist Dressings

Wounds managed in a moist environment covered by an occlusive dressing do not form a scab, so epidermal cells are able to move rapidly over the surface of the dermis through the exudate that collects at the wound-dressing interface. Figure 20.1 diagrams moist wound healing. The application of a totally occlusive or semipermeable dressing to the wound can also prevent secondary damage as a result of dehydration. Moist wound healing also promotes autolytic debridement, the natural removal of slough and nonviable tissue by enhancing the action of enzymes released by the neutrophils of wound. It facilitates wound cleaning, since wound exudate is part of the healing cascade and has been shown to carry a number of growth factors essential to the healing of wounds. It also protects granulating tissue and encourages epithelialization. Dressings are used directly on the wound as the primary dressing or over the primary dressing to hold it in place or to help absorb exudate as a secondary dressing. Early research into the functions of occlusive dressings began in 1948 with the publication by J.P. Bull of a paper in the *Lancet* entitled "Experiments with occlusive dressings of a new plastic."[1] Bull's work examined the physical

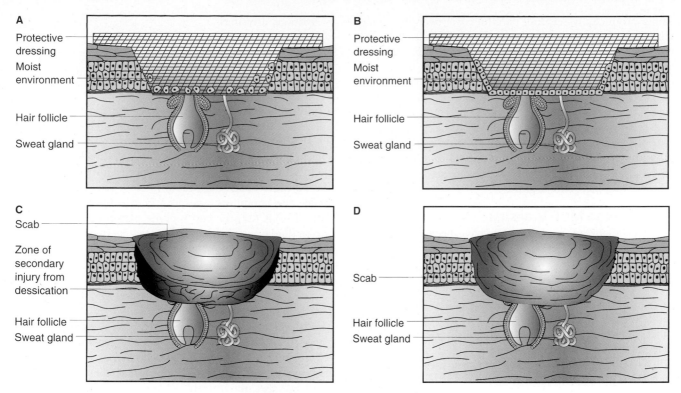

FIGURE 20.1 A–D: Moist wound healing.

properties of a film derived from nylon. He concluded that the film was an effective barrier against microorganisms and that its physical properties, in particular the water vapor permeability of the film, was important as this was the first time this property was demonstrated as a suitable material for wound dressings. He tested it on human skin to find out whether the film's permeability to water vapor would be sufficient to prevent the skin from becoming soaked and found that the bacterial flora of healthy skin under the dressing became modified, *Staphylococcus aureus* disappeared, and the presence of a variety of organisms was reduced.

Schilling published a study of the use of the nylon-derivative film in a specifically industrial setting, conducting a comparative trial with a waterproof dressing in common use at the time.[2] The study concluded that the healing times of wounds treated with the nylon-derivative film were significantly shorter. Twelve years later, George D. Winter was able to pinpoint specific differences between the healing of wounds left open to the air and those kept under an occlusive dressing in his study "Formation of the scab and the rate of epithelialization of superficial wounds in the skin of young domestic pigs."[3] His experiment showed that wounds healing under moist conditions healed 50% faster than wounds open to the air and healing under dry conditions. Winter's work has since formed the basis of the principles of modern moist wound management.

This work was extended in 1963 by Cameron D. Hinman and others from the Division of Dermatology at the University of California, who published a study on the "Effects of air exposure and occlusion of experimental human skin wounds."[4] In effect, Hinman repeated Winter's work, but this time with healthy adult male volunteers. He again used a sterile polyethylene film in artificially made wounds that were then either occluded or allowed to heal open to the air. Occluded wounds

in Hinman's study showed the same rate of healing as those in Winter's work, confirming the earlier results.

Limitations and Appropriate Use of Inert Wound Dressings

Examining their continued use as described by Turner,[5,6] it is clear that they are still important as they set the standard for future product development and use. Inert wound dressings are simple absorbent or nonabsorbing dressings that play no part in the wound environment other than exudate absorption and wound coverage. There are a number of drawbacks to the use of passive products, particularly gauze. First, because it's a fibrous material, gauze tends to shed very readily and, as such, will contaminate the wound. Second, gauze is highly absorbent and, as a primary dressing, will tend to dry the surface of a wound rapidly. Third, gauze is permeable to bacteria, and moist gauze tends to be an environment that promotes bacterial growth. These bacteria can subsequently penetrate and ultimately contaminate the wound. Fourth, gauze is adherent and will traumatize the wound further on removal, risking pain and damage to granulating tissue. New alternatives to gauze, such as nonwoven swabs that do not shed fibers, are now available both for cleaning wounds and for primary dressings.

In recent years, other simple, modified absorbent pads have been developed. These are typically covered with a perforated plastic film to prevent adherence to a wound. These products include Melolin™ and Telfa™, which are used as both primary and secondary dressings and in minor wounds and wounds with low exudate.

Paraffin (petrolatum) gauze dressings, developed by Lumiere in World War I, were among the earliest modern dressings. Many variations have been developed over the years by changing the loading of paraffin in the base. In general, these dressings produce a waterproof paraffin cover over the wound, which can lead to maceration because paraffin may not allow water vapor and exudate to pass through. These products are permeable to bacteria and are known to adhere to the wound, causing trauma on removal. Their use is limited to simple, clean, superficial wounds and minor burns. They are also used over skin grafts. They need to be changed frequently to avoid drying out and always require a secondary dressing.[7]

One alternative to paraffin dressings is products made from synthetic fibers tightly meshed and impregnated with an emulsified base, lipid-colloid, or silicone. Examples are Adaptic™, Cuticerin™, Mepitel™, and Urgotul™.[8–10]

Properties of an Ideal Dressing

The properties of an ideal dressing have been described as follows[5]:

- Will remove excessive exudates from the wound but will not allow the wound to dry out, maintaining a moist environment
- Will allow gaseous exchange so that oxygen, water vapor, and carbon dioxide can pass into and out of the dressing
- Will be thermally insulating, maintaining the wound core temperature at approximately 37°C
- Will be impermeable to microorganisms, minimizing contamination from outside the wound
- Will be free from either particulate or toxic contamination
- Will be nontraumatic and will not adhere to the wound, so that no damage is done to granulating tissue on removal

In addition, the following properties should be considered when selecting the appropriate dressing:

- Will provide the proper environment for healing
- Will be user-friendly (to ensure compliance)
- Will have ease of application and removal
- Will simplify treatment (minimal changes of dressing)
- Will be cost-effective (i.e., total management cost)
- Will be compatible with the wound
- Will have minimal need for secondary dressings
- May be suitable for combined use with compression therapy
- May be used in infected wounds
- Will remain in place

INTERACTIVE WOUND DRESSINGS

Interactive wound dressings provide the wound environment for healing to take place. The term interactive is used because they are not passive but feature the ability to work actively with wound properties like wound fluid, tissue, cells, and growth factors within the wound to enhance healing. Thus, they provide an ideal wound environment for healing. Different dressing characteristics are exploited by choosing dressings based on the wound properties to be addressed. The various interactive dressings do have different properties and are classified into six specific groups accordingly. For example, these dressings vary in their ability to absorb exudates: some have no ability to absorb, some will cope with low levels of exudates, and some are able to absorb large volumes of exudate.

The six types of interactive dressings are

- Film dressings
- Foam dressings
- Hydrogel dressings
- Hydrocolloid dressings
- Alginate dressings
- Hydroactive dressings

Film Dressings

Film dressings are thin membranes coated with a layer of acrylic adhesive. They are moisture vapor-permeable and oxygen-permeable. These properties vary in only minor ways from brand to brand. One important difference in selecting a dressing is moisture vapor permeability. The moisture vapor permeability is measured with the moisture vapor permeability test.[11] This test is performed under the conditions specified in the *British Pharmacopoeia 1980*. In this test, the cup is either placed upright, so that any loss of fluid occurs by evaporation, or inverted, so that the liquid comes in contact with the membrane. It should be noted that the loss of water vapor from intact skin is 240 to 1920 g/m²/24 hours, and the water vapor loss from an open wound is about 4800 g/m²/24 hours. Table 20.1 identifies several film dressing products and their vapor permeability.

Although films are permeable to both oxygen and moisture vapor, they are impermeable to microorganisms and moisture. Thus, film dressings are flexible, elastic, extensible, and allow easy assessment of the wound because they are transparent. They are also impermeable to microorganisms. They do not have the ability to absorb any exudate. There are films available with very high moisture vapor permeability; as such, they can be used on more highly exuding wounds. Film dressings are elastic and extensible.[11,12]

Effects

The effects of film dressings include the following:

- Provide a moist environment
- Assist with autolytic debridement
- Provide protection from chemicals, friction, shear, and microbes
- Transmit oxygen into and carbon dioxide and water vapor out of the dressing
- Function as a secondary dressing

Indications for Use

Film dressings are indicated in the management of minor burns and simple injuries (e.g., scalds, abrasions, and lacerations),

TABLE 20.1	Comparison of Moisture Vapor Permeability of Different Wound Dressings	
Dressing Brand	**Cup Upright g/m²/24 h**	**Cup Inverted g/m²/24 h**
OpSite	839	862
Bioclusive	547	605
Ensure	436	436
Opraflex	456	477
DermaFilm	422	472
Tegaderm	794	846

and as a postoperative dressing over suture lines. They are also used as a protective layer over intravenous catheters, and for the prevention and treatment of superficial pressure areas.[13,14] A film dressing enables autolytic debridement and provides a moist wound healing environment.

Indications for Discontinuation
An increased level of exudation that causes pooling under the dressing can lead to maceration of both the wound and the surrounding skin. The dressing should be discontinued in such cases. Use of the dressing should also be discontinued if the wound becomes clinically infected.

Method of Application
An appropriately sized piece of film should be chosen to cover the wound and provide an overlap of at least 4 to 5 cm from the edge of the wound. It is important to ensure that the skin around the wound is dry and free from oils or cream, because these may reduce adherence to the skin. Remove the bottom backing paper, and carefully apply the film dressing over the wound, while maintaining light but firm stretching of the edges of the film to prevent it from sticking to itself. Once the dressing is in place, remove the upper cover.

Film dressings are also used as a secondary dressing over hydrogels and alginates, as an alternative to tape for holding a dressing in place, and to provide a waterproof covering. In addition to standard film dressings, island versions are now available, comprising a simple absorbent pad covered by the film. These products are able to absorb small amounts of wound exudate and can be used in wounds with low exudates. Simple, small versions of these dressings can also replace plastic first aid strips, with the advantage of not causing the maceration common with plastic strips.[15–21]

New Absorbent Film Dressings
Tegaderm™ Absorbent Dressing has an acrylic polymer absorbent pad differing from other island film dressings in that the pad for absorption is not cotton wool–based. Wound exudate moves through perforations in the bottom layer of Tegaderm™ Transparent Film, which is coated with a moist-skin adhesive. Through the process of diffusion, wound exudate is absorbed into the patented, clear, acrylic polymer pad. Moisture vapor is released through the top, breathable, waterproof layer of Tegaderm™ Film, which also provides a barrier to outside contaminants.

OpSite Post-Op Visible™ is a transparent film with a lattice foam structure allowing monitoring of the progress of the wound without unnecessary dressing changes. This reduces disturbance to the wound bed. The film has a high MVTR controlling moisture, absorbing wound discharge, and preventing buildup of fluid underneath the dressing.[22]

Antibacterial Film Dressings
Tegaderm Plus™ consists of a thin polyurethane membrane coated with a layer of an acrylic adhesive that contains 2% available iodine in the form of an iodophor. In contact with skin, the iodophor slowly releases iodine, which has bactericidal activity and provides protection against infection.[22]

Tegaderm™ chlorhexidine gluconate (CHG) IV Securement Dressing™ is a transparent, antimicrobial dressing used to cover and protect catheter sites and to secure devices to skin.[15–21]

Precautions and Contraindications
Film dressings may remain in place for up to 1 week or even longer. Changing of the dressing will depend on the position, type, and size of the wound. It is important to remove film dressings with care. Do not pull the dressing back across itself. Care should be exercised in applying film dressings to damaged or frail skin and in those with fine and dry skin. Because of the risks of further damage on removal, the film should be carefully pulled away from itself while applying light pressure to the center of the film dressing until it has been entirely removed.

Film dressings are not recommended for use over deep-cavity wounds, full-thickness burns, and wounds showing signs of clinical infection. They should be used only with caution in patients with damaged or frail skin and in those with fine and dry skin, because of the risks of skin damage on removal.

Expected Outcomes
Film dressings provide a transparent, flexible, waterproof, and gas-permeable dressing that can protect simple wounds and encourage healing. They can be left in place for 1 week or longer and are cost-effective; only one application of the dressing may be needed to manage the wound. When they are used postsurgically over sutures, they can remain in place until the sutures are removed.

Foam Dressings
Foam dressings are produced from polyurethane as soft, open cell sheets, and can be composed of one layer or multiple layers. They are also available impregnated with charcoal and with a waterproof backing.[12] Foam dressings meet many of the standard requirements of the ideal dressing. They absorb exudate, thereby protecting the surrounding skin from maceration; raise the core temperature of the wound; and maintain a moist environment. Many polymer products are similar in appearance to foam dressings; however, these are hydroactive dressings or foam-like dressings that adsorb moisture into their structure and swell up. They are absorbent dressings, but they are not interchangeable with foam dressings in every situation. Foams are useful as both primary and secondary dressings.

Effects
The effects of foam dressings include the following:
- Provide a moist environment
- Provide high absorbency
- Conform to body shape
- Provide protection and cushioning
- Produce no residue
- Do not adhere to the wound
- Provide thermal insulation
- Transmit moisture vapor out of the dressing
- Require no secondary dressings

Indications for Use
Foams are indicated for a wide range of minor and major wounds, including exuding wounds (both superficial and cavity types), leg ulcers, decubitus ulcers, and sutured wounds. They can be used over skin grafts, donor sites, and minor burns. They also may be used as secondary dressings over amorphous hydrogels. Foams improve the functioning of amorphous hydrogels by removing excess exudate from the wound and raising its core temperature. This assists with autolytic debridement. Foams

TABLE 20.2	Foam Dressings	
Dressing Brand	**Main Constituent**	**Forms**
Allevyn	Polyurethane	Three layers film/hydrophilic foam/plastic net
Curafoam	Polyurethane	Single uniform structure
Hydrasorb	Polyurethane	Single uniform structure
Lyofoam	Polyurethane	Two layers hydrophobic foam/hydrophilic contact layer
Lyofoam Extra	Polyurethane	Three layers film/hydrophobic foam/hydrophilic contact layer

can also be used around tracheostomy tubes and other drainage tubes and catheters.[23–25] Table 20.2 compares the forms of foam dressings used by different manufacturers.

Indications for Discontinuation

Foam dressings should be discontinued when the level of exudation cannot be absorbed into the dressing in less than a 24-hour period.

Method of Application

Place the foam dressing over the wound, allowing for a margin at least 3 to 4 cm greater than the size of the wound. Secure the dressing in place with one of the following:

- In patients with fine or easily damaged skin:
  1. Lightweight cohesive bandage
  2. Tubular bandage
- In other patients:
  1. Adhesive tape (hypoallergenic)
  2. Tubular or lightweight cohesive bandage

Foam dressings can be used under compression bandaging and as a secondary dressing for amorphous hydrogels and alginates. For a wound with a cavity, select the appropriately sized device to fit comfortably into the cavity and insert it into the wound. It may remain in place for 1 to 4 days or until saturated with exudate. A sheet foam dressing can remain in place for up to 7 days or until the exudate has saturated to the edge of the dressing.

You can cut foam dressings in shapes to allow better application to specific parts of the body. For instance, foams can be cut in an "L" shape for application to fingers or toes. The method is to wind the shaft of the L shape around the finger or toe and secure with tape. Then fold over the foot of the L to complete the dressing and secure it in place with tape. To form a cup that can be used over a healing wound, cut a square piece of foam diagonally to the center and fold the cut edges inward so they overlap to form a cup that can be used over a healing wound.[26–28]

Precautions

Foam dressings are of little value on dry wounds with a scab or eschar. They also should not be used alone in a dry cavity, but they may be used with an amorphous hydrogel. There are no specific contraindications for the use of foam dressings. The author has clinical experience with a local reaction causing erythema, but this may have been due to an allergic reaction or to the increased blood flow caused by the thermal effect of the dressing.

Expected Outcomes

Foam dressings provide a satisfactory primary and secondary dressing for a wide range of wounds. They aid in the removal of exudate, raise the core temperature of the wound, and protect the wound from external irritation. They will also protect the healthy skin around the wound from becoming macerated by the wound exudate.

Hydrogels

Hydrogels are a group of complex organic polymers with high water content, from 30% to 90%. These broad classes of polymers are swollen extensively in water, but they do not dissolve. They are three-dimensional, water-swollen, cross-linked structures formed from hydrophilic homopolymers or copolymers. There are two types of hydrogels: amorphous and sheet.

Amorphous hydrogels are nonfixed macrostructures that absorb water, progressively decreasing viscosity. They are free-flowing and will easily fill a cavity space. Table 20.3 shows a comparison of the water content of some amorphous hydrogel products.

TABLE 20.3	Water Content of Amorphous Hydrogel Products	
Dressing Brand	**Chemical Type**	**Water Content (%)**
Carrasyn Gel	Triethanolamine, Carbomer 940, Acemannan	95
DuoDERM Gel	Sodium carboxy-methylcellulose, Pectin, Propylene glycol	81.5
IntraSite Gel	Modified carboxymethyl-cellulose, Propylene glycol	78
Purilon Gel	Carboxymethyl-cellulose, Calcium Alginate	90
Solugel	Propylene Glycol Saline	75
Saf-Gel	Carbomer Propylene Glycol Sodium/ Calcium Alginate	86

Sheet hydrogels are usually manufactured in the form of a thin, flexible sheet. These gels swell, increasing in size until the gel is saturated; they do not change their physical form as they absorb fluid.

Effects

Hydrogels provide moisture to dry wounds, but they are also able to absorb fluid. They have the following useful effects:

- Provide a moist environment
- Aid in autolytic debridement
- Conform to body shape
- Do not adhere to the wound
- Provide moisture and absorb moisture
- Relieve pain

Indications for Use

Amorphous hydrogels are generally indicated for dry and sloughy wounds to rehydrate the eschar and enhance autolytic debridement. They are used on leg ulcers, pressure wounds, extravasation injuries, simple-thickness and partial-thickness burns, and infected wounds and necrotic wounds. They facilitate granulation and epithelialization by preventing the wound from drying out. Hydrogels are used to prevent the drying out of such tissue as tendon. Hydrogels are also a useful carrier of topical drugs to be applied to wounds, such as metronidazole and proteolytic enzymes. Amorphous hydrogels are also used for management of the lesions of chickenpox and shingles.[13,29–32]

New Antibacterial Hydrogels

Flaminal® hydrogels are based upon gelled alginate and not on other polymers. Flaminal® hydrogels use the enzymes glucose oxidase and lactoperoxidase to control the bioburden in a similar way to honey. Flaminal® contains lactoperoxidase, which is an enzyme extracted from milk and acts as an important natural antimicrobial. It has been shown to be bacteriostatic against gram-positive organisms and exhibits pH-dependent bactericidal action against gram-negative organisms in the presence of hydrogen peroxide and thiocyanate. Peroxidases are enzymes that belong to the natural nonimmune defense systems found in milk and in the secretions of exocrine glands such as saliva, tears, intestinal secretions, cervical mucus, and the thyroid. From the available laboratory and clinical evidence, it is clear that the Flaminal® products are safe and effective both clinically and microbiologically though some studies have shown MRSA is not always cleared.

The major difficulty is that there is little published evidence other than case studies and very little in the way of studies in the major wound or medical literature.[33,34]

Indications for Discontinuation

Use of amorphous hydrogels should be discontinued if exudate from a wound is excessive. It is generally advised that the use of sheet hydrogels should be stopped if a wound is clinically infected.

Method of Application

Amorphous hydrogel should be applied to a wound to a minimum thickness of 5 mm and covered with a secondary dressing. The choice of secondary material depends on the type and position of the wound, as well as availability and cost. The author has found that foams are the most satisfactory secondary dressings, by virtue of their properties of exudate absorption, thus maintaining the integrity of the gel for a longer time, protecting the surrounding skin from maceration, and raising the core temperature to aid in autolysis. Other products, such as film dressings, hydrocolloids, and simple nonadherent dressings, may be used. Gauze is also a suitable secondary dressing.

Hydrogels can remain in place for a clean wound for up to 3 days; they should then be removed by irrigation with water or saline. When used for the lesions of chickenpox, they should be applied four or five times a day.

Place sheet hydrogels over the wound with at least 3 to 4 cm coverage greater than the wound. Hold the sheet in place with tape or a light cohesive bandage, depending on the skin of the patient. In difficult areas, hold them in place with a retention sheet, such as Hypafix™, Fixomull™, or Medipore™ Sheet hydrogels do not cause maceration of the surrounding tissue. They can therefore be left in place, depending on the wound type and on the amount of exudation, for up to 3 to 4 days. For some superficial burns, they may remain in place for up to 7 days. When removed, they cause no discomfort and leave no residue on the skin.

Precautions and Contraindications

Because of their occlusive nature, sheet hydrogels should not be applied to clinically infected wounds unless the patient is taking systemic antibiotics. Amorphous hydrogels containing propylene glycol should not be used in patients known to be sensitive to propylene glycol. Sheet hydrogels should not be applied over small deep-cavity wounds. They should also not be used in heavily exuding wounds.

Expected Outcomes

Hydrogels aid in the rapid removal of necrotic tissue and rehydrate dry wounds, thereby assisting in granulation and reepithelialization. In burns, they reduce heat and pain. The thicker sheet hydrogels, when used in the management of superficial pressure wounds, also reduce pressure by reducing friction and shear forces.

Hydrocolloids

Hydrocolloid dressings are a combination of gel-forming polymers with adhesives held in a fine suspension on a backing of polyurethane film or foam. The dressing mass contains, in most cases, sodium carboxymethyl cellulose (CMC) and other gel-forming agents, such as pectin, gelatin, and elastomers.[12] These products are also available as granules, powder, and paste. When applied to an exuding wound, exudate combines with the polymers to form a soft gel mass in the wound. This gel will vary in viscosity, depending on the brand of dressing. The dressing does not adhere to the wound itself, only to the intact skin around the wound.

Hydrocolloids were originally introduced as Stomahesive™ to protect good skin around ileostomies and colostomies. They vary from being occlusive to being semipermeable.

Hydrocolloids come in a wide range of shapes, sizes, and types. These include regular thickness, thin, bordered, padded, and in combination with alginates, as well as for cavity use as pastes, granules, and powder. When removed, the gel remaining is yellow and malodorous, but not infected. The presence of bacteria under hydrocolloid dressings does not retard healing.

TABLE 20.4	Comparison of Hydrocolloid Dressing Products		
Dressing Brand	**Main Component**	**Backing**	**Forms**
Comfeel	Sodium carboxymethyl-cellulose	Polyurethane film	Standard, thin
DuoDERM	Carboxymethyl-cellulose	Polyurethane foam/film	Standard, thin
Tegasorb	Polyisobutylene	Polyurethane film	Standard, thin
Restore		Polyurethane film	Standard, thin

Effects

Hydrocolloids have the following effects[35,36]:

- Provide a moist environment
- Aid in autolytic debridement of wounds
- Conform to body shape
- Protect from microbial contamination
- Provide a waterproof surface
- Require no secondary dressing

Table 20.4 compares hydrocolloid dressing products.

Indications for Use

Hydrocolloids are indicated in the management of superficial leg ulcers, burns, donor sites (when hemostasis has been obtained), and pressure wounds. They may be used in small-cavity wounds, in combination with hydrocolloid paste, powder, or granules. Thin versions can be used as dressings over sutures after minor and major surgeries.[13,24,37–39]

Indications for Discontinuation

Hydrocolloids should be discontinued on surface granulation of the wound or if hypergranulation occurs.

Method of Application

Hydrocolloids on a superficial wound should be applied to the wound with a margin of at least 3 to 4 cm greater than the wound size. The skin should be dry to ensure good adhesion, and it is preferable to place one-third of the dressing above the wound and two-thirds below the wound; this will prolong the wear time of the dressing. The dressing may remain in place for 5 to 7 days or until strikethrough has occurred (i.e., exudate has migrated to the outside edge of the dressing). Then, carefully remove the dressing and irrigate the wound with warm saline before applying a new dressing.

In the case of small-cavity, relatively moist wounds, fill the cavity with hydrocolloid paste, powder, or granules and cover it with a sheet of hydrocolloid dressing. With a minimally to moderately exuding cavity, insert hydrocolloid paste carefully and then cover the wound with a sheet of hydrocolloid dressing. Change the dressing after 3 to 4 days. Irrigate the cavity with warm saline and gently remove any remaining product before applying the new dressing.

Apply thin hydrocolloid dressings after surgical wound suturing. In most cases, these dressings can remain in place until removal of the sutures, clips, or Steri-Strip. For surgical wounds, these dressings have the advantage of being both flexible and waterproof. They require no secondary dressing, and help to appose wound edges by distributing tension at the suture line across the surface area of the dressing.

Precautions and Contraindications

When using these dressings on patients with thin and fragile skin, take care that the dressings do not cause further skin damage on removal. There are no absolute contraindications for use of hydrocolloids, but they are not indicated for use in heavily exuding wounds or in clinically infected wounds. They also are not considered suitable for deep-cavity wounds.

Expected Outcomes

Hydrocolloids help to remove necrotic tissue and slough from a wound and encourage angiogenesis and granulation of the wound. The presence of colonized bacteria in a wound does not contraindicate the use of these dressings.

Alginates

Alginates are the calcium or calcium/sodium salts of alginic acid and are composed of mannuronic and guluronic acids obtained from seaweed, primarily the genus *Laminaria*. They are available as a mixture of sodium alginate and calcium alginate in textile fiber sheets or as a loose packing ribbon. When applied to a wound, sodium ions present in the wound exchange for the calcium ions in the dressing, producing a hydrophilic gel and providing calcium ions to the wound. Since calcium acts as a clotting factor (factor IV), this mechanism enables some alginates to act as a hemostat.

Sodium alginate has a complex structure consisting essentially of two uronic acids, D-mannuronic acid and L-guluronic acid. The ratio of these isomers varies, depending on the species of seaweed from which the alginate is extracted and the method of production. Gels that are rich in mannuronic acid form soft amorphous gels that partially dissolve or disperse in solutions containing sodium ions. Alginates that are rich in guluronic acid tend to swell in the presence of sodium ions, while retaining their basic structure.[12,40]

Effects

Alginates have the following useful effects:

- Provide a moist environment
- Provide a high absorptive capacity
- Conform to body shape
- Protect from microbial contamination
- Provide hemostasis
- Do not adhere to the wound

Table 20.5 compares the chemical composition of different alginate products.

Indications for Use

Alginates are used in exuding wounds, such as leg ulcers, cavity wounds, and pressure wounds, and at donor sites (as a

TABLE 20.5	Comparison of Alginate Chemical Composition			
Name	Guluronic Acid (%)	Mannuronic Acid (%)	Calcium Alginate (%)	Sodium Alginate (%)
Algoderm	58	42	100	
Curosorb	68	32	100	
Kaltostat	66	34	80	20
CarboFlex	66	34	80	20
Sorbsan	34	63	100	
TegagenHG (discontinued)			100	
Tegagen HI			100	
Cutinova Alginate	70	30	90	10
Calgicare	65	35	80	20

hemostat postsurgically) and other bleeding sites. They may be used in infected wounds.[13,25,41–44]

Indications for Discontinuation
Alginates should be discontinued if the amount of exudate is insufficient to cause the fiber to gel. They should not be premoistened with saline to promote gelling.

Method of Application
Sheet alginates should be placed in and conformed to the shape of the wound, and covered with a secondary dressing, such as a foam, or a nonadherent dressing. Depending on the condition of the patient's skin, the sheets can be held in place with tape or a light cohesive bandage. If the wound is extremely exudative, add an extra covering with a simple absorbent pad. In the case of a cavity wound, gently place rope or packing alginate material in the cavity, taking care not to pack the material tightly into the space. When used on a donor site, apply the sheet alginate to the donor area after skin harvesting and cover it with a film dressing or foam. This aids in rapid hemostasis and provides an environment conducive to reepithelialization of the skin.

In general, the dressing should remain in place in clean wounds for no longer than 7 days or until the gel loses its viscosity (this will vary, depending on the level of exudation from the wound). Change dressings on clinically infected wounds daily. Remove the alginate by simple irrigation of the wound or cavity with warm saline. Freeze-dried alginates may be applied not only to the wound but also to cover the periwound skin because they gel only over the wound, thus protecting the periwound skin from maceration.

Precautions and Contraindications
For clinically infected wounds, the dressing should be changed daily and the concurrent use of systemic antibiotics is typically necessary. There are no known contraindications for the use of alginates; however, they are not suitable for use in dry wounds or in wounds with thick, black eschar.

Expected Outcomes
Alginates absorb exudate and provide a moist environment for granulation. They are suitable for use in infected wounds and are very effective in the management of bleeding, particularly in postnasal surgery, post biopsy, and when applied to donor sites. They provide a comfortable dressing, and rapid healing of the skin is expected.

Alginate dressings have known hemostatic properties: factors such as wound type, position, and depth will determine the best dressing to apply over a bleeding wound. One study examined the absorption of blood by moist wound healing dressings and confirmed the action of some alginate dressings.[45]

Combination Alginates
Manufacturers have combined alginates with other products to enhance the effects of each.

Alginate and Charcoal Combination
CarboFlex is a combination of calcium and sodium alginate and Aquacel in a fiber sheet, bonded to a layer of activated charcoal and an outer layer of viscose. This product is a highly absorbent dressing with the ability to absorb odor. It is indicated in infected, malodorous wounds, fungating neoplasms and ulcers, and superficial pressure wounds.

The sheet should be applied to the surface of the wound, ensuring that the white alginate layer is in contact with the wound, and that the dark charcoal layer is on the outside. Cover the product with a secondary dressing and hold it in place with tape or a light cohesive bandage. Change the dressing every few days, depending on the level of exudate and extent of infection. The dressing is easily removed, and removal may be assisted by irrigation with warm saline. This dressing, as with other alginates, is of no value in a dry wound with thick, dark eschar.

Alginate/Hydrocolloid Combination
The combining of hydrocolloids and alginates in one dressing, such as in the Curaderm™ and Comfeel Plus™ products, enhances the dressings' properties and allows them to be used in more excessively exudative wounds. They are similar in appearance to standard hydrocolloid sheets, and are used in a manner similar to that of hydrocolloids. The combination dressings, however, can remain in place for a longer period of time because of their superior absorptive properties.

Hydroactive Dressings

Hydroactive dressings have some similarities to hydrocolloids; however, they are not gel-forming products. Instead, they act by absorbing exudate into the structure of the dressing, swelling as the liquid is absorbed. They thereby maintain a moist environment at the interface of the wound.

Hydroactive dressings consist of multiple layers of highly absorbent polymer gel with an adhesive backing. These dressings are composed of an outer polyurethane film membrane, combined with a polyurethane gel and other absorbents (e.g., sodium polyacrylate). They are semipermeable and adhere to the skin. They are available in a number of forms, including cavity fillers, foam-like, and thin types.[12]

Effects

Hydroactive dressings have the following useful effects:

- Provide a moist environment
- Provide high absorbency
- Provide a waterproof surface
- Regain their shape when stretched
- Aid in autolysis
- Leave no residue
- Are semipermeable to moisture vapor

Indications for Use

Hydroactive dressings are indicated for use on exuding wounds, including leg ulcers, pressure wounds, minor burns, and exuding cavity wounds. They are of particular use over joints, such as the elbows, knees, fingers, toes, and ankles, because of their ability to expand and contract without causing constriction.[46–48]

There are foam-like forms of hydroactive dressings. These should not be confused with typical foam dressings, because they react to exudate in a different manner, by absorbing (this type of dressing attracts the liquid into its surface and absorbs the fluid into the spaces in the sponge-like structure) the exudate into their structure. This can be observed by their change of shape. Hydroactive dressings absorb exudates rapidly, regardless of the amount of exudation.

Indications for Discontinuation

Use of hydroactive dressings should be discontinued for wounds with little or no exudation, or if the dressing is unable to absorb the amount of exudate being produced by the wound.

Method of Application

The method application of hydroactive dressings varies, depending on the brand of dressing used.

- Place Tielle over the wound so that the central island of dressing completely covers the wound. Allow for a margin 2 to 3 cm greater than the wound size, and then adhere it to the surrounding skin.
- Apply Cutinova Hydro™ directly to the wound, allowing for a margin of 3 to 4 cm of dressing around the wound. It's a good idea to warm the edges of the dressing slightly with your hands to aid adhesion.
- Allevyn plus Cavity™, because of its ability to absorb exudate and expand, should be placed carefully into the cavity, not occupying more than 33% of the space. Cover the outer wound with a suitable dressing, such as Allevyn Thin™ or Cutinova Hydro™.
- Biatain™ and PolyMem™ are hydroactive dressings available as both a standard and an adhesive sheet. Apply them in a manner similar to the other hydroactive dressings.

These dressings may remain in place for up to 7 days, depending on the amount of exudation. Use great care when removing them in patients with thin or easily damaged skin. When removed, they will leave no residue; however, you may still need to irrigate the wound with warm saline before redressing if there is exudate present on the surface.

Precautions and Contraindications

Hydroactive dressings are not considered suitable for use on clinically infected wounds or nonexuding wounds. There are no known contraindications to their use; however, it's essential to work slowly and gently when using these products on fine and easily damaged skin.

Expected Outcomes

Hydroactive dressings absorb exudate and provide a moist environment for granulation and epithelialization. They provide a comfortable dressing that will remain in place and have a good wear time.

MISCELLANEOUS DRESSINGS

With ongoing research and development, new products regularly enter the market that do not fit into any of the standard groups mentioned. These products may have properties resembling those of existing groups but are composed of different materials. We can discuss here only a few of these many innovative products.

Matrix Dressings

Matrix products include Promogran™ and Oasis™. Promogran is a freeze-dried matrix composed of collagen and oxidized regenerated cellulose (ORC) formed into a sheet. When applied to a moist wound, it forms a soft biodegradable gel. It binds growth factors and inactivates matrix metalloproteinases (MMPs). Promogran is used in partial-thickness and full-thickness wounds and is applied every 2 to 3 days.

Oasis™ is derived from porcine small intestinal submucosa. It acts as an extracellular matrix and can be used in a range of wound types including ulcers, pressure wounds, and minor burns. It is reapplied at each dressing change on areas no longer covered by the previous application.

Nonadherent Pads

Exu-dry™ is a nonadherent absorbent pad composed of an outer layer of perforated polyethylene-laminated rayon and an inner layer of absorbent rayon/polypropylene blend. The pad has a cellulose backing that wicks wound exudate and holds large quantities of fluid. It is indicated in highly exudative wounds, particularly burns.[49]

Mepore™ is a similar nonadherent pad with greater absorbency than simple nonadherent dressings due to their thickness and greater surface area for absorption.

CombiDERM™ is a multilayer absorbent pad combining a semipermeable hydrocolloid border with absorbent padding of hydrocolloid particles and a nonadherent cover against the wound. This product is highly absorbent and is able to hold the exudate within the dressing, preventing maceration to the surrounding skin. It maintains a moist environment. It is indicated on highly exuding wounds, pressure wounds, leg ulcers, and surgical wounds. It can be used as a secondary dressing over cavity wounds.

Hydrofibers

Hydrofibers are similar to alginates in appearance; however, though fibrous, they are composed of the polymer CMC. Hydrofiber dressings are activated by moisture in the wound and they are able, as polymers, to absorb and trap within their structure the moisture from the wound. While they have a similar ability to absorb exudates as do alginates, they do not have the hemostatic property of alginates.

Presently only one type of hydrofiber is available. Aquacel is composed of nonwoven, 100% sodium CMC spun into fibers and manufactured into sheets and ribbon dressings. This product mirrors the properties and actions of alginate dressings, but it rapidly absorbs exudate vertically and does not absorb laterally. It thereby retains fluid within the structure of the fibers, which convert into a gel sheet as they swell. Aquacel™ is indicated in heavily exuding wounds, such as leg ulcers, pressure wounds, cavity wounds, minor burns, and donor sites.

When applying the dressing to the wound, allow a dressing margin 2 to 3 cm greater than the wound size or wound cavity. The dressing can remain in place for 1 to 3 days, depending on the exudate amount and when the product is saturated. Like freeze-dried alginates, Aquacel can be applied to the periwound skin and the wound without the risk of maceration.

Products containing a hydrofiber component include Versiva Dressing™ and Alione™. Versiva Dressing™ is a sterile wound dressing consisting of a thin, perforated adhesive layer, a nonwoven layer with a hydrofiber blend, and a top polyurethane foam-film layer. The dressing absorbs wound fluid, creates a moist environment, and aids in autolytic debridement. Alione™ is a hydrocapillary dressing consisting of a number of fibers combined in the capillaries of the dressing. The capillaries transport the exudate away from the wound, keeping it moist but not wet. The top surface is film, and the core is a hydrocapillary pad; a wound contact layer and either an adhesive hydrocolloid or a microporous skin protection layer complete the dressing.

Silicone

Silicone is a manufactured polymer that includes the element silicon. Dressings containing silicone are used to reduce hypertrophic and some keloid scars. These dressings (Table 20.6) should be applied as soon as possible after sutures or clips are removed from the incision site. They are changed every 1 to 3 days, after which the area is washed and the dressing is reapplied. The same piece of dressing may be used for about 7 days, and then a fresh piece is applied.

Silicone is also used as the surface layer on a number of other types of dressings including tulles and foam dressings. The silicone helps maintain adhesion of the dressing onto the skin; however, silicone does not stick and thus allows nontraumatic removal. The dressing also reduces pain at the wound interface and on removal of the dressing.[9,10,50,51]

TABLE 20.6	Silicone Dressings	
Brand	**Manufacturer**	**Type**
Mepetil	Molnlycke	Tulle
Mepilex	"	Foam
Mepilex border	"	Combination
Mepilex Transfer	"	Foam
Mepilex Thin	"	Foam
Cica Care	Smith & Nephew	Scar reduction dressing
Mepiform	Molnlycke	"
Allevyn Gentle	Smith & Nephew	Foam
Allevyn Gentle Border	"	Foam

Charcoal

Charcoal is used in combination with a number of dressings, including foam and alginates. It is also available in specific dressings (e.g., Actisorb Plus). The main function of charcoal dressings is to absorb odor.

Collagen

Collagen is a vital structure in wound healing; when crosslinked, it is essential to the tensile strength in a wound. Dressings composed of a collagen matrix, either bovine collagen or avian collagen, stimulate fibroblast activity and improve the healing cascade. Although many other collagen products are on the market, their clinical role has yet to be clarified.

Hyaluronic Acid Derivatives

Hyaluronic acid is a carbohydrate component of the extracellular matrix that plays an important role in the healing cascade. Derivatives of hyaluronic acid are in use clinically, but their role in wound healing is not yet clear. For example, Hyalofill™ is a hyaluronic acid derivative being used in the management of nonhealing neuropathic ulcers and other chronic wounds. It is available in the form of a sheet or ribbon. Hyalofill™ should be applied to the entire surface of the wound, where it will absorb wound exudate and form a hyaluronic acid gel. The dressing is left in place for 3 days.[52]

Proteolytic Enzymes

Proteases are proteolytic (protein-splitting) enzymes that have both positive and negative actions on wounds. Proteolytic enzymes are applied topically to wounds to aid in the removal of slough and breakdown of nonviable tissue. This method of debridement has been used clinically for many years. The enzymes used in commercial products include papain in Accuzyme™ and Panafil™, and collagenase in Santyl™.

Hypertonic Saline

Hypergranulation develops when epithelium fails to cover the granulating tissue and continues to grow beyond the surface of the wound. Traditionally this tissue has been reduced by the application of silver nitrate or copper sulfate solutions; however, these solutions are toxic. Thus, hypertonic saline dressings are now used to stop the exuberant tissue growth and encourage new epithelium. They are composed of an inert fabric impregnated with sodium chloride.

The action of hypertonic saline is to draw fluid from surface cells by setting up an osmotic gradient between the highly concentrated solution in the dressing and the lower concentration of the cells. Examples of hypertonic saline are Mesalt™ and Curasalt™.

Hypertonic saline is used on hypergranulating and necrotic wounds. The dressing should be applied only to the wound area, and changed every 24 hours until the tissue returns to normal surface depth. Discontinue the dressing if the patient experiences pain on application or if the wound is dry.

TOPICAL ANTIMICROBIALS

Excessive bioburden on the surface of a wound can retard healing, but difficulties also arise when topical antimicrobials (antiseptics and antibiotics) are applied that can have a negative effect on wound healing. Although there is little research on the effects of antiseptics on open wounds, one of the most prolific researchers in this area has claimed that antiseptics for wound healing may be harmful, in that they damage healing tissue, thus allowing infection to gain a foothold.[53–57] As early as 1919, Alexander Fleming cautioned that it is essential when estimating the value of an antiseptic to study its effects on the tissues, rather than its effect on bacteria. Unfortunately, Fleming's wise counsel has tended to be ignored in modern practice.

It is known that the surface of open wounds does not need to be sterile for healing to take place. There is also no evidence to support the notion that dressing changes performed once or twice a day with antiseptics guarantee protection from invasive infection. There is, however, sufficient in vitro evidence indicating tissue injury with the prolonged use of antiseptics in chronic wounds.[58] The exceptions are patients with major arterial circulation deficiencies, such as diabetic patients and immunocompromised, neutropenic patients. A decision should be made for the individual patient, taking into account all of the positive benefits and risks.

In this section, we discuss a variety of topical antimicrobials currently in use.

Hypochlorites

In general, the concern with antiseptics is their toxicity. This is especially true for hypochlorite antiseptics (recall that sodium hypochlorite is a bleach). A number of studies with hypochlorites have shown major problems, including cell toxicity, depression of collagen synthesis, localized edema, hypernatremia, hyperthermia, and burns. There have also been reported cases of renal failure associated with topical application of chlorinated solutions to pressure sores. This has been attributed to the release of a toxic lipid from bacteria, causing the bacteremia or endotoxic shock known as Schwartzman reaction.[59]

Hypochlorites are chemically unstable, have a short shelf life, and are rapidly deactivated by organic material. They also are not cost-effective, requiring frequent changes of dressing.

Superoxide Solutions

A new development is the production of a superoxide solution by the electrolysis of water and sodium chloride; the resultant solution is a pH-neutral superoxide solution.

This solution has been used in the management of infected diabetic wounds and leg ulcers and burns. The solution has shown antibacterial activity in vitro including being bactericidal, fungicidal, virucidal, and sporicidal. There are limited published studies on the use of this product. The registered name of this product is Microcyn.[60,61]

Chlorhexidine

Chlorhexidine is commonly used as a hand or skin disinfectant. It is bactericidal, with activity against both gram-positive and gram-negative organisms. It is ineffective against acid-fast bacteria, bacterial spores, fungi, and viruses. Antimicrobial activity is best at neutral or slightly alkaline pH. Chlorhexidine is incompatible with soap; the presence of blood and organic material also will decrease its activity. Skin sensitivity is reported.

Polyhexamethylene biguanide (PHMB) is a polymeric cationic antimicrobial agent that has been deployed in consumer applications for over 40 years. While it shares many attributes with the simpler cationic agents, it has additional action mechanisms that render it unique among this generic class of antimicrobials. PHMB was recognized as possessing superior antimicrobial effect to other cationic biocides, but it could only be poorly defined chemically. Early attempts to rationalize the PHMB mixtures were unsuccessful and precluded their use in pharmaceutical products. Nevertheless, PHMB was marketed as a broad-spectrum antimicrobial agent in a number of diverse applications. As with the bisbiguanides, PHMB was shown to bind rapidly to the envelope of both gram-positive and gram-negative bacteria and in doing so displaces the otherwise stabilising presence of Ca^{2+}. This binding is to the cytoplasmic membrane itself, and also to lipopolysaccharide and peptidoglycan components of the cells wall.

The toxicity profile of both the biguanides and the polymeric biguanides is excellent. Neither molecule is a primary skin irritant or a hypersensitizing agent. With respect to the deployment of PHMB as part of a wound care system, there is little or no evidence to suggest that this would lead to the emergence of PHMB resistant.

Use of the agent within a barrier wound dressing such as Kerlix AMD would impair both the growth and the penetration through the dressing of adventitious pathogens from the environment to the dressed wound.

Prontosan is a solution containing polyhexanide, a biguanid antiseptic related to chlorhexidine, and undecylenamidopropyl betaine. Betaine is a very mild, active surfactant with a dual water and oil solubility. A highly pure betaine based on undecylenic acid was developed for the special demands of the personal care industry. This betaine is exceptionally mild and its action is to reduce surface tension and allow wound contaminants to lift. Surfactants are wetting agents that lower the surface tension of a liquid, allowing easier spreading, and lower the interfacial tension between two liquids. The action of a surfactant on a wound is to assist in the separation of loose nonviable material on the surface of a wound. The product is also available as a hydrogel.[62,63]

Quaternary Ammonium Compounds

Quaternary ammonium compounds can be used alone (an example is Cetrimide) or in combination with the chlorhexidine preparations (an example is Savlon). These preparations are bactericidal against gram-positive and gram-negative organisms. They are relatively ineffective against bacterial spores, viruses, or fungi, and some strains of *Pseudomonas aeruginosa* and *Mycobacterium tuberculosis* are resistant. They can also cause hypersensitivity reactions.

Silver

Silver is one of the oldest elements known. It is found independently in nature and also associated with copper and gold, or as the ore argentite. Metallic silver exists as two isotopes and is inert in this form. In the presence of fluid, silver ions are present as charged ions Ag^+, Ag^{++}, and Ag^{+++} and can form some soluble and mostly insoluble compounds. Silver is used in an elemental form, such as nanocrystalline or foil, in inorganic compounds, such as silver oxide and silver nitrate, and as organic complexes. A number of these forms are used in silver dressings and contrast with silver sulfadiazine, delivered as a cream or tulle. The decreased size of silver particles leads to an increased proportion of surface atoms compared with internal atoms. It is believed that the nanocrystalline structure is responsible for the rapid and long-lasting action. The significance of the forms of silver used in dressing products is discussed below.

Silver has been used clinically for many years, and it has proven antimicrobial activity. It is broad spectrum and inactivates almost all known bacteria, including methicillin-resistant *Staphylococcus aureus* (MRSA) and vancomycin-resistant enterococci (VRE). No cases of bacterial resistance have been documented.

Silver sulfadiazine cream is used in the treatment of burns. Although this cream has also been applied to some wounds, it can lead to the development of mucilaginous slough. A range of new combination silver dressings overcomes this difficulty by delivering varying levels of silver directly from the dressing. The base dressings include hydrocolloids, alginates, and tulles. Tulles are used in many parts of the world and were first introduced as paraffin tulles, a gauze piece saturated with yellow soft paraffin. There are many tulles in use e.g. Jelonet™, Bactigras™, hydroactives, foams, gels, and other polyethylene mats (this is the base of the product Acticoat). Contemporary silver dressings allow for continued release for up to 7 days.

Several factors influence the ability of a dressing to kill microorganisms.[64] These include
- Silver content and distribution in the dressing
- Chemical and physical form (metallic, bound or ionic)
- Dressing's affinity to moisture

The level of silver content contained in dressings varies greatly. The mode of action also varies; that is, some release silver into the wound, others partly release the silver and hold some in the dressing, and others keep the silver within the dressing. Dressings with the silver content concentrated on the surface or those with the silver in ionic form have performed well in tests due to the level of ionic silver released from the dressing.

Indications for Use

Silver dressings are indicated for the reduction of bioburden in surface or cavity wounds in colonized and infected wounds. They may also be used to reduce the risk of infection over skin grafts, burns, and injection sites. The choice of silver dressing will depend on the wound type, level of exudate, and depth.

Indications for Discontinuation

In general, silver dressings are for short-term use to reduce the bioburden. They are then discontinued to allow other products, depending on the wound, to assist in the healing of the wound.

Method of Application, Precautions, and Contraindications

Table 20.7 identifies the use, precautions, and contraindications for a wide variety of silver dressings. Bear in mind that the decision about whether or not to use a silver dressing depends on the wound itself, the clear presence of high levels of colonization, and if the wound is clinically infected. Silver should not be the automatic choice in all wounds. Once the decision to use a silver dressing has been made, the product type must reflect the wound environment itself, the tissue, depth, and level of exudate.

Iodine

Iodine in its various forms has been used as a topical antiseptic since 1840. The newer forms of iodophors have been used since the 1950s. Most of these new forms combine iodine in a complex with a polymer (e.g., povidone, cadexomer), which slowly releases the iodine (Table 20.8). There is no evidence of resistance to iodine.

Povidone-iodine comes in many forms, including skin paints, throat gargle, scrub wash, and ointments. It is a combination of povidone (PVP) and elemental iodine. It is effective against bacteria, mycobacteria, fungi, protozoa, and viruses.

Cadexomer iodine is the combination of the polysaccharide polymer cadexomer and iodine at low strength. When this product is applied to a wound, the exudate is absorbed into the polymer structure, forming a gel and slowly releasing the iodine at about 0.1% continuously over 72 hours. The product will reduce the level of slough in the wound and absorb exudate. It is antibacterial and stimulates inflammatory growth factors. Iodosorb and Iodoflex are two forms of this product.

Indications for Use

Povidone-iodine is typically used in a 10% solution as a skin prep before a procedure. It can also be applied to a wound. Cadexomer iodine is used on sloughy leg ulcers, pressure wounds, and other nonhealing wounds.

Indications for Discontinuation

Some patients experience pain on initial application of the product. In most cases, this subsides after 1 to 2 hours. Some patients with a low pain threshold may find it necessary to discontinue use of the product.

Method of Application

Povidone-iodine should be diluted to 1% or, if used in full strength, leave it in place for only 3 to 4 minutes and then wash it off. It can also be applied as a cream at 5%, or diluted to 0.5% to use as a gargle. Cadexomer iodine is applied directly to the

TABLE 20.7	Silver Dressings		
Product name	**Acticoat 3 & 7**	**Acticoat Absorbent**	**Acticoat Moisture Control**
Product Type	High-density polyethylene	High-density polyethylene	Three layer silver coated foam with a semi-permeable polyurethane film outer layer
Manufacturer	Smith & Nephew	Smith & Nephew	Smith & Nephew
Silver Type/Content	Nanocrystalline silver Acticoat 107 mg/100 cm² Acticoat 7 120 mg/100 cm² Held in two layers of polyethylene mesh enclosing a single layer of rayon and polyester; silver is released into the wound Acticoat-7 has an additional layer of silver-coated polyethylene mesh silver; released silver 24 h 60 ppm	Calcium alginate coated with nanocrystalline silver 144 mg/100 cm² Released silver at 24 h 60 ppm as exudate is absorbed into the dressing; silver is released into the wound	Nanocrystalline Silver Acticoat 0.75–2.01 mg/cm² Held as the outside layer of polyurethane Foam silver is released into the wound Released Silver 70–100 ppm for up to 7 d
Method of Use	Before application, moisten with water (must not be saline, as this will react with the silver). Dressing trimmed to wound size; darker blue surface is placed in contact with the wound. Cover with a secondary dressing depending on the level of exudate	Applied to moderately to highly exudating surface or cavity wounds; covered with a secondary dressing depending on the level of exudate	The dressing is applied to the wound allowing a 2–3 cm greater than the wound with the silver layer in contact with the wound and the blue layer on the out side. The dressing is held in place with tape or a bandage
Frequency of changing	Every 3 d (A-3) Maximum of 7 d (A-7)	Every 3 d	The dressing may remain in place for up to 7 d or until the exudate comes within 1–2 cm of the edge
Contraindications	Patients with known hypersensitivity	Patients with known hypersensitivity	Patients with known hypersensitivity, patients undergoing MRI
Warnings	Do not use with oil-based adproducts or topical antimi-crobials; if applied to lightly exudating wounds, may need to be re-moistened with water	Do not use in cavity wounds where sinuses are present	**Do not use with oil based products or topical antimicrobials**
Uses	Partial- and full-thickness wounds, e.g., burns, donor sites, and ulcers covered with a secondary dressing	Partial- and full-thickness, moderate to highly exudating wounds	Partial and full thickness wounds, e.g, burns, donor sites, ulcers and diabetic wounds

Product Name	Allevyn Ag / Allevyn Ag Adhesive	Allevyn Gentle Ag/ Allevyn Ag Gentle Border	Aquacel Ag
Product Type	Three layer silver containing polyurethane foam The outer layer is a semi-permeable polyurethane film The adhesive version has a polyacrylate adhesive to hold the dressing in place	Three layer silver containing polyurethane foam The outer layer is a semi-permeable polyurethane film The adhesive version has a soft silicone adhesive to hold the dressing in place For use in patients with fragile skin. The border version has an extra layer of film	Hydrofiber
Manufacturer	Smith & Nephew		ConvaTec
Silver Type/Content	Silver sulfadiazine at 0.087 mg/cm² is held in the structure of a polyurethane foam The silver is released at 79–45 ppm into the wound as the foam absorbs exudate	Silver sulfate 1.2 mg/cm²	Sodium carboxymethylcellulose containing silver 8.3 mg/100cm² Released silver at 24 h 20 ppm; silver is released into the wound
Method of Use	The dressing is applied to the wound allowing a 2–3 cm greater than the wound with the silver layer in contact with the wound and the pink layer on the outside. The dressing is held in place with tape or a bandage and the adhesive version is applied and is held in place by the products adhesive.	The dressing is applied to the wound allowing a 2–3 cm greater than the wound with the shinny silver layer in contact with the wound and gray layer on the outside. The dressing is held in place with tape or a bandage.	Apply to the surface or lightly packed (no more than 80%) into moderate to highly exudating wounds
Frequency of changing	The dressing may remain in place for up to 7 d or until the exudate comes within 1–2 cm of the edge	The dressing may remain in place for up to 7 days or until the exudate comes within 1–2 cm of the edge	Depending on the wound, may need to be daily, every third day, or up to 14 d in burns
Contraindications	Patients with known hypersensitivity. should not be used on females at or near term pregnancy or lactating or premature new born infants	Patients with known hypersensitivity must be removed before x-ray or similar procedures	Patients with known hypersensitivity; little value in lightly exudating or dry wounds
Warnings	**Do not use with oil based products or topical antimicrobials**	**Do not use with oil based products or topical antimicrobials**	Should not be used with other wound care products
Uses	Partial and full thickness wounds, e.g., burns, donor sites, ulcers	Partial and full thickness wounds, e.g., burns, donor sites, ulcers, infected wounds	Partial- and full-thickness wounds, e.g., burns, donor sites, ulcers, and wounds covered with a secondary dressing, depending on the level of exudate

(continued)

TABLE 20.7 Silver Dressings (continued)

Product Name	Allevyn Ag / Allevyn Ag Adhesive	Allevyn Gentle Ag/ Allevyn Ag Gentle Border	Aquacel Ag
Product Type	Foam	Tulle	Silver-impregnated activated charcoal
Manufacturer	SSL	Hartmann	Johnson & Johnson
Silver Type/Content	Silver zirconium phosphate 1.59 mg/100 cm² Released silver at 24 h 0 ppm; silver is held in the dressing	Metallic silver 35 mg/100 cm² Released silver at 48 h 100 µg/100 cm²; silver is released into the wound, although mostly held in the dressing	Silver 2.43–2.95 mg/100 cm² Released silver 24 h 0 ppm; silver is held in the dressing
Method of Use	The foam is applied on and around the surface in lightly to moderately exudating wounds	Apply to the wound and peri-skin, and cover with a secondary dressing, depending on the level of exudate	Apply to the wound and peri-skin, and cover with a secondary dressing, depending on the level of exudate
Frequency of changing	Every 3 d	Every 3–7 d	Up to 7 d
Contraindications	Patients with known hypersensitivity	Patients with known hypersensitivity	Patients with known hypersensitivity and lightly exudating wounds
Warnings	Should not be applied to wounds covered with dry scab or hard black necrotic tissue; do not cover with occlusive film, as this reduces water vapor loss	Should not be used in combination with paraffin-containing dressings or ointments	Must be used intact; do not cut. Should not be used in conjunction with topical preparations or paraffin-containing products
Uses	Partial- and full-thickness wounds, e.g., burns, donor sites, ulcers	Complementary use in infected or contaminated partial-thickness wounds, e.g., burns, donor sites, ulcers	Used to reduce bacterial colonization in partial- and full-thickness chronic wounds
Product Name	Arglase	BIATAIN Ag	Contreet-H
Product Type	Impregnated film	Hydroactive	Hydrocolloid
Manufacturer	Unomedical	Coloplast	Coloplast
Silver Type/Content	Polymer silver 100 µg/100 cm² Released silver 24 h 8 ppm	Silver complex 47mg/100 cm² on contact with exudate provides sustained release of the silver 70% of the silver is released within 7 d. The silver is released into the wound	Silver complex 32 mg/100 cm² 30% of the silver is released within 7 d; silver is released into the wound
Method of Use	The film dressing is applied to the intact skin or to the wound; film is adhesive and will stick to the peri-skin	Applied on and around surface wounds and lightly packed into cavity wounds	Applied to light to moderately exudating surface wounds.
Frequency of changing	Up to 7 d	Up to 7 d	Every 4–7 d

Contraindications	Patients with known hypersensitivity and greater than lightly exudating wounds		Patients with known hypersensitivity; use with caution on arterial, diabetic lower leg/foot wounds that need review daily
Warnings	Should be used on dry or lightly exudating wounds only		Potential allergic reaction to adhesive or components; must be removed prior to radiotherapy
Uses	Postoperative suture lines, securing IV lines		Partial- and full-thickness wounds, e.g., burns, donor sites, ulcers, pressure sores
Product Name	**Contreet**	**Polymem Silver**	**Silvercel**
Product Type	Hydroactive	Hydroactive	A non-woven fibre of alginate and carboxylmethylcellulose impregnated with elemental silver
Manufacturer	Coloplast	Ferris	Systagenix
Silver Type/Content	Silver complex 47 mg/100 cm^2 on contact with exudate provides sustained release of the silver; 70% of the silver is released within 7 d. Silver is released into the wound	Nanocrystalline silver 12.4 mg/100 cm^2; released silver at 48 h 50 µg/100 cm^2; silver is released into the wound, although mostly held in the dressing	Elemental Silver 8%w/w held in the fibrous base releasing silver over 7 d
Method of Use	Applied on and around surface wounds and lightly packed into cavity wounds	Apply to the surface or lightly packed (no more than 80%) into moderate to highly exudating wounds	The fibre is applied to the wound or packed in the wound cavity and covered with a secondary dressing depending on the level of exudate
Frequency of changing	Up to 7 d	Every 3 d	The dressing may remain in place for up to 7 d or until the dressing is saturated by the exudate
Contraindications	Patients with known hypersensitivity; should not be used with hydrogen peroxide, hypochlorite solutions, or over exposed muscle or bone		Patients with known hypersensitivity, must be removed before x-ray or similar procedures
Warnings	May cause transient discoloration of wound bed; should be removed prior to radiation therapy, x-rays, etc.	None provided	**Do not use with oil based products or topical antimicrobials**
Uses	Partial- and full-thickness wounds, e.g., burns, donor sites, ulcers, pressure sores; use in moderately to high exudating wounds	Partial- thickness or cavity wounds, lightly exudating wounds	Partial and full thickness wounds, e.g., burns, donor sites, ulcers covered with a secondary dressing

TABLE 20.8	Iodine Dressings	
Brand	**Manufacturer**	**Type**
Betadine	MudiPharma	Povidone-iodine
Povidone-iodine	Various	Solution, cream, paint, gargle
Iodosorb	Smith & Nephew	Cadexomer iodine paste/powder
Inadine	Johnson & Johnson	Iodine gauge (tulle)

wound as powder, paste, or dressing. Cover it with a simple nonadherent dressing and leave it in place for up to 3 days. At dressing changes, you will notice that the product, initially brown in color, has become a white, paste-like gel. Wash this gel away, and apply fresh product to the wound.

Precautions and Contraindications

Povidone-iodine may cause local irritation and sensitivity, and if applied to denuded areas, it may cause burns. It should not be used on patients with goiter. Its absorption may also interfere with thyroid function tests. It is incompatible with alkalis. Cadexomer iodine should not be used on children younger than 12 years of age, or on patients with a known allergy to iodine. No more than 50 g as a single dose or 150 g in a week should be used.

Expected Outcomes

The dressing should reduce bioburden, odor, level of slough, and pain. The wound should show increased granulation and a decrease in size.[65]

Indications for Use of Antibiotics in Chronic Wounds

If a wound is clinically infected, the use of systemic antibiotics should be considered as the most appropriate action. The decision to use topical antibiotics in chronic wounds should be based on an understanding of certain general principles. First, topical use of antibiotics is not recommended generally because of the development of resistance and sensitization. However, in surface anaerobic contamination of some wounds, especially fungating wounds, the use of metronidazole gel (MetroGel) is appropriate, and there have been cases of methicillin-resistant *Staphylococcus aureus* in which topical mupirocin (Bactroban) has been used with success. Another topical antibiotic used in clinical practice is silver sulfadiazine cream (see Table 20.7). It is indicated in some infected ulcers in which *Pseudomonas* has been found to be present.[66–68]

Use of Topical Antimicrobials for Acute Wounds

The use of topical antimicrobials for acute wounds is entirely different from their use in chronic wounds. In a traumatic wound, the risk of infection from contamination at the time of wounding is very high. Also, in the case of major burns, the presence of necrotic tissue is a focus for infection, and topical management is mandatory. In both cases, the goal is to reduce the level of bacteria in the wound and allow the body's own mechanisms to destroy the rest. The use of povidone-iodine, chlorhexidine, and chlorhexidine/cetrimide products is appropriate in the early management of acute traumatic wounds. The use of products such as silver sulfadiazine cream (Silvadene, SSD) in burns is part of the early management of this type of wound.

DRESSING CHOICE

Wounds are dynamic and, as such, the choice of dressing will vary and change as the wound changes. That choice should be based on the three major aspects of any wound: *color, depth, and exudate* (Table 20.9). Color will vary from pink (epithelializing), to red (granulating), to yellow (sloughy), to black (necrotic). Depth will include superficial, shallow, and deep cavity. Exudation will be none, minimal, moderate, or high. Other aspects to consider are the presence of infection, the tissue surrounding the wound, the need to add graduated compression, the fragility of the skin, and any medical condition that may have an impact on the dressing choice. For example, a patient who has serosanguineous exudate may benefit from use of an alginate dressing that has hemostatic properties, or a patient with an infected wound may benefit from a silver or cadexomer iodine dressing.

Secondary Dressings

The choice of secondary dressing depends on the nature, position, and level of exudate. In general terms, film dressings and nonadherent dressings are suitable for lightly exuding wounds, but not for high levels of exudation. Foam dressings are useful over amorphous hydrogels and alginates (this does not apply to the foam-like hydroactive dressings). The use of gauze as a secondary dressing is limited, especially over hydrogels or alginates, because it reduces the ability of the dressing to function at its optimum level.

Another important consideration is the method of dressing retention. If the surrounding skin is healthy, the dressing can be held in place with high-quality tape. If the skin is dry, thin, fragile, or otherwise poor, a tubular bandage or a lightweight cohesive bandage is suitable.

Wound Cleansing

The approach to cleansing a wound at the time of dressing changes depends on the nature of the wound. In general, if the wound is clean with little or no residue from the dressing, simple irrigation with water or saline is the most appropriate. If there is dressing residue, slough, or dry or scaly tissue, the use of a skin wash with surfactant properties in addition to water or saline will aid in the removal of the debris. It is critical to minimize direct contact with the granulating wound. It is considered best to use the cleansing materials at body temperature, because the application of a cold solution reduces the temperature of the wound and can affect blood flow. The use of antiseptic cleansers is of little value in chronic wounds; however, they are of benefit in the initial cleaning of an acute wound.[69]

Another issue in relation to the use of any skin cleanser is the pH of the product. It is important to maintain an acid pH level of 5 to 6 in the wound and the periwound skin. It should

TABLE 20.9	Dressing Choice			
			Wound Depth	
Wound Type (Color/Exudate)	**Aim**	**Superficial**	**Cavity**	
Black/low exudate	Rehydrate and loosen eschar. Surgical debridement is the most effective method of removal of necrotic material. Dressings can enhance autolytic debridement of eschar.	Amorphous hydrogels Hydrocolloid sheets Proteolytic enzymes		
Yellow/high exudate	Remove slough and absorb exudate. Hydrocolloids, with or without paste or powder, for the deeper wounds. Hydrogels, alginates, and enzymes will aid in the removal of the slough and absorb the exudate.	Hydrocolloid Alginate Enzymes Hydroactive Cadexomer Iodine	Hydrocolloids with paste, granules, or powder Hydrogel enzymes Alginates Hydroactive cavity Hydrocolloid/alginate Foam cavity dressing Cadexomer iodine	
Yellow/low exudate	Remove slough, absorb exudate, and maintain a moist environment. Hydrogel, in particular, will rehydrate the slough. Hydrocolloids, films, and enzymes also will aid in autolysis.	Amorphous hydrogels Sheet hydrogels Hydrocolloids Film dressings Cadexomer iodine	Amorphous hydrogels Hydrocolloids with paste Enzymes Hydrocolloid/alginate Cadexomer iodine	
Red/high amounts of exudate	Maintain moist environment, absorb exudate, and promote granulation and epithelialization. Foam dressings, alginates, and hydroactive dressings help to control exudate; use hydrocolloids with paste, powder, or granules for deeper areas.	Foam Alginates Hydroactive	Foam cavity dressing Alginates Hydrocolloid/alginate Hydrocolloid with paste, powder or granules Hydroactive cavity	
Red/low exudate	Maintain moist environment and promote granulation and epithelialization. Hydrocolloids, foams, sheet hydrogels, and film dressings will maintain the environment. It is possible to use a combination of amorphous hydrogels with a foam cavity dressing in deeper wounds.	Hydrocolloids Foams Sheet hydrogels Films In addition, the use of zinc paste bandages in superficial granulating venous ulcers is appropriate.	Hydrocolloids with paste, powder, or granules Amorphous hydrogels Foam cavity dressing	
Pink/low exudate	Maintain moist environment, protect, and insulate. Foams, thin hydrocolloids, thin hydroactives, film dressings, and simple nonadherent dressings will provide the necessary cover.	Foams Films Hydrocolloids (thin) Hydroactive (thin) Nonadherent dressing In addition, zinc paste bandages may also be used.		
Red unbroken skin	To prevent skin breakdown. Hydrocolloids and film dressings provide the best protection.			

be noted that most soaps are significantly alkaline and will have a negative effect on the wound and the periwound skin.

Wounds should be cleansed with care; health professionals must consider the temperature of the cleansing product (it should be at body temperature) and the pH of the products to avoid any unnecessary damage to the wound and the periskin and avoid vigorous cleaning of the wound.

CONCLUSION

The products applied to a wound at each stage of wound healing play a vital role in controlling the wound environment. The choice will depend on the many factors that relate to the wound itself, such as wound type, level of exudates, and presence of bacteria and/or infection.

REVIEW QUESTIONS

1. A problem associated with traditional wound care theory is:
   A. A scab increases the risk of scarring and poor cosmetic results.
   B. Exposure to air increases the surface temperature of the wound.
   C. Exposure to air decreases fluid loss.
   D. A scab assists with the movement of epidermal cells.
2. Moist wound healing:
   A. While promoting granulation, slows epithelialization.
   B. Hinders growth factors reaching the wound bed due to exudate.
   C. Enhances the action of enzymes released by neutrophils.
   D. Complicates wound cleansing due to exudate on the surface.

3. Cadexomer iodine:
   A. Has no effect on the level of slough.
   B. Inhibits inflammatory growth factors.
   C. Is antibacterial.
   D. Is nonabsorbent.
4. A factor that can influence silver dressings ability to kill micro-organisms is:
   A. The distribution of silver in the dressing.
   B. The dressing's resistance to moisture in the wound.
   C. Whether the wound is colonized or infected.
   D. The bacterial resistance of the micro-organisms.
5. Alginate dressings:
   A. Adhere to the wound
   B. Do not conform to the body hape.
   C. Are not used in infected wounds.
   D. Provide hemostasis.

REFERENCES

1. Bull JP. Experiments with occlusive dressings of a new plastic. *Lancet.* 1948;213–215.
2. Schilling RSF. Clinical trial of occlusive plastic dressings. *Lancet.* 1950;293–296.
3. Winter GD. Formation of the scab and the rate of epithelization of superficial wounds in the skin of the young domestic pig. *Nature.* 1962;193:293–294.
4. Hinman CD. Effect of air exposure and occlusion on experimental human skin wounds. *Nature.* 1963;200:377–378.
5. Turner TD. Products and their development in wound management. *Plast Surg Dermatol Aspects.* 1979;75–84.
6. Turner TD. Surgical dressings in the drug tariff. *Wound Manage.* 1991;1:4–6.
7. Thomas S. Pain and wound management: Community outlook. *Nurs Times.* 1989;85(suppl):19–15.
8. Bernard FX, Juchaux F, Laurensou C, et al. Stimulation of the proliferation of human dermal fibroblasts in vitro by a lipid colloid dressing. *J Wound Care.* 2005;14:215–220.
9. Bourton F. An evaluation of non-adherent wound contact layers for acute traumatic and surgical wounds. *J Wound Care.* 2004;13:371–373.
10. Terrill PJ, Varughese G. A comparison of three primary non-adherent dressings to hand surgery wounds. *J Wound Care.* 2000;9:359–363.
11. Thomas S, Loveless P, Hay NP. Comparative review of the properties of six semipermeable film dressings. *Pharm J.* 1988;240:785–788.
12. Thomas S. *Handbook of Wound Dressings.* London: Macmillan; 1994.
13. Golledge CL. Advances in wound management. *Mod Med Aust.* 993;36:42–47.
14. Myers JA. Ease of use of two semi-permeable adhesive membranes compared. *Pharm J.* 1984;233:685–686.
15. Mizuguchi K, et al. Analysis of special features of various film dressings. *Wound Repair Regen.* 2008;16(1):102–107.
16. Terrill P. The split thickness skin graft donor site; have we found the perfect dressing. *ANZ J Surg.* 2007;77(suppl 1):62.
17. Pittman J. Comparative study of the use of antimicrobial barrier film dressing in postoperative incision care. *J Wound Ostomy Continence Nurs.* 2005;32(3S)(suppl 2):S25–S26.
18. Aindow D. Films or fabrics: is it time to re-appraise postoperative dressings. *Br J Nurs.* 2005;14(19):S15–S16, S18, S20.
19. Jones V. When and how to use adhesive film dressings. *Nurs Times.* 2000;96(14 suppl):3–4.
20. Fletcher J. Using film dressings. *Nurs Times.* 2003;99(25):57.
21. Dornseifer U. The ideal split-thickness skin graft donor site dressing: rediscovery of polyurethane film. *Ann Plastic Surg.* 2009;63(2):198–200.
22. Thomas S. SMTL Dressings Datacard Revision No. 1.3 Revision date 1997/12/16.
23. Loiterman DA, Byers PH. Effects of a hydrocellular polyurethane dressing on chronic venous ulcer healing. *Wounds.* 1991;3:178–181.
24. Myers JA. LYOfoam: a versatile polyurethane foam surgical dressing. *Pharm J.* 1985;235:270.
25. Foster AVM, Greenhill MT, Edmonds ME. Comparing two dressings in the treatment of diabetic foot ulcers. *J Wound Care.* 1994;3:224–228.
26. Jones V. When and how to use foam dressings. *Nurs Times.* 2000;96(36):2.
27. Majno G. *The Healing Hand.* Cambridge, MA: Harvard University Press; 1991.
28. Sussman G. Wound dressings: removing the confusion. *Aust J Podiatr Med.* 1998;32(4):145–148.
29. Sussman GM. Hydrogels: a review. *Prim Intention.* 1994;2:6–9.
30. Smith RA, Rusbourne J. The use of Solugel in the closure of wounds by secondary intention. *Prim Intention.* 1994;2:14–17.
31. Thomas S, Jones H. Clinical experiences with a new hydrogel dressing. *J Wound Care.* 1996;5:132–133.

32. Thomas S. Comparing two dressings for wound debridement. *J Wound Care*. 1993;2:272–274.

33. White R. Flaminal: a novel approach to wound bioburden control. *Wounds*. 2006;2(3):64–69.

34. Sollie P. Evaluation of alginate gels with antimicrobial enzyme system technology for leg ulcer healing. *Wounds*. 2007.

35. Thomas S, Loveless P. A comparative study of the properties of six hydrocolloid dressings. *Pharm J*. 1991;247:672–675.

36. Rousseau P, Niecestro RM. Comparison of the physicochemical properties of various hydrocolloid dressings. *Wounds*. 1991;3:43–45.

37. Marshall PJ, Eyers A. The use of a hydrocolloid dressing (Comfeel transparent) as a wound closure dressing following lower bowel surgery. *Prim Intention*. 1994;2:39–40.

38. Banks V, Bale SE, Harding KG. Comparing two dressings for exuding pressure sores in community patients. *J Wound Care*. 1994;3:175–178.

39. Thomas SS, Lawrence JC, Thomas A. Evaluation of hydrocolloids and topical medication in minor burns. *J Wound Care*. 1995;4:218–220.

40. Thomas S. Observations on the fluid handling properties of alginate dressings. *Pharm J*. 1992;248:850–851.

41. Sussman GM. Alginates: a review. *Prim Intention*. 1996;4:33–37.

42. Miller L, Jones V, Bale S. The use of alginate packing in the management of deep sinuses. *J Wound Care*. 1993;2:262–263.

43. Thomas S. Use of a calcium alginate dressing. *Pharm J*. 1985;235:188–190.

44. Thomas S. Alginates: a guide to the properties and uses of the different alginate dressings available today. *J Wound Care*. 1992;1:29–32.

45. Terrill P, Sussman G, Bailey M. Absorption of blood by moist wound healing dressings. *Prim Intention*. 2003;11:7–10,12–17.

46. Williams C. Treating a patient's venous ulcer with a foamed gel dressing. *J Wound Care*. 1993;2:264–265.

47. Achterberg VB, Welling C, Meyer-Ingold W. Hydroactive dressings and serum protein: an in vitro study. *J Wound Care*. 1996;5:79–82.

48. Collier J. A moist odor-free environment. *Prof Nurse*. 1992;7:804–807.

49. Brown-Etris M, Smith JA, Pasceri P, et al. Case studies: considering dressing options. *Ostom Wound Manage*. 1994;40(5):46–52.

50. Dykes PJ, Heggie R, Hill SA. Effects of adhesive dressings on the stratum corneum of the skin. *J Wound Care*. 2001;10:7–10.

51. Hollingworth H, Collier M. Nurses' views about pain and trauma at dressing changes: result of a national survey. *J Wound Care*. 2000;9:369–374.

52. Foster AVM, Edmonds M. Hyalofill: a new product for chronic wound management. *Diabetic Foot*. 2000;3:29–30.

53. Sleigh JW, Linter SPK. Hazards of hydrogen peroxide. *Br Med J*. 1985;291:1706.

54. Brennan SS, Leaper DJ. The effects of antiseptics on the healing wound: a study using the rabbit ear chamber. *Br J Surg*. 1985;72:780–782.

55. Lawrence CJ. Dressings and wound infection. *Am J Surg*. 1994;167(suppl):21S–24S.

56. Brennan SS, Foster ME, Leaper DJ. Antiseptic toxicity in wounds: healed by secondary intention. *J Hosp Infect*. 1986;8:263–267.

57. Leaper DJ. Antiseptics and their effect on healing tissue. *Nurs Times*. 1986;82(22):45–46.

58. Lawrence JC. Wound infection. *J Wound Care*. 1993;2:277–280.

59. Morgan DA. Chlorinated solutions: (E) useful or (e) useless. *Pharm J*. 1989;243:219–220.

60. Gutierrez A. The science behind stable super-oxide water. *Wounds Suppl*. 2006;18:7–10.

61. Wolvos TA. Advanced wound care with stable super-oxide water. *Wounds Suppl*. 2006;18:11–13.

62. Valenzuela AR, Perucho NS. The effectiveness of a 0.1% polihexanide gel. *Rev Enferm*. 2008;31(4):7–12.

63. Andriessen A, Eberlein T. Feature: assessment of a wound cleansing solution in the treatment of problem wounds. *Wounds*. 2008;6S:171–175.

64. Thomas S, McCubbin TS. A comparison of the antimicrobial effects of four silver-containing dressings on three organisms. *J Wound Care* 2003;12:101–107.

65. Sundberg JA. Retrospective review of the use of cadexomer iodine in the treatment of chronic wounds. *Wounds*. 1997;3:68–86.

66. Leaper DJ, Brennan SS, Simpson RA, et al. Experimental infection and hydrogel dressings. *J Hosp Infect*. 1984;5:69–73.

67. Young JB, Dobrzanski S. Pressure sores: epidemiology and current management concepts. *Drugs Aging*. 1992;2:42–57.

68. Brown CD, Zitelli JA. A review of topical agents for wounds and methods of wounding. *J Dermatol Surg Oncol*. 1993;19:732–737.

69. Dire JD, Welsh AP. A comparison of wound irrigation solution used in the emergency department. *Ann Emerg Med*. 1990;704–707.

CHAPTER 21

Management of the Wound Environment with Advanced Therapies

Craig J. Pastor, Matthew J. Trovato, Mark S. Granick, Nancy L. Tomaselli, and Barbara M. Bates-Jensen

CHAPTER OBJECTIVES

At the completion of this chapter, the reader will be able to:

1. Describe criteria for defining a refractory wound.
2. Identify three advanced wound therapies.
3. Compare and contrast advanced wound therapies.
4. Describe and explain indications for each advanced wound therapy.

Advanced wound therapy includes topical wound products and devices. Therapy in this category does not fall into other wound treatment categories and typically costs more than other wound therapies. Examples of advanced wound therapy include living skin equivalents (LSEs); topical growth factors; devices that directly change the local wound environment, such as negative pressure wound therapy (see Chapter 28 on "Negative Pressure Wound Therapy") and temperature therapy; and synthetic skin dressings. This chapter focuses on topical growth factors, LSEs, and synthetic skin dressings.

The debate about when the use of advanced wound therapies is appropriate centers around the ability of the clinician to define the appropriate wound candidate. One suggestion is to use advanced therapies only on wounds that fail to heal with standard approaches. Another suggestion is to use them immediately on wounds identified as being potentially harder to heal. Some wound therapies provide specific guidelines for appropriate use, and others provide more general indications. It is accepted that advanced wound therapies are particularly useful for refractory wounds.

Merriam-Webster's Collegiate Dictionary defines *refractory* as "(1) Resisting control or authority, stubborn or unmanageable, (2) resistant to treatment or cure, (3) unresponsive to stimulus, immune, insusceptible, (4) difficult to fuse, corrode, or draw out."[1] The term *refractory* is typically used to define wounds that have not healed, despite appropriate treatment. It has come to be used to define difficult-to-heal wounds and wounds that do not progress toward healing. Wounds may be considered refractory when they present with certain characteristics such as extensive necrosis, undermining, or tunneling. Some studies have found that undermining present on initial wound assessment was associated with poor wound healing outcomes.[2,3] Others did not find undermining at baseline assessment to be a significant predictor of healing.[4] The presence of necrotic

tissue in wounds provides a physical impediment to healing, and, not surprisingly, several have found that healing outcomes in necrotic wounds are fewer than those without necrotic tissue.[5,6] These studies suggest that the presence of necrotic tissue is associated with slower healing times[6] and a decreased proportion of improving ulcers.[5]

Specific comorbidities that are known to compromise wound healing, such as immunosuppression,[7,8] diabetes mellitus,[9,10] vascular disease,[11] or hypovolemia,[12] may determine whether the wound is diagnosed as refractory. There may be an additional significant host burden that impairs healing, such as infection,[13,14] wounds of prolonged duration, or extensive wounds.[5,15–18] Finally, a wound may be diagnosed as refractory when it fails to meet research-based temporal healing expectations. For example, in pressure ulcers, clean full-thickness pressure ulcers should show signs of improvement within 2 to 4 weeks,[5,18] partial-thickness ulcers should improve in 1 to 2 weeks,[19] and those that do not decrease in size with improvement at 1 week may not progress to healing.[4] Time frames and surface area changes have also been identified for diabetic foot ulcers and venous ulcers. Exhibit 21.1 presents a proposal for diagnostic criteria for the "refractory" wound to assist clinicians in determining those wounds that may benefit from early use of advanced wound therapy.

GROWTH FACTORS

Several growth factors have been identified as regulatory polypeptides that coordinate the complex interaction of cellular and biochemical events that control wound healing. Growth factors participate in the regulation of cell proliferation, differentiation, and organ growth. Several growth factors, including recombinant human (rh) platelet-derived growth factor (PDGF), epidermal growth factor (EGF), and basic fibroblast growth factor

EXHIBIT   21.1

Refractory Wound Criteria

Wound characteristics present: undermining, tunneling, extensive necrotic tissue

Host burden present: extensive wounding, multiple wounds, prolonged wound duration, infection

Healing risk factors present: diabetes, vascular disease, immunocompromise, hypovolemia

Inadequate movement toward healing present: full-thickness wounds fail to improve with appropriate treatment in 2 to 4 weeks; partial-thickness wounds failure to improve in 1 to 2 weeks

(bFGF), have been produced and are available for use. Only rh-PDGF has been approved by the United States Food and Drug Administration (FDA) for use in wound therapy.[20]

Platelet-Derived Growth Factor

PDGF and its relative proteins were the first approved proteins for promoting diabetic foot healing and other refractory ulcers. In 1986, Knighton et al. reported their successful treatment of chronic ulcers with autologous platelet-derived wound healing factor (PDWHF).[21] In their study, 49 patients with 95 chronic wounds were treated with PDWHF, resulting in a mean time to 100% healing of 10.6 weeks. Patients received 198 weeks of conventional wound care without healing before PDWHF application. Recombinant PDGF was first reported in the treatment of pressure ulcers in a 1992 phase I/II prospective, controlled clinical trial of 20 patients in which 100 µg/dL of topical rh-PDGF increased the rate of wound closure compared with other groups.[22] In the phase II follow-up multicenter trial of 45 patients with pressure ulcers, the Mustoe group again reported that topical application of rh-PDGF accelerated the rate of wound closure. Ulcers receiving 100 µg/dL of rh-PDGF showed a 71% decrease in area over 28 days, and those treated with 300 µg/dL showed a 60% decrease. The report concluded that only a certain dose of growth factors is necessary to facilitate wound healing. Rees et al. completed a phase II, multicenter, double-blind, parallel group, placebo-controlled trial using rh-PDGF-BB (becaplermin) 300 µg/g daily, 100 µg/g twice daily, and placebo resulting in complete healing in 19%, 23%, and 0%, respectively.[23] Approved by the FDA in 1997, becaplermin is used for pressure, lower extremity diabetic, and neuropathic ulcers.

Description and Effects

Regranex Gel is a topical gel that contains the active ingredient becaplermin formulated in an aqueous sodium carboxymethyl cellulose–based (NaCMC) gel. Each gram of Regranex Gel contains 100 µg of becaplermin. The biologic activity of becaplermin includes promoting recruiting (chemotaxis) and proliferation (mitosis) of cells involved in wound repair, and enhancing granulation production (synthesis), which is similar to that of endogenous PDGF.

Indications for Use

Regranex Gel 0.01% is indicated for use in the treatment of diabetic neuropathic ulcers that extend into the subcutaneous tissue or beyond and have adequate blood supply.[24] When used in conjunction with good wound care, it increases the incidence of complete wound healing. The cornerstones of good wound care include

• Sharp debridement at all office encounters
• Control of infection
• Off-loading of pressure from the affected area
• Maintenance of a moist, clean wound environment

Recently, Calhoun described the use of Regranex Gel™ 0.01% for the treatment of mucosal wounds in two patients who had corticocancellous bone grafts following mandibular bone loss. Both patients' wounds showed increasing granulation tissue, with one patient proceeding to a fully healed wound with minimal bone loss. The second patient was lost to follow-up before full healing had occurred.[25] The efficacy of becaplermin for the treatment of other types of wounds is currently being evaluated.[23]

Indications for Discontinuation

Regranex should be discontinued if the patient has extensive necrosis, untreated active infection, or ischemia. Once the ulcer is debrided, infection is treated, or the area is revascularized, the gel may be used. Continued treatment with becaplermin gel should be reassessed if the ulcer does not decrease in size by approximately 30% after 10 weeks of treatment or if complete healing has not occurred in 20 weeks.[24]

Method of Application

Regranex Gel is available in a 15 g multidose tube as a clear, colorless to straw-color, topical gel. The dosage of gel to be applied will vary, depending on the size of the ulcer area. The formula to calculate the length of gel to be applied daily is length × width divided by 4.[24]

CLINICAL WISDOM

Becaplermin Gel Application

To apply the becaplermin gel, squeeze the calculated length of gel onto a clean surface, such as wax paper. Then transfer the gel from the clean surface with an applicator, such as a cotton swab or tongue blade, and spread over the entire ulcer area at approximately 1/16 of an inch in thickness. Cover the gel with a saline-moistened gauze dressing and leave in place for approximately 12 hours. Remove the dressing and rinse the ulcer with saline or water to remove the gel and then cover the ulcer again with a second saline-moistened dressing without the gel for the next 12 hours. Apply the gel to the ulcer once daily until complete healing occurs. If the ulcer does not decrease in size by approximately 30% after 10 weeks of treatment or if complete healing has not occurred in 20 weeks, reassess continued treatment with the gel. Store Regranex in the refrigerator.

Precautions and Contraindications

Becaplermin gel is contraindicated in patients with known hypersensitivity to any component of the product or known neoplasms at the application site. Erythematous rashes occurred in 2% of patients treated with Regranex Gel. Wounds that close by primary intention should not be treated with Regranex because it is a nonsterile, low-bioburden, preserved product. The effects of becaplermin on exposed joints, tendons, ligaments, and bone have not been established in humans. Carcinogenesis and reproductive toxicity studies have not been conducted. It is not known whether Regranex can cause fetal harm when administered to a pregnant woman, can affect reproductive capacity, or is excreted in human milk. The safety and effectiveness in patients younger than 16 years has not been established. It is also not known whether Regranex Gel interacts with other topical medications applied to the ulcer site.[24]

Expected Outcomes

When becaplermin gel is used in conjunction with good ulcer care, including regular sharp debridement, pressure relief, and infection control, the gel increases the incidence of complete healing of diabetic ulcers.[26]

Alternative Growth Factor Options

Basic Fibroblast Growth Factor

bFGF has also been used in clinical trials to treat chronic ulcers. Robson et al.[27] completed randomized, blinded, placebo-controlled human trials of bFGF for pressure sores. Three concentrations of bFGF in five dosing schedules were tested for safety. No toxicity, significant serum absorption, or antibody formation was detected. The slopes of the regression curves of volume decrease with initial pressure sore volume showed a greater healing effect in the bFGF-treated patients. Histologically, bFGF-treated wounds showed an increase in fibroblasts and capillaries. Treatment with bFGF achieved more than 70% wound closure.[24] Fu et al.[28] evaluated the safety and efficacy of topical application of recombinant bFGF on the healing of chronic cutaneous wounds resulting from trauma, diabetes mellitus, pressure, and radiation in a prospective, open-label crossover trial. Thirty-three wounds that failed to heal within 4 weeks with conventional therapies were locally treated once daily with 150 AU/cm^2 rbFGF and showed improved healing. Eighteen wounds were completely healed within 2 weeks, four healed within 3 weeks, and another eight completely healed within 4 weeks. The remaining three wounds healed on days 30, 40, and 42 with continued treatment of rbFGF, yielding a 90.9% 4-week efficacy. Histologically, capillary sprouts were more abundant and fibroblasts were more differentiated in wounds treated with rbFGF. No adverse effects were observed. An optimal formulation has not yet been established.

Keratinocyte Growth Factor-2

Robson et al.[29] conducted a phase II A multicenter, randomized, double-blind, placebo-controlled trial that investigated the effect of keratinocyte growth factor-2 (KGF-2) on chronic venous stasis ulcers of 3 to 36 months duration. The 94 study subjects were otherwise treated with standard compression therapy. Compression dressings were changed twice a week, with placebo or 20 or 60 µg/cm^2 of KGF-2 (repifermin) applied topically during dressing changes. When both active dose groups were pooled, there was a significant improvement in the proportion of wounds that were 75% and 90% healed at 12 weeks. Based on these results, a phase II B trial was undertaken. However, the percentage of patients treated with repifermin who achieved complete wound closure within 20 weeks of treatment was not statistically significantly different from the placebo groups, nor were there any favorable trends in the treatment group. As a result, manufacturers have ceased development of repifermin for chronic wound therapy, though Kepivance, palifermin, was approved in December 2004 for the prevention of chemotherapy-induced mucositis in patients with hematologic malignancies.

Macrophage-Colony Stimulating Factor

Colony-stimulating factors (CSF) enhance a general wound healing response, working directly on macrophages and monocytes, as opposed to fibroblasts, keratinocytes, or endothelial cells. This is the basis for the rabbit ear chronic wound model study by Wu et al.,[30] which hypothesizes that macrophage-CSF (M-CSF) accelerates healing as a result of generalized macrophage activation, thereby increasing TGF-β transcription and granulation volume.

Marques da Costa et al.[31] used compression dressings for a randomized, double-blind, placebo-controlled trial of human granulocyte/ M-CSF for treatment of venous stasis ulcers. The selected ulcers were less than 30 cm^2 and well-perfused. The ulcers were treated with rhGM-CSF using four equidistant injections near the poles of the target wound. The treatment was placebo or 200 or 400 µg of rhGM-CSF, administered once a week for 4 weeks or until wound healing occurred. Using standard wound care, the percentage of ulcers with complete closure at 13 weeks was 61%, 57%, and 19% for 400, 200 µg, and placebo, respectively. Further clinical investigations are necessary for FDA approval.

AutoloGel

Lastly, an autologous, patient-specific topical preparation, AutoloGel, is available. PDWHF tries to seal the wound with the patient's own blood products, initiates coagulation, and provides growth factors that accelerate the patient's own wound repair cascade. The inflammatory, proliferative, and maturation phases of wound repair are mediated by the autologous tissue coagulum that is applied topically by a physician and redressed after 5 days with an alternative wound dressing for the next 7 days. This is repeated until the wound heals. A large retrospective study of PDWHF revealed significantly increased effectiveness for healing diabetic neuropathic ulcers over standard treatment particularly in larger wounds involving deeper structures (e.g., tendon and fascia).[32] A recent broad literature search revealed clear evidence supporting palifermin use in the treatment of hematopoietic stem cell transplant recipients with hematologic malignancies. Data supporting its use in other oncologic conditions are less clear.[33] Since AutoloGel is derived from the patient's own blood, its application does not require FDA approval.

Combined Growth Factors

The use of topical cytokines/growth factors in wound healing does not always lead to positive results. Reasons for failure include the use of a single growth factor, the application in nonpharmacologic doses, peptide degradation, and poor wound bed conditions. Recent multicenter studies have looked at the role of amnion-derived cellular cytokine solution (ACCS) in wound healing. This solution, made up of PDGF, vascular endothelial growth factor, angiogenin, transforming growth factor β2, tissue inhibitor of metalloproteinase-1, and tissue inhibitor of metalloproteinase-2, is obtained by collecting the proteins produced by amnion-derived multipotent progenitor cells. Since this solution contains multiple cytokines at physiologic levels[34] it improves upon some of the shortcomings of previous products. Xing looked at the effects of amnion-derived multipotent cells (AMPs) on wound-breaking strength in the acute wound. In an animal model, he found that injecting AMP cells into the load-bearing layer of rat abdominal walls prior to laparotomy reduced the incidence of wound failure.[35] Franz similarly found ACCS to improve healing in acute and chronic wounds in an animal model. His group found that priming laparotomy incisions with ACCS led to increased breaking strength, fewer acute wound failures, and fewer incisional hernias when compared with phosphate-buffered saline and unconditioned media. Likewise, the ACCS led to an accelerated rate of wound closure in chronic wounds when compared with unconditioned media.[35]

BIOLOGICAL SKIN SUBSTITUTES

For more than a century, there has been a need for alternatives in the treatment of full-thickness or deep partial-thickness life-threatening burn injuries. Though an invaluable reconstructive tool, there are problems and limitations with skin grafting. The donor site can be painful or unsightly. The graft does not always take and heal the wound. In very large wounds or burns, the need for grafts can necessitate the use of reharvested donor sites, unusual donor sites, wide meshing of the grafts, and other creative strategies for obtaining wound coverage. The need for an off-the-shelf skin substitute that can promote healing, eliminate the donor site, be quickly and easily accessible, minimize contracture and scarring, and be immunologically compatible has resulted in the evolution of tissue-engineered skin equivalents and skin substitutes. Currently approved tissue-engineered skin equivalents include Biobrane, *AWBAT*, Apligraf, and Integra (see Table 21.1).[36]

Biobrane/*AW*BAT

Biobrane, a bilaminate membrane comprising a thin semipermeable silicone membrane bonded to a thicker nylon fabric mesh, was developed in 1979 by Dr. Aubrey Woodroof. A coating of type I porcine collagen to the nylon mesh encourages wound adherence by allowing for fibrin ingrowth.[37] Biobrane has been shown to possess good wound adhesion, vapor transmission, flexibility, elasticity, and transparency for wound observation.[38]

*AW*BAT, *Advanced Wound Bioengineered Alternative Tissue*, was cleared by the FDA in 2009 as the latest temporary skin substitute. As an extension of the design of Biobrane, *AW*BAT has significant design changes including increased porosity of the silicone layer and continuity of the 3D nylon structure. In addition, the type I collagen peptide is not crosslinked to the silicone-nylon membrane. These changes are proposed to improve acute wound adherence, reduce fluid accumulation, increase permeability to topical antimicrobials, and reduce the potential for punctate scarring. *AW*BAT can remain sterile and stable at room temperature for 3 years.[39]

CASE STUDY

Growth Factor

The patient is a 55-year-old Hispanic female with a 12-year history of type 2 diabetes; a 2-year history of Charcot deformity of the right foot; hypertension; peripheral neuropathy; nonhealing diabetic, neuropathic ulcer on the plantar surface of the right foot for 8 months; and tinea pedis of the toe webs. Figure 21.1 shows the ulcer predebridement, and Figure 21.2 shows the ulcer after debridement and initial application of becaplermin gel. The patient was using a walker and crutches to off-load pressure from the ulcer. Figure 21.3 shows improvement in the ulcer, with a decrease in size from 2.8 × 2.2 × 1.8 cm to 1.8 × 1.1 × 0.7 cm. Figure 21.4 shows further decrease in the ulcer size at 1.1 × 0.6 × 0.4 cm. Figure 21.5 shows complete wound closure, which took 14 weeks after the ulcer was treated with becaplermin gel after weekly debridement. The patient is now in custommolded shoes with no recurrence of the ulcer. (For basic information on growth factors and physiology of wound healing, see Chapter 2.)

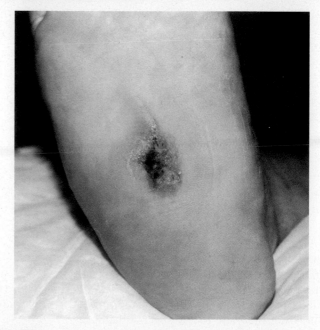

FIGURE 21.1 Ulcer predebridement. (Copyright © Nancy Tomaselli.)

CASE STUDY

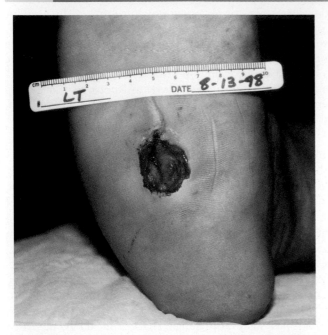

FIGURE 21.2 Ulcer postdebridement, Regranex growth factor treatment started. (Copyright © Nancy Tomaselli.)

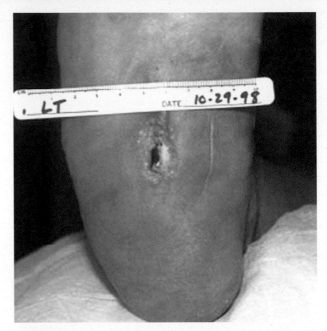

FIGURE 21.4 Ulcer 10 weeks after Regranex growth factor treatment started. (Copyright © Nancy Tomaselli.)

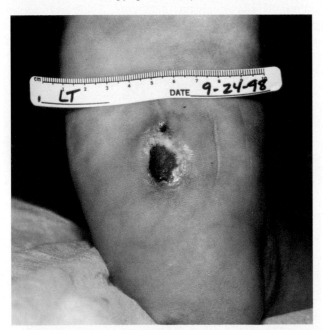

FIGURE 21.3 Ulcer after 6 weeks on Regranex growth factor treatment. (Copyright © Nancy Tomaselli.)

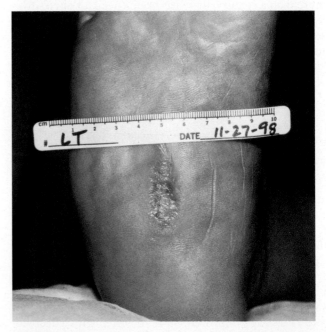

FIGURE 21.5 Complete wound closure. (Copyright © Nancy Tomaselli.)

Indications for Use

Biobrane and *AWBAT* are indicated for the treatment of superficial and moderate-depth partial-thickness burns. Barrett performed a prospective randomized control study comparing Biobrane to 1% silver sulfadiazine in 20 pediatric patients with partial-thickness burns. Biobrane was found to significantly reduce pain, pain medication requirements, healing time, and length of hospital stay.[40] Biobrane has also been shown to be effective in the treatment of skin-graft donor sites, providing superior pain control, reduced exudate accumulation, and faster healing compared to Scarlet Red,[41] though in one study there was some increase in the rate of infection.[42] Similarly, when compared with Xeroform and Duoderm, Biobrane provided superior pain control at the cost of increased infection risk.[43] There is additional literature on the use of Biobrane in axillary reconstruction, CO_2 laser resurfacing of the face, mechanical dermabrasion, and toxic epidermal necrolysis.[37]

TABLE 21.1	A Guide to Biological Skin Substitutes				
Trade Name	**Schematic Representation**	**Layers**		**FDA Approval**	**Cost**
*AW*BAT		1. Silicone (altered porosity) 2. Nylon mesh 3. Collagen (modified from Biobrane)		Yes	$$
Biobrane		4. Silicone 5. Nylon mesh 6. Collagen		Yes	$
TransCyte		1. Silicone 2. Nylon mesh 3. Collagen seeded with neonatal fibroblasts		Yes	$$$
AlloDerm		1. Acellular deepithelialized cadaver dermis		n/a	$$
Integra		1. Silicone 2. Collagen and glycosaminoglycan		Yes	$$
Dermagraft		1. Dexon or Vicryl seeded with neonatal fibroblasts		Yes	$$$
Apligraf		1. Neonatal keratinocytes 2. Collagen seeded with neonatal fibroblasts		Yes	$$$$$
CEA (Epicel)		1. Cultured autologous keratinocytes		n/a	$$$$$$
CAK (Laserskin)		1. Cultured autologous keratinocytes 2. Hyaluronic acid with laser perforations		n/a	$$$$$$

Indications for Discontinuation

Nonadherence and infection are indications to discontinue Biobrane. If the Biobrane is loose and there is purulent discharge beneath it, remove that portion of the dressing and begin local wound care. Biobrane should also be discontinued in instances of allergic reaction.

Method of Application

Biobrane should be applied wrinkle-free with the fabric or dull side down on a freshly debrided or excised, or meshed autograft wound containing less than 10^6 bacteria per gram of tissue. It should be secured under slight tension with sutures, skin staples, tape, or skin closure strips and then wrapped with dry gauze. Twenty-four to thirty-six hours postapplication, the outer dressing should be removed. Nonpurulent drainage should be rolled out or aspirated and a new gauze dressing should be placed. At 48 to 72 hours post application, the outer dressing can be discontinued if the Biobrane is adherent to the underlying tissue. The Biobrane should be removed when the underlying tissue is healed.

Precautions and Contraindications

Biobrane should only be applied to clean or thoroughly debrided wounds. It will not adhere to dead tissue. Rare complications associated with Biobrane include contact dermatitis, punctate scarring, and toxic shock syndrome.[37]

Expected Outcomes

The use of Biobrane in the treatment of burns is strongly supported in the literature.[40,44] Further research is necessary to support its use in other conditions. More research is needed to explore clinical applications and results of *AW*BAT.

Apligraf

Invented in 1981 at MIT by Eugene Bell as the first medical device containing living cells to receive FDA approval, Apligraf (formerly known as Graftskin) is a bilaminar construct consisting of a simulated dermal phase and a simulated epidermal layer.[45] The dermal component is a bovine collagen mesh, seeded with living neonatal fibroblasts. The fibroblasts are a pure cell culture, derived from neonatal foreskin. The epidermal layer is a pure keratinocyte culture, similarly derived from neonatal foreskin. Histologically, it closely resembles normal skin without the rete ridges. The technical difficulties in creating pure cell cultures free of contamination and being able to deliver them to remote sites on demand for clinical use are incredible.

CLINICAL WISDOM

Wound Cleansing with Apligraf

During Apligraf use, avoid all cytotoxic substances, such as Dakin's solution, chlorhexidine, or povidone-iodine.

Indications for Use

Apligraf was FDA approved in 1998 for venous leg ulcers of greater than 1 month duration that are refractory to conventional therapy, and in 2000 for treating diabetic foot ulcers of greater than 2 weeks duration, without tendon, muscle, capsule, or bone exposure.

Indications for Discontinuation

There are few indications for discontinuation of the product. The presence of infection or allergic reaction would be strong indicators for discontinuing treatment with Apligraf. Failure of the wound to improve significantly after two applications would be another reason to cease further treatment with the product.

Method of Application

The product arrives in a thermally controlled box. It must be incubated until it is used, which needs to be soon after it is received. The graft is 7.5 cm in diameter. It is packaged on agarose media that is colored with a pH indicator in a Petri dish. The graft is gently lifted and placed on the wound with overlapping edges. A compression wrap is used to fix it in place.[46] Apligraf is indicated only for use on wounds that are free of infection and necrotic debris, so it may be necessary to pretreat the wound with mechanical debridement or topical antibiotics.

Precautions and Contraindications

Apligraf is contraindicated in infected wounds or in people who are allergic to bovine collagen or the agarose shipping media.

Expected Outcomes

Initially, the Apligraf sticks to a clean wound and looks like a skin graft. After about a week, the material loses its appearance as a graft and takes on a gelatinous look. It is important not to disrupt the "living skin equivalent" during the initial 2 to 3 weeks. Because of these changes, it can be easily washed away. The healing process for the LSE differs significantly from that of a skin graft, despite its initial appearance. The LSE cells are rapidly replaced by the patient's own cells. The wound, typically bearing a chronically indolent, inactive surface, becomes biologically more active as the wound healing cascade is stimulated. The LSE acts as a biologic growth factor factory, as well as a biologic occlusive at the surface. This increased activity continues for 6 to 8 weeks. With full healing there is minimal contracture, and it achieves a remarkably normal appearance. In fact, the patient's own melanocytes repopulate the healing area to obtain a confluent color. If additional treatment is required, a new LSE may be applied.

TransCyte

TransCyte uses human neonatal fibroblasts cultured for 17 days onto the nylon mesh component of Biobrane to secrete extracellular matrix (ECM; fibronectin, type I collagen, proteoglycan, and matrix-bound growth factors) into the mesh. The cells are no longer viable in the final product.

Indications for Use

TransCyte was FDA approved in March 1997 as a temporary wound covering for surgically excised full-thickness and partial-thickness thermal burns in patients requiring coverage prior to autografting. This was based on a 66-patient trial in which comparable full or deep partial-thickness burn sites on each patient were randomized to TransCyte or cadaver allograft.[47] The label expanded in October 1997 to include partial-thickness burns mid-dermal to indeterminate depth that may be expected to heal without autografting.

Indications for Discontinuation

The product is applied to a freshly debrided wound. It adheres to the wound and lasts for up to 100 days. If infection or fluid accumulation occurs under the TransCyte, it must be removed.

Method of Application

The product is stored at −70°C. A specific thawing protocol must be followed for TransCyte to work. The product is applied to the wound and placed under a pressure dressing or negative pressure.

Expected Outcomes

Kumar et al. showed that, when used in partial-thickness burns in children, TransCyte promotes faster reepithelialization and requires fewer overall dressings than Biobrane or Silvazine. Patients who received Silvazine or Biobrane required more autografting than those treated with TransCyte in the study.[48] Currently off the market, TransCyte is licensed to Advanced Biohealing where production and marketing are ongoing.

Integra

Originally dubbed "Artificial Skin," Integra is a membrane bilayer. The silicone outer layer temporarily provides the sealant properties of the epidermis, and the collagen and

CLINICAL WISDOM

TransCyte Storage

TransCyte is 3 to 13 times more expensive than allograft. It is 16 times more expensive than Biobrane and 2 to 3 times more expensive than Integra. It is also more difficult to store and handle than Biobrane or Integra. It must be stored between −70°C and −20°C. When stored correctly, it has a shelf life of 18 months. It is, however, an extremely effective method for treating partial-thickness burns or large surface area wounds.

Apligraf

The patient illustrated in Figures 21.6 to 21.8 has chronic venous disease in her leg. She has been treated with chronic compression, with which she has been poorly compliant. Several years ago, she underwent a skin graft that healed an ulcer. She reappeared with a recurrence in the middle of her old skin graft. She was treated with Apligraf. Initially, it had the appearance of a healed skin graft. A gelatinous phase followed. Within 8 weeks, the wound healed and has remained so for more than 1 year.

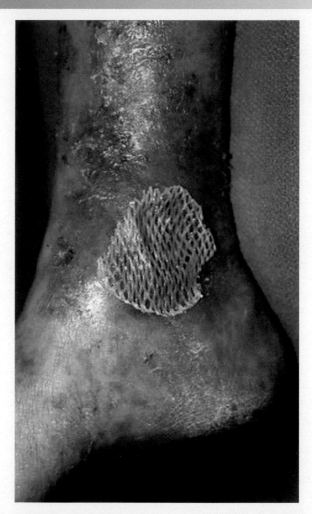

FIGURE 21.7 Apligraf living skin equivalent in place. (Copyright © Mark S. Granick, MD, FACS.)

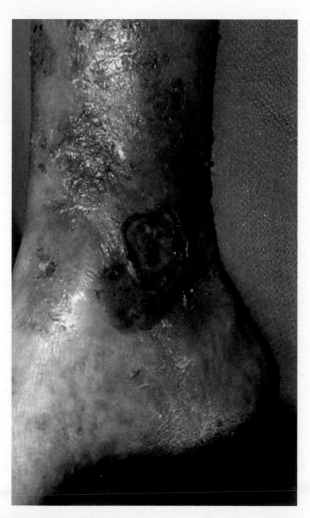

FIGURE 21.6 Recurrent venous ulcer. (Copyright © Mark S. Granick, MD, FACS.)

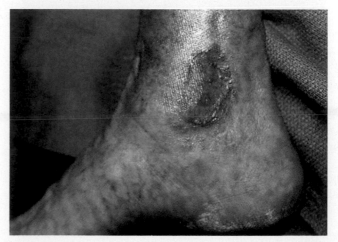

FIGURE 21.8 Complete wound closure within 8 weeks of therapy. The wound has remained healed for over 1 year. (Copyright © Mark S. Granick, MD, FACS.)

chondroitin-6-sulfate layer, after being placed on a wound, is infiltrated by fibroblasts that lay down their own ECM and subsequently remodel the collagen and glycosaminoglycan. Over 3 to 6 weeks, the inner layer takes on the properties of dermis, and the synthetic outer layer is then removed and replaced with ultrathin split-thickness skin grafts (STSG). A postapproval study involving 216 burn injury patients who were treated at 13 burn care facilities in the United States showed that the incidence of invasive infection at Integra-treated sites was 3.1% and that of superficial infection 13.2%. The mean take rate of Integra was 76.2%. The mean take rate of epidermal autograft was 87.7%.[49]

Indications for Use

Integra was FDA approved in 1996 for the postexcisional treatment of life-threatening full-thickness or deep partial-thickness thermal injury where sufficient autograft is not available at the time of excision or not desirable due to the physiologic condition of the patient. The label was subsequently expanded based on retrospective uncontrolled studies to include "the management of wounds including: partial and full-thickness wounds, pressure ulcers, venous ulcers, diabetic ulcers, chronic vascular ulcers, surgical wounds (donor sites and grafts, post-Mohs surgery, postlaser surgery, podiatric, wound dehiscence), trauma wounds (abrasions, lacerations, second-degree burns, and skin tears), and draining wounds."

Integra has also been successfully employed for scar reconstruction, including scar resurfacing and keloids. Evaluation of Integra in 89 patients for contracture release (127 procedures) indicated that at 76% of the release sites, range of motion or function was rated as good (significant improvement in range of motion or function) or excellent (maximal range of motion or function possible) by physicians. Responding patients expressed satisfaction with the overall results of treatment at 82% of sites. No recurrence of contracture at 75% of the sites was observed during follow-up monitoring.[50]

Integra benefits the treatment of necrotizing fasciitis by allowing for a height build-up via layering.[51] Several studies have now focused attention on the use of cultured epidermal autografts (instead of STSG) combined with Integra. This use allows for the early physiologic closure of large wounds with decreased donor site morbidity and deals with the challenge of little to no donor site availability.[52,53] A head and neck full-thickness burn injury was reconstructed with Integra and early implantation of microdissected hair follicles through the silicone epidermis 12 days after the injury resulted in complete reepithelialization and a hair-bearing scalp without the need for STSG.[54]

Indications for Discontinuation

Infection or lack of adherence to the wound bed is indication for removal.

Method of Application

Standard burn center protocol for topical agents and antibiotics should be employed. Early and complete excision of burn eschar and necrotic and contaminated tissue should be performed, ensuring a viable graft bed, such as white dermis, pure yellow fat, or glistening fascia. Meticulous hemostasis must be achieved to prevent hematoma or seroma formation, and the graft bed should be smooth and flat to ensure good contact with the Integra. The product should be meshed or fenestrated to minimize fluid collection under the graft. If complete excision is not possible, a barrier must be in place to separate Integra from unexcised skin and place an allograft.

The FDA requires physicians to be trained prior to using Integra. In the operating room, Integra may be applied as a sheet or meshed at a 1:1 ratio and fixated with staples or sutures. The meshed product should not be expanded. The advantages of meshing are that it decreases the risk of fluid accumulation and hematoma formation, allows antimicrobials to penetrate the wound bed, and improves conformability. The disadvantages of the meshed Integra are that it does not allow for physiologic closure, is a pathway for bacteria to enter the wound, and may guide granulation tissue to form a mesh pattern.

Postoperatively, compressive elastic net dressing, or negative pressure wound therapy (which promotes good contact of the product with the wound bed, prevents shearing forces, and provides visibility) should be used. An antimicrobial layer that may include moistened Acticoat or burn roll is necessary over the seams if nonmeshed and over the entire wound surface if meshed. Xeroform or petrolatum products are to be avoided. Compressive Kerlix and Ace wrap are then added for compression. Occupational and physical therapy may begin after 3 to 5 days.

Precautions and Contraindications

Integra is contraindicated in patients with a known hypersensitivity to bovine collagen or chondroitin materials (the components of the dermal replacement layer). The product is also contraindicated in the presence of wound infection because it is more vulnerable than a standard skin graft and will partially or completely fail.

Expected Outcomes

The silicone layer is removed 14 to 21 days after application when the deposition of new dermal tissue and resorption of the collagen-glycosaminoglycan matrix has occurred. The neodermis has formed when it blanches under compression, there is separation/wrinkling of the silicone layer, and the color is peachy/pink or yellow. Do not remove the silicone layer until

---

CLINICAL WISDOM

Integra

Integra should be monitored daily for infection, seromas, and hematomas. These areas should be aspirated or removed immediately. Otherwise, the elastic net that allows for observation of the operative site should be left intact. Outer dressings may be changed every 4 to 5 days. Do not allow immersion in water.

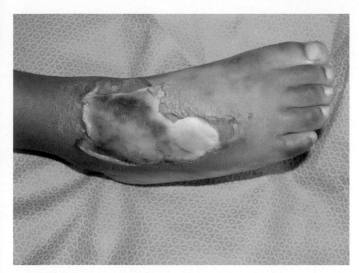

FIGURE 21.9 Full-thickness wound on dorsum of foot. (Courtesy of Mark S. Granick, MD, FACS.)

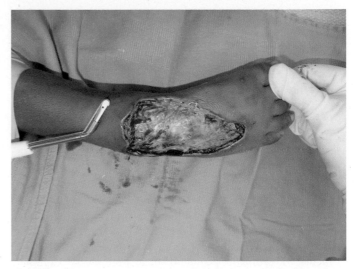

FIGURE 21.11 Debridement with Versajet. (Courtesy of Mark S. Granick, MD, FACS.)

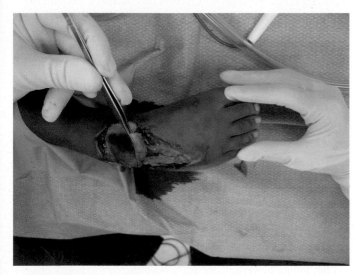

FIGURE 21.10 Sharp debridement. (Courtesy of Mark S. Granick, MD, FACS.)

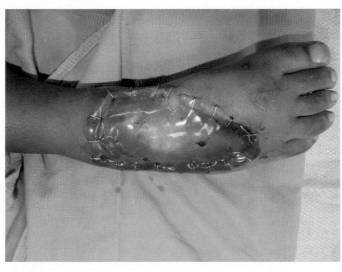

FIGURE 21.12 Integra™ Bilayer Wound Matrix Dressing placed on clean wound bed. (Courtesy of Mark S. Granick, MD, FACS.)

neodermis has formed completely. It should be easy to remove at this point. A thin epidermal graft of 0.003 to 0.007 inch is harvested. The grafts may be placed as a sheet or a mesh and should be attached per standard protocol.

Integra has increasingly shown promising uses in off-label applications because it is well tolerated, does not elicit a rejection reaction,[55] is thought to result in superior cosmesis with reduced donor site morbidity, and is readily available with a shelf life of 2 years at room temperature (see Figs. 21.9–21.13).

Dermagraft

Dermagraft is a composite of neonatal foreskin fibroblasts cultured onto bioresorbable glycolic acid mesh (polyglactin 910, i.e., Vicryl). The cells deposit ECM (collagens, vitronectin, GAG, and growth factors) prior to cryopreservation at −70°C. In contrast to TransCyte, the cells initially remain metabolically active in Dermagraft, though they are eventually lost. In this respect, Dermagraft is biologically active, stimulating healing through ingrowth of fibrovascular tissue.

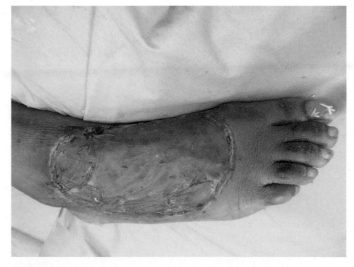

FIGURE 21.13 Healing partial-thickness skin graft following removal of silicone layer. (Courtesy of Mark S. Granick, MD, FACS.)

CLINICAL WISDOM

Dermagraft

A second application at 1 to 2 weeks is usually required.

Indications for Use

Dermagraft was FDA approved in September 2001 for use in the treatment of full-thickness diabetic foot ulcers of greater than 6 weeks duration that extend through dermis but without exposed tendon, muscle, joint capsule, or bone. The pivotal study was a 314-patient controlled, randomized clinical trial including Dermagraft plus conventional therapy versus conventional therapy alone (sharp debridement, saline-moistened gauze, pressure-reducing footwear) in plantar diabetic foot ulcers. Complete wound closure by week 12 revealed that 30% of Dermagraft patients healed compared with 18% of control patients.[56] Prior clinical trials had failed to support an FDA approval.[57]

Indications for Discontinuation

If infection occurs or the wound regresses, additional applications should not be placed.

Method of Application

The product is thawed according to protocol and placed directly onto the freshly debrided wound. The overlying dressings keep the Dermagraft in place. The dressings should be changed in 5 to 7 days postapplication.

Precautions and Contraindications

The wounds must be properly debrided prior to each application.

Expected Outcomes

Healing usually takes place within 1 month.

SUMMARY

Impaired wound healing can be a burden to the patient, practitioner, and society in general. Advanced therapies, including topical products and devices, are now available to assist with the healing of wounds refractory to traditional means of treatment. These therapies range from growth factors that stimulate wound healing to biologic skin substitutes. As more becomes known about the pathophysiology of these refractory wounds, new products will be developed. Currently, products that are individualized to patients' specific wound type and characteristics are emerging.

REVIEW QUESTIONS

1. Which growth factor has been approved by the Unites States Food and Drug Administration for the use in wound therapy?
   A. Basic fibroblast growth factor
   B. Epidermal growth factor
   C. Recombinant human platelet-derived growth factor
   D. Keratinocyte growth factor
2. Regranex Gel is approved for use in the treatment of which type of wound?
   A. Diabetic neuropathic ulcers
   B. Vascular insufficiency ulcers
   C. Ischemic ulcers
   D. Sacral pressure ulcers
3. AWBAT, *Advanced Wound* Bioengineered Alternative Tissue, is an updated and modified version of which material?
   A. Integra
   B. Apligraf
   C. TransCyte
   D. Biobrane
4. Integra is composed of
   A. human acellular dermis
   B. a silicone membrane bonded to a nylon mesh
   C. a bovine collagen mesh seeded with living neonatal fibroblasts and a pure keratinocyte culture
   D. a silicone layer attached to collagen and chondroitin-6-sulfate matrix
5. Amnion-derived cellular cytokine solution consists of all of the following except
   A. platelet-derived growth factor
   B. transforming growth factor β2
   C. basic fibroblast growth factor
   D. tissue inhibitor of metalloproteinase-1

REFERENCES

1. *Merriam-Webster's Collegiate Dictionary*. 10th ed. Springfield, MA: Merriam-Webster; 1993.
2. Allman RM, Walker JM, Hart MK, et al. Air-fluidized beds or conventional therapy for pressure sores: a randomized trial. *Ann Intern Med.* 1987;107:641–648.
3. Bates-Jensen BM. The pressure sore status tool a few thousand assessments later. *Adv Wound Care.* 1997;10(5):65–73.
4. Bates-Jensen BM. A quantitative analysis of wound characteristics as early predictors of healing in pressure sores. Dissertation Abstracts International, Vol. 59, No. 11, University of California, Los Angeles; 1999.
5. Van Rijswijk L. Full-thickness pressure ulcers: patient and wound healing characteristics. *Decubitus.* 1993;6(1):16–30.
6. Xakellis GC, Chrischilles EA. Hydrocolloid versus saline-gauze dressings in treating pressure ulcers: a cost-effective analysis. *Arch Phys Med Rehabil.* 1992;73(5):463–469.

7. Barbul A, Lazarou SA, Efron DT, et al. Arginine enhances wound healing and lymphocyte immune responses in humans. *Surgery.* 1990;108(2):331–336.

8. Mosiello GC, Tufaro A, Kerstein M. Wound healing and complications in the immunosuppressed patient. *Wounds.* 1994;6(3):83–87.

9. Bagdade JD, Root RK, Bulger RJ. Impaired leukocyte function in patients with poorly controlled diabetes. *Diabetes.* 1974;23(1):9–15.

10. Pecoraro RE, Ahroni JH, Boyko EJ, et al. Chronology and determinants of tissue repair in diabetic lower extremity ulcers. *Diabetes.* 1991;40:1305–1313.

11. Coleridge-Smith PD, Thomas P, Scurr JH, et al. Causes of venous ulceration: a new hypothesis. *Br Med J Clin Res Educ.* 1998;296(6638):1726–1727.

12. Hartmann M, Jonsson K, Zederfeldt B. Effect of tissue perfusion and oxygenation on accumulation of collagen in healing wounds. Randomized study in patients after major abdominal operations. *Eur J Surg.* 1992;158(10):521–526.

13. Sapico FL, Ginunas VJ, Thornhill-Hoynes M, et al. Quantitative microbiology of pressure sores in different stages of healing. *Diagn Biol Infect Dis.* 1986;5(1):31–38.

14. Robson MC, Stenberg BD, Hegger JP. Wound healing alterations caused by infections. *Clin Plast Surg.* 1990;17(3):485–492.

15. Allman RM. Pressure ulcers among the elderly. *N Engl J Med.* 1989;320(13):850–853.

16. Gorse GJ, Messner RL. Improved pressure sore healing with hydrocolloid dressings. *Arch Dermatol.* 1987;123:766–771.

17. Gentzkow GD, Pollack SV, Kloth LC, et al. Improved healing of pressure ulcers using dermapulse, a new electrical stimulation device. *Wounds.* 1991;3(5):158–169.

18. Van Rijswijk L, Polansky M. Predictors of time to healing deep pressure ulcers. *Ostomy/Wound Manage.* 1994;40(8):40–50.

19. Ferrell BA, Osterweil D, Christenson P. A randomized trial of low-air-loss beds for treatment of pressure ulcers. *JAMA.* 1993;269:494–497.

20. Fu X, Li X, Cheng B, et al. Engineered growth factors and cutaneous wound healing: Success and possible questions in the past 10 years. *Wound Rep Reg.* 2005;13:122–130.

21. Knighton DR, Ciresi KF, Fiegel VD, et al. Classification and treatment of chronic nonhealing wounds. *Ann Surg.* 1986;204:322–330.

22. Robson MC, Phillips LG, Thomason A. Recombinant human platelet-derived growth factor-BB in the treatment of pressure ulcers. *Arch Surg.* 1994;129:213–219.

23. Rees R, Robson MC, Smeill JM, et al. Becaplermin gel in the treatment of pressure ulcers: a phase II randomized, double-blind, placebo-controlled study. *Wound Repair Regen.* 1999;7:141–147.

24. *Regranex (becaplermin) Gel 0.01% (product labeling).* Raritan, NJ: Ortho-McNeil Pharmaceutical, Inc.; 1998.

25. Calhoun CC, Cardenes O, Ducksworth J, et al. Off-label use of becaplermin gel (recombinant platelet-derived growth factor-BB) for treatment of mucosal defects after corticocancellous bone graft: report of 2 cases with review of the literature. *J Oral Maxillofac Surg.* 2009;67(11):2516–2520.

26. Steed DL, Donohoe D, Webster MW, et al. The Diabetic Ulcer Group. Effect of extensive debridement and treatment on the healing of diabetic foot ulcers. *J Am Coll Surg.* 1996;183:61–64.

27. Robson MC, Phillips LG, Lawrence WT, et al. The safety and effect of topically applied recombinant basic fibroblast growth factor on the healing of chronic pressure sores. *Ann Surg.* 1992;216:401–406.

28. Fu X, Shen Z, Guo Z, et al. Healing of chronic cutaneous wounds by topical treatment with basic fibroblast growth factor. *Chin Med J.* 2002;115:331–335.

29. Robson MC, Phillips TJ, Falanga V, et al. Randomized trial of topically applied repifermin (recombinant human keratinocyte growth factor-2) to accelerate wound healing in venous ulcers. *Wound Repair Regen.* 2001;9:347–352.

30. Wu L, Yu YL, Galiano RD, et al. Macrophage colony-stimulating factor accelerates wound healing and upregulates TGF-beta 1 mRNA levels through tissue macrophages. *J Surg Res.* 1997;72:162–169.

31. Marques da Costa R, Jesus FM, Aniceto C, et al. Double-blind, randomized, placebo-controlled trial of the use of granulocyte-macrophage colony-stimulating factor in chronic leg ulcers. *Am J Surg.* 1997;173:165–168.

32. Margolis DJ, Kantor J, Santanna J, et al. Effectiveness to platelet releasate for the treatment of diabetic neuropathic foot ulcers. *Diabetes Care* 2001;24:483–488.

33. Sonis ST. Efficacy of palifermin (keratinocyte growth factor-1) in the amelioration of oral mucositis. *Core Evid.* 2009;4:199–205.

34. Steed DL, Trumpower C, Duffy D, et al. Amnion-derived cellular cytokine solution a physiological combination of cytokines for wound healing. *Eplasty.* 2008;8:157–165.

35. Xing L, Franz MG, Marcelo CL, et al. Amnion-derived multipotent progenitor cells increase gain of incisional breaking strength and decrease incidence and severity of acute wound failure. *J Burns Wounds.* 2007;7:39–52.

36. Jones I, Currie L, Martin R. A guide to biological skin substitutes. *Br J Plast Surg.* 2002;55:185–193.

37. Whitaker IS, Cantab MA, Prowse S, et al. A critical evaluation of the use of Biobrane as a biologic skin substitute: a versatile tool for the plastic and reconstructive surgeon. *Ann Plast Surg.* 2008;60(3):333–337.

38. Yang JY, Tsai YC, Noordhoff MS. Clinical comparison of commercially available Biobrane preparations. *Burns.* 1989;15:197–203.

39. Woodroof EA. The search for an ideal temporary skin substitute: AWBAT. *Eplasty.* 2009;9:95–104.

40. Barret JP, Dziewulski P, Ramzy PI, et al. Biobrane versus 1% silver sulphadiazine in second degree pediatric burns. *Plast Reconstr Surg.* 2000;105:62–65.

41. Zapata-Sirvent R, Hansbrough JF, Carroll W, et al. Comparison of Biobrane and Scarlet Red dressings for treatment of donor site wounds. *Arch Surg.* 1985;120:743–745.

42. Prasad JK, Feller I, Thomson PD. A prospective controlled trial of Biobrane versus Scarlet Red on skin graft donor areas. *J Burn Care Rehabil.* 1987;8:384–386.

43. Feldman DL, Rogers A, Karpiniski RH. A prospective trial comparing Biobrane, Duoderm and Xeroform for skin graft donor sites. *Surg Gynaecol Obstet.* 1991;173:1–5.

44. Klein RL, Rothman BF, Marshall R. Biobrane: a useful adjunct therapy in outpatient burns. *J Pediatr Surg.* 1984;19:846–847.

45. Falanga V, Sabolinski M. A bilayered living skin construct accelerates complete closure of hard to heal venous ulcers. *Wound Rep Regen.* 1999;7:201–207.

46. Falanga V. How to use Apligraf to treat venous ulcers. *Skin Aging.* 1999;Feb:30–36.

47. Purdue GF, Hunt JL, Still JM Jr., et al. A multicenter clinical trial of a biosynthetic skin replacement, Dermagraft-TC, compared with cryopreserved human cadaver skin for temporary coverage of excised burn wounds. *J Burn Care Rehabil.* 1997;18(1 pt 1):52–57.

48. Kumar RJ, Kimble RM, Boots R, et al. Treatment of partial-thickness burns: a prospective, randomized trial using TransCyte. *ANZ J Surg.* 2004;74:622–626.

49. Heimbach DM, Warden GD, Luterman A, et al. Multicenter postapproval clinical trial of Integra dermal regeneration template for burn treatment. *J Burn Care Rehabil.* 2003;24(1):42–48.

50. Frame JD, Still J, Lakhel-LeCoadou A, et al. Use of dermal regeneration template in contracture release procedures: A multicenter evaluation. *Plast Reconstr Surg.* 2004;113(5):1330–1338.

51. Orgill DP, Strauss FH II, Lee RC. The use of collagen-GAG membranes in reconstructive surgery. *Ann NY Acad Sci.* 1999;888:233–248.

52. Loss M, Wedker V, Kunzi W, et al. Artificial skin, split-thickness auto-graft and cultured autologous keratinocytes combined to treat a severe burn injury of 93% TBSA. *Burns* 2000;26(7):644–652.

53. Boyce ST, Kagan RJ, Meyer NA, et al. The 1999 clinical research award. Cultured skin substitutes combined with Integra Artificial Skin to replace native skin autograft and allograft for the closure of excised full-thickness burns. *J Burn Care Rehabil.* 1999;20(6):453–461.

54. Navsaria HA, Ojeh NO, Moiemen N, et al. Reepithelialization of a full-thickness burn from stem cells of hair follicles micrografted into a tissue-engineered dermal template (Integra). *Plast Reconstr Surg.* 2004;113(3):978–981.

55. Michaeli D, McPherson M. Immunologic study of artificial skin used in the treatment of thermal injuries. *J Burn Care Rehabil.* 1990;11(1):21–26.

56. Marston WA, Hanft J, Norwood P, et al. Dermagraft Diabetic Foot Ulcer Study Group. The efficacy and safety of Dermagraft in improving the healing of chronic diabetic foot ulcers: Results of a prospective randomized trial. *Diabetes Care.* 2003;26(6):1701–1705.

57. Pollak RA, Edington II, Jensen JL, et al. A human dermal replacement for the treatment of diabetic foot ulcers. *Wounds.* 1997;9(1): 175–183.

CHAPTER 22

Management of Wound Pain

Carrie Sussman and Barbara Bates-Jensen

CHAPTER OBJECTIVES

At the completion of this chapter, the reader will be able to:

1. Explain the relationship between neuroanatomy, mechanisms of pain physiology and chronic wound pain.
2. Discuss the consequences of wound pain on wound healing.
3. Characterize wound pain in relation to vascular (venous and arterial), diabetic (neuropathic), and pressure ulcers and burn etiologies.
4. Use validated tools/methods for assessing wound pain.
5. Choose appropriate wound pain management, including pharmaceutical and nonpharmaceutical strategies.
6. Educate patients and caregivers about pain and wound healing.

The International Association for the Study of Pain has defined **pain** as "An unpleasant sensory and emotional experience associated with actual or potential tissue damage or described in terms of such damage."[1] This definition emphasizes that pain involves two components: physical and emotional. The World Union of Wound Healing Societies defines wound-related pain as "a noxious symptom or experience directly related to an open skin ulcer."[2]

These components are present in patients with different wound pain etiologies, whether operative pain associated with surgery or pain from debridement and dressing changes associated with chronic wounds, burns, or cancer. For example, cancer patients who reported high-intensity pain levels also reported correspondingly high levels of frustration and exhaustion.[3]

Pain is typically assessed using pain scales, which are one-dimensional and measure only the physical component, intensity of pain.[4] Multidimensional scales, such as the McGill pain questionnaire, that measure both physical and emotional components are used less often. Thus, frequently the clinician or caregiver interprets the patient's pain experience in accordance with his or her own personal perspectives and biases.[5] As a result, the patient's pain experience, especially in the case of chronic wound pain, may be marginalized, and the pain may be poorly controlled.[6,7] Pain is not inconsequential. Recent research shows that patients can develop chronic/persistent pain problems as a result of improper and ineffective wound care. This finding increases our responsibility as clinicians to understand pain and its management in the context of wound care.[6] Current understanding of wound pain is largely drawn from studies related to the pain associated with other painful conditions like

cancer and burns. The burn literature has historically addressed procedural pain at dressing changes and debridement, and what has been learned there is relevant to treatment of other wounds as well.[8] That is changing with the publication of observational and descriptive studies looking at the patient's quality of life and the wound pain problem.[9–11] In acute care settings, the Joint Commission for Accreditation of Health Care Organizations (www.JCAHO.org) considers pain management a quality indicator. The JCAHO pain standards for acute care include appropriate assessment of pain, aggressive and effective pain management, and regular reassessment of pain.[12] Most healthcare institutions comply with these JCAHO standards.

In long-term care facilities, the Medicare minimum data set (MDS) assessment includes items about pain. As one of the MDS quality measures, pain prevalence is reported for all US nursing homes that participate in the Medicare program, and that information is listed on a Web site available to consumers (http://www.hhs.gov).

Pain management requires highly individualized, skilled medical care, as well as patience, compassion, and commitment. Pain management experts are not available in most settings, and many clinicians are inadequately prepared to develop pain management plans of care.[6] Clinicians need guidelines on management of acute and chronic wound pain. The purpose of this chapter is to provide these guidelines. We begin by reviewing pain physiology and pathophysiology, and the relationship of pain to acute and chronic wounds and wound healing. This is followed by information on assessment and interventions to manage or prevent pain and guidelines for referrals and patient self-care.

PHYSIOLOGY AND PATHOPHYSIOLOGY OF WOUND PAIN

The pain experience depends on the interaction and modulation of the biologic and psychosocial characteristics of the individual.[4,13] Biologic considerations include genetics, sex, and endogenous pain control (e.g., cortisol and endorphins). Psychological characteristics include anxiety, depression, coping skills, behavior, and cognitive status. Pain is also a consequence of the individual's history of disease and present disease status. Environmental factors also are part of the individual's pain responses. Examples of environmental factors are socialization, lifestyle, traumas, and cultural background (expectations, upbringing, and roles).

Understanding and recognizing the nervous system response and adaptation to pain are critical to understanding a patient's pain experiences and selecting appropriate treatment interventions that will address these mechanisms.[14] Clinically, pain management is moving from empiric therapies toward a mechanisms-based approach.[4] The following section examines the function of pain, neurophysiology and anatomy, and emerging information about the mechanisms of pain. Table 22.1 is a glossary of pain-related terms.

Positive and Negative Aspects of Pain

As defined earlier, pain is an unpleasant experience that occurs in response to actual or potential tissue injury. Pain has many beneficial functions, but it can also have negative consequences.

On the positive side, pain is protective and serves as a warning sign of imminent or actual danger and triggers an appropriate response within the body to avoid or minimize injury. Although most of us fear pain and would prefer avoiding the sensation, the inability to feel pain and respond to danger or injury—such as occurs in neuropathy resulting from diabetes, alcoholism, or chemotherapy, or with spinal cord injury or multiple sclerosis—puts the individual at risk for serious bodily harm.

Following injury, the pain signal also initiates the release of chemical mediators, as described in Chapter 2, necessary to start the healing cascade. Another benefit of acute pain in inflamed tissues is that pain provokes hypersensitivity of the injured tissues, causing the individual to guard the damaged tissue while healing occurs.[15] Typically, as healing occurs, pain intensity subsides, as does guarding. Pain can also be a signal of the presence of infection.[16,17]

On the negative side, pain can interfere with the immune response, influence the healing process, and delay wound closure.[6] Pain is not beneficial when it is "out of control" and triggers an emotional response that includes excessive release of hormones, such as cortisol and epinephrine, which interfere with healing processes.[18] The effects of cortisol and epinephrine on healing are explained in Chapter 2. Inflammatory mediators and cytokines are helpful following initial injury, but if they are released frequently following repetitive procedures such as sharp or mechanical debridement, or dressing changes, they lower the firing thresholds and decrease the baseline sensitivity of nociceptors (pain receptors) in such a way that they begin to respond to normally innocuous thermal and mechanical stimuli, resulting in hyperalgesia (exaggerated pain response).[19] The pain experience begins as acute pain and over time—3 to 6 months depending on the source—is learned by the nervous

system and becomes chronic or persistent pain that can even be prompted by the patient's expectation of pain; this illustrates the complex and dynamic interactions that make up the pain experience.[4,13] The term *chronic pain* has a negative connotation associated with futility of treatment; it has recently been suggested to change the term to persistent pain to foster a more positive attitude by patients and health-care professionals.[6] This will be the terminology used here. Although many researchers believe that persistent pain offers no biologic advantage, another point of view is that persistent pain can be the biologic way of protecting tissues at risk of injury, such as painful joints associated with rheumatoid arthritis and osteoarthritis (OA). In these cases, the pain is protective of further injury.[20]

Neurophysiology, Anatomy, and Mechanisms of Pain

This section biologizes the pain experience by considering the structures and physiology involved in the experience of pain. This presentation does not account for the multidimensional aspects of pain; instead, our goal is to demonstrate the involvement and interaction of the components, and, where appropriate, how pain mechanisms are affected by wound care interventions and how that may affect healing. The neuroanatomic structures involved are the peripheral nervous system (PNS) including the sympathetic nervous system (SNS) and components of the central nervous system (CNS) including spinal cord, medulla, thalamus, and cerebral cortex.[23] The body's other protective systems triggered by pain include the motor, endocrine, and immune systems.

Peripheral Nervous System Involvement

We begin with discussion of the PNS's) nociceptive system. Nociceptive pain physiology is the easiest to explain and understand. It is a stimulus/response relationship and essential survival mechanism that dominates an individual's attention and drives action.

Nociceptive pain

Nociceptive pain is when there is excitation of the nociceptor terminals in the skin. Nociceptors are triggered by different stimuli producing three overlapping nociceptive pain patterns: mechanical, ischemic, and inflammatory (Fig. 22.1). These patterns are usually time limited.

> ## RESEARCH WISDOM
>
> ### Epidural Anesthesia and Heel Pressure Ulcers
>
> Anesthesia during surgery has both beneficial and detrimental effects. Trauma unrelated to the surgery can occur when pain is absent. For example, case reports and communications in several medical journals discuss the complication of heel pressure ulcers in healthy, young adults after epidural analgesia.[21] Epidural blocks can reduce blood pressure, produce immobility of the lower limbs, and block the nociceptive sensory inputs from the periphery that warn of impending tissue damage.[22]

TABLE 22.1	Glossary of Pain-Related Terminology and Characteristics

Pain Terminology	Characteristics
Allodynia	Increased sensitivity such that stimulation, which would normally not be perceived as painful, becomes painful
Acute pain	Pain present for 4 wk or less[21]
A "beta" (Aβ)	Nerve fibers that sense touch and pressure
A "delta" (Aδ)	Large nerve fibers that rapidly transmit sharp acute pain
Afferent	A nerve that conducts a signal from the periphery toward the CNS
Background pain	Persistent pain at rest
Breakthrough pain	Transient exacerbations of pain occurring in the background or continuous pain that is otherwise satisfactorily controlled[63]
C fiber	Small, slow-acting nerve fibers that transmit dull aching pain; unmyelinated
C-nociceptors	Respond to stimuli that are potentially noxious Release a complex mix of pain and inflammatory mediators
Central sensitization (wind-up)	Central mechanisms involved in maintaining and generating pain[27]
Chronic wound pain	Pain present for 6 mo; usually persistent and occurs without manipulation of tissues such as the throbbing of an abdominal wound when a patient is just lying in bed[68]
Cyclic or episodic acute pain	Is periodic acute wound pain that recurs due to repeated treatments or interventions such as daily dressing changes or turning and repositioning[68]
Disinhibition	Injury to peripheral nerves may reduce the amount of inhibitory control (also called disinhibition) over dorsal horn neurons through various mechanisms
Efferent	A nerve that conducts a signal from the CNS back to the periphery
Hyperalgesia	Exaggerated pain response produced by noxious stimuli[59]
Incident pain	Frequent, predictable pain episodes brought on by certain activities (e.g., wound care procedure); may occur on a background of continuous pain or the patient may otherwise be pain free[63]
Myelin sheath	A fatty sheath that covers the axon nerve fiber, acts like insulation, and assists in rapid transmission of the signal
Neuropathic pain	Damaged nerves cause signals to travel in abnormal pain pathways
Nociceptive pain	Noxious stimuli (chemical, mechanical, and thermal) detected by free nerve endings (nociceptors) perceived as pain
Noncyclic or incident acute pain	A single episode of acute wound pain, for example the pain of surgical debridement or of drain removal[68]
Opioids	Drugs that exert analgesic activity by binding to endogenous (opioid) receptors and that elicit the characteristic stereospecific actions of natural morphine-like ligands[63]
Pain mediators	Activated at time of cell damage. Include: arachidonic acid (Aa), potassium (K^+), bradykinin (BK), prostaglandin (PG), histamine (HS)
Peptides (substance P)	Activates the immune system with further release of histamine
Peripheral sensitization	Nociceptors become sensitized and have a lowered firing threshold
Persistent pain	Pain that has been present for more than three months; the pain may be continuous or intermittent[63]
Primary hyperalgesia (wind-up)	Increased sensitivity of neurons to repeated stimulus, especially small stimuli that are perceived as painful
Secondary hyperalgesia	May be accompanied by secondary increase in sensitivity in nearby uninjured tissues perceived as painful
Unmyelinated nerve fiber	Nerve fibers that are unsheathed with myelin Slower conductors of neuronal signals

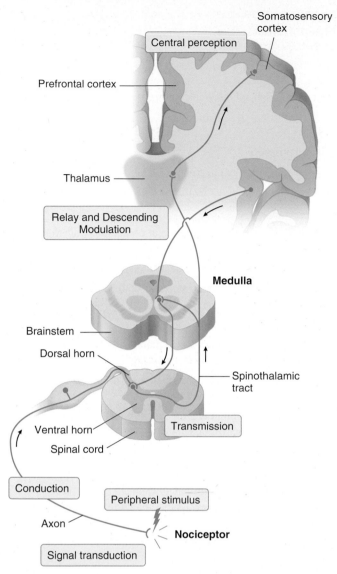

FIGURE 22.1 Nociception.

Mechanical nociception is triggered by mechanical distortion of the tissues such as during repositioning, pressure, or scar tissue manipulation.

- Ischemic nociception occurs when there is interruption of blood flow and resulting alteration of the chemical environment of the tissues. Ischemic tissues become more acidic, are hypoxic, and are rich in nociceptor-sensitizing chemicals: bradykinin, potassium ions, and prostaglandins. An example of ischemic pain is intermittent claudication that occurs during walking and then subsides when the activity ceases.
- Inflammatory nociception is related to the inflammatory processes following tissue injury and the chemical mediators involved and will reduce as the tissues heal[20] (see Chapter 2). Inflammatory pain is also the pain called neuritis due to irritation of nociceptive nerve endings, axons, or nerve processing circuits.

When peripheral nociceptors are in a continuous inflammatory state, such as occurs with repeated procedural traumas like dressing changes, they become sensitized and release a mixture of endogenous pain and inflammatory mediators whose presence lowers the threshold for nociceptor firing and enhances

the response to any further stimulus. This is referred to as *peripheral nerve sensitization.*[24]

Acute nociceptive pain following perturbation of nociceptors is easy to localize and only lasts a limited amount of time because the A-delta nerve fibers have quick onset and recovery. The large, thinly myelinated A-delta and small unmyelinated C nerve fibers transmit pain and other sensations over pathways, chemically and electrically, from the peripheral tissues along the axons to the neurons in the dorsal horn of the spinal cord. This is afferent stimulation. The efferent response could be a local withdrawal reflex mediated at the spinal cord level. However, the afferent information continues traveling to higher centers in the brain via neuronal pathways where additional actions occur.

The endogenous inflammatory mediators usually remain for a period of time following the initial tissue trauma and are responsible for perpetuating pain through repetitive signaling of the abundant C fibers transmitting afferent pain sensations reported as dull, throbbing, aching, or burning or tingling or tapping to the CNS. Intensity depends on the type of tissue and area involved.

Two types of sodium channels are found in sensory nerves. The first type is sensitive to tetrodotoxin, a potent puffer fish toxin, and the second type is insensitive to the same toxin. Whereas the channels that are sensitive to the tetrodotoxin are responsible for the initiation of the action potential and exist in all sensory neurons, those that are *insensitive* are found only on nociceptor sensory neurons and are implicated in pathologic pain states.[19] New analgesic medications are being developed that target this type of sodium channel. If this sodium channel can be blocked peripherally, pain impulses will be blocked from reaching the spinal cord and brain. One pharmaceutical product that has shown efficacy in blocking this sodium channel peripherally without adverse effects is lidocaine patch 5%.[25,26] The use of lidocaine patch 5% for wound pain will be discussed later. This is an example of how the concept of targeting a specific pain mechanism for treatment instead of using empirical therapies is applied. This is one of the major changes occurring in pain management.[4,27]

Sympathetic Nervous System

SNS is a component of the autonomic nervous system (ANS) that is concerned with glandular secretions, smooth muscle action, and cardiac muscle. SNS responds to all injuries and pain by releasing catecholamines, epinephrine, and norepinephrine from SNS receptors causing increased heart rate, vasoconstriction, increased blood pressure, enhanced pain perception, sweating, and slower wound healing. During a painful experience, heart rate increases in response to the intensity of the pain even if there is no apparent change in affect.[15] Monitoring heart rate during treatment would be useful clinically for monitoring pain but should not be used in lieu of the patient's self-report of pain.[28] Catecholamines increase with fear, anxiety, anger, and frustration and are suppressed and their action ameliorated with relaxation techniques and visual imagery. The catecholamines from SNS nerves affect the same cluster of neurons in the CNS as do inputs from nociceptors associated with damaged tissue and thus create a like perceptual pain experience.[20] Thus, cognitive factors like family financial issues or illness, not injured tissue, may be the cause of the pain experience or intensifying it and quarrying of patient or family about psychosocial issues is warranted (see Chapter 3 about psychophysiologic stress).

Cognitive Pain Suppression

Ann was preparing for a much anticipated 7-day cruise with friends from Florida to the Bahamas when the hurricane lamp she was holding broke in her hand, and a shard of glass fell and pierced the tendon of her left great toe on the dorsum of her foot. She carefully removed the glass and cleaned her wound. She says that she did not experience pain. Not wanting to disrupt her plans, she proceeded to enjoy her trip. She cared for the wound by cleansing with water and bandaging. Pain was not an issue, although she used ice, took some pain medication, and enjoyed alcoholic drinks in case the pain should increase. During her cruise, she danced in high heels, walked in the sand, and bathed in the ocean. The foot did not show any significant signs of inflammation; however, the toe was beginning to show signs of toe drop. When she returned to the mainland, she visited an urgent care clinic podiatrist who was amazed that the foot was not inflamed, pain was minimal, and the wound was uninfected since the tendon of the great toe had been severed. Immediate surgery was performed, and after this, she experienced pain and required pain medication.

The immune system is provoked by pain impulses and initiates vigorous and highly organized neuroimmune interactions that are implicated in initiating persistent neuropathic pain. Therefore, a cycle of pain is initiated and has the unintended consequence of promoting widespread nervous system sensitization. The following case study is an example of cognitive inhibition of inflammation, pain and the immune system.

Spinal Cord Involvement

Neurons in the spinal cord act as relay stations receiving and delivering signals to and from the PNS and to and from the brain. The gray matter of the spinal cord is shaped like a butterfly. The shoulders of the wings are called horns. One horn faces forward and that is the anterior or ventral horn, and the other horn faces backward and is the dorsal or posterior horn (Fig. 22.1). Each half of the butterfly represents the same side of the body. Each has neurons with specific functions. The dorsal horn neurons of the spinal cord receive inputs from neurons that process and transfer information about peripheral stimuli and transfer the information to the ventral horn via interneurons that synapse with neurons of the spinothalamic, spinoreticulothalamic, and spinohypothalamic tracts. The name indicates the end points of the spinal cord, thalamus or hypothalamus, or reticular system. Of these three pathways, the spinothalamic system is the major ascending pain pathway with two divisions: (1) ipsilateral, which carries mechanosensory inputs to the brain on the side of the stimulus and (2) contralateral, which carries both fast and slow pain signals and temperature sensations to the opposite cerebral hemisphere.[29] The end points are relay stations that dispatch the signals to appropriate brain areas or receptor organs for perception, localization, and action. Figure 22.1 shows the directions of flow of stimulation. The spinal cord is divided into segments that correspond to the vertebral column segment; however, the nerve has branches that transmit signals, (Fig. 22.2) via interneurons between segments as well as via cerebrospinal tracks up to the brain or up or down to another segment. The firing of these neurons can be either excitatory or inhibitory. Inputs from injury to peripheral nerves may reduce the amount of inhibitory control (also called disinhibition) over dorsal horn neurons through various mechanisms. Descending nerve input can modulate the incoming pain signals to the spinal cord, but anxiety and depression can inhibit this action. Conversely, increased inhibition will reduce the activity in dorsal horn neurons and act as a spinal "gate." One important concept to learn here is that pain can spread between segments as well as up to the brain unless there is a "gate" used to block the transmission. Use of transcutaneous electrical nerve stimulation (TENS) to block pain activates segmental inhibitory pathways.[19] The expected result of the TENS is to prevent or manage sensitization and spread of the pain pattern.

Brain Involvement

Neuroimaging techniques, such as positron emission tomography and functional magnetic resonance imaging (fMRI), are noninvasive or minimally invasive indirect measurement techniques used to observe and track regional blood flow and metabolic activity sweeping through specific regions linked with function-related changes in neuronal firing levels.[30] Using this information, brain pain regions have been mapped (Fig. 22.3). Brain maps show how electrical storms are activated by stimulation of receptive fields of neuronal populations in the skin and then encoded and translated into thoughts, emotions, sensations, and memories and stored in the cortex.[13,30–32] Based on brain mapping research, pain perception appears to involve several brain regions collectively called the "pain matrix."

Pain Matrix

The term "pain matrix" is used to describe a set of brain regions involved in processing pain. Major structures of the "pain matrix" are the thalamus, hypothalamus, anterior conjugate cortex, insular cortex, somatosensory cortex, somatomotor cortex, and prefrontal cortex (Fig. 22.4).[13,30,33] The thalamus is

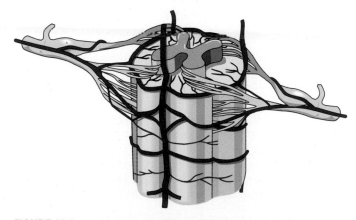

FIGURE 22.2 Anterior sectional view of the spine showing the spinal cord, spinal nerves and arterial blood supply. Notice that the fibers of the spinal nerve extends to the next spinal segments above and below.

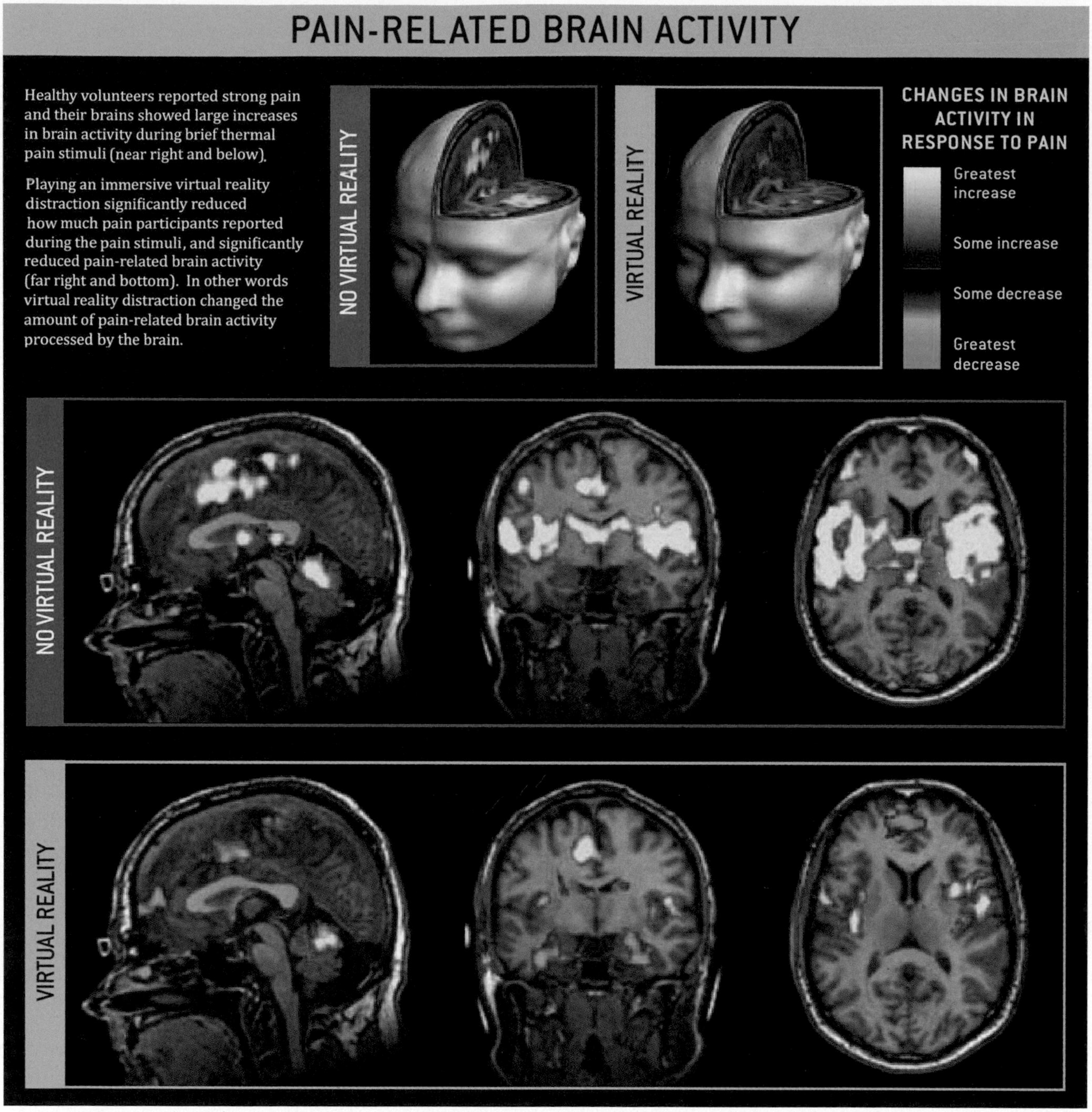
PAIN-RELATED BRAIN ACTIVITY
Healthy volunteers reported strong pain and their brains showed large increases in brain activity during brief thermal pain stimuli (near right and below).
Playing an immersive virtual reality distraction significantly reduced how much pain participants reported during the pain stimuli, and significantly reduced pain-related brain activity (far right and bottom). In other words virtual reality distraction changed the amount of pain-related brain activity processed by the brain.
NO VIRTUAL REALITY
VIRTUAL REALITY
CHANGES IN BRAIN ACTIVITY IN RESPONSE TO PAIN
Greatest increase
Some increase
Some decrease
Greatest decrease
NO VIRTUAL REALITY
VIRTUAL REALITY

FIGURE 22.3 Pain Related Brain Activity. Top line: the cutaway figure of the brain shows a whole brain imaged to show how the pain matrix is activated in one hemisphere during severe burn related pain next is a brain where a technique called virtual reality is used to alter brain input through distraction. Middle Line shows heightened brain activity shown on a fMRI scan without intervention during burn debridement. The bright yellow and red distributions indicate severe pain. Bottom line: virtural reality distraction is employed and these are fMRI scans from the pain matrix during sharp debridement. The brain activity has greatly reduced. (Copyright Hunter Hoffman used with permission.)

the critical relay site where nociceptive afferent input is received and then transmitted to cortical and subcortical structures.[13,33] Precisely how the thalamus relays nociceptive impulses is still poorly understood. Activation of areas within this set of "pain matrix" components, by a nociceptive signal, is believed to be sufficient to generate a perception of pain.[13]

Primary Somatosensory and Somatomotor Cortex

The brain region responsible for receiving the pain input from the thalamus and interpreting the signal source is the primary somatosensory cortex. Anatomically, it is located at the precentral gyrus (Fig. 22.4) alongside of the somatomotor cortex with which it directly communicates and which closely corresponds in representation.

Wilder Penfield mapped the somatomotor cortex and created an image of the body known as *cortical homunculus*.[34] The cortical homunculus shows a pictorial representation of how much of each cortical area innervates what proportion of the body. There are homunculi in several areas of the brain, but the two types of homunculi of interest to our discussion of

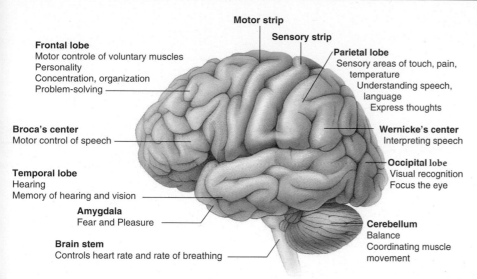

Frontal lobe
Motor controle of voluntary muscles
Personality
Concentration, organization
Problem-solving

Broca's center
Motor control of speech

Temporal lobe
Hearing
Memory of hearing and vision

Amygdala
Fear and Pleasure

Brain stem
Controls heart rate and rate of breathing

Motor strip

Sensory strip

Parietal lobe
Sensory areas of touch, pain,
temperature
Understanding speech,
language
Express thoughts

Wernicke's center
Interpreting speech

Occipital lobe
Visual recognition
Focus the eye

Cerebellum
Balance
Coordinating muscle
movement

FIGURE 22.4 Anatomical representation of brain areas.

pain are sensory representing the *primary somatosensory cortex* and motor representing the *primary somatomotor cortex*. The homunculus image is a grotesquely disfigured human with huge hands, lips, and face and disproportionately small body and extremities (Fig. 22.5). The homunculus has been called the "brain's map of the body."[35] These are the portions of the human brain directly responsible for exchange of sensory (namely touch: sensitivity, cold, heat, pain, etc.) and motor information. The exaggerated representation of these body parts occurs because the size of the represented area is proportional to how richly innervated and sensitive are receptors or the number of muscle and motor units within that region, not the size of the body area. Since the face and hands are richly innervated with sensory and motor units needed for fine motor skills, they have largest representation. It is important to recognize that the homunculus representation is an oversimplification of what is going on in the body. Instead, you should think of the represented areas as a "library" of sensations and movements.[35]

The representation is unique to each person and develops over the life span. For example, the hand of an infant is different from that of professional pianist. A pianist will have larger representation of the hand than a football player who may have a proportionately larger representation of the leg. Thus we can see that the functional organization of the somatosensory and somatomotor cortex is plastic, that it can learn and change in response to external stimuli, experience, or damage.[36] This phenomenon is called neuroplasticity. Neuroplasticity is a concept that provides an understanding about how neural circuitry can change in both function and number as a result of inputs from the environment and deliver multiple different outputs to the whole body. Repetitive stimulation of one area of the body can change, distort, and alter the representation of that portion of the homunculus and create a body integrity disorder like phantom limb pain or neglect of a body area after a stroke.

Cerebrospinal Tracts

As you will recall, pain information is transmitted multidirectionally between the periphery and the brain along spinal nerve tracts. Nociceptive pain impulses reach the brain through spinal nerve tracts ascending through the brainstem, the medulla,

and the thalamus. The thalamus appears to be the critical relay site for nociceptive input before impulses are transmitted to cortical and subcortical structures.[13,33] How thalamus processing of nociceptive impulses occurs is still relatively poorly understood.

Following perception, the pain impulse is modulated by input from the higher centers of the brain pain matrix and then transmitted via descending inhibitory and facilitatory cerebrospinal tracts to the ventral horn of the spinal cord. Dysfunction in the descending pain modulation network of the CNS has been implicated in central sensitization and associated with chronic pain. *Central sensitization* refers to increased responsiveness of nociceptive neurons in the CNS to normal or subthreshold afferent input.[24] Central sensitization amplifies transmission of input from peripheral tissues and produces secondary hyperalgesia.[37] This is an increased pain response evoked by stimuli applied to tissue outside the area of injury. The dysfunction may be either an impaired descending inhibitory system or an enhanced descending facilitatory system.[13]

Pain Threshold

The least amount of pain that can be recognized is called the "pain threshold."[13,24] Pain threshold can be modulated, raised or lowered, in different ways. Lowering the response threshold preprograms the nervous system to respond more quickly and efficiently to danger. Repetitive injury to the peripheral tissue lowers the threshold of peripheral nociceptors that results in abnormal processing of nociceptor input, changes the patterns of pain and the pain threshold, causing peripheral and central sensitization of nociceptors in the CNS at the spinal cord level, and affects the brain circuitry.[13,15,38]

Pain Perception

Perception of pain occurs when the pain signal is received by the amygdala in the brain; the signal then is relayed to the interpretive brain center and response(s) initiated. How this pain signal is interpreted depends on many factors. In a normally functioning nervous system, the arrival of an unpleasant stimulus is recognized as pain, and the response, usually withdrawal from the activity, follows. If that signal is interrupted, such as

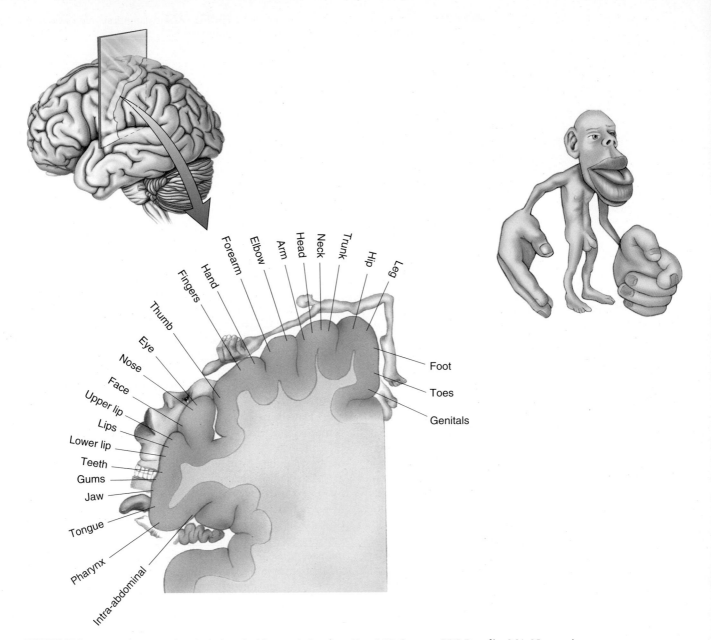

FIGURE 22.5 Sensory homunculus. (Reprinted with permission from Bear MF, Conners BW, Paradiso MA. Neuroscience: Exploring the Brain. 3rd ed. Baltimore: Lippincott Williams & Wilkins, 2007.)

occurs in patients with peripheral neuropathy, no protective action follows. In addition, the higher brain centers may block or enhance the message completely or partially through behavioral, cognitive, psychological (e.g., anxiety, memory), biologic (e.g., sex hormones), or pharmacologic activities.[4] The result is that individual differences account for different perceptions and interpretations and responses to the same painful stimulus delivered to the peripheral tissue.

Pain is a conscious event and nociception is not necessary nor sufficient for the perception or expectation of pain to occur. In a qualitative study, 41 healthy adults used mental concentration and visualization of pain as a cognitive stimulus, and 66% reported pain symptoms, including numbness, pins and needles, and moderate aching or definite pain, thus demonstrating

that prolonged mental stimulation may have induced the learning of pain symptoms.[39] Cognitive changes come into play in many ways. For example, Moseley et al. reported that viewing the magnification of a painful extremity enhances the pain experience and increases local edema while minifying the same minifies the pain experience and reduces edema. The distorted visual input results show a cortical effect of body image on body tissues, thus demonstrating that the link between body image and the tissues is bidirectional.[40]

Degradation

Repeated stimulation either closely (e.g., dressing changes) or intermittently delivered (e.g., maintenance debridement) also causes cortical changes in the somatosensory and somatomotor areas by increasing the cortical area representing the skin surface area engaged. The skin area experiencing pain enlarges, and the ability to localize the pain is diminished or lost. Over time, there is a cortical reorganization and the representation on the homunculus is changed, and this is called *representation degradation*. Phantom limb pain is an example of representational degradation. Almost all patients with amputations experience phantom limb pain.[41,42] After amputation, altered inputs and synaptic changes occur that are associated with resprouting of nerve endings in the stump and loss of connections in cortical areas. In complete or partial amputation, the loss of tissue integrity results in severed nerves trying to reconnect with their counterparts in adjacent tissue but, when unable to do so, forming neuronal end buds or neuromas that send abnormal, ectopic nerve signals into the CNS and up to the primary somatosensory cortex.[32,43] Altered inputs and synaptic changes probably began long before the amputation since patients who require amputation as a result of chronic vascular disease are often elderly and have extended periods of preamputation pain due to ulceration, often requiring extensive wound care including debridement. During wounding and subsequent debridement, nerve endings are severed and repeatedly resprout. These patients complain of persistent rest pain and pain at dressing changes probably related to the ectopic firing of these resprouted nerve endings. More about vascular ulcer pain will be presented shortly.

After amputation, there is nociceptive pain associated with the surgery, and this further alters pain signals to the somatosensory cortex, and for some individuals, this establishes the conditions for development of phantom limb pain.[43]

Unintended Consequences of Pain

Neuroscience research has documented unintended consequences of chronic pain for different persistent pain conditions such as chronic back pain, fibromyalgia, peripheral nerve injury, and phantom limb pain.[42,44–47]

There is no reason to suppose that the consequences of chronic wound pain are different. In this section, we discuss six unintended consequences of persistent pain:

1. Hyperalgesia
2. Allodynia
3. Wind-up
4. Cerebral atrophy
5. Pain memories
6. Delayed wound healing

Hyperalgesia
Primary Hyperalgesia

Three types of hyperalgesia are recognized according to the type of stimulus that provokes the response: thermal, mechanical, chemical, and cognitive. They can occur singularly or in combinations, depending on the nociceptor that has been sensitized[14]:

- Thermal hyperalgesia is provoked by a slight change in temperature, such as being touched with a cool hand or cool fluid, which is perceived as severe pain.
- Mechanical hyperalgesias are subdivided into brush evoked (dynamic) and pressure evoked (static) and punctate (pin prick).[19] As with thermal stimuli, very mild mechanical

stimulation such as a gentle breeze is perceived as excruciating pain. Hyperalgesia is not confined to nociceptors. Neuromas such as occur at the end of an injured nerve (e.g., amputated limb or chronic wound edges) resprout new axons, and these may exhibit exquisite sensitivity to mechanical perturbation because of altered membrane properties of both C and A fiber axons.
- Chemical hyperalgesia refers to exposure to endogenous chemical mediators such as cytokines, chemokines, and other inflammatory mediators. The nociceptors may become further sensitized to heat and mechanical stimuli after chemical stimulation.[14] For example, after a sunburn, inflammatory mediators are released in the skin, and when the skin is exposed to hot water in the shower, the nociceptors which are already sensitized respond excessively to the heat.

Secondary Hyperalgesia—Wind-up and Central Sensitization

A further complication following peripheral injury is increased pain response both of intensity and duration and the involvement of the surrounding uninjured tissues. Reaction in the surrounding skin depends on CNS recruitment and is termed *secondary hyperalgesia*.[14] Earlier central sensitization was mentioned as a consequence of repetitive injury (noxious stimuli) to the peripheral tissue lowering the threshold of peripheral nociceptors. Even repetitive application of identical nonnoxious stimuli to the tissues at a certain rate can induce a progressive buildup in the response at the level of the spinal cord dorsal horn interneurons and is a normal response of the undamaged nervous system to repetitive or sustained application of nonnoxious stimuli without any tissue damage.[14] Thus, secondary hyperalgesia is initiated by a stimulus peripherally, and then the sensation is transmitted along the sensory axons of the C fibers centrally to the dorsal horn of the spinal cord. There complex plastic changes or "Wind-up" occurs in spinal cord dorsal horn cells. The C fibers release glutamate that acts on three receptor types, one of which is the *N*-methyl-D-aspartate (NMDA) receptor. NMDA receptor activation, through a complex cascade of intercellular events, results in dorsal horn neuron hyperexcitability or central sensitization.[19,48] NMDA antagonist drugs such as ketamine are now available to block the pain pathway at this point.[21] However, ketamine should be used only by a pain specialist.

Over time, the plastic changes increase, the size of the receptive field within the dorsal horn grows, and the interneurons transform by adding fast pain receptors that amplify the pain signals that are then sent via the spinothalamic tract up to the thalamus and somatosensory cortex. Modifier pathways in the brain attempt to modulate the signals through the release of endogenous opioid peptides (e.g., enkephalins, and Beta (β)-endorphins) and other neurotransmitters (norepinephrine, serotonin) but are defeated when the modulating descending signal is received by the hypersensitive neurons in the ventral horn and is blocked. A feedback loop occurs and sends pain signals continuously to the brain where it is perceived as severe unrelenting pain. Theoretically, repeated handling of a wound even gently over a prolonged period of time would have the potential to create such a wind-up effect.

As wound care clinicians, we will see patients with patterns such as those described by Gifford and Butler that are suggestive of central sensitization.[20] These patterns include ongoing pain after expected tissue healing time; unfamiliar anatomic pain patterns; secondary allodynia and hyperalgesia; latency (delayed response) to sensory input; atypical pain behaviors; pain that has "a mind of its own;" pain exacerbated by emotional and physical stress, often significant affective (emotional) and cognitive components; variable responses to passive treatment; and poor response to medication, even opioids.[20] Over time these physiologic conditions will reverse unless there has been significant tissue injury or nerve damage.[14]

Although central sensitization was first described in the dorsal horn, as discussed, similar synaptic changes occur in structures involved in the emotional aspects of pain such as the amygdala, anterior cingulate gyrus, and prefrontal cortex.[49]

Allodynia

Allodynia is a subclassification of hyperalgesia. *Allodynia* refers to the production of pain (including reflex withdrawal) by a stimulus that does not normally provoke pain, such as the breeze described above[1] and is a common type of pain associated with chronic wounds. It can last as long as 12 months after the wound is healed.[50] Allodynia can occur in two ways:

1. When the large-diameter, low-threshold mechanoreceptors, A-delta fibers, are activated following central sensitization produced by C fiber activity. Then the Aß fibers become capable of responding to noxious stimuli and activating CNS pain-signaling neurons, resulting in increased perception of pain from benign stimuli that would not normally be perceived as painful.
2. By a reduction in the threshold of nociceptor terminals in the periphery.[14]

Cerebral Atrophy

In a studies of patients with chronic low back pain and fibromyalgia, it was found that there is atrophy of neocortical grey matter (massive loss of brain cells) related to pain.[47,49] Cerebral atrophy occurs due to altered brain neurochemistry, changes in dopamine and opioid availability, and a reduction of receptors in the forebrain. Patients also report change in mental functions like forgetfulness.[46,47,49,51,52] Even after nociceptive input ceases, such brain changes may be irreversible and this perhaps explains why the persistent pain condition exists.[13]

Pain Memories

There is evidence that pain can become "imprinted" in unique CNS pathways similar to those of memories.[23] The CNS learns to recognize a sensory experience from the repetitive pairing of environmental cues with sensory stimuli. Pain-related information is "learned" and stored in pain matrix areas of

---

RESEARCH WISDOM

Increased sensitivity of nociceptors to repetitive stimuli can cause benign sensations to become painful.[14] Patients with chronic wounds experience repetitive stimulation to the wound and the surrounding tissues and are often hypersensitive to handling.

---

the cerebral cortex such as the somatosensory cortex and the insula. The consequence of this imprinting is the formation of a "pain memory;" that is, movements or sensations that elicit pain eventually elicit *anticipation* of pain. There is evidence that these pain expectations become a patient's reality; that is, the stored information preprograms the CNS pain expectation.[15,53] Thus, anticipation of pain remembered from a previous procedure determines the individual's future pain experience for that same procedure (e.g., sharp debridement or dressing change) and is called nocebo hyperalgesia,[54] which is the opposite of placebo analgesia. The expectation or anxiety about impending pain triggers activation of cholecystokinin that facilitates pain transmission.[55] The perceived intensity of a painful stimulus then becomes amplified by the anxiety so that perceived pain is greater than in the absence of negative expectations—an effect associated with activation of specific brain regions such as amygdala. Conversely, when there is a low expectation of pain, there is a reduction in perceived pain that rivals the effects of an analgesic dose of morphine.[15]

Patients report that cleansing and dressing removal are the most painful procedures, and the higher the anticipatory level of pain, the greater the pain reported during treatment. Anxiety was a significant predictor of mean pain scores.[56,57]

The patient is usually unaware of these pain memories; moreover, patient responses to pain medications and other interventions differ when pain memories are present. These factors make extinguishing pain memories very difficult.[23] However, some success has been reported using patient education to teach about the anatomy and pathophysiology associated with the inappropriate action of the nervous system and its relationship with the pain problem. This increases the awareness of the patient of the mechanism causing the problem, and those individuals show increased pain thresholds.[23]

Imprinting (learning) of the CNS for pain expectation is demonstrated by an experience common to many people: having a childhood injury that was treated with an adhesive bandage and later having the bandage removed, with the pulling of the hair and skin causing noxious pain. Following this experience, whenever an adhesive bandage has to be removed from hairy skin, the person immediately recalls that pain and anticipates another experience of intense pain. A common response is both withdrawal and grimacing even before the adhesive bandage is removed. However, if a new adhesive bandage is used that doesn't cause pain when removed, the person's expectation of pain is changed centrally, and anticipation is reduced at the next bandage removal.

Delayed Wound Healing

Another example of perceived expectations effecting outcomes is the measurement of stress levels in presurgical patients. Patients who worried most about the effects of the surgery before the event had the lowest levels of proinflammatory cytokines and metalloproteinase concentrations in wound fluid after surgery, demonstrating that the expectation of difficulties (e.g., pain) associated with the surgery (stress) produced the reality of an impaired inflammatory stage of wound repair.[18] Pain is psychophysiological stress, and as we learned in Chapter 2, stress negatively affects wound healing. For more discussion, refer to Chapter 2.

Wound care requires many procedures that can cause pain. By preventing or decreasing the pain experience—for example, by using less aggressive bandage adhesives or other means of dressing placement—you will simultaneously reduce the patient's pain expectations and anxiety about procedures.

Pruritus (Itch)

Closely related to pain is the sensation of itch, or *pruritus*. The sensation can be as severe as or exceed pain in intensity. It is discussed along with pain because both phenomena are often experienced at the same time.

Research into the pathophysiology of pruritus is very difficult because the nature of the condition is capricious.[58] What is known is that diffuse itch sensation is induced and transmitted by a specific set of nonmyelinated C fibers that originate in the skin. Nonmyelinated "itch receptors" are presumed to be located in the lower epidermis and possibly at the dermal-epidermal junction. This group of receptors is polymodal, responding to mechanical, thermal, and chemical stimuli. Like pain, they can be stimulated by proinflammatory (pruritogenic) mediators. The resulting signals, also like pain, are transmitted via nonmyelinated C fibers to the dorsal root ganglia, to the dorsal roots, and into the spinal cord, from which the impulses are sent via spinothalamic tracts through the brainstem to higher centers in the thalamus and hypothalamus.

Peripheral and central mechanisms of pruritus are not fully understood but are believed to be related to altered peripheral excitation and central disinhibition. The act of scratching is thought to partially restore central inhibition. Endogenous agents are thought to be involved in a causal role, but only histamine has been directly linked as a causative agent. Perhaps it is the repeated release of histamine from trauma during wound care procedures that predisposes these individual to pruritus.

Pruritus is reported by patients with underlying medical conditions including chronic renal disease, primary biliary cirrhosis, endocrine disorders (e.g., diabetes), and malignant disease (e.g., lymphoma).[59] Patients with a history of thermal injury often experience severe itching during healing; this may continue after the wound is completely closed. In elderly patients, dry skin is associated with pruritus. Scratching to relieve the itching contributes to excoriation of the skin.

Itch is included in the list of pain quality items evaluated with pain scales.[60] Topical agents like 5% doxepin cream applied after wound closure have been shown to reduce itching,[61] and recently gabapentin has been shown to reduce itching in children recovering from burn wounds.[62] Colloid and oatmeal baths are effective in treating dry skin to relieve itch.

Summary

Multiple components of the nervous system are involved with pain. The action and response are associative and interactive. The nociceptors receive a pain signal, which is the provocation to transmit the signal to other parts of the nervous system, and the reaction is withdrawal from the activity, or the brain may perceive a painful experience before it occurs and warn the individual to react. Tissue damage and inflammation increases the sensitivity of the nociceptors that transmit the

pain signals. Central sensitization of the spinal neurons occurs when actual tissue damage has ceased and the pain persists after healing, as it does in many patients who have experienced chronic wounds. Pruritus, while not exactly pain, is a common occurrence in patients with a history of chronic wounds such as venous ulcers or burns. It can be categorized with and is treated similarly to pain.

PERSISTENT (NEUROPATHIC) PAIN

Persistent pain is clinically referred to as **neuropathic pain**. Rather than arising from stimulation of nociceptors, it reflects an abnormal functioning of the peripheral or central nerves themselves. In short, it is a disease of the nervous system, not a symptom.[38] Neuropathic pain is clinically defined as pain being present for more than 3 months, whether continuous or intermittent.[63] An example is *background pain*, which is pain at rest, and is often associated with venous ulcers and burns.[64,65]

Classification of Neuropathic Pain

Clinicians classify neuropathic pain into two categories: in *central* neuropathic pain, the lesion or dysfunction affects the CNS; in *peripheral* neuropathic pain, the lesion or dysfunction affects the PNS.[1,66] Peripheral neuropathic pain is sometimes further subdivided into stimulus-evoked pain or stimulus-independent pain (spontaneous pain)[19]:

- *Stimulus-evoked pain* is a heightened reaction to a painful stimulus, as described previously for hyperalgesia and allodynia, that occurs when the peripheral nerve is damaged or altered.[4,19]
- *Stimulus-independent pain* arises from spontaneous activity in the spinal cord, brainstem, or thalamic/cortical areas. It is less common and may have many mechanisms.[19]

With an initial injury, these conditions tend to be acute and reversible, and the symptoms usually resolve in about 12 months.[50] With persistent injury, the peripheral nerves can be permanently damaged, and the pain can become constant.

Clinicians also distinguish between acute and chronic neuropathic pain. Sensations associated with acute neuropathy characteristically occur independent of a stimulus. The pain can be shooting, lancinating, or burning. Other terms describing acute neuropathic sensations are electric shock, squeezing, throbbing, knife-like, and allodynia. As noted, acute cases resolve.

Sensations associated with chronic neuropathy include numbness, tingling, and prickling. These symptoms may be present continuously or intermittently, but they do not resolve. Rather, they remain after the period of tissue healing, disrupting sleep and normal living, and no longer providing any protective function.[66]

Etiology of Neuropathic Pain

Neuropathic pain may be related to a primary lesion, an unresolved injury, or other neurological disease. It may be inflammatory (e.g., postherpetic neuralgia), metabolic (e.g., diabetes), or ischemic (e.g., arterial insufficiency), and often reflects multiple pathophysiologies.[4,19]

In 99% of persons with chronic neuropathic pain, there is some underlying derangement or abnormal function of the nervous system that resulted from an acute incident.[38]

For example, a patient may experience a wide area of discomfort surrounding a wound or a stump that healed long ago. Although unpleasant, this pain reflects natural changes in the nervous system's response to the signals it receives.[14] As mentioned earlier, patients with chronic wounds experience significant amounts of repetitive handling and trauma, resulting in sensory stimulation that can be sustained within the CNS.

Chronic neuropathic pain can also arise from other etiologies, such as spinal compression, spinal stenosis, cerebral vascular accident, complex regional pain syndrome (formerly called reflex sympathetic dystrophy), distal polyneuropathy (human immunodeficiency virus [HIV] and diabetes), phantom limb, postherpetic neuralgia, fibromyalgia, and multiple sclerosis. Similarly, certain pharmaceuticals, such as those used to treat cancer or HIV, insult the nervous system and can permanently damage nerves.[38] Chemotherapy and radiation-associated neuropathies are becoming more common as people are living longer following a cancer diagnosis and many undergo several courses of chemotherapy or radiation with drugs that are toxic to the nervous system.[38]

Mixed Pain

Many patients with wounds experience nociceptive pain mixed with neuropathic pain. The mixed pain may be caused by both acute injury and secondary effects or chronic comorbidities. Examples of painful conditions found in populations that also experience chronic wound pain include

- Degenerative joint disease
- Spinal stenosis pain syndromes
- Musculoskeletal problems
- Fracture
- Surgical wounding
- Lower extremity arterial insufficiency
- Infection

In some cases, complaints of diffuse pain can mask significant problems. For example, a blocked artery developed in a resident of a long-term care facility who had multiple regions of musculoskeletal pain and intermittent claudication with walking.[67] When the other pain complaints were addressed and pain was cleared in those areas, it became apparent that the cause was visceral and warranted further investigation. Thus, it is essential to distinguish which condition is causing which pain picture, and whether the pain is nociceptive or neuropathic or both, so that the pain can be treated effectively.

RESEARCH ON CHRONIC WOUND PAIN

This section discusses two models of chronic wound pain, an international survey of wound care clinicians, and behavioral studies on the effect of pain on wound healing.

The Experience of Chronic Wound Pain

Krasner called attention to the chronic wound pain experience (CWPE) in 1995 when she presented an empirically and inductively derived visual schematic model she called the CWPE (Fig. 22.6).[68] Krasner's model relates the occurrence of pain to timing rather than to physiologic aspects. The model does not address psychosocial and behavioral aspects of the pain experience. From her personal and clinical experience, Krasner pointed out that at different times, patients with chronic wounds will experience all three types of pain: noncyclic, cyclic, and chronic. She suggested using the CWPE model to guide wound assessment to plan strategies related to the prevention and relief of wound pain and evaluate the outcomes.[7] The three types of pain are described below.

1. Noncyclic acute wound pain occurs intermittently, for instance with sharp debridement or drain removal, and is nociceptive. The plan of care suggested for pain management includes both pharmacologic and nonpharmacologic interventions such as topical anesthetics, local anesthetics, or anti-anxiety medication prior to debridement. Nonpharmacologic interventions are not indicated for this pain type.
2. Cyclic acute wound pain, which occurs in a regular time cycle like daily dressing changes or turning or repositioning, is also nociceptive. The plan of care in addition to the previously listed interventions could include use of nontraumatic dressings, soaking dressings before removal, or time-outs and use of appropriate repositioning devices.
3. Chronic wound pain, which is persistent neuropathic pain, is felt by the patient all the time (e.g., background pain), even without manipulation. The plan of care is as previously suggested for the other pain situations with the addition of nonpharmaceuticals like transcutaneous nerve stimulation or warmth and pharmaceuticals like tricyclic antidepressants (TCAs).[6,68]

Additional information about use of the mentioned interventions is presented later in this chapter.

Woo and Sibbald Chronic Wound Pain Model

Woo and Sibbald developed an evidence base scheme for addressing chronic wound pain. The purpose of this scheme was to raise awareness and promote a systemic approach to managing pain.[57] This scheme has evolved over a number of years and has been published in multiple iterations.[6,17,69,70] The iteration from 2007 is called the Chronic Wound-Associated pain (WAP) model: the wound, the cause, the patient. As in earlier models, three key components are included.[69,70] The three factors are in the current scheme are

1. Pain-causing factors by wound etiology (venous, arterial, pressure, diabetic foot, other)
2. Local wound care factors (débridement, bacterial balance, infection and inflammation, and moisture balance)
3. Patient factors (anxiety, depression, anticipation of pain)

Key elements of this model are: identification and addressing the three factors in a systematic manner. All wound etiologies share common elements associated with wound pain including procedural trauma, infection/inflammation, and moisture balance, too little or too much. However, the structure of the scheme focuses around the most significant common element: patient-centered concerns. Wound pain is often described as unrelenting, disabling, and devastating and the patient's number one concern.[70] In the following section, we examine variations in the experience of pain according to wound etiology.

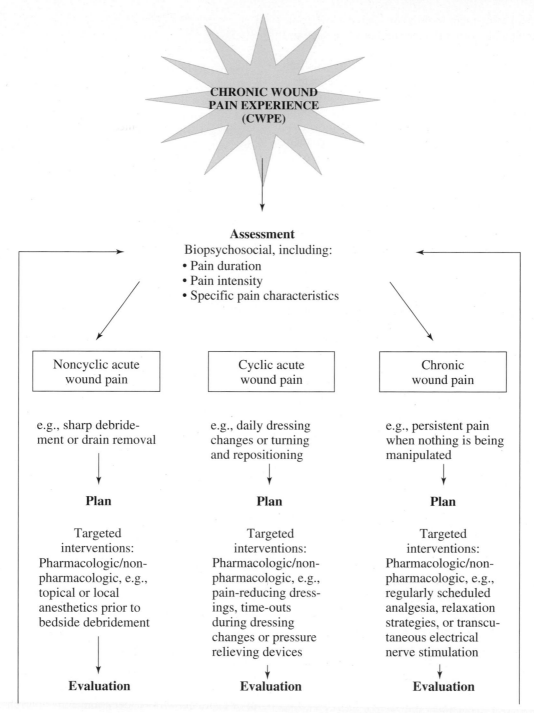

FIGURE 22.6 Krasner chronic wound experience. (Copyright Diane L. Krasner.)

Clinical Survey of Wound Pain

An international two-part survey of health-care practitioners from 11 countries explored the understanding of pain and trauma at wound dressing.[71] Part one of the survey looked at causes of wound pain related to dressings, and part two was a questionnaire that asked clinicians to rate the patient's pain experience at dressing changes based on their perceptions and experience.

The key findings of the survey related to wound dressings were as follows:

1. Dressing removal is the time of the most pain.

2. Dried-out products and adherent products are most likely to cause pain and trauma at dressing changes.

3. A main consideration at dressing changes is prevention of wound trauma and prevention of pain, infection, and skin damage, in that order.

4. Gauze is most likely to cause pain; new products such as hydrogels, hydrofibers, alginates, and soft silicone dressing are least likely to cause pain (see Chapter 20).

5. Awareness of the products available and the range of and ability to select dressings is highly variable between countries.

6. Use of valid pain assessment tools is considered a low priority in assessment with greater reliance on body language and nonverbal cues.[71]

Clinicians' perceptions of pain as determined by this survey were as follows: The most often listed wound pain experience was reported to be for patients with leg ulcers, followed by superficial burns, infected wounds, and pressure ulcers. Other wounds were ranked as less painful. However, the authors caution that this may reflect the practitioner's lack of assessment and experience rather than a true estimate of pain perceived by patients.

Behavioral Studies of Wound-Related Pain

Franks and Moffatt[9] did a qualitative study of the effects of pain on leg ulcer healing and patients' quality of life. They found that the risk of poor healing for venous ulcers can be predicted based on the pain intensity level at baseline. Overall healing rates declined with increasing levels of pain and with daily use of analgesics. Quality of life in the area of wound pain and healing has shown that with effective treatment interventions, levels of pain decrease significantly.[9]

Reddy et al.[6] recommend a patient-centered approach to wound pain management. They recognize that pain is related to a multitude of factors that affect an individual's psychological state, which include the attitude, beliefs, and knowledge of the caregiver, the patient, and family. The wound needs to be treated holistically. Dressing changes, for example, need to be viewed not just as a task but also in terms of their impact on the patient. To ensure that care is patient-centered, they recommend the following:

1. Consider all aspects of the patient: physical, psychological, social, familial, and spiritual.
2. Enlist the patient in treatment decisions and the process.
3. Take time to assess the patient's pain and determine quality-of-life issues.
4. Provide pain relief.
5. Ensure that the patient's right to pain relief and treatment that minimizes trauma and pain is provided.

VARIATIONS IN THE EXPERIENCE OF PAIN ACCORDING TO WOUND ETIOLOGY

Different wound etiologies are associated with specific pain syndromes. It is helpful if you identify these syndromes as part of your initial and subsequent clinical assessments. In the next section, wound pain syndromes that commonly present for arterial, diabetic foot, venous, and pressure ulcers will be described.

Arterial Ulcers

Peripheral ischemia is responsible for wound pain in patients with arterial insufficiency. The pain of arterial insufficiency is nociceptive and changes with position (increased with elevation and decreased with dependency or incurred with walking). The latter is intermittent claudication, relieved with 10 minutes of rest. It may also be neuropathic; that is, nocturnal, or occurring at rest even without elevated positioning. The following

> ### CLINICAL WISDOM
>
> Temporary resolution of ischemic pain of a leg or foot may be achieved when the activity is stopped or the legs are placed in a dependent position (e.g., dangling legs down at the edge of the bed). If the cause of the pain has not been evaluated, this would be an indication for referral to a vascular specialist.

assessments for indicators of limb ischemia are recommended (see Chapter 6 for instructions and test significance).[72]

1. Palpation of pulses. If not palpable, proceed to Doppler examination.
2. Doppler examination for ankle-brachial index of ankle pressure and/or toe pressure if there are calcified vessels. Finding of ankle pressure less than 40 mm Hg or finding of toe pressure less than 30 mm Hg are signs of critical limb ischemia and ischemic pain used to determine if there is adequate blood supply for healing.
3. Signs/symptoms
   a. Rest pain that requires analgesics
      i. Less than 2 weeks' duration is defined as subcritical limb ischemia
      ii. Greater than 2 weeks' duration is defined as critical limb ischemia[72]

After the assessment is complete, if there is critical limb ischemia and ischemic pain, the following interventions should be considered.

Exercise

Based on considerable research that exercise is beneficial in reducing claudication pain, exercise is recommended as an intervention for lower extremity arterial disease.[72]

Pharmacologic Therapy

Pharmacologic agents should be included in the treatment regime. See Chapter 11 for management of vascular ulcers.

Diabetic Foot Ulcers

Painful diabetic neuropathy is quite common and is a harbinger of loss of sensation. These following symptoms are reported by individuals with diabetic and other peripheral neuropathy etiologies. A minority of persons with chronic diabetic foot ulcers may experience tingling, burning, stabbing, or shooting sensations related to peripheral neuropathy.[73] Subcritical and critical peripheral ischemia is a complication of diabetes, and ischemic pain is frequently encountered during physical activities such as walking.[74]

Deep compartment infection can cause pain even in persons with severe neuropathy.[73] The typical signs of infection will most likely be blunted or absent in this population, but even mild edema or erythema are signals to pay attention and act. If a patient with a previously painless foot reports pain, *urgent* referral is required because it may signal limb-threatening complications of infection.[73] Refer to Table 22.2 for management strategies.

TABLE 22.2	Differential Diagnosis for Diabetic Foot Pain	
Diagnosis	**Clinical/Investigation**	**Comments**
Ischemia	Pain with walking (claudication) or positional (elevated position relieved with dependency)	Not a candidate for compression
	TcPO$_2$ ankle pressure < 40 mm Hg	Risk for nonhealing
	Toe pressure	
	<30 mm Hg	
Neuropathic pain	Sensations	Persistent or intermittent
	Numbness	Allodynia
	Tingling	Hyperalgesia
	Burning = nerve irritation	
	Shooting or stabbing = nerve damage	
	Throbbing	
	Paresthesia	
	Electric shock	
Deep compartment infection	Sudden onset	Needs systemic treatment
	Mild dermal erythema > 2 cm	Refer for medical treatment
	Mild swelling > 2 cm diameter	
	New wound or increased wound size	
	Temperature increase of 4°F	
	Probes to bone	
Charcot arthropathy	Hot temperature increase of 4°F	Offload (total contact cast or other)
	Swollen	Monitor change in temperature; offload until temperature normalizes
	Very painful foot	
	Biochemical markers of bone formation	

Adapted from Sibbald GR, Armstrong DG, Orsted HI. Pain in diabetic foot ulcers. *Ostomy Wound Manage.* 2003;49(suppl 4A):24–29.

Venous Leg Ulcers

Studies of leg ulcer pain reported in the literature point to a significant prevalence of ulcer pain ranging from 50% to 87%, which until recently has been ignored.[65,75] Pain relief for venous ulcer pain is of concern for most patients but is of greatest concern for those between the ages of 60 and 70 years.[65] It is widely recognized and reported that patients with venous leg ulcers have both nociceptive and neuropathic pain, the latter expressed as constant background pain.[76,77]

Pruritus was reported in 50% of leg ulcer patients.[78] Dermatitis, another complication associated with venous disease, often affects the skin surrounding the ulcer and is a reaction to the use of products that contain allergens and irritants such as topical lubricants, emollients, topical antibiotics, and other wound care products. The complaint is usually in the area of distribution of product use and is usually associated with pruritus and burning sensations.[65] Pain may be constant or intermittent and vary in intensity from severe to mild, with many patients suffering from night pain. Many patients are

using analgesics with reported efficacy in most cases.[67,75] The most frequently used medication for management of leg ulcer pain in one study was nonsteroidal anti-inflammatory drugs (NSAIDs) (70%).[10] The profile of the patient with pain is likely to include the presence of other comorbid painful conditions, including OA, a foot ulcer,[75] or a combination of venous and arterial insufficiency. Characteristics that are associated with venous pain include pitting edema, superficial phlebitis, deep vein thrombosis, acute lipodermatosclerosis, chronic lipodermatosclerosis, and wound infection. Figure 22.7 shows a patient with edema and trophic changes associated with lipodermatosclerosis. Cellulitis, scarring (atrophy blanche), and acute contact dermatitis are also useful in development of differential diagnosis of venous pain.[65] Table 22.3 lists clinical presentation, treatment choices, and comments about the differential diagnosis of venous pain.

Many patients with venous leg ulcers have lived with the condition for more than 10 years.[75,76] In these patients, central and peripheral sensitization are highly probable. Persistent

FIGURE   22.7 Lipodermatosclerosis.   (*1*)
Edema leakage through wounds (*2*) Scaling
and crusting (tropic changes). (Copyright
B.M. Bates-Jensen.)

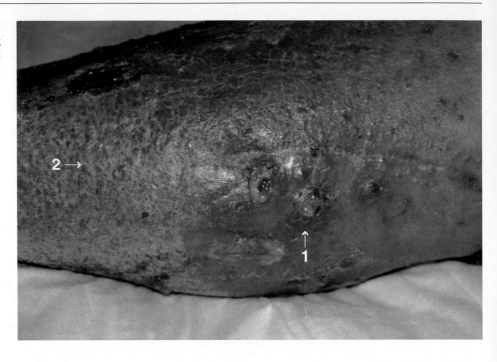

pain in the leg should be evaluated thoroughly. Pain characteristics most frequently reported by patients with leg ulcers
are divided into three categories that correspond to the McGill
pain questionnaire—sensory, affective, and evaluative. Surveys
reveal that the most frequently reported pain is in the sensory
category and includes throbbing, drilling, burning, stabbing,
sharp, pressure, aching, sharp, tender, and stinging. These
reported sensations are consistent with abnormal nervous
system function associated with persistent neuropathic pain.
Affective pain descriptors commonly used include nagging, tir-
ing, sickening, troublesome, and unbearable.[10,76,79] Aggravating
factors for pain that patients and clinicians listed most frequently include dressing changes, both during and between
changes, followed by movement.[71,79] Suggestions for the relief
of pain at dressing changes is offered in the section on nonpharmacologic methods of pain relief. The current standard
of care for treatment of venous leg ulcers is compression, but
the relationship of compression to venous leg ulcer pain has
been minimally evaluated. Nemeth et al.[76] reported on the
effect of compression on leg ulcer pain and found that, among
patients using compression over a 5-week period, there was a
trend toward decreased pain scores but pain persisted throughout the study. See Chapter11 for more information about
venous disease and Chapter 19 for management of edema and
compression.

Pressure Ulcer Pain

Pressure ulcer pain has been attributed to ischemia, friction/
shear, moisture related to incontinence (feces and urine), deep
tissue injury, deep infection, periulcer irritation, poor nutritional status, neuropathy, muscle spasm, and immobility. All
should investigated for wounds with this etiology.[70,76,80]

Pressure ulcer pain is related to tissue ischemia caused
by pressure and the response by inflammatory mediators.
Descriptions of pressure ulcer pain include burning, stabbing,
stinging, tugging, throbbing, and sharp, suggesting mixed nociceptive and neuropathic pain.[70]

Over a period of more than 10 years, several studies have
shown that patients with pressure ulcers experience excruciating pain. Szor and Bourguignon evaluated pain at rest and
during dressing changes in patients with stage II, III, or IV pressure ulcers and found that 18% reported pain at the highest
level (e.g., "excruciating"), 84% reported pain at rest, and 42%
reported pain both at rest and during dressing changes. Yet,
only 6% of those persons reporting pressure ulcer pain received
any medication for their pain.[81] Eriksson et al reported that
in 186 persons identified with pressure ulcers, 12% reported
continuous pain and 54% reported occasional pain or dressing change pain.[82] Roth et al.[83] examined persistent pain in
patients who received a tissue flap procedure for stage III or IV
pressure ulcers or diabetic ulcers and found that 35% of those
with stage III or IV pressure ulcers reported pain as compared
with 17% of those with stage II pressure ulcers. Manz and colleagues examined pressure ulcer pain in cognitively impaired
and unimpaired nursing home residents with mild to moderate
pain. Stage II pressure ulcers were the most painful. Manz also
was able to show that both cognitively intact and cognitively

CLINICAL WISDOM

Not everyone can tolerate elastic compression because of
pain related to the high levels of compression at rest. An
alternative treatment plan that may relieve pain is an inelastic compression system that does not have high pressure at
rest like that shown in Figure 22.8. It is also easier to apply
than elastic compression products, which facilitates patient
acceptance.[65]

TABLE 22.3	**Differential Diagnosis of Venous Pain**		
Diagnosis	**Clinical/Investigation**	**Treatment**	**Comments**
Pitting edema	Dull ache at end of day	Compression bandaging	Nonelastic stockings or compression bandaging may initially be preferred as they are less likely to cause pain at rest
	Press thumb into skin and not degree of depression	Support stockings	
	Grade 1+ to 4+	Ambulation, exercise	
		Improve calf muscle pump	
Superficial phlebitis	Pain and tenderness along affected vein—usually saphenous	Compression	Risk of associated underlying DVT is low, especially if affected area is below the knee
		Ambulation	
		NSAID therapy	
Deep phlebitis (DVT)	Acute, red, tender, swollen calf—almost too painful to touch	ASA, unfractionated heparin	Suspect a DVT in patients with a sudden increase in calf pain, with risk factors such as immobilization, recent surgery, oral contraceptives, etc.
	Doppler necessary to confirm diagnosis	Warfarin	
		Low-molecular weight heparin	
		Bed rest	
Acute lipodermatosclerosis	Diffuse, purple-red, swollen leg resembling cellulitis, aching and tenderness is common	Compression bandaging	Usually bilateral, though may be more prominent in one leg
		Support stockings	Compression therapy essential
		NSAIDs	
Chronic lipodermatosclerosis	Diffuse brown sclerotic pigmentation with widespread chronic pain	Same as with acute lipodermatosclerosis but with topical steroids and lubricants	Support stockings may have to be custom made to accommodate for leg shape
		Pentoxifylline	
Wound infection	Change in pain character associated with other clinical signs of infection	Topical antimicrobial agents and oral antibiotics, if indicated	Maintain bacterial balance, and watch for increase in pain, size, exudates, odor, or granulation tissue as signs of infection
Cellulitis	Diffuse bright red, hot leg, usually unilateral associated with tenderness and often fever	Oral antibiotics, with IV antibiotics needed for severe episodes or with low host resistance	Venous ulcers make individuals more prone to cellulitis
Atrophie blanche	Pain, stellate, white, scar-like areas associated with pain at rest and standing	NSAID therapy	May be seen in association with scars of healed ulcers, or may be an independent clinical feature
		Other analgesics	
Acute contact dermatitis	Itching, burning red areas on leg corresponding to area of use of topical product	Remove the allergen	Lanolin, colophony, latex, and neomycin are some of the more likely agents involved
		Apply topical steroids	

Ryan S, Eager C, Sibbald RG. Venous leg ulcer pain. *Ostomy/Wound Manage*. 2003;49(4A suppl):18.

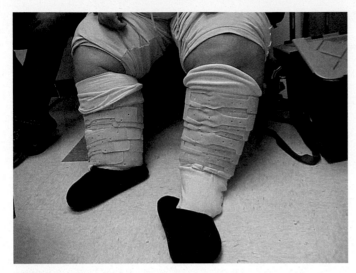

FIGURE 22.8 CircAid™ compression system. The Circaid (tm), non-elastic compression system is adjustable, easy to don and more comfortable for patients with painful, or restricted joints. (Photo used with permission of E. Fowler.)

impaired persons could differentiate pressure ulcer pain from other pain.[84]

In addition to studies specifically examining pressure ulcer pain, treatment studies often report on pressure ulcer pain. For example, Van Rijswijk in a study of hydrocolloid dressings reported that 21 (37%) ulcers were not at all painful and 14 (25%) were very painful during dressing changes.[85] Positioning and transfers often stimulate tissue pain receptors. Table 22.4 presents strategies for managing pressure ulcer pain. Chapters 9 and 10 have additional strategies for pressure ulcer prevention and management.

Burn Pain

Unfortunately, the amount of pain and suffering experienced by patients during wound care remains a worldwide problem for burn victims as well as a number of other patient populations. During wound care such as daily bandage changes, wound cleaning, staple removals etc., opioids are not enough, not even close, to managing procedural pain. Over 86% of the burn patients report having severe to excruciating pain during wound care even when standard levels of opioids were used. The pain management techniques in use are not goodenough. Patients are suffering.[86]

ASSESSMENT OF WOUND PAIN

Wound pain assessment is not really different from other types of pain assessment, but there are factors related to wounds that are unique and should be considered during the assessment. For example, wound pain may be caused by an as yet undetected infection, or it may be related to specific wound care procedures. In all cases, focus your assessment on the cause of the pain, and develop your pain management plan accordingly.

Focus subsequent assessments on the efficacy of the pain management plan. If the patient's pain is not relieved,

determine the cause of the plan failure and develop a new plan. Plan failure may be related to a new treatment intervention or to a change in the wound or the host status, or to a combination of factors, including psychosocial factors.

Elements to include in the initial pain assessment are divided in to the following four categories[28]:

1. Detailed patient history, including pain intensity and character
2. Physical examination, including neurologic component
3. Psychosocial assessment
4. Appropriate diagnostic workup to determine the cause and type of pain

Patient History

The screening for wound pain begins with a review of the patient's medical history and an interview. Use a pain questionnaire with a body diagram to speed the interview process and the pain diagnosis (Fig. 22.9). The answers to the questionnaire will help you determine quickly if there is a pain pattern and develop a diagnosis about the type of pain.[38] Pain scales, described shortly, should be part of the assessment process.

Include the following items in your pain assessment interview:

Onset and temporal pattern: Determine the onset of the wound and the pain problem to focus attention on whether the pain is related to an acute event like a dressing change or is there constantly. For example, patients with wounds of long duration such as venous ulcers are likely to have developed hyperalgesia, and the pain is persistent background pain that is aggravated at dressing changes.

Other comorbidities and wound procedures: Consider the relationship of wound pain to other comorbidities (e.g., peripheral vascular disease, venous insufficiency or diabetic neuropathy, musculoskeletal disease or cancer) and procedures (e.g., surgery, debridement, negative pressure therapy, pulsed lavage) to narrow the index of suspicion as to the etiology of the pain and to differentiate wound pain from other pain sources.

Location and distribution: Critical information needed to make a differential diagnosis of the type of wound pain includes the location and distribution of the pain.

Description of the type of pain: Reported sensations like sharp, deep, burning, tingling, and light touch help differentiate the type of pain (e.g., local nociceptive, acute hyperalgesia, or central sensitization, persistent).

Quality and intensity: Measure the quality and intensity of the pain with validated pain scales (discussed shortly). There is agreement that the best assessment of pain is the patient's self-report.[28] The self-reporting pain scales presented below are designed to be used with patients with all types of pain etiologies. While subjective, they are validated. Not all patients do well with the same scale, so there are different ones available to meet different needs.

Aggravating and relieving actions: Part of the patient's self-report should include aggravating and relieving pain actions. For example, intermittent wound debridement, regular dressing changes, and infection have been identified as aggravating factors, whereas use of topical analgesics, protective dressings, and systemic and local treatment of infection are identified as relieving factors.[69]

TABLE 22.4	Pressure Ulcer Pain Management Strategies		
Cause of Pain	**Definition**	**Treatment**	**Comments**
Pressure	A force applied to the skin and underlying tissues that inhibits blood flow when it ↓ pressures within the capillary: capillary closing pressure (CCP) = 32 mm Hg (average value)	Special surface:	Consider:
		Pressure reduction ↓ pressure, but not necessarily below CCP, e.g., high density foam, standard hospital mattresses	Pressure mapping
		Synthetic (not sheepskin) heel booties	Wheelchair assessment
		Pressure Relief ↓ pressure below CCP, e.g., dynamic flow beds	
		Turning schedules crucial	
Friction	Created by movement of the patient over a surface	Heel booties, e.g., sheepskin booties (do not reduce pressure but may decrease friction)	On its own, friction doesn't usually cause ulcers. However, friction in addition to pressure greatly ↑ risk of ulcer development.
		Careful with patient transfers (use turning sheet)	
		Hydrocolloid over bony prominences	
Shear	Adjacent body surfaces slide across each other (as happens when a patient slides down in bed)	Keep head of bed ≤30 degrees tilt seating, rather than recline (may need some recline if slumping is a problem)	Again, more dangerous when combined with pressure
Moisture	Imitation and maceration from sweating, stool, urine, wound drainage	Prevention	Can also use film-forming topical acrylate liquids
		If urine incontinence, bladder training, urinary catheter (in and out rather than permanent, if possible)	Watch for secondary yeast, especially in folds
		Change undergarment pads frequently	
		Local wound care to keep surrounding skin from maceration	
		Absorbent surface next to skin	
		Treatment	
		Barriers to wound edges (e.g., zinc oxide, petrolatum, occlusive dressing)	
		May need antidiarrhea medications	
		If surrounding dermatitis, may need steroid cream/ointment	
Periulcer irritation	Can be due to dermatitis, maceration, and/or infection (e.g., candida)	To reduce periulcer irritation can apply either Vaseline, zinc oxide; film-forming liquid (e.g., acrylate); occlusive dressings (picture frame technique) and if candida suspected, hydro-cortisone in Canesten cream BID	If hydrocortisone in Canesten is being easily wiped off with body positioning and move-movement, then can cover with zinc oxide

Do you have pain? _____ Yes _____ No
Location of the pain _____
Intensity of the pain
Pain scale: Visual Analog (1-10), Numeric Pain Scale, or Faces Pain Scale
Pain distress scale: _____

Describe the pain

_____ Sharp	_____ Stabbing	_____ Burning
_____ Shooting	_____ Cramping	_____ Dull
_____ Heavy	_____ Aching	_____ Tender
_____ Splitting	_____ Tiring	_____ Exhausting
_____ Throbbing	_____ Difficult to localize	_____ Easily localized

Pain in the legs after walking a short time (claudication)?   _____ Yes _____ No
Pain when legs are hanging down (dependent pain)?   _____ Yes _____ No
Pain when legs are elevated?   _____ Yes _____ No
Pain during the night when you are in bed sleeping?   _____ Yes _____ No
Does the pain wake you up during the night?   _____ Yes _____ No

Duration of the pain
Is the pain constant (continuous)?   _____ Yes _____ No
Is pain intermittent (come and go)?   _____ Yes _____ No
How long does it last?   _____ Minutes _____ Hours _____ Constant
Is the current pain management: _____ Adequate _____ Inadequate

Current Pain Medications:	What Kind	How Much	How Often	Result
_____ Acetaminophen	_____	_____	_____	_____
_____ Aspirin	_____	_____	_____	_____
_____ NSAIDS/Cox 2	_____	_____	_____	_____
_____ Steroids	_____	_____	_____	_____
_____ Narcotic (codeine, morphine)	_____	_____	_____	_____
_____ Patch	_____	_____	_____	_____
_____ Other?	_____	_____	_____	_____

Functional Capacity (as affected by pain)
Sleep: _____ Adequate _____ Restful _____ Inadequate _____ Restless
Appetite   _____ Adequate _____ Poor
Bladder continence: _____ Yes _____ No
Bowel continence: _____ Yes _____ No
Toileting   _____ Independent _____ Assistance _____ Dependent
Dressing: _____ Independent _____ Assistance _____ Dependent
Bathing: _____ Independent _____ Assistance _____ Dependent
Relationship with others: _____ Okay _____ Irritable _____ Other
Emotions: _____ Okay _____ Irritable _____ Other
Work: _____ Able _____ Not able
Drive: _____ Able _____ Not able
Hobbies: _____ Able _____ Not able

Adapted from Fowler E. Plain talk about wound management. *Ostomy Wound Management* November 2005, Volume 51, Issue 11A (Suppl).

FIGURE 22.9 Pain experience assessment form. (Adapted from Fowler E. Plain talk about wound management. *Ostomy Wound Manage.* 2005;51:11A (suppl):292.)

Associated features or secondary signs and symptoms: Evaluate change in the character of the wound pain associated with signs and symptoms such as increased size of the wound, odor, and cellulitis, which can indicate clinical infection.

Associated factors: Factors like sleep patterns, mood, depression, and anxiety can be related to pain. Pain often varies with stress and activities during the day and from day to day. A pain diary can pinpoint the time of day and the activity associated with pain relief and aggravation. Then the timing for pain relief can be chosen. An example of a pain diary is shown in Exhibit 22.1. *Treatment response*: Evaluate medication or nonpharmaceutical treatment for its effect on the pain. Is it effective? For how long? How does it affect activities of daily living? Again, a pain diary is a useful tool to monitor and assess treatment responses.

Neuropathic Wound Pain Assessment

A simple neurologic physical examination is used to confirm diagnosis and distribution of neuropathic pain.[27,38] The diagnosis of neuropathic pain is made clinically by interpreting the results of negative (e.g., absences of tactile, protective sensation, or diminished reflexes) as well as positive (e.g., report of burning or shocking) findings during the exam along with review of a validated pain questionnaire such as the neuropathic pain scale (NPS). Sophisticated technology tests do not add information needed to diagnose neuropathic pain.[38] Simple clinical tests like testing for protective sensation, vibration testing, and thermal testing as described in Chapters 3 and 12 are appropriate and valid.

> **CLINICAL WISDOM**
>
> Invite the patient's significant other to be present during the pain assessment to help identify how and what contributes to the patient's pain, treatment response, and how the pain interferes with daily activities.

EXHIBIT 22.1

Wound Pain Diary

Date	Time	Location	Sensation	Activity	Pain Intensity Rating (0-10)	Medication, Treatment	Results
10/20	1 pm	Lower leg	Burning	Dressing change by nurse	4	None	None
10/20	9 pm	Lower leg	Throbbing	Resting	2	NSAID	Reduced pain to 0 Able to sleep through the night

Directions for using the toolkit, items tested and the associated pain mechanisms and guidelines for conducting a neurologic physical examination and interpreting results are found in Table 22.5.

Pain Scales

It is best to use brief, easy-to-use assessment tools that reliably document pain intensity and pain relief.[33] Pain scales meet these criteria. A variety of pain scales are described below. These are of two types. Unidimensional pain scales assess only the intensity of the patient's pain. Multidimensional scales like the PAINAD scale rate multiple behaviors such as breathing, independent vocalizations, negative vocalization, facial expression, body language, and consolability.

Unidimensional Pain Scales

Although intensity is only one aspect of a patient's pain, unidimensional pain scales are useful for evaluating pain relief interventions. Pain intensity is commonly measured quantitatively using a visual analog scale (VAS), FACES scale, numerical rating scale (NRS), or verbal descriptor scale (VDS). All are useful for evaluating the intensity of wound pain. In general, as pain reaches the higher levels on pain intensity scales (such as 7 or 8 out of 10 on an NRS), it interferes with mood, sleep, work, and enjoyment of life and motivates the person to seek help. In contrast, pain felt at lower levels on pain intensity scales (such as 2 or 3 on an NRS) might not be reported by patients as pain at all.[38]

Visual Analogue Scale

The VAS is a 0 to 100 mm number line with ratio scale properties (Fig. 22.10A). It has demonstrated high validity and reliability when used with hospitalized patients.[87,88] Following the instructions for use of the VAS may be difficult for children and frail elders with or without cognitive impairment. A VAS using a color scale has been found to be valid and reliable when tested with cognitively impaired elders.[89] The colored VAS has a visual depiction of pain intensity on one side, which is shown to the patient, and the 0 to 100 mm NRS on the other side for the clinician.

FACES Scale

The FACES scale consists of six cartoon faces ordered from smiling to crying (Fig. 22.10B).[90] The FACES scale has been used extensively with pediatric populations. A version for use with adults and cognitively impaired elders uses oval-shaped faces, without tears, that are more adult-like in appearance. Advantages of FACES scales are the ease and quickness of administration, simplicity, the correlation with VAS, and little mental energy required by the patient.[91]

Numerical Rating Scale

The NRS uses two number anchors, most typically 0 and 10, in which 0 represents no pain and 10 represents the worst pain imaginable.[92] The NRS is administered verbally, allowing for use over the phone and with those who have visual or physical impairments such that use of other tools is difficult or not possible. The NRS has demonstrated sensitivity to treatments that influence pain intensity and is easy to score and use.

Verbal Descriptor Scale

The VDS uses adjectives that reflect extremes of pain and are ranked in order of severity.[83] Each adjective is given a number that constitutes the patient's pain intensity. In general, a VDS is easy to administer and understand. However, the patient must pick one word to describe his or her pain even if no word choice accurately describes it. Furthermore, individuals with limited English and those who are illiterate may have difficulty with this tool.[93]

Pain Distress Scales

If patients express or exhibit signs of anxiety or other emotional distress during the screening interview, they should be asked to separately rate their emotional distress. A variety of pain distress scales are available that are similar to the pain intensity scales.[28] Three pain distress scales are shown in Figure 22.11.

Use of Unidimensional Pain Scales with Special Populations

Assessing pain intensity in patients who cannot communicate verbally, are cognitively impaired, or have a form of dementia, can be challenging. Mild to moderately impaired patients can respond to simple direct yes/no questions.[87] For those who cannot communicate verbally but who can understand and respond, cue with direct yes/no questions such as: Does it hurt more than 5? Or with words that correspond to the items on the pain distress scale. Is the pain annoying? Is it dreadful? You can

| TABLE 22.5 | Assessment of Sensory Symptoms or Signs in Neuropathic Pain[27] | |

Tool Kit for a Neurologic Exam

A simple tool kit is recommended for performing a quick neurologic exam to confirm diagnosis of neuropathic pain and its distribution.[23,28] Items in the kit include: a piece of dry gauze, a reflex hammer, a 5.7 g monofilament (some come attached to a reflex hammer), and a tuning fork.

Sensory Symptoms and Signs	Clinical Exam	Mechanism
Negative signs are diminished responses:		
A. Touch	Brush skin with gauze	Aβ fibers
B. Pin	Poke area of pain with monofilament point	Aδ fibers
C. Cold	Place cold tuning fork on painful area	Aδ and C fibers
D. Vibration	Strike tuning fork and place on lateral malleolus	Aβ fibers
Positive Signs:		
Spontaneous activity		
a. Paresthesia	These are present and graded (from 0 to 10)	Aβ afferents
b. Dysesthesia		C/A δ afferents
c. Superficial burning pain		C nociceptors
d. Deep pain		Joint/muscle nociceptors
Evoked		
Touch: dynamic hyperalgesia	Brush skin with gauze	Central sensitization
Pressure: static hyperalgesia	Gentle mechanical pressure	Central sensitization
Punctate hyperalgesia	Pricking skin with monofilament	Aδ fiber input
Punctate repetitive hyperalgesia (wind-up like pain)	Pricking the skin with monofilament 2×/s for 30 s	Central sensitization
		Central sensitization
After sensation	Time pain duration after stimulation	Aδ fiber input
Cold hyperalgesia	Place cold tuning fork on skin	Central sensitization

Adapted from Jensen TS, Baron R: Translation of symptoms and signs into mechanisms in neuropathic pain. *Pain* 2003;102:1–8.

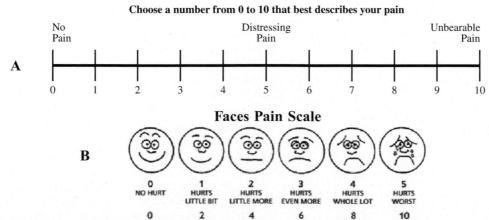

Visual AAA Log (VAS) Pain Assessment Scale

Choose a number from 0 to 10 that best describes your pain

FIGURE 22.10 Pain intensity scales. **A.** Reprinted from Jacox A, et al. Agency for Health Care Policy and Research (AHCPR). Publication No. 94-0592, 1994, U.S. Department of Health and Human Services, Rockville, Maryland. p. 295. **B.** From Wong DL, Hockenberry-Eaton M, Wilson D, et al. *Wong's Essentials of Pediatric Nursing.* 6th ed. St. Louis, MO: 2001:1301. Copyrighted by Mosby, Inc. Reprinted by permission. p. 295.

Simple Descriptive Pain Distress Scale[1]

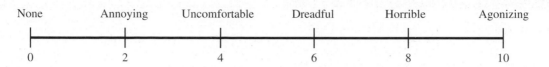

None	Annoying	Uncomfortable	Dreadful	Horrible	Agonizing
0	2	4	6	8	10

0 to 10 Numeric Pain Distress Scale[1]

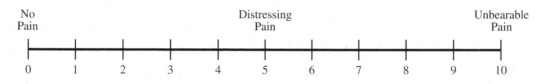

No Pain   Distressing Pain   Unbearable Pain

0	1	2	3	4	5	6	7	8	9	10

Visual Analog Scale (VAS)[2]

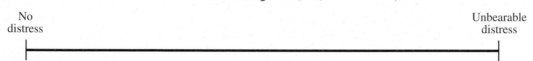

No distress   Unbearable distress

FIGURE 22.11 Three Pain distress scales. (Reprinted from Acute pain management Guideline Panel. Acute pain management: operative or medical procedures and trauma. Clinical Practice Guidelines Agency for Health Care Policy and Research (AHCPR), Publication Pub. 92-0032 1992, U.S. Department of Health and Human Services, Rockville, Maryland. p. 296.)

then record the corresponding number on an intensity scale. Additionally, several studies have demonstrated the ability of elders with mild to moderate levels of cognitive impairment to respond to the FACES scale and VAS.[94,95] You should also look for behaviors indicating pain intensity such as suggested in the PAINAD scale described below.

Multidimensional Pain Scales

As noted earlier, multidimensional pain scales assess not only the intensity of the patient's pain but also a variety of other qualities. One of the most commonly used is the multidimensional long-form McGill pain questionnaire. It provides information about pain quality based on 20 descriptor scales.[96] Each scale contains a variable number of words as a list ranked in intensity. The scales are divided into four main dimensions: sensory, affective, evaluative, and miscellaneous. The patient is asked to choose one word from any relevant list. A short-form McGill pain questionnaire is also in use.

A nonverbal multidimensional pain assessment instruments is the PAINAD scale. The PAINAD has been tested in people with advanced Alzheimer disease and other progressive dementias. It requires minimal training and may be useful for detecting wound pain in persons with cognitive impairment. PAINAD rates five behaviors on a 0 to 2 scale, in which 0 indicates normal or none present and 2 indicates the most severe behaviors observed.[97,98] These five behaviors are

- Breathing independent of vocalizations
- Negative vocalization
- Facial expression
- Body language
- Consolability

The American Geriatrics Society (AGS) Panel on Persistent Pain in Older Persons recommends looking for the following

behaviors.[93] Notice that many of these correspond with the items on the PAINAD.

- Facial expressions: frowns, sad frightened face, grimacing, wrinkled forehead, closed or tightened eyes, any distorted expression, rapid blinking
- Verbalizations or vocalizations: sighing, moaning, groaning, calling out, grunting, chanting, noisy breathing, asking for help, verbally abusive
- Body movements: rigid, tense body posture, guarding, fidgeting, increased pacing, rocking, restricted movement, gait or mobility changes
- Changes in interpersonal interactions: aggressive, combative, resisting care, decreased social interactions, socially inappropriate, disruptive, withdrawn
- Changes in activity patterns or routines: refusing food, appetite change, increase in rest periods, sleep, rest pattern changes, sudden cessation of common routines, increased wandering
- Mental status changes: crying or tears, increased confusion, irritability, distress

The AGS Persistent Pain Panel cautions that some patients exhibit little or no specific behaviors with pain. The heterogeneity of pain symptoms in the cognitively impaired is what makes pain detection in this population so difficult.

DIAGNOSIS OF WOUND PAIN

After the history review, determine if there is a specific pain pattern that can suggest a probable source of the wound pain. Goodman and Snyder suggest that four pain patterns should be considered.[101] The following have been adapted to illustrate relationships to wound-specific pain.

1. Cutaneous (related to the skin). The pain may be superficial or related to subcutaneous tissue. This type of pain pattern

RESEARCH WISDOM

Use the Patient's Facial Expression to Monitor Pain

The Facial Action Coding System is used in the psychological field to analyze emotional states.[99] As we have discussed, the ANS is effected by emotions with release of hormonal secretions like cortisol. The same changes occur in the ANS activity with changes in facial expressions.[100] When healthy adults were asked to remember, to relive, or to make a facial expression that represents a stressful experience, all showed the same ANS physiological responses. The explanation is that associative learning had occurred at an earlier time. Associative learning is the pairing of experiences like Pavlov ringing the bell for the dog when presenting food. Remember the anticipation of pain with bandage removal that we experienced earlier? Associative learning can help explain why the faces pain scales are valid and reliable for measuring pain. The patient pairs the look on the face with prior emotional experience. With the faces scale the patient reads and interprets the "facial expression." You can become familiar with common facial expressions that evoke emotions for sadness, anger, pain, and fear. You can then read the patient's facial expression to see if you can interpret the patient's emotions. For instance, if you are about to do a dressing change, what is the look on the patient's face? However, always confirm the emotions with the patient.[32]

Finally, the NPS is a multidimensional scale using a 0 to 10 NRS to rate ten domains of pain. Two global measures (intensity and unpleasantness) and eight specific ratings that assess both pain location (deep and surface) and pain quality (sharp, hot, dull, cold, sensitive, and itchy) are scored. Individual item scores and composite scores (determined by summing all items) can be used to determine the overall effects of pain treatments. A subscale (e.g., the NPS-6) specific to the quality of pain sensation is also useful in evaluating pain relief. The NPS has been shown to be sensitive to changes in pain condition associated with pain treatment, is easy to administer, and reflects both neuropathic and nonneuropathic pain symptoms.[60]

often is localized, although skin tenderness may occur in both referred and somatic pain. Infection is an example. If the pain is acute, the intensity should be consistent with the problem, and patients may describe the pain as sharp, sudden, or intense. With neuropathic pain, the pain pattern may be inappropriate and different in character than would be expected, and descriptors may include burning, throbbing, or shocking. Cutaneous pain perception is individual probably due to different pain mechanisms, gender, or ethnicity.

2. Somatic (emotional). Emotional distress produces physical symptoms that are apparent briefly or that recur or have multiple manifestations. Some manifestations of distress include anxiety about wound treatment and not keeping clinic appointments. Depression about a wound can manifest as poor acceptance of treatment or interpersonal conflict.

3. Visceral (related to internal organs). Visceral disease may be accompanied by hypersensitivity to touch, pressure, and temperature. The pain is usually poorly localized and diffuse because the innervation of the viscera is multisegmental and both visceral and somatic afferents converge.

Lower extremity ischemic pain, for example, is characterized by burning and boring, and is usually worse at night and relieved in the dependent position. The patient with an arterial ulcer often will report disturbed sleep.

4. Referred (related to irritation or deep somatic or visceral structures). Referred pain typically occurs in tissues supplied by the same or adjacent nerves as an area of injured tissue. The patient can usually point to the area that hurts. Pain can be present in adjacent tissue after a wound has healed. This type of pain could indicate secondary hyperalgesia.

MANAGEMENT OF WOUND PAIN

After the wound pain assessment and the pain diagnosis are made clinically, the next step is to develop a treatment plan to reduce acute pain by treating any underlying conditions such as infection, using wound care procedures that are less painful, and addressing the emotional consequences of having a wound and adequately treating any persistent pain problems the patient may have. The first part of this section focuses primarily on nonpharmaceutical treatment to mitigate pain from wound care procedures and the emotional consequences of having a wound. The second part focuses on pharmaceutical options. Either option may be used separately, or they can be used together.

As a guideline, severe to moderate pain should be managed primarily with medication (e.g., opioid oral medication for severe pain) and nonpharmacologically as the secondary treatment (e.g., pain-reducing dressings). Low levels of pain may be manageable with nonpharmaceutical methods such as pain-reducing wound dressings, relaxation techniques, and topical analgesia for procedural pain. Figure 22.12 shows a clinical wound pain decision tree to guide selection of treatment intervention based on the type of wound pain, the pain characteristics, and its causes.

Nonpharmaceutical Options

We chose to discuss nonpharmaceutical options first because they have great potential to mitigate pain and are minimally invasive and thus have minimal systemic effects and adverse responses.

Positioning

Positioning is a readily available means to help reduce wound pain. Chapters 10 and 12 provide specific suggestions about positioning. The positioning intervention is mentioned here briefly to call attention to the potential for pain relief. For example, offloading of bony prominences will reduce ischemic pain from pressure and traumatic pain from friction and shear. Elevation of the legs will reduce edema-related pain in the lower extremities associated with venous insufficiency. With surgical wounds, offloading will reduce tissue tension and contact with surgical wounds and reduce pain.

Specific examples of positioning interventions for pain management include the following: Use a bed cradle to lift the weight of bedcovers off hypersensitive tissues. Provide immobilization via splinting so that painful tissues are not manipulated. Use transfer-assist devices to minimize pain when moving a patient in and out of bed or on and off a stretcher. Reposition a patient in bed with lift sheets, not draw sheets, to avoid friction and shear that can lead to painful ulceration.

Wound Dressings

Appropriate dressing choice is one of the best nonpharmacologic wound pain treatments. Use dressings less likely to cause

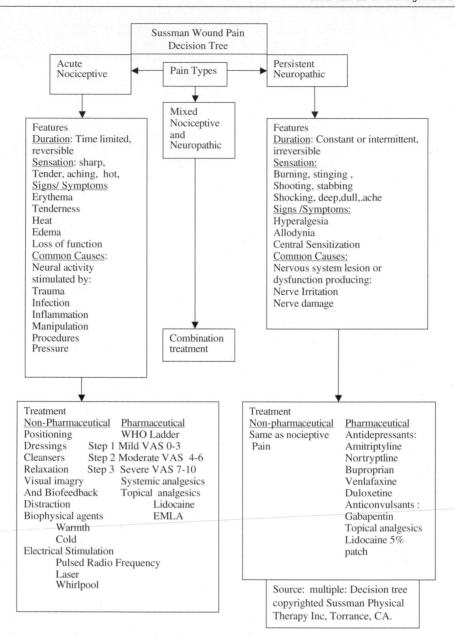

FIGURE 22.12 Wound pain decision tree. (Source: Multiple: decision tree copyrighted Sussman Physical Therapy, Inc., p. 297.)

pain and/or those that require less frequent dressing changes.[102] Gauze dressings are more likely to cause pain. Of 5,850 patients, approximately half with acute and half with chronic wounds, nearly 80% reported moderate to severe pain at dressing changes. When the usual dressing was changed to a nonadherent dressing, pain was reduced during dressing changes in 88% of patients with chronic wounds and 95% of patients with acute wounds.[103] The clinician must be aware of the absorptive capacity, adhesiveness, pain reduction properties, and appropriate use of dressings for specific wound healing goals. Chapter 19 provides detailed information about wound dressings. Here the focus is on selecting the proper dressing to reduce pain. For example, dressings useful for autolytic and enzymatic debridement also retain moisture that bathes exposed nerve endings in moist warm wound fluid, soothing them and reducing pain.

Choose dressings with an adhesive that is aggressive enough to keep the dressing in position but not so aggressive that the surrounding skin or wound bed is traumatized. Self-adhesive dressings have been implicated in aggravating leg ulcers.[104] Use of other methods for dressing placement such as Montgomery straps or nonadhesive netting can help decrease pain related to dressing adhesives. In general, thin film dressings have no absorptive capacity or aggressive adhesive, and they minimize pain by covering exposed nerve endings. Thin film dressings are adherent to the skin surrounding the wound and sometimes the wound itself, making dressing removal more likely to be painful. Thin film dressings have been shown to decrease wound pain when used to dress surgical incisional wounds.[105]

Hydrocolloids, hydrogels, and foam dressings typically have a minimal to moderate absorptive capacity. Hydrocolloid dressings are occlusive and reduce pain by preventing exposure of the wound to air; however, they have aggressive adhesive properties and can cause pain if removed improperly. Foam dressings are moderately absorptive, warmth retentive, which is soothing, and nonadherent, resulting in reduced pain during dressing changes. But they can dry out if the wound is minimally exudative. Hydrogel dressings are cool and soothing and particularly effective in wounds that have a burning sensation. Hydrogel dressings are nonadherent, thus reducing wound pain during dressing changes. Soft silicone dressings absorb minimal amounts of drainage but also are nonadherent and reduce pain associated with dressing changes.

Calcium alginates, alginate collagen dressings, and exudate-absorbing beads, flakes, pastes, or powders absorb large amounts of drainage. Dressings with a large absorptive capacity reduce pain related to maceration of surrounding tissues and to pressure caused by excess exudate. Calcium alginates and exudate-absorbing products are generally nonadherent and easily removed from the wound during dressing changes. However, like gauze and foam dressings, they can dry out if left in the wound for a prolonged period. Thoroughly soak dried dressings, especially the edges, to avoid trauma and pain when they are removed. (For information and instructions about using dressings, see Chapter 20).

Avoid packing wounds too tightly, as this can traumatize tissues and stimulate pain receptors. Granulation tissue can grow into wound-packing materials, and there is minimal benefit reported from soaking to ease removal.[92] For wound pain related to use of negative pressure wound therapy, line the wound with a low-adherent liner to avoid trauma when removing the packing or the sponge used in the therapy. Decrease the pressure incrementally until pain diminishes, and switch foam types or sponges used in the therapy. (See Chapter 29 for more information on negative pressure wound therapy).

In general, perform dressing changes as infrequently as required depending on the wound characteristics, as this reduces risk of infection by environmental contaminants and stunning

CLINICAL WISDOM

Patient-Centered Concerns

Patients have good reasons to express fear of dressing changes and debridement procedures. Use gentle hands and acknowledge the patient's pain and fear.[7] Use of the pain-reducing wound care strategies identified in Exhibit 22.2, along with reassurance, will reduce anxiety and fear and improve trust and outcomes.

of the cells of repair on dressing removal. Also, be aware that just the provision of a dressing or wrapping may be enough to reduce wound pain without the use of medication.[65] A dressing removes the visible reminder of the wound and thereby the psychological pain, while it simultaneously reduces the risk of external stimulation such as pressure, friction, and shear.[106] Exhibit 22.2 lists ways to alleviate pain at dressing changes.

Wound Cleansing

Wound cleansing should be gentle. To limit the patient's pain during this procedure, limit the pressure you apply. Use just enough fluid and pressure to flush out debris and necrotic tissue from the wound to reduce the risk of infection. Pressure irrigation such as pulsed lavage with suction (see Chapter 28) can be painful, and premedication and time limits are recommended. If the wound is irrigated, select low pressures (e.g., 4–15 psi).

Your choice of irrigant solution or cleansing agent can affect wound pain. Choose topical agents and wound cleansers that are nontoxic and nonirritating (e.g., hypoallergenic) to wound tissues

---

 EXHIBIT 22.2

Ways to Alleviate Pain at Dressing Changes

- Maintain moisture balance so nerve endings are bathed in moist wound fluid, which is soothing.
- Thoroughly soak dried dressings, especially the edges, to avoid trauma and pain when they are removed. Alginates as well as gauze and foam products can dry out.
- Protect surrounding skin from wound exudate irritation and maceration with skin sealants, ointment, or barriers to prevent or minimize skin damage and pain.
- Avoid packing wounds too tightly and using dressing products that can traumatize tissues and stimulate pain receptors.
- Line the wound with a low-adherent liner such as safe silicone to avoid trauma when removing the packing or the sponge that accompanies negative pressure therapy.
- Select wound adhesives that are aggressive enough for positioning the dressing but not so aggressive that tissue is damaged when removed.
- Perform dressing changes as infrequently as required depending on the wound characteristics.
- Avoid any unnecessary stimulation to the wound during dressing changes such as a draft from open windows or air conditioning, prodding and poking of the wound or surrounding tissues.
- "Time-outs" and self-dressing changes are recommended to reduce patient anxiety and improve tolerance for the dressing change procedure.
- Position the patient and the wound site so the dressing change can be performed in the most comfortable position for both patient and clinician.
- Premedicate 30 to 90 minutes before dressing changes to reduce anxiety and pain.

and surrounding skin. As examples, hydrogen peroxide is caustic to viable tissue cells and surrounding skin, causing a burning sensation; acetic acid, often used to treat *Pseudomonas aeruginosa* wound infection, can cause severe stinging; and silver nitrate sticks used to remove hypergranulation tissue can cause pain.[65,107,108]

Use fluids warmed to at least room temperature when cleansing wound tissues to prevent shocking the cells of repair, startling the patient, and initiating pain. Wound cells interpret the shock as trauma, and cell mitosis is halted for up to 3 hours after dressing change.[109] Further, for patients with hyperalgesia the shock of a cold fluid can set off a pain cycle. To avoid shocking the patient, always alert the patient before applying the cleansing solution. Even room temperature fluid can startle the patient and set off a destructive SNS response with release of catecholamines, epinephrine, and norepinephrine, all of which interfere with wound healing. Warm cleansing fluids by placing the solution container in a warm water bath while preparing other wound dressing supplies. Always test the temperature of the wound cleansing solution prior to administering to a patient's wound.

Reframing

Reframing teaches the patient to evaluate negative thoughts and images and replace them with positive or neutral self-talk that facilitates coping.[28] Like the nocebo effect we discussed, negative self-talk such as "This pain is driving me crazy!" or "I don't know if I can stand this pain much longer!" will intensify the output of pain impulses from the brain. Whereas a positive statement like "I have taken my pain medication and that will help me cope with the dressing change today" will have a positive effect by lowering the anxiety and anticipation of pain. Another suggestion for coping with wound procedures is for the patient to control the situation with time-outs or helping with dressing removal.

Distraction and Virtual Reality

Distraction means turning attention to something other than "the pain." Examples include watching TV or listening to music or the radio. Distraction is useful to temporarily relieve pain such as when it is not yet time for another pain pill or during the time it takes for the medicine to take effect. It is a myth that if the person can be distracted, the pain is not severe. Distraction is just one method to temporarily relieve even intense pain. There are situations where very focused distraction is required such as with burn patients. Such focused distraction is provided by a technological advance called Virtual Reality (VR) Procedural pain and other acute traumatic pain can be significantly relieved by distraction as shown in in fMRI studies shown in Figure 22.3

SnowWorld, developed at the University of Washington HITLab in collaboration with Harborview Burn Center, was the first immersive virtual world designed for reducing pain. (Figure 22.13) SnowWorld was specifically designed to help burn patients. Patients often report re-living their original burn experience during wound care, SnowWorld was designed to help put out the fire. The logic for why VR will reduce pain is as follows. Pain perception has a strong psychological component. The same incoming pain signal can be interpreted as painful or not, depending on what the patient is thinking. Pain requires conscious attention. The essence of VR is the illusion users have of going inside the computer-generated environment. Being drawn into another world drains a lot of attentional resources, leaving less attention available to process pain signals. Conscious attention is like a spotlight. Usually it is

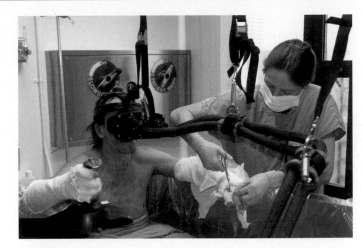

FIGURE 22.13 Patient in tub receiving procedure wearing virtual reality goggles B the virtual reality image being viewed. Cold scene was chosen because it promotes thoughts of cool. Hoffman, H Virtual Reality Pain Reduction University of Washington Seattle and U.W. Harborview Burn Center, website vrpain.com used with permission.

focused on the pain and wound care procedure. VR is luring that spotlight into the virtual world. Rather than having pain as the focus of their attention, for many patients in VR, the wound care becomes more of an annoyance, distracting them from their primary goal of exploring the virtual world. This works especially well for children.[110]

Relaxation

Relaxation is used to achieve physical and mental relaxation. Relaxation reduces muscle tension that puts stress on the painful tissues around the wound. For some people, relaxing may make them more aware of their wound problems. If this happens, suggest that the patient talk to someone about those feelings. An individual's ability to relax can change over time, and it may take up to 2 weeks of practice to feel the first results of relaxation.

Relaxation can be practiced throughout the day by taking a couple of deep breaths, holding your breath, and then blowing out the air. If the patient has lung problems, check with the doctor before advising deep breathing relaxation. Deep breathing may at first make the patient feel light-headed. If this is a problem, ask the patient to take shallow breaths and/or breathe more slowly. Breathing in deeply and slowly will also help bring more oxygen to the lungs and to the tissues that need to heal. Relaxation can be done anyplace, anytime. However, for it to be most successful, it should to be done for 5 for 10 minutes twice a day on a regular schedule in a quiet place in a comfortable position. In the relaxed state, the patient should be asked to visualize something pleasant that will help distract him or her from pain.

Visual Imagery

Like relaxation, visual imagery is used to achieve physical and mental relaxation. Visual imagery is a powerful method to plant helpful messages deep within the mind and body. During visual imagery the patient is asked to consider directing messages to the body to relax, ease pain, and direct blood flow and healing cells to the tissues for healing. Relaxation with guided imagery has been shown to help postsurgical patients to relax, reduce anxiety levels, and lower cortisol levels and erythema following surgery.[111] In a randomized controlled trial of patients with chronic nonhealing diabetic foot ulcers, biofeedback with muscular relaxation was attributed to promoting significantly increased blood flow and healing in the treatment group as compared with placebo.[112] In an fMRI study of patients who experience phantom limb pain, imagination of moving a phantom hand by upper extremity amputees showed activation in the contralateral primary motor and somatosensory areas of the brain and tracked their ability to reorganize the brain and reduce phantom limb pain.[42]

Psychological Interventions

Psychological interventions are another way to address the emotional component of the pain and the wound. They are used in conjunction with other methods, both nonpharmaceutical and pharmaceutical. As has already been explained, evidence shows that how people think about pain can change their sensitivity to it as well as their feelings and reactions.

One effective psychological intervention is cognitive/behavioral therapy (CBT). Classic CBT techniques have been associated with restoring a sense of self-control in cancer patients, which is often lost.[28] They can also help the patient coping with a chronic wound and all the associated pain.

Other psychological interventions can be as simple as holding a patient's hand, offering reassurance, and acknowledging the pain and suffering associated with the wound pain. Referral to a clinical psychologist may be useful.

Biophysical Agent

Part IV of this book, Chapters 23 to 30, presents biophysical agents that are used for wound healing and also have indications for analgesia. These nonpharmaceutical interventions include electrical stimulation, pulsed radio frequency (induced electrical stimulation), laser, and hydrotherapy. Transcutaneous nerve stimulation (TENS), for example, is recommended to treat wound pain and has the additional benefit of reducing the need for pain-relieving medications (though it cannot replace them).[28,68,102] The evidence to support the efficacy and utility for pain management of these agents is presented in those chapters. No adverse reactions are reported using these agents in conjunction with pharmaceutical or other nonpharmaceutical interventions.

Biophysical agent interventions are usually provided by physical therapists who have the knowledge and skills needed for successful application and outcomes. Occupational therapists also use biophysical agents and strategies for pain relief and prevention.

Two biophysical agents not discussed in Section IV are the use of topical warmth and cold. These interventions can be used by patients or caregivers at home. Both distract from pain but have many other pain-mitigating properties.

Heat is soothing, induces relaxation, and causes vasodilation and increased blood flow that can help with healing. However, prolonged heating brings more blood to the area, along with the chemical mediators associated with pain, histamine, bradykinins, and prostaglandins. Thus, heat should be limited to no more than 10 minutes. Patients with allodynia may be unable to tolerate even shorter sessions of mild heat.

Cold, or cryotherapy, may directly or indirectly reduce pain sensations and produce an immediate reduction in pain. Cold applied immediately following a trauma has the ability to reduce capillary permeability and thus block release of substances like histamine and other chemical mediators associated with pain. An example would be to use a cold pack applied to adjacent tissues after a dressing change. Do not apply directly so as not to cool the wound. A 10- to 15-minute application of a cold pack can control pain for 1 or more hours.[113] If there is tissue ischemia, cold would be contraindicated because it would further restrict blood flow to the ischemic tissues. As with heat, patients with allodynia probably will find cold intolerable.

Pharmaceutical Interventions

Accurate diagnosis of the pain type is critically important before selecting a pharmaceutical intervention. Recommended treatment for nociceptive pain is usually antiinflammatory or analgesic medications; neuropathic pain is treated with medications that influence neurotransmitters, such as antidepressants and antiepileptic drugs.[114] Recommendations for pharmaceuticals for management of chronic wound pain are not wound pain–specific but are based on evidence about treatment of pain associated with etiologies like cancer, burns, low back pain, fibromyalgia, OA, postherpetic neuralgia, and diabetic neuropathy. One such example is the guidelines of the World Health Organization (WHO) analgesic ladder[115] described in this section, which is well validated as an effective method for pain relief in 90% of cancer patients.[34] (Table 22.6).

Guidelines for Analgesic Use

Guidelines for the use of analgesics are provided by the WHO analgesic ladder and presented in Table 22.6.[115] The WHO approach is to measure the pain on a pain intensity scale and then match the patient's pain intensity with the potency of analgesic to be prescribed, beginning with nonopioids and progressing to stronger medications if pain is not relieved, adding adjuvants as the ladder is climbed.[116] Mild pain would be indicated by a pain score of 1 to 3 and be treated with nonopioids such as aspirin, other NSAIDS, or acetaminophen. If pain persists or worsens, move to the next level. Moderate pain would be indicated by a pain score of 4 to 6 and be treated with a mild opioid such as codeine. In general, it is always better to combine opioids with other analgesic agents such as NSAIDS or acetaminophen. This produces an additive analgesic effect while minimizing the dose of opioids required and thus minimizes undesirable side effects. This "opioid sparing" strategy is the backbone of the WHO ladder. Severe pain would be indicated by a pain score of 7 to 10 and be treated with strong opioids such as morphine hydromorphone and transdermal fentanyl.

NSAIDS

NSAIDS such as aspirin or ibuprofen are used routinely for common pain complaints like headache, sore muscles, or menstrual cramps, and are more effective than acetaminophen for treatment of inflammatory conditions such as arthritis. They are also beneficial *following* extensive procedures; however, they are not useful during debridement, and there are differing opinions about whether or not they are useful as premedication for debridement.[117] Some clinicians follow the WHO recommendations, which do include NSAIDS 30 to 90 minutes before sharp or mechanical debridement.[80]

NSAIDS should not be used for extensive periods because of adverse reactions; they are also contraindicated in patients with gastric ulceration.[118] Caution is needed for NSAID use in the elderly because of the risk of complications such as gastrointestinal bleeding. These drugs are best avoided in this patient population.

The effect of NSAIDs on wound healing is controversial. NSAIDS inhibit cyclooxygenase, thus decreasing the synthesis of prostaglandins. NSAIDS also blunt the inflammatory process

TABLE 22.6	WHO Ladder			
WHO Step	**Treatment**	**Pain Mechanism**	**Advantages**	**Disadvantages**
1. Mild pain 1–3	Nonopioid	Target: the peripheral nerves to block painful impulses	–Useful for mild to moderate pain	–Ceiling effect to analgesia
			–Widely available	–Side effects (GI, Renal or Liver)
			–Low cost	–Caution in elderly
			–Additive when used with opioids	
			–Patient or caregiver administration	
2. Mild to moderate pain 4–6	Opioid for pain ± nonopioid or adjuvant	Target: CNS to alter the perception of pain and peripheral nerves to block painful impulses	–Effective for local and general pain	–Prescription is regulated
			–Ceiling to analgesic effectiveness limited by only by side effects	–Side effects limit analgesic effectiveness
			–Patient or caregiver administration	–Fear of dependency
			–Long acting controlled release forms	
			–Some are low cost	
3. Moderate to severe pain 7–10	Opioid for pain ± adjuvant	Target: CNS to alter the perception of pain	Same as above	–Side effects limit analgesic effectiveness
				–Withdrawal symptoms likely
				–Need to taper off dosage gradually
				–Subject to substance abuse
				–Psychologic dependence

by deactivation of platelet aggregation, which can impair the wound healing process, depending on how early in the inflammatory phase it is administered.[119,120] In contrast to NSAIDs, acetaminophen does not interfere with platelet function. An explanation of the effects of NSAIDS on wound healing bioactivity is found in Chapter 2.

Opioids

Opioids such as codeine or tramadol are added to the pain management regimen when pain persists or increases. Whereas nonopioids work on the peripheral nerves to block painful impulses, opioids work on the CNS to alter the patient's perception of pain.[116] Because these drugs work synergistically, combining drugs such as a nonopioid (e.g., gabapentin) and an opioid (codeine), pain relief can be enhanced and decrease the need to progress to higher doses of opioids.[28] Examples of combination products are acetaminophen with codeine, acetaminophen with oxycodone, and acetaminophen with dihydrocodeine. The combination of acetaminophen and codeine is recommended for relief of pain associated with procedures such as débridement. Acetaminophen with oxycodone is not recommended for individuals with gastrointestinal disease and heart disease because of serious side effects.

In some cases, generalized puritis has been attributed to use of opiates. In these cases there is no visible dermatosis. The cause is attributed to nonimmunological mast cell degranulation, releasing histamine and other inflammatory mediators. Itch may last for some days afterwards, and is frequently incorrectly diagnosed.[121]

Use of combination drugs is not recommended by all clinicians.[6] Of concern is the fact that combination drugs are often administered in fixed-dose combinations that may be determined by the content of acetaminophen or NSAID. This may produce dose-related opioid toxicity. The guideline for use of combination analgesics is "start low and go slow."[6] Moreover, the dosage of these combination drugs needs to be tapered off gradually so that the patient does not experience withdrawal symptoms.

If pain is not managed at this level, the third step on the WHO ladder is used. At this step, separate dosages of the opioid and nonopioid drugs should be used.[28]

RESEARCH WISDOM

The maximum dose of acetaminophen for patients with normal renal and hepatic function and no history of alcoholism is 4,000 mg/d.[6]

Adjuvants

Additional drugs, or *adjuvants*, should be used if the pain cannot be controlled with the primary drugs.[115] Adjuvants are drugs that are not primarily analgesic but that research has shown to have independent or additive analgesic properties.[28] Examples are TCAs. TCAs are tertiary amines that can provide pain relief within 24 hours.[118] Neuropathic pain can be treated with antidepressants and the effect is independent of any effect on depression.[122] The most well studied (10 RCT) is amitriptyline. At least one or more out of three patients has moderate pain relief or better with global improvement for conditions like diabetic peripheral neuropathy. A newer TCA, venlafaxine, is showing similar effectiveness. These drugs modulate pain transmission by interacting with specific neurotransmitters and ion channels.[114] A systematic review found level A evidence in support of TCAs usefulness for treatment of both chronic neuropathic and nonneuropathic pain syndromes; this is independent of antidepressant effects.[123] Compared with anticonvulsants, TCAs are more cost-effective and have fewer safety concerns for elderly patients.[114] TCA drugs are classified into first and second generation. The second-generation group of TCAs has fewer adverse reactions. Adverse effects commonly related to use of these adjuvants include sedation and weight gain; elderly patients should not be treated with tertiary amines because of anticholinergic effects.[114] TCAs in combination with electrical stimulation (TENS) have shown enhanced efficacy in treatment of neuropathic pain.[111] In addition to efficacy in treatment of persistent neuropathic pain, TCAs have documented efficacy in treatment of nociceptive pain. TCAs should be considered as a pain adjuvant to promote sleep and alleviate muscle spasm. Successful outcome for pain relief is considered to be a 30% to 50% reduction in pain.[114]

Antiepileptic drugs are also classified into first and second generation. According to one systematic review by European Federation of Neurological Societies Task Force, the second-generation antiepileptic drug gabapentin (Neurontin) also has level A patient-related evidence of efficacy in treatment of diabetic neuropathy and when combined with TCAS and opioids (also level A) it enhances the effects.[123] However, another systematic review by Wiffen et al. found that although anticonvulsants are used widely in chronic pain, surprisingly few trials show analgesic effectiveness. There is no evidence that anticonvulsants are effective for acute pain. In chronic pain syndromes other than trigeminal neuralgia, anticonvulsants should be withheld until other interventions have been tried."[124]

Patients are also making decisions about using both TCA and anticonvulsants because of adverse effects. One patient in five discontinues use of antidepressants (amitriptyline) due to adverse effects[122] such as dizziness, drowsy, dysgeusia (taste disorder), headache disorder, increased appetite, weight gain, and xerostomia (dry mouth).[125] Adverse effects frequently reported by users of gabapentin include ataxia, blurred vision, diplopia, dizziness, drowsiness, impaired cognition, nausea, nystagmus, myalgia, peripheral edema and/visual changes.[126] This controversy is likely to continue until more studies confirm or refute efficacy. In the meantime, individual practitioners will be challenged to make decisions that will be best for patients.

Another adjuvant treatment, also with level A evidence, is the lidocaine dermal delivery patch 5% (Lidoderm), mentioned previously.[123] The release of lidocaine blocks sodium channels and

---

> ### CLINICAL WISDOM
>
> A common problem with opioid analgesia is loss of analgesic effectiveness over time. Use of adjuvants not only can improve analgesia but may make it possible to lower the dosage of opioids and reduce adverse opioid reactions such as nausea, vomiting, constipation, pruritus, sedation, and respiratory depression.[118]

has been approved for postherpetic neuralgia. The lidocaine 5% patch is also used generally for neuropathic pain. It has shown effectiveness in reducing neuropathic pain in both randomized and open label clinical trials.[26,127] It was also used in an open label study for nociceptive as well as neuropathic pain with good results.[60] In this study, the lidocaine 5% patches were applied by the patient once daily to cover the area of maximal pain and showed no adverse effects. It is suggested that the patches be applied at the same time each day and be used in conjunction with other analgesic medications.[26] A benefit of using the lidocaine 5% patch is that it delivers the medication directly to the site of the pain and thereby reduces the risk of systemic adverse events and drug interactions.[26,60] Clinical application of the lidocaine 5% patch could be useful for control of persistent background pain, promoting function and improving quality of life.

Principles for Using Pain Control Medications

To maintain freedom from pain, administer drugs "by the clock"; that is, every 3 to 6 hours rather than "on demand." Use the least invasive route for administration first. By starting with low doses, monitoring frequently, and titrating as needed, you will determine the safe and effective dose. Be patient, as this process may take 1 to 2 days for short-acting drugs and up to a week for longer-acting drugs.[6] Reassess and adjust the dosage as frequently as needed to achieve optimal pain relief, and monitor and manage side effects.[128]

> ### CLINICAL WISDOM
>
> #### Timing Application of Topical Analgesics
>
> Apply topical analgesics according to manufacturer's directions (usually 20 to 30 minutes and up to 60 minutes prior to procedures) to allow adequate time for action. Topical analgesic peak time for action to relieve pain is 30 to 60 minutes post administration.[102]
>
> Use of a lidocaine soak has been recommended as a quick and efficient way to reduce local wound pain during debridement procedures.[129] The procedure for a lidocaine soak is presented in Exhibit 22.3. Another option is EMLA cream (eutectic mixture of lidocaine 2.5%, prilocaine 2.5%), which reduces debridement pain scores and might have a vasoactive effect cutaneously.[130,131] It should be used only on intact adjacent skin. Apply before sharp or mechanical debridement. Low-dose topical morphine has been used in two small pilot studies to successfully control pressure ulcer–related pain.[132,133]

EXHIBIT 22.3

Lidocaine Soak Procedure[137]

1. Ask about allergies

2. Lidociane 2%: insert needle and withdraw 5–10 cc of the medication

3. Cleanse the wound after removing the dressing with water, saline, or wound cleanser

4. Place clean dry gauze over the wound

5. Saturate the wound and the periwound skin edges with lidocaine

6. Allow the soaked cause to sit on the wound for 3 to 5 minutes

7. Check if pain sensation and if anesthetized; begin débridement procedure

Adapted from Fowler E. Plain talk about wound pain. *Ostomy.* 2005;51(11A suppl):6.

Procedural Medications

Sequential debridement procedures, such as involved in acute burn care or treatment of chronic wounds, release inflammatory mediators that sensitize the peripheral nociceptors and produce peripheral sensitization and set the stage for central sensitization. Mitigation of sensitization at both levels should be given high priority. The following suggestions have demonstrated efficacy for local anesthesia but have not been studied for preemptive effects for sensitization.

Specific medication regimes that are useful for noncyclic and cyclic nociceptive wound pain associated with procedures include providing opioids or benzodiazepines 30 minutes prior to the procedure and less than 30 minutes or immediately afterwards, and administering topical anesthetics, including topical opioids using hydrogels as a transport media. Topical opioid gels (diamorphine or benzydamine 3%) provide a significant degree of analgesia for patients with a variety of painful skin ulcers. They provide relief by acting on opioid receptors in peripheral nerves that are activated during inflammation.[102]

Procedural sedation and analgesia (PSAA) is used to produce a suppressed level of consciousness adequate for painful or unpleasant procedures such as extensive sharp debridement.[134] Medications currently used as first-line agents for PSAA are ketamine for children and etomidate for adults. Alternatives are fentanyl and midazolam.[131] Benzodiazepines are commonly used for PSAA in US burn centers, where it is recognized that the patient's pain is exacerbated by anxiety. Benzodiazepines reduce anxiety while helping to wean patients from opioids or combination products being used for pain control. Because PSAA suppresses consciousness, the physician must be aware of the potential complications, including the potential for respiratory failure from airway obstruction or hypoventilation. Careful monitoring for respiratory complications is critical because the risk of respiratory problems is higher when using PSAA than when using either a sedative or analgesic separately.[117,134]

REASONS FOR REFERRAL

If the patient's wound pain is not remitting and is unrelieved, consider referral for a more complete pain evaluation. The presence of wound pain that is suggestive of serious complications such as infection, ischemia, or severe tissue tension warrants an urgent referral to a physician for further evaluation. If the patient is demonstrating weight loss and decreased or absent appetite due to pain, early referral to a dietitian or nutritionist in addition to the physician would be indicated.

SELF-CARE TEACHING GUIDELINES

Wound pain management is a collaborative effort between the patient and his or her caregiver/family member and the healthcare provider. Patients and caregivers must be active healthcare consumers and active participants in their own care. To foster collaboration, bring the patient into the process from the beginning by determining the patient's pain problem and the patient's goal for management. Determine the patient's motivation and ability to be part of the process. Empower the patient by letting him/her know that adequate pain relief is a right and that the pain management plan can change if the pain is not under control. Your goals should be to provide the patient with a feeling of personal control over the pain situation, to dispel myths about pain management, and to demonstrate willingness to be equal partners in the process. You also need to show real concern about what the patients say and empathize and sympathize with their feelings. Patients need to be empowered to express their pain, anxiety, and fears. Some patients will catastrophize their pain and show signs of anxiety and fear. Explain how this will be addressed.

Many patients have been socialized to believe that "no pain equals no gain," "no pain, no change," or "no pain, no

CLINICAL WISDOM

Clinicians often believe that dead tissue cannot hurt during debridement. Sibbald rates debridement pain severity as follows: surgical and mechanical, moderate to severe and autolytic and enzymatic, mild to moderate.[6] However, wound margins and underlying tissues contain functioning pain receptors that are easily stimulated by a sharp instrument or chemicals used for the debridement procedure.

Protecting Neuropathic Feet

History

BF was a 69-year-old woman who had a reoccurrence of breast cancer and was treated with several courses of chemotherapy. She was ambulatory and well nourished.

Reason for Referral

BF developed a pressure ulcer over the fifth metatarsal head that she found when she was putting on her stockings. Skin was black but unpainful. She sought medical care.

Tests

Tactile sensation was negative and monofilament for protective sensation; findings were negative for 5.7 mg.

Diagnosis and Treatment Interventions

Black skin was diagnosed as eschar necrosis and peripheral neuropathy related to her chemotherapy. She was treated with debridement and wound care measures and patient education.

The cause of the ulcer problem: Shoes that were too narrow had applied pressure to the soft tissue over the fifth metatarsal head. The condition was not detected because of the patient's neuropathy and loss of protective sensation.

Outcome of Care

Once the diagnosis of pressure ulcer secondary to chemotherapy-related neuropathy was explained to her, the patient replaced her narrow shoes with wider shoes, and began to examine her feet regularly. The wound healed uneventfully in 2 weeks. There were no further foot ulcers.

---

problem." All are myths or misconceptions about pain because (1) pain may not be a sign of gain but (a) a sign that something is terribly wrong like an infection and (b) it impairs wound healing; (2) pain is *not* a sign of active healing; (3) *no* pain can be a problem when the patient has peripheral neuropathy, cannot recognize pain, and will not seek help at the early signs of a problem. Patients may also value stoicism and prefer not to talk about their pain, don't want to bother others or sound like a complainer, and believe that the health-care provider should know when they are in pain.

Moreover, misconceptions exist about pain medicine always causing addiction, confusion, or sleepiness. The lessons to be taught here is that all pain medication may have adverse effects and may require adjustment. Appropriate use should not be harmful. Less than 1% of patients develop addiction taking pain medications. The risk of having debilitating pain is more significant.[70] Fear of overmedication may take precedence over the fear of pain, and rather than taking pain medication "by the clock" to prevent pain, patients may reach for pain medication only when they are in agony. Patients need to understand that preventing pain "round the clock" requires less medication and is more efficient and effective than chasing it when it is agonizing. Also, multiple regimens are available to ease pain including topical treatments.

Here are some tips to share with patients about communicating wound pain.[135]

1. Remember that you have the RIGHT to adequate pain relief.
2. The relationship between patient and health-care provider is an equal partnership.
3. A pain management plan is a collaborative effort between the health-care provider, the patient, and the caregiver. If the plan isn't working, tell your health-care provider.
4. Get "more mileage" out of a pain pill by taking it on a regular schedule, setting an alarm as a reminder if necessary.
5. Provide details about your pain when you communicate with your health-care provider. Be specific about where it hurts and when. Draw a picture of a figure and mark the spot(s) where it hurts if that is easier than using words.

6. Use a number to indicate the intensity (how much it hurts). The usual number system rates no pain as 0 and the worst pain as 10. It may not be possible to reach a zero pain level, but it should certainly be possible to get down to a number that is tolerable.
7. If a number doesn't tell your pain story, make a face about how much it hurts or point to a picture of faces in pain.
8. Use words like sharp, hot, stinging, throbbing, aching, and dull to describe your pain.
9. How does the pain affect your mood? Prickly as a porcupine? Mad as a bear with a thorn in his paw? Helpless? Crabby? Crawling into a shell? Sad?
10. Keep track of what you have done to ease the pain and whether it is effective. A pain diary can help.
11. Share with your health-care provider your beliefs about showing or talking about pain: Is it a sign of weakness? Or a taboo?
12. Sudden or increasing pain is often a signal that the wound needs help. Contact your health-care provider right away.
13. Tell your health-care provider about ANY pain that won't go away or gets worse.
14. Medical language is a lot like a foreign language to most people. Ask your health-care provider to define any words you don't know in terms that you can understand.
15. Explaining pain management choices to the patient and caregiver is another way to collaborate.

Here are some suggestions to use when explaining drug and nondrug treatment of pain.

DRUG TREATMENT

- Drug treatment and nondrug treatment can be successful to control and prevent pain. Don't worry about getting "hooked" on pain medicines; this is a rare event unless you already have a problem with drug abuse.
- Pain medicine may be given as a pill or liquid, as a shot, or as a topical application such as a patch. Do NOT be reluctant to take the pain medicine. Take it to PREVENT the pain, not to chase the pain.

- Take action to relieve pain as soon as it starts. It is harder to ease the pain once it starts.
- Pain medicine will take 30 to 60 minutes to take effect. It will not stop pain immediately.
- A medication schedule can prevent breakthrough pain. Taking pain medication 30 to 60 minutes before a wound care procedure (dressing change or debridement) is a good plan.

NONDRUG TREATMENT

- Nondrug treatment options include use of warmth, relaxation, music, pastimes that distract you from thinking about the pain, positive thinking, and electrical nerve stimulation. These techniques can be used alone or in conjunction with pain medication.
- Pain at dressing changes is NOT inevitable. Manufacturers have designed dressings and tapes that do not hurt the wound or skin when they are removed.
- Participate in your dressing changes so you can help control the procedure.
- There are lots of pain relief choices; if one isn't working, tell your health-care provider that you would like to try something else.

The term *noncompliant* has been overused to describe such patients. Such labeling is unfortunate, because lack of adherence to a pain management plan may be due to any of the above-mentioned misperceptions, as well as several other valid reasons. These include

- Complexity—that is, the plan is too difficult to follow or too complicated to understand, or the patient is confused by the medical terminology
- Financial limitations—the patient has difficulty getting the medicine because of cost
- Side effects—the medication may have unpleasant side effects such as drowsiness or confusion which the patient finds less tolerable than the pain of treatment, and confusion over medical terminology

In addition, patients with peripheral neuropathy experience painless wound trauma. They need to be taught to fear the pain that they DO NOT feel and how to care for and protect their feet from trauma (see Chapter 12.)

CONCLUSION

The mnemonic ABCDE summarizes a routine clinical approach to pain assessment and management[28].

Ask the patient about pain regularly. Assess pain systematically.

Believe the patient and family in their reports of pain and what relieves it.

Choose pain control options appropriate for the patient, family, and setting.

Deliver interventions in a timely, logical, and coordinated fashion.

Empower patients and their families. Enable them to control their course to the greatest extent possible.

CASE STUDY

Medical History

Mrs. F, a 65-year-old woman with a history of 3 months of right lower leg edema, with weeping skin, lipodermatosclerosis along the calf and an open ulcer above the medial malleolus was referred to physical therapy for wound pain management because she was experiencing persistent pain in her leg and wound that increases when she moves and at wound dressing changes. She had a medical history of chronic obstructive pulmonary disease, hypertension, and OA of her knees. She had been limiting her mobility (walking) and activities outside the home because of the pain and the weeping skin problems. She was taking NSAIDS for her OA knee pain and wound pain with some efficacy. She was wearing a foam wound dressing with a secondary dressing and netting to hold it in place and then compression bandage wraps over the dressings.

Pain Assessment
Patient Screening
Can you point to where your pain is located?

Can you rate your pain on a scale of 0 = no pain and 10 = maximal pain?

What is your pain level at the low and high times of the day and when is that?

Responses
Pain Location: Pain is from the knee down on the right lower leg and at the knee on the left.

Duration: Persistent but fluctuates in intensity during the day. Pain is worst in the knees in the morning when I get up or after I have been sitting for a while.

Intensity: Patient's VAS rating related to above questions: 3/10 at the low pain time of day, which is in the afternoon and 7/10 at the high period in the morning. Pain increases to 10/10 during dressing changes. She has persistent background pain of 3/10.

Description of Sensation: Can you describe how the pain feels in words?

Response: Pain is throbbing and aching pain, and at times it is burning.

Emotional status: Evaluated with the simple descriptive pain distress scale: What word on the line best describes how distressed you feel about your wound or wound care?

Response: Dreadful. She explained that she dreaded coming to her wound care appointments because of her expectation of intense pain during the wound care procedures.

Prior treatment results: What have you done to relieve you pain and what was the result?

Response: Taking NSAID three times a day.

Result: Reduced pain level for several hours.

Functional activities: What effect has the wound and pain had on your activities?

Response: I don't walk very much. My knees are very stiff and painful in the morning when I get up and the pain goes all the way to my toes.

Findings and Clinical Decision Making

1. Pain diagnosis: Based on the reported type of pain sensations: throbbing and aching pain and at times, which are signs of acute pain and it is burning, signs of nerve irritation, with periods of heightened leg pain in the morning and at dressing changes, there appears to be a mixed pain pattern:
   a. Acute wound pain around the venous ulcer. The wound and surrounding tissues have become hyperalgesic.
   b. Cyclic nociceptive pain related to wound care procedures and OA. Patients with OA typically have stiffness and pain in the morning or after a period of inactivity lasting usually less than 30 minutes. Pain and stiffness typically follow periods of inactivity and decreases during the day with activity.[136]
   c. Tissue tension from edema causing pressure on the nociceptors is adding to hyperalgesia.
   d. Psychosomatic pain based on her experience and learned expectation of severe pain with wound procedures causing dread, and so severity of pain (10/10) is probably related to this as well as the nociceptive cyclic pain from the procedure.
2. Evaluation of current plan of care:
   a. Current regime of wound care has probably contributed to her hyperalgesia.
   b. Compression is not effective in controlling tissue congestion, allowing weeping of nonulcerated adjacent skin and stimulation of the nociceptors of the leg, adding to the pain problem.
   c. Foam dressings, a nonpharmacological strategy, have not been effective for reducing local wound pain and may be drying out.
   d. Her NSAID pain medication is not controlling the background pain.

Prognosis and Revised Interventions

1. Reduce her anxiety and expectation of pain during dressing changes by using a gentle wound dressing.
   a. Selected Intervention: A soft silicone-type dressing Mepilex™ border would meet these criteria (Mölnlycke Health Care Ltd. Norcross, GA).
2. Prevent development of central sensitization of her wound pain.
   a. Intervention: Ask her physician about use of a lidocaine 5% patch to control her hyperalgesia and early symptoms of persistent pain along with continued use of NSAIDS for her OA pain.
3. Improve efficacy of compression to control edema, stop weeping, and reduce tissue tension.
   a. Intervention: Evaluate an inelastic compression device instead of the compression wraps since they do not seem adequate to control edema and weeping (see Chapter 19).
4. Improve her mobility, which will help with her edema management and knee stiffness.
   a. Intervention: Instruction in appropriate exercises by a physical therapist. Exercise has been shown to improve OA pain.

Outcome of Care

After a 7-day trial with the new plan of care, Mrs. F returned to the clinic and was delighted to report that she could now rate her pain as 0 at rest and her pain was 3/10 at that dressing change. Edema was reduced and weeping stopped. She asked to continue treatment with the soft silicone product and inelastic compression. The wound went on to heal in 2 weeks. She continued with her compression regime due to the recurrent nature of her pathology and started a program of physical therapy to improve her mobility. Early intervention with a pain management program probably prevented her pain from progressing to central sensitization and persistent neuropathic pain that is commonly reported in patients with venous ulcers.

REVIEW QUESTIONS

1. Past experience of pain effects pain expectations by
   A. decreasing actual pain
   B. forming a pain memory
   C. causing a placebo analgesia
   D. inhibiting the activation of cholecystokinin

2. Two probable causes of persistent neuropathic wound pain are
   A. abnormal function of the nervous system from an acute incident and sympathetic dystrophy
   B. phantom limb and fibromyalgia
   C. cerebral vascular accident and multiple sclerosis
   D. all of the above
3. Sensations associated with chronic neuropathic wound pain include
   A. burning, tingling, electric shock
   B. numbness, squeezing, throbbing
   C. prickling, numbness, tingling
   D. knife-like, electric shock, throbbing

REVIEW QUESTIONS *(continued)*

4. Which group of nonpharmaceutical methods used to treat either nociceptive or neuropathic pain is incorrect?

A. Offloading wound area, use of bed cradle, and immobilization via splinting

B. Dressing designed for autolysis, self-adhesive dressings, and hydrogel dressings

C. Nonadhesive netting, Montgomery straps, and hydrocolloid dressings

D. Elevation of wound area, foam dressings, and film dressings

5. After pain has been measured on a pain intensity scale The WHO ladder recommends which of the following treatments?

A. Mild pain with nonopioids, moderate pain with mild opioids, severe pain with strong opioids, and uncontrolled pain with a combination of drugs with analgesic properties

B. Mild pain with nonpharmacologic methods, moderate pain with a mild opioid, severe pain with a strong opioid, and uncontrolled pain with a combination of drugs with analgesic properties

C. Mild pain with nonopioids, moderate pain with combination of mild opioids, severe pain with mild opioids and NSAIDS, and uncontrolled pain with a combination of strong opioids

D. Mild pain with NSAIDS or acetaminophen, moderate pain with mild opioids, severe pain with strong opioids, and uncontrolled pain with combination of strong opioids and nonpharmacologic methods

REFERENCES

1. IASP Task Force on Taxonomy. Pain terminology. In: Merskey H, Bogduk N, eds. *Classification of Chronic Pain*. Seattle, WA: IASP Press; 1994:209–214, http://www.iasp-pain.org/terms-p.html#Neuropathic%20pain.

2. World Union of Wound Healing Societies. Principles of best practice: Minimising pain at wound dressing-related procedures. Toronto, Canada June 2008.

3. Sela RA, Bruera E, Conner-Spady B, et al. Sensory and affective dimensions of advanced cancer pain. *Psycho Oncol*. 2002;11(1):23–34.

4. Holdcroft A, Power I. Recent developments: Management of pain. *BMJ*. 2003;326:635–639.

5. Rae C, Gallagher G, Watson S, et al. An audit of patient perception compared with medical and nursing staff estimation of pain during burn dressing changes. *Eur J Anaesthesiol*. 2000;17:43–45.

6. Reddy M, Kohr R, Queen D, et al. Practical treatment of wound pain and trauma: A patient-centered approach. An overview. *Ostomy/Wound Manage*. 2003;49(4A Suppl):2–15.

7. Krasner D. Caring for the person experiencing chronic wound pain. In: Krasner D, Rodeheaver G, Sibbald GR, eds. *Chronic Wound Care: A Clinical Source Book for Healthcare Professionals*. 3rd ed. Wayne, PA: HMP-Communications; 2001:79–88.

8. Carrougher GJ, Ptacek J, Sharer SR, et al. Comparison of patient satisfaction and self reports of pain in adult burn-injured patients. *J Burn Care Rehabil*. 2003;24(1):1–8.

9. Franks PJ, Moffatt C. Who suffers most from leg ulceration? Paper presented at: Journal of Wound Care; September 1998.

10. Goncalves ML, Conceicaode, G, Santos VL, et al. Pain in Chronic Leg Ulcers. *J WOCN*. 2004;31(5):275–283.

11. Evonne F. Wound pain during dressing changes. Paper presented at: How to Decrease Trauma and Pain at Dressing Changes—Satellite Symposium—Symposium For Advanced Wound Care; April 30, 2001, Las Vegas, NV.

12. (JCAHO) JCoAoHO. Pain management standards (Standard RI 2.8 and PE 1.4). In: JCAHO, ed. *Comprehensive Accreditation Manual for Hospitals*; 2001.

13. Tracey I. Nociceptive processing in the human brain. *Curr Opin Neurobiol Sens Syst*. 2005/8 2005;15(4):478–487.

14. Wulf H, Baron R. The theory of Pain. Paper presented at: European Wound Management Association Position Document; 2002, London, UK.

15. Tetsuo K, McHaffie JG, Laurienti PJ, et al. The subjective experience of pain: Where expectations become reality. *Proc Natl Acad Sci*. 2005;102(36):12950–12955.

16. Cutting KF, Harding KG. Criteria to identify wound infection. *J Wound Care*. 1994;3(4):198–201.

17. Sibbald R, Williamson D, Orsted H. Preparing the wound bed—debridement, bacterial balance, and moisture balance. *Ostomy/Wound Manage*. 2000;46(11):14–35.

18. Broadbent E, Petrie KJ, Alley PG, et al. Psychological stress impairs early wound repair following surgery. *Psychosomatic Med*. 2003;65:865–869.

19. Woolf CJ. Neuropathic pain: aetiology, symptoms, mechanisms and management. *The Lancet*. 1999;353:1959–1964.

20. Gifford L, Butler D. The integration of pain sciences into clinical practice. *J Hand Therapy*. 1997;10:86–97.

21. Pediani R. What has pain relief to do with acute surgical wound healing? *World Wide Wounds (on line publication)*. March 2001.

22. Shah JL. Lesson of the week: postoperative pressure sores after epidural anaesthesia. *BMJ*. 2000;321(7266):941–942.

23. Hampton T. Pain and the brain: researchers focus on tackling pain memories. *JAMA*. 2005;293(23):2845–2846.

24. Loeser JD, Treede RD. The Kyoto protocol of IASP basic pain terminology. *Pain*. 2008;137:473–477.

25. Galer B, Sheldon E, Pate N. Development and preliminary validation of a pain measure specific to neuropathic pain: the neuropathic Pain Scale. *Neurology*. 1997;48:332–338.

26. Argoff Charles E, Galer Bradley S, Jensen Mark P, et al. Effectiveness of the lidocaine patch 5% on pain qualities in three chronic pain states: assessment with the Neuropathic Pain Scale. *Curr Med Res Opin (r)*. 2004;20(suppl 2):S21–S28.

27. Jensen TS, Baron R. Translation of symptoms and signs into mechanisms in neuropathic pain. *Pain*. 2003;102:1–8.

28. Jacox A, Carr DB, Payne R, et al. *Management of Cancer Pain*. Rockville, MD: The Agency for Health Care Policy and Research (AHCPR) now Agency for Health Care Research and Quality (AHRQ); 1994.

29. Purves D, Augustine GJ, Fitzpatrick D, et al., ed. *Neuroscience*. 2nd ed. Sinauer Associates; Sunderland, MA 2001.

30. Rossini PM, Forno GD. Integrated technology for evaluation of brain function and neural plasticity. *Phys Med Rehabil Clin N Am*. 2004;15:263–306.

31. Holdcroft A, Power I. Management of pain. *BMJ*. 2005;326:635–639.

32. Sussman C. Preventing and modulating learned wound pain. *Ostom Wound Manage*. 2008;54(11):38–47.

33. Wager TD, Rilling JK, Smith EE, et al. Placebo-induced changes in fMRI in the anticipation and experience of pain. *Science*. 2004;303(5661):1162–1167.

34. Jasper H, Penfield W, eds. *Epilepsy and the Functional Anatomy of the Human Brain*. 2nd ed. Little, Brown and Co.; 1954.

35. http://en.wikipedia.org/wiki/Cortical_homunculus rf. *Wikipedia* December 8, 2010. Accessed December 11, 2010.

36. Boyd LA, Vidoni ED, Daly JJ. Answering the call: the influence of neuroimaging and electrophysiological evidence on rehabilitation. *Phys Ther*. 2007;87(6):684–703.

37. Dahl JB, Kehlet H, eds. Postoperative pain and its management. In: McMahon SB Koltzenberg M, ed. *Wall and Melzack's Textbook of Pain*. Elsevier Churchill Livingstone; Philadelphia, PA 2006.

38. Nicholson BD. Neuropathic pain: new strategies to improve clinical outcomes. Paper presented at: The National Initiative on Pain Control; January 2005, online: www.Medscape.com.

39. McCabe CS, Haigh RC, Halligan PW, et al. Simulating sensory-motor incongruence in healthy volunteers: implications for a cortical model of pain. *Rheumatology*. 2005;44(11):509–516.

40. Moseley Lorimer G, Timothy P, Charles S. Visual distortion of a limb modulates the pain and swelling evoked by movement. *Curr Biol*. 2008;18(22):R1047–R1048.

41. Flor H, Denke C, Schaefer M, et al. Effect of sensory discrimination training on cortical reorganisation and phantom limb pain. *Lancet*. 2001;357(9270):1763–1764.

42. Lotze M, Flor H, Grood W, et al. Phantom movements and pain: an FRMI study in upper limb amputees. *Brain*. 2001;1124:2268–2277.

43. Flor H, Nikolajsen L, Jensen TS. Phantom limb pain: a case of maladaptive CNS plasticity? *Nat Rev Neurosci*. 2006;7:873–881.

44. Flor H. Remapping somatosensory cortex after injury. *Adv Neurol*. 2003;93:195–204.

45. Moseley GL. Evidence for a direct relationship between cognitive and physical change during an education intervention in people with chronic low back pain. *Eur J Pain*. 2004;8:39–45.

46. Garzione J. Brain atrophy associated with chronic pain. *Phys Ther Pract*. 2009;21(3):110.

47. Buckalew N, Haut MW, Morrow L, et al. Chronic pain is associated with brain volume loss in older adults: preliminary evidence. *Pain Med*. 2008;9(2):240–248.

48. University Health Network Toronto, CA. *Effects of N-Methyl-D-Aspartate (NMDA) Receptor Antagonism on Hyperalgesia, Opioid Use, and Pain After Radical Prostatectiny*, 2006.

49. Burgmer M, Gaubitz M, Konrad C, et al. Decreased gray matter volumes in the cingulo-frontal cortex and the amygdala in patients with fibromyalgia. *Psychosom Med*. 2009;71(5):566–573.

50. Boulton AJM. Management of Diabetic Peripheral Neuropathy. *Clin Diab*. 2005;23(1).

51. Schmidt-Wilcke T. Variations in brain volume and regional morphology associated with chronic pain. *Curr Rheumatol Rep*. 2008;10(6):467–474.

52. Schmidt-Wilcke T, Hierlmeier S, Leinisch E. Altered regional brain morphology in patients with chronic facial pain. *Headache*. 2010;50(8):1278–1285.

53. Raij T, Numminen J, Narvanen S, et al. Brain correlates of subjective reality of physically and psychologically induced pain. *Proc Natl Acad Sci*. 2005;102(6):2147–2151.

54. Colloca L, Sigaudo M, Benedetti F. The role of learning in nocebo and placebo effects. *Pain*. 2008;136:211–218.

55. Colloca L, Benedetti F. Nocebo hyperalgesia: how anxiety is turned into pain. *Curr Opin Anaesthesiol*. 2007;20(5):435–439.

56. Enck P, Benedetti F, Schedlowski M. New insights into the placebo and nocebo responses. *Neuron*. 2008;59(2):195–206.

57. Woo K. Meeting the challenges of wound-associated pain: anticipatory pain, anxiety, stress and wound healing. *Ostomy Wound Manage*. 2008;54(9):10–12.

58. Arthur R, Shelley W. The peripheral mechanism of itch in man. Paper presented at: Pain and Itch: Nervous Mechanisms; March 1959, London.

59. Basbaum AI. Distinct neurochemical features of acute and persistent pain. *Proc Natl Acad Sci*. 1999;96(14):7739–7743.

60. Jensen MP, Dworkin RH, Gammaitoni AR, et al. Assessment of pain quality in chronic neuropathic and nociceptive pain clinical trials with the Neuropathic Pain Scale. *J Pain*. 2005;6(2):98–106.

61. Demling R, DeSanti L. Topical doxepin cream is effective in relieving severe pruritis caused by burn injury: a preliminary study. *Wounds: Compend Clin Res Pract*. 2001;13(6):210–215.

62. Mendham JE. Gabapentin for the treatment of itching produced by burns and wound healing in children: a pilot study. *Burns*. 2004;30(8):851–853.

63. British Pain Society RCoA, Royal College of General Practitioners, Royal College of Psychiatrists. *Recommendations for the appropriate use of opiods for persistent noncancer pain*. March 2004.

64. Meyer III, Walter J, Nichols Ray J, et al. Acetaminophen in the management of background pain in children post-burn. *J Pain Symptom Manage*. 1997;13(1):50–55.

65. Ryan S, Eager C, Sibbaid RG. Venous leg ulcer pain. *Ostomy/Wound Manage*. 2003;49(4A suppl):16–23.

66. Berry PH Chapman C, Covington EC, et al. Pain: current Understanding of Assessment, Mangement and Treatments. *Am Pain Soc [online]*. July 19, 2004. Accessed May 5, 2005.

67. Sliwa JA Wiesner S, Novick AK, et al. Concurrent musculoskeletal pain in a patient with symptomatic lower extremity arterial insufficiency. *Arch Phys Med Rehabil*. 1989;70:848–850.

68. Krasner D. The chronic wound pain experience. *Ostomy /Wound Manage*. 1995;41(3):20–27.

69. Sibbald RG. Pain in general. Paper presented at: How to decrease trauma and pain at dressing changes-Satellite Symposium, Symposium for Advanced Wound Care; April 30, 2001, Las Vegas, NV.

70. Woo KY, Sibbald R. Chronic wound pain: a conceptual model. *Adv Skin Wound Care*. 2008;21(4):175–188.

71. Moffatt CJ, Franks PJ, Hollinworth H. Understanding wound pain and trauma: an international perspective. Paper presented at: Pain at Wound Dressing Changes; Spring 2002, Europe.

72. Bonham PA, Flemister BG, Ratliff CR. *Guideline for Management of Wounds in Patients with Lower-Extremity Arterial Disease*. Glenfiew, IL: Wound Ostomy Continence Nurses Society (WOCN); 2002.

73. Sibbald RG, Amstrong D, Orstead H. Pain in diabetic foot ulcers. *Ostomy/Wound Manage*. 2003;49(4A suppl):24–29.

74. Miscavige M. Considering patient priorities when choosing a dressing. *Ostom Wound Manage*. 2004;50(11):16,18.

75. Nemeth KA, Harrison MB, Graham ID, et al. Pain in pure and mixed aetiology venous leg ulcers: a three-phase point prevalence study. *J Wound Care*. 2003;12(9):336–340.

76. Nemeth KA, Harrison MR, Graham ID. Understanding venous leg ulcer pain: results of a longitudinal study. *Ostom Wound Manage*. 2004;50(1):34–46.

77. Shimizu T, Kosaka M, Fujishima K. Human thermoregulatory responses during prolonged walking in water at 25, 30 and 35 degrees C. *Eur J Appl Physiol Occup Physiol*. 1998;78(6):473–478.

78. Lindholm C, Bjellerup M, Christianson O, et al. Quality of life in chronic leg ulcer patients. An assessment accordeing to the Nottingham Health Profile. *Acta Derm Venereol*. 1993;73(6):440–443.

79. Shukla D, Tripathii AK, Agrawal S, et al. Pain in acute and chronic wounds: a descriptive study. *Ostom Wound Manage*. 2005;51(11):47–51.

80. Reddy M, Keast D, Fowler E, et al. Pain in pressure ulcers. *Ostomy/ Wound Manage.* 2003;49(4A suppl):30–35.

81. Szor JK, Bourguignon C. Description of pressure ulcer pain at rest and at dressing change. *JOWCN.* 1999;26(3):115–120.

82. Eriksson E, Hietanen H, Asko-Seljavaara, S. Prevalence and characteristics of pressure ulcers: a one-day patient population in a Finnish city. *Clin Nurs Spec.* 2000;14:19–25.

83. Roth RS, Lowery JC, Hamill JB. Assessing persistent pain and its relation to affective distress, depressive symptoms, and pain catastrophizing in patients with chronic wounds A pilot study. *Am J Phys Med Rehabil.* 2004;83:821,827–834.

84. Manz BD, Moser R, Nusser-Gerlach MA, et al. Pain assessment in the cognitively impaired and unimpaired elderly. *Pain Manage Nurs.* 2000;1(4):106–115.

85. vanRijswijk L. Full-thickness pressure ulcers: patient and wound healing characteristics. *Decubitus.* 1993;6(1):16–21.

86. Hoffman H. Virtual Reality Pain Reduction University of Washington Seattle and U.W. Harborview Burn Center, website vrpain.com used with permission.

87. Scott J, Huskisson EC. Graphic representation of pain. *Pain.* 1976;2:175–184.

88. Wewers ME, Lowe NK. A critical review of visual analogue scales in the measurement of clinical phenomena. *Res Nurs Health.* 1990;13:227–236.

89. Freeman K, Smyth C, Dallam L, et al. Pain measurement scales: a comparison of the visual analogue and faces rating scales in measuring pressure ulcer pain. *J Wound Ostomy Continence Nurs.* 2001;28(6):290–296.

90. Wong D, Baker C. Pain in children: comparison of assessment scales. *Pediatr Nurs.* 1988;14:9–17.

91. Stuppy DJ. The Faces Pain Scale: reliability and validity with mature adults. *Appl Nurs Res.* 1998;11:84–89.

92. Paice JA, Cohen FL. Validity of a verbally administered numeric rating scale to measure cancer pain intensity. Validity of a verbally administered numeric rating scale to measure cancer pain intensity. *Cancer Nurs.* 1997;20:88–93.

93. Fink R, Gates R. In: Ferrell, BR, Coyle, N, eds. *Pain Assessment in Textbook of Palliative Nursing.* 2nd ed. New York: Oxford University Press; 2006:97–127.

94. Taylor LJ, Herr K, Paice JA. Pain intensity assessment: a comparison of selected pain intensity scales for use in cognitively intact and cognitively impaired African American older adults. *Pain Manage Nurs.* 2003;4:87–95.

95. Galloway S, Turner L. Pain assessment in older adults who are cognitively impaired. *J Gerontol Nurs.* 1999;25:34–39.

96. Melzack R. The short-form McGill Pain questionnaire. *Pain.* 1987;30(2):191–197.

97. Lane P, Kuntupis M, MacDonald S, et al. A pain assessment tool for people with Advanced Alzheimer's and other progressive Dementias. *Home Healthcare Nurse.* 2003;21(1):33–37.

98. Pautex S, Herrmann F, Le Lous P, et al. Feasibility and reliability of four pain self-assessment scales and correlation with an observational rating scale in hospitalized elderly demented patients. *J Gerontol A Biol Sci Med Sci.* 2005;60(4):524–529.

99. Ekman P, Friesen WV, Ellsworth P. *Emotions in the Human Face.* Elmsford, NY: Pergamon Press; 1972.

100. Levenson RW, Ekman P, Friesen WV. Voluntary facial action generates emotion-specific autonomic nervous system activity. *Psychophysiology.* 1990;27(4):363–384.

101. Goodman CC, Snyder-Kelly TE. Pain types and viscerogenic pain patterns. In: *Differential Diagnosis for Physical Therapists: Screening for Referral.* 4th ed. United States: Saunders, an imprint of Elsevier; 2007:124–131.

102. Panel NPUAP,EPUA. *Prevention and Treatment Of Pressure Ulcers: Clinical Practice Guideline.* Washington, DC: National Pressure Ulcer Advisory Panel; 2009.

103. Meaume S, Téot L, Lazareth I, et al. The importance of pain reduction through dressing selection in routine wound management: the MAPP study. *J Wound Care Republished Ostomy Wound Manage.* 2004/2008;13/54(10/4):409–413/410–402.

104. Karlsmark T, Zillmer R, Agren M, et al. Will self-adhesive dressings cause trauma to periwound skin? Paper presented at: The 7th Annual Conference of the Canadian Association of Wound Care; November 2001, London, Ontario, Canada.

105. Briggs M. Surgical wound pain: a trial of two treatments. *J Wound Care.* 1996;5(10):456–460.

106. Briggs M, Torra I, Bou JE. Pain at wound dressing changes: a guide to management. Paper presented at: EWMA Position Document; 2002, London, UK.

107. Hollinworth H, Collier M. Nurses' view about pain and trauma at dressing changes: results of a national survey. *J Wound Care.* 2000;9(8):369–373.

108. Hollinworth H. *Pain and Wound Care.* Ipswich, UK: Wound Care Society; 2000.

109. Yang Q, Berghe D. Effect of temperature on in vitro proliferative activity of human umbilical vein endothelial cells. *Experientia.* 1995;51(2):126–132.

110. Hoffman Hunter G, Chambers Gloria T, Meyer III Walter J, et al. Virtual Reality as an Adjunctive Non-pharmacologic Analgesic for Acute Burn Pain During Medical. *Procedures. Ann Behav Med.* 2010; DOI 10.1007/s12160-010-9248-7. 2010.

111. Holden-Lund C. The effects of relaxation with guided imagery on surgical stress and wound healing. *Res Nurs Health.* 1988;11(4):235–244.

112. Rice B, Kalker A, Schindler J, et al. Effect of biofeedback-assisted relaxation training on foot ulcer healing. *J Am Podiatr Med Assoc.* 2001;91(3):132–141.

113. Cameron MH. Thermal agents. In: Cameron MH, ed. *Physical Agents in Rehabilitation.* Philadelphia, PA: WB Saunders; 1999:134–135.

114. Maizels M, McCarberg B. Antidepressants and antiepileptic drugs for chronic non-cancer pain. *Am Fam Phys.* 2005;71:483–490.

115. Committee WHOE. *World Health Organization. Cancer Pain Relief and Palliaive Care.* Geneva, Switzerland: World Health Organization; 1990.

116. Dallam LE, Barkauskas C, Ayello E, et al. Pain management and wounds. In: Baranoski S, Ayello E, eds. *Wound Care Essentials: Practice Principles.* Philadelphia, PA: Lippincott Williams and Wilkins; 2003:217–236.

117. Kennedy KL, Tritch DL. Debridement. In: Krasner D, Kane D, eds. *Chronic Wound Care: A Clinical Sourcebook for Healthcare Professionals.* Wayne, PA: Health Management Publications; 1997:227–235.

118. Goldstein F. Adjuncts to opioid therapy. *J Am Osteopath Assoc.* 2002;102(9 suppl):15S.

119. Salcido R. Do antiinflammatories have a role in wound healing. Paper presented at: Clinical Symposium on Advances in Skin and Wound Care; October 23–26, 2005, Las Vegas, NV.

120. Schafer AI. Effects of nonsteroidal antiinflammatory drugs on platelet function and systemic hemostasis. *J Clin Pharmacol.* 1995;35(3):209–219.

121. Szarvas S, Harmon D, Murphy D. Neuraxial opioid-induced pruritus: a review. *J Clin Anesth.* 2003;15: 234–239.

122. Saarto T, Wiffen PJ. Antidepressants for neuropathic pain. *Cochrane Database Syst Rev.* 2007(4):Art. No.: CD005454. DOI: 005410.001002/12651858.CD14005454.pub14651852.

123. Attal N, Cruccu G, Baron R, et al. EFNS guidelines on the pharmacological treatment of neuropathic pain: 2010 revision. *Eur J Neurol.* 2010;17:1113–1123.

124. Wiffen PJ, Collins S, McQuay HJ, et al. WITHDRAWN. Anticonvulsant drugs for acute and chronic pain. *Cochrane Database Syst Rev.* Jan 20 2010(1):CD001133.

125. Medscape. Amitriptyline. *Medscape* [Internet WWW.Medscape.com]. 2010 Accessed December 26, 2010.

126. Medscape. Gabapentin *Medscape* [online WWW.Medscape.com accessed December 26, 2010].

127. Galer B, Jensen M, Ma T, et al. The lidocaine patch 5% effectively treats all neuropathic pain qualities: results of a randomized, double-blind, vehicle-controlled, 3-week efficacy study with use of the neuropathic pain scale. *Clin J Pain.* 2002;18(5):297–301.

128. Lawhorne L, Passerini J, Harlan M. *Chronic Pain Management in the Long-Term Care Setting.* American Medical Directors Association; 1999.

129. Jones KG, et al. Inhibition of angiogenesis by nonsteroidal antiinflammatory drugs: insight into mechanisms and implications for cancer growth and ulcer healing. *Nat Med.* 1999;5(5):1418–1423.

130. Hafner HM, Thomma SR, Eichner M, et al. The influence of Emla cream on cutaneous microcirculation. *Clin Hemorrheol Microcirc.* 2003;28:121–128.

131. Briggs M, Nelson EA. Topical agents or dressings for pain in venous leg ulcers. *Cochrane Database Syst Rev.* April 14 2010; CD001177(4).

132. Zeppetella G, Paul J, Ribeiro M. Analgesic efficacy of morphine applied topically to painful ulcers. *J Pain Symptom Manage.* 2003;25:555–558.

133. Flock P. Pilot study to determine the effectiveness of diamorphine gel to control pressure ulcer pain. *J Pain Symptom Manage.* 2003;25:547–554.

134. Brown T, Lovato L, Parker D. Procedural sedation in the acute care setting. *Am Fam Physician.* 2005;71(1):85–90.

135. Sussman C. Pain doesn't have to be a part of wound care. *Ostom Wound Management.* 2003;49(3):10–12.

136. Boissonnault W, Goodman C. Bone, joint and soft tissue disorders. In: Goodman C, Fuller K, Boissonnault W, eds. *Pathology: Implications for the Physical Therapist*; 2nd. Saunders Philadelphia PA, 2003;965–967.

137. Fowler E. Plain talk about wound pain. *Ostom Wound Manage.* 2005;51(11A suppl):4–6.

PART IV

Management of Wound Healing with Biophysical Agent Technologies

Carrie Sussman

Management of wound healing with biophysical agent technologies is presented in Part IV, Chapters 23 to 30. Biophysical agents included are electrical stimulation, radio frequency/electromagnetic fields (a variant of electrical stimulation), phototherapy (ultraviolet and laser light), ultrasound (high and low frequency, therapeutic and diagnostic), hydrotherapy (including whirlpool and soaking), pulsed lavage with suction, negative pressure therapy, and hyperbaric oxygen. Biophysical agents use physical energies to change cellular and tissue responses to affect healing. Chapters 23 to 30 describe the physical science associated with each technology, what is currently known about the science and clinical efficacy, the safety and rationale for its use, devices, procedures for application, and case studies. Each device mentioned in Part IV has the ability to affect one or more of the barriers (e.g., ischemia, infection or moisture balance) to healing. How to choose between them remains a key question. This introduction provides some guidelines about why, when, for whom, and how to choose a biophysical agent. The individual chapters discuss the same questions specific to each device and how to use them.

BIOPHYSICAL AGENTS AND THE ELECTROMAGNETIC SPECTRUM

One purpose of this introduction is to look at the physical relationship between the different biophysical agents and the electromagnetic spectrum (EMS) and to shed some insight into why there is so much interest in them, why they are useful for wound healing, and why many of the effects appear to be so similar (see Fig. IV.1). Chapters 23 to 25 deal with technologies that exploit the properties of the EMS frequency or wavelength signal. However, no optimal wavelength signal has as yet been identified. Patient characteristics, clinician intervention expertise, and device availability in addition to evidence are often the deciding points.

Why Exploit the EMS?

Exposure to electromagnetic radiation is ongoing for all living systems. Sources of exposure are both natural (e.g., sunlight and earth's electromagnetic field) and man-made (e.g., cell phones, power lines, computers, and sunlamps). Man recognized long ago that the sun had healing properties and has tried to take advantage of those properties by harnessing the energy of the sun in different way to exploit those properties. As science has progressed, scientists have been able to analyze the components of the electromagnetic radiation and develop a scale to describe the relationship between them. EMS is the whole range of wavelengths or frequencies of electromagnetic radiation, extending from very short gamma rays to visible light and the longest radio waves (see Fig. IV.1). Further scientific advances have led to the development of technologies that use segments of the EMS for biologic purposes. The EMS is categorized according to frequency and wavelength. As the frequency increases, the wavelength decreases. All EMS wavelengths share the property of passing through space (e.g., body tissue or wound dressings) without requiring a medium for transmission. The different wavelengths are like family members that differ from each other only in their wavelength or frequency, and there is often overlap between the neighbors. At low frequencies, 30 to 300 kHz, there are the long radio waves that are used in the radiofrequency stimulators and electric stimulators. In the middle are the midfrequency wavelengths, shorter than radio or microwaves but longer than visibile light, infrared radiation (IR) (75-10-6 cm). These wavelengths overlap the radio waves of the long end and have the same properties as visible light on the short end. Laser and monochromatic light are components of this segment of the EMS.

One of the properties of IR is thermal radiation. This feature is used in thermography and also to heat superficial tissues such as with hydrotherapy. The rainbow is the visible light part of the EMS, and this part of the spectrum stimulates many body cellular systems including the system that produces vitamin D. Beyond the visible light segment is the still shorter wavelengths of ultraviolet (UV) light (UV A, B, C), which is a component of sunlight and has the ability to heal as well as burn the skin. The frequency of UV is 1013 to 1017 Hz or wavelengths of 400 to 4 nm. Low frequencies through UV range are considered to be nonionizing radiation and cannot break molecular bonds or produce ions, which makes them safe for therapeutic applications.

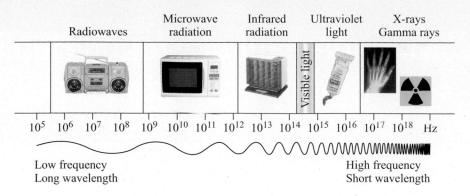

FIGURE IV.1 The electromagnetic spectrum.

Shortest wavelength relatives of the EMS family are the x-rays and gamma rays, which are ionizing and have the potential to inhibit cell growth or have the ability to damage cells. They are used therapeutically to exploit those properties in treatment of cancer, for example, but are avoided for purposes of wound healing.

It has been firmly established that each of these EMS members presented here have abilities to affect complex cellular process and influence tissue growth. This should not be a surprise since the body is continuously bombarded with wavelengths from the EMS in the environment. Cells over time have learned to respond to signals from the environmental bombardment. Now as a result of extensive research efforts, the effects of the EMS component on cellular systems are being applied clinically through the use of complex delivery systems to trigger responses needed for wound healing. Details about the physical properties of each segment of the EMS used in the different technologies are described in the individual chapters in Part IV, along with the results of research efforts.

BIOPHYSICAL AGENTS UNRELATED TO EMS

Chapters 25 to 30 discuss other biophysical agents, unrelated to EMS, including ultrasound, hydrotherapy, pulsatile lavage with suction (negative pressure), negative pressure wound therapy, and hyperbaric oxygen therapy. Ultrasound (US) is also nonionizing but it is not a part of the EMS; it is high-frequency sound waves that, unlike EMS waves, require a medium for transmission of the energy into tissues (see Chapter 26). Each chapter describes the physical properties of each therapy intervention, the different technologies, and physiological effects of the energy.

Regulatory Approval

The devices described in Part IV are all FDA approved for medical application but most are not specifically approved for wound healing applications. Individual chapters have information about FDA premarket approval for specific application of that technology. All have best-practice methods that will provide effective outcomes, and some do have significant health risks if used improperly. Any adverse medical events that result from using any of these products should be reported to the FDA. Prior reports can be viewed at the FDA Web site; this is the link to MAUDE, the database on devices and adverse events: http://www.access-data.fda.gov/scripts/cdrh/cfdocs/ cfMAUDE/search.CFM

CANDIDACY FOR INTERVENTION

The interventions discussed in Part IV chapters are often classified as adjunctive or advanced therapies. There is a new paradigm called "multimodal therapy" where more than one biophysical agent are used together or in sequence for specific reasons.[1] Eaglstein suggested adding new, alternative, or adjunctive therapies at four "points" in the course of care[2]:

1. Initially when predictors such as ulcer size and duration indicate a likely failure of standard care
2. When the rate of healing with standard care predicts failure
3. After failure to heal in the "magic" time (2–4 weeks)
4. Under special circumstances such as unusual diagnosis or patient demand

The mode of intervention best suited to the patient, the treatment setting, and the wound will be determined by the clinical wound manager (e.g., MD, PT, or WOCN) and recommended to the wound management team.

As a guide, patients should be referred for intervention with a biophysical agent when the additional following candidacy criteria are met:

- Medical comorbidities exist that predict that a wound needs extra help to heal (e.g., arterial occlusive disease, spinal cord injury, diabetes, venous insufficiency, hematoma, or deep tissue injury).
- Healing will be speeded by the therapy.
- The wound has a large size or is of long duration.
- The wound has been recalcitrant to other methods of healing.
- There is an acute wound in a patient with a comorbidity such as chronic obstructive pulmonary disease or atherosclerosis, or diabetic neuropathy, indicating a high probability of delayed healing.
- The acute traumatic wound(s) is associated with neuromuscular or musculoskeletal problems that may require immobilization.
- The wounds extend into subcutaneous tissue and deeper underlying structures and interfere with functional activities

(e.g., the patient is unable to sit up in a wheelchair because of the wounds over the ischial tuberosities or coccyx).

- The patient's functional status is impaired by slow wound healing (e.g., gait will be helped if the wound is healed more rapidly, or the patient may be able to return to work).
- Patient or family preference.

Each chapter has a section about candidacy for that specific biophysical intervention. Based on research presented in the individual chapters, optimal time for intervening with biophysical agents is during the first 72 hours immediately after injury, when cellular events are most likely to be positively influenced to produce a successful healing cascade (see Chapter 23, 24, and 26). However, in reality, more chronic wounds than acute wounds are referred for these advanced therapies, in spite of evidence from several studies, reported in the following chapters, showing that early intervention soon after onset of the problem reduces cost and the consequences of costly health problems. As a reflection of clinical reality, most of the clinical research, except for healing of acute surgical wounds, has focused on healing chronic wounds. Research results provide evidence of healing of chronic wounds or favorable alteration of factors related to chronic wound healing such as circulation, tissue oxygenation, cellular processes, pain, and edema. Expected outcomes would be based on identified and targeted problems.

Although biophysical agents are efficacious for healing, the dosing regimens remain largely empirical because the science of the interactions at the cellular level is only just being discovered. Innovative scientists, engineers, designers, and manufacturers are working continuously to discover the underlying science and clinical effects and to develop products that will deliver these biophysical signals to target tissues and exploit them for therapeutic benefit. Biophysical treatments are alternatives to pharmacologic interventions with benefits theoretically of sustained increases in cellular processes at the local and, in some cases, systemic levels, without risk of local or systemic toxicity.

PRIMARY OR ADJUNCTIVE THERAPY

Are all the treatment interventions in this section considered adjunctive rather than primary treatment modalities? Negative pressure wound therapy and pulsed lavage with suction usually are used as primary treatment interventions. Photo stimulation and ultrasound are used on a case-by-case basis determined by the health-care professionals treating the patient. Electrical stimulation is now considered a primary advanced treatment modality rather than adjunctive therapy by some experts. However, Medicare still considers it adjunctive for purposes of reimbursement. The Center for Medicare and Medicaid Services (CMS) coverage policy, for example, does not reimburse for ES or PRF for wound healing until the wound shows chronicity of at least 30 days and is a full-thickness or deeper ulcer (stage III or IV). Patients need to be informed that they have this treatment option early but that reimbursement by the Medicare program will probably not be paid. See the CMS Web site for details, www.hhs.cms, and search for electrical stimulation coverage policy.

Choosing Between Interventions

A frequently asked question is, "How do I know which biophysical agent to choose?" The purpose of presenting information about many different biophysical interventions in this section is to provide the clinician with choices and enough information about each intervention to determine if the presenting patient is a candidate for one or more of them.

The rules for selection of treatment interventions include consideration of the patient's medical status, the status of the wound healing phase, and all treatments used to achieve the expected outcome. Wounds receive multimodal treatments, (e.g., topical agents, dressings, and a biophysical agent) requiring that all treatment interventions be compatible with the patient, one another, and the wound. This will require collaboration of the team members—nurse, physician, pharmacist, and PT. Exhibit IV.1 lists three rules of treatment selection, an example of how each is used, and a formula for selection of treatments to achieve a desire outcome in a prescribed period. The letters "A," "B," and "C" in the formula represent three treatment interventions. The number of treatments usually given is often three but is not limited to three. The chapters in Part IV address the issue of treatment interactions and compatibility with other interventions.

If more than one of the technologies affects the same aspect of the healing phase, other criteria would be used to choose the modality. For instance, most devices described have the ability to increase tissue perfusion. What differs is the mechanism by which it acts, but the expected treatment outcomes of progression through the phases of healing are similar for each of the therapies.

Reimbursement Issues

The payer often must be agreeable to paying for the biophysical intervention selected. For example, Medicare has an exclusion policy for payment of UV light to treat wounds. However, there is now evidence that UV light is a useful treatment to control infection and reinitiate an inflammatory response. At this time, the cost of the UV treatment cannot be billed separately. However, other rationale need to be considered besides reimbursement to justify its selection such as the very short treatment time (e.g., <30 seconds) and rapid wound disinfection that could speed healing and reduce long-term costs. Electrical stimulation and pulsed radiofrequency as described in Chapters 23 and 24 are other examples of Medicare coverage policy restrictions. However, reimbursement restrictions should not preclude advising patients of their availability as a choice if the patient would benefit from their use.

Treatment Availability

Treatment availability is a practical reality. If the preferred intervention is not available and cannot be obtained, another choice must be made. Medical contraindications exist for all of the different biophysical technologies, but the medical contraindication that rules out the use of one will not necessarily rule out the use of others. For example, a semicomatose patient should not be referred for whirlpool, but wound cleansing with pulsatile lavage with suction at bedside would be an appropriate alternative. Sometimes treatment availability leads to overuse of a particular intervention and restricts choice of other possibilities. Such practice needs to be rethought for better, more effective outcomes.

CASE STUDY

Choosing the Appropriate Treatment Intervention

Multiple factors had to be considered when making a choice of intervention for E.F. E.F., an elderly lady, lived in a nursing home because of Alzheimer disease. She had venous disease and a history of recurrent venous ulcers of the lower leg. A new episode of venous insufficiency with subcutaneous hemorrhaging occurred and the patient was referred immediately to physical therapy. The physical therapist performed a history and systems review and learned that the patient had a pacemaker, would not stay in bed or in a wheelchair for 5 minutes, and would not tolerate dressings or compression devices. The venous insufficiency diagnosis ruled out whirlpool, which probably would not have been tolerated either. The pacemaker ruled out any form of electrotherapy. The low tolerance for compression ruled out compression devices. Pulsatile lavage with suction was not available and would not have been tolerated by the patient. The only choice remaining was ultrasound because she could be kept still and amused for the 5 minutes required for a peri-wound direct contact high-frequency ultrasound treatment. This was also an appropriate choice because ultrasound is particularly effective during the acute inflammatory phase and promotes thrombolysis and absorption of hemorrhagic materials (see Chapter 26). This patient is included as one of the case histories in Chapter 26 along with photographs of her condition and progress.

The following case study illustrates how thoughtful evaluation of the history and systems review narrowed down the choice of treatment intervention to one appropriate technology after considering all the factors.

FUNCTIONAL WOUND COST OUTCOMES MANAGEMENT

How do costs for treatment with biophysical agents for wound healing compare? Does this group of interventions provide good value for the money spent?[3]

Health-care professionals including the entire team and program directors need to understand the information required to predict and manage cost for proper utilization of services. The necessary information to predict cost and outcome are available from several sources: clinical trials, program evaluation reports, the facility's clinical database, evidence-based clinical practice guidelines, and payer data–based reports.

Does your clinic know your cost outcomes? Cost outcomes are differentiated from the technical outcome for the wound (e.g., closure). Cost outcomes are what it costs to provide a course of care compared with the billed charges. This determines the cost to the provider as differentiated from the charges to the payer. The cost outcome is based on all the related costs for providing the service: labor cost, supply cost, and equipment cost. To determine the cost of treating a wound, the clinical manager needs to predict the number of expected visits to achieve a specific outcome. For example, if an outcome of closure is expected in 49 visits, a cost analysis can be done as follows:

Labor cost at $30/visit × 49 = $1,470
Supply cost at $6.25/visit × 49 = $306.25
Equipment cost at $0.50 × 49 = $24.50
Total cost = $1,800.75
Billed charges at $60/visit × 49 = $2,940
Net profit = $1,139.25

The cost for a different outcome to convert the wound to clean and stable may take half the time to closure. Cost to the payer would be reduced by half, to $1,470. The case manager for the payer may be more willing to authorize an interim step for a known cost than an unknown outcome at unmanaged cost.

UTILIZATION REVIEW AND COST OUTCOMES MANAGEMENT

Utilization review and cost outcomes management mean that continued ongoing evaluation of patient candidacy for the advanced therapy intervention be reviewed. Candidacy determined at the initial evaluation may change as the patient experiences a course of care.

References

1. Frykberg RG, Martin E, et al. A case history of multimodal therapy in healing a complicated diabetic foot wound: negative pressure dermal replacement and pulsed radio frequency energy therapies. *Int Wound J.* 2011;8(2):132–139.
2. Eaglstein W. What is standard care and where should we leave it? In: *Evidence Based Outcomes in Wound Management.* Dallas, TX: ConvaTec; 2000.
3. Swanson G. Use of cost data, provider experience, and clinical guidelines in the transition to managed care. *J Ins Med.* 1991;23(1):70–74.

CHAPTER 23

Electrical Stimulation for Wound Healing

Carrie Sussman

CHAPTER OBJECTIVES

At the completion of this chapter, the reader will be able to:

1. Explain the physical properties of electrical stimulation used for wound healing treatment, including their significance.
2. Describe the applied physiologic effects of electrical stimulation on body systems: cellular, circulatory, and neuronal.
3. Discuss the current research into the effectiveness of electrical stimulation in promoting wound healing.
4. Describe the results of animal and clinical studies using different types of electrical stimulation waveforms.
5. Select the appropriate candidates for wound healing with electrical stimulation.
6. List the contraindications and precautions of electrical stimulation for wound healing.
7. Apply electrical stimulation for different wound healing situations, including home self-care, and evaluate outcomes of care.

Electrical stimulation (**ES**) for wound healing, as used here, is defined as the use of direct contact (capacitive) electrodes applied to the skin or wound surface. Use of ES to promote healing of chronic recalcitrant ulcers of many etiologies has been reported in the literature for almost 50 years. Although initially there was skepticism about the use of this intervention, it is now recognized as an evidence-based tool for tissue healing. That recognition is demonstrated by recommendation of ES as a treatment choice in clinical practice guidelines,[1–5] reimbursement of ES by the Center for Medicare and Medicaid Services,[6] and its frequent mention in the wound healing literature. However, not all reviewers are in agreement with this recommendation for pressure ulcers, and many believe that larger and higher quality studies are needed.[7]

In 2009, the National Pressure Ulcer Advisor Panel and the European Pressure Ulcer Advisor Panels reviewed the evidence about the use of ES and other adjunctive therapies for treatment of pressure ulcers. Therapies considered by the panel were ES; induced ES; infrared, ultraviolet, and low-energy laser irradiation; ultrasound; negative pressure; and hyperbaric oxygen (see Chapters 23–25, 28, and 29). Of these therapies, ES received the highest rating. The recommendation reads: "Consider the use of direct contact (capacitative) ES in the management of recalcitrant Category/Stage II pressure ulcers as well as category/

Stage III and IV pressure ulcers to facilitate wound healing. Strength of evidence = Level A."[5] Findings about the other therapies are considered in following chapters.

Pressure ulcers are not the only wound etiology that has been investigated for wound healing with ES. Additional studies also support a positive effect of ES treatment for wounds of different etiologies.[8–11] Taken together, there is an accumulated body of research data about ES efficacy. This research data will be presented in this chapter for your better understanding.

For over 50 years, researchers have explored many aspects of ES effects. Thus the amount of information available is proportionally larger than provided in other chapters. It is important to have this background information to skillfully use the technology to achieve the desired outcomes.

ES has its own terminology and principles that effect tissue physiology and healing. Since they are used throughout this chapter, Chapter 23 begins by introducing them. The author then examines applied physiology of ES for explanation of the therapeutic effects of ES on body and wound. Next the author defines and describes the extensive research evaluating the therapeutic effects of ES for wound healing. This is followed by a discussion of the use of ES in clinical practice. Before closing, the chapter provides self-care teaching guidelines for ES application as a treatment intervention that can be taught to patients and caregivers.

THERAPEUTIC ELECTRICAL CURRENTS: CHARACTERISTICS AND TERMINOLOGY

Familiarity with the characteristics and terminology of electrical currents (ECs) will help you understand the interrelationships between the various stimulation characteristics and the clinical effects demonstrated. The terminology used in this section follows the recommendations adapted by the Section on Clinical Electrophysiology and Wound Management of the American Physical Therapy Association. The purpose of the recommendations is to "facilitate communication in electrotherapy."[12] Unfortunately, the literature on this subject is inconsistent in its use of EC characteristics and terminology. The following is not meant to be a comprehensive description of all EC characteristics but instead emphasizes those that have a demonstrated role in wound healing. After studying this chapter, you will be able to apply what you learn here to comprehend the information you encounter in the rest of this chapter and in the literature you read about EC. Table 23.1 is a list of EC terms and definitions. Most of the parameters listed on the panel are described in the following sections.

TABLE 23.1 **Electrical Stimulation Terminology**

Name	Alternate Name(s)	Definition
Amperage, milliamperage, microamperage	A, mA, µA	A unit of current that represents the rate at which charge flows past a fixed point.
Amplitude	Intensity	Measure of the magnitude of the voltage.
Anode	Positive pole	Positive pole of an electric circuit.[12]
Biological current		The flow of charge in biological tissues.
Biphasic current	Alternating, Bidirectional, or Bipolar. Figure 23.3 lines 2 and 3.	The waveform shape may be square, sinusoidal, or triangular and has two phases. The biphasic waves are constantly changing.
Capacitively coupling		Involves the transfer of electric current through an applied surface electrode pad that is in wet (electrolytic) contact (capacitively) coupled with the external skin surface and/or wound bed.
Cathode	Negative pole	Negative pole of an electric circuit.[12]
Charge	Q	Quantity of electricity that flows in electric currents.
Charge density		The amount of electric charge in a line, surface, or volume.
Conductance, conductor		The inverse of resistance and represents the ease with which current can flow. Conductor allows passage of current.
Coulomb, microcoulomb	C, µC	It is the quantity of electricity transferred by a current of one ampere in 1 s. Quantity of electricity transfer by a µA current in a millionth of a second.
Current		The flow of charge from one place to another.
Current density		The electrical charge per cross-sectional area of the electrodes.
Current of injury		Current flow through the ionic fluids of the tissues between the outer and inner layers of the skin
Direct current	DC, Galvanic Current	Always continuous, unidirectional, and is a flow of charged particles from one pole to the other lasting 1 s or longer.
Duty cycle		The ratio of *on time* to the *total cycle time*, including both the on and off time.
Electrical circuit		Is a path that transmits electric current. Electrons flow from the negative pole to the positive pole.
Electrical potential		A surplus of electrons in one lead or electrode of a stimulator (negative potential) and a deficiency in electrons (positive potential) in a second.
Electrical stimulation	ES	The conductance of electricity through a conductive medium for the purpose of inducing *direct* influence on both excitatory and nonexcitatory systems and *indirect* effects associated with circulatory response.[13]
Electrodes		The means by which the electric current is conducted from the stimulator device to the tissues.
Galvanotaxis		Unidirectional electrical current flowing in the tissues attracts the cells of repair by a signaling mechanism.

TABLE 23.1	Electrical Stimulation Terminology *(continued)*	
Name	**Alternate Name(s)**	**Definition**
High-voltage monophasic pulsed current	See Figure 23.5	Monophasic electrical stimulators that deliver pulsed DC current via short monophasic pulses at amplitude from 100 to 500 V.
Impedance	I	Frequency dependent opposition to EC flow and is expressed in ohms.
Interpulse interval	See Figure 23.4	The time between pulses.
Ion (negative)		An atom that has lost electrons and it has a net negative charge (–).
Ion (positive)		An atom that has gained electrons and it has a net positive charge (+).
Low voltage pulsed current	LVPC, Low Intensity Direct Current (LIDC)	It is a proprietary waveform that is monophasic and has a square wave shape.
Microampere	μA	Is a millionth of an ampere.
Microelectronic nerve stimulation	MENS	A pulsed monophasic low-voltage form of electrical stimulation.
Milliamp	Ma	One thousandth of an ampere.
Microamp	μA	One millionth of an ampere
Monophasic pulsed current	See Figure 23.3 line one and Figure 23.5	Unidirectional, pulsed current that deviates from baseline and returns to baseline after a designated period. This current does not oscillate between poles and its shape may be square, triangular or twin peaked. All phases will be either positive or negative.
Negative direct current		Current flows from the negative to the positive pole.
Ohm's law		Voltage equals resistance times current (V = RI).
Oscillation		The periodic change from one direction to another.
Phase		Point in the wave cycle where the oscillation begins.
Phase charge	Q	Is represented by the area under the curve and is expressed as the product of the phase duration (t) and the peak current amplitude (I).
Phase duration	T	The length of time that the pulse is on.
Polarity		Property of having two oppositely charged poles.[12] It refers to the direction of electron flow toward a magnetic pole.
Positive direct current	DC(+)	Current flows from the positive to the negative pole.
Pulsatile currents	PC or PES	DC that is pulsed so current amplitude increases for a period of time and then returns to baseline.
Pulse	See Figure 23.4	Is a single electrical event separated by a finite time from the next event.
Pulse duration or width	See Figure 23.4	Is the time elapsed between the beginning and end of all phases including the interpulse interval.
Pulse rate	Frequency (pps)	Is the number of pulses delivered per unit of time. It is measured in pulses per second (pps).
Pulsed current	PC or PES	Is the emission of a train of pulses that are repeated at regular intervals.
Resistance	R	Is the property of a conductor that limits the movement of current through it (e.g., electrodes and body tissues).
Sine/sinusoidal/ alternating waveform	Alternating or biphasic. See Figure 23.2	A mathematical function that describes a smooth repetitive oscillation of current. Usually oscillation between positive and negative.
Transcutaneous electrical nerve stimulation	TENS	Stimulators usually using biphasic or modified AC currents.
Voltage	V	An electromotive force capable of moving ions through a conductor, i.e., electrodes, skin or wound tissue.
Waveforms	See Figure 23.2	The graphic representations of current flow on an amplitude/time or voltage/time plot.
Window of charge		Represents a range of charge intensity, between 200 and 600 μC that has been determined to be effective for wound healing.

Instrumentation

Electrical stimulators have three basic components: a source of power, an oscillator circuit, and an output amplifier. There are two size ranges: clinical models and portable models. The latter can be as small as a mobile phone. Two basic power sources are used: batteries and house line current. Batteries are used in portable stimulators; house line current is usually used in the clinic setting. Batteries need to be fully charged to deliver the output expected. A spare battery should be kept on hand. Rechargeable batteries may be more cost-effective than single-use types. However, over time they will need to be replaced.

Charge Density

The size of the electrode will determine the amount of charge density or concentration of charge delivered per unit area of the electrode. The purpose of the treatment is to deliver adequate charge density to a specific tissue. There is an inverse relationship between charge density and electrode surface area.[12] Two electrodes are used to conduct a current. They may be of equal or unequal size depending on how much and where the charge density should be delivered to the tissues for specific objectives. A large electrode will disperse the charge across a greater surface area and thus have less charge density per unit area. This is usually called the dispersive or indifferent electrode. The patient will experience less sensation under the larger electrode. This will be explained in the treatment section.

Electrodes

Electrodes are the means by which the electric current is conducted from the stimulator device to the tissues. The path taken by the current is dependent on a number of factors including the type and size of the electrode and the method of coupling the electrode to the skin. Electrodes must be good electrical conductors. Pre-gelled self-adhesive electrodes, carbon rubber electrodes, and aluminum foil meet this criterion. Capacitively coupled ES involves the transfer of electric current through an applied surface electrode pad that is in wet (electrolytic) contact (capacitively) coupled with the external skin surface and/or wound bed as shown in Figure 23.1. The rubber and foil electrodes need a conductive medium (i.e., hydrogel-impregnated gauze) added to enhance the uniform conductivity at the electrode skin interface. When capacitively coupled ES is used, at least two electrodes, one representing the negative pole and one

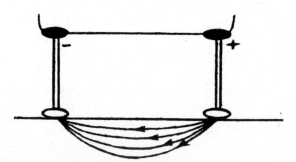

FIGURE 23.1 A pair of direct-contact electrodes used for HVPC and placed over the skin, showing the resultant current flow through the skin. (Nelson RM, Currie DP. *Clinical Electrotherapy*, 2nd Edition, © 1991, 390, 391. Reprinted by permission of Pearson Education, Inc., Upper Saddle River, NJ.)

the positive pole, are required to complete the electric circuit. Surface transmission of EC is called transcutaneous electrical nerve stimulation (TENS).

Current

The flow of charge from one place to another is called *current*. The flow of charge in biological tissues is called a "biological current." Current can only flow from one place to another when there is difference in electrical potential. Electrical potential refers to a surplus of electrons in one lead or electrode of a stimulator (negative potential) and a deficiency in electrons (positive potential) in a second. This difference must be present for the current to flow. When the electrical difference is transferred to the tissues, the electrons begin to move. The force that moves the current is the voltage, which is described soon.

Current Density

Current density is the second measurement of dosage that indicates the electrochemical effects of stimulation.[14,15] The current density is defined as the electrical charge per cross-sectional area of the electrodes. As with charge density, the larger the size of the electrode, the less the current density, and conversely, the smaller the electrode, the greater the current density.

RESEARCH WISDOM

Measuring ES Dosage Delivered

Reich et al. reviewed 17 studies of pulsed stimulation and computed the absolute spatial (precise area) current density for each of them.[16] The findings indicated the parameters obtained by multiplying the average spatial current density by the effective duty cycle (duty cycle = 1 for DC) (duty cycle is explained nearby) by the total duration of treatment is essential in measuring dosage delivered to the tissues. To perform this calculation, it is essential to know the size of the electrode or to have a report of current density (A/cm^2) as part of the study methods. A follow-up calculation of importance is to multiply the absolute current density by the time of the treatment. This gives the total amount of charge delivered per unit area (coulombs/centimeter squared).[15] Unfortunately, most researchers fail to provide all of the data needed for these calculations. Most notably, the electrode size is omitted.[15,17] These authors went the extra mile and contacted some of the researchers or manufacturers to obtain the information needed to perform the calculations.[16] Why would the clinician want to know this information? A question that comes up when preparing for treatment is what size electrodes and parameters should I use? For those who want to ensure that the value of the current density is an adequate dose for wound healing and not excessive, a calculation would be useful. Too much current or charge density can damage tissue.[18] Too little will not have the desired treatment effect. Many manufacturers are presetting wound healing protocols and presumably make these calculations, but the size of the electrodes would be unknown.

Amperage

Ampere (A) is a unit of current defined as the rate at which charge flows past a fixed point. One A is a large unit of current. In the context of therapeutic applications, devices that generate smaller units of current are usually used. A milliampere (mA) is one thousandth of an ampere. A microampere (μA) is a millionth of an ampere. Therefore, if an electrical stimulator is rated as mA stimulator or if that is what is reported in the literature, the amount of charge delivered to the tissues will be a million times greater than a μA stimulator. More current and/or charge are not necessarily better for desired physiological effects. More will soon be learned about physiological effects of ES at different amperes.

Impedance

Impedance is the frequency-dependent opposition to EC flow within the circuit and is expressed in ohms. Skin impedance can limit current penetration. A change in skin impedance occurs when the skin is broken. This is explained when we discuss physiological responses to ES in the next section. Impedance decreases as the pulse rate or cycle duration decreases. Conversely, increasing the frequency (pps) increases current penetration. *Resistance* (**R**) is the property of a conductor that limits the movement of current through it (e.g., electrodes). *Conductance* is the inverse of resistance and represents the ease with which current can flow. Current amplitude can also be used to alter tissue resistance.

Voltage

Voltage is an electromotive force capable of moving ions through a conductor, that is, electrodes, skin, or wound tissue. You will remember that electrical potential difference between two points in an electrical field is the force that causes charged particles to move. Thus, the electrode with a positive charge donates electrons to the negatively charged electrode and the current flows through the skin or wound tissue to the opposite electrode. This potential difference is measured in volts (V). The relationship between voltage and current is expressed as Ohm law. The formula is voltage equals resistance times current ($V = RI$, where V is voltage, I is current, and R is resistance).

Amplitude

Amplitude refers to the measure of the magnitude of the **voltage** (**V**), which is a measure of the *force* of the flow of electrons and is a more accurate term than *intensity*.[19] The higher the amplitude, the higher the voltage. Similarly, when voltage is turned up, the current (amperage) will also go up, and vice versa. Some stimulators provide a readout of voltage and some a readout of amperage. In order for current to flow, there must be a pathway that will conduct and support the passage of the charged electrons. An electrode and leads along with biological fluids or other liquids fill this requirement. However, when the current reaches the conductor skin interface, the resistance can be considerable. The current amplitude along with other factors including frequency, phase and pulse duration will affect tissue resistance.[20] In order to keep the stimulation tolerable, the amplitude must be kept as low as possible, forcing the duration of the stimulus to be longer. The benefit of high-voltage pulsed current (HVPC) is that the short pulse duration allows use of higher amplitude (V) that is tolerable.

Polarity

Electrical polarity (positive and negative) is present in every *electrical circuit*. An electrical circuit is a path that transmits electric current. Electrons flow from the negative pole to the positive pole.

Electrical stimulators are usually designed so that polarity can be selected. Polarity appears to effect healing directly. For example, research[16] has concluded that alternating polarity (negative initially) for a specific period of days followed by a period with positive was more effective in promoting wound healing than maintaining either positive or negative polarity throughout the course of treatment. Examples of how polarity is used in research and for clinical applications are discussed throughout this chapter.

Waveforms and Phase

Waveforms are the graphic representations of current flow on an amplitude/time or voltage/time plot.[12] Direct current (DC) has no waveform and only one phase because once the current is initiated from the zero line, it flows in one direction for at least one second. Pulsed currents (PCs) and alternating currents (ACs) use descriptors of the shape of the wave including the terms sinusoidal, rectangular, and twin spiked to define and describe the period of on and off time for the current. The *sine wave* or *sinusoidal* waveform is a mathematical function that describes a smooth repetitive *oscillation* of an AC and a biphasic current (Figure 23.2). Oscillation refers to the periodic change from one polar direction to another or the *phase*. Zero current line is the baseline or starting point for each oscillation.

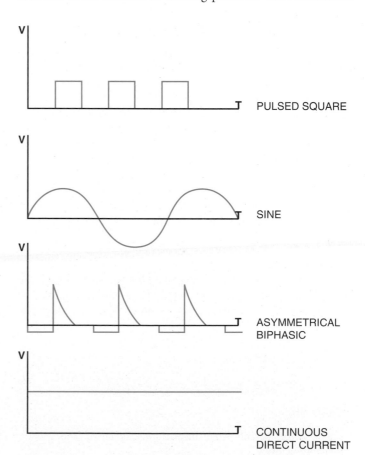

FIGURE 23.2 Waveform characteristics.

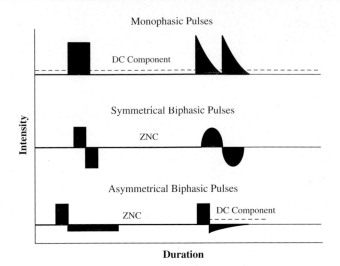

FIGURE 23.3 Representation of typical monophasic and biphasic waveforms. (Reprinted from Alon G, De Dominico G. *High Voltage Stimulation: An Integrated Approach to Clinical Electrotherapy.* 1st ed. Hixson, TN: The Chattanooga Group; 1987:62, with permission.)

The current line above the baseline always represents positively charged flow, and the current line under the baseline is negatively charged. The phase specifies where in its cycle the oscillation begins. Figure 23.2 shows representation of a sine wave. Waveforms used in therapeutic stimulators can be classified by one of two waveform groups: monophasic and biphasic[13] (Figure 23.3).

Types of Electric Currents used in Rehabilitation

There are two types of therapeutic currents used in rehabilitation. They are DC and PC.[20] *DC* (historically called *galvanic current)* is always continuous, is unidirectional, and is a flow of charged particles from one pole to the other lasting one second or longer. DC polarity is classified by the direction of current flow. If the current flows from the positive to the negative pole, it is a *positive* current. If reversed, it is *negative* current. The positive pole is called the *anode* and the negative pole the *cathode*. Pulsed or pulsatile currents may be unidirectional or bidirectional. In PC, there is a periodic interruption in the current during which no ions flow. Bidirectional current refers to the periodic reversal of the ion flow as in biphasic current (Figure 23.3).

Monophasic

Monophasic current does not oscillate between poles. The shape of the monophasic wave may be square, triangular, or twin peaked, but all phases will be either positive (above the

CLINICAL WISDOM

Pulse Shape

Pulse shape is the least important aspect of the pulse physiologically.[21]

zero line) or negative (below the zero line). A choice can be made by the clinician. Monophasic PC flow is always unidirectional, meaning that it will have a single phase that will be either positive or negative. The shape of the waveform may be designed so that the phases occur at different frequencies or may be equal as in twin-peaked pulses or a square single wave as shown in Figure 23.3. (Figure 23.3 illustrates the concept of phase for monophasic and biphasic waveforms.)

Biphasic

Biphasic current waveforms are also referred to as *alternating, bidirectional,* or *bipolar.* The waveform shape may be square, sinusoidal, or triangular. All biphasic current has two phases. Biphasic waves are such that the polarity is constantly changing. They are opposite at any moment in time. When using biphasic current, polarity considerations can generally be ignored. However, the waveform can be biased so that one polarity is emphasized. Biphasic waveforms may be symmetric, in which the shape and size of the waveform are always balanced, or asymmetric, in which the shape and size of the waveform can be either balanced or unbalanced (Figure 23.3). One of the most common outputs from an electrical stimulator is balanced asymmetric current. A balanced asymmetric waveform is typical of TENS used for pain modulation.

Several studies of biphasic current for wound healing have been conducted. The best wound healing effects seem to be achieved when a biphasic waveform is asymmetric and biased, so that the polarity at one pole predominates, which is usually the negative pole (cathode). Pain modulation and edema reduction in patients with diabetic neuropathy have been reported with a biphasic waveform.[22,23] Biologic effects like pain and edema modulation and effect on wound healing of biphasic stimulation are discussed further in following sections.

Pulse Characteristics

Pulse characteristics to know include:

1. The *pulse* is a single electrical event separated by a finite time from the next event.
2. *PC or pulsed electrical stimulation (PES)* emits a train of pulses that are repeated at regular intervals.
3. The *pulse rate,* or *frequency,* is the number of pulses delivered per unit of time. It is measured in pulses per second (pps).[24] The unit of measurement for pulse rate is Hertz (Hz).
4. The pulse duration also called the pulse width is the time elapsing between the beginning and end of all phases including the interpulse interval. It is usually measured in μs. The greater the pulse duration, the more current will be delivered to the tissues. Short duration is more comfortable than long duration. Short-duration pulses also have less chemical change under the electrodes, which is why the very short HVPC pulse duration is very comfortable.
5. The time between pulses is the *interpulse (interphase) interval* (Figure 23.4). The longer the interpulse interval, the lower the average current delivered to the tissues.
6. The *phase duration* is the length of time that the pulse is on. (Figure 23.4)
7. The more pps, the shorter the pulse duration.

For monophasic waveforms, the phase duration and pulse duration are synonymous. For biphasic waveforms, since there

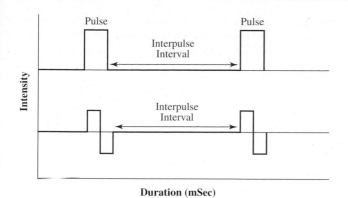

FIGURE 23.4 Pulse characteristics. (Reprinted from Alon G, De Dominico G. *High Voltage Stimulation: An Integrated Approach to Clinical Electrotherapy*. 1st ed. Hixson, TN: The Chattanooga Group; 1987:35, with permission.)

are two phases, the pulse duration may be the same for both phases or can be configured, by device manipulation, to favor one phase or the other by changing the phase duration.[20]

Phase and Pulse Charge

Phase Charge

In symmetric waveforms, the phase charges for each phase are equal (Figure 23.3 line one and two). An asymmetric waveform's phase characteristics are unequal with respect to the baseline (Figure 23.3 line 3). These waveforms may be either phase charge balanced or unbalanced.[19] The phase charge (Q) is represented by the area under the curve and is expressed as the product of the phase duration (t) and the peak current amplitude (I).[13] It makes no difference what type of current shape is used (high or low voltage, monophasic, or AC time, or amplitude modulated); biphasic, or as long as there is sufficient phase charge for a given phase duration, excitation of the nerve and physiologic cellular effects will occur[13] and are the reasons for administering ES. Kloth presented evidence to the Center for Medicare and Medicaid Services Medical and Surgical Procedures Panel that the phase charge quantity (dosage) needed to enhance soft tissue healing can be computed for monophasic (triangular) HVPC and square wave (PES or low-voltage PC [LVPC]) pulses using the formula described here to quantify the dose (phase charge) delivered to the tissues across a number of studies, regardless of device used.[25]

Pulse Charge

The pulse charge of a sine wave can be compared with the pulse charge of a square wave by doubling the charge delivered by one phase. The result is that the charge delivered by the square wave is significantly greater than that of the sine wave. Thus, more pulse amplitude is required to provide the same charge with a sine wave than a square wave, making it less efficient for excitation.[13]

In his review of the literature, Kloth found that four studies[18,26-28] reported the pulse charge information. Two of the studies used HVPC[26,27] and two[18,28] used PES or LVPC. He then went on to calculate the charge quantity per unit for other studies using the data in those reports. Based on the calculations derived from his review of these studies, Kloth found that the charge quantity varied somewhat, but that the effective "window of charge" dosage is between 200 and 600 µC.[25]

Pulsatile Currents

PC or *PES* is defined as an EC that has a very short pulse duration (millisecond or µs). If the current flows for less than 1 second, for example, a few milliseconds (ms) or less, it is no longer DC but is a PC or PES.[13] PC is an interrupted current that flows in phases as opposed to continuously. It may be unidirectional or bidirectional. The waveforms that are classified as pulsatile currents include monophasic, biphasic, and polyphasic (alternating). This type of current has many names, which leads to much confusion when trying to review and understand reports in the literature.

PC devices can be identified based on voltage levels and pulse durations. Such devices are divided into two voltage ranges: LVPC devices that are capable of delivering either a monophasic or biphasic waveform with pulse duration up to 1.0 second and require lower voltages between 0 and 150 V and HVPC devices that are capable of delivering monophasic twin triangular pulses with durations of typically 10 to 60 µs. Due to the short pulse duration, it is necessary to use higher voltages in the range of 150 to 500 V to drive the currant.[29] If authors, vendors, and clinicians identified the waveform or shape used in their documentation, the confusion would be greatly reduced.[13] All of these configurations of PC are used to achieve therapeutic effects.

Monophasic Pulsed Current

Monophasic pulsed current is defined as a unidirectional, PC that deviates from baseline and returns to baseline after a designated time period. Monophasic pulses and phases are identical (Figure 23.5). Monophasic waves are such that one electrode, or pole, is positive, and the other pole is negative. This polarity stays constant throughout the treatment unless changed by the clinician. The monophasic pulse rate most frequently used for wound healing is 50 to 120 pps (0.83–1.25 milliseconds). Each

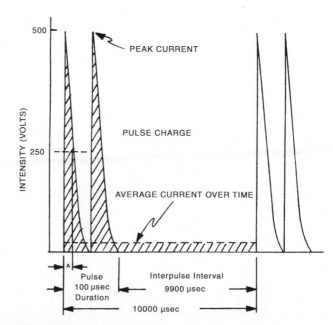

FIGURE 23.5 The effect of waveform on charge accumulation (*darkened area*). (Adapted from Alon G, De Dominico G. *High Voltage Simulation: An Integrated Approach to Clinical Electrotherapy*. 1st ed. Hixson, TN: The Chattanooga Group; 1987:41, with permission.)

peak or spike has an effective 5- to 20-μs phase duration. There is a long interpulse interval between pulses that makes an overall low average current.

High-Voltage Monophasic Pulsed Current

HVPC devices are defined as those that deliver from 100 to 500 V. The amplitude selected for wound healing is usually between 80 and 200 V. It has a high peak current of very short duration (5–20 μs) which overcomes skin resistance. Thus the twin-peaked (triangular-shaped) pulses are able to penetrate deep into tissue.[20] (Figure 23.5). A typical high-voltage stimulator has a maximum pulse charge of only 10 to 15 μC, which is very low and within safety limits.[23] The high-voltage stimulator can cause threshold excitation of sensory, motor, and pain-conducting fibers because at very short phase duration, thus less charge is needed to cause threshold excitation.[13]

Low-voltage Pulsed Current

LVPC is a proprietary waveform that is monophasic and has a square wave shape. It is also called low-intensity direct current (LIDC).[30] Two devices, the Varipulse and its successor Dermapulse, were formerly manufactured between 1989 and 1997 by Stayodyne, Inc. (Longmont, CO, USA). An ES stimulator identical to the Stayodyne Dermapulse is now manufactured by a company called woundEL (Hamburg, Germany).[29] The waveform for this current has the following properties: 140 μs pulse duration, peak pulse amplitude of 30 to 35 mA, and a fixed frequency of either 64 or 128 pps.[29]

Phase Modulation

Phase modulations are possible and useful for rehabilitation purposes including wound healing. Modulation possibilities include change of phase duration, change of phase, change of pulse amplitude, and change in pulse frequency or rate. Monophasic waveforms may be modulated into pulsatile currents with specific phases. Pulse duration affects biologic responses. For example, DC has a continuous pulse duration that can raise tissue temperature and change the pH under the electrode, which can produce blisters under the electrode. However, a short pulse duration (5–100 μs), typical of monophasic-type ES shown in Figure 23.5, produces insignificant changes in both tissue pH and tissue temperature.[14,20,31] Such a current is therefore very safe but raises questions about the effect of polarity when the pulse duration is so short.

Microcurrent Electrical Nerve Stimulation

A pulsed monophasic low-voltage form of ES is *microcurrent electrical nerve stimulation* (MENS). With MENS, the amplitudes of the PC are less than 1 mA (1–999 μA), and the voltage is less than 100 V. These amplitudes have minimal detectable sensation and are incapable of motor nerve stimulation.

MENS typically has a single modified monophasic square waveform. The pulse duration of these devices ranges from 0.1 to 999 Hz, equivalent to an on time of 1 μs to 10 seconds. The pulse duration is inversely related to the frequency. Microcurrent stimulation has a prolonged pulse duration at lower frequencies, which will have a different tissue polarity effect than a shorter-duration pulse, most typically used in high-voltage stimulation. For example, a low-voltage pulsed stimulus at 0.1 Hz is on for 10 seconds, whereas the high-voltage monophasic simulators are used at 80 to 120 pps and are on for only 0.83 to 1.25 milliseconds. Thus, pulsed low-voltage current of at least 1 pps can maintain the polarity effect delivered to the tissues under the electrode. The peak amplitude is usually 600 μA/60 V. The average amplitude commonly used is 200 to 300 μA for soft tissue.[32] MENS has been used in bone healing; however, in this clinical application, the amplitude recommended is 20 to 50 μA[33–40]

When pulsed slowly, MENS produces cellular and tissue polarity effects under the electrodes.[41] There is some concern that the voltage may be too low to push the current through the resistance of the skin and the subcutaneous tissues, but no specific studies confirm this.

Device Parameters

Manufacturers of electrotherapeutic devices in general, *low-voltage* devices produce peak voltages ranging from 60 to 100 V. At an amplitude above 100 V, the devices are categorized as *high-voltage*, not to be confused with high-voltage power lines. These devices can generate a voltage in the range from 100 to 500 V at peak amplitude. The term *peak amplitude* refers to the highest amplitude of the current or voltage; for example, a low-voltage device might have a peak amplitude of 100 V. This is important in wound care because voltage is used to deliver a dose of charge to the tissues; it must be sufficient to overcome resistance but not too high. Amplitude is chosen depending on the status of the wound healing phase and the physiologic rationale for the treatment.

Duty Cycle

The *on/off ratio* is the ratio of the time the current is on to the time the current is off. A *duty cycle* is the ratio of *on time* to the *total cycle time*, including both the on and off time. A ratio is used to express the relative proportion of the on and off time and can be expressed as a percentage. For instance, if the total cycle is 60 μs, then on time is 20 μs, and the off time is 40 μs, there is a 1:2 on/off ratio, and the duty cycle is a 1:3 ratio, or a 33% duty cycle. The calculation for duty cycle is pulse duration in seconds frequency (Hz) = fraction of time during which current is actually applied.

Transcutaneous Electrical Nerve Stimulation

Except for true DC, most clinical stimulators are *TENS* devices. In TENS, the electrodes are applied transcutaneously, with the physiologic objective of exciting peripheral nerves. As long as surface electrodes are used and peripheral nerves are excited, the stimulator is a TENS unit, regardless of the names used by commercial companies or the waveforms.[24] However, for clarification, the studies that report use of TENS stimulators are usually using biphasic or modified AC currents.

Neuromuscular Electrical Stimulation

Neuromuscular electrical stimulation (NMES) is used to stimulate intact peripheral motor nerves and induces isometric and isotonic muscle contraction. However, factors that can compromise its effect include peripheral neuropathies, partial innervation from peripheral nerve injuries or entrapment, and muscle pathology (myopathy and dystrophy). Why include this form of ES application in a chapter on wound healing? First, prevention/risk reduction for integumentary disorders is one aspect of patient management provided by physical therapists.[42] Next, there is a body of evidence (reported soon in this chapter) where use of NMES reduces risk of pressure ulcers for patients with permanent loss of voluntary motor control (e.g., SCI patients, stroke patients).[43,44] For long-term management, surface stimulation may not be functional due to variability of electrode placement and skin irritation from prolonged use. A better permanent option is the implantation of a stimulator that functions similar to a pacemaker. However, this is not always possible due to medical factors and patient preference. What is required is a current waveform with a high peak current to achieve greater depth of stimulation and a high frequency rate to maximize the firing rate of recruited motor units. The physical therapist should be familiar with these requirements, which are beyond the scope of this discussion.

PHYSIOLOGIC EFFECTS OF ELECTRICAL STIMULATION

The body has its own bioelectrical system. This system influences wound healing by attracting the cells of repair, changing cell membrane permeability, enhancing cellular secretion through cell membranes, and orienting cell structures. The concept of adding exogenous EC to the body is to support and augment the body's own bioelectric system. Evidence about the effects of ES on physiologic components of wound healing will be presented in this section including the following topics (Table 23.2):

- Impedance
- Current of injury
- Galvanotaxis

TABLE 23.2	Applied Physiologic Effects of Electrical Stimulation			
Effects	**Attraction Pole**	**Cells and Charge**	**Type of Current**	**Researcher**
Inflammatory phase: autolysis and phagocytosis	Cathode	Macrophages (+)	DC	Orida and Feldman[53]
	Cathode	Macrophages (+)	Sinusoidal, 1 Hz, 2 V/cm	Cho et al.[54]
	Anode/cathode	Neutrophils (±)		
	Cathode	Lymphocytes, platelets (+)		Bassett and Becker[34]
	Anode	Mast cells (decreased) (−)	DC	Fukushima et al.[55]
			PES, 35 mA, 128 pps	Kloth,[56] Weiss et al.,[57] Gentzkow and Miller[49]
Proliferative phase: fibroplasia (collagen formation)	Cathode	Fibroblasts (+)	HVPC, 50 V,100 pps	Bourguignon and Bourguignon[58]
	Cathode	Fibroblasts (+)		Bassett and Becker[34]
	Cathode	Fibroblasts (+)	DC, 10–100 mV/cm	Erickson and Nuccitelli[59]
	Cathode	Fibroblasts (+)	DC,1,500 mV/cm	Yang et al.[60]
Wound contraction	Alternating (±) every 3d	Myofibroblasts (+)	HVPC	Stromberg[61]
Epithelialization phase	Cathode	Epidermal cells (+)	DC 50 mV/mm	Cooper and Schliwa[62]
	Cathode	Keratinocytes (+)		Nishimura et al.[63]
↓ Edema (animal studies)	Negative		HVPC	Mendel and Fish[107]
	Negative		HVPC	Reed[106]
	Negative		HVPC	Ross and Segal[112]
Thrombolysis	Negative		DC	Sawyer and Deutch[116–118]
Thrombosis	Positive		DC	Williams and Carey[182]
Oxygen (tcPO$_2$)	Anode		MENS, 100 µA low volt	Byl et al.[143]
Oxygen (tcPO$_2$)	Negative Bias		Asymmetric biphasic	Baker et al.[183]
Tendon repair	Positive		HVPC	Owoeye et al.[184]
Bacteriostatic effects	Anode/Cathode		DC	Barranco et al.[120]
			DC	Rowley et al.[121]
			HVPC	Kincaid and Lavoie.[122]
			HVPC	Szuminsky et al.[123]

- Wound healing phases
- Circulation (blood flow [BF] and oxygenation)
- Edema
- Thrombosis, thrombolysis, and débridement
- Bacteriostasis
- Electroanalgesia
- Neuropathic pain
- Burns and grafts

Impedance

When there is a break in the skin, there is a significant lowering of the skin impedance to current. As you will recall, impedance is the opposition to current flow. Different body tissues have different impedances to current flow. Skin, bone, and subcutaneous adipose tissue as well as necrotic tissue have high impedance and are poor electrical conductors. Since subcutaneous adipose tissue has a high level of impedance, this affects density of current penetration into deeper tissues of patients with a thick subcutaneous adipose layer. A sine wave has better penetration than a square wave. To overcome the impedance, a higher amplitude, to patient tolerance, or a different waveform is needed to overcome the resistance.[45] When necrotic tissue resists current flow, the current then shifts to an area of low resistance.[46] BF will follow the current path as well. Therefore, there will be little increase in BF in the area of necrotic tissue.

Changes in BF around a wound such as with local heating of a segment of the skin reduces electrical impedance and permits increased current flow to the area.[47] This treatment method is described in the treatment section. Other techniques to reduce skin impedance include abrasion of the skin surface to remove the hard layers of keratin on the surface, tissue warming, and hydration. High-voltage currents of approximately 100 V have the demonstrated ability to cause sudden, spontaneous breakdown in skin impedance.[48] Because of the fluid in muscles and blood vessels, these tissues are good electrical conductors, and it can be expected that current will flow directly through them, with little impedance.

Current of Injury

When there is a break in the skin surface, current can flow through the ionic fluids of the tissues between the outer and inner layers of the skin (Figure 23.6).[49] The break causes an electrical current in the skin that short-circuits the epidermal battery, allowing the current flow out of the wound.[50] This distinct pattern of unidirectional current flow in broken skin is referred to as the *current of injury*. If the wound is allowed to dry, wound impedance increases and blocks the flow of current.[50]

The surface of intact skin maintains an average constant electronegative charge of approximately −23 mV with respect to the deeper epidermal layers. The negative charge on the surface is created by negatively charged chloride ions (Cl^-), which stay on the surface after positively charged sodium ions (Na^+) are pumped into the inner layers of the epidermis by the sodium ion pump. Thus, the skin has electrical potentials across it; in a sense, it acts as a battery. This is an **endogenous** current.

Regenerating tissues show a distinct pattern of unidirectional current flow and polarity switching (e.g., positive to negative and reverse). Indeed, as healing is either completed or *arrested*, the current of injury disappears. For example, when ulcers become dry, the voltage gradient is eliminated, and the current disappears,[41] suggesting an explanation of why moist wounds heal better than dry wounds. One rationale for applying exogenous ES is that it mimics the natural current of injury and will jump-start or accelerate the wound healing process.[28] A significant body of research demonstrates that *polarity*—the condition in which a given region of tissue has an overall positive or negative charge relative to that of another region—influences healing in different ways at different phases. Table 23.2 lists the Applied Physiologic Effects of ES on several aspects of biologic systems related to wound healing.

Electrical Potentials as Healing Marker

Can electrical potentials be used as an indirect marker for wound healing? The electrical field in the epidermis close to the wound edge exceeds 100 mV/mm, which is a large electric field. Under such conditions, galvanotaxis (cellular attraction) appears be enhanced. To test the hypothesis that ulcers kept moist maintain a higher electrical potential than do dry wounds, Cheng[51] measured the electrical potentials of partial-thickness wounds treated with occlusive dressings. During the 4 days that it took for the wound to epithelialize, he measured the electrical potential with a voltmeter. The device was placed with one electrode in the center of the wound and a second electrode placed on the adjacent normal skin surface. He compared the changes in electrical potential between wounds that were occluded to retain

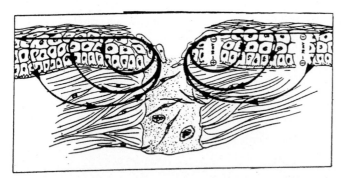

FIGURE 23.6 Current of injury. Disruption in the epidermis has provided a return path for current driven by transepithelial potential. (Reprinted from Jaffe LF, Vanable JW. *Clinics in Dermatology*, Vol. 2, Electric Fields and Wound Healing. 1984, with permission from Elsevier Science.)

CLINICAL WISDOM

Moist Wounds Promote the "Current of Injury"

Keeping a wound moist with normal (0.9%) saline (sodium chloride) maintains the optimal bioelectric charge because it simulates the electrolytic concentration of wound fluid. Dressings such as amorphous hydrogels and occlusive dressings help to promote the body's "current of injury" by keeping the wound environment moist. One rationale for applying ES is that it mimics the natural current of injury and will jump-start or accelerate the wound healing process.[28]

moisture and those that were air exposed and allowed to dry out. On day 0, day of wounding, both groups had the identical electrical potential (35–38 mV). The occluded wounds **maintained** a high electrical potential (current of injury) of 29.6 mV for the 4-day period. The air-exposed wounds electrical potential **dropped** to 5.2 mV. After epithelialization was completed in the occlusion group, the electrical potential returned to a similar potential to that of the air-exposed group. This work supports the hypothesis that occlusive dressings can help to promote the current of injury and that the electrical potential disappears with epithelialization.

In recalcitrant wounds, the current of injury appears to disappear. Sumano and Mateos[52] applied a protocol of modified biphasic stimulation ES that was delivered for 20 minutes on a daily or every-other-day to recalcitrant wounds and burns. Part of the protocol called for the wounds and burn injuries never to be closely covered with heavy dressings or gauzes, and the patients were instructed to allow air contact to the wounds in the home and minimal coverage outdoors. Of the 44 wounds treated, 41 (93%) had greater than 90% healing, and 3 (7%) had greater than 60% to 90% healing. None of the wounds healed less than 60%. Perhaps the ES treatment imitated the current of injury sufficiently that, even with the dry wound environment, the wounds progressed toward healing. These studies suggest the possibilities of using the electrical potential as a marker for nonhealing.[50] Further investigation is needed to test the measurement of electrical potential as a marker for stunned wound healing (see Chapter 3 regarding stunned wound healing).

Galvanotaxis

Unidirectional EC flowing in the tissues attracts the cells of repair by a signaling mechanism called *galvanotaxis*. The effects of galvanotaxis are distributed across all phases of wound healing. Polarity is a key factor in what cells are attracted to the wound site and when. As we just learned, the current of injury changes polarity during the healing process. Therefore, it is not unexpected that a significant number of studies find that polarity influences specific cells in an organized and predictable way at different phases of healing.[49,53–63]

Role of Polarity in Three Wound Healing Phases

Table 23.2 summarizes the galvanotactic cellular effects by phases of wound healing. Here we will review how polarity plays a role in all wound healing phases. Chapter 2 reviews in detail the roles of cell types in the wound repair and regeneration process.

Inflammatory Phase

As you have learned in several chapters, neutrophils, lymphocytes, platelets, epidermal cells, keratinocytes, and macrophages are early responders following injury and play significant roles in development of the inflammatory response. An applied electrical field in the physiologic range can induce directional cell migration. Neutrophils are attracted to the negative pole if the wound is infected and to the positive pole if not infected.[55] Lymphocytes and platelets are attracted to the negative pole[65] as are epidermal cells[63] and keratinocytes.[66] These cells fight infection and produce chemotactic and growth-stimulating cytokines needed to repair or regenerate the tissue. One class of lymphocyte is the T cell, and movements of the T cell can

be directionally controlled by an electric field and the rate of migration increased.[67]

As we reviewed in Chapter 2, macrophages are a key cell during the inflammatory phase. Studies have found that, in the presence of an electric field, the organization of macrophages is improved and random movement is suppressed. Orida and Feldman found that macrophage migration is enhanced by ES, as macrophages are attracted to the positive pole.[53] Cho et al. have now shown that macrophage motility occurs in a 1-Hz low-amplitude (2 V/cm) sinusoidal electric field.[54] Laminin- or fibronectin-coated substrates need to be present for the macrophage migration to proceed. Ferrier recognized that different cell types, when subjected to the same electrical signal, can react differently,[68] and that has implications for concepts of galvanotaxis that remains to be developed.

Proliferative Phase

Fibroblasts are the key cells during the proliferative phase. They are attracted by the negative pole to proliferate and synthesize collagen and to contract the wound.[59,65] Protein and DNA synthesis, building blocks of tissue regeneration, are also enhanced by negative stimulation. When an EC pulsates, a force is created on the cell, in this case the fibroblast, that causes the cell to expand and contract. It has been suggested that this effect accounts for increased collagen deposition.[69,70]

Negative polarity also effects *calcium ion* function. Calcium ion (Ca^{2+}) uptake by fibroblast cells is increased. This effect in turn produces an increased exposure of insulin receptors on the fibroblast cell surface. If insulin is available to bind, the additional receptors on the fibroblasts will significantly increase protein and DNA synthesis. Thus if insulin is administered after exposure to negative pole stimulation, further increase in Ca^{2+} uptake and a twofold increase in protein and DNA synthesis will occur. Therefore, timing of insulin delivery and ES treatment to diabetic patients with wounds should be coordinated. Conversely, the same receptors are inhibited by Ca^{2+} channel blocker medications; thus, expect slower healing in patients taking these medications. Studies with guinea pigs showed that pulsed low-voltage microamperage direct current (LIDC) causes a rapid calcium flux in the epidermis. The researchers concluded that the growth of fibroblasts and keratinocytes may be enhanced by pulsed LIDC, due to changes in calcium homeostasis.[30] LIDC clinical study results are presented in Table 23.3.

Fibroblasts morph into myofibroblasts as part of the process of wound contraction at the end of the proliferative phase. Stromberg[61] found that alternating polarity using monophasic current, every 3 days, at 128 pps and amplitude at 35 mA accelerated wound contraction during the first 4 weeks after start of treatment. Conversely, he found that constant polarity, either negative or positive, was less effective. Thoughtful application should be considered in areas where rapid wound contraction would not be desirable, such as in the hand or neck.

Epithelialization Phase

The generation of an electric field has also been associated with the upregulation of epidermal growth factor receptors, which is significant for early response to injured tissue. However, for this to occur, there needs to be an aqueous serum available for the cellular migration and the presence of substrates, fibronectin,

TABLE 23.3	**LIDC Clinical Study Protocols and Results**

Investigator	Type of Study	Polarity	Amplitude/ Rate	Frequency and Duration	Disease State	Mean Healing Times
Wolcott et al.[96]	Uncontrolled clinical trial	3 d cathode followed by anode; reversed daily or every 3 d if wound plateaus	200–800 μA	2 h twice or three times daily	Ischemic dermal ulcers	9.6 wk
						10.4%/wk
Gault and Gatens[127]	Uncontrolled clinical trial	3 d cathode followed by anode; reversed daily or every 3 d if wound plateaus	200–800 μA	2 h twice or three times daily	Ischemic skin ulcers	5.0 wk
						20%/wk
Carley and Wainapel[138]	Randomized controlled clinical trial	3 d cathode followed by anode; reversed daily or every 3 d if wound plateaus	200–800 μA pulsed	2 h twice daily	Pressure ulcers	8 wk for 58% of group treatment
						12.5%/wk
Katelaris et al.[152]	Comparative clinical study	Negative throughout	20 μA	Not stated	Venous leg ulcers	8.2% /wk. No significant difference between groups.
						ES povidone-iodine group took longer to heal 12.2 wk
Wood et al.[30]	Randomized clinical trial	Starting negative	300–600 μA; .8 Hz	3 times/wk, duration not stated	Pressure ulcers	6.5–7 wk
						14.3%/wk

Note: Calculations of mean healing times based on study data.
Source: Data from references listed in the table

and laminin.[66] Animal studies demonstrate that, in the early acute inflammatory phase of healing, the rate of epidermal cell migration in dermal wounds is enhanced by 3 days of ES with a negative pole, followed by stimulation with the positive pole for 4 days. Epithelialization was achieved in 100% of the treatment group and in only 87% of the control group. Comparison of tensile strength and mitotic activity between the treated and control groups was comparable. This corresponds to a 0- to 3-day inflammatory phase and a 4- to 7-day repair phase of healing.[71,72]

CLINICAL WISDOM

During your review of the patient's medical history, evaluate data from the pharmaceutical history with these factors in mind. Drug effects could change the prognosis for healing with ES.[28]

Collagenase is linked to wound epithelialization. Hydrogel dressings enhance collagenase levels in burn wounds, but the addition of PC increases collagenase level twofold ($p = .001$) above hydrogel alone in pigs during the initiation of epithelialization.[73]

Remodeling Phase

Wolff law[74,75] states that, under conditions of repetitive stress, collagen is remodeled. One type of stress on a tissue is a mechanical force, which can be created when electricity is delivered to the tissue. A pulsatile current creates a mechanical force that perturbates cells, causing them to contract and expand, creating a piezoelectric effect that is thought to increase collagen deposition independent of polarity effects.

The final step in remodeling is a scar whose characteristics are most like the original skin. Mast cells regulate this process throughout the healing cycle. An excessive number of mast cells in the healing wound, however, is associated with diseases of abnormal fibrotic healing, such as keloid and hypertrophic scar formation (see Chapter 16). In one study, following exposure to positive polarity ES (PES 150 μs, 128 pps, peak current 35 mA), a decrease in mast cells, decreased scar thickness, softer scar, and better cosmetic results were observed in donor sites used for partial-thickness skin grafts. By contrast, the control scars on the same patient showed evidence of hypertrophy. A side benefit of the ES treatment was the reduction in pruritus in the treated wounds, compared with intense pruritus in the control scar on the same patient.[57]

Effect of Electrical Stimulation on Circulation

We have discussed throughout this text the importance of maintaining perfusion of healing tissues. BF study results using ES are reported in two ways in the literature: kinetic measurement of BF using devices like laser Doppler imaging (LDI) and the measurement of the partial pressure of oxygen (tcPO$_2$) measured in millimeters of mercury (mm Hg). We will begin with a discussion of BF and follow with tcPO$_2$. Numerous studies in the literature have looked at the effects of ES on BF in animals and humans, both healthy and with disease. When reading studies evaluating changes in BF using ES, the results reported may appear inconsistent. Reasons for the inconsistencies are related to the dissimilarity of study populations, EC characteristics (polarity, frequency, waveform), and methods of recording measurements. Standardization from one study to another is lacking. While this is a problem, the studies do give us the opportunity to see what is being done in the research world in this area. For details about treatment parameters for BF and oxygen studies, see cited cases (Table 23.4).

You will recall from Chapter 2 that endothelial cells line the walls of the arteries and when BF increases, they are repeatedly exposed to shear stress. Reaction to the stress includes release of nitric oxide. Nitric oxide (NO) as discussed in Chapter 2 has bactericidal effects and is an essential ingredient in wound healing. Chapter 27 also has a discussion of the effects of increased BF on endothelial cells and NO.

BF (Perfusion)
Animal Studies

We begin this portion of the section by looking at animal studies about effects of exogenous EC on BF. Animal studies precede human testing or allow testing of different protocols and theories that would not be acceptable to explore in people. The findings often lead to develop of treatment for us.

Polarity and Pulse Rate Findings

1. **Testing of rat BF when exposed to HVPC.**[64]
   - Negative polarity induced greater BF volume than did positive polarity.
   - BF volume was increased nearly instantaneously at the pulse rates tested: 2, 20, 80, and 120 pps.
   - BF volume was enhanced by increasing the amplitude of the current (up to stimulating muscle contraction).
   - In a small number of cases, BF volume increased without visible muscle contraction.
   - BF velocity remained elevated from 4 to 20 minutes after treatment.

2. **Skin Vascular Reactivity in Old Rats**
   Mehri et al.[76] showed that there is an age-related decline in skin vascular reactivity by the sensory nerves that correlates with a decline in wound repair efficacy. They used low-frequency TENS (20 V, 5 Hz for 1 minute) and compared the effect on BF, using laser Doppler flowmetry (LDF), with high frequency (20 V, 15 Hz for 1 minute). At the high frequency, the vascular response in old rats was significantly reduced (46%) compared with young controls. At low frequency, however, older rats produced similar vascular responses to the young. Results suggest that sensory nerves respond preferentially to low-frequency ES, and this may be useful in selecting treatment parameters for older adults.

3. **Skin Flap Survival in Pigs**
   Necrosis of skin flaps and free full-thickness skin grafts are a major problem following plastic surgery. Two skin flap studies in rats and pigs showed greater BF increases and improved survival of anode-treated flaps than did controls or those treated with the cathode.[77-79] Another study with pigs used PES (128 pps, 35 mA, 30 minutes twice daily) and a protocol of alternating polarity every 3 days.[80] Treated flaps that were given PES twice on the first day postoperatively had a 92% survival rate, compared with those treated only once on that day (19% survival). None of the control flaps survived.

Human Studies

LDI, intravital video microscopy, and computerized image analysis technologies have made it possible to evaluate and quantify circulatory changes induced by ES at the microcirculatory levels. Researchers have used a variety of methods to report results of BF studies as a consequence of ES application including photoplethysmography (PPG), cutaneous thermistors, transcutaneous oxygen partial pressure (tcPO$_2$) measurement, and laboratory tests for vasodilator substances.

Peripheral Blood Flow in Healthy Adults

1. It is useful to know about responses in a healthy population so as to make comparison with sick individuals. Hecker et al.[81] chose to look at the effects of 1 hour at each of five frequencies—2, 8, 32, 64, and 128 Hz— of pulsed ES on peripheral BF in 10 healthy adult volunteers. They systematically varied both current polarity and frequency to maximize the likelihood of observing BF and/or temperature effects. The electrodes were placed over the left brachial artery in the axilla, negative polarity, and over the left radial artery at the wrist, positive polarity. Stimulation was given for 1 hour and a 30-minute period between changes in frequency was allowed to return to baseline. Current amplitude was adjusted to the highest level attainable, not exceeding the subjects' perceived discomfort. Testing was repeated on two separate occasions. On the second test, polarity was reversed. Measurements were made with thermistors attached to fingers and PPG, a noninvasive measurement of the efficiency of the musculovenous pump of the lower leg. Results showed that current frequency, polarity, and varying combinations of the two had no significant effect on BF. A trend toward greater BF corresponded to the highest frequencies (32, 64, 128 Hz) with negative polarity. No significant temperature variations, compared with baseline, were found. The authors postulated that healthy individuals may have transient BF increases but that they rapidly return to baseline.

TABLE 23.4   Effects of Electrical Stimulation on Circulation in Human Subjects

Researcher	Hecker et al.[81]	Cramp et al.[82]	Dodgen et al.[185]	Forst et al.[100]	Gilcreast et al.[188]	Peters et al.[101]	Kaada[84]	Cosmo et al.[86]	Mawson et al.[88]	Goldman et al.[11]
Type stimulator	PES	TENS	TENS HVPC	TENS	HVPC	DC	TENS	TENS	HVPC	HVPC
Frequency										
Low	2 Hz, 8 Hz	4 Hz	Not stated	Not stated		N/A	2 Hz	2 Hz		
High	32 Hz, 64 Hz, 128 Hz	110 Hz	Not stated	Not stated	100 pps			Not tested	10 pps	100 Hz
Polarity	Negative/positive	Biphasic	Biphasic positive/negative	Biphasic	Negative		Biphasic	Biphasic	negative	Negative
Amplitude	Mean 22.56 mA	Not stated	Not stated	Not stated	100 V	Not stated	15–30 mA	10–45 mA	75 V	Sensory or max 360 V
Duration of stimulation	60 min at each FQ	15 min	30 min	Not stated	30 and 60 min	4, 60-min periods	30 min 3 times daily	60 min	30 min	1h daily ×14 wk
Effect during Rx	High ↑ BF trend at 32, 64, 128 Hz, negative polarity; no temperature variations from baseline	Low ↑ BF / High, no change; no change skin temp	Both stimulators produced ↑ tcPO₂ levels / Response not polarity dependent	↑ BF / ↓ axon reflex vasodilation in neuropathic group; induced hyperemia associated with suppressed sweat response in all groups	Bimodal response ↓ BF (73%) (N = 35) / Oxygen response higher at baseline than later responders: olders with neuropathy ABI <	No significant increase unless PVD present; transient rise in PVD group	Widespread vasodilation; release of vasoactive polypeptide	35% ↑ BF in ulcer / 15% ↑ BF periwound skin	35% ↑ sacral / TcPO₂ supine	↑ tcPO₂ from10mmHg to 30mmHg and laser Doppler flow threefold increased in dermal periwound perfusion increased perfusion compared to controls

2. Cramp et al.[82] compared the sensitivity to change in blood perfusion during treatment with TENS, using LDF and a skin thermistor. Double-blind conditions were implemented. Low- and high-frequency (4 and 110 Hz) TENS was applied to the forearm skin of 30 healthy human volunteers. BF and skin temperature readings were recorded before, during, and for 15 minutes after TENS application. Analysis of the results showed significant increases in blood perfusion during the treatment period in the low-frequency group, when compared with the other two groups, and no significant changes in skin temperature.

3. The blister wound is a new standard wound used for clinical studies. Wikstrom et al.[83] quantified BF changes at two different frequencies (2, 100 Hz, and sham) when TENS was applied to nine healthy adults. Changes in BF were measured, using LDI every 5 minutes. Results showed mean BF increases of 40% during low-frequency TENS, compared with a 12% increase at high frequency and no change during sham stimulation. In the second part of this study, Wikstrom and associates looked at circulatory changes in blister wounds of the leg induced in the same nine healthy adults before and during a 45-minute application of TENS (2 and 100 Hz). Microcirculatory BF was measured, using intravital video microscopy and computerized image analysis, as red blood cell velocity (RBC-V) in 5 to 14 individual capillaries in each wound. Mean RBC-V increased by 23% during low-frequency TENS ($N = 6$) and by 17% during high-frequency TENS ($N = 8$). More investigation about frequency is warranted to develop protocols for best treatment results.

Peripheral Blood Flow in Adults with Ulcers

Kaada[84,85] reported a causal relationship between TENS and mechanisms involved in widespread microvascular cutaneous vasodilatation. Results showed that a 15- to 30-minute period of TENS-induced vasodilatation produced a prolonged vascular response with a duration of several hours or longer, potentially indicating the release of a long-lasting neurohumoral substance or metabolite. Kaada attributed the effects to three possible modes of action: inhibition of the sympathetic fibers supplied to skin vessels; release of an active vasodilator substance, vasoactive intestinal polypeptide; or a segmental axon reflex responsible for affecting local circulation. The Kaada studies included reports of clinical results, wherein patients served as their own controls of stimulation-promoted healing in cases of chronic ulceration of various etiologies.[84]

Chronic Lower Leg Ulcers

LDF was used to study the effects of TENS in and around chronic lower leg ulcers. Cosmo et al.[86] enrolled 15 older adult patients with chronic leg ulcers of various causes in the study. Duration of the ulcers ranged from 3 months to 16 years. Low-frequency TENS (2 Hz, 10–45 mA) was applied for a 60-minute period. The changes in BF were measured every 5 minutes by LDF. After the treatment period, mean BF had increased in the ulcer by 35% and in the intact skin surrounding the ulcer by 15%. Mean BF increases of 29% in the ulcer and 9% in the skin were measured 15 minutes after the cessation of TENS treatment.

Oxygen Delivery

Transcutaneous partial pressure of oxygen ($tcPO_2$) measurements taken at the skin level are a reflection of the oxygen available to the tissues. In wounds, constant delivery of oxygen is required to meet high metabolic demands of the tissues, oxidative killing of infectious organisms, protein and collagen synthesis, and hydroxylation of proline to make useful collagen (see Chapter 2). Thus, it is obvious that there is a direct correlation between increasing BF and enhancing oxygen delivery to the tissues. This section relates to measurement of oxygen as a consequence of ES application in three special populations: spinal cord–injured (SCI), diabetics (DM), and ischemic. Chapter 6 has more information about $tcPO_2$ measurements.

Spinal Cord Injury

SCI problems, including decreased muscle bulk and reduced capillary network associated with the bulk loss over the sitting surfaces reducing blood volume that could be supplied to the tissues, as well as loss of blood pumping function, decreased sympathetic nervous system activity resulting in decreased blood pressure, and vascular patency that makes the blood vessels in the area less capable of withstanding normal tissue load and maintaining BF.[43] The result is decreased tissue health below the level of the injury, resulting in increased risk for pressure ulcer development. In paralysis where disuse atrophy has occurred, stimulation "exercises" can be used to enhance muscular force, build muscle bulk, and improve vascular performance. The muscular force changes occur due to changes in muscular fiber diameter and improved cardiovascular fitness.[44] This application is termed functional ES due to the fact that it improves function of critical systems to support health. This author has observed clinically that muscle hypertrophy can be achieved with SCI patients but the stimulation must be done on a regular basis or there is a reversal of the effects. The required stimulation parameters are those needed to provide motor excitation leading to evoked intermittent tetanic muscle contraction. The following studies report on the outcomes of research about use of ES for functional circulatory improvement.

1. Mawson et al. did several studies on the SCI population.[87,88] Individuals with SCI are at risk for pressure ulcers especially in the area of the sacrum, so they focused on studying the $tcPO_2$ levels. The following is a summary list of their findings.

   a. SCI subjects whose $tcPO_2$ values were above and below the median supine levels were compared in terms of presence or absence of pressure ulcers.

   b. Five of the 10 (50%) of SCI subjects with $tcPO_2$ levels below the median supine $tcPO_2$ level had a pressure ulcer, compared with one among the 11 (9%) SCI subjects with $tcPO_2$ levels above the median ($p = .055$). These findings suggest the need for further studies on the role of reduced oxygen in the etiology of pressure ulcers.[87]

   c. Another study looked at the possibility of developing a new way of preventing pressure ulcers in SCI individuals. They chose to study whether HVPC could increase sacral $tcPO_2$ levels in SCI persons lying prone and supine. They conducted four experiments, with the following results:

d. When HVPC was applied to the back at the spinal level T6, dose-related *increases* in sacral tcPO$_2$ were measured in three subjects lying prone.

e. In the second experiment, carried out on 29 subjects lying supine on egg-crate mattresses, HVPC (75 V, 10 Hz) produced a 35% increase in sacral tcPO$_2$ from baseline level (mean ± SD) or 49 ± 21 to 66 ± 18 mm Hg after 30 minutes of stimulation (p = .0001).

f. Simulated HVPC was found to have no effect on sacral tcPO2 in five subjects lying supine.

g. HVPC applied as in (a) was repeated on 10 subjects, and its effects were found to be highly reproducible. The mode of action attributed by the researchers to these effects is that the HVPC restores the sympathetic tone and vascular resistance below the level of the spinal cord lesion, thereby increasing the perfusion pressure gradient in the capillary beds.

2. Bogie et al. employed a NEMS system of implants to provide muscular stimulation to the gluteal muscles. Results were 50% increased gluteal muscle bulk and change in ischial pressure distribution plus a secondary benefits of increased tcPO$_2$ levels in the ischial region, in the unloaded state, after 8 weeks.[43]

3. Kim et al tested sensory (submotor threshold) ES as a preemptive pressure ulcer measure for six SCI patients in a controlled clinical trial in the manner described by Mawson.[87,88] Findings were that there was transitory increase in tcPO2 levels, but there did not appear to be any sustained effects on tissue health status indicative of reduced pressure ulcer risk for individuals with SCI.[89] This research group was also involved in the prior study by Bogie et al., and their opinion is that a contractile muscle response is critically important to achieving sustainable increase in tcPO$_2$ and that sensory stimulation is not appropriate prevention strategy for patients with SCI.

Conclusions

Use of NEMS as a preventive treatment has been investigated, and results indicate that it may be useful for initiating muscle pump function in situations in which the motor pump function is lost, due to paralysis or other lifestyle situations.[43,44,89–95]

Diabetes

Lack of adequate tissue oxygenation is a partial explanation why diabetics have difficulty healing neuropathic ulcers.[96] Another explanation is constriction of vascular smooth muscle that is regulated by vascular endothelial cells. Diabetics have vascular endothelial system damage that interferes with vasodilation and thus BF.[97] Numerous researchers have investigated use of ES in this population with mixed results. The following is a review of some of their reports:

1. Monophasic-paired spikes with negative polarity and a compensated monophasic waveform were used in this study. Stimulation was introduced with the cathode over the wound. Age-matched older normal adults and diabetics were the subjects. Baker et al.[98,99] took oximetry readings of tcPO$_2$ 30 minutes prior to stimulation, during 30 minutes of stimulation, and 30 minutes after stimulation. The older normal adults showed higher tcPO$_2$ levels at the end of 30 minutes of stimulation than the diabetics, regardless of waveform used. However, there were differences in response time for the diabetics. The normal adults showed increased oxygen levels earlier in the treatment period than did the diabetics. Diabetic subjects showed measurable but not significant increases in tcPO$_2$ at the end of the 30 minutes of stimulation but did show significant increases 30 minutes after cessation of the stimulation with the monophasic and submotor-compensated monophasic waveforms. The authors' analysis of the study was that diabetic subjects demonstrate a compromised ability to increase transcutaneous oxygen during submotor stimulation, *regardless* of the waveform used. When trace level muscle contraction was elicited with the compensated monophasic waveform, there was no change in the tcPO$_2$ levels in the diabetics. For some reason, the trace muscle contraction blunted the tcPO$_2$ response in the diabetics. The same effects were found for both waveforms and with stimulation by either the positive or the negative pole

2. Comparison of the microvascular response to TENS and postocclusive ischemia in the diabetic foot was reported by Forst et al.[100] LDF was used to measure the "flare" response (hyperemia) following TENS and to compare this axon reflex vasodilatation with postischemic hyperemia in the skin of the foot of diabetic and nondiabetic subjects. Twenty-one control subjects and 57 diabetic subjects were enrolled. The diabetics were stratified into four groups:
   1. 24 without complications
   2. 14 with neuropathy and without retinopathy
   3. 8 with retinopathy and without neuropathy
   4. 21 with both neuropathy and retinopathy

3. Following TENS, there was increased skin BF across all groups. However, compared with the control group, axon reflex vasodilatation was significantly reduced in groups 2 and 4. All groups had equivalent increased BF after arterial occlusion. There was a good association observed between postocclusive and TENS-induced hyperemia at the dorsum of the foot, but poor association at the base of the big toe. An observation reported was that the TENS-induced hyperemia was associated with a diminished sweat response but not with pathologic cardiovascular function tests. The conclusion reached was that electrical axon reflex vasodilatation is diminished in diabetic patients suffering from peripheral autonomic C-fiber injury, especially in skin rich in thermoregulatory BF. The diminished neurovascular response is independent of vascular alteration due to diabetes mellitus.

4. Peters et al.[101] evaluated the effects of galvanic ES on vascular perfusion in 19 diabetic subjects. Eleven of these were diagnosed with impaired peripheral perfusion, based on their initial tcPO$_2$ values (<40 mm Hg). Stimulation was given at the lateral side of one leg, and measurements were taken at the dorsum of the foot and at the base of the great toe of *both* feet. On the first day, one foot was treated with ES for four 60-minute periods and vascular perfusion assessed before and after the stimulation session. Measurements were taken for 1 hour on day 1 of the experiment. Methods of measurement were transcutaneous oximetry (tcPO$_2$) and LDF. Findings were that, during the first 5 minutes of stimulation, there was a significant rise in tissue oxygenation as

compared with the control measurements in the group of diabetics with impaired vascular perfusion. However, for those without vascular disease (tcPO$_2$ levels > 40 mm Hg), there was no significant increase, compared with baseline. Also, after the stimulation periods, the stimulated feet did not show any significant increase in BF over the control feet. The data suggest to the researchers that external subsensory ES induces a transient rise in skin perfusion in persons with diabetes and impaired peripheral perfusion.

5. Gilcreast et al.[188] tested the effect of HVPC (100 pps, 100 V, negative polarity) on foot skin perfusion in diabetics at risk for foot ulceration. A sample of 132 subjects was tested. Baseline tcPO$_2$ levels were obtained, stimulation applied, and repeat tcPO$_2$ measurements recorded at 30- and 60-minute intervals. Initial tcPO$_2$ levels were significantly higher than subsequent readings. However, the oxygen response was distributed bimodally: 35 (27%) subjects showed increased tcPO$_2$, and 97 (73%) experienced a *decreased* tcPO$_2$ reading. This treatment appears to increase BF in a subset of diabetics.

Ischemia

1. *Ischemia.* Byl et al.[102] found that, when supplemental oxygen was given by mask prior to and during microamperage stimulation (100 µA for 45 minutes), there were significant increases in subcutaneous oxygen measured. Maximal oxygen saturation may be necessary prior to and during ES to facilitate the dissociation of oxygen from the hemoglobin.[102]

2. *Ischemic Leg Ulcers.* Ischemic wounds not only do not heal but also often increase in size unless reperfused with bypass surgery. However, many patients do not meet the criteria for reperfusion surgery, including patients with diabetes and end-stage renal disease. For these individuals, amputation may be required. tcPO$_2$ levels below 20 mm Hg, is a predictor of poor healing outcomes of lower extremity wounds.

3. *Ischemia and Diabetic Ulcers*: Goldman et al. reported a six-subject case series that showed that HVPC *induced a slow persistent increase in tcPO$_2$*, levels in the periwound skin of patients with diabetes. After tcPO$_2$ levels exceeded 20 mm Hg, four of the six wounds eventually healed.[103]
Junger found that after 4 months of treatment with pulsed LIDC patients with severe ischemia (20 mm Hg) and venous leg ulcers had a significant increase in tcPO$_2$ levels in the forefoot (p-.0006).[104] However, there was not significant healing reduction in wound size compared to controls.

4. *Critical Ischemia*: This case series prompted them to do a chart review of retrospective data to determine patients with critical ischemia (tcPO$_2$ < 10 mm Hg) with arteriosclerosis and who were high-risk nonsurgical candidates with ischemic wounds.[105] They located 22 patients (the six cases mentioned were among this group) that met the inclusion criteria of *critical* ischemia. Half had only standard wound care, and the others had taken a course of HVPC. Those in the HVPC group tended to rise out of the critical ischemic range (5 ± 8 mm Hg initial values elevated to 26 ± 20 mm Hg). The control group also had increased tcPO$_2$, but not as great. The wounds in the HVPC group closed by 32 weeks after the start of treatment. By contrast, the control group wound area increased more than three times the initial area by 16 weeks.

5. *Small RCT.* The nature of the case studies and retrospective analysis have potential for bias. Goldman et al realized this and based on the preliminary trends observed, undertook a pilot investigation of this special population, a small prospective RCT (N = 8) lasting 14 weeks. In this study, by week 14, the HVPC-treated wounds averaged 30 mm Hg in the periwound tissues, well above the ischemic range, and the control group had an increase in tcPO$_2$ averaging 15 mm Hg. Laser Doppler evaluation of these two groups showed a threefold significant increase in dermal periwound perfusion in the HVPC group by week 8, compared with controls.

6. *Long-Term Effects on Ischemia.* Although a number of the studies reviewed here looked at changes in tcPO$_2$ levels before and up to 15 to 30 minutes after treatment, they did not look at the long-term effects of regular ES over a period of weeks. The increased tcPO$_2$ levels in ischemic tissues over time (8–14 weeks), as reported by Goldman et al.[102] and Bogie and Reger[43] in these small studies using HVPC, suggests that it takes more than a few minutes of ES treatment time to have a carryover effect on oxygen transport in ischemic tissues. So far, this application has had limited prospective study with small sample size. Further study with larger sample sizes could be useful in determining if this approach would be beneficial as primary care for prevention as well as healing.

Venous System

As yet, ES is not used extensively for management of venous circulation problems but merits inclusion in this section for thoughtful application. There is no support for intervention in the acute phase of varicose hemorrhage or deep vein thrombosis, but ES can effectively treat chronic conditions, including deep vein thrombosis and venous stasis that often precede ulceration. The required stimulation parameters are those needed to provide motor excitation leading to evoked intermittent tetanic muscle contraction. When muscle groups in the calf and posterior thigh are stimulated to produce intermittent tetanic muscle contraction, there is very effective enhancement of venous return in cases of venous insufficiency or deep vein thrombosis contraction. Augmentation of the venous return initiates a response of vasodilatation of the arterioles to bring BF to the muscles. Motor stimulation of an SCI patient with acrocyanosis (cyanosis of the extremity) also reversed some circulatory problems of the lower extremity.[90] Rationale for this application is that ES restores the sympathetic tone and vascular resistance below the level of SCI (refer to Case Study). Vasodilator polypeptides have also been identified in the blood following ES.[84,85] Gastrocnemius muscle stimulation produces muscle pump activation and ankle joint mobilization of patients with venous insufficiency, especially those with limited mobility. Best results are realized when NMES is used in conjunction with compression (see Chapter 19). Outcomes reported include improved cardiovascular performance, range of motion, and pain relief.[95] In SCI individuals, there is a loss of normal vasomotor tone in the abdomen and lower extremities. Peripheral edema and a high incidence of deep vein thrombosis have been associated with the circulatory stasis that occurs.

RR, a 50-year-old male, 15 years post-SCI quadriplegic, has had two flap procedures for ischial tuberosity pressure–related ulcers. Wounds healed slowly. Acrocyanosis over the ischial tuberosity occurred when sitting on his pressure relief cushion in his wheelchair for 1 hour and took about 2 hours to resolve. He had been confined to very short trips out of the house to see the doctor. Now he has an ulcer in the area (see Figure 23.16A,B).

Reason for the referral: (1) concern that he would have a reoccurrence of skin breakdown, and (2) bed-bound status was interfering with his social interaction with family and friends and ability to go out into the community.

A program of ES was initiated to resolve the cyanosis, heal the ulcer, and increase tissue perfusion and oxygen. After 5 days of 60-min/d ES with HVPC using the procedure described here, up time in his wheelchair increased to 3 hours, and cyanosis was 50% to 75% less intense and resolved in about 30 minutes. By day 10, he was able to be up in the wheelchair for 6 hours with pressure relief of 5 min/h, and resolution of the cyanosis occurred consistently within 30 minutes.

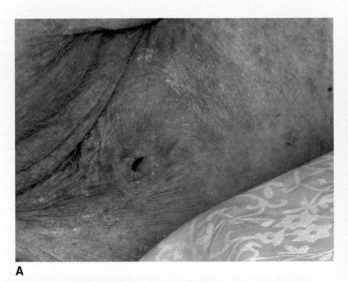
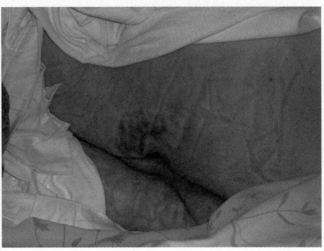

A   **B**

FIGURE 23.16 A. Acrocyanosis at the gluteal fold of a patient with SCI. B. After treatment with biphasic stimulation. Same wound and tissues as (A).

One case study of a patient with edema, cyanosis of the feet, and toe ulcers demonstrated the benefits of using computer-controlled NEMS to stimulate numerous muscle groups, resulting in reduced edema, improved skin color, and healed ulcers by the fifth week of the treatment regimen.[90] The use of the ES-induced leg muscle contractions in individuals with paraplegia to augment cardiovascular responses, probably via reactivation of the skeletal muscle pump and resulting increased venous return, has been reported in several studies.[91–93] Benefits include ameliorating blood pooling in the lower extremities and prevention of edema in the extremities by promoting lymph flow (see Chapter 19).

If the arterioles are severely occluded, the vasodilatation response may not occur, and electrically evoked muscle contraction may not be desired. In fact, the muscle contraction may cause severe pain by curtailing limited BF to the area, leading to ischemia. There are very limited clinical data to support specific protocols for this effect. Therefore, it is up to the PT to evaluate the vascular impairments, based on the diagnostic process, and to select a protocol to support the desired effect. The section on protocols and procedures provides an example for guidance.

Edema

Edema is a consequence of disruption in circulation and BF to the tissues. Following traumatic injury, initially there is hemostasis, clotting, and margination to halt bleeding followed by edema (see Chapter 2). Others are systemic breakdown, such as loss of valvular competency in venous disease or loss of autonomic nervous system function in SCI.

ES is believed to relieve edema via a process called *cataphoresis*, the movement of positively charged particles under the influence of an electrical field towards the negative pole (cathode). In a healing wound, cataphoresis causes the movement of nondissociated colloid molecules, such as droplets of fat, albumin, particles of starch, blood cells, bacteria, and other single cells, all of which have an electrical charge. For example, albumin, a colloidal protein found in blood, is negatively charged, and is repelled by negative polarity, causing a fluid shift and, thereby, a reduction of edema. In animal studies, ES has been shown to reduce edema by reducing blood vessel permeability.[64,106] While there are many anecdotal reports, evidence of the efficacy of ES to reduce or prevent edema is limited to a few animal studies, some human studies, and limited clinical trials. What is known is presented here for your guidance.

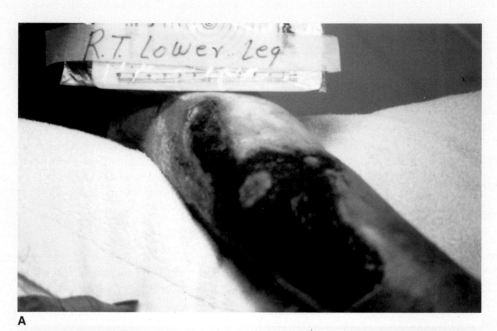

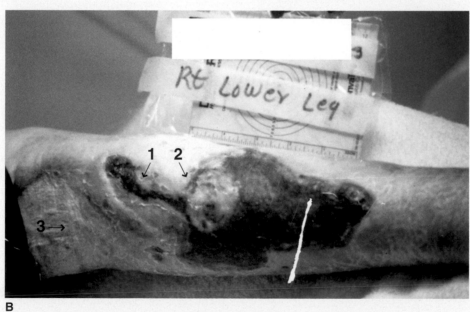

FIGURE 23.17 A. Note beefy, red granulation tissue and island of epidermal tissue in full-thickness wound. The wound was in the acute proliferative phase on 12/28. B. Same wound as in (A). Note: (1) Epidermal migration from wound edges, island, and wound shape changes. (2) Progression to the acute epithelialization phase by 2/17. (3) Hyperkeratotic skin changes due to old burn wounds and poor circulation. (Copyright © C. Sussman.)

Initial Assessment

Reason for Referral

The patient came to the PT because a vascular ulcer on the posterior right calf would not heal. The patient and his wife reported that they had been caring for the ulcer for more than 6 months, and they wanted it to heal so they could resume their usual activities in the community.

Medical History

The patient has a history of severe arterial vascular occlusive disease of the lower extremities. Old World War II burn

(continued)

scarring covered the surrounding area of the calf, with hyper-keratotic scarring that kept breaking down. The recurrent skin breakdown on his leg resulted in protracted periods of healing (e.g., more than 1 year). One ulcer had healed in 6 months after a course of care using ES (HVPC). The previous ulcer took more than a year and did not heal. The patient was ambulatory and alert, with mild confusion. His wife reported that any moisture left on the surrounding skin caused maceration and skin breakdown. A femoral angioplasty had been done the week before the patient was seen in the outpatient clinic.

Functional Diagnosis and Targeted Outcomes

Integumentary Examination
Adjacent Skin
Hyperkeratosis; scar tissue; flaky, friable, dry skin; and pallor are present.

Functional Diagnosis
The patient has loss of functional mobility due to integumentary impairment.

Targeted Outcome
The patient will have improved skin texture and integrity; due date: 6 weeks.

Wound Tissue Examination
The wound edges are poorly defined. There is necrotic tissue along the margins. There is a small island of skin in the middle of the wound bed. The wound has partial-thickness skin loss with moderate exudate. The wound is about 200 cm^2.

Functional Diagnosis
There is absence of an inflammatory phase.

Targeted Outcome
Acute inflammation will be achieved; due date: 2 weeks.

Associated Impairment
Necrotic tissue is present.

Targeted Outcome
A clean wound bed will be achieved; due date: 4 weeks.

Functional Diagnosis
There is absence of a proliferative phase.

Targeted Outcome
The wound will exhibit granulation tissue and be ready for grafting; due date: 6 weeks.

Vascular Examination
Medical Diagnosis
The patient has severe arterial vascular occlusive disease, status postangioplasty.

Functional Diagnosis
The patient has vascular impairment contributing to impaired healing.

Targeted Outcome
Perfusion will be enhanced; due date: 2 weeks.

The patient's loss of function in these systems is responsible for the undue susceptibility to skin breakdown on the legs and inability to heal without integumentary intervention. The patient has improvement potential. The wound will heal partially, and the wound bed will be prepared for grafting following intervention.

Need for Skilled Services

The patient has failed to respond to treatment with wound dressings and conservative management of the leg ulcer. It requires débridement of necrotic tissue to initiate the healing process and HVPC to initiate the healing phases and to enhance perfusion so that the wound bed is prepared for grafting.

Treatment Plan

- The patient and wife instructed to perform HVPC as a daily home treatment program with a portable HVPC rental unit.
- Wound débridement performed by PT to remove necrotic tissues; methods will include autolysis, sharp débridement, and enhanced perfusion with the use of HVPC.
- The wife instructed in wound dressing changes with alginate to absorb moderate exudate, including how to cut the dressing to fit the wound to avoid maceration.

Discharge Outcomes

- Start of care mid-December.
- The wound was necrosis-free.
- The wound phase changed to both proliferative and epithelialization. The wound size was reduced to less than half the original area.
- The wound was grafted at the end of February.
- The wound graft was successful. A smaller graft was needed than originally expected because of the epithelialization. Surrounding integumentary integrity was improved: the skin was softer and smoother, and no new hyperkeratosis developed in the scar tissue area.

General Comments

The patient and his wife complied with the home treatment regimen. The femoral angioplasty apparently opened the vessels enough to permit the enhanced perfusion from the HVPC to reach the tissues or possibly the 2 months of regular HVPC treatment effected the microcirculation as described in the clinical studies by Goldman et al.[11,103,105] Grafting was the best option for this couple because it provided faster closure and allowed them to live more functional lives without having wound care duties. It also provided a better covering with healthier skin from the opposite thigh to cover the open area. New scar tissue was better-quality tissue than that surrounding older scars, possibly because of the improved collagen organization and vascularization associated with the HVPC.

Animal Studies

Several attempts have been made to learn how edema reduction occurs with application of HVPC.[106]

1. Vascular permeability
   a. Reed[106] reported reduction of posttraumatic edema in hamsters following HVPC and attributed the effect to reduced microvessel leakage
   b. Posttraumatic edema was curbed in frogs treated with HVPC when the cathode was used. There was no effect if the anode was applied. Treatment effect was significant from the end of the first treatment session until the end of data recording 17 hours later.[107]
   c. A similar study using HVPC on rat hind paws found significant treatment effects after the second 20-minute treatment with the cathode.[64]
   d. Thornton and colleagues[108] found that edema formation was curbed in Zucker-Lean and Brown Norway rats but not in Sprague-Dawley rats when cathodal HVPC (120 pps) at 10% less than needed to induce visible muscle contraction was applied. The fact that not all species of rat react the same way suggests a caveat in extrapolating data to human subjects.
   e. Matylevich et al.[109] observed the effect of 40 mA DC on plasma albumin extravasation after partial-thickness burn injury in Sprague-Dawley rats. Silver nylon wound dressings were used as the anodes. Burn rats with no treatment or treated with silver-nylon dressing without current were used as controls. Quantitative analysis of fluorescein isothiocyanate (FITC) albumin leakage and accumulation in the wound tissue was performed using confocal fluorescence microscopy. When DC was applied, leakage was reduced by 30% to 45% and approached normal rates by 8 hours post burn. FITC-albumin concentration peaked at 4 hours post burn, was 18% to 48% less than in burned control, and approached the level observed in unburned control by 18 hours postburn. The conclusion of the study was that DC has a beneficial effect in reducing plasma protein extravasation after burn injury.
   f. Chu et al.,[110] who worked with the Matylevich group on the study reported above, then considered the effect of DC on wound edema after full-thickness burn injury in the same rat species. Using the same study design as described, the main results were that continuous DC reduced burn edema by 17% to 48% at different times up to 48 hours postburn. Neither reversal of electrode polarity nor change in current density had any significant effect on the results of treatment. Starting treatment during the first 8 hours post burn produced the least edema accumulation, but the reduction was significant even when DC was applied 36 hours after burn. If started immediately after injury, treatment had to be continued for a minimum of 8 hours to be most effective.
2. *Effectiveness on animals:* A systematic review of the literature from 1966 to 2010 produced 11 studies that met the inclusion criteria for the review.[111] The available evidence indicates that HVPC administered using negative polarity, pulse frequency of 120 pps, and intensity of 90% visual motor contraction may be effective at curbing edema formation. In addition, the evidence suggests that treatment should be administered in either four 30-minute treatment sessions (30-minute treatment, 30-minute rest cycle for 4 hours) or a single, continuous 180-minute session to achieve the edema-suppressing effects. These findings suggest that the basic science literature provides a general list of treatment parameters that have been shown to successfully manage the formation of edema after acute injury in animal subjects.

Human Studies

There are few studies showing positive effects of the use of ES for edema in humans. Those reporting efficacy are described. Investigation on a larger scale on the efficacy of ES in reducing edema in humans is needed to verify this phenomenon and to determine the effective treatment parameters.

Postoperative Edema

Ross and Segal[112] claimed benefit in treating postoperative edema, healing, and pain with HVPC in 25 postoperative patients. Believing that the effects of DC on edema were attributed to cataphoresis, a protocol based on the use of the cathode to reduce edema was chosen. The treatment parameters were negative polarity, four paired pps for 15 minutes. After 15 minutes, the polarity was switched to positive and pulse rate increased to 80 paired pps for another 15 minutes. Treatment was over the surgical site.

Burn Wound Edema

1. Fakhri and Amin[113] reported that, if edema was present around a burn wound, there was an immediate discharge of pus and tissue fluids during application of the low-voltage DC (LVDC) that ceased when the current was terminated.
2. Sumano and Mateos[52] included a case study as part of their clinical trial report. Using modified biphasic stimulation on a patient with a second-degree burn wound, there was significant reduction of the signs of inflammation, including edema and pain, after three treatments.
3. Edgar et al. found that local acute hand burn edema is reduced ($p = .02$), and active hand motion increased ($p = .0003$), using ES along with other usual physical therapy.[114]

Posttraumatic Edema

Griffin et al.[115] compared the efficacy of intermittent pneumatic compression (IPC) and HVPC in reducing chronic posttraumatic hand edema in an RCT. Thirty patients were assigned to one of three groups (10 to each) to receive a single treatment for 30 minutes of IPC, HVPC, or sham HVPC. Chronic edema was defined as edema following traumatic injury persisting for 14 to 21 days. The HVPC stimulator was set at 8 pps, with a reciprocal mode of stimulation alternating between the ulnar and median nerves at the elbow. Intensity was adjusted to produce minimal muscle contraction of thumb flexion and finger abduction, and polarity was set at negative for the active sites. The results reported were that there was no significant difference between HVPC and IPC ($p = .446$), and the difference between the HVPC and placebo HVPC groups did not quite reach statistical significance. The single 30-minute IPC session produced significant reductions in edema. There was also wide variability reported between the HVPC and IPC groups.[115]

There appears to be a trend suggesting that cathodal ES has a potential benefit for treatment of burn and wound edema. No harm has been reported using this intervention. However, based on the limited amount of human reports of edema prevention or reduction, it is not possible to make a recommendation. More and larger human studies are needed.

Thrombosis, Thrombolysis, and Débridement

Wounding, as we have discussed throughout this text, is followed by clot formation or thrombosis in the wound space, and that is often surrounded by ecchymosis due to associated subcutaneous bleeding in the adjacent tissues. You will remember that necrotic tissues are made up of coalesced blood elements. ES using negative current can produce *thrombolysis* (solubilization of clotted blood).[116–118]

The beneficial effects of ES on profusion have just been documented. Reperfusion is known to be rapidly followed by autolytic débridement. For example, two studies reported that on average there was nearly complete débridement of pus and necrotic tissue with cathode stimulation during the first 2 weeks of treatment.[9,119]

Another example of thrombolysis with the negative electrode is reversal of clumping and thrombotic effects.[28] This may explain an clinical observation by this author, in which hematoma and hemorrhaging at the wound margin or on granulation tissue are lysed and reabsorbed following application of HVPC with the negative pole. This is of clinical importance because hemorrhagic material goes on to necrosis if not lysed and reabsorbed quickly. Figure 23.7 is an example of such trauma. Studies to support these initial findings are needed.

Bactericidal Effects of ES

Bactericidal effects have been attributed to ES, and research suggests that there is evidence to support this contention. In vitro and in vivo studies applying DC have both been shown to inhibit bacterial growth rates at the cathode for organisms commonly found in chronic wounds.[120–124] It is not clear whether these results are due to polarity or to another mechanism

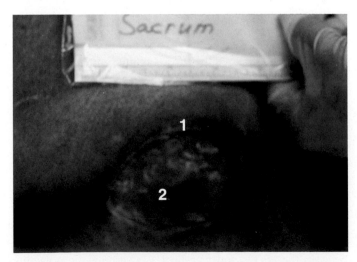

FIGURE 23.7 Wound is in chronic proliferative phase. Note: (1) Trauma to granulation tissue caused hemorrhagic spot that may go on to necrose; (2) Hemosiderin staining from prior bleeding surrounds ulcer. (Copyright © C. Sussman).

RESEARCH WISDOM

Deep tissue injury involves hemorrhage of capillaries and initiation of the clotting cascade. If tissues are not reperfused early, ischemia reperfusion injury may occur, along with cell death. More on deep tissue injury and ischemia reperfusion injury is presented in Chapter 3.

such as increased subcutaneous oxygen from enhanced perfusion, which has bactericidal effects.[125] After review of the cases reported, further investigation of the use of ES for bactericidal effects in human subjects is warranted. Here we review some case studies and basic science reports.

1. ***Case Study Reports.*** The following published case studies reported that patients with infected wounds had positive outcomes following treatment with ES: Thurman and Christian,[126] Gault and Gatens,[127] Webster et al.,[128] Fitzgerald and Newsome,[129] and Sumano and Mateos.[52] Organisms mentioned in these studies included *S. aureus* and *P. aeruginosa*. Infectious conditions reported included septic abscess, chronic osteomyelitis, infected burn, and thoracic spinal infection. Stimulation types used were low-intensity pulsed direct current, constant current, HVPC, and modified biphasic. Wound asepsis was normally accomplished within 3 to 7 days, using negative polarity.[127] Concurrent use of antibiotics and alternating the polarity during the treatment session with HVPC (negative 20 minutes, followed by 40 minutes of positive polarity) was mentioned by Fitzgerald and Newsome.[129]

   Under laboratory conditions, all biofilm bacteria within the electric fields are readily killed by an antibiotic on all areas of the active electrodes. The benefit of the bioelectric effect is the reduction in the concentration of antibacterial agents needed to kill biofilm bacteria to levels very close to those needed to kill planktonic, floating bacteria of the same species. However, this killing effect has not been seen in the electric field alone but during dual treatment.[130] Polak[9] reported cleansing ulcers of "pus" and necrotic tissues during the first 2 weeks of care using HVPC at the negative pole. No organisms were mentioned.[9]

2. Sumano and Mateos[52] reported that use of antiseptics and antibiotics was precluded in all cases enrolled in their study and attributed the reduction in observable signs of infection to the ES treatment. One case included was a patient who had recurrent osteomyelitis. The patient response to the ES protocol was fair (>60%–90% healing), but complete recovery was not achieved. These authors suggest that, under these circumstances, ES may be regarded as beneficial and harmless, and may even have a preparatory role for further medical care. Presence of osteomyelitis has long been considered a contraindication for ES therapy.

ES with Silver Nylon Dressing

1. Chu et al.[131] used microamperage current (0.4–40 μA) conducted through a silver nylon dressing placed in the burn wound of male Sprague-Dawley rats. Chu induced burn wounds in rats and then inoculated them with a lethal dose

of *P. aeruginosa* bacteria followed by treatment with the silver nylon dressing as the anode and learned that it was effective as a barrier to infection. Even the silver nylon dressing alone, without the current applied, had a significant protective barrier effect. However, when the silver nylon dressing was used with the cathode or just the nylon cloth without a metal coating, an effective protective barrier did *not* occur.

2. Webster used electrically activated silver dressings with the dressing as the anode to treat chronic osteomyelitis wounds. Sixteen (64%) of the cases resulted in closed, stable, pain-free wounds, and nine of twelve cases, complicated by non-union, achieved union. The authors suggest that the silver anode dressing is an effective treatment for chronic bone infection, when combined with surgical débridement, and reduces the need for prolonged systemic antibiotics.

   Current thinking is that treatment of wounds with a history of osteomyelitis can be treated with ES if the osteomyelitis is being or has been treated with antibiotics.

3. Huckfeldt et al used silver nylon dressings moistened with sterile water as conductive medium for an RCT ($N = 31$) to treated burn patients who received skin grafts postoperatively with anodal microcurrent ES. Controls were just treated with the silver dressing protocol. The treatment group showed significantly faster healing ($p \leq 001$) than controls.[132]

4. In another RCT ($N = 16$) of patients with pressure ulcers, silver nylon dressings moistened with either tap water or hydrogel were used as a contact medium in the wound while HVPC was applied, and the results showed 69% healed in 4.5 months and remained healed at follow-up.[133]

Biofilms

Biofilms are colonies of microorganims, usually bacteria, that adhere to surfaces such as wound beds, and produce a slimy matrix of proteins and polysaccharides that gives them heightened resistance to conventional antibiotics. For obvious reasons, wound bed biofilm colonization is a significant healing problem (see Chapter 17).

Although biofilms are not readily affected by biocides and antibiotics or ES individually, when these therapies are combined, low-intensity DC electric fields (1.5–20 V/cm and current

The Bioelectric Effect

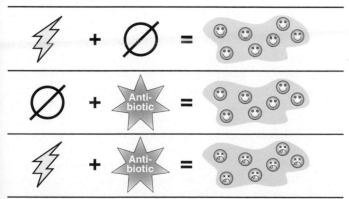

FIGURE 23.8 The bioelectric effect of combining ES and an antibiotic to kill biofilms. (Photo used with permission by the Center for Biofilm Engineering. MSU. Bozeman, MT.)

Source	Infection Type	Stimulation Type Used	Results
Thurman and Christian[126]	Abscess in diabetic	HVPC	Healed
Fitzgerald and Newsome[129]	Spinal wound with *Staphylococcus aureus*	HVPC	Healed
Webster et al.[128]	Chronic osteomyelitis	DC	Healed
Sumano and Mateos[52]	Osteomyelitis	Modified biphasic	Improved
	Infected burn		Healed

TABLE 23.5 — Case Study Reports of Beneficial Results of ES on Infected Wounds

Data from references listed in the table.

density 15 µA/cm²) have been shown to completely override the inherent resistance of biofilm bacteria to biocides and antibiotics.[130] ES enhances the efficacy of the antibiotics against the biofilm bacteria within the electric field (Figure 23.8).

Costerton called this the "bioelectric" effect.[130] However, very low-current density ES along with antibiotics is unable to effectively destroy bacteria in biofilm communities except when administered at intolerably high doses. As was mentioned earlier in this chapter, current density and charge dosage must be adequate for biological responses to occur. The potential for clinical application of this dual approach to treat chronic wounds that are colonized with bacteria biofilms needs to be researched clinically. Chapter 17 describes biofilms and their significance for chronic wounds.

Table 23.5 summarizes the beneficial results of ES on infected wounds.

Electroanalgesia

A large body of literature supports the use of TENS to provide electroanalgesia, for both acute and chronic wound pain management. Treatment with PES, also, effectively reduces pruritus associated with healing of donor sites.[57]

Neuropathic Pain

Chapter 22 was totally devoted to the discussion of pain but you were referred to this chapter as a source for evidence about use of ES for electroanalgesia. The following studies were chosen because they are related to the types of etiologies seen in patients who need wound management.

1. Kumar et al.,[22] in a randomized controlled, single-blinded trial with biphasic TENS and amitriptyline (Elavil, Etrafon, Limbitrol) ($N = 23$), found that there was a beneficial effect from TENS for relief of painful diabetic neuropathic pain beyond the effect of the amitriptyline. The treatment unit used was a proprietary device called *H-wave* (Electronic Waveform Laboratory, Huntington Beach, CA), with characteristics of biphasic exponentially decaying waveform with pulse widths of 4 milliseconds, <35 mA, <35 V, and

2 to 70 Hz. Treatment was applied at the knee region, and treatment effect occurred in the foot. Results of the study showed that 41 patients (44%/ ± 4%) using H-Wave TENS reported subjective reduction in pain; 13 patients had no improvement.[23] Those who had no improvement also reported a significantly higher incidence of foot ulcers than did the responder group. Nineteen patients reported swelling over the ankles. Twelve reported some decrease in the swelling with the TENS treatment, six claimed no change, and one had an increase. Only one of the 12 responders was using compression stockings. However, four of six of those who reported no change were wearing compression stockings. Data from this RCT suggest that the beneficial effects of electrotherapy for neuropathic pain continue with prolonged usage. Why the nonresponders had more foot ulcers than the responders deserves further investigation.

2. A recent meta-analysis located 3 RCTs involving 78 patients comparing the effectiveness of TENS on diabetic peripheral neuropathy that met the study inclusion criteria. The reduction in pain scores was significantly greater for the TENS group at 4 and 6 weeks' follow-up. At 12 weeks follow-up, there was significant subject improvement in overall neuropathic symptoms. No adverse effects were found. Thus, TENS was deemed a safe and effective treatment for relief of diabetic peripheral neuropathic pain. However, this is a very small sample, and larger studies are necessary to further evaluate effectiveness.[134]

3. Surface electrode PC nerve stimulation has not been well received by patients, clinicians, or manufacturers. Many have switched to electrical implants. Recently, there is a renewed interest in using the surface electrode methodology for neuropathic pain. Some people are well served by this treatment methodology as is apparent in the look-back study by Kupers et al. of five patients who have used PC for a 20-year period of home treatment for neuropathic pain following peripheral nerve injury.[135] Of 11 patients in the original study (1988), six were still using PC for pain management at home (2009). One did not participate in the review due to travel distance. Patients reported using the PC stimulator as needed, weekly or daily. Evaluations showed subjectively reduced pain ratings and improved quality of life on days stimulation was used. Objectively, positron emission tomography showed decreased activation in the pain matrix at rest, and during thermal stimulation, PC use led to increased BF not only in the primary somatosensory cortex but also in the other structures of the pain matrix (anterior cingulate and insular cortices, caudate nucleus, thalamus, and prefrontal cortex), see Chapter 22. Based on these findings, we learn that PC can provide long-term pain relief in a select group of patients. Patients must have a strong belief in the value of the treatment to adhere to it for so long. This may be a placebo effect, but as we discussed in Chapter 22, a placebo effect can be as powerful as a dose of morphine.[136] An unanswered question is whether the increased BF to the cortex prevented loss of grey matter, which we learned is a common finding in chronic pain patients.

4. *Persistant Venous Leg Ulcer Pain.* In a DBRCT study of painful venous leg ulcers ($N = 39$), pulsed LIDC, provided significant ($p = .049$) rapid, lasting pain relief.[104] In another open RCT of venous leg ulcers, pain ($N = 35$ with 43 painful ulcers), as measured by VAS scores, decreased significantly ($p = .0001$) after 2 months of irregularly pulsed LIDC.[137]

Burns and Grafts

In animal and human studies, flaps and grafts treated with monophasic PC ES heal without ischemia and result in flatter, thinner, and more resilient scars than in controls.[61,71,138] Pulsed ES was used to stimulate healing of burned rat skin.[139] The repaired skin of the electrostimulated group had an appearance similar to that of the control skin, and the overall appearance of the repaired skin was compatible with a well-organized healing process.

Adamian et al.[140] reported that 12 patients with slow healing postburn wounds received local ES treatment. Morphologic and biochemical studies confirmed marked stimulating effects of local ES-associated acceptance of dermal autografts and healing. Fakhri and Amin[113] reported a descriptive study in which they treated 20 indolent burn wounds with DC stimulation twice a week for 10 minutes per session until healed or ready for regrafting. All patients had failed one or two surgical skin grafts and served as their own controls. The wounds were deep dermal wounds or full-thickness or mixed. Epithelialization began by day 3 after start of the ES treatment. The largest wounds took the longest to heal (up to 3 months). Autologous skin grafts were successful after 2 to 4 weeks of ES treatment. The paper particularly cites the appearance of islands of epithelial cells in full-thickness skin burns that would have been expected to be destroyed. Benefits to scar formation from the treatment were better elasticity, more durability to stress, better cosmesis, and better regeneration of the skin pigments.

From case studies and clinical trials, evidence is being compiled to look at the outcomes of the treatments with ES on all phases of wound healing. Currently, there is a positive trend to treatment with ES, with an expected outcome of a functional, improved quality scar. More studies with human subjects are needed to compare different current waveforms and treatment parameters and their effects on collagen formation and scar.

Monophasic, Biphasic, and Microcurrent Stimulation Effects

Few comparative studies have been published about different effects based on the type of waveform used for treatment.

Animal Studies

A comparison of biphasic with monophasic stimulation of acute incisional wounds in rats by Bach et al.[141] showed that both types of current caused a significant increase of collagen content around the incision line, compared with controls, but did not affect the tensile strength or the energy absorption of the collagen formation in the early postoperative period. Reger et al.[142] also compared biphasic and monophasic stimulation of wounds induced in new monoplegic pigs with wounds in normal pigs and denervated controls. When compared with controls, both biphasic- and monophasic-stimulated wounds showed reduced healing time and increased perfusion in the early phases of healing. Monophasic stimulation reduced the wound area more rapidly than did biphasic, but biphasic stimulation reduced the wound volume more rapidly than did monophasic. Their impression was that the applied current appears to orient new collagen formation, even in the absence of neural influences. Collagen organization is considered an important factor in improved tensile strength of the scar. This study found that the ES did not reduce the strength of the healing wounds below those of the nonstimulated controls.

TABLE 23.6	Treatment Effects of Monophasic and Biphasic Electrical Stimulation		
Investigator	Subjects and Disease States	Direct Current	Alternating Current (Biphasic)
Stromberg[61]	Healthy pigs	Faster wound contraction if polarity alternated	
Reger et al.[142]	Spinal cord injury, pigs	Faster wound contraction	Faster volume reduction
Stefanovska et al.[145]	Spinal cord injury, humans	Less effective for deep wounds	Less effective for large wounds
Frantz[146]	Pressure ulcers, humans		Fast volume reduction; slow wound contraction
Huckfeldt[132]	Skin grafts humnas	Faster closure	

Data from references listed in the table.

Microcurrent stimulation has been studied in animal models in which current was applied only one or two times per day for 30 minutes for 1 to 2 weeks; no significant clinical effects were demonstrated on wound healing.[143,144] In another study, there were significant increases in subcutaneous oxygen measurements when supplemental oxygen was given by mask during the MENS stimulation.[102] There was no acceleration in healing.

Human Studies
Pressure Ulcers

Stefanovska et al.[145] compared the efficiency of monophasic (600 µA, 2 hours daily) and biphasic (40 Hz, 15–25 mA to produce minimal muscle contraction, 2 hours daily) in healing pressure ulcers in 150 patients with SCIs. Treatment was applied across the wounds using a bipolar technique. As in the Reger study,[142] monophasic was less effective for reducing the depth of deep wounds than was biphasic, and biphasic was less effective for reducing the wound area of large wounds. Frantz[146] reported that full-thickness pressure ulcers had a statistically significant reduction in depth but not in surface area when treated with biphasic.[49]

Huckfelt et al.[132] used continuous anodal microcurrent (50–100 mA dependent on wound resistance) for a monopolar technique with a silver nylon contact dressing as an electrode to speed time to stable wound closure of burn wounds postoperatively after graft placement. Findings of this RCT ($N = 31$) showed a 36% decreased time to closure in treatment group compared to controls. Table 23.6 summarizes the treatment effects attributed to biphasic and monophasic.

CLINICAL TRIALS

Since the 1960s, a series of clinical trials have been undertaken to evaluate the effect of ES on wound healing. In this section we review clinical trials by current waveform categories. The early studies are classics in this field.

Monophasic Pulsed Current Clinical Trials

Nine randomized controlled clinical (RCT) prospective studies were found in a literature review reporting the use of HVPC for wound healing. Reporting investigators included Franek et al.,[119] Goldman et al.,[11] Griffin et al.,[26] Gogia et al.,[147] Houghton et al.,[10,133] Kloth and Feedar,[27] Peters et al.,[148] and Polak et al.[9] A brief summary of each study follows.

Table 23.7 summarizes the data for all of them.

The above study populations were heterogeneous, but subsequent studies have been homogenous or stratified by etiology of the population and separate results reported.

Pressure Ulcers

- Kloth and Feedar[27] studied pressure ulcer healing and found a mean healing time of 7.3 weeks, and 100% of the treatment group healed. Positive polarity was used initially and then switched to negative if the wound plateaued.
- Gogia et al.[147] treated for 20 minutes following a 20-minute whirlpool session five times a week, beginning with 4 days of negative polarity, then switched to positive polarity. The rate of healing in the experimental group was particularly high during the first 2 weeks of treatment (31.45%), then slowed considerably, and was not statistically different from the control group after 5 weeks. The above study populations were heterogeneous, but are stratified by etiology of the population and separate results reported.
- Gentzkow et al.[28] reported a study of 40 ulcers in 37 patients. Nineteen pressure ulcers were stimulated, and 21 were sham stimulated. The trial lasted for 4 weeks. The treated ulcers healed more than twice as much as the sham-stimulated ulcers (49.8% versus 23.4%), healing at a rate of 12.5% per week, compared with 5.8% for the sham-stimulated group. Crossover results for 15 of the 19 sham-treated ulcers showed a fourfold greater healing during the 4 weeks of stimulation, compared with 4 weeks of sham treatment. This difference was statistically significant.[27]
- Feedar et al.[18] published a study on pressure ulcers. The 61 patients served as their own controls. The treatment phase of the study was preceded by a 4-week control phase of optimal nonelectrically stimulated wound care. Only the Stage III or IV ulcers with need of surgical débridement, necrotic/purulent drainage, or exudate seropurulent drainage that did not improve during the control phase went on to the treatment phase. After 4 weeks of treatment, 58.8% of the wounds had improved. After a mean of 8.4 weeks, 23% completely healed and 82% improved significantly.

TABLE 23.7 Monophasic Clinical Studies

Population, No. of Patients, Study Type	Polarity	Amplitude/Rate	Frequency and Duration	% Healed	Mean Time To Heal
Alon et al.[150] Diabetic foot ulcers; N = 15 treated, 0 controls; clinical trial	Anode	80 pps	3×/wk	80% (12/15)	10.4 wk (9.6%/wk)
Kloth and Feedar[27] Pressure ulcers; RCT; N = 16 9 treated, 7 controls, 3 crossovers	Anode switched to cathode then alternated daily	100–175 V, 105 Hz 50 μs on 100 μs interpulse interval (1.6 μC)	45 min 5×/wk;	100%	TG 7.3 wk (13.7%/wk) CG: no change
Griffin et al.[26] Pressure ulcers; DBRCT; N = 17; 8 treated, 9 controls	Cathode	200 V, 100 pps	1 h/× 20 d	80% Reduction in size	TG Stage II healed 100%
Feedar et al.[18] Chronic dermal ulcers (mixed etiologies: 35 pressure, 9 surgical, 1 vascular, 5 traumatic; DBRCT (N = 50); partial and full thickness (Stages: II = 2, III = 39, IV = 9)	Cathode until clean; then alternated daily until healed	35 mA, 128 pps 132 μs × 3 d; 64 pps 132 μs until healed or 3.5 wk	30 min 2× daily, × 4 wk	TG ↓ 66%	TG Stage III ↓ <25%; stage IV ↓ 67% in surface area; 4-wk treatment period healing (20%/wk) CG Stage II healed 100%; Stage III ↑ area; Stage IV ↓ 14%; Healing rate/week
				CG ↓ 34% (p < .02)	TG: 14%; CG 8.25%
				5 CG increased in size	14 After crossover
				CG crossover: × 4wk = ↓ 88,7% in area	12.8% p = .005
Gentzcow et al.[189] Pressure ulcers; DBRCT (N = 61)	Cathode until clean then switched to positive until healed or plateaued, then reversed again.	35 mA, 128 pps 140 μs (1.78 C/h/d)	30 min 2× daily	TG ↓ 60% by wk 2, 82 % by week (mean) 7.3 wk 100% (23%)	23 % healed (Stage IV 13.2% and 34.8 Stage III)
Stage III N = 23					
Stage IV N = 38					

Study	Population/Design	Electrode/Technique	Parameters	Dose	Results	Outcome
Unger[170]	Mixed; uncontrolled N = 223 treated, 0 controls				89.7%	10.85 wk (9.27%/wk)
Unger et al.[171]	Pressure ulcers; CT (N = 179 treated, 8 controls				88.9%	7.3 wk (13.7%/wk)
Gogia et al.	Mixed, RCT N = 12	Cathode × 4 tx; anode × 16 tx = 20 tx	250 V, 100 pps, 5–8 µs	20 min 5×/wk × 20 treatments	Area reduction	20 d (20%/wk)
	6 Treated with sterile whirlpool and HVPC				TG ↓ 35% (ES with whirlpool) versus CG ↓ 28% (whirlpool only)	
	6 Controls treated with sterile whirlpool				Depth reduction	
					TG ↓ 30% (ES with whirlpool)	
					CG ↓ 58%	
Polak et al.[9]	Venous leg ulcers; clinical trial, N = 42; 22 treated, 20 controls treated with medications	Cathode initially until clean; switch to anode for rest of period; monopolar technique	100 V, 100 Hz, 0.1 ms	50 min/d, 6 d/wk × 7 wk	TG ↓ area 73%; and 91% ↓ volume	7 wk treatment
					CG Controls reduction: area: ↓ 47% volume ↓ 68%	6.5 wk controls
						Number healed not reported
Houghton et al.[10]	Leg ulcers: diabetic, venous, arterial; RCT N = 42 ulcers 27 patients; 3 groups by eticlogy	Cathode	150 V, 100 Hz, 100 µs	45 min 3×/wk × 4 wk	TG 44 ± 8.8% ↓ mean size	CG treated with topical agents and dressings use of compression not mentioned; TG 8 infected ulcers
					CG 16% ± 8.9% ↓ mean size.	CG 4 infected ulcers
						4-Week study (healing rate 11%/wk)
						TG healed 2× faster than CG

(Continued)

TABLE **23.7** Principal Mechanisms of Primary and Secondary Intention Healing *(continued)*					
Population, No. of Patients, Study Type	Polarity	Amplitude/Rate	Frequency and Duration	% Healed	Mean Time To Heal
Houghton et al.[133]	Pressure ulcers—SCI; SBRCT; *N* = 34 SCI Stage II *N* = 5; Stage III *N* = 10; Stage IV *N* = 17; Stage X = 2.	Initially cathode, monopolar, alternate polarity weekly	50–150 V contractile threshold; 50 μs, 100 and 10 Hz	20 min 100 Hz; 20 min 10 Hz, 20 min rest/each hour × 8 h.	TG 70 ± 25% healed
				CG 36 ± 61% healed (*p* < .048)	
Goldman et al.[105]	Ischemic ulcers retrospective, observational (TG *N* = 11) SC *N* = 7	Not stated	80–330 V, 100 pps	60 min/d, 5–7 d/wk at home × 1 y; SC 1 y + 28 d	TG: 9/11 healed, 1 patient died, 1 amputation; SC 2/7 healed, 5 not healed
Goldman et al.[11]	Quasistable ischemic ulcers (tcPO$_2$ > 10 mm Hg), SBRCT *N* = 8	Cathode, monopolar technique	Sensory threshold or max 360 V	60 min/d × 7 d × 14 wk	TG wk 14 tcPO$_2$ 30 mm Hg	4 wk CG ↑ 50% in area
				CG wk 12 tcPO$_2$ 15 mm Hg (*p* < 0.05)	1 y TG ¾ healed; 1 expired
					CG ¾ healed 1 amputation
Adegoke and Badmos[190]	Pressure ulcers SCI RCT *N* = 7	Not stated	30 Hz, rectangular square wave; below muscle contraction	45 min 3×/wk × 4 wk	TG ↓ 22%	4 wks most change occurred in 2 wks
					CG ↓ 2.6 %	

Source: Data from references listed in the table.

- Griffin et al.[26] demonstrated an 80% reduction in size of pressure ulcers in SCI-injured patients in 4 weeks, when treated with negative polarity, but ulcers were not treated until healed.
- Franek et al reported in a prospective RCT ($N = 58$) of Stage I, II, III pressure ulcers using HVPC treatment that after a 6-week treatment period of stimulation five times weekly for 50 minutes per session, the treatment group healed twice as fast as the controls.[149] During the treatment period, 8/29 ulcers healed versus 4/29 controls. Results were not stratified by pressure ulcer stage making it difficult to determine effects on different stages. Volume reduction occurred simultaneously with area reduction. There was more efficient reduction in necrotic tissue and enhanced growth of granulation tissue in treatment group but not of statistical significance.
- Adegoke and Badmos used monophasic PC in an RCT to study effects on an SCI pressure ulcer population. This very small study, originally seven and then six subjects, found that in 4 weeks, the treatment group healed 22% compared to 2.6% for the control group.

Venous Leg Ulcers

- Houghton et al.'s[10] RCT focused on treatment of vascular leg ulcers ($N = 27$ subjects, 42 ulcers). The study time was not intended to take the wounds to closure but to evaluate the effect of HVPC on size and tissue appearance over a 4-week period. The vascular leg ulcers were stratified into three groups: diabetic, arterial, or venous. Then the ulcers were randomly assigned to one of two treatment groups. One group received HVPC treatment and the other placebo treatment. All HVPC treatment was given at negative polarity, three times weekly treatment of 45 minutes per session. Outcome measures reported included percentage reduction in surface area and wound tissue appearance as evaluated with the photographic wound assessment tool (PWAT). (Chapter 5 describes this assessment tool.) Surface area for the total experimental group decreased 44.3% ± 8.8%, or 11% per week during the 4 weeks of the study, and the ulcers in the control group did not decrease. Seven patients had bilateral venous ulcers and they were used as their own controls. Data were stated in two ways: combined healing for the combined group of vascular ulcers (above) and separately for the seven. In patients who were their own controls, the treated ulcer had a surface area reduction that was significantly greater (57% ± 15) than the control ulcer (20% ± 18.16%) and PWAT scores reduction over the time of the study.
- Polak et al.[9] also reported an RCT using HVPC for venous leg ulcers. English translation of the Polish published study was provided by the first author as a personal communication. In this study, 22 patients were enrolled for treatment and 20 as controls. The study lasted 7 weeks. Treatment was six times weekly for 50 minutes per session. Outcomes were reported two ways: percentage of healing and weekly healing rate of both volume and surface area. Findings were that the treated ulcer had a 73.4% reduction of area compared with 47% reduction for control. Volume reduction for the experimental group was 91.3% versus 68%. Weekly healing rate was a volume reduction of 1 cm³ for treated ulcers and 0.6 cm³ for controls. The number of healed or percentage of healed ulcers was not reported.[9] Likewise, the rate of area reduction was faster for the experimental group (1.4 versus 1.0 cm²/wk).

- A second RCT from Poland by Franek, Polak, and Kucharzewski also investigated the effect of HVPC on venous ulcers. Three groups were used: group A ($N = 33$) received HVPC treatment and compression bandaging., group B ($N = 32$) received topically applied medicine and compression therapy, and group C ($N = 14$) received Unna boot compression. Outcome measures analyzed were rate of healing, rate of "pus" débridement/cleansing, and degree of granulation formation after 2 weeks. Findings were that the rates of wound healing and pus cleansing were highest in group A. An inclusion criterion was ankle-brachial index ABI greater than 0.8. Negative polarity was used until wound was clean of pus, typically 1 to 3 weeks, and then changed to anode for the rest of the study.

Diabetic

- Alon et al.[150] used positive polarity and stimulated diabetic wounds three times a week for 1 hour; 12 of the 15 (80%) of the ulcers treated healed. One patient died, one did not respond, and the ulcer in one decreased significantly in size but did not heal in 21.6 weeks.
- Peters et al. reported a 12-week RCT study of ES efficacy on healing of diabetic foot ulcers ($N = 40$) using an unusual protocol.[148] All patients received off-loading, débridement as needed, and moist wound healing dressings that were changed twice daily. Treatments and dressing changes were performed by the patient or a family member. The object was to test outcome as related to compliance using a unique treatment schedule. The treatment took place in the patient's home during night sleep, the purpose being to improve compliance because the patient's regular schedule of activities would be minimally impacted. The device used was a small microcomputer strapped to the leg and the electric current was delivered through a Dacron mesh silver nylon stocking. The device used compliance metering. Current was delivered as twin peak pulses at 50 V amplitude in three phases: high pulse rate (80 pps) for 10 minutes followed by low pulse rate (10 pps) for 10 minutes, then a 400-minute rest period. Polarity was not reported. Programming of the computer allowed for this sequence to be repeated throughout the night, presumably for seven to eight cycles per night. Conductivity was assured with a slowly evaporating electrolyte fluid applied to the skin.

Compliance was evaluated and the findings were that (1) compliance from both groups was essentially the same; (2) compliant patients only used the device correctly 50% of the time; and (3) compliant patients in both groups had better outcomes than both noncompliant groups. Two dropouts occurred in each group. Healing outcomes were as follows: 75% of treatment group healed and 35% in placebo group healed. Among the healers in both groups, the average healing times were essentially the same: 6.8 ± 3.4 weeks and 6.9 ± 2.8 weeks. Conclusion: Patients who used the ES protocol for 20 hours or more per week were more likely to heal than those who used placebo or less than 20 hours of stimulation per week.

Ischemic Ulcers

Goldman reported a small RCT pilot study ($N = 8$; four in each group) of patients with ischemic ulcers. Ischemic ulcers have a predisposition to be unstable and rapidly expand into gangrenous eschar.[11] Patient inclusion criteria for this study was critically ischemic wounds occurring below the knee diagnosed by vascular study that had not healed in at least 4 weeks. The groups were appropriately matched. Risk was evaluated by the clinical team; expectation that the wound would not increase in size over the 14-week study period was another inclusion criterion. A significant finding from this small study was that both $tcPO_2$ levels and laser Doppler flow measurements were increased out of the ischemic range in the treatment group and not in the controls.

At the 1-year follow-up, there were was one unrelated death but no amputations in the HVPC group. There was one amputation in the control group even though the controls elected to transfer to HVPC after the 14-week trial period. Motivation for conducting this RCT prospective pilot study was a 5-year retrospective RCT observational study previously reported by the same principal author. In that study, they identified criteria met by 22 patients with ischemic wounds below the ankle who were poor candidates for revascularization. Eleven subjects had received HVPC plus standard care and the other eleven subjects received only standard care. At the end of 1 year from start of treatment, 90% of wounds (9/10) were healed in the HVPC group, compared with 29% (2/7) who only received standard care. In addition, there were observations of a marked increase in $tcPO_2$ levels in the HVPC-treated group of patients over the study period and that ulcer healing tended to improve after the start of ES (see the section on ES and oxygen earlier in this chapter). The study authors recognized correctly that a small number of subjects have the ability to skew the results and calculated an N of 24, 12 each group, to test their hypothesis about increasing microcirculation with an ES phase 2 study.[105]

Unknown Etiologies

Akers and Gabrielson[151] published a study that compared (1) HVPC direct application to the wound; (2) application of HVPC using the whirlpool as a large electrode; and (3) whirlpool alone. The direct application of the active electrode to the wound site had the best outcome, followed by HVPC using the whirlpool as an electrode. Whirlpool alone was the least effective.

In all the studies except the Gogia, Houghton, and Peters studies, the treatment frequency was five to seven times per week for 45 to 60 minutes. At this time, it is hard to state what is the optimal amount of stimulation needed to effect healing. However, it does seem apparent that HVPC is an effective adjunct to standard wound care for the populations studied.

Low-Voltage Pulsed Electrical Current (LIDC) Studies

Two RCTs of treating pressure ulcers with LVPC, labeled PES, were located in the literature.

CLINICAL WISDOM

Best Method for Effective HVPC Treatment

Apply HVPC directly to the wound for best expected outcome.

Low-Voltage Microamperage Direct Current (LVDC) Clinical Trials

LVDC was used in six clinical studies. Wolcott et al.,[96] Gault and Gatens,[127] Carley and Wainapel,[138] Katelaris et al.,[152] and Wood et al.[30] studied treatment of ischemic and indolent ulcers. In the first three studies, a positive (anode) polarity was used after a period of 3 or more days at the cathode. The polarity was reversed every day or every 3 days if wound healing did not progress. Rationale for initial cathode application was the solubilization of necrotic tissue[56] and bactericidal effects.[120,121] All studies except the Katelaris study used an amplitude of 200 to 800 µA. Duration of treatment was very long: 2 hours, two or three times per day, or 42 h/wk for the first two studies, and 20 h/wk for the third study. Treatment in the Wood study was administered three times per week, but length of treatment was not stated. Katelaris et al. incorporated ES treatment with dressings, did not state how long current was applied, and used negative polarity throughout. A combined total of 225 patients were treated, and 75 served as controls. In most cases, the patient served as his or her own control. Mean healing times reported were 9.6, 4.7, 5.0, 8, and 6.5 to 7 weeks, respectively, for the five studies (see Table 23.3).

The difference in healing time between these studies is not clear. Perhaps in the Wolcott et al study, the wounds were more extensive. Carley and Wainapel[138] noted that the pulsed LIDC treatment group healed 1.5 to 2.0 times faster than did the control subjects, who were treated with wet to dry dressings and whirlpool. Katelaris et al.[152] found no statistical difference in healing times between normal saline, normal saline with electrode, and povidone-iodine–treated wounds. However, results when povidone-iodine was used with the negative electrode showed that the mean healing rate was statistically longer, 85.3 days (12.2 weeks). The researcher theorized that the retardation effect may be due to the negative pole ionization of the iodine and forcing iodine ions down an electrochemical gradient into the cell, where they act as intracellular toxins.

Biphasic Stimulation Studies
Controlled Animal Study

Khalil and Merhi[153] decided to test the effect of frequency on wound healing in aged rats. Aged rats were wounded and then divided into an active treatment group and a sham treatment group. Low-frequency TENS (20 V, 5 Hz for 1 minute) was applied twice daily to the treatment group, and sham treatment was applied to the controls. The active group required 14.7 ± 0.2 days for complete healing, which was a significant improvement over the sham group (21.8 ± 0.3 days). The conclusion reached was that wound healing in aged rats can be accelerated by peripheral activation of sensory nerves, using low-frequency parameters. Most patients sent for ES intervention are elderly so perhaps similar mechanisms control wound healing in human elders and that is why we see so many reports of good results for this population.

Human Studies

There are reports in the literature by Kaada,[84] Lundeberg et al.,[8] Stefanovska et al.,[145] Baker et al.,[154,155] Barron et al.,[156] Petrofsky[46,47,157,158] of clinical trials of wound healing with biphasic waveforms. Benefits were found in patients with SCI who had pressure ulcers[145,154] and in patients with diabetic ulcers, including those with peripheral neuropathy[155] and venous

TABLE 23.8	Clinical Studies Using Biphasic Protocols							
Researcher	Phase Duration	Pulse Rate	Waveform	Amplitude	Frequency/ Duration	Location	Population/Study Type	Treatment Results
Kaada[84]	Not reported	100 Hz	Symmetric	15–30 mA muscle contraction	Daily; three 30-min sessions (off 45 min between sessions)	Negative electrode	Mixed, case series	Healing
						Web between 1st and 2nd metacarpal bones		
Lundeberg et al[8]	1 ms	80 Hz	Symmetric	15–25 mA evoking parasthesias	Twice daily × 20 min	Wound edge	Diabetics with venous stasis ulcers (N = 64) RCT	TG Healed: 42% 7% ↓/week versus CG healed 15%
								4.25% ↓/week
Stefanovska et al.[145]	0.25 ms	40 Hz	Asymmetric, charge balanced	15–25 mA below contraction	Daily for 2 h	Wound edge	Spinal cord injury with pressure ulcers (N = 150) RCT	TG 25.2%/↓week
								CG 15.4 ↓/week
Baker et al.[154,155]	100 μs	50 Hz	Asymmetric	24–25 mA below contraction	Daily three 30 min sessions (short break between sessions	>1 cm from wound edge; proximal and distal to ulcer	(1) SCI PU N = 185 / RCT	1 and 2 significantly improved healing rates 60 % > controls
							(2) Diabetic ulcers N = 80/RCT	
Frantz[146]	15 μs	85 Hz	Symmetric square	10 mA	Three times daily 30 min	(1) web space both hands	Pressure ulcers (N = 37) RCT	TG 28 d; CG 53 d median time to closure (using wound volume measurements)
						(2) + proximal to wound edge		
						(3) − distal to wound edge		

(continued)

TABLE 23.8	Clinical Studies Using Biphasic Protocols *(continued)*							
Researcher	Phase Duration	Pulse Rate	Waveform	Amplitude	Frequency/ Duration	Location	Population/Study Type	Treatment Results
Barron et al.[156]	Not stated	0.5 Hz	Modified square	600 μA/50 V	Three times per week	0.2 cm from ulcer edge, moved around wound edge	Pressure ulcers (N = 6)	Healing and decreased size
Sumano and Mateos[52]	Not stated	65 Hz	Symmetric square	0.04 mA; current charge density 0.4–0.8 C	Daily or every other day 20 min	Wound edge	Mixed wounds(34) and burns(10)/case series	Healing in organized manner
Lawson et al.[97]		30 Hz	Sine + warm room (32°C)	20 mA	30 min 3×/wk × 4 wk	Bipolar	Diabetic (TG) nondiabetic (CG)	TG 70% ± 32.3%
							Stages III and IV grade (N = 20) RCT	PG 38.4 ± 22.3, $p < .01$; ↑BF TG 215 % versus 49% PG
Petrofsky et al.[158]	250 μs		Sine + local heat (37°C)	20 mA	30 min 3×/wk × 4 wk	Wound edge	Wagner Grade 2 Diabetic (N = 20)/ RCT	TG ↓ 68.4%±28.6 area; 69.3 ± 27.1 volume ($p < .05$)
								BF↑ 152,3 ± 23,4 versus ↑ 102,3 ± 25 CG
Suh et al.[191]	200 μs	30 Hz	Symmetric biphasic	20 mA	3×/wk × 4 wk	3 electrodes around wound	Mixed patient own control	TG ↓ 43.4% ± 44.5%
							CCT (N = 18)	Area; 57.0 ± 27.9 % volume

stasis.[8] Another research finding is that more rapid reduction in wound depth occurs when biphasic is used.[146] One animal RCT[142] and two human RCTs[145,146] have noted this observation. In all of the studies except Kaada, stimulation was delivered to the skin at the wound perimeter, rather than into the wound bed. An advantage of the perimeter stimulation was less disruption of the wound bed, less cross-contamination of the wound, and less interference with the dressing. Table 23.8 summarizes the protocols used and results for all of the biphasic studies.

Diabetic/Venous Ulcers

- Lundeberg et al.[8] conducted an RCT on 64 patients with chronic diabetic ulcers due to venous stasis. All patients received standard treatment with paste bandage, in addition to the sham or TENS treatment. Asymmetric biphasic stimulation was determined to produce significant wound healing effects, whereas the other waveforms did not increase the healing rate.
- In two RCTs, Baker et al.[154,155] compared asymmetric biphasic, symmetric biphasic, and microcurrent (DC) in two sets of patients, one with diabetic ulcers and the second with pressure ulcers. The asymmetric biphasic waveform has a potential for some polar effect that should not be discounted. The polar effect may explain why it was more effective than the symmetric biphasic waveform. However, another likely explanation of the effects just mentioned is stimulation of neural mechanisms that effect healing.[154]
- Petrofsky and his work group reported several different aspects of biphasic treatment for diabetic wounds.[46,97,159] Global and local heating of the skin to 35°C releases vascular skin vasoconstriction and increases skin BF. When ES follows skin heating, there is a further large BF increase (35%) at the wound margins in the diabetic population compared to nondiabetics (18%). However, heating in a 32°C (90°F) room presents some practical difficulties. Thus, an alternate method was tested by Petrofsky et al. using a combination of local dry heat (infrared heat lamp) and ES (biphasic, 30 Hz, PW 250 milliseconds, about 20 mA). The results measured with LDF images showed that BF increased from rest of 102.3 ± 25.3 to 152.3 ± 23.4, and there was significantly decreased wound area and wound volume ($p < .05$) in a 1-month period in a group of 20 diabetic subjects. Preheating was done locally to the periwound and wound area after removing the dressing and cleansing the wound with an infrared heat lamp placed 35 cm above the tissues to raise tissue temperatures 37°C. Preheating was found to reduce skin resistance so that when ES was added there was a synergistic effect on BF that increased the release of vasodilator NO. They found that area and volume of combination-treated ulcers reduced significantly in area and volume (68.4 ± 28, 63% versus) in a 4-week period. Treatment given three times per week.[158]

Their conclusion was that the addition of local heating, raising tissue temperature to 37°C, appeared to be a relevant part of the healing equation.

Pressure Ulcers

The RCT study by Stefanovska et al.[145] compared DC and asymmetric biphasic current. Barron et al.[156] reported a study of six patients with pressure ulcers who were treated three times a week for 3 weeks, for a total of nine treatments with microcurrent stimulation. The waveform was a modified biphasic square wave. The treatment characteristics were 600 μA, 50 V, and 0.5 Hz. The electrode probes were placed 2 cm away from the edge of the ulcer and then moved circumferentially around the ulcer. Each successive placement of the probes was 2 cm from the prior placement. In this small study, two ulcers healed 100%, three healed 99%, and one decreased in size 55%.

Mixed Etiologies

Kaada[84] reported results of TENS on 10 subjects, who served as their own controls, with recalcitrant ulcers of different etiologies. Stimulation was provided indirectly over the web of the thumb daily (HoKu point) during three 30-minute sessions with rests of 45 minutes between, for a total of 1½ hours of stimulation. Stimulation was below visible muscle contraction.

Sumano and Mateos[52] reported the use of acupuncture-like ES for the treatment of unresponsive wounds of mixed etiologies and burns. In this clinical trial, in which patients served as their own controls, the device used had the parameters of 300 mV, 67 Hz, 0.04 mA, and a calculated absolute charge density of 0.4 to 0.8 C/cm². The method of delivery for most wounds was via electrodes clipped to stainless steel acupuncture filiform needles that were inserted subcutaneously along the edges of the lesion and placed to form an almost complete, closed peripheral circuit. In very large burn wounds, the current was applied by means of covering the wound with saline-soaked gauze, and then randomly attaching alligator clips from the stimulator to the gauze, maximally separating the positive and negative electrodes. Delivery of current through the gauze in this manner without a conductor is problematic. Treatments were administered either daily or every other day, based on the severity of the lesion and compliance of the patient.

Throughout the course of the treatment protocol, no local antiseptics or antibacterials (either systemic or local) were administered. Dry wound healing methods, as described in an earlier section, were used. Only normal saline was used to cleanse wounds. Forty-four wounds (34 wounds/10 burns) were treated. Patients and wounds were assessed using a stratified classification method of lesion and medical condition severity. When wounds were classified according to their severity, as well as the overall condition of the patient, a closer statistical correlation between the lesion grade and number of treatments to total cure was observed ($r = 0.98$). Number of treatments were less (8.4 ± 2.3) for grade I severity lesions ($N = 10$) than for those of grade III severity ($N - 17$)(41.38 ± 6.58). The authors reported a positive correlation between the severity grade and the time of the first visit for alternative treatment. Mean time from lesion identification to first presentation was 11.8 ± 4.49 days for grade I, 15.44 ± 8.58 for grade II, and 24.5 ± 5.21 days for grade III.

All patients in the study requested this alternative type of medical treatment when their wounds/burns did not heal quickly (2–4 weeks) with conventional wound healing procedures and drugs. Although this procedure uses acupuncture needles, it is not an orthodox acupuncture procedure. Authors reported that the patients were compliant with the treatment and attributed the compliance to high patient satisfaction, with the evident improvement seen from the first treatment session. Early intervention with the ES procedures seems to have accelerated the healing process, reduced risk for increased wound severity, and required fewer treatment interventions to achieve an excellent outcome. In all patients, healing proceeded in a thoroughly organized manner, almost regardless of the severity of the type of wound or burn treated.[52]

Meta-Analysis of Effect of ES on Chronic Wound Healing

Gardner and Frantz[160] used meta-analysis to average quantitatively the findings across multiple ES studies. The meta-analysis for ES for wound healing was undertaken by the authors for three purposes:

1. To quantify the effect of ES as an adjunctive therapy for chronic wound healing
2. To explore the influence that the type of ES may have on efficacy of the ES treatment
3. To explore the influence that the wound etiology may have on ES effectiveness for healing

To achieve these goals, the meta-analysis estimated the rate of healing of chronic wounds treated with ES. To be included in the meta-analysis, the following criteria had to be met:

1. The study was on the use of ES for ulcer or periulcer stimulation
2. The subjects were humans
3. Reports would include all types of chronic wounds (arterial, diabetic, pressure, and venous)

The outcome measure chosen for evaluation was the percentage of healing per week because it was the most common measurement either reported or that could be calculated from study data. Fifteen studies, which included 24 ES and 15 samples, were analyzed and the average rate of healing per week calculated for each sample. The 15 studies included have been described in the preceding text. Ninety-five percent confidence intervals were also calculated. The 95% confidence intervals of the ES (18%–26%) and control samples (3.8%–14%) did not overlap. Then the samples were grouped by type of ES device and chronic wound, and reanalyzed. The rate of healing per week was 22% for ES samples and 9% for control samples. The net effect of ES was 13% per week. Net increase in rate of healing was 10.9%. DC healing rate was 12.6% per week versus PC healing rate net increase of 15.5%. ES treatment was most effective for treatment of pressure ulcers (net effect = 13% per week). Findings regarding the relative effectiveness of different ES devices were inconclusive. The authors felt that the problem was extensive overlap in the confidence intervals.

The conclusion reached by these authors was that ES produces a substantial improvement in the healing of chronic wounds, and further research is needed to identify which ES devices are most effective and which wound types respond best to this treatment. Evaluation of the meta-analysis showed that the studies chosen for the meta-analysis were both published and unpublished, randomized and nonrandomized clinical trials, and descriptive studies. Only three were reports of TENS, alternating was classified separately, and the rest were either DC or pulsed DC. Many of the studies chosen for this analysis had very small subject samples (3–7). Controls received a variety of treatments, including moist dressings (13), antiseptics (4), and whirlpool (4). However, the evidence of effectiveness of this adjunctive therapy compares favorably or surpasses treatment with other interventions used for wound healing.

Summary

The previous section evaluated the efficacy of ES on many aspects and components of wound prevention, including clinical trials of wound healing. Electrical stimulation studies reviewed in this section vary from continuous waveform application with DC to pulsed short-duration monophasic pulses to biphasic pulses. What is known and acknowledged is that ES seems to have positive effects on wound healing or on the aspects and components necessary for wound healing (e.g., BF and oxygen uptake, DNA, and protein synthesis), but there is still ambiguity about the type of ES characteristics that are most important or critical. For instance, polarity has played an important role in protocols used, even though the likelihood of polarity effects of currents with pulses of very short duration is questionable. Now we are learning that prewarming and concurrent warming substantially decrease vasoconstriction and appear to have a synergistic effect that enhances BF and thus ES treatment efficacy. One possible reason for the wound healing effects of ES with any type of current may result from the effect of low-level sensory stimulation on the peripheral nerves, which is not wholly dependent on the polar nature of EC. Kaada[85] describes effects that include inhibition of sympathetic input to superficial vessels, release of an active vasodilator, and axon-reflex stimulation. Study results are beginning to show evidence that stimulation with DC, AC, and PC have somewhat different physiologic effects. As identification of the specific effects of different currents' aspects is more thoroughly tested, the clinician will be able to choose the type of stimulation and a protocol to derive a specific outcome for prevention or healing.

CHOOSING ES AS AN INTERVENTION: CLINICAL REASONING

Selection of ES for wound healing is not dependent on the wound etiology or the patient's medical diagnosis. ES is appropriate when there are impairments to the systems that interfere with healing at one or more levels: cellular, tissue, or organ. Functional loss at any of these levels suggests that the wound will not or has not healed with the current level of intervention. In such cases, refer the patient to PT for the consideration of additional strategies to facilitate healing. The use of externally applied currents is one such strategy. Physical therapists have unique education and skill set that makes them the most skilled providers of electrotherapeutic interventions and the most likely to have predictable results.

Wound attributes that respond positively to ES include necrotic tissue and pus, inflammation, wound contraction, infection, and wound resurfacing. Wounds of all depths, from partial-thickness to full-thickness and deeper (e.g., Stage II to IV pressure ulcers) have been treated successfully with ES. Table 23.9 identifies wounds appropriate for treatment with ES.

TABLE 23.9	**Apropriate Wound Types for Electrical Stimulation**
Level of tissue disruption (wound severity)	Superficial, partial thickness, full thickness, subcutaneous, and deep tissues
Etiologies/diagnostic groups	Burns, neuropathic ulcers, pressure ulcers, surgical wounds, vascular ulcers (venous and arterial)
Wound healing phase	Inflammatory phase: acute, chronic, absent
	Proliferative phase: acute, chronic, absent
	Epithelialization phase: acute, chronic, absent
	Remodeling phase: acute, chronic, absent
Age	Older than 3y

Subjects selected for clinical trials with ES typically had nonconforming wound healing with long chronicity. The chronic wounds were the reason for referral for ES. Still, there is significant scientific evidence that early intervention with externally applied ECs will also accelerate healing for the acute healthy wound. Early intervention with ES could be a useful method to prevent chronicity and return the individual to a functional status earlier.

Precautions

Signs of adverse effects using ES for wound healing were evaluated in the various clinical trials. The only two adverse signs were some skin irritation or tingling under the electrodes in a few cases and pain in some other cases. Patients with severe peripheral vascular occlusive disease, particularly in the lower extremity, may experience some increased pain with ES, usually described as throbbing. An alternative acupuncture protocol has been suggested in these cases—placing the active electrode on the web space of the hand between the thumb and first finger instead of over the ulcer located on the leg.[84,85]

Children less than 3 years of age should not be considered candidates for intervention with ES. Healing mechanisms for this group are not well understood and, although there are no known adverse effects, the benefits are not defined. However, older children may benefit from use of an ES intervention to stimulate sensory nerves and accelerate the rate of healing.[161]

RESEARCH WISDOM

Remove Iodine Products before ES

Make certain that any form of iodine, if used to treat a wound, is thoroughly removed before application of electrotherapy.[152]

Contraindications

Contraindications for the use of ES fall into the following categories[56,162]:

- When stimulation of cell proliferation is contraindicated (e.g., malignancy)
- Where there is evidence of osteomyelitis
- Where there are metal ions
- Where EC could affect the function of an electronic implant
- Where the placement of electrodes for treatment with ES could adversely affect a reflex center
- When severe cardiac arrhythmia is present
- During pregnancy unless used during labor for pain management

Carefully evaluate the medical history and review body systems when considering candidates for use of this intervention (see Chapter 2).

Presence of Malignancy

ES should not be used when there is presence of a malignancy (e.g., malignant melanoma, basal cell carcinoma) in the area to be treated. This is because ES stimulates cell proliferation and could lead to uncontrolled cell growth. If the malignancy is distant from the wound (e.g., breast cancer in a patient with a pressure ulcer on an ankle), local use of ES should be considered, weighing the risks and the perceived benefit of the treatment, mindful that ES has demonstrated systemic effects.[85,163] In such a case, it would be a precaution but not a contraindication. (Note, however, that this is not consistent with required manufacturer labeling.)

Active Osteomyelitis

There has been concern that stimulation of tissue growth with ES may cause superficial covering of an area of osteomyelitis. This could blind the site from observation. Thus, a history of a bone infection should prompt you to conduct an investigation of the current status of the infection. The osteomyelitis may be resolved but not noted as such in the medical record. If the osteomyelitis is being treated actively with antibiotic therapy, some clinicians are recommending that treatment with ES be started. In many published case studies, patients with active osteomyelitis were treated successfully with ES (see section above about bactericidal effects); thus, in such cases, consult with the patient's physician. Controlled clinical trials are indicated to evaluate the benefits of ES for treating wounds in which there is evidence of osteomyelitis.

CLINICAL WISDOM

Identification of Osteomyelitis

If a wound penetrates to the bone, as determined by inserting a probe, it must be assumed that osteomyelitis is present and the patient should not be treated with ES. An immediate referral to a surgeon for evaluation must be initiated.[164]

Topical Substances Containing Metal Ions

Topical substances containing metal ions (e.g., povidone-iodine, zinc, Mercurochrome, and silver sulfadiazine [Silvadene, SSD] that might be used as part of the wound treatment regimen) should be removed before the application of ES. Direct-current ES has the ability to transfer ions into the tissues by iontophoresis. Heavy metal ions may have toxic properties when introduced into the body. If removal of the topical substance is not appropriate, you could still use ES on other areas of the skin where the topical agent has not been applied.

Electronic Implants

Demand-type cardiac pacemakers and other electrical implants raise concerns regarding the use of EC. ES is contraindicated *over* electrical implants because the current and electromagnetic fields could disrupt function of the implant. Use of ES with a demand-type cardiac pacemaker is one of its contraindications. Studies to evaluate safe utilization of TENS in the presence of a cardiac pacemaker report mixed results.[165,166] Thus, although patients with cardiac pacemakers should not be excluded from the use of TENS, these patients do require careful evaluation and extended cardiac monitoring. The risks and benefits of using ES for wound healing need to be carefully weighed.

Natural Reflex Centers

The natural reflex centers of the body are particularly sensitive to any stimulation. These include the carotid sinus, the heart, the parasympathetic nerve ganglia, the laryngeal muscles, and the phrenic nerve. ES can interfere with the function of these vital centers and be harmful to the patient, for example by creating a vasospasm, some type of vasoconstriction that could lead to a vasovagal response, or some other type of adverse neural response. Thus, ES is contraindicated in situations when the current would need to run through the upper chest and anterior neck.

Choosing and Testing the Equipment

Select a stimulator based on the available waveforms, pulse characteristics, and ability to adjust amplitude and polarity and to manually control the settings. A desirable stimulator should allow for flexibility to set up and deliver a variety of protocols, based on changes dictated by clinical trials and current concepts of physiologic rationale. Manufacturers are an important source of helpful information about the characteristics of their devices.

Expect to find an FDA-mandated instruction manual accompanying each electrical stimulator. Listed in the manual are labeled indications, contraindications, warnings, and precautions (Exhibit 23.1). When selecting a protocol with ES (discussed in the next section), consider all such restrictions, and use thoughtful clinical judgment. Here, we discuss regulatory approval of ES, devices available, and equipment testing.

Regulatory Approval

Under what is called *premarket approval* (PMA), manufacturing companies are allowed to make claims of effectiveness and safety about medical devices. PMA requires extensive clinical trials, typically 2,000 to 3,000 cases for approval. No electrical stimulators have received PMA by the FDA for wound healing. Externally applied currents for wound healing are considered as

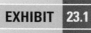

EXHIBIT 23.1

FDA Indications and Contraindications for Electrical Stimulation

FDA indications
- Relaxation of muscle spasms
- Prevention or retardation of disuse atrophy
- Increasing local blood circulation
- Muscle re-education
- Immediate postsurgical stimulation of calf muscles to prevent venous thrombosis
- Maintaining or increasing range of motion
- Pain
- Edema

FDA contraindications
- Should not be used on patients with demand-type cardiac pacemakers
- Should not be used on persons known to have cancerous lesions
- Should not be used for symptomatic pain relief unless etiology is established or unless a pain syndrome has been diagnosed
- Should not be used over pregnant uterus
- Electrode placements must be avoided that apply current to the carotid sinus region (anterior neck) or transcerebrally (through the head)

"off-label" use at this time; that is, not FDA approved. Off-label use for medical devices is an accepted and common practice in medicine as innovative therapy, as long as the clinicians are not closely associated with the manufacturer.[167]

Testing Equipment

It is important to test for current flow between two electrodes. Use the meter that comes with the device if available; if no meter is available on the stimulator, pursue other options. You can also check the electrode pads by placing a wet contact on both positive and negative electrodes, and then resting your forearms on each pad. Ask a colleague to turn up the device until you feel a sensation of prickling. Patient sensation is always a good indicator, if the patient can give a report. Patients who are insensate or unable to communicate, or who have deep wounds below the level of sensation, will not be able to indicate whether or not the current is flowing. Another test method is to position the large electrode over a muscle motor point to determine whether there is a muscle twitch or tingling under the electrode.

Electrical stimulation equipment should also have regular calibration checks by a trained service technician. In between checks, use a multimeter for spot checking to see that the equipment is functioning properly. Multimeters, which are a combination of volt-ohm-milliammeter, have the ability to determine current flow. They are inexpensive, easy to use, and readily available. A broken lead wire, weak battery, or resistant electrode may not be apparent because the stimulation in the wound bed is below the level of sensation or the patient is insensate or cognitively impaired and cannot report changes in sensation. Checking for good electrical conduction is the responsibility of the clinician.

Electrodes

As noted earlier, the electrode is the contact point between the electrical circuit and the body. The electrode must be a good conductor, provide very little resistance to the current, and conform well to the surface. Carbon/rubber electrodes over time become resistant to current flow and need to be replaced when this occurs.

Active/Treatment versus Inactive/Dispersive Electrodes

For monophasic stimulation, the small electrode is commonly referred to as the *active or treatment electrode*, and the large electrode is called the *inactive or dispersive electrode*. If the two are of nearly equal size or have equal current, the current will be divided between the two, with the current density at the two sites the same. If the two are not of equal size, the larger electrode will disperse the current over the surface of the electrode, and then it will have less current density and charge per unit area than the smaller electrode and not enough to do active treatment. Thus, the other term *inactive* electrode is used. As a rule, the combined area of the active electrodes should not exceed the overall area of the dispersive/inactive electrode. Another benefit of using a larger size dispersive/inactive electrode is more comfort for the patient, since the charge density and perception are lower underneath it.

Electrode Materials

All metals are good conductors of electricity. Aluminum foil is an excellent conductor to use for electrodes (Figure 23.9). It is nontoxic, inexpensive, disposable, conformable, and can be sized as needed. Carbon-impregnated electrodes are sold to go with most electrotherapeutic devices. They are designed for multiple uses and are relatively inexpensive, but they need to be disinfected between uses, even if restricted to a single patient. They are less conformable than aluminum foil and will become resistive over time as they lose carbon and accumulate body oils and cleaning products. Self-adhesive electrodes can be used for bipolar techniques but not for direct wound applications.

> ### CLINICAL WISDOM
>
> **Benefits of Aluminum Foil Electrodes**
>
> Aluminum foil electrodes are very cost-effective and time efficient for treatment of open wounds. They are easily made from household aluminum foil, are good conductors, can be molded to fit the body part, can be sized for maximum current density to the wound, and are disposable. Saline-soaked gauze packed in the wound and covered with an aluminum foil electrode is also cost-efficient and is particularly good on deep lesions.

A novel approach to electrodes is an electro-mesh conductive silver nylon garment (stocking and glove, etc.) (Prizm Medical, Inc.; Oakwood, GA www.prizm-medical.com) A slowly evaporating electrolyte fluid is applied to the skin under the garment to reduce skin resistance and allow conduction of the current to the tissues.[148] This application allows delivery of the stimulation over a large surface area without concern about size, shape, or electrode placement around the wound. It is particularly useful in treating ulcers on toes and other boney prominences of the feet.[133] The company makes an HVPC and TENS stimulator that interfaces with the garment electrodes (Figure 23.10). Recommendation is that the sock be worn at night since the stimulator has a specific cycling on and off pattern that works best during that type of regimen.

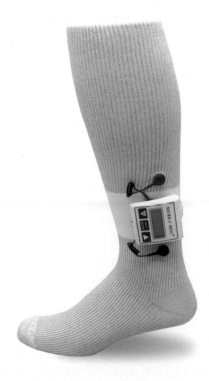

FIGURE 23.10 Silver Nylon Stocking Garment. (Courtesy Prizm Medical, Inc., Oakwood, GA. www.prizm-medical.com).

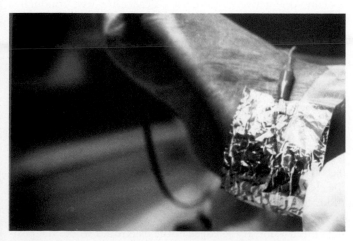

FIGURE 23.9 Aluminum foil electrodes with alligator clips.

Electrode Size, Shape, and Arrangements

Size, shape, and arrangement of electrodes affect the current density and depth. As you will recall from the beginning of this chapter, current density is the amount of current flow per unit area. It is a measure of the quantity of charged ions moving through a specific cross-sectional area of body tissue. The unit of measurement is mA or mA/cm². This measure will affect the reaction of the tissues being stimulated. Two determinants of current density are *size* of the electrode and the *amplitude* of the current applied,[48] and for PCs, it is also important to know the duty cycle. Small electrodes concentrate the current for local effects more than do larger electrodes, which tend to disperse the charge. Also, the farther apart the electrodes, the deeper the current penetrates but the current density is reduced the greater the distance.

Tangential Electric Fields

The effects of the tangential electric field, the electrical field acting along or in the direction of a tangent away from the electrode, extends and affects events from 2 to 3 cm up to 11+ cm beyond the edge of the stimulating electrodes.[168] Maximum tangential electric fields occur on the body surface in the edge regions where the two electrodes of opposite polarity faced each other, and maximum tangential fields are stronger than the perpendicular fields directly under the stimulating electrodes.[168] Therefore, to achieve polarity effects, avoid placement of the active and inactive electrodes so that they touch each other or are too close so as to avoid the possibility that the wound is receiving stimulation from both poles. Current amplitude in the center of the electrodes and the tangential fields at different depths is dependent on several variables including the size of the electrode and the distance of separation between the electrodes.[169] Wounds treated with tangential fields and those treated with perpendicular fields have nearly the same rate of healing.[51] Studies that report patients having two wounds, one of which is used as the control and the second treated with ES, may report results that are better than studies when external controls are used because of influence of the tangential electrical field.[127]

Electrode Placement

Attempts have been made to apply scientific findings to electrode placement. Most studies use monopolar technique with the active electrode directly applied to the site,[10,27,170,171] (Figure 23.11) but some use the bipolar technique at the wound edges.[8,145,154,155] The inactive/dispersive electrode placement has more variation. For example, in two similar studies, the dispersive electrode was placed differently. In one study,[27] it was placed cephalad on the neural axis, whereas in the second study it was placed 30.5 cm from the wound.[2] One study on SCI patients with pressure ulcers in the pelvic region used a protocol in which the dispersive was always placed on the thigh. Another method is to place the dispersive proximal to the wound.[170,171] Current thinking suggests that the dispersive should be moved around the wound to induce the current to enter the wound from different sides. At this time, there is not an established, proven method that has been shown to change the effect of the treatment. All reported treatment methods had statistically significant treatment results. The significant amount of separation of the poles may have been contributory to these effects.

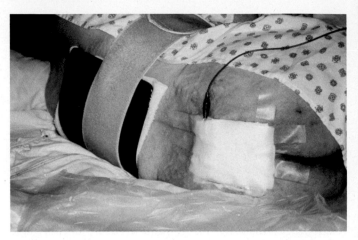

FIGURE 23.11 Monopolar technique. (Copyright © C. Sussman).

Because of the fluid in muscles and blood vessels, these tissues are good electrical conductors, and it can be expected that current will flow directly through them, with little impedance. It is important to understand these principles of tissue impedance and current flow and then to apply them correctly to derive the optimal benefits from treatment with ES. For example, if the dispersive electrode is to be placed on the back, place it *below* the scapula to avoid impedance by the bone to current flow. Patients with thick layers of callus on the feet will have high impedance to current. Paring the callus should precede ES treatment, or another placement must be found where the electrode does not lie on callus. The muscular tissue of the thigh is a good placement for the dispersive electrode when treating wounds of the lower leg or foot. One suggestion is to switch the dispersive electrode for each treatment so that the current flows into the wound from each side of the wound through different surrounding tissues and through a different wound edge.[168,187] It is not only the active electrodes that can be bifurcated; the dispersive electrode can also be bifurcated. This allows use of a pair of smaller electrode pads that can be made to conform to smaller body parts, such as an arm or a lower leg

Monopolar Technique: Exploiting Polarity

Use monopolar technique with monophasic continuous or pulsed waveforms to exploit the polarity at the wound site. Usually, one active electrode is placed on a wet, conductive medium in the wound bed, and the inactive electrode, in a wet conductive medium at a distance from the wound site, is placed on the intact skin (Figure 23.11). Polarity for the two electrodes will be opposite. The poles are usually set up in parallel fashion, enabling current to flow between the positive and negative electrodes, no matter how many electrodes are used at either pole. Current will flow through the intervening tissues between the two electrode poles. The current under the active electrode will reflect the polarity selected on the stimulator, provided that there is adequate separation of the poles. There is a uniform electrical potential with a strong electrical field at the edges of the electrodes and perpendicular to them. However, the amplitude of the electrical field has been found to decrease as the distance between the electrodes increases. The electrical field has maximum value at the edges of the electrodes where the positive and negative stimulating electrodes face each other.[168]

RESEARCH WISDOM

For polar effects, separate the active and dispersive electrode poles by at least 10 to 30 cm.[169]

The electrodes can be arranged to target the stimulation to specific tissue sites. Remember to visualize the path of the current flow when placing the inactive electrode.

Multichannel Electrode System

Research is currently being undertaken and reported about use of a three- or four-electrode system to overcome an inherent problem of the common two-electrode system of uneven current flow and distribution.[47,191] Three or four electrodes are placed around the wound similar to the bipolar setup, and the active electrode is rotated every few seconds between the three. The result of using a three-channel delivery system, with the same current between the electrodes, the BF was significantly higher than a two-channel system. With a four-channel system, the BF in the wounds was even higher. Thus, it would appear that current delivery was better in the four-channel system. Presumably, this would be an aid to wound healing.[157]

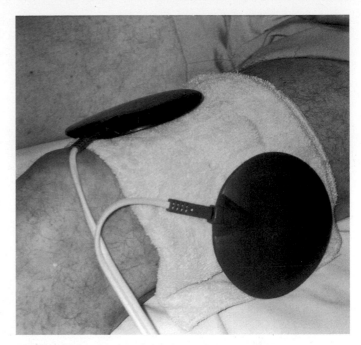

FIGURE 23.12 Bifurcated leads.

Current and Charge Density

Two points to weigh in your decision about electrode sizes are having adequate current and charge density under active electrodes (1) when treating multiple wounds and (2) when treating deep and undermined wounds.

1. Some patients have multiple wounds that you will want to treat during the same treatment session. When the surface area of all the electrodes is unequal, the current density will not be the same under each site. The problem with this is that, if there is a difference in the total surface area of the electrode(s) connected to one lead compared with the other, the stimulation will be stronger under the electrode with the smaller total surface area because there will be greater current density under that electrode. So as to ensure an adequate but not excessive charge, you can do this by adjusting the electrode sizes to correspond with the wound size.
2. Depth and undermining can make the effective electrode size of a small wound significantly larger than the surface area appears (see Chapter 3).
3. Petrofsky et al showed that the majority of the current on the skin flows in the midline between two electrodes with a 10-cm separation distance; the current density in the center of the electrodes is significantly greater (p 0.01) in comparison to the locations further apart and tangential to the center. As the electrodes were moved further apart (15 and 20 cm), the curves flattened and there was more even distribution of the current density across the electrode independent of the size of the electrodes.[169]

The PT must do some calculations to ensure that the charge and current densities are within the parameters of the "window of charge" for the number and size of wounds being treated.[12,16,25] Earlier we discussed this concept and learned that the "window

of charge" represents a range of charge intensity, between 200 and 600 µC, that has been determined to be effective for wound healing.[25] It may be advantageous to increase the inactive/dispersive electrode area size so that this electrode is larger than the combined area of the active electrodes. Another strategy is to bifurcate the inactive electrode and use 2. Otherwise, it may be prudent to use a stimulator with two channels or two stimulators to have two concurrent treatment sessions if there are multiple wounds with a large discrepancy in wound sizes or if the wounds are in different phases of healing.

Monopolar use of Multiple Electrodes with Bifurcated Leads

At times in clinical practice, it is necessary to treat multiple wound sites with a single electrical circuit, using one or two bifurcated lead wires (Figure 23.12). The advantage of bifurcation is that more sites can be treated simultaneously. A disadvantage is that, although the same amount of current and charge per phase passes through all the bifurcated leads, the physiologic responses can vary significantly because of the different tissue impedances. Physiologic reactions can be different when subliminal stimulation is perceived under one electrode and the sensory stimulation under the other. Also, significant levels of stimulation may affect the healing results of wounds that are distant from each other but on the same body.[16] Given these caveats, an important consideration is patient and clinician convenience and adherence since, as you will learn soon, each treatment session needs to be 45 to 60 minutes daily.

Bipolar Technique

The bipolar technique is the placement of two oppositely charged electrodes (cathode and anode) on either side of the wound near the wound edge. The bipolar technique is used with either monophasic or biphasic waveforms. In this

CLINICAL WISDOM

Managing Multiple Wounds on One Patient

1. **Enlarging the Inactive/Dispersive Electrode**
   If the wound area size is nearly as large as or larger than the skin area under the dispersive electrode, it will be more comfortable for the patient to enlarge the inactive electrode surface area.
2. **Applying Bifurcated Leads Using One or Two Stimulators**
   The author has treated multiple wound sites on one patient using the bifurcated lead method with good results in all lesions (See Figure 23.13A–C). A bifurcated lead wire is a single lead connected to the stimulator that bifurcates at a point along the wire into two divisions. That allows each division to be connected to an electrode, and two wounds can be treated at the same time. Another approach the author has employed is two simulators each with bifurcated leads, for the same patient. This allows different protocols to be selected for each set of electrodes.

application, both electrodes are active treatment electrodes and should be placed over the target areas to be affected by stimulation. This technique has the advantage that it can be used without disrupting the wound dressing. It brackets the wound as shown in Figure 23.14 so the current charge flows across the wound area.[24] The two poles should not be too close together so that the polarity effects of the two electrical fields will not overlap. This is a reasonable choice for superficial or partial-thickness wound disruptions but may not be as effective for deep ulcers.

An application of the bipolar technique is to place the electrodes on either side of the wound (bracket the wound) or to place the active electrode in the wound and use four bifurcated dispersive electrodes placed around the wound so that current will flow through the wound from all sides at once. Finally, one active electrode could be placed in the middle of the wound and a dispersive electrode fashioned like a donut, made from aluminum foil, slipped over the treatment electrode with an intervening space between so that stimulation would flow into the wound bed from all sides of the wound edges simultaneously. The foil electrode would connect to the dispersive lead with an alligator clip, just like the active leads (Figure 23.9).

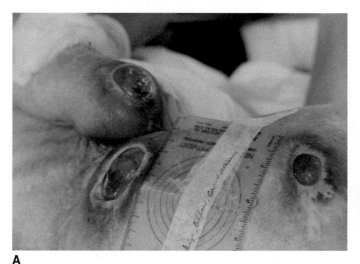

A

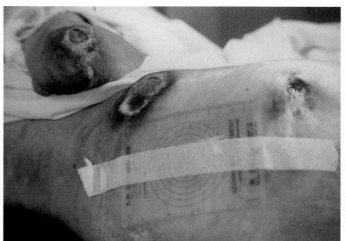

B

FIGURE 23.13A–C. A patient with multiple pressure ulcers treated with ES. (Copyright © C. Sussman).

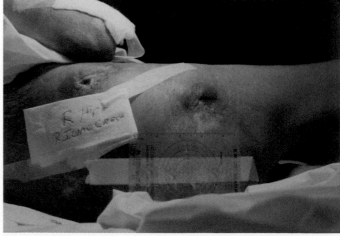

C

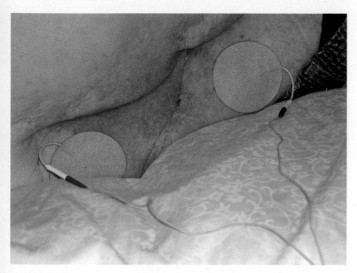

FIGURE 23.14 Bipolar technique. (Copyright © C. Sussman.)

TABLE 23.10	Selecting an Evidence Based Waveform for Treatment	

Waveform	Evidence Based Treatment Utility
Biphasic (TENS)	Impaired skin vascularity
	Impaired blood flow
	LE chronic ulcers
	Diabetic ulcers
	Pressure ulcers
	Venous ulcers
	Diabetic neuropathic pain
HVPC	Pressure ulcers
	Diabetic ulcers
	Venous ulcers (with compression)
	Burns
	Grafts
	Pressure ulcers prevention
	Impaired BF and tcPO$_2$
	Impaired sympathetic tone and increased vascular resistance
	Ischemia and atherosclerosis
	Edema
	Infection
NEMS	Pressure ulcers
	Impaired BF and tcPO$_2$
	Venous (with compression)
	Edema
LIDC	Diabetic ulcers
	Pressure ulcers
	Burns
	Grafts
	Biofilms and infection
	Enhance efficacy of antibiotics

CLINICAL WISDOM

Aluminum foil may be used as the dispersive as well as active electrode material. It can be cut to size and conforms easily to all body contours.

ELECTRICAL STIMULATION TREATMENT METHODS FOR WOUND HEALING

Selecting the Device and Treatment Protocol

With today's use of interdisciplinary wound teams, different clinicians from different disciplines are using ES for wound treatment. Yet, as previously mentioned, it is the physical therapist who is the best-educated and trained practitioner in the physical properties of different ES devices, and the bioelectric and physiologic effects of each. As such, the PT has the unique qualifications to select equipment and protocols, to be responsible for accurately predicting outcomes, and to instruct others in the proper use of the ES equipment. Table 23.10 provides a listing of devices and waveforms and their evidence-based treatment utility as discussed in this chapter.

New ES devices are coming to market and are being evaluated by clinical studies. Each device has its own proprietary waveform and/or delivery system. For example, there is a device with 2, 3, or 4 electrode channels that sequentially changes the active electrode during the treatment so that the active polarity is delivered around the wound perimeter.[157] Another device changes the treatment parameters every 20 minutes.[133] A third device uses sequences of modulated electrical stimuli that vary automatically in terms of pulse frequency and duration.[104] Therefore, these devices do not fit conveniently into the categories of devices and the studies described earlier. The PT needs to be aware of the changing marketplace and investigate the claims of manufacturers about a new proprietary device, to read carefully the specification sheets that come with the device, and to read studies about ES therapy with this in mind. There are many different ES protocols for wound healing. This section first describes some of the aspects of the protocols as described in clinical research. It then discusses selection of the device and protocol.

Aspects of ES Protocols

Tables 23.3, 23.7, and 23.8 present protocols used in research studies with three different types of ES, LIDC, HVPC, and biphasic. This section discusses aspects of ES protocols including polarity switching, pulse frequency (pps), and amplitude for monophasic current followed by aspects of biphasic current.

Polarity Switching
Monophasic

Polarity must be considered when using galvanic and monophasic PC. Electrode polarity varies, depending on the protocol selected. Most researchers studying ES for wound healing start their protocols with the negative pole as the active electrode and then change the polarity after a period of treatment.[61,71,112,138] Some advocate maintaining negative polarity to the wound site throughout the assessment period of 4 weeks or longer.[10,11,26] Other researchers recommend using negative polarity for 3 to 7 days, then changing polarity. Another recommendation is to use negative polarity until the wound is cleansed of necrotic tissue and drainage is serosanguineous, and then to continue with the negative polarity for three additional days or change to the positive pole.[9,119,170,171] If the wound is not infected, positive polarity can be used to start the treatment.[27] Some researchers suggest that the polarity should be changed back to negative for 3 days when the wound plateaus.

Another method is to change the polarity every 3 days until the wound is healed to a partial-thickness depth. Once that outcome is achieved, change the polarity by alternating daily until the wound is closed. Several animal studies demonstrate better healing when polarity is initiated at the negative pole and then switched to positive.[71,72,172]

Usually, the negative electrode is used as the active electrode when infection is suspected. The polarity is often switched back and forth during the course of healing. Electrode polarity switching accommodates the variability in the skin battery potentials that occurs during the course of healing. Thus, electrode polarity may need to be alternated during treatment to achieve an optimal rate of healing. Additional research is needed to ascertain whether wound healing with ES is dependent on matching treatment electrode polarity with fluctuations in wound injury potential polarity.[27] So far, studies have not reported on this important issue. Still, the idea of polarity switching has some demonstrated merit.

Biphasic Current

When a symmetric biphasic waveform is used, the polarity switches constantly so no polar effect is registered. However this waveform can be made asymmetric so that one phase can be biased towards one specific pole. Protocols demonstrating significant benefit for wound healing with biphasic current are now appearing regularly in the literature.[8,51,127,145,154–156] The eight studies reported in this chapter have similar protocols, except that the two studies by the Baker et al.[154,155] research group found that the best outcome was achieved when the biphasic waveform was asymmetric and biased toward the negative pole. Sumano and Mateos[52] used filiform needles to conduct the current and not carbon electrodes. Biphasic treatment protocols and the results are shown in Table 23.8.

Pulse Frequency

Pulse frequency, or pulse rate, is another variable that varies from study to study without much explanation. Several studies used a pulse rate of 100 to 128 pps for treatment with HVPC.[26,27] Another investigator started treatment at 50 pps.[170,171] The author uses 30 pps based on the effect of lower frequency on BF. In several studies, lower-frequency pulse rates produced higher mean BF velocity than did higher pulse rates and had a longer mean recovery time following cessation of ES, compared with control levels.[64] Frequency rate switching during the healing process is also not well understood but becomes more relevant as more information about pulse charge is discovered. For example, in one study, the rationale given for reducing the pulse rate for the final phase of healing from 128 to 64 pps was "because we believed the higher pulse frequency might be harmful to the newly healed tissue."[18] This concern is probably due to the higher pulse charge delivered to the tissue at the higher pulse rate.

Device Selection

Depending on the stimulator selected, the protocol for treatment will vary. In some cases, the characteristics of ES for different current type may not always be based on the wound healing phases. For example, asymmetric biphasic stimulation parameters are not varied during the progression through the phases of healing.[154,155] The protocols are based initially on the wound healing phase diagnosis (Chapter 3). There are changes in polarity and pulse rate as the wounds progress through the phases of healing. The most common stimulator used for wound healing today is probably the HVPC neuromuscular stimulator. The protocols presented below are based on use of the HVPC stimulator.

However, now there are more RCTs and CCTs showing efficacy using biphasic and LIDC (TENS) than using HVPC. See Table 23.8. Depending on the wound status (full versus partial thickness), different stimulator current effects should be considered. The protocol parameters and dosage are similar to those reported in the studies with low-voltage pulsed EC.[18,28] Thus, this protocol would also be appropriate to use with those stimulators.

Selection of Amplitude

Earlier we learned that amplitude is measured in volts (V), milliamperes (mA) or microamperes (µA). High-voltage protocols report amplitudes as V. Typically, the range of treatment amplitude is 100 to 200 V. This is what the readout on the stimulator will show. LVDC (LIDC) or pulsed EC (PES) report amplitude as mA. Typical LIDC amplitude is 35 mA, and µA devices use less than 1 mA. These devices usually do not have a readout.

In wound care, the amplitude of an ES device is adjusted until the patient with sensation can feel a tingling sensation (paresthesia) at the edge of the wound. Insensate individuals, of course, cannot respond to this sensation. In that instance, the voltage is usually turned up until there is a mild muscle contraction or fasciculation, and then backed down until that muscle contraction is no longer visible.

Adjust the amplitude to patient comfort. The ability of the patient to tolerate high-intensity current will depend on the sensory perception of the individual. For example, in superficial or partial-thickness wounds, if there is intact sensation, an amplitude above 100 V may be very uncomfortable. In deeper wounds or in cases of impaired sensation, these higher amplitudes are well tolerated. It has been suggested to test the amplitude by stimulating until there is a visible muscle contraction under the electrode. This is not a practical test if the active electrode is located in a wound within a muscle because the sensory nerves will not be stimulated

CLINICAL WISDOM

Perform Sharp Débridement before HVPC Treatment

Complete sharp débridement of necrotic tissue before setting up the patient for HVPC treatment so that the wound packing will act as a pressure dressing to control any bleeding and so that the wound environment will not have to be disturbed again after HVPC treatment.

Conclusion

Clearly, more investigation is needed to achieve an optimal treatment protocol with ES. In the meantime, the protocols and dosage presented in this chapter are for use with low- and high-voltage monophasic and biphasic waveforms, which represent this author's interpretation of the literature and the application to clinical treatment. The author has used these protocols for several years, with good clinical results. Protocols are listed for wound healing for the three phases of repair and for the treatment of an edematous limb in which the edema extends beyond the wound area. Protocols change for each phase of repair and have expected outcomes for each. Expected outcomes are based on the literature and clinical experience.

Sussman Wound Healing Protocol

Table 23.11 identifies the Sussman Wound Healing Protocols for HVPC for all four phases of wound healing and edema control. Using this method, you would initiate an HVPC treatment protocol based on the assessed aspect of the wound healing phase diagnosis and predict an expected outcome for that protocol. Because the polarity of the healing wound changes during the phases of healing, treatment characteristics differ as wound healing progresses. In the protocol given below, the stimulation selected for treatment is a monophasic current and monopolar technique used with HVPC.

For wounds in the acute inflammatory phase, with an absence of the aspects of the inflammation phase, or in a chronic inflammatory phase, start treatment with parameters to stimulate circulation and cellular responses for healing that induce aspects of an inflammatory phase. The protocol calls for a change of parameters as the wound healing phases progress. Likewise, for a wound healing phase, diagnosis of the repair (proliferative) phase, and a wound in the remodeling phase, the PT would start treatment using a different set of parameters, as outlined.

Predictable Outcomes with Sussman Wound Healing Protocol

Predictable outcomes are expected for each protocol, and are equivalent to a change in the aspects of the wound phase characteristics. For example, if the aspects of the wound healing phase diagnosis is *acute inflammatory phase*, the *expected outcomes* are hemorrhage free, necrosis free, erythema free, edema free, exudate free, red granulation, and progression to the next phase—the proliferative phase. These aspects of the wound correspond to the items on the Sussman Wound Healing Tool shown in Chapter 5. If there is absence of inflammation or chronic inflammation, an acute inflammatory phase needs to be initiated, to restart the healing process. Expected outcomes would indicate change to an acute inflammatory phase, described as increased erythema (change in skin color), edema, and warmth. The phase change outcome predicted is *initiation of acute inflammatory phase*. Each wound healing phase has its own diagnosis and expected outcomes that are independent of wound etiology.

Figure 23.15A–D illustrates a pressure ulcer that progressed through the three phases of healing under treatment with HVPC.

TABLE **23.11**	**Protocols for HVPC Treatment**					
Parameters	Edema	Inflammation	Proliferation	Epithelialization	Remodeling	Venous Return2
Polarity	Negative	Negative	Alternate negative/positive every 3 d	Alternate daily	Alternate daily	Not critical; adjust for patient comfort
Pulse rate (frequency)	30–50 pps	30 pps	100–128 pps	60–64 pps	60–64 pps	40–60 pps
Intensity	150 V or less depending on patient tolerance	100–150 V	100–150 V	100–150 V	100–150 V	Surge mode on time, 3–15 s; off time, 9–40 s (1:3 on/off ratio) to motor excitation
Duration	60 min	60 min	60 min	60 min	60 min	5–10 min, progress to 20–30 min
Treatment frequency	5–7 times/wk for first week, then 3 times/wk for 1 wk	5–7 times/wk, once daily	5–7 times/wk, once daily	3–5 times/wk, once daily	3 times/wk, once daily	Daily; modify to biweekly

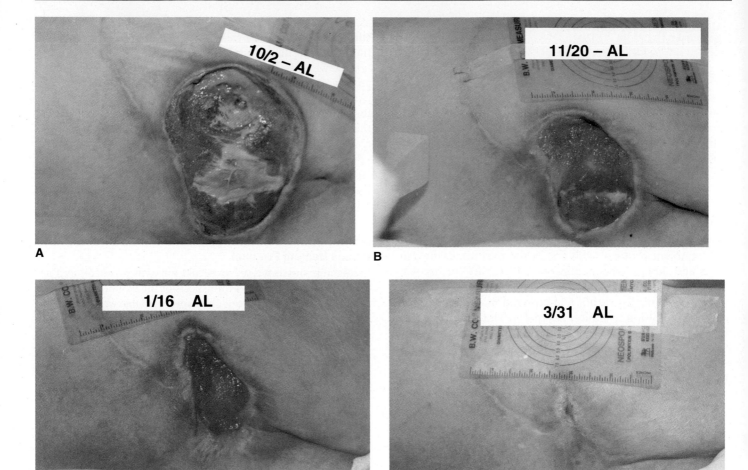

FIGURE 23.15A–D. A pressure ulcer that progressed through the three phases of healing under treatment with HVPC. A. Chronic wound: converted to acute proliferative phase. This is a sacral wound with stringy, yellow slough evident. Note example of epidermal ridge formation. Predominant wound healing phase diagnosis: proliferative phase. Wound severity diagnosis: Impaired integumentary integrity secondary to skin involvement extending into fascia, muscle, and bone. (Stage IV pressure ulcer). Same wound as in (A), progressing through the proliferative phase. The wound is contracting and proliferating. Note changes in size, shape, and depth, as well as new healthy granulation tissue compared with (A). B. Note sustained wound contraction evident here and in (B). Note epithelialization and proliferative phases. The wound is completely resurfaced and is in the remodeling phase. (Copyright © Sussman.)

PREPARING AND ADMINISTERING ES PROCEDURES

The procedure section of this chapter is outlined in a step-wise fashion to help you deliver ES in a systematic and time-efficient way. Treatment with ES requires a number of supply items and steps. Consider having an assistant set up the treatment station where the equipment and supplies are available (see list of equipment and supplies needed). The same set of instructions would be useful to give to a patient or caregiver for home treatment. Make sure that all supplies are ordered and available in the department. Always have enough supplies on hand so that treatment is not delayed while someone is running around chasing down the needed equipment.

Protocol for Use of HVPC for Wound Healing
Equipment Needed
- Normal saline (0.9%)
- Clean gloves
- Irrigation syringe, 35 mL with 19-gauge needle or angiocatheter
- Clean gauze pads
- Aluminum foil electrode or carbon electrode
- Alligator clips if using foil
- Electrode leads
- Bandage tape
- Nylon stretch strap
- Wet washcloth
- Dispersive pad (carbon or gel)
- HVPC machine leads
- Infectious waste bag

CLINICAL WISDOM

Suggestions for Setup to Maximize Treatment Effectiveness and Efficiency

- Assemble the setup supplies into kits before the start of the treatment day to make the delivery of service more time efficient.
- Precut and shape the aluminum foil electrodes. Size and shape should be close to the size of the wounds. Precut foil electrodes are available from various vendors.
- To make an electrode, cut a strip of household aluminum foil the width of the electrode. Fold the strip in half and turn in the edges to make a smooth pad.
- To make a packing strip from gauze, open a gauze pad, pull on the bias or diagonal, and twist to make a spaghetti strip or use stretch gauze strips.
- Warm saline or a package of amorphous hydrogel by placing bottle between a folded hot pack before use to avoid chilling the wound tissue and slowing mitotic activity. Check the temperature with a digital thermometer. The temperature should not be greater than 98°F to avoid burns.
- Myer[175] reported keeping a 16-oz bottle of saline warm for 3 to 4 hours by placing it in a hydroculator tank. She observed that warming of the saline before ES treatment resulted in brighter redness of granulation tissue and contributed to reduction of pain. The increased redness was probably due to vasodilation and enhanced BF associated with the warmth.
- Room temperature where treatment is to be given should be very warm, and the patient should be warmed for 10 to 15 minutes if possible before, during, and 15 minutes after the ES treatment to improve circulatory results. In cold climates, warming may take longer.

Instructions for Patient and Caregiver

1. Explain the procedure, the reason for treatment, and how long it will last. Explain that a mild tingling will be felt and where it will be felt.
2. Advise the patient not to handle, replace, or remove electrodes during the treatment. Patients who cannot understand these directions or will not cooperate need to be monitored closely.
3. Give patient a call light to use.
4. Cover patient with a blanket to maintain warmth.

Procedure for Setting Up the Patient for HVPC Wound Treatment

1. Have supplies ready before undressing the wound.
2. Position the patient for ease of access by staff and for the comfort of both.
3. Remove the dressing and place in infectious waste bag (usually a red bag).
4. Cleanse wound thoroughly to remove slough, exudate, and any petrolatum products.

5. Sharply debride necrotic tissue, if required, before HVPC treatment.
6. Open gauze pads and fluff, then soak to moisten in normal saline solution; squeeze out excess liquid before applying.
7. Fill the wound cavity with gauze, including any undermined/tunneled spaces. Gauze pad can be opened to full size and then pulled diagonally to form a thin "spaghetti" strip. Insert into undermined/tunneled spaces like roller gauze. Pack gently.
8. Place electrode over the gauze packing; cover with a dry gauze pad and hold in place with bandage tape.
9. Connect an alligator clip to the foil.
10. Connect the stimulator lead to the electrical stimulator.
11. Place the dispersive electrode.
    a. The dispersive electrode is usually placed proximal to the wound (see section on electrode placement for alternative locations).
    b. Place over soft tissues; avoid bony prominences.
    c. Place a moist washcloth under the dispersive electrode against the skin and hold it in good contact at all edges with a nylon elasticized strap. If placed on the back, the weight of the body plus the strap can be used to achieve good contact at the edges.
       Covering the wet dispersive setup with a plastic sheet to separate it from the bed and the patient's clothing to keep them dry will be appreciated by the patient and the nursing staff.
    d. The dispersive pad should be larger than the sum of the areas of the active electrodes and wound packing. If the size of a self-adhesive electrode is large enough to disperse the current, it can be used instead of a carbon dispersive pad.
    e. Dispersive and active electrodes should be at least 10 cm apart but no more than 15 to 20 cm apart for monopolar effects as shown in Figure 23.11.

Additional Treatment Methods

Two wounds can be set up with a single-channel stimulator, using bifurcated leads from the stimulator to the electrodes. For a patient with multiple wounds, it is not practical to run several series of treatments. An alternative is to use two HVPC stimulators, if available. Electrode placement will require careful planning so that the current flows through target tissues. For example, if there is a wound on the right hip, coccyx, left foot, and right heel, the dispersive electrode should be placed on either the right or left thigh. The thigh has a good blood supply and good conductivity. This setup will send the current flowing through the deep tissues to the feet, the hip, and the coccyx.

- Alternate placement of the inactive/dispersive electrode for each treatment, if possible, to DC flow to opposite sides of the wound.[152] This will be more difficult when wounds are located in the feet. This would be a situation where the electrical nylon stocking shown in Figure 23.10 could be considered as the current would flow around the entire wound perimeter and adjacent tissues. If a limb is involved, the circumference may be too small to wrap with the large dispersive electrode and maintain good contact. An alternative is to use bifurcated leads and two dispersives. When using this setup, attach two round, carbon-impregnated electrodes or make a foil electrode that increases the surface area of the dispersive electrode, making it larger than the active electrode. If using the bifurcated leads, place the electrodes on either side of the limb. It is easier to conform two pads or a foil electrode to a small limb segment than the large rectangular dispersive electrode, standard with most stimulators. Usc wct gauze under the electrodes; if a greater conductive surface is required, use a larger piece of foil. Hold the dispersive electrode in place with nylon elasticized straps or tape with weak adhesive. If the patient complains of excessive tingling under the dispersive setup, check for good contact.

Aftercare

After the ES treatment is complete, slip the active electrode out from between the wet and dry gauze. The wound can be left undisturbed. If saline-soaked gauze is the conductive medium, it should be changed before it dries or be covered with an occlusive dressing. If additional topical treatments are required, such as enzymatic debriding agents or antibiotics, the packing will need to be removed. Frequent dressing change is discouraged because it disturbs the wound healing environment by removing important substances in wound exudate and cooling the wound. It takes 3 hours for a chilled wound to rewarm. Cooling slows leukocytic and mitotic activity.[176–178] If dressing is to be changed, redress the wound in the warm room environment immediately following ES treatment.

Alternative Methods of Conducting Current Using Wound Dressings

Alternative methods of conducting current to the wound using dressing products have been of interest for many years. Studies of conductivity of different wound dressings report that, although transparent films are poor conductors, silver dressings have benefits, and fully hydrated hydrocolloids, alignates, and hydrogel amorphous gels and sheet forms are good conductors.[179,180]

Silver Dressings

As reported earlier, silver dressings have demonstrated benefits when used in animal and human studies for bactericidal effects, reduction of edema that has been enhanced with the addition of anodal DC EC and also, in a RCT, as the active electrode for treatment of pressure ulcers.[109,110,133] Some clinicians believe that silver dressings should be discontinued when infection is controlled; and they are not an appropriate dressing choice for wounds with eschar. The eschar must be débrided first (see Chapter 20 for indications and contraindications and evidence about the application of silver dressings). Actions that speeds the healing of burn wound grafts have the potential for decreasing length of hospital stay and reducing health-care costs. Perhaps now that clinical trials are demonstrating utility of silver nylon dressings as conductors and their safety and efficacy when used with ES more applications will adopted.

Hydrogels

Use an amorphous hydrogel-impregnated gauze to conduct current. This type of dressing is used for partial-thickness, full-thickness, and subcutaneous lesions extending into deep tissue wounds. Hydrogels can be left in the wound for up to 3 days. This product class can benefit the wound management by:

- Conducting EC when covered with an electrode
- Promoting the "current of injury"
- Absorbing light to moderate wound exudate
- Maintaining a moist wound environment
- Gradually absorbing wound moisture (is also a moisture donor to the wound)
- Retaining the cell growth factors in the wound bed
- Reducing trauma and cooling of the wound, through less handling
- Reducing product and labor costs by serving a dual purpose

It is also possible that hydrogels promote collagen synthesis. An animal study demonstrated that PES delivered through a hydrogel dressing increased the levels of collagenase during the critical period of epithelialization initiation.

Hydrogel sheets also have high water content and can also be used to conduct current when placed under the electrode.[180] They have benefits similar to the amorphous hydrogels, except that they should not be left on an infected wound. They are used for lightly exudating wounds and are best used for superficial partial-thickness wounds, such as donor sites after skin grafting.

Amorphous hydrogel-impregnated gauze or a hydrogel sheet can be used as the wet contact coupler under an electrode. Although manufacturers say that all that is required is to clip the alligator clips to the dressing to conduct current, Alon[181] explained that this will focus the current at one small area of the dressing and not disperse it throughout the wound area unless the entire dressing surface is covered with a conductive electrode. Follow the setup steps described above, but substitute the saline-soaked gauze with the amorphous hydrogel-impregnated gauze or hydrogel sheet. Dressings may be left in place for up to 3 days. The amorphous hydrogel should be warmed before application, but be careful not to overheat the product and cause burns. Check temperature with a digital thermometer. Temperature should not be greater than 97°F. If wound conditions permit, cover with a moisture/vapor-permeable transparent film or another dressing to retain moisture without maceration and to maintain body warmth. For amorphous hydrogel-impregnated gauze, on the second day, lift the secondary dressing and slip an aluminum foil electrode underneath; connect an alligator clip lead to the dressing and the stimulator. Replace secondary dressing. Repeat on the third day. The same approach would apply to the hydrogel sheet.

CLINICAL WISDOM

Remove Petrolatum Before Stimulation

All petrolatum products, including enzymatic débriding agents such as collagenase (Santyl) and Papain urea (Accuzyme), which are petrolatum-based products (Healthpoint Biotherapeutics, Ft. Worth, TX, www.healthpointbio.com), must be removed before treatment or current will not be conducted into the wound tissues.

Infection Control and Disinfection of ES Equipment

The use of aluminum foil electrodes is a good method of controlling infection and eliminates the need for disinfection. If carbon electrodes or electrodes with sponges are used over the wound, they need to be disinfected between each use, even if used for a single patient. Check with the infection control agent for your facility to select a cold disinfection solution that will disinfect for all organisms in a short time period (e.g., 10 minutes).

Disinfection of other items:

- The dispersive pad, which is placed on intact skin, should be cleaned between uses with soap and water followed by an alcohol wipe.
- Alligator clips that come in contact with wound contaminants should be disinfected between uses. One company furnishes alligator clips with packs of hydrogel-impregnated gauze that can be kept for single patient use.
- Over time, the carbon electrodes will absorb oil and detergent products used for disinfection and will become resistant to current flow. A periodic check (e.g., every 30 days) of the conductivity of the electrodes is highly recommended.

SELF-CARE TEACHING GUIDELINES

HVPC stimulation and biphasic TENS type units are very safe and easy-to-apply treatments that a patient or caregiver can be taught for self-treatment at home. HVPC and biphasic stimulators, as described in this chapter, are available as portable, battery pack units. Some units come with compliance meters and would be recommended for home patient use.

Selecting the Candidate for Self-Care

Although ES is a simple treatment, it requires the capacity to follow instructions over several sequential steps. Review the procedures with the person who will deliver the care to ensure that adequate instruction will be given to achieve the predicted outcomes. Select the patient or caregiver who is alert, motivated, and able to learn the directions for application. If you do not believe that the patient or caregiver is capable of performing the procedure properly and safely, document this finding, and consider a referral for skilled services or another intervention.

To achieve success in self-care, psychosocial concerns need to be addressed as well. Your support and encouragement can help convince the patient/caregiver to accept the responsibility for self-care. Patients and caregivers are accustomed to receiving medical care at the clinic or by a home care practitioner, rather than doing self-care. The concept of sharing the problem between patient and clinician is new to many people. It takes a step-by-step process to gain patient acceptance and cooperation.

Whether in the clinic or at the home visit, begin by encouraging and teaching the patient and/or the caregiver to participate in the setup process. Many people are repulsed by the sight of a dirty, smelly, ugly wound. That is often the first hurdle. Take it slowly, with patience and acceptance of these feelings. Explain in simple language why the wound is dirty, smelly, and ugly, and how the treatment will improve the problem. Wound measurements and photographs can be used as motivation to encourage continued participation. "Before and after" photographs of other clients treated in this way are particularly effective ways of showing the patient/caregiver how other wounds improved. Move the patient or caregiver increasingly into the role of treatment provider as soon as possible. Observe, instruct, and offer words of support and praise.

Instructions

Independence in the treatment routine must be established before dispensing electrical stimulator for self-care at home. Although it may seem overwhelming to give five steps of instructions for a single treatment protocol, understanding the five steps of instructions listed here will ensure that the patient or caregiver is able to achieve the goal of independence in the treatment routine. Keep instructions as simple as possible so that the responsible party will not be overwhelmed. Because of the number of steps required, prepared instruction sheets listing the five steps would be helpful. Simple drawings can be helpful in teaching the proper placement of the electrodes. Don't assume that the patient will know where to place the electrodes or how to put on the dressing when he or she arrives home. Two or three visits may be necessary to complete the instruction. Schedule regular follow-up assessments, usually weekly, to evaluate outcomes and change protocols.

The five steps of instruction are as follows:

1. The list of needed supplies: Make sure that the patient can acquire all the necessary items or help make arrangements to acquire those that are needed (e.g., a portable HVPC stimulator and electrodes).
2. Setup of the patient and the wound for treatment, including all the steps listed: Review what is on paper, then do a demonstration and return demonstration to confirm understanding.
3. The treatment protocol: Review the treatment protocol by dialing in the characteristics for the selected protocols on the stimulator to be used. The dials can be left at the correct setting to help the patient, but they may be moved and should be rechecked at each treatment session. Give *only* the treatment protocol for the current wound healing phase. Tell the patient or caregiver what outcomes to expect and what findings should be reported promptly. Change instructions as the wound heals.
4. The aftercare procedures: Aftercare procedure instructions should include how to apply the prescribed dressing product and disposal of the disposable waste products from the treatment in the home setting (see Chapter 20). Make sure that the patient or caregiver understands the proper use of the prescribed aftercare dressing products. Damage to the wound and failure to achieve predicted outcomes can be avoided by instruction in use of products. Again, practice and a return demonstration are proven methods of teaching new techniques.
5. A list of expected signs and symptoms: The patient and the caregiver need to be aware of the importance of any expected changes in signs and symptoms related to the treatment and must know when to report any undesirable results.

1. Wound attributes that have responded positively to electrical stimulation include
   A. Necrotic tissue and pus
   B. Inflammation and infection
   C. Wound contraction and resurfacing
   D. All of the above
2. The positive pole attracts
   A. Lymphocytes
   B. Platelets
   C. Macrophages
   D. Neutrophils
3. Biphasic Current is also known as
   A. Alternating
   B. Galvanic
   C. LVPC
   D. HVPC
4. Healing can be initiated and facilitated when using
   A. Positive current
   B. Negative current
   C. Neither current
   D. Alternating between currents
5. Which statement regarding monopolar technique is correct?
   A. Current will flow through the path of greatest tissue resistance.
   B. Current has the most difficulty flowing through muscles, nerves, and deeper tissues.
   C. Decreasing the distance between electrodes is a good choice if the wound are deep.
   D. The farther apart the two electrode poles are, the deeper the current will flow into the intervening tissues.[182–187]

REFERENCES

1. Bergstrom N, Allman RM, Alvarez OM, et al. *Clinical Practice Guideline: Treatment of Pressure Ulcers AHRQ Publication No. 95-06-0652*. Rockville MD: US Department of Health and Human Services Public Health Service Agency for Health Care Policy and Research (AHCPR) now Agency for Health Care Research and Quality (AHRQ);1994:15.
2. Taler G, Bauman T, Breeding C, et al. *Pressure Ulcers: Clinical Practice Guideline*. Columbia, MD: American Medical Directors Association; 1996.
3. Ovington LG. Dressings and adjunctive therapies: AHCPR Guidelines Revisited. *Ostomy Wound Manage* 1999;45(suppl 1A):94s–106s.
4. Garber SL, Biddle AK, Click CN, et al. *Pressure Ulcer Prevention and Treatment Following Spinal Cord Injury: Clinical Practice Guideline for Health-Care Professionals*. Jackson Heights, NY: Paralyzed Veterans of America; 2000.
5. National Pressure Ulcer Advisory Panel and European Pressure Ulcer Advisory Panel (EPUAP) (2009). *Pressure Ulcers Prevention and Treatment: Clinical Practice Guideline*. Washington, DC: National Pressure Ulcer Advisory Panel.
6. National Coverage Decision for Electrical Stimulation (ES) and Electromagnetic Therapy for the Treatment of Wounds. Vol 270.1; 2004.
7. Reddy M, Gill SS, et al. Treatment of pressure ulcers a systematic review. *JAMA* 2008;300(22):2647–2662.
8. Lundeberg TCM, Eriksson SV, Mats M. Electrical nerve stimulation improves healing of diabetic ulcers. *Ann Plast Surg* 1992;29(4):328–330.
9. Polak A, Franek A, Hunika-Zurawinska W, et al. High voltage electrostimulation in treatment of venous crural ulceration. *Wiadomosci Lekarskie* 2000;LIII:7–8.
10. Houghton PE, Kincaid CB, Lovell M, et al. Effect of electrical stimulation on chronic leg ulcer size and appearance. *Phys Ther* 2003;83(1):17–28.
11. Goldman R, Rosen M, Brewley B, et al. Electrotherapy promotes healing and microcirculation of infrapopliteal ischemic wounds: a prospective pilot study. *Adv Skin Wound Care* 2004;17:284–290.
12. Kloth L, Alon G, Baker L, et al. Electrotherapeutic terminology. In: *Physical Therapy*. Alexandria, VA: Section on Clinical Electrophysiology, American Physical Therapy Association; 1990.
13. Alon G. Principles of electrical stimulation. In: Nelson R, Hayes KW, Currier DP, eds. *Clinical Electrotherapy*. 3rd ed. Stamford, CT: Appleton & Lange; 1999:55–124.
14. Newton RA, Karselis TC. Skin pH following high voltage pulsed galvanic stimulation. *Phys Ther* 1983;63(10):1593–1596.
15. Reich J, Tarjan P. Electrical stimulation of skin. *Int J Dermatol.* 1990;29(6):395–400.
16. Reich J, Cazzaniga A, Tarjan P, et al. The reporting and characterization of exogenous electric fields. In: Brighton C, Pollack SR, eds. *Electromagnetics in Biology and Medicine*. San Francisco, CA: San Francisco Press, Inc.; 1991:355–360.
17. Mertz PM. Electrical stimulation and wound healing: commentary. *Wounds Compend Clin Res Pract* 2000;12(6):172–173.
18. Feedar JA, Kloth LC, Gentzkow GD. Chronic dermal ulcer healing enhanced with monophasic pulsed electrical stimulation. *Phys Ther* 1991;7(19):639–649.
19. Alon G, Robinson AJ, Spielholz N, et al. *Electrotherapeutic Terminology in Physical Therapy*. 2 ed. Alexandria, VA: American Physical Therapy Association; 2000.
20. Alon G, De Domenico G. High voltage stimulation: an integrated approach to clinical electrotherapy. *Hixton,* TN: The Chattanooga Group; 1987.
21. Alon G. lecture "Current Classification" 1986.
22. Kumar D, Alvaro MS, Julka IS, et al. Diabetic peripheral neuropathy effectiveness of electrotherapy and amitriptyline for symptomatic relief. *Diabetes Care* 1998;21(8):1322–1325.
23. Julka IS, Alvaro MS, Kumar D. Beneficial effects of electrical stimulation on neuropathic symptoms in diabetes patients. *J Foot Ankle Surg*1998;37(3):191–194.
24. Alon G. Principles of electrical stimulation. In: Nelson R, Currier D, eds. *Clinical Electrotherapy* Norwalk, CT: Appleton & Lange; 1991:35–114.
25. Medical and Surgical Procedures Panel. *Medicare Coverage Policy-MCAC: Electrical Stimulation for the Treatment of Wounds*. Baltimore, MD: Health Care Financing Administration; 2000:1–73.
26. Griffin JW, Tooms RE, Mendius SK, et al. Efficacy of high voltage pulsed current for healing of pressure ulcers in patients with spinal cord injury. *Phys Ther* 1991;71:433–444.
27. Kloth L, Feedar J. Acceleration of wound healing with high voltage, monophasic, pulsed current. *Phys Ther* 1988;68:503–508.

28. Gentzkow G, Pollack S, Kloth L, et al. Improved healing of pressure ulcers using dermapulse, a new electrical stimulation device. *Wounds* 1991;3(5):158–170.

29. Kloth LC Wound Healing with conductive electrical stimulation. It's the dosage that counts. *Wound Technology* 2009;6:30–37.

30. Wood JM, Evans PE III, et al. A multicenter study on the use of pulsed low intensity direct current for healing chronic Stage II and Stage III ulcers. *Arch Dermatol* 1993;130(5):660–661.

31. Newton RA. High-voltage pulsed current: theoretical bases and clinical applications. In: Nelson R, Currier D, eds. *Clinical Electrotherapy*. Norwalk, CT: Appleton & Lange. 1991:201–220.

32. Gersh M. Microcurrent electrical stimulation: putting it in perspective. *Clin Manage* 1989;9(4):51–54.

33. Bassett CAL, Pawluk RJ, Becker RO. Effects of electric currents on bone in vivo. *Nature* 1964;204:652–654.

34. Bassett CAL, Becker RO. Generation of electric potentials by bone in response to mechanical stress. *Science* 1962;137:1063.

35. Friedenberg B, Roberts PG, Didizian NH, et al. Stimulation of fracture healing by direct current in the rabbit fibula. *J Bone Joint Surg* 1971;53A:1400–1408.

36. Bassett CAL. Electromechanical factors regulating bone architecture. In: Fleish R, Backwood HJJ, Owen M, eds. *Third European Symposium on Calcified Tissues*. New York: Berlin, Springer-Verlag; 1966:78.

37. Friedenberg ZB, Kohanim M. The effect of direct current on bone. *Surg Gynecol Obstet* 1968;127:97–102.

38. Friedenberg ZB, Harlow MC, Brighton CT. Healing of nonunion of the medial malleolus by means of direct current: a case report. 1971;11:883–885.

39. Brighton CT. Current concepts review: the treatment of nonunions with electricity. *J Bone Joint Surg* 1981;63-A:847–851.

40. Goh JCH, Bose K, Kang YK. et al. Effects of electrical stimulation on the biomechanical properties of fracture healing in rabbits. *Clin Orthop* 1998;223:268–273.

41. Jaffe LS, Vanable JW. Electric fields and wound healing. *Clin Dermatol* 1984;3:34.

42. American Physical Therapy Association. Guide to physical therapist practice. *Phys Ther* 2001;81(1):S695.

43. Bogie KM, Reger SI, Levine SP, et al. Electrical stimulation for pressure sore prevention and wound healing. *Asst Technol.* 2000;12(1):50–66.

44. Baker LL, ed. Electrical stimulation to increase functional activity. In: *Clinical Electrotherapy*. Stamford, CT, Appleton and Lange; 1999.

45. Petrofsky JS. The effect of the subcutaneous fat on the transfer of current through skin and into muscle. *Med Eng Phys* 2008;30:1168–1176.

46. Petrofsky J, Schwab E, et al. Effects of electrical stimulation on skin blood flow in controls and in and around stage III and IV wounds in hairy and non hairy skin. *Med Sci Monit* 2005;11:CR309–CR316.

47. Petrofsky J, Suh H, et al. A multi-channel stimulator and electrode array providing a rotating current whirlpool for electrical stimulation of wounds. J Med Eng Technol 2008;32(5):371–384.

48. Cook T, Barr JO. Instrumentation. In: Nelson R, Currier D, eds. *Clinical Electrotherapy*. Norwalk, CT: Appleton & Lange; 1991:11–33.

49. Gentzkow G, Miller K. Electrical stimulation for dermal wound healing. *Clin Podiatr Med Surg* 1991;8:827–841.

50. Byl N. Electrical stimulation for tissue repair: basic information. In: Nelson R, Hayes KW, Currier DP, eds. *Clinical Electrotherapy*. Samford, CT, Appleton & Lange; 1999.

51. Cheng K, Mertz PM, Tarjan P. Theoretical study of rectangular pulse electrical stimulation (RPES) on skin cells (in vivo) under conforming electrodes. Paper presented at: Biomedical Sciences Instrumentation; April 23, 1993.

52. Sumano H, Mateos G. The use of acupuncture-like electrical stimulation for wound healing of lesions unresponsive to conventional treatment. *Am J Acupunct* 1999;27(1/2):5:14.

53. Orinda N FJ. Directional protrusive pseudopodial activity and motility in macrophages induced by extracellular electric fields. *Cell Motil* 1982;2:243–255.

54. Cho MR, Thatte HS, Lee RC, et al. Integrin-dependent human macrophage migration induced by oscillatory electrical stimulation. *Ann Biomed Eng* 2000;28(3):234–243.

55. Fukushima, Senda N, Inui H, et al. Study of galvanotaxis of leukocytes. *Med J Osaka Univ* 1953;4:195–208.

56. Kloth LC. Electrical stimulation in tissue repair. In: McCulloch J, Kloth L, Feedar J, eds. *Wound Healing Alternatives in Management*. 2nd ed. Philadelphia, PA: FA Davis; 1995:275–310.

57. Weiss D, Eaglestein W, Falanga V. Exogenous electric current can reduce the formation of hypertrophic scars. *J Dermatol Surg Oncol* 1989;15:1272–1275.

58. Bourguignon GJ, Bourguignon LYW. Electric stimulation of protein and DNA synthesis in human fibroblasts. *FASEB J* 1987;1:398–402.

59. Erickson CA, Nuccitelli R. Embryonic fibroblast motility and orientation can be influenced by physiological electrical fields. *J Cell Biol* 1984;98:296–307.

60. Yang W, et al. Response of C3H/10T1/2 fibroblasts to an external steady electric field stimulation. *Exp Cell Res* 1984;155:92–104

61. Stromberg BV. Effects of electrical currents on wound contraction. *Ann Plast Surg* 1988;21(2):121–123.

62. Cooper MS, Schliwa M. Electrical and ionic controls of tissue cell locomotion in DC electrical fields. *J Cell Physiol* 1995;103:363–370.

63. Nishimura KY, Isseroff R, Nuccitelli R. Human Keratinocytes migrate to the negative pole in direct current electric fields comparable to those measure in mammalian wounds. *J Cell Sci* 1996;109:199–207.

64. Mohr T, Akers T, Wessman HC. Effect of high voltage stimulation on blood flow in the rat hind limb. *Phys Ther* 1987;67:528–533.

65. Bourguignon GJ, Jy W, Bourguignon LYW. Electric stimulation of human fibroblasts causes an increase in Ca2+ influx and the exposure of additional insulin receptors. *J Cell Physiol* 1989;140:379–385.

66. Zhao M, Pu J, Forrester JV, Et al. Membrane lipids, EGF receptors, and intracellular signals colocalize and are polarized in epithelial cells moving directionally in a physiological electric field. *FASEB J* 2002;16(8):857–859.

67. Lin F, Baldessari F, et al. Lymphocyte electrotaxis in vitro and in vivo. *J Immunol* 2008;181:2465–2471.

68. Ferrier J, Ross SM, Kanehisa J, et al. Osteoclasts and osteoblasts migrate in opposite directions in response to a constant electrical field. *J Cell Physiol.* 1986;129:283–288.

69. Byl NN, McKenzie A, Wong T, et al. Incisional wound healing: a controlled study of low and high-dose ultrasound. *J Orthoped Sports Phys Ther* 1993;18(5):619–627.

70. Byl NN, McKenzie A, West JM, et al. Low-dose ultrasound effects on ultrasound healing: a controlled study with Yucatan pigs. *Arch Phys Med Rehabil* 1992;73:656–664.

71. Brown M, McDonnell M, Menton DN. Polarity effects on wound healing using electrical stimulation in rabbits. *Arch Phys Med Rehabil* 1989;70:624–627.

72. Alvarez O. The healing of superficial skin wounds is stimulated by external electrical current. *J Invest Dermato* 1983;8(12):144–148.

73. Agren MS, Engel MA, et al. Collagenase during burn wound healing: influence of a hydrogel dressing and pulsed electrical stimulation. *Plast Reconstr Surg* 1994;94(3):518–524.

74. Wolf J. Das *Gesetz der Transformatin der Knochen*. Berlin, Germany: Hirschwald; 1897.

75. Forrester JC, et al. Wolf's law in relation to the healing of skin wound. *J Trauma* 1970;10:770–778.

76. Mehri M, Helme R, Khalil A. Age related changes in sympathetic modulation of sensory nerve activity in rat skin. *Infamm Res* 1998;47(6):239–244.

77. Politis MJ, Zankis MF, Miller JE. Enhanced survival of full-thickness skin grafts following the application of DC electrical fields. *Plast Reconstr Surg* 1989;84(2):67–72.

78. Pollack S. The effects of pulsed electrical stimulation on failing skin flaps in Yorkshire pigs. Paper presented at the Meeting of the Bioelectrical Repair and Growth Society, Cleveland, OH; 1989.

79. Lundeberg T, Kjartansson J, Samuelsson U. Effect of electrical nerve stimulation on healing of ischemic skin flaps. *Lancet* 1988;2:712–714.

80. Im MJ, Lee WPA, Hoopes JE. Effect of electrical stimulation on survival of skin flaps in pigs. *Phys Ther* 1990;70:37–40.

81. Hecker BCH, Schwartz DP. Pulsed Galvanic Stimulation: Effects of current frequency and polarity on blood flow in health subjects. *Arch Phys Med Rehabil* 1985;66:369–371.

82. Cramp A, Gilsensan C, Lowe A, et al. The effect of high and low frequency transcutaneous electrical nerve stimulation upon cutaneous blood flow and skin temperature in healthy subjects. *Clin Physiol* 2000;20(2):150–157.

83. Wikstrom S, Svedman P, Svensson H, et al. Effect of transcutaneous nerve stimulation on microcirculation in intact skin and blister wounds in healthy volunteers. *Scand J Plastic Reconstr Surg Hand Surg* 1999;33(2):195–201.

84. Kaada B. Promoted healing of chronic ulceration by transcutaneous nerve stimulation (TNS). *Vasa* 1983;12:262–269.

85. Kaada B. Vasodilation induced by transcutaneous nerve stimulation in peripheral ischemia (Reynaud's phenomena and diabetic polyneuropathy). *Eur Heart J* 1982;3(4):303–314.

86. Cosmo P, Svensson H, Bornmyr S, et al. Effect of transcutaneous nerve stimulation on the microcirculation in chronic leg ulcers. *Scan J Plast Reconstr Surg Hand Surg* 2000;34:61–64.

87. Mawson A, Siddiqui F, Connolly G, et al. Effect of high voltage pulsed galvanic stimulation on sacral transcutaneous oxygen tension levels in the spinal cord injured. *Paraplegia* 1993;31(5):311–319.

88. Mawson AR, Siddiqui FH, Connolly B, et al. Sacral transcutaneous oxygen tension levels in the spinal cord injured: risk factors for pressure ulcers. *Arch Phys Med Rehabil* 1993;74(7):745–751.

89. Kim J, Ho CH, et al. The use of sensory electrical stimulation for pressure ulcer prevention. *Physiother Theory Pract* 2010;26(8):528–536.

90. Twist D. Acrocyanosis in a spinal cord injured patient-effect of computer-controlled neuromuscular electrical stimulation: a case report. *Phys Ther* 1990;70:45:49.

91. Thomas AJ, Davis GM, Sutton JR. Cardiovascular and metabolic responses to electrical stimulation-induced leg exercise in spinal cord injury. *Methods Med* 1997;36(4–5):372–375.

92. Raymond J, Davis GM, Bryant G, et al. Cardiovascular responses to an orthostatic challenge and electrical-stimulation-induced leg muscle contractions in individuals with paraplegia. *Eur J Appl Physiol Occup Physiol* 1999;80(3):201–212.

93. Phillips W, Burkett LN, Munroi R, et al. Relative changes in blood flow with functional electrical stimulation during exercise of the paralyzed lower limbs. *Paraplegia* 1995;33:90–93.

94. Faghri PD, Votto JJ, Hovorka CF. Venous hemodynamics of the lower extremity in response to electrical stimulation. *Arch Phys Med Rehabil* 1998;79:842–848.

95. Moloney CM, G. Lyons, et al. Haemodynamic study examining the response of venous blood flow to electrical stimulation of the gastrocnemius muscle in patients with chronic venous disease. *Eur J Vasc Endovasc Surg* 2006;31:300–305.

96. Wolcott L, Wheeler P, Hardwicke H, et al. Accelerated healing of skin ulcers by electrotherapy: preliminary clinical results. *South Med J* 1969;62:795–801.

97. Lawson D, Petrofsky J. A randomized control study on the effect of biphasic electrical stimulation in a warm room on skin blood flow and healing rates in chronic wounds of patients with and without diabetes. *Med Sci Monit* 2007;13(6):CR258–CR263.

98. Baker LL. The effect of electrical stimulation on cutaneous oxygen supply. *Rehabil Res Dev Prog Rep* 1988;176.

99. Baker LL, Chamber R, Merchant L, et al. The effects of electrical stimulation on cutaneous oxygen supply in normal older adults and diabetic patients. *Phys Ther* 1986;66:749.

100. Forst T, Pfutzner A, Bauersachs R, et al. Comparison of the microvascular response to transcuteinous electrical nerve stimulation and post occlusive ischemia in the diabetic foot. *J Diabetes Complications* 1997;11(5):291–297.

101. Peters EJ, Armstrong DG, Wunderlich RP, et al. The benefit of electrical stimulation to enhance perfusion in persons with diabetes mellitus. *J Foot Ankle Surg* 1998;37(5):396–400.

102. Byl N, McKenzie A, West J, et al. Microamperage stimulation: effects on subcutaneous oxygen (II). Presented at the Annual Conference of the California Chapter of the American Physical Therapy Association, San Diego, CA; 1990.

103. Goldman RJ, Brewley BI, Golden MA. Electrotherapy reoxygenates inframalleolar ischemic wounds on diabetic patients: a case series. *Adv Skin Wound Care* 2002;15:112–120.

104. Junger M, Arnold A, et al. Local therapy and treatment costs of chronic, venous leg ulcers with electrical stimulation (Dermapulses): a prospective, placebo controlled, double blind trial. *Wound Rep Reg* 2008;16:480–487.

105. Goldman R, Brewley B, Zhou L, et al. Electrotherapy Reverses Inframalleolar Ischemia: a retrospective observational study. *Adv Skin Wound Care* 2003;16:79–89.

106. Reed BV. Effect of high voltage pulsed electrical stimulation on microvascular permeability to plasma proteins: a possible mechanism in minimizing edema. *Phys Ther* 1998;68:491–495.

107. Mendel F, Fish D. New perspectives in edema control via electrical stimulation. *J Athlet Train* 1993;28:63–74.

108. Thornton RM, Mendel FC, Fish DR. Effects of electrical stimulation on edema formation in different strains of rats. *Phys Ther* 1998;78:386–394.

109. Matylevich NP, Chu CS, McManus AT, et al. Direct current reduces plasma protein extravasation after partial thickness burn injury in rats. *J Trauma* 1996;4(3):424–429.

110. Chu CS, Matylevich NP, McManus AT, et al. Direct current reduces wound edema after full-thickness burn injury in rats. *J Trauma* 1996;40(5):738–742.

111. Snyder AR, Perotti AL, et al. The influence of high-voltage electrical stimulation on edema formation after acute injury: a systematic review. *J Sport Rehabil* 2010;19(4):436–451.

112. Ross C, Segal D. HVPC as an aid to post-operative healing. *Curr Podiatry* 1981;50:19–25.

113. Fakhri O, Amin MA. The effect of low-voltage electric therapy on the healing of resistant skin burns. *J Burn Care Rehabil* 1987;8(1):15–18.

114. Edgar DW, Fish JS, et al. local and systemic treatments for acute edema after burn injury: a systematic review of the literature. *J Burn Care Res* 2011 (Ahead of publication).

115. Griffin JW, Newsome LS, et al. Reduction of chronic posttraumatic hand edema: A comparison of high voltage pulsed current, intermittent pneumatic compression and placebo treatments. *Phys Ther* 1990;70:279–286.

116. Sawyer PN. Bioelectric phenomena and intravascular thrombosis: the first 12 years. *Surgery* 1964;56:1020–1026.

117. Sawyer PN, Deutch B. The experimental use of oriented electrical fields to delay and prevent intravascular thrombosis. *Surg Forum* 1995;5:163–168.

118. Sawyer PN, Deutch B. Use of electrical currents to delay intravascular thrombosis in experimental animals. *Am J Physiol* 1956;187(473–478).

119. Franek A, Polak A, Kucharzewski M. Modern application of high voltage stimulation for enhanced healing of venous crural ulceratio. *Med Eng Phys* 2000;22:647–655.

120. Barranco S, Spadaro J, Berger TJ, et al. In vitro effect of weak direct current on staphylococcus aureus. *Clin Orthop* 1974;100:250–255.

121. Rowley BA McKenna J, Chase G. The influence of electrical current on an infecting microorganism in wounds. *Ann NY Acad Sci* 1974;238:543–551.

122. Kincaid CB, Lavoie K. Inhibition of bacterial growth in vitro following stimulation with high voltage, monophasic, pulsed current. *Phys Ther* 1989;69:29–33.

123. Szuminsky NJ, Albers AC, Unger P, et al. Effect of narrow, pulsed high voltages on bacterial viability. *Phys Ther* 1994;74:660–667.

124. Kloth LC. Bactericidal effect of passing an electrical current through a silver wire [poster presentation]. Presented at the Symposium on Advanced Wound Care; Atlanta, GA; April 1996.

125. Knighton DR, Halliday B, et al. Oxygen as an antibiotic: the effect of inspired oxygen on infection. *Arch Surg* 1984;119:199–204.

126. Thurman BF, Christian E. Response of a serious circulatory lesion to electrical stimulation. *Phys Ther* 1971;51(10):137–140.

127. Gault W, Gatens, PF. Use of Low intensity direct current in management of ischemic skin ulcers. *Phys Ther* 1976;56(3):141–145.

128. Webster DA, Spadaro JA, Becker RO, et al. Silver anode treatment of chronic osteomyelitis. *Clin Orthop Relat Res* 1981;161:106–114.

129. Fitzgerald GK, Newsome D. Treatment of a large infected thoracic spine wound using high voltge pulsed monophasic current. *Phys Ther* 1993;73(6):355–360.

130. Costerton JW, Ellis B, Lam K, et al. Mechanisms of electrical enhancement of efficacy of antibiotics in killing biofilm bacteria. *Antimicrob Agents Chemother* 1994;38(12):2803–2809.

131. Chu CS, McManus AT, Pruitt BA Jr, et al. Therapeutic effects of silver nylon dressings with weak direct current on Pseudomonas aeruginosa-infected burn wounds. *J Trauma* 1998;28(10):1488–1492.

132. Huckfeldt R, Flick A B, et al. Wound closure after split-thickness skin grafting is accelerated with the use of continuous direct anodal microcurrent applied to silver nylonwound contact dressings. *J Burn Care Res* 2007;28: 703–707.

133. Houghton PE, Campbell KE, et al. Electrical stimulation therapy increases rate of healing of pressure ulcers in community-dwelling people with spinal cord injury. *Arch Phys Med Rehabil* 2010;91:669–678.

134. Jin DM, Xu Y, et al. Effect of transcutaneous electrical nerve stimulation on symptomatic diabetic peripheral neuropathy: a meta-analysis of randomized controlled trials. *Diabetes Res Clin Pract* 2010;89(1):10–15.

135. Kupers R, Laere KV, et al. Multimodal therapeutic assessment of peripheral nerve stimulation in neuropathic pain: five case reports with a 20-year follow-up. *Eur J Pain* 2010;15(2):161–169.

136. Koyama T, McHaffie JG, et al. The subjective experience of pain: where expectations become reality. *Proc Natl Acad Sci* 2005;102(36):12950–12955.

137. Jankovic A, Bini I. Frequency rhythmic electrical modulation system in the treatment of chronic painful leg ulcers. *Arch Dermatol Res* 2008;300:377–383.

138. Carley PJ, Wainapel SF. Electrotherapy for acceleration of wound healing: low intensity direct current. *Arch Phys Med Rehabil* 1995;66(7):443–446.

139. Castillo E, Sumano H, Fortoul TI, et al. The influence of pulsed electrical stimulation on the wound healing of burned rat skin. *Arch Med Res* 1995;26(2):185–189.

140. Adamian AA, Shloznikov BM, Muzykant LI, et al. Clinicomorphological changes in a burn wound after electric stimulation with pulsatile current. *Khururgiia(Mosk)* 1990;1990(6):77–81.

141. Bach S, Bilgrave K, Gottrup F, et al. The effect of electrical current on healing skin incision. An experimental study. *Eur J Surg.* 1991;157(3):171–174.

142. Reger SI, Hyodo A, Negami S, et al. Experimental wound healing with electrical stimulation. *Artif Organs* 1999;23(5):460–462.

143. Byl N, McKenzie A, West J, et al. Pulsed micro amperage stimulation: a controlled study of healing of surgically induced wounds in Yucatan pigs. *Phys Ther* 1994;74:201–218.

144. Leffmann DJ, Arnall DA, Holmgren PR. Effect of microamperage stimulation on the rate of wound healing in rats: a histological study. *Phys Ther* 1994;74:195–200.

145. Stefanovska A, Vodovnik L, Benko H, et al. Treatment of chronic wounds by means of electrical and electromagnetic fields, 2: value of FES parameters for pressure sore treatment. *Med Biol Eng Comput* 1993;31:213–220.

146. Frantz RA. Nursing intervention: healing pressure ulcers with TENS, submitted.

147. Gogia P, Marquez R, Minerbo G. Effects of high voltage galvanic stimulation on wound healing. *Ostomy/Wound Manage* 1992;38(1):29–35.

148. Peters EJ, Lavery LA, Armstrong DG, et al. Electric stimulation as an adjunct to heal diabetic foot ulcers: a randomized clinical trial. *Arch Phys Med Rehabil* 2001;82:721–725.

149. Franek A, Kostur R, et al. Effect of high voltage monophasic stimulation on pressure ulcer healing: results from a randomized controlled trial. *Wounds Compend Clin Res Pract* 2011;23(1):15–23.

150. Alon G, Azaria M, Stein H. Diabetic ulcer healing using high voltage TENS. *Phys Ther* 1986;66:77. Abstract.

151. Akers T, Gabrielson A. The effect of high voltage galvanic stimulation on the rate of healing of decubitus ulcers. *Biomed Sci Instrum J* 1984;20:99–100.

152. Katelaris PM, Fletcher JP, Little JM, et al. Electrical stimulation in the treatment of chronic venous ulceration. *Aust NZ J Surg* 1987;57(9):605–607.

153. Khalil Z, Merhi M. Effects of aging on neurogenic vasodilator responses evoked by transcutaneous electrical nerve stimulation: relevance to wound healing. *J Gerontology biol Sci Med Sci* 2000;55(6):B257–263.

154. Baker LL, Rubayi S, Villar F, et al. Effect of electrical stimulation waveform on healing of ulcers in human beings with spinal cord injury. *Wound Rep Reg* 1996;4:21–28.

155. Baker LL, Chambers R, Demuth S, et al. Effects of electrical stimulation on wound healing in patients with diabetic ulcers. *Diabetes Care* 1997;20(3):1–8.

156. Barron JJ, Jacobson WE, Tidd T. Treatment of decubitus ulcers. *Minn Med* 1985;68(2):103–106.

157. Petrofsky J, Lawson D, et al. Effects of a 2, 3, and 4 electrode stimulator design on current dispersion on the surface and into the limb during electrical stimulation in controls and patients with wounds. *J Med Eng Technol* 2008;32(6):485–497.

158. Petrofsky J, Lawson D, et al. Enhanced healing of diabetic foot ulcers using local heat and electrical stimulation for 30 min three times per week. *J Diabetes* 2009;2:1–6.

159. Petrofsky JF, Lawson D, et al. The influence of local versus global heat on the healing of chronic wounds in patients with diabetes. *Diabetes Technol Ther* 2007;9(6):535–544.

160. Gardner SE, Frantz RA, Schmidt FL. Effect of electrical stimulation on chronic wound healing: a meta-analysis. *Wound Repair Regen* 1999;7(6):495–503.

161. Alon G, Smith GV. Kid Care: helping heal with E-Stim. *Adv Directors Rehabil* 1999(March):47–50.

162. Barr JO. Transcutaneous electric nerve stimulation for pain management. In: Nelson R, Currier D, eds. *Clinical Electrotherapy*. Norwalk, CT: Appleton & Lange; 1991:280.

163. Chen D, Philip M, Phillip PA, et al. Cardiac pacemaker inhibition by transcutaneous electrical nerve stimulation. *Arch Phys Med Rehabil* 1990;71(1):27–30.

164. Donayre C. Diagnosis and management of vascular ulcers: arterial, venous and diabetic. Presented at Wound Care Management 96; Torrance, CA; October 1996.

165. Shade SK. Use of transcutaneous electrical nerve stimulation for a patient with a cardiac pacemaker. A case report. *Phys Ther* 1985;65(2):206–208.

166. Sliwa JA, Marinko MS. Transcutaneous electrical nerve stimulatorinduced electrocardiogram artifact. A brief report. *Am J Phys Med Rehabil* 1996;75(4):307–309.

167. Eaglestein W. Off-label uses in wound care. Paper presented at the Symposium on Advanced Wound Care; Atlanta, GA; April 1996.

168. Brown M. Electrical stimulation for wound management. In Gogia PP, ed. *Clinical Wound Management*. Thorofare, NJ: Slack, Inc.; 1995:176–183.

169. Petrofsky J, Prowse M, et al. Estimation of the distribution of intramuscular current during electrical stimulation of the quadriceps muscle. *Eur J Appl Physiol* 2008;103:265–273.

170. Unger PC. A randomized clinical trial of the effect of HVPC on wound healing. *Phys Ther* 1991;71(suppl):S1118.

171. Unger PC, Eddy J, Raimastry S. A controlled study of the effect of high voltage pulsed current (HVPC) on wound healing. *Phys Ther* 1991;71(suppl):S119.

172. Kloth LC. Electrical stimulation for wound healing. Exhibitor presentation at American Physical Therapy Association Conference; Minneapolis, MN; June 1996.

173. Burdge J, Hartman JF, Wright L. A retrospective study of high voltage, pulsed current as an adjunctive therapy in limb salvage for chronic diabetic wounds of the lower extremity. *Ostom Wound Manage* 2009;55(8):30–38.

174. Davis S. The effect of pulsed electrical stimulation on epidermal wound healing. *J Invest Dermatol* 90:555.

175. Myer A. Observable effects on granulation tissue using warmed wound care products. Presented at Symposia, "Future Directions in Wound Healing"; American Physical Therapy Association Scientific Meeting; June 1997; San Diego, CA.

176. Lock P. The effect of temperature on mitosis at the edge of experimental wounds. In: Lundgren A, Sover A, eds. *Symposia on Wound Healing: Plastic, Surgical and Dermatologic Aspects*. Sweden: Molndal; 1980.

177. Myers JA. Wound Healing and use of modern surgical dressing. *Pharm J* 1982;229:103–104.

178. Thomas ST. *Wound Management and Dressings*. London: The Pharmaceutical Press; 1990.

179. Selkowitz DM. Electrical currents. In: Cameron MH, ed. *Physical Agents in Rehabilitation*. Philadelphia, PA: WB Saunders; 1999;402.

180. Bourguignon GL, et al. Occlusive wound dressings suitable for use with electrical stimulation. *Wounds* 1991;3(3):127.

181. Alon G. Antibiotics enhancement by transcutaneous electrical stimulation. Presented at Symposia, "Future Directions in Wound Healing"; American Physical Therapy Association Scientific Meeting, San Diego, CA; June 1997.

182. Williams RD, Carey LC. Studies in the production of "standard" venous thrombosis. *Ann Surg* 1959;149:381–387.

183. Baker L, Dogen P, Johnson B, et al. The effects of electrical stimulation on cutaneous oxygen supply in diabetic older adults. *Phys Ther* 1987;67:773.

184. Owoeye I, Spielholtz NI, Fetto J, et al. Low intensity pulsed galvanic current and the healing of tenotomized rat Achilles tendons: preliminary report using lead to break measurements. *Arch Phys Med Rehabil* 1987:415–418.

185. Dodgen PW, Johnson BW, Baker LL, et al. The effects of electrical stimulation on cutaneous oxygen supply in diabetic older adults. *Phys Ther* 1987;67(5):S4.

186. Rasmussen MJ, Hayes DL, Vlieststra RE, et al. Can transcutaneous electrical nerve stimulation be safely used in patients with permanent cardiac pacemakers? *Mayo Clin Proc* 1998;63:443–445.

187. Petrofsky JS, Lawson D, et al. Enhanced healing of diabetic foot ulcers using local heat and electrical stimulation for 30 min three times per week. *J Diabetes* 2010;2(1):41–46.

188. Gilcreast D, Stotts N, Baker L. Effect of electrical stimulation on foot skin perfusion in persons with or at risk for diabetic foot ulcers. *Wound Repair Regen* 1998;6(5):434:441.

189. Gentzkow GD, Alon G, Taler G, et al. Healing of refractory stage III and IV pressure ulcers by a new electrical stimulation device. *Wounds Compend Clin Res Pract*. 1993;5(3):160–172.

190. Adegoke B, Badmos KA. Acceleration of pressure ulcer healing in spinal cord injured patients using interrupted direct current. *Afr J Med Sci* 2001;30(3):195–197.

191. Suh HJ, Petrofsky JS, Takkin L, Lawson D, et al. The Combined Effect of a Three-Channel Electrode Delivery System with Local Heat on the Healing of Chronic Wounds. *Diabetes Technology and Therapeutics*. 2009;11(10):681–688.

CHAPTER 24

Radio Frequency and Electromagnetic Energy

Carrie Sussman

CHAPTER OBJECTIVES

CHAPTER OBJECTIVES

At the completion of this chapter, the reader will be able to:

1. Describe the physical properties of electromagnetic energy that render an electromagnetic field signal bioeffective.
2. Identify and differentiate between the physiologic effects of thermal and nonthermal use of electromagnetic energy for wound healing.
3. Evaluate electromagnetic energy device potential efficacy based on their potential benefits for wound healing based on the evidence gathered and analyzed from animal and human studies.
4. Evaluate a patient's candidacy for application of electromagnetic energy based on medical history, wound indications, precautions, and contraindications.
5. Prepare a patient for treatment with thermal and nonthermal electromagnetic devices and evaluate outcomes of care.

Electromagnetic energy in medicine has a greater than 100-year history. At the turn of the 20th century, an electromagnetic device using electromagnetic energy from the short radio wave segment of the EMS was developed and was called *diathermy*. Diathermy was a first-generation continuous electromagnetic wave device that used an induced electrical field to generate heat in tissues. The term *diathermy*, introduced by Nagelschmidt, was meant to describe the relatively uniform deep heating (heating through) produced in tissue by the conversion of high-frequency electromagnetic currents into heat.[1] In the following decades, diathermy was the common name and it was used to treat all types of illnesses and injuries including wounds. However, the heating properties were not always beneficial or the only useful aspects. Therefore, engineers in the late 1950s and 1960s designed the second generation of devices so as to virtually eliminate the heating aspect and deliver primarily nonthermal electromagnetic energy. In early studies, this was labeled as *diathermy athermal*, but this is incorrect based on the law of physics that says when you convert one form of energy to another some heat is produced. Thus we have another term, *diathermy nonthermal*, to indicate that heating of the tissues is not measurable. This technology has even more names, which will be sorted out in the first chapter section.

One extremely important finding, reported by Erdman in 1960, showed that the application of pulsed electromagnetic field (PEMF) induced electrical current in the body could increase blood flow to the tissues without the necessity of heating the tissues.[2] Pulsed diathermy (electromagnetic field [EMF]) devices, also electrotherapy devices, were an improvement over devices based on continuous waves. These devices used less power, had a limited radiofrequency (RF) radiation pattern due to improved antenna and circuit design, and did not interfere with other electrical devices such as those used in hospitals. Electromagnetic therapy must not be confused with the static magnets, or bar magnets, that have recently become so popular for pain treatment and which lack evidence for the purposes of wound care.[3]

During the 1960s and 1970s, many clinical studies used animals and biologic systems to determine the possible biologic mechanisms of the action of electromagnetism on tissue. Most were labeled athermal diathermy or by manufacturer name (e.g., Diapulse Therapy, Diapulse Corporation of America, Great Neck, NY). Unfortunately, many of these studies were not blinded, controlled, or randomized. In the past 30 years, there have been case studies, clinical trials, and some randomized clinical trials with both animal and human subjects designed to determine the effects of electromagnetic stimulation on the biologic aspects of wound healing and wound closure.

As a result of this work, a series of third-, and now fourth-generation nonthermic RF devices have been developed that use microelectronics that allow the generators to be miniaturized, programed, battery operated, single patient use and disposable, that are inexpensive while at the same time delivering directed, concentrated energy to the tissues based on research findings.

In this chapter, we are going to examine the use of this biophysical technology as a clinical tool for wound healing. We begin the first chapter section with the biophysical properties and terminology of EMF to facilitate your searching and reading of the chapter and the literature. Next step is to explain the interrelationships between the various stimulation properties and research questions and results, followed by clinical decision making and treatment.

BIOPHYSICAL PROPERTIES OF ELECTROMAGNETIC FIELDS

It is the goal in this section to make the terminology comprehensible, and to connect it with demonstrated effects in wound healing, we begin by defining the biophysical properties of EMFs: carrier frequency and waveforms, pulse rates and duration, duty cycle, and amplitude/intensity (see Table 24.1).

Electromagnetic Fields

The energy we are studying in this chapter comes from one small portion of the electromagnetic spectrum (EMS) (sometimes referred to as the *radio, radiation,* or *radio frequency spectrum*) (see Fig. 24.1). In its entirety, the spectrum ranges in energy from below power transmission waves (very low frequency) to above cosmic rays (very high frequency), and includes radio waves, microwaves, visible light, infrared, ultraviolet light, and x-rays. All frequencies within the spectrum have certain characteristics in common. For example, they all travel at the speed of light, which is 300,000 km (186,000 mi) per second. They all travel unimpeded through a vacuum. They

are "pure energy" and do not have any mass. They all consist of two parts, a magnetic field and an electrostatic field, traveling at right angles to each other. A radio wave is induced when an alternating current (AC) flows through a coil or antennae and generates an EMF suitable for wireless broadcasting and/or communications or medical applications.[4]

One of many important differences between waves from different portions of the spectrum is what happens when they encounter an object. Are they absorbed (like infrared heat waves)? Are they reflected (like light waves striking a mirror)? Do they have some other effect on the object (like tissues or cells)? Or do they fail to affect the object at all (like cosmic rays passing through Earth)?

Carrier and Waveform Frequencies

In this chapter, the focus is on RF portion of the EMF. When studying RF energy, used by diathermy equipment thermal and nonthermal, the two frequencies to be aware of are the *carrier* (radio band) *frequency* and the *waveform* (or modulation) frequency.

Carrier Frequency

The *carrier frequency* is the transmitted RF (like the frequency transmitted by your local FM radio station) and similarly authorized by the Federal Communications Commission. The authorized RF, used by RF medical equipment, typically operates at a carrier frequency of 27.12 MHz and was chosen in order not to interfere with radio communication. The term *short wave* is applied to this frequency because of its short wave length (30 m) compared to radio waves of greater length (3 km for long radio waves) that are also part of the EMF.[5] (See Fig. 24.1 Graphic of RF portion of the EMF.)

TABLE 24.1	**EMF Terminology and Definitions**
Term	**Definition**
Athermal	Old incorrect term for not heating
Bioeffective	Effecting biologic actions or processes
Bioelectric current	A self-propagating endogenous bioeffective current made up of ions rather than electrons that flow in the body effecting and signaling cells
Carrier frequency	Transmitted radio frequency (27.12 Hz)
Diathermy	Heating through, deep heating
Electromagnetic Field (EMF)	Simultaneous periodic variations of electric and magnetic field intensity
Nonthermal	Refers to insignificant tissue heating of <1°C
Pulsed electromagnetic field (PEMF)	Pulse modulated RF waveforms
Pulsing	A time varying, interrupted or modulated signal consisting of either rectangular or arbitrary and low frequency sinusoidal waveforms
Radio frequency	One small portion of the EMS (sometimes referred to as the *radio, radiation,* or *frequency spectrum*)
Short radio wave	10–100 MHz frequency and 3–30 m wavelength
Transmission	Signal transmission is not impeded by nonmetallic structures (i.e., can travel through the body relatively unhindered)
Waveform (or modulation) frequency	The frequency at which the carrier frequency is modulated (i.e., the music from the radio station)

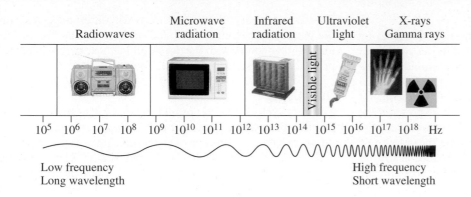

FIGURE 24.1 Electromagnetic spectrum.

Waveform (Modulation) Frequency

The RF signal is broadcast either (1) as a continuous signal (e.g., *continuous short wave* or RF) or (2) as a time varying, interrupted, or modulated signal consisting of either rectangular or arbitrary and low-frequency sinusoidal waveforms (<100 Hz also called pulsing [e.g., *pulsed short wave* or *pulsed radio frequency* (PRF)]). Another term for the pulsed signal is *PEMFs* and is applied to pulse modulated RF waveforms, particularly in the 15 to 40 MHz range.[6] However, you can see from the diagrams of the bursts of pulses, shown in Figure 24.2, two distinct examples showing modulation of EM wave frequency. Both modulate the 27.12-MHz carrier frequency with square or pulsed bidirectional (sinusoidal) waveforms. PRF was introduced in the late 1950s.

EMF Frequency Transmission

Like all radio wave signals, the 27.12-MHz signal travels through air and is not impeded by nonmetallic structures (otherwise, your radio would not play indoors). The same radio waves can travel through the body relatively unhindered, without requiring contact between the applicator and the body.

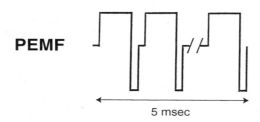

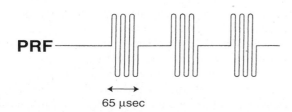

FIGURE 24.2 PEMF signal was designed for bone growth stimulation, whereas PRF waveform is mainly used in treatment of soft tissues. Note: PEMF signal is asymmetric, whereas PRF represents rectangular envelope of pulse burst of 65 μs. (Reprinted from *Wounds: A Compendium of Clinical Research and Practice*, Vol. 7, No. 4, 1995, Health Management Publications, with permission.)

Tissue Penetration

The depth of penetration by the EMF is not impeded by skin, bone, wound dressings, or cast materials. Since the EMF bypasses the sensory pain receptors, application is painless. At 27.12 MHz, the EMF is unable to depolarize motor nerves or produce muscle contraction because the signal is only 36 ns in duration, which is not long enough for migration of ions through cellular membranes of nerve or muscle.[5]

Biophysics of Thermal and Nonthermal Effects

When RF energy is transmitted as a continuous wave or signal, enough energy can be absorbed by an object to cause noticeable heating. In the body, RF induces bioelectric currents in deep body tissues where the absorbed energy is converted to heat. Thus, we have the derivation of the term "diathermy," heating through the tissues. When we put this term together with the frequency of the radio wave, we have "short-wave diathermy" (SWD), a common term used for medical devices of this class. We see this heating effect, for example, in a microwave oven. Like microwaves, the radio waves go rapidly to the inside of the material, which is heated first and then is reflected back to the surface. Absorption and reflection depend on the nature of the material (e.g., muscle or bone) being radiated. To control heating effects with the microwave, we adjust the power output, so that at full power heating occurs quickly or we adjust the power to a lower lever to slow or reduce the amount of heating. To control heating effects of the EMF stimulation, manufacturers developed generators that deliver bursts or trains of short-wave RF pulses such as that you see in Figure 24.2 that modulate the duration of the signal applied to the tissues. Both the geometry of the coil through which the current is passed and the nature of the tissue also effect the distribution of the current flow and therefore the heating effects.[7]

> ### CLINICAL WISDOM
>
> #### Clarifying use of the term Radio Frequency Ablation
>
> *RF* as discussed in this chapter is the same type of energy used for *RF ablation*, which is a treatment where high-amplitude radio waves are used to create sufficient heat to destroy a part of a nerve to relieve joint pain or to treat cancer tumors. However, for wound healing and associated biologic effects of heating to destroy tissue is not part of the therapy.

Depth of EMF Penetration

The depth of penetration of the magnetic field decreases by approximately the square of the distance as it moves away from the surface of the applicator. Markov and Pilla[8] found that the magnetic field of 27.12 MHz radio waves is 30% of the initial value at 5 cm distance from the applicator, 10% at 10 cm, and 3% to 5% at 15 cm. Treatment effects would be expected to be altered by the distance of the applicator from the target tissues. Therefore, another method of controlling the amount of RF energy delivered to the tissues and thus reduce heating is to change the proximity of the magnetic field source and the target tissue. For example, as the gap between the tissues and the applicator head increases, a portion of the magnetic field is dispersed away from the target. One clinical application to reduce the heating created by a RF device is by increasing the gap between the applicator head and the tissue for patients with heat sensitivity, or when only mild heating is required. On the other hand, when using PRF equipment that has been modulated to reduce heating, any gap should be very small, 0.5 cm, in order to avoid reducing the energy too much.

Pulse Rate and Pulse Duration Effect Heating

Pulsing the radio waves did not solve all the problems of creating a truly nonthermal device. The next modification was to change the signal so that the signal was pulsed at lower rates and longer intervals. While the pulse is on, the signal is delivered during the interval it is not. The pulse rates for PRF vary from 1 to 7,000 pps. The pulse duration (or width) varies from 65 to 400 microseconds (μs) (1 μs = 10^{-6} s). This is a significant difference between PEMF (upper scan) and PRF (lower scan) shown in Figure 24.2. Long pulse duration, coupled with high-frequency pulse rate, results in short interpulse intervals, and heat builds up in the tissues because the short interpulse interval does not allow heat to dissipate giving the diathermy effect. For example, pulsed short-wave diathermy (PSWD) has a typical pulse duration of 95 μs.

Nonthermal PRF medical devices generally have a short fixed pulse duration of 65 μs (of the basic 27.12-MHz wave), with pulse rates that can vary from 80 to 600 pps are classified as low frequency. A short pulse duration (which means a long interpulse interval), coupled with a low-frequency pulse rate, produces insignificant or nonthermal tissue effects.

It is important to become familiar with the device you intend to use. Some devices offer a large range of variability of pulse rates and pulse durations from which to choose others are

CLINICAL WISDOM

Testing Thermal and Nonthermal Effects at Different Settings

Try combinations of different on/off times and pulse rates on normal subjects over superficial tissues. Evaluate their effects before and after treatment and over various time intervals by measuring changes to the surface temperature of the skin with a liquid crystal skin thermometer, or to deeper tissue with an infrared scanner.

fixed at the factory. Treatment effects will differ, depending on the parameters selected. Read and understand the instruction manual that comes with the device and choose parameters that provide the physiologic response required.

Duty Cycle

The duty cycle is the ratio of on time to total cycle time, which includes both the on and off times. As an example, at a pulse duration having an on time of 65 μs and a pulse rate of 600 pps, each complete period lasts 1/600 s or 1,667 μs. The interpulse interval, or off time, is then 1.667 to 65 = 1,602 μs. At 600 pps, the duty cycle is 65 μs/1,667 μs = 3.9%.[8] This means that, in a 30-minute treatment (30 $\times$ 60 seconds $\times$ 3.9%), a total of only 70 seconds of energy is delivered.[8] This information is important because most clinical studies use a 30-minute treatment time period. Therefore, adjustment of treatment time would need to be carefully considered in order to make sure that there was an adequate but not excessive amount of energy delivered to the tissue.

Amplitude

Looking at the power output of the device generator does not show the actual power delivered to the tissues because of the way the instruments are engineered. For example, 1,000 watts (W) of generated power is transferred to the drum applicator, where it undergoes significant transformation into the EMF that is then delivered to the patient. Until the transformation into an EMF, it is appropriate to speak of power, but at the last step, it is more correct to speak of the amplitude of the EMF delivered to the tissues. The power driving the applicator coil can be measured either as peak pulse power (which for the Diapulse® [Diapulse Corp of America, Great Neck, NY) ranges from 185 to 275 W] or as mean power, which [for both Diapulse and Provant (Regenesis Biomedical, Scottsdale, AZ) devices] ranges from 7.5 to 38 W. These values are determined by settings of peak power and pulse frequency. The benchmark for measurement of heating effects is 38 W or more. Less than 38 W mean power is, therefore, used as an indicator of minimal heating or nonthermal therapy.[5] The heating effect of a PSWD device is related to the magnitude of the mean power output and can be adjusted to achieve appropriate treatment effects by either direct or indirect application. Treatment outcome can be gauged by measuring the skin temperature where heating is desired or by measuring skin blood flow with a laser Doppler.

The amplitude of the EMF is described in terms of flux density with the units in gauss (G) or tesla (T), where 10,000 Gauss (G) = 1 T. *Flux density* is a measure of the strength of a magnetic field at a given point. Also called *magnetic induction*.[9] For example, the magnetic resonance imaging (MRI) devices achieve desired depth of tissue penetration when it operates on the order of 1 to 5 T or 10,000 to 50,000 G.[4,10]

For wound healing medical applications, Gordon has learned from studying the phenomena and a review of the literature that a magnetic field strength less than 30 G and frequency of greater than 100 Hz, called extremely low frequency, are most effective in modulating cellular responses.[10]

Manufacturers include tables in their instruction manuals, listing the approximate values of average output power in watts at different pulse rates and widths and field strengths. This information should be used only as a guide, not as a definite

RESEARCH WISDOM

Electropollutant and Medical PEMF

EMFs are studied extensively as electropollutants, for example, cell phones, as well as a therapy, under the general heading of PEMF technology. Electropollutants are manifestly different in field strength and frequency in comparison to therapeutic applications, yet the USFDA (2002) considers them the same and lists therapeutic devices as "potentially dangerous" by association. World Health Organization convened scientists from around the world that found field strengths less than 20,000 G, that is low field MRI, free of adverse side effects[10]

amount of power delivered to the tissues because while the electric or magnetic field itself can be measured, it is not yet possible to measure the intensity *received* by the tissues.

Nonionizing Radiation

Another property of RF is nonionizing radiation, meaning that there is insufficient energy concentration to dislodge orbiting electrons from atoms.[5] Therefore, EMF do not exhibit polar properties as occurs when using direct contact electrical stimulation. You can think of RF as noncontact *induced* electrical stimulation as opposed to direct contact electrical stimulation discussed in Chapter 23. Since RF induces a bioelectric current, it appears to have similar effects as other currents on the cells of wound healing that are similar to those of direct contact electrical stimulation (see Chapters 2 and 23).

COMPARISON OF ELECTROMAGNETIC FIELD DEVICES

We have discussed the physical properties of some EMF devices and explained how they got their names. However, more names and acronyms of EMF are found in the literature besides PEMF, PRF, and PSWD including pulsed electromagnetic induction, pulsed electromagnetic energy including time varying electromagnetic field, and designed electromagnetic pulsed therapy. The last term was chosen to reflect the penetration we see clinically, the need to specifically design the pulse for maximal bioefficacy, and the general understanding that pulsed fields demonstrate increased efficacy over static designs.[10] Therefore, it is important to recognize that the acronym *PEMF* is not generic

CLINICAL WISDOM

Electromagnetic waves and Ultrasonic waves

It should also be noted that the electromagnetic waves discussed here do not include sound or ultrasonic waves that require a physical medium through which to travel and are discussed in Chapter 26.

for all EMF devices, and that there are important differences between the therapeutic modalities. For example, signal characteristics differ in several ways. The main differences are the signal shape, pulse rate, duration and depth of penetration. Keep these distinctions in mind when reviewing studies reporting on the use of the different EMFs and when selecting therapeutic devices. If you are considering acquiring such a device, the vendor should be able to provide this information. In this chapter, terms used will be continuous short-wave diathermy (CSWD), PSWD, PRF, and PEMF as previously defined.

Electromagnetic Field Devices used for Wound Healing

All of the terms for EMF devices are very confusing. Adding to the confusion is that studies and manufacturers use the terms PEMF and PFR as if they are identical. In this section, we will examine some of the differences. EMF devices used for wound healing purposes can be categorized into two groups: (1) PEMF and (2) PRF. They differ in the following ways:

1. The PEMF waveform typically has a relatively low frequency, pulse duration 1 to 100 μs, and a repetition rate of 1 to 100 pps, as shown in Figure 24.2. The PEMF signal duration may be longer than that of PRF.[8] The signal amplitude of the PEMF is in the mV/cm range.[8] A PEMF waveform is typically an asymmetric train of pulses (Fig. 24.2). Asymmetry of the stimulus pulse was at one point thought to be necessary to achieve a therapeutic effect. Asymmetric pulses require significant electrical energy, however, constraining clinical delivery systems to suboptimal designs. The results of a study on rabbit fibula osteotomy suggest that asymmetry is not in fact necessary for clinical therapeutic effect.[11] PEMF studies have primarily been conducted or reported in the literature outside of the United States, and only since communication has improved across borders, as a result of the Internet and clinical databases, has this information become available to other clinicians. PEMF devices have been used in the United States primarily for osteogenesis, but several studies on soft tissue repair for venous ulcers have been reported (these are reviewed in the clinical section).[12–17] Magnatherm electromagnetic (PEMF) unit (Meditea Electromedica, Buenos Aires), operating at 3 to 50 Hz and an amplitude of up to 200 G, was the type of equipment used by researchers in some of the animal studies discussed in this chapter.

2. The PRF signal represents a burst of pulses within a rectangular envelope of sinusoidal waves with a duration of 65 μs (Fig. 24.2). The PRF repetition rate varies between 80 and 600 pps, and are classified as high frequency. The duty cycle is less than 4%.[8] The signal amplitude of the PRF is in the V/cm range.[8] PRF is used mainly for the treatment of pain, edema, and soft tissue injuries as well as cellular stimulation.

Although PSWD and PRF are alike in most ways, their effects are based on two different physiologic phenomena. PSWD has the ability to heat the tissues, whereas PRF is nonthermal and mostly affects the tissues at the cellular level. Both PSWD and PRF penetrate deeply into the tissues and most affect those tissues with good conductivity. Because PSWD energy penetrates deeply, it heats from the inside out, just as, when cooking food in the microwave the center is heated first. Heating effects may continue even after the stimulation is removed. Delayed

EXHIBIT 24.1

PSWD/PRF Characteristics

- 27.12-MHz radio waves.
- Modulation waveform square or pulse bidirectional.
- Signal travels through air.
- Not impeded by nonmetallic structures.
- Pulse rates: 1 to 7,000 pps maximum; PR = maximum average intensity.
- 200 pps →moderate to vigorous heating.
- 90 to 200 pps →mild heat.
- <90 pps →nonthermal.
- Applicator: wire coil covered by housing.
- Uniform magnetic field.
- Induce electric current in tissues.
- Deep penetration 5 to 6 cm up to 15 cm (MF value decreased by approximately the square of the distance)

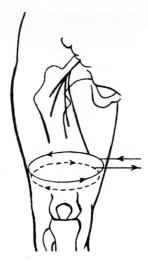

FIGURE 24.3 A PSWD or PRF coil placed over the anterior thigh, showing the exciting current (*solid line*) and the resultant induced current (*broken line*). (Nelson RM, Currie DP. *Clinical Electrotherapy,* 2nd Edition, © 1991, 390, 391. Reprinted by permission of Pearson Education, Inc., Upper Saddle River, NJ.)

response to stimulation is an important concept to remember; the patient may not report heating right away because the skin is not heated first, such as when a hot pack is applied (see Exhibit 24.1). Follow the guidelines listed in the protocols for treatment parameters. Heating effects are adjusted by changing the pulse rate and intensity. Higher pulse rates have greater thermal impact. Low pulse rates, in the 90- to 200-pps range, produce mild heating and are nonthermal at lower rates. Both transmit radiation from a coil contained in the drum head to the target tissues. This method of energy transfer to the tissues is called *induction.* An electrical current is induced in the tissues, as described above.

Pulsing the radio waves did not solve all the problems of creating a truly nonthermal device. The next modification was to change the signal so that the signal was pulsed at lower rates and longer intervals. PRF was introduced in the late 1950s.

PRF and High-Voltage Pulsed Current Fields

As we have just learned, PRF induces electrical currents in the body through the action of an EMF. As such, it has no positive or negative poles, and the current goes in concentric circles (see Fig. 24.3).[4] This induced AC is not related to intervening tissue, but is related to the distance from the coil, with the current intensity being greatest just beneath the coil edges.

For treatment purposes, high-voltage pulsed current (HVPC) has, in general, the same amplitude as do PSWD/PRF (see Chapter 23). HVPC, however, has a unidirectional flow, with a specific polarity,[18] whereas the electromagnetically generated current is a circular flow of current without polarity, as shown in Figure 24.4. The mechanism of action for PSWD/PRF is a direct effect of the magnetic field and induced electric current in the cells. HVPC, on the other hand, has a negligible magnetic field, and the method of cellular stimulation is by electric current. The direct effect of magnetic and electrical fields in the tissues cannot be distinguished because they come together with high-frequency fields. The methods of delivery are different for PSWD/

PRF and HVPC. PSWD/PRF is delivered without skin contact, and the signal is "broadcast" through the air. HVPC by contrast is delivered by capacitive coupling from an electrode, through a wet contact medium applied to the skin. HVPC has a negligible magnetic field (Fig. 24.4), and its stimulation is mainly by electric current. PRF delivers a more uniform and predictable signal to the tissues than do capacitive coupled electrodes.[8]

Summary of Properties and Effects of EMF Devices

The effects of both PSWD and PRF stimulation are detailed in Exhibit 24.2, and the attributes that make them useful for the treatment of wounds are as follows:

1. The penetration of the magnetic field into the tissues is not restricted by impedance from intervening structures, such as skin, bone, or plaster. However, metal (e.g., rings) will alter penetration and/or localized heating (see Safety Issues below).
2. Stimulation at the skin level is not sufficient to depolarize the pain nerve endings in the skin and is therefore painless.
3. Treatment is nondisruptive and compatible with other interventions. For instance, treatment may be delivered over a bandaged wound or over a splint or cast.
4. There is relative uniformity of the induced magnetic field in the entire volume of the wound.[8]
5. Relatively good dosimetry can be achieved because the magnetic field lines are essentially parallel and remain in this alignment throughout the healing process.[8]

The cellular effects of PSWD have not been reported in the literature, but ongoing research is being conducted using radio frequency in the thermal range for treatment of tumors; there are, however, numerous reports concerning the cellular effects of PRF and PEMF. This is not to say that PSWD does not have similar effects on cells that are as yet unknown. CSWD and PSWD are considered thermotherapy, but PRF and PEMF are classified as nonthermal induced electrotherapy.

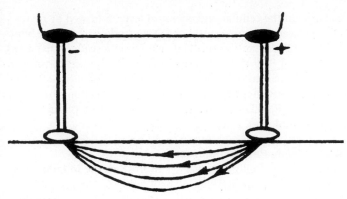

FIGURE 24.4 A pair of direct-contact electrodes used for HVPC and placed over the skin, showing the resultant current flow through the skin. (Nelson RM, Currie DP. *Clinical Electrotherapy*, 2nd Edition, © 1991, 390, 391. Reprinted by permission of Pearson Education, Inc., Upper Saddle River, NJ.)

PHYSIOLOGICAL EFFECTS OF EMF

This section presents a synopsis of the physiologic effect of PRF and PEMF on some cellular systems. Care must be taken when attempting to extrapolate findings in the laboratory to the human body.

Electromagnetic field Modulation of Biologic Phenomena

In order for an EMF signal to be effective, it must be detected by the cells or tissues that have the ability to respond to the

EMG signal and modulate biologic phenomena.[6,8] EMF signal transmission, transduction, and modulation occur by means of intercellular junctions where the activities of the individual cells that make up tissue are coordinated, enabling each tissue system to function as a whole. There are gaps between junctions, and the gap junction forms pathways for direct intercellular communication and electrical coupling. Cellular activity can be modified by induced changes in the electrical status of the cell, the cell membrane, and the cell-to-cell communications via electrically conducting gap junctions. Gap junctions, present in all tissues, provide pathways for ionic and molecular intercellular communication without which disorders in growth control and tissue repair including neoplastic transformation could occur.[7] Thus, this pathway is a key to changing cell dynamics and it is through this mechanism that the EMF signal sensitivity is increased by several orders of magnitude versus a single cell exposed to the same EMF source.[6,8] *EMF modulation* of biologic processes depends first on the physiologic state of the injured tissues and whether or not a physiologically relevant response can be achieved and, second, on the use of an effective dose of EMF to the injury (target) site.[6,8] Effective dosimetry is achieved by configuring the frequency waveform to satisfy the target response time and minimum amplitude required for.[6,8]

Signal Transduction

The processes involved in cellular membrane signal transduction affected by an applied electric field of specific strength and form are receiving considerable research attention. Normally, cell membranes are impermeable to all ions carrying a charge. However, ions can move through specific protein membrane channels, when exposed to relatively small strength ($[10^3–10^4$ Vm^{-1} range] at frequency below 150 Hz) EMF. For example, there is supporting research that applied EMF opens Na$^+$ and Na$^+$/K$^+$ channels. Enhanced Na$^+$ inflow causes an action potential resulting in the depolarization of the cell.[19] The opening of the calcium ion (Ca^{2+}) channels also occurs with EMF, which causes an increase of Ca^{2+} influx that is released from intracellular stores.[19,20] Inflow of Ca^{2+} into the cells will activate numerous cellular processes through the binding to calmodulin, which will then activate calmodulin-dependent kinases whose function is to phosphorylate proteins using ATP. What ensues is a biochemical cascade that has the potential to have far-reaching effects on cells, including cell orientation and migration, immune-cell functions, cell proliferation, cell shape changes, and ultimately on the optimal function of the body. The PEMF signal also modulates Ca^{2+} binding kinetics, stimulates all types of cell proliferation, affects the cell membrane diffusion and/or permeability, and moves negatively charged plasma proteins toward lymph capillaries, which may explain edema reduction as described in section of inflammatory phase effects.[19,21]

PEMF exposure stimulates mRNA expression of several bone morphogenic proteins and upregulates TGF beta mRNA. It has been suggested that the increase in TGF Beta-1 mRNA protein synthesis in osteoblast cultures is a direct result of the effect of the EMF on calcium/calmodulin-dependent pathways.[22] TGF Beta-1 is instrumental in the cascade of

---

EXHIBIT 24.2

Wound Healing-Related Effects with PSWD/PRF

- Perfusion of tissues is increased, either directly or indirectly.
- Deep tissue heating with PSWD allows heating within deep wounds and tunnels, including areas with abscess or infection.
- PSWD raises tissue temperatures.
- Painful wounds and associated soft tissue can be treated without direct contact.
- PSWD and PRF provide analgesia of pain endings.
- PSWD and PRF produce edema reduction.
- PRF stimulates cellular activity and cell membrane signal transduction mechanisms.
- PRF stimulation can take place over clothing, wound dressings, elastic wraps, splints and casting materials.
- No disruption of the wound healing environment is needed with PRF.
- Stimulation of deep structures with PSWD, including nerves and blood vessels, can effect physiologic changes.
- PSWD and PRF provide relative uniformity of the induced magnetic field in the entire volume of the wound.
- PSWD and PRF provide relatively good dosimetry.

regulatory events involved in extracellular matrix formation, cell growth, and accelerated chondrogenesis. This process has been identified as one mechanism involved in the stimulation of osteogenesis.

Another cellular study looked at the effect of EMFs on transduction pathways that regulate lymphocyte proliferation, and found that 0.1 mT, 60 Hz EMFs can induce a 20% mean increase in the anti-CD3 binding to T-cell receptors of Jurkat cells. There was a relationship between cell proliferation and the amount of energy given. T cells are key modulators of inflammation, and potentially EMF technology can be used to treat inflammatory diseases.[23]

To test these effects of low-frequency (60 Hz) EMF on patients, a before-after design study of recalcitrant leg ulcers ($N = 26$ patients; 18 patients with 25 chronic venous and 8 patients with 17 chronic arterial ulcers) was performed. EMF was applied to the arm placed inside a EMF chamber to promote healing based on the concept that the EMF will interact with peripheral blood mononuclear cells (PBMC) via Ca^{2+} channels activating signal transduction cascades, promoting cytokine synthesis, and changing cell proliferation patterns.[24] More details of this study are found in the section on Wound Healing Clinical Studies and Table 24.5.

Signal Dosimetry

Originally, the exogenous application of PEMF was designed to mimic the asymmetric waveform that is detected when bone is dynamically deformed.[25] Now that the mechanism of PEMF effects is better understood, it is clear that waveform configuration plays an important role in dosimetry.[20] PEMF thresholds appear to encompass more factors than dose response alone. Frequency, amplitude, and timing, singly or in combination, appear to be involved in the results of many of the experimental studies.[20,21,25] At this time, we do not know optimal or best parameters to make a recommendation based on such a level of evidence. That being said there is information from studies about protocols and the results to provide guidance for current practice.

Growth Factor Regulation

Both electric and EMFs have demonstrated ability to produce a sustained upregulation of growth factors. A mechanism ascribed to stimulating cells with EMF is the induction of growth factors that in turn stimulate cell replication through a Ca^{2+} pathway.[21] EMF stimulate and regulate the expression of genes and the synthesis of growth factors in connective tissues for structural extracellular matrix (ECM) constituents, and dosimetric relationships have been described.[26]

Effects on Attributes of the Inflammatory Phase

Inflammation is the most painful stage of wound healing and can have profound effects including delaying repair and repair complications such as fibrosis, scaring, keloid formation.[27] In this chapter section, we will look at the evidence for effects of PRF and PSWD cytokine production, growth factor production, and antioxidant efficacy to control-free radical activity and on two of the attributes of the inflammatory phase, pain and/or edema. First, we will get an overview of anti-inflammatory

activities at the cellular and chemical levels followed by reviews of the efficacy on pain and edema. Two studies are double blind RCT (DBRCT) and controlled five clinical studies that used nonthermal PRF as the treatment intervention are considered next. The final study in this section used mildly thermal PSWD. Each study asked questions and reports results about the ability of PRF and PSWD to influence the inflammatory phase for different pathologies.

Anti-Inflammatory Modulation

We will review cellular responses to EMF in the inflammatory phase; here we are looking at new fields of interest, electrochemistry, and electrogenomics that regulate the inflammatory phase. Inflammatory cytokines are considered as causative factors in pain. Therefore, measuring levels of cytokines in acute wound fluid along with pain scores provides quantitative measurements of the mechanisms attributed to PEMF efficacy for pain reduction. Rohde et al measured levels of interleukin (IL)-1β from acute wound fluid in postoperative patients, described in a study below, and found that levels were approximately $27\% \pm 36\%$ lower in those treated with PEMF compared to sham group. There was also a direct correlation between the reduction in cytokines and pain levels in this group.[27]

Ionescu et al.[28] observed that, when burn wounds were treated with PRF, there was prevention of edema formation, pain, and reduction in local symptoms. These observations led to further investigation to understand the mechanisms involved and to demonstrate objective proof. Local skin enzymatic activity was chosen as an indicator of the viability of the tissue. Samples of proteins and some principal enzymes in normal and burned tissue were compared before and after PRF therapy. Enzymatic activities of the skin usually decrease when traumatized or burned. The study data showed that, compared with normal skin, the enzymatic activity was significantly modified after the treatment. The earlier the application of treatment, the sooner the normal enzymatic activities were restored.

The reports indicate that there is upregulation of growth and restoration genes that can accelerate the healing cascade up to four times more efficiently than in untreated cases by quenching the escalation of free radical that degrade organs and tissues to levels of stunning and death.[10,26] Free radical and ischemia reperfusion injury are explained in Chapter 2.

Edema and Pain

Edema and pain restrict function and slow healing responses so therapy that can mitigate these physiological phenomena are welcome parts of the wound healing armamentarium. Here we will look at several studies where PEMF/PRF were used and evaluated for efficacy against both.

Traumatic Injury

Results: PRF treatment for 20 to 30 minutes reduced soft tissue edema following trauma that has persisted for several hours after treatment. The mechanism by which this occurs is postulated to be the effect of PRF on sympathetic nervous system outflows, inducing vasoconstriction and restriction of blood flow from blood vessels to the interstitial areas around the wound site.[8]

Hand Injuries

Early intervention with PRF (Diapulse) in the treatment of hand injuries was studied by Barclay et al.[29] to compare the effects on edema, pain, and improvement of function with untreated pairs. Sixty matched pairs of patients who had hand injuries were evaluated within 36 hours of admission.

Results: In the treated group, with the exception of two cases, there was a complete resolution of edema by the third day, compared with the control subjects, whose swelling greatly increased. The 17 patients in the treated group were symptom free by the third day, and by day 7, only one in the treated group had slight loss of function; the 29 other patients had been discharged. By contrast, in the control group of 30 patients, 3 had been discharged and the remaining 27 were still symptomatic with edema, pain, and loss of function.[29]

Acute Ankle Sprains

Acute ankle sprains have a rapid onset of edema and pain and are common injuries in athletes and in the military. Pennington et al.[30] studied the effect of PRF (Diapulse) on 50 patients with grade I and II ankle sprains of military personnel at 1 to 24 hours, 25 to 48 hours, and 49 to 72 hours after injury.

Results: A statistically significant decrease in the edema (0.95% versus 4.7%) was observed. Reduced pain was reported for 64% of the treated patients, compared with 33% for the control group. Because of the small sample size in the three different time-elapsed groups, no analysis was performed on this component but, overall, those patients who were treated within the 72-hour time frame had a statistically significant effect, including a significant decrease in the time lost from military training.[30]

Acute Head Trauma

In another study, 200 acute head trauma patients with a Glasgow Coma Scale of 8 or less were alternately assigned to treatment with PRFS or to serve as controls.[31] The patients in this category had diffuse brain damage, multiple contusions, and brain edema, and were in poor states of consciousness. Except for the addition of the PRF stimulation, the same management protocol was followed in the intensive care unit (ICU). PRF stimulation at 600 pps for 30 minutes was given every 12 hours, with the drum alternating on the right and left sides of the head. Treatment began at the time of admission into the ICU. Serial computed tomography scans were done to evaluate the outcomes and for comparison with controls. In all cases, on the first day of admission to ICU, there was clear evidence of edema, and the ventricles appeared slit like.

Results: By the 10th day, for those in the PRF treatment group, the edema had disappeared, and the ventricles were seen well. However, in the control cases, it took 12 to 15 days to see the ventricles. Another measure reported for 20 cases was intracranial pressure (ICP). In the 10 cases receiving PRF, the ICP diminished by the fifth day after injury and by day 7 came to near normal levels. Controls' ICP began to diminish by day 7. Mortality at the end of 1 month for the PRF group was 24% in the PRF group and 29% among controls.[31]

CLINICAL WISDOM

Some PSWD devices can be set at a protocol that is mildly thermal. The Magnatherm (International Medical Electronics, Kansas City, MO) and the Curapulse (Enraf Nonius, Delft, The Netherlands and Henley International, Sugarland, TX) are such devices and there may be others on the market.

Postsurgical Wound Pain

Two DBRCTs looked at postoperative pain of breast surgical patients who received PEMF immediately after surgery.

1. Heden and Pilla[32] used DBRCT to examine the efficacy of a PEMF device (SofPulse®, Ivivi Health Sciences San Francisco, CA) with an induced EMF parameters of 2 milliseconds burst, magnetic field 0.05 G, electrical field 32 ± 6 mV/cm to effect pain patients in patients who had breast augmentation surgery. The device is a battery powered, single subject use, light weight device. For bilateral breast augmentation surgery, two coils attached to a single generator were used one placed over each breast. The device was left in place 24 hours per day and used twice daily for 30 to 60 minutes starting 3 to 5 hours post surgery. Outcome measure for pain was the 100 mm Visual Analog Scale (VAS) and postoperative medication pill count.

   Results: VAS. Postoperative day 1 VAS (0–100 mm) score was 53 ± 3 mm for both groups. Active Treatment group: Postoperative day 3 score was 28.5 ± 4 mm; decrease 87% ($p < .001$) versus sham group 40.2 ± 3.5; 2.7 times greater pain reduction for treatment group. Narcotic medication: Postoperative day 1: 6.2 ± 0.4 pills; Treatment group postoperative day 3: 3.1 ± 0.3 ($p < .001$); Sham group day 3: 4.9 ± 0.5. Pain decreased significantly in PEMF group.

2. Rohde et al.[27] used the same Ivivi device as in the Heden study for a DBRCT to measure postoperative pain plus IL 1B levels in 24 patients who had breast reduction surgery. Again the VAS was used to measure pain. The treatment was provided automatically, 20 minutes every 4 hours for the first 3 days, then once every 8 hours for next 3 days and then twice daily.

   Results: Active treatment group: 1 hour postoperatively mean pain scores were 57% less than controls ($p < .01$), 5 hours postoperatively 300% less ($p < .001$) and pain levels remained low for the next 48 hours. There was a 2.2-fold lower use of narcotics in the active group compared to the sham group ($p = .002$). Measurement of the IL-1B concentrations in exudate was 275% higher in wound fluid from the active versus the control group. Conclusion was that EMF was effective in more effective than the use pain pumps for reducing pain and contributed to hastening inflammation.

Podiatric Surgery

A controlled study of 25 podiatric surgical patients was conducted by Santiesteban and Grant[33] using PSWD at a dosage of 700 pps and a power setting of 12, or approximately 120 W.

This intensity is now called *mildly thermal*, but was reported in the study as *athermal*. A control group of 25 did not receive this treatment. Two electrodes were used: one over the plantar aspect of the postoperative foot and the other on the inguinal region. If both feet were operated on, the electrodes were placed over the plantar aspects of both feet. Two treatment sessions were given. One was given as soon after surgery as possible and the other 4 hours later.

Results: Nurses noted the number and types of pain medications used and the length of the hospital stay, measured in hours. There were significant differences between the treatment group and the control group. The former had a length of stay that was on average 8 hours shorter, and used weaker analgesic medication.[33]

Conclusion from Studies

Intervention during the acute inflammatory phase—the first 72 hours after injury (e.g., trauma including burns, pressure, contusion)—with PRF has demonstrated reductions of edema, pain, and enhanced perfusion of the tissues, with resulting acceleration through the phases of repair, and consequent early return to work.[27–30,32]

Effects on Cellular Systems during the Proliferative Phase

Researchers have been focusing on its effects on different cellular systems that are involved in the biological cascade of healing. In this subsection, we will examine the effects of PRF and PEMF on the cells primarily associated with the proliferative phase of wound healing.

Cellular Changes

Cellular changes following treatment with PRF have been observed to alter processes that are essential to tissue repair, including proliferation of parenchymal and connective tissue cells, synthesis of ECM proteins, collagenization, and acquisition of wound strength.[6,8]

Dosimetry

The purpose of this study was to determine the influences of different PRF dosages applied to human fibroblasts and chondrocyte cells in vitro. Different parameters were used for each experiment. One experiment used a mean input power to the applicator of 13.8 W (<1 W in situ) and exposure for 10 minutes with the result of significantly increased fibroblast proliferation compared with control groups. In another experiment, lower power to the applicator (6 W) for 10 minutes increased proliferation of chondrocyte cells. From the results of these experiments, it was learned that response is dose and, most important, time dependent.[34] In a different experiment, 24 hours after PRF treatment, fibroblasts that were exposed to 10 minutes of radiation at a dose of 32 mW/cm^2 showed half-maximally enhanced proliferation, but those subjected to longer durations of 15 to 60 minutes showed maximal cell proliferation.[21] Under the same treatment dose parameters, epithelial cells also showed maximal mitogenesis with treatment durations of 30 minutes.

Manufacturers also read the literature and then can be motivated to change their device parameters based on new information. For example, one company, Ivivi Health Sciences (CA), has reduced the peak input power to the applicator from 300 W to less than 10 W for the Ivivi SofPulse®. However, since this change there is only one published case study.[35] This is not much on which to base new treatment protocols. More evidence is needed.

THERMOTHERAPY WITH SHORT-WAVE DIATHERMY

The practice of warming wounds to promote healing has been performed since ancient times, and warm soaks and warm compresses are still used for healing. From the time of its introduction, diathermy has been used to heat tissue and influence circulation. In the interim time, parameters for heating have been revised along with delivery systems. Only recently have scientists begun to understand and explain why wounds respond to warmth. Warmth changes hemodynamics through suppression of vasoconstriction, enhancement of vasodilation, and increasing blood flow along with vascular endothelial stress that triggers the nitric oxide production system all of which are needed for successful wound healing. Hemodynamics is explained more fully in Chapters 23 and 27, so please refer to those chapters for details.

Another discovery is that heat can counter the inhibitory effects of chronic wound fluid on fibroblasts (see Chapter 2). Thus, raising the temperature of the wound by a degree or more could reduce the wound fluid inhibitory activity and assist in the healing of chronic wounds.[36]

Clinically, CSWD and PSWD are widely available but not widely used for wound healing in the United States. Diathermy units, which as we know are part of the EMF group of interventions, are available and used for treatment in many places outside the USA. For example, a survey of 41 hospital-based physical therapy departments in Ireland found that PSWD was the preferred mode of treatment, often used more than once daily. Treatment efficacy was reported anecdotally for soft tissue injury and hematomas as well as other inflammatory conditions.[37] This book is intended to guide international wound practice. Thus, we want to provide guidance in this section about the use of SWD thermotherapy and nonthermal therapies to aid in wound healing.

Circulatory Effects of Diathermy

Increased blood flow benefits wound healing by autolytic debridement of necrotic tissue, delivering critically needed oxygen and nutrients and removing metabolites. Local application of heat causes vasodilation of the vasculature and allows for increased blood flow. Infection rates are inversely proportional to blood flow and oxygen levels because, in this situation, oxygen functions equivalent to an antibiotic by oxygenation of the leukocytes, which are critical to fighting infection.[38] All of the processes of wound healing are oxygen dependent, including collagen deposition. Heat is a simple and effective method to enhance blood flow.[18,39] For example, if blood flow can increase to the lower extremities without elevating body heat and if it can be maintained, it can then be applied as a helpful treatment of vasospastic PVD and could be beneficial in controlling infection. Treatment interventions that can increase perfusion to the tissues are important tools. The following studies report the effects of CSWD, PSWD, and nonthermal PRF on blood flow to the extremities. Table 24.2 summarizes studies on circulatory effects.

TABLE 24.2	Clinical Studies of the Effects of PSWD and PRFS on Circulation				
Researcher	**Silverman and Pendleton**[43]	**Santoro et al.**[45]	**Erdman**[2]	**Mayrovitz and Larsen**[46]	**Mayrovitz and Larsen**[47]
Type of study	Case series	Uncontrolled	Case series	Controlled	Controlled
Type of stimulator	PSWD	PSWD	PRFS (Diapulse)	PRFS (MRT sofpulse)	PRFS (MRT sofpulse)
Frequency	80–2,600 pps	7.000 pps 90 μs 700 pps 95 μs	400 pps; 500 pps; 600 pps 65 μs	600 pps 65 μs	600 pps, 65 μs
Amplitude	Average high power 65 W Average low power 15 W	Maximum power	Moderate power level (4) to peak (6) Av power 16 W at (4) Max of 40 W at (6)	Peak power 35 W Peak power	1 G at skin surface
Duration of stimulation	20 min indirect heating at abdomen	20 min max amp indirect heating 10 min mod amp direct heating	Indirect stimulation at epigastrum	45 min 1 × direct stimulation at the arm	45 min 1 × direct stimulation of lower limb
Effect of Rx	Average increases tissue temp with pulsed high power at abdomen 5.8°C	Insignificant temp increase in tx limb; significant temp increase contralateral limb	↑ Av temp at foot 2.0°C	Blood flow: Mean group increase: 29% in treated limb	↑ Blood flow volume at tx site; No increase at contralateral control site (Note: at baseline the ulcerated limb had higher BFV than contralateral)
	At foot 2.2°C	Increased tcPO$_2$ both limbs (Note: Temp peaked at 20 min)	↑ Volume increase of 1.75 at max power	Untreated: no change	No increase in skin temp
	Increase of 165% at foot			Skin Temp: Mean Group 1.8°C ↑ skin temp treated limb	
	Average increases tissue temp at low power at abdomen			Untreated limb: 0.5°C ↑ skin temp	
	3.1°C–3.4°C at foot no significant change				
Effect post Rx (15–30 min)	Not reported	Not reported	↑ Volumetric change Returned to baseline within 30 min post	Not reported	Not reported
Method of Measurement	Temperature	Temperature tcPO$_2$	Volumetric plethysmography Skin temperature readings	Skin temperature (thermistor) Laser Doppler Flowmetery	Skin temperature (thermistor) Laser Doppler Flowmetry
Health Status Tested and N	Healthy adults N not stated	Arterial PVD $N = 10$	Healthy young adults $N = 20$	Healthy adults $N = 9$	Diabetics $N = 15$ with foot ulceration, 9 with PVD

Data from references listed in the table.

Tissue Heating

Early experimental and clinical research of CSWD was focused on the effects associated with tissue heating that can occur when tissue temperatures are raised, 5°C, from 41°C–45°C in the deep tissue structures.[40,41] More recent experimental testing confirmed that PSWD can also raise tissue temperature, 3 cm below the surface over a large surface area, with a treatment of 15 to 20 minutes duration by 4°C. Raise and decay were both linear.[41] It is the only way to heat tissue greater than 2 cm below the surface and effect a large area. A temperature rise of 1°C can reduce mild inflammation and increase tissue metabolism, 2°C to 3°C raise can decrease pain and muscle spasm. This is clinically meaningful.[41] This is a safe tissue temperature range when the patient could respond to pain stimuli (e.g., overheating), and when there is a sufficient reservoir of blood with adequate cooling capacity to dissipate the heating through blood flow. Where circulatory occlusion is present heating may be contraindicated because, in limited circulatory systems, there is poor heat dissipation and consequently a higher risk for burns.[42] Alternative methods then need to be considered. Alternative heating methods have been studied and are reviewed here.

Continuous Short-Wave Diathermy and Circulation

Because of concerns about overheating of ischemic tissues, researchers from the 1930s to 1960s tested indirect diathermy applications (to the abdomen epigastric and sacrum) to evaluate tissue heating and the effect on peripheral blood flow dynamics in the feet and hands, resulting in several published studies. For instance, irradiated tissues treated with low frequency (8 MHz) high intensity (1.5 kW) CSWD for 30 to 60 minutes show an increase in blood flow and cell membrane permeability, resulting in increased ability to revascularize, repair, and prevent ischemia and fibrosis.[43] One study of blood flow changes in normal adult women was published by Wessman and Kottke.[44] The parameters of the treatment were not stipulated, unfortunately. They did find statistically significant heating at the hands and toes, but less marked effects in the calf, from 13 to 37 minutes after CSWD, with effects lasting up to approximately 80 minutes after application of the diathermy. Heating was noted in the calf later than in the foot and in a two-step pattern. Researchers attributed the results to the ways that circulatory control of the two areas functions. In the foot, there are many arterioanastomoses, allowing greatly increased blood flow to occur in the foot. This shunting with indirect heating occurs to a lesser extent in the calf. It was apparent that changes of blood flow in the hand and foot do not represent changes of cutaneous flow throughout the body, nor do changes of blood flow to the calf or forearm indicate changes of muscular flow only.[44] Perhaps the explanation is that warmed blood initiated vasodilation of the peripheral vascular system and improved blood flow. Just like there is continued heating and cooking of microwaved food after the power is turned off, indirect heating effects with CSWD last an average of 80 minutes after application, which demonstrates that there is a long-lasting effect on the peripheral blood flow and metabolism of the limbs.[44] Clinical application of these findings suggests that the use of indirect heating to increase peripheral blood flow in patients with peripheral arterial insufficiency may be useful to improve healing of foot and leg ulcers as shown in the Case Study of a patient with pressure ulcers (see Fig. 24.10A–C).

CASE STUDY

Pressure Ulcer Treated with Pulsed Short-wave Diathermy

Patient ID: S.D. Age: 86 years.

Functional Outcome Report: Initial Assessment

Reason for Referral

The patient is minimally mobile and has developed a pressure ulcer on the left heel and fifth metatarsal head. She is alert but lacks the ability to reposition. Autolytic debridement with occlusive dressing has not been successful (see Fig. 24.10A).

Medical History and Systems Review

The patient experienced a left fractured hip with open reduction and internal fixation 3 years ago. She never regained the ability to ambulate after the hip fracture. She also has a history of multiple cerebrovascular accidents that suggests that her circulatory system is impaired. She is placed in a wheelchair for a few hours a day. She takes food orally and eats most of the diet offered. There has been no recent loss of weight. She is incontinent of bowel and bladder and has a Foley catheter in place.

Evaluation

The patient has an impaired healing response that is due to impairment of the circulation and loss of the muscle pump function due to immobility of the lower extremities. These functional losses contribute to the inability of the wounded tissue to progress through the phases of repair without intervention. The patient has improvement potential for the wounds, but will remain at risk for future pressure ulceration. The following examinations are indicated:

- Mobility: muscle function and joint integrity
- Circulatory status function
- Integumentary system: surrounding skin and wound

Examination Data Muscle Function and Joint Integrity

The patient has a fixed varus deformity of the leg, and no active mobility of the left hip joint exists. There is minimal mobility of the left knee, and a knee flexion contracture at 75 degrees limits function of the left leg. The hip and knee deformities have created a positioning problem, with the left ankle crossing over the right leg and the lateral aspect of the foot, from toes to heel, in a position that is subject to pressure. Ankle joint range and mobility is also severely impaired.

Mobility

The patient is immobile. She does not attempt to self-reposition in either bed or wheelchair.

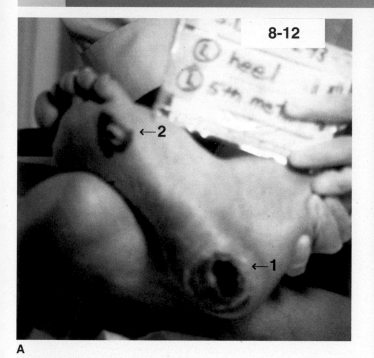

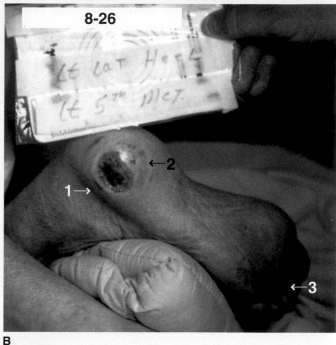

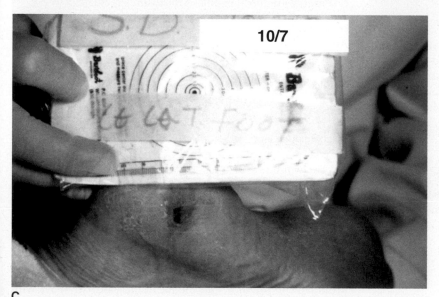

FIGURE 24.5 Case study wound healing with pulsed short-wave diathermy. **A:** Patient with pressure ulcers. PSWD was begun on 8/16. Note: (1) Black eschar on heel wound surrounded by partial-thickness skin loss; there is an absence of inflammatory phase (2) Black eschar over the fifth metatarsal head; there is an absence of inflammatory phase. **B:** Same ulcer as seen on heel in Figure 24.5A, 10 days after start of PSWD. Note: (1) Eschar removed to soft necrosis (2) Reepithelialization of partial-thickness skin loss (3) Eschar removed fifth metatarsal, and wound healed. **C:** Same heel ulcer as in Figure 24.5A and B, on 10/7. The ulcer healed and is shown in the remodeling phase. (Copyright © C. Sussman.)

Circulation

There is edema of the left foot, extending to the ankle. The foot is warm (98.6°F), with 1+ palpable pulses. No dependent rubor is noted when the patient is seated in a wheelchair.

Integumentary System

There is an ulcer on the left lateral heel; it has eschar necrosis, inflammatory signs of changes in skin color (red), warmth (98.6°F), and local edema. The whole foot to the ankle is edematous. There is an ulcer on the left fifth metatarsal head with eschar necrosis, signs of mild inflammation, no pain, changes in skin color (red), and warmth (98.6°F) and edema.

It is 6.9 cm². (See Fig. 24.5A,B of the wounds at evaluation and during treatment.)

Functional Diagnosis

- Undue susceptibility to pressure ulceration on the feet
- Both wounds chronic inflammatory phase
- Tissue impairment due to presence of eschar

Need for Skilled Services: The Therapy Problem

The patient has failed to respond to interventions with dressing changes for the last 2 weeks. She now requires debridement of the eschar from both wounds to determine the extent

CASE STUDY *(continued)*

of tissue involvement and to initiate the healing process; PSWD would be of benefit to enhance circulation to the foot, facilitate debridement, and restart the process of repair; and she requires therapeutic positioning to avoid trauma from pressure to the foot.

Targeted Outcomes

- The wound bed will be clean.
- There will be an enhanced inflammatory response: erythema, edema, and warmth.
- The patient will progress through the phases of healing from inflammation to epithelialization.
- The patient will be properly positioned to remove pressure from the left foot.

Treatment Plan

Debridement Strategy
Score eschar and use an enzymatic debriding agent and occlusion for autolysis. Sharply debride when eschar is softened. Apply PSWD for perfusion and cellular stimulation

Prognosis
Clean wound bed; due date: 21 days

PSWD Protocol
Apply PSWD for increased circulation to the foot, using the protocol of one applicator over the abdomen and the second applicator over the plantar surface of the foot. Sussman in this case study followed the parameters proposed by the manufacturer (International Medical Electronics) of the Magnatherm:

1. a short initial phase (5 minutes) of heating at a high pulse rate (5,000 pps) and peak power output, for vigorous heating to warm the blood
2. followed by a reduction in the pulse rate to the lowest level (700 pps), at peak power output for mild heating effect. The lower pulse rate was maintained for 25 minutes. The total treatment time was 30 minutes.

TABLE 24.9	**Magnatherm Protocol Used by Sussman for Case Study**	
Magnatherm Settings	**Duration**	**Effect**
PR 5,000 pps power level 12 (thermal)	5 min	Vigorous heating—warm up
PR 700 pps power level 12 (nonthermal)	25 min	No perceived sensation of heat

The rationale was that the effects of the high-dose heating treatment would rapidly raise the tissue temperature and cause vasodilation. The lower pulse rate produced mild heating, and the longer interpulse interval would allow for heat dissipation. Additional rationale for this setting was that this would sustain the vasodilation effects of the high heating phase throughout the duration of the treatment (see Table 24.9).

Prognosis
- Acute inflammation; due date: 14 days
- Progression through phases to closure; due date: 8 weeks

Frequency
Apply PSWD daily seven times per week, twice daily for 30 minutes.

Therapeutic Positioning
Use therapeutic positioning with pillows to eliminate pressure on the left foot; instruct nurses' aides in proper positioning.

Discharge Outcome
The wound on the fifth metatarsal head was healed by day 15. The wound on left heel had full-thickness skin loss after removal of eschar and necrotic tissue. The wound had a clean wound bed by week 4. Closure was achieved by week 7 (see Fig. 24.10C).

Pulsed Short-Wave Diathermy and Circulation
The idea of indirect tissue heating was also tested using PSWD. As we have learned, PSWD can heat both deep and superficial tissues. Silverman and Pendleton[43] and Santoro et al.[45] wanted to know whether indirect tissue heating in the abdomen and lumbosacral areas would increase peripheral blood flow and raise the distal tissue temperature in the foot and the calf. In both studies, PSWD, CSWD, and a placebo were used to treat young adults by placing the treatment head over the lower abdomen. Silverman and Pendleton's treatment protocol used two treatment machines: one set at a high average power setting of 65 W and one at low average power of 15 W for 20 minutes. To achieve the high power, the pulse rate was set at 2,400 pps, and the low power pulse rate was 600 pps. Peripheral circulation was then measured in the calf and in the foot. The result was that the change in circulation was most prominent in the foot, and the mean increase was 165% with pulsed high power and 195% with continuous high power. No circulatory effects were found in the foot with low power using either PSWD or CSWD. Temperatures were recorded under the treatment head. The mean increase in local skin temperature was 5.3°C with continuous treatment and 5.8°C with pulsed treatment. The foot temperature increased to 1.9°C and 2.2°C, respectively. Local heating occurred on the abdomen of the subjects who received low power, with mean changes of 3.1°C and 3.4°C, respectively, for PSWD and CSWD. Subjects reported a comfortable sensation under the treatment heads. These are statistically significant changes in temperature and blood flow overall, but not significantly different between the pulsed and continuous generators, confirming the ability of a PSWD generator to increase blood flow with less heating of tissues.

EXHIBIT 24.3

Summary of Effects of PSWD

↑Perfusion
↑Local tissue $tcPO_2$
↑Tissue metabolism
↑Antibiotic delivery to tissue
↑O_2 antimicrobial effect
↑Cellular processes

In Santoro's study,[45] 10 patients with moderate to severe arterial peripheral vascular disease were treated with PSWD 5 days a week for 20 days, spread over a period of 1 month. The treatment consisted of a 30-minute, two-part protocol. During the first 20 minutes, the treatment was at maximum amplitude for the unit, which was a high-dose heating level, 95 μs at a rate of 7,000 pps. During the last 10 minutes, the intensity was reduced to a low heating level, 95 μs at a rate of 700 pps, in what was called a *cooling phase*. Two applicator heads were used, with one placed over the plantar surface of the foot and the second over the area of the anterior thigh. In cases in which both limbs were affected, both applicators were placed over the plantar surfaces of the feet. Variables measured included surface temperature, transcutaneous partial pressure of oxygen ($tcPO_2$), segmental Doppler blood pressure, superficial blood flow (measured with a laser Doppler flowmeter), and patient perceptions. Findings were that temperature peaked at the end of the 20 minutes of high heat, and then gradually reduced. The $tcPO_2$ readings increased in the treated and the untreated limbs. They were insignificant in the treated limbs but significant in the untreated limbs, possibly because of reflex vasodilation from the warm circulating blood and sympathetic nervous system activity. Sixty percent of the patients reported subjectively that they felt that the treatment had improved their quality of life. No adverse effects were reported.[36]

Exhibit 24.3 lists the effects of PSWD, and Table 24.2 summarizes clinical study reports on the effects of PSWD and PRF

CLINICAL WISDOM

Radio Frequency Interference

One problem with RF signal is that it is not confined to the treatment target tissue and radiation is dispersed into the environment and may effect signals from other electronic equipment such as electronic implants. However, with reduced power output, there is negligible radio frequency interference on monitoring and life-sustaining electronic equipment that might otherwise be effected.

on circulation. Further study is needed to determine the efficacy of thermotherapy (CSWD and/or PSWD) in prevention of tissue fibrosis and enhancement of healing of irradiated tissues.

Good quality controlled studies of PSWD meeting current standards are needed to test its effects on chronic wound healing. At this time, the reports of successful outcomes for wound healing remain anecdotal such as the Case Study at the end of this chapter.

Nonthermal PRF Effect on Circulation

Erdman[2] studied the effect of PRF with the inductive head placed over the epigastrium, in a study measuring changes in blood flow to the feet of 20 normal young adults. The findings included a mean increase in foot temperature of 2.0°C and an average volume increase of 1.75-fold at the maximum generated power. Rectal temperatures did not change, nor did pulse rates. Furthermore, in all 20 cases, increased blood flow was directly proportional to the energy applied at the three highest settings. A short period of effect followed cessation of the treatment. Mayrovitz and Larsen[46] reported that treatment with PRF increased skin blood perfusion in the treated region. PRF stimulation with the MRT SofPulse® (Electropharamacology now disbanded) at 65 μs at a pulse rate of 600 pps and peak power, applied for 40 minutes on the forearm skin of nine healthy men and women, produced enhanced microvascular perfusion, averaging 30% compared with pretest levels. Skin temperature was increased by an average of 1.8°C, but the rise occurred ahead of

CASE STUDY

Postsurgical Use of PRF

R.J., a 74-year-old male, had hand surgery to remove a synovial mass located between the first and second metacarpal bones of his left (dominant) hand. There were incisions on both the dorsum of the hand and the palm because of the extent of the mass. Surgery was carried out with a regional anesthetic block. Numbness prevailed for several hours after the surgery. Approximately 3 hours after surgery, a battery-operated PRF coil (SofPulse®) was used over the wound pressure dressing for a 30-minute treatment. The treatment was repeated about 4 hours later. At bedtime, R.J. reported that the anesthetic had worn off, he took two plain acetaminophen 500 mg tablets as

a prophylactic for possible pain during the night and went to bed. Those were the only pain medications that he took. He continued to use the PRF device several times daily for 30- to 60-minute sessions. When the pressure dressing was removed 5 days later, the incision was tender to pressure but otherwise the hand was free from pain. Edema was present in all the fingers and did not seem to be affected by the PRF. He was able to use the hand functionally for self-care (dental hygiene, eating, dressing) from the first postoperative day. He continued to use the PRF device for 3 weeks to facilitate the healing process and potentially improve the quality of the scar. There were no complications.

the measured increased perfusion. This is similar to the Erdman study. Mayrovitz and Larsen[47] conducted another study using the MRT SofPulse®, also to study effects on perfusion. Laser Doppler red blood cell perfusion, volume, velocity, and skin temperatures were evaluated for 15 subjects, each of whom had had diabetes for at least 5 years and each of whom had an ulcer on the foot or toe of one limb. Ulcer duration was a minimum of 8 weeks. The contralateral limb was intact and served as the control. Nine subjects had PVD, as confirmed by noninvasive vascular testing. Baseline data were collected for the multiple variables. The ulcerated limb had pretreatment perfusion and volume much greater than the control limb. A single treatment was administered at the periulcer site. The result was an increase in perfusion, measured by a laser Doppler, and increased skin temperature related to PRFS treatment. These preliminary findings suggest that, if the resting perfusion is marginally inadequate for healing, giving this small boost in perfusion may be sufficient to aid the healing of the ulcer. The parameters of the stimulation were 65 μs, 600 pps, at peak power, with the head 1.5 cm above the surface of the ulcer.[47]

Pulsed Radio Frequency Effect on Hematoma and Thrombolysis

A high level of concern about the issue of deep-tissue injury and hematoma exists, but there is limited information about tested methods for thrombolysis of clotted blood associated with hematoma. Information presented here is a starting place for more study, both to validate the current findings and to develop clinical procedures. Clinicians can begin gathering data about wounds or soft tissue areas that are treated in the clinic that have hemorrhagic areas and report results.

"Deep tissue injury," viewed symptomatically as a hemorrhagic area beneath the skin that later manifest as an open ulcer, has been recognized as frequent sequelae of pressure that are referred to as "purple ulcers."[48–50] More information about hematoma and deep tissue injury is found in Chapter 3 and 4 In the usual healing process, thrombolysis occurs automatically. However, when there is a lot of blood or when the host is unable to adequately lyse the clotted blood, necrosis of the tissues often follows. Therefore, the ability to promote thrombolysis and absorption of the clotted blood products is a desirable attribute of therapy. The following studies show the effects of PRF on thrombolysis.

Basic Science and Animal Studies

Fenn[51] found that hematoma absorption in rabbit ears was accelerated compared with the control group, and that the acceleration became statistically significant on the sixth day after initiation of treatment with PRF. In an attempt to explain what happened, researchers looked at a nonthermal phenomenon observed after application of PRF that they called a *pearl chain phenomenon*. When fat globules in milk were exposed to nonthermal PRF, the fat globules aligned into an order array of pearl chains and remained in that formation until the energy was removed. A second test using thermal energy caused agglomeration of the fat particles that was irreversible. This pearl chain phenomenon was also reproducible with blood and lymph cells.[52]

Cameron[53] looked at wound healing in 20 dogs, comparing a control group of untreated animals with a PRF-treated group.

He took specimens from 24 hours to 10 days after wounding and studied the tissues under the microscope. At 48 hours, the hematoma had been absorbed and replaced by fat that was arranged in strands migrating toward the ends of the wounds. By comparison, the control animals had minimal fat activity by the fourth day after wounding.

Human Clinical Trials

Sambasivan[31] treated four cases of extradural hematomas with PRF. Treatment was applied twice daily for 10 days at a maximum pulse rate of 600 pps and a 65-μs duration for 30 minutes per session, alternating right and left sides of the head. The treated cases showed clearance of their hematoma. If the results are reproducible, this could have tremendous potential for shortening healing times.

Neuropathic Pain

Neuropathic pain (NP) often accompanies neuropathic wounds. Chapters 12 and 22 discuss NP more fully. Here we are looking at some attempts to determine if EMF therapy (PEMF/PRF) can be used to improve nerve conduction velocities (NCVs) and reduce NP in patients with diabetic peripheral neuropathy (DPN). Results from the following clinical trials are mixed.

Graak et al. reported that in a DBRCT of 30 patients with early stages of DPN, they looked at two different outcome measures at two different frequencies using a PRF 600 and 800 Hz compared to controls who received standard wound care. PRF treatments were provided for 30 minutes daily for 12 days. Outcome measures were pre- and post-NCVs including latency of the peroneal nerve and VAS scores.

Results: Group 1 treated at 600 Hz NCV scores: before 36.23 ± 2.09 seconds and after 39.44 ± 2.83 seconds, which was faster than Group 2 treated at 800 Hz. Latency also improved more for Group 1, which was significant ($p < .05$). There were significant differences in decreases in VAS scores: Group 1 66.6%, Group 2 63.25%, and Control Group 22.5%.

Musaev et al.[54] chose PEMF to see if it had the ability to modulate nerves pain and degeneration in 121 patients with DPN. The PEMF device used a complex time-varying pulse regimen modulating both the frequency and the sequencing of the pulses. Two sets of treatment parameters were tested: Group 1 ($N = 62$) device had a PEMF carrier frequency of 100 Hz and a modulation frequency of 1 Hz. Group 2 had a PEMF carrier frequency of 10 Hz and a modulation frequency of 0.5 Hz. Intensity for both groups was 8 mT. Both groups received 10 daily sessions.

Pretrial testing included a battery of quantitative tests to determine the grade of neuropathy of the lower extremities, NCV, VAS scores, clinical signs of sensory and autonomic nervous system (ANS) involvement. Testing showed that 19% of the patients had early clinical signs, 63% showed moderate DPN, 13% DPN with paresis of the dorsal toe extensors, 5% had disabling DPN. Treatment was applied to multiple areas: the spinal segmental nerves for the region of neuropathy and both the upper and lower extremities that corresponded to the same spinal segmental zones of innervation. Each area received 10 to 15 minutes of stimulation.

Results: Group 1: 54.8% has significant analgesia and 37.1% insignificant. The most improved subgroup were those with moderate PN and sensory and ANS involvement.

Group 2: 67.8% had significant improvement, 23% insignificant, 8% no change and again those with moderate involvement were most improved. Those in initial disease state showed marked changes in NCV of the large motor nerve fibers of the lower leg muscles, they had improved amplitude of the H neurologic reflex and there was evidence of greater spinal cord motor neuron excitability. The conclusions from this study were that 10 Hz is the closest to the rhythm of major physiological process in tissues. The conclusions from this study were that 10 Hz is the closest to the rhythm of major physiological process in tissues. Recommendation was to start PEMF therapy at the earliest stages of disease before irreversible structural changes occur in peripheral nerves and spinal cord motor neurons.

WOUND HEALING CLINICAL STUDIES

Several double-blind, and/or randomized, or nonrandomized controlled, and case study reports on PRF efficacy for wound healing in animals and humans are reviewed. A significant problem with the studies that was identified while reviewing the literature on electromagnetic radiation therapy for wound healing and related systemic factors was the inability to compare or combine the results of these studies because, in most cases, the study results reported are subjective, observational, qualitative data, rather than quantitative, and not statistically analyzed data. For example, most of the studies reviewed did not have data about the percentage of change in wound size per unit of time reported or data from which that information can be calculated. Systematic reviews of the literature are often quantitative. In 2009, the National Pressure Ulcer Advisory Panel (NPUAP) and the European Pressure Ulcer Advisor Panel (EPUAP) published evidence-based clinical practice guidelines for the Prevention and Treatment of Pressure Ulcers. Using criteria for evaluation of levels evidence, which for PRF were found to be II, III, IV, and V evidence and a recommended grade of "B" was chosen.[55] This was based on two small RCT using PRF for pressure ulcers both of which are included in the NPUAP/EPUAP evidence tables and reported here. Another small DBRCT is reported here. Likewise, there are small RCT for treatment of leg ulcers, mostly venous using PEMF.

Pulsed Electromagnetic Field Studies

Researchers have branched out from investigating the effect of PEMF on osteogenesis to also look at its effects on soft tissue healing in animals and human subjects. However, stimulation periods using very low-frequency devices that demonstrate efficacy have been much longer than other treatments, up to 3 or 4 hours per day. Treatment at higher frequency and shorter duration had similar effects. The need for longer treatment periods or higher frequency and shorter duration is probably due to the need to accumulate sufficient pulse charge in the tissues to have a biologic effect on the target tissues (see Chapter 23).

Several studies located were performed in countries outside of the United States, some were reported in peer-reviewed US journals, and others were published in the journals of other countries. There is a positive trend to the results for healing of venous ulcers. They are presented here for thoughtful consideration.

Cutaneous Surgical Wounds: Animal Studies

a. Randomized controlled studies of the effects of PEMF on healing of cutaneous surgical wounds in animals (rats,[56,57] dogs,[58] rabbits[59]) demonstrate that PEMF significantly enhances wound epithelialization and provides significant short-term changes in other variables indicative of healing.

b. PEMF was able to significantly reverse the impaired healing effect of corticosteroids.[56]

c. In a study comparing PEMF and pulsed magnetic field (PMF) therapy (17 Hz), there was better collagen alignment in repaired tendons and better suppression of extravascular edema during early inflammation in the PMF (17 Hz) group than in a group treated with PEMF.[60]

d. Ligament tissue stimulated by PEMF showed earlier increases in capillaries and fibroblasts, with better organization of collagen than controls. Amongst three intensities tested, the group treated with 50 G consistently had the best results during the study period.[60]

Human Clinical Studies of Soft Tissue Healing

Human clinical studies reported in this section have been sorted by etiology of the wounding and include pressure ulcers, postsurgical wounds, venous ulcers, and diabetic foot ulcers. Studies within each subsection are described in chronologic order, from oldest to most recent. Venous leg ulcer studies all have the use of PEMF in common. However, the parameters for treatment vary. Table 24.3 (Pressure Ulcer Clinical Studies), Table 24.4 (Postsurgical Clinical Studies), and Table 24.5 (Venous Ulcer Clinical Studies with PEMF) summarize the studies for each section.

Pressure Ulcers

Wound etiology of pressure was the criterion for participation in the following clinical studies.

a. Itoh et al.[61] studied the effect of PRF on stage II partial-thickness and stage III full-thickness pressure ulcers. Comorbidities included cerebrovascular accidents, multiple sclerosis, organic brain syndrome, spinal cord tumor, diabetes, spinal cord injury, and spinal stenosis. Conventional treatments, dressings and topical agents, were continued. In all, 22 patients were included during the 9-month study. Treatment was provided using the Diapulse PRF device at a setting of 600-pps pulse frequency and a setting of 6 (peak power) for 30 minutes twice daily. Treatment sessions were scheduled at approximately 8-hour intervals.[61]

Results: All ulcers healed. Stage II ulcers healed in 1 to 6 weeks (mean 2.33 weeks), and all stage III ulcers healed in 1 to 22 weeks (mean 8.85 weeks).

b. Wilson[62] reported on results of recalcitrant pressure ulcers treated with PRF (Diapulse). Twenty-five stage II, eleven stage III, and fourteen stage IV pressure ulcers affecting 32 patients were enrolled in the uncontrolled study. Duration of ulcers was reported to be up to 2 years. Ages ranged from 77 to 88 years. All received conventional treatment for several weeks up to 2 years prior to inclusion in the PRF study.

Results: Significant wound healing was observed in the most difficult ulcers in 3 to 7 days. Initially, wound exudate increased for 1 to 2 days, then ceased by the third day. All but one patient

| TABLE 24.3 | Pressure Ulcer Clinical Studies | | | | |

Researcher	Itoh et al.[61]	Wilson[62]	Salzberg et al.[64]	Seaborne et al.[65]	Gupta et al.[66]
Type of study and N	Uncontrolled (N = 22)	Uncontrolled (N = 25; 11 stage II; 14 stage IV)	DB-RCT (N = 20 (SCI) 10 stage II; 10 stage III)	B-RCT	DB-RCT (N = 12)
	Unblinded	Observational			
	Observational				
Type of stimulator	PRFS (Diapulse)	PRFS (Diapulse)	PRFS (Diapulse)	ES versus PEMF	PEMF
Frequency	600 pps	Not stated	600 pps	20 pps ES	1 Hz
	65 μs		65 μs	110 pps ES	
				20 pps PEMF	
				110 pps PEMF	
Amplitude/ Intensity	Peak power	Not stated	Peak power		30 mA
Duration of stimulation	30 min BID	Not stated	30 min BID × 12 wk		45 min 5×/wk × 30 sessions with standard wound care Sham group same protocol but PEMF not turned on
Effect of Rx	All patients healed	Significant healing in 3–7 d	Stage II mean healing time of 13 d versus sham group 31.5 d; stage III also healed	All groups showed highly significant reduction in surface area size. No statistical difference between groups	Significant healing in both groups
	Stage II in 1–6 wk mean 2.33 wk; stage III in 1–22 wk mean 8.85 wk	Initial increase in wound exudate (1–2 d) ceased by day 3			TG: p = .008 and sham p = .014
					Not significant difference

Data from references listed in the table.

completely healed, and that individual's wound showed marked improvement before the patient died from other causes.[63]

c. Salzberg et al.[64] used a RCT with an N = 20 of patients with spinal cord injuries, 10 of whom had stage II pressure ulcers and 10 who had stage III pressure ulcers. The group was randomized to 10 treated and 10 sham-treated groups. The device tested was the PRF (Diapulse). Although the study did not list the treatment parameters, an inquiry to the principal author and the Diapulse Corporation provided the information that the settings were 600-pps pulse frequency and 6, peak power. The treatment lasted for 30 minutes twice daily for 12 weeks or until the ulcers healed.

Results: Active treatment group with stage II ulcers had a shorter mean time to complete healing than did the control group (13 versus 31.5 days). The stage III ulcers also healed faster than the controls, but the size of the group was very limited. The study authors' conclusion was that the treatment significantly improved healing.[64]

d. Seaborne et al.[65] randomized 20 nonambulatory individuals with pressure ulcers of the trochanter and sacrum into four groups of five subjects each for a study with PSWD. Allocations were concealed and assessors blinded. Each group was treated with one of four different protocols. Protocols were electrostatic field (electrical stimulation) at 20 and 110 pps, and PEMF nonthermal at 20 and 110 pps. An ABAB repeated measures experimental design was used, with each treatment regimen lasting one calendar week.

Results: Multifactorial analysis showed highly significant reduction in the pressure ulcer surface area in all treatment groups, without significant difference between the groups.[65]

e. Gupta et al.[66] studied PEMF efficacy on NPUAP stage III and IV pressure ulcers using a DBRCT with an N = 12. Admission criteria specified only clean uninfected, debrided pressure ulcers of these stages. Patients were all spinal cord injured persons aged 12 to 50 years. Outcome measures were change in the Bates Jensen Wound Assessment Tool (BWAT)

TABLE 24.4	Postsurgical Clinical Studies					
Researcher	**Goldin et al.**[68]	**Cameron**[67]	**Santiesteban and Grant**[33]	**Kaplan and Weinstock**[69]	**Aronofsky**[70]	**Cornorosan et al.**[72]
Type of study	DB-RCT	Study I	RCT	DB-RCT	CT (nonrandomized, unblended)	CT
		DB Controlled				
		Study 3				
		Uncontrolled				
Type of stimulator	PRFS (Dispulse)	PRFS (Dispulse)	PSWD	PRFS (Diapulse)	PRFS (Diapulse)	PRFS (Diapulse)
Frequency	400 pps/600 pps	400 s	700 pps	400 pps/600 pps	600 pps	400 pps/600 pps
	65 µs	55 µs	95 µs	65 µs	65 µs	65 µs
Amplitude	25.3 W/38 W	Med power(4)	120 W (max power setting)	Peak power (6)	Peak power	Peak power (6)
				Med power(4)		Med power (4)
Duration of stimulation	10 min (hepatic) 20 min (wound) every 6 h × 7 d	Study I	30 min after surgery and 4 h later	Before surgery 20 min BID post 15 min to wound and 15 min epigastrium (hepatic)	Gr 1: 15 min 24 h preop and 10 min just preop	10 min (hepatic)
		20 min (hepatic) 20 min over wound BID × 4 d				15 min (wound)
		Study 2			Postop: 24, 48, 72 h	
		Same as in study 1			Gr 2: 10 min postop	
					Postop: 24, 48, 72 h	
					Gr 3: no PRFS	
Rx Effect	90% or greater healing for 59% of tx group	Study 1	Active group had 8 hr shorter length of hospital stay than controls and significantly less pain medication	Postop d 3:	Inflammation and pain 72 h post:	Plasma; fibronectin concentrations ↑ on postop d 7 in tx group; lower than baseline in control group
	29% healing for sham group	Tx group little improvement for abdominal incision with regard to suture removal; sutures removed on day 5 postop		Severe/moderate edema	Gr 1: None 75%	

(continued)

TABLE 24.4   Postsurgical Clinical Studies (continued)

Researcher	Goldin et al.[68]	Carneron[67]	Santiesteban and Grant[33]	Kaplan and Weinstock[69]	Aronofsky[70]	Cornorosan et al.[72]
		Study 2		Placebo 80%	Mod 20%	
		Shorter hospital stay for tx group		PRFS 58%	High 3.3%	
					Gr 3: None 2%	
					Mod 57%	
					High 37%	
					Pain:	
					Gr 1: None 63%	
					Mod 30%	
					High 6.7%	
					Gr 3: None 7%	
					Mod 57%	
					High 37%	
					Healing in group 1: 3–5 d postop	
					Group 3: 10–12 postup	
Method of measurement	Degree of pain	Retrospective review of medical records	Retrospective review of medication and length of stay records	Likert-like scale grading for edema, erythema, and pain		Observation of inflammatory and infectious process and scarformation
		Subjective measurements				Lab measurements
Etiology tested and N	Split-thickness skin graft donor sites N = 29 active 38 sham	Heterogenous surgical patients	Post podiatric foot surgery	Postsurgical podiatric patients	Oral surgery	Heterogenous surgical wounds
		Study 1 N = 100	N = 25 active		N = 90 (30/group)	N = 15 active
		Study 2 N = 81	25 control			10 control

Data from references listed in the table.

TABLE 24.5	Venous Ulcer Clinical Studies with PEMF

Researcher	Ieran and Zaffuto[73]	Todd et al.[75]	Duran et al.[74]	Stiller et al.[76]	Kenkre et al.[77]
Type of study	DB CT	DB-RCT	Observational	DB-RCT	DB-RCT
Type of stimulator	PEMF	PEMF	PEMF	PEMF	PEMF
Frequency	75 Hz	5 Hz	Not available	25% duty cycle	600 Hz 800 Hz
Amplitude	28 mT	Field strength 60	Not available	0.06 m V/cm 22 G	25 µT
Duration of stimulation	4 h daily × 90 consecutive d	15 min twice weekly	15 min × 10 treatments	3 h daily × 8 wk	30 min 5×/wk × 30 d
Effect during Rx	Healing of exp group Av 71 d 30% decrease in size of ulcers in controls	• Mean reduction of ulcer size:	33% reduction in mean surface area	• Wound surface area:	Wound surface area:
		7% was the same for treatment and control groups		47.1% decrease for active	Gr A Placebo
		• Girth of affected leg:		48.7% increase for placebo	↓ 14.2% (20 d)
		Active: decrease 2.77%		• Wound depth decrease: 46% for active; 3.8% for placebo	↓ 21.8% (30 d)
		Control: increase 1.16%		• Granulation tissue: quantity and quality	Gr B1 600 Hz
				14.1% decrease in unhealthy granulation in active	↑ 28.15% (20 d)
				0% decrease for placebo	↑ 76% (30 d)
				• Clinical Assessment based on 8-pt scale:	Gr B2 800 Hz
				50% of active group healed or markedly improved	↓ 24.7% (20 d)
				54% of placebo group rated worse	↓38% (30 d)
				0% of active group rated worse	
Effect post Rx	Healing continued post-tx period for the tx group versus 50% in controls				4 wk observation period.
					D 50 B2 800 Hz group had significantly greater healing (63% versus 34% Gr A) + improved mobility
Method of Measurement	Healing	Reduction in surface area size	Reduction in surface area of ulcer	Wound characteristics	Reduction in surface area size
					Pain reduction; QOL
Etiology tested and N	Venous ulcers N = 44	Venous leg ulcers N = 19	Venous ulcers N = 18	Venous ulcers N = 31	Venous leg ulcers N = 19

Data from references listed in the table.

score and reduction in the "stage" (using "reverse staging methodology") (see Chapter 5). The device used was a body size set of coils that surrounded the entire body. Parameters were 1 Hz and 30 mA current for 45 minutes five times per week for 30 sessions or until healed.

Results: BWAT scores showed no significant differences but there was a trend to significant healing ($p = .008$). This was a very small sample of patients and so results cannot be generalized.

Postsurgical Wounds

Postsurgical wounding was the pathogenesis of wounds treated in the following studies. Two additional studies of postsurgical wounding are found in an earlier section pain.

a. Cameron[67] undertook three studies on the effect of PRF (Diapulse) on postsurgical wound healing. Study 1 was a 100-patient, double-blind study of postsurgical patients, study 2 was an observational uncontrolled study of 81 postsurgical and orthopedic patients, and study 3 was a 465-patient observational uncontrolled study of nonsurgical orthopedic patients. In studies 1 and 2, each patient was treated twice daily for 20 minutes over the liver and 20 minutes over the wound (400 pps, 4-inch penetration) for 4 days after their operation. Patients in the third study were outpatients and were given the regimen twice daily 3 days a week for 2 weeks, then twice a day on Monday and Friday, then once weekly (twice a day). The PRF was used as an adjunctive treatment to other standard methods of care.

Results: Outcomes were evaluated by the surgeon, who was asked to complete a questionnaire rating whether the patient's condition was the same, better, or worse, as compared with other patients in their experience. The groups analyzed by same, better, or worse showed no statistically significant difference in the treatment and control groups. There was a moderate reduction in length of hospital stay in the treatment group except in those with back surgery. The 81-patient study results demonstrated short hospital stays, despite the fact that some of the patients had osteomyelitis. The outpatient study of 465-patient results showed that acute trauma and inflammatory processes responded the best, but less than 20% recovered within 3 to 4 weeks, which is what would have been expected normally. There also appeared to be no significant benefit from the PRF treatment of chronic cases. There were some methodologic problems with the Cameron studies. Too much emphasis was placed on subjective clinical findings. Use of other treatment modalities along with the PRF did not allow for an accurate evaluation of the PRF efficacy, and absence of inferential statistics further compounds the methodologic problems associated with this study.

b. A double-blind, controlled clinical trial by Goldin et al.[68] used PRF (Diapulse) to study the effects on healing a pain in medium-thickness split-skin grafts. The patients were randomized into two groups, 29 in the active treatment group and 38 in the sham treatment group. The parameter for the treatment group was peak output frequency, 400 pps. The average pulse was fixed at 65 seconds. Mean energy output was nonthermal, 25.3 W. Treatment was given preoperatively and postoperatively every 6 hours for 7 days. Two variables were evaluated: the stage of healing and the degree of pain during the healing phase.

Results: Healing rates on day 7 were 90% or greater healing for 59% of the treatment group and 29% of the sham-treated group. Mechanisms of healing are not clear. Theories to explain the results include increased blood flow and reduced incidence of edema. The stimulation of the cells of repair and repolarization of the depolarized cell membranes of damaged cells that reversed the "injury potential" and the electrical field were thought to be the mechanisms of action.[68]

c. A double-blind randomized clinical evaluation of PRF (Diapulse) following foot surgery in 100 patients was reported by Kaplan and Weinstock.[69] The average number of surgical procedures performed was slightly less than five. As in other studies with Diapulse, the protocol called for 400 pps over the epigastrium and 600 pps over the surgical site. Power level was at 4 for 15 minutes and 6 for 15 minutes to the respective areas. Treatment began before surgery with a 10-minute treatment. A Likert-type scale was used to grade the tissue for symptoms of edema, erythema, and pain.

Results: Statistically significant reduction in severe to moderate edema in the treatment group at the third postoperative day (80%) versus controls (58%); however, the data were reported descriptively.

d. Dental surgery procedures are often the cause of pain, edema, ecchymosis pressure, and disfigurement. In a nonrandomized controlled clinical trial, 90 dental surgery patients were divided into three groups of 30 each.[70] They were treated with PRF (Diapulse) at 600 pps peak power 72 hours preoperatively and postoperatively, only postoperatively 72 hours, or with placebo.

Results: Statistically significant absence of inflammation and pain at 72 hours postoperatively for the pre/postoperative treatment group.

e. Children undergoing orchidoplexy were treated in a double-blind clinical trial. A total of 50 paired boys were involved in the trial. Circumferential measurements of the scrotum were made before and after surgery and treatment of the scrotum, and photographs were taken to measure edema and bruising. Repeat measurements and photographs were taken, with the objective of reducing subjective observation reports of edema and bruising. Treatment was with PRF (Diapulse) at 500 pps and level 5 intensity for 20 minutes over the scrotum and at 500 pps level 4 intensity over the epigastrium for 10 minutes. The treatment regimen was repeated three times daily for the first 4 postoperative days. Matched pairs of boys were used, with one as the control. Investigators chose this operation as a model because of its classic edema and bruise formation.

Results: Suggestive of a trend toward less edema formation, and significantly accelerated resolution of posttraumatic bruising was found.[71]

f. Comorosan et al.[72] treated postsurgical wounds with PRF (Diapulse) over the wound site and over the hepatic area. For the controlled clinical trial, fifteen patients were selected for treatment and 10 served as the control group. The local application was at 600 pps at maximum power output for 20 minutes and the hepatic application at 400 pps at a power setting of 4 for 10 minutes. Treatment started on the second postoperative day and continued for 5 days.

Results: Comorosan et al. reported that the results of this protocol were evaluated by looking at the clinical criteria for wound healing, including the resolution of edema, hematoma, and parietal seroma; lack of inflammatory and infectious processes; suppleness and presence or absence of keloids in the scar; and the degree of postoperative sensitivity. All clinical wound attributes evaluated showed clear-cut improvement. An additional analysis of the effects of the hepatic stimulation showed another measure of healing, increased fibronectin levels, in the treated patients and lower fibronectin levels in the controls.[72]

Leg Ulcers

Presence of venous or other chronic leg ulcers were the criteria for admittance to the following studies. All but one used PEMF. The last and most recent study was a retrospective review of PRF.

a. Ieran and Zaffuto[73] carried out a double-blind study of 44 patients with skin ulcers of venous origin using a coil electrode to generate a PEMF with 75 Hz and 2.8 mT intensity for 4 hours daily for 90 consecutive days.

Results: Healing was within 71 days, on average. Success was significantly higher in the experimental group, both on day 90 and in the follow-up period. Twenty-five percent of the patients in the experimental group and 50% in the control group experienced recurrence of the ulcer.[73]

b. Duran et al.[74] reviewed 18 cases with venous ulcers who were treated 10 times with PEMF, each session lasting 15 minutes.

Results: A significant reduction in the mean surface area of 33% by reepithelialization following treatment with PEMF.

c. Todd et al.[75] reported that the results of double-blind randomized controlled clinical trial of 19 patients with venous ulcers used a protocol applying PEMF two times weekly over a 5-week period. Treatment parameters were field strength of 60, 5-Hz intensity, and duration of 15 minutes. Treatment was carried out by placing coils on either side of the ulcer over the wound dressings. Parameters measured were ulcer size, lower leg girth, degree of pain, and presence of infections.

Results: The findings were that there was no statistically relevant difference noted between the active and inactive treatment groups. However, there was a trend in favor of a decrease in ulcer size and lower leg girth in the active treatment group and no proliferation of bacterial populations. No effect was noted on report of pain. One patient in the study in the active treatment group had an initial ulcer size that was so large that it skewed the mean ulcer pre- and posttreatment areas. Removing this patient's ulcer from the study group reflected truer results that showed a trend toward improved healing but was not statistically significant (17.5% in active treatment versus 7.1% in sham treatment). Another study defect was the mean initial duration of the venous ulcer, which ranged from a mean 3.5 years for the active treatment group to a mean of 18.3 years for the sham group.[75] The results of this pilot study are inconclusive, due to the small sample size and lack of rigor in selecting the patients. Also, the duration and frequency of the treatment were perhaps too minimal to have a more statistically significant treatment effect.

d. Stiller et al.[76] reported that 31 patients were enrolled in a prospective, randomized, double-blind, placebo-controlled multicenter study of venous ulcer healing to determine the efficacy of PEMF treatment. Treatment was provided using a portable home device that the patient or caregiver applied for 3 hours daily for 8 weeks or until the ulcer healed, if prior to 8 weeks. Treatment parameters were 3.5-milliseconds pulse width, bidirectional delta B of approximately 22 G. The protocol was derived from the study of PEMF used effectively to treat nonunion fractures.

Results: Recalcitrant venous ulcers showed after 8 weeks that the active treatment group of 18 had a 47.7% decrease in wound surface area versus 42.3% for the placebo group of 13 ($p<.0002$). A global evaluation of the wounds indicated that 50% of the ulcers in the active group healed or markedly improved versus 0% in the placebo group. None of the active group of ulcers worsened versus worsening in 54% of the placebo group ($p<.001$). Likewise, there were statistically significant decreases in wound depth and pain intensity in the active group. Researchers concluded that PEMF is a safe and effective nonsurgical therapy for recalcitrant venous leg ulcers. The subjects in this trial may have done better than the earlier group they tested because the duration of the stimulation, given on a daily basis, allowed for enough pulse charge accumulation to reach the target tissues and produce a biologic effect. (See Chapter 23 for information about pulse charge accumulation.)

e. Kenkre[77] reported the results of a study with 19 patients with venous leg ulcers enrolled in a prospective, randomized, double-blind controlled clinical trial. Outcome measures were rate and scale of ulcer healing, changes in pain levels, quality of life, degree of mobility, side effect profile, and acceptability to patients and staff. The device used was the Elmedistraal electromagnetic device (available in the United Kingdom) that delivered perpendicular electric and magnetic fields through a pulse generator, creating frequencies of 100, 600, and 800 Hz. The magnetic field produced was 25 µT. These parameters appear to be similar to PRF, although the study is called "electromagnetic therapy."

Results: Sixty-eight percent of the active treatment group achieved improvement in ulcer size, and twenty-one percent of those experienced complete healing. Reduction of pain levels was also statistically significant, despite the chronicity of the ulcers. Those treated at 800 Hz were found to have statistically greater healing and pain relief than either those in the 600-Hz group or the control group at day 50. However, when the treatment phase ended at day 30, the trend for healing was better in the control group and the 800-Hz group, compared with the 600-Hz group but reduction of pain scores was greatest in the 600-Hz group. In all three groups, some ulcers with a long history of chronicity healed. It appears that, as in the Ieran study,[73] the effects of the treatment continued after cessation of the treatment. Adverse effects reported were sensations of heat, tingling, pins and needles in the lower half of the limb, and headaches (unusual for two patients), but patients who experienced these sensations continued with the study. Psychosocial benefits of improved mobility and community activity were reported.

f. Canedo-Dorantes et al.[24] evaluated healing of patients with chronic arterial and venous leg ulcers that were resistant to medical and surgical treatment. The subjects were grouped as follows: group 1, 8 patients with 17 ulcers of predominantly arterial origin, and group 2, 18 patients with 25 chronic leg ulcers of predominantly venous origin. Systemic treatments for pain, rheumatoid arthritis, arterial hypertension, and diabetes were continued but other systemic medications and preventive treatments were discontinued. Local wound care was limited to wound cleansing with soap and water and covering with an unspecified dressing. The team of researchers used a novel approach, applying the EMF to either *arm* not the ulcer directly. The purpose of this alternative application was to determine whether the EMF could alter systemic effects by interaction with EMF action potentials at a peripheral location. The hypothesis was that PBMCs could be induced in the body of the patients with chronic leg ulcers by using EMF frequencies that were previously tested on normal human blood samples. The treatment method described was to place an arm into an exposure chamber so as to achieve a homogeneous magnetic field. Average exposure time was 2 to 3 hours per day three times a week for a 4-month period. EMF strength of 36.36 G was generated inside the chamber. Wound surface area size and appearance were documented at baseline and during follow-ups photographically and the information digitized and processed electronically.

Results: reported by groups:

Group 1 "responders" fully healed or experiencing a greater than 50% reduction. Responders, with 29 previously unresponsive ulcers, began to heal by week 2 and by the end of the study period 15 arterial and 14 venous ulcers were in the responder group. Responders healed at the same rates, the arterial ulcer group showed the development of visible vascular networks and increased periwound temperatures after 4 to 8 weeks of treatment. In the responders with venous ulcers, pain, edema, and weeping reduced significantly or were eliminated 3 to 6 weeks after start of care.

Group 2 "nonresponders" had at least one ulcer that experienced a less than 50% reduction or increase in size. Two arterial and 11 venous ulcers were in the nonresponder groups. Nonresponders in the venous group had higher body mass index, nonpitting edema, and severe lipodermatosclerosis. The arterial group had severe arterial occlusion and/or uncontrolled arterial hypertension. Pain among nonresponders only partially reduced in 4 to 6 weeks of treatment.

Healing or deleterious effects were observed in all patients within the first 2 weeks after initiation of the treatment. No negative secondary effects were reported either during treatment or the follow-up period.

g. Frykberg et al.[78] did a retrospective descriptive study of cases in a wound registry established and maintained by Regenesis Biomedical, Inc. (Scottsdale, AZ) to determine outcomes of lower extremity ulcer cases from 100 geographically diverse US medical facilities. Criterion for evaluation was record of outcome of care after 4 weeks treatment. There were no exclusions based on comorbidity, wound type, wound, or prior medical history. Analysis of 113 patient records of 128 chronic wounds was performed. The wound etiologies in the distribution were 25% diabetic foot ulcers, 30% venous ulcers, 25% pressure ulcers stages II to IV, and 20% other wound types.

Treatment parameters were the RF signal, 27.12 MHz, 42 μs pulse width at 1,000 pps. Regenesis sells the Provant Therapy System, which is the PRF device used for treatment.

Results: Mean percent reduction in wound area after 4 weeks was pressure ulcers 49% ± 6% ($p < .0001$); diabetic foot ulcers 38% ± 6% ($p < .0001$); venous ulcers 44% ± 5% ($p < .0001$); other wound types 39% ± 9% ($p = .0001$). The healing trend suggested that treated wounds would have healed with ongoing therapy.

Diabetic Foot ulcers

No large RCT or controlled trials for this patient population were identified. Some of the patients in the retrospective study above had diabetic ulcers. These case studies show a positive trend continuing.

Larsen and Overstreet[79] used PRF for treatment of two patients with diabetes.

a. Case Study:1. Patient with uncontrolled diabetes and a foot ulcer was at high risk for amputation. Other treatment interventions including growth factors and other advanced therapies had failed to heal. He received good standard wound care plus PRF.

Results: wound closure in 16 weeks and remained closed at 9-month follow-up. The healing rate was 1.56 mm² per day.

b. Case Study:2. Patient had prior transmetatarsal amputation, besides diabetes there were multiple comorbidities. The wound had a toe infected with osteomyelitis. Besides standard wound care, the foot was offloaded, debrided, and silver dressings were used.

Results: closure in 16.7 weeks, healing rate 6.0 mm² per day.

Conclusions from Leg Ulcer Studies

All of these studies represent a small sample of patients with leg ulcers, but there seems to be a trend that shows wound healing efficacy with PEMF and PRF. The preliminary work presented shows that there is potentially significant benefit from use of EMF for leg ulcer healing but additional high-quality studies are warranted to evaluate efficacy and best treatment parameters.

CLINICAL DECISION MAKING

Several patient intrinsic and extrinsic factors must be taken into consideration when considering a treatment with thermal PSWD, nonthermal PRF, or PEMF. Therefore, begin your decision making as you would care any planning with a comprehensive patient history, systems review, and examination and wound examination. Review the history and systems for information about sensation, circulation, edema, metal and electronic implants, acute osteomyelitis, cancer, mental status, and pregnancy, all of which will be used to guide proper choice of this therapy.

Selection of Candidates

Age should be considered when selecting candidates for PRF or PSWD. Application of PRFS or PSWD over growth plates is probably not harmful because of the short duration of the wound healing treatment application, compared with the lengthy period of stimulation required to alter bone formation in bone healing studies using PEMFs.

Special Populations

Special populations are discussed next because each group requires special consideration depending on unique factors. Special needs populations include children, the elderly, and patients with implants.

Children and Elderly

Children have growth plates until about 16 years of age, depending on race, sex, and the bone involved (use over immature bone is a listed contraindication). Children usually do not have the underlying comorbidities that lead to chronic wounding, but forced immobility due to pain would be detrimental to a child. Some of the most common wounds in children are burns. A child with burn wounds would benefit from PRFS early intervention to normalize skin enzymes and to eliminate edema and reduce pain, resulting in less scarring and quicker return to play and school activities. If the benefit of accelerated wound healing outweighs the small risk of interference with a bone plate, prudent judgment should be used. Elderly must always be evaluated for circulatory impairments and changes in sensory perceptions and mentation.

Patients with implants, electronic, or metal (including intrauterine devices)

Metals reflect radio frequency energy common to all EMF devices, so application over metal implants will reflect the energy back into the tissues, creating more intense energy levels in the tissues over the implant than usual, disregulation of electronic circuit function or the energy may be blocked from reaching the target tissues. Location of the metal should guide you to consider an alternative method of application, such as moving the applicator head above or below the area of metal (whichever is closest to the wound) to treat the surrounding wound tissues.

Exhibit 24.4 shows a list of contraindications, warnings, and cautions to be taken when using PSWD and PRF equipment. PRF has fewer precautions and contraindications because it does not heat tissues, osteomyelitis, cancer, or pregnancy. Avoid using this intervention in the presence of any of these conditions.[8,80]

Precautions and contraindications for the two classes of EMF equipment, thermal and nonthermal, are listed separately in each category.

Pulsed Short-Wave Diathermy Precautions and Contraindications

- Review the patient's vital signs. Patients who are febrile should not be treated with additional heat.
- Check the pharmacy history for blood-thinning medications and tendency for hemorrhage.
- Do not treat patients in the first 24 to 48 hours after traumatic injury because the treatment can increase bleeding and edema, hemorrhaging tendency, including heavy menstruation.
- Change the parameters of the treatment to modify the amount of heating. If wound examination findings are acute

---

EXHIBIT 24.4

FDA Contraindications, Warnings, and Cautions for PSWD and PRF

PSWD	PRF
• Do not treat over ischemic tissue with inadequate blood flow	• Do not use as a substitute for treatment of internal organs
• Do not treat over or near metallic implants	• Do not use over metal implants
• Do not use with patients with cardiac pacemakers	• Do not use with patients with cardiac pacemakers
• Do not treat in any region where presence of primary or metastatic malignant growth is known or suspected	• Do not use with patients who are pregnant
• Do not treat over immature bone	• Do not treat over immature bone
• Do not treat over acute osteomyelitis without adequate drainage or before adequate drainage has been established	
• Do not treat patients who have a tendency to hemorrhage (including menses)	
• Do not treat over pelvic or abdominal region or lower back during pregnancy	
• Do not treat transcerebrally	
• Do not use over anesthetized areas	
• Avoid situations that could concentrate the field, including moist dressings, perspiration, adhesives	
• Use caution when treating patients with heat sensitivity	
• Use caution when treating patients with inflammatory processes	

Data from International Medical Electronics, *Magnatherm® Model 1000 Instruction Manual* and Electropharmacology (company disbanded), *MRT® sofPulse™ User's Manual*.

inflammation, direct heating should be avoided, but indirect heating could be useful (e.g., inflammation in the foot can be treated with PSWD or PRF applied over the abdomen or sacrum).

According to required manufacturer's labeling requirements, PSWD is contraindicated for all conditions for which heat is contraindicated.

- Do not use areas of insensitivity that prevent the patient from reporting a sensation of heating.
- Do not use over ischemic tissue (e.g., an ankle-brachial index of <0.8) because the body requires adequate perfusion to regulate tissue temperature. If circulatory perfusion is obstructed, it may not allow for the heat to dissipate and result in burning.
- Do not use PSWD over metal, including surgical metal hardware; foreign bodies, such as shrapnel, bullets, or metallic sutures; or intrauterine devices. The metal may become heated and reflect high levels of energy that will cause burns.
- Do not use PSWD if the patient has electronic implants or is connected to electrical or electronic equipment because the EMF of the PSWD may cause interference with these electronic devices.
- Do not use over any area where there is primary or metastatic malignant tissue growth or over organs or tissues containing high fluid volumes (e.g., the heart, edematous extremity, and over the abdomen and lumbar areas during pregnancy). Even though pulsed radio frequency is used for cancer treatment, as mentioned earlier, this is a specialized heating procedure used under radiographic guidance by a skilled practitioner.
- Do not treat over areas with acute osteomyelitis without adequate drainage or before drainage has been established.
- Do not use if there is diagnosis of active tuberculosis.
- Do not use if there is acute hemorrhaging or acute inflammation.

Safety Issues

- **PSWD.** One way to mitigate the heating effect of PSWD is to leave a greater air gap or more toweling between the applicator and the tissues. Check pulses and perform other visual examinations to detect circulatory deficits. If findings show diminished circulation, noninvasive vascular testing may be required.
- Examination for wound drainage is important. If PSWD is used, wounds that have a heavy amount of wound exudate would require special handling to absorb all of the moisture before treatment, to avoid burns.[8,81] Consider indirect heating with PSWD or nonthermal PRF over the lumbar area or the abdomen that will produce reflex vasodilation in areas remote from the site of heating, for example, the foot.[2,47] This is also suggested for patients with vasospasm.
- Contact with any metal (e.g., jewelry, zippers, brassiere fasteners, and brassiere underwires) should be avoided when using PSWD because of the risk of burns and distortion of the EMF is possible from metal objects placed near the cables. Also avoid contact with metal furniture or parts (e.g., mattress springs). PSWD should not be used over synthetic materials that may melt and cause burns.[1] Electronic devices (e.g., hearing aids, watches) should not be worn during treatment with these devices because the EMF may cause disruption of the device. Hearing aids may produce annoying noise feedback.

- **PRF.** Electronic devices (e.g., hearing aids, watches) should not be worn during treatment with PRF devices for the same reasons cited above. Do not administer PRF directly over metal (e.g., jewelry, zippers) because the energy will be reflected and not reach the target tissues.
- **PEMF.** PEMF safety appears to be well established. No toxicologic or teratologic effects have been demonstrated by in vitro or in vivo safety testing.[25,26]
- **Therapist Safety.** Many sources of EMFs are present in the environment, and most do not affect the human body. By the nature of the PSWD and PRF devices described in this chapter, although shielded from EMF radiation, the EMFs do not pass 100% of the energy into the tissues being treated. Some energy is dissipated into the area close to the equipment. Operators and persons close to the equipment will absorb a small amount of an EMF. EMFs from PSWD at distances of 0.5 m from the cables and 0.2 m from inductive applicators are low at low and medium pulse settings. A study of physical therapist work habits found that most remain at least 1 m from the applicator and 0.5 m from the cables during the operation of PSWD equipment. At those distances, there is little danger of excess absorption.[82] However, some older model PSWDs may not have shielded cables. The device should be checked for leakage of EMF energy. For personnel working with this equipment who have electronic implants, however, it would be prudent not to be exposed to the EMF because the stray radiation may affect the operation of those devices. The same holds true for other patients or family members occupying the same treatment areas. A timer is usually part of the equipment, and it will turn the equipment off automatically, but if the patient needs to be assisted during the treatment, the staff member can approach the console without standing close to the cables. Several studies have attempted to measure the effects of EMFs on personnel working in areas where frequent exposure to SWD occurs. An epidemiologic study looked at the risk of birth defects, perinatal deaths, and late spontaneous abortions affecting fetuses of female therapists working with SWD. The result of this retrospective study showed that the risk of a miscarriage was not associated with reported use of SWD.[83] Patients, except as mentioned, have no measurable risk from the EMF associated with this equipment, and the benefits probably outweigh any negative effects. Of current concern are PEMF such as radiate from cell phones or the small printed circuit devices used for medicine, but at this time there are no proven negative effects.

EQUIPMENT

In the introduction of this chapter, you were told that EMF equipment has undergone 4 iterations. SWD equipment manufactured and many devices like the Curapulse (Enraf Nonius, Delft, The Netherlands and Henley International, Sugarland, TX), the Megapupilse (Electromedical Supplies, Ltd., UK, and PTI Corporatio, Topeka, KS), and Magnatherm™ (International Medical Electronics Ltd., Kansas City, MO) shown in Figure 24.7 are on the market. These are best suited for use in the clinic setting. Some lighter portable models are also manufactured. When PRF was first introduced as a separate piece of equipment by the Diapulse Corporation of America (Great Neck, NY), it

Nonthermal PRF and PEMF

Equipment classified as nonthermal diathermy (PRF) was designed to allow for dissipation of heat, and to reduce its accumulation by lowering the power settings and by means of pulsing the current wave. Several studies report the effects of nonthermal PRF using commercially available PRF devices. The way in which manufacturers handle the technical specifications for their devices is the way in which the outputs are reported. Diapulse is constructed with vacuum tubes. Provant and MRT SofPulse® (Electropharmacology company disbanded) were both solid-state analogues of Diapulse. Diapulse, Provant devices use fixed pulse duration, 65 μs for the former and 42 μs for the latter. The FDA has designated these devices as equivalent. Based on recent research and a change in product

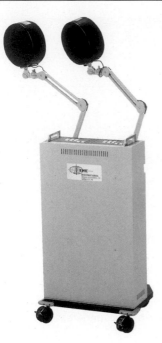

FIGURE 24.6 Shortwave diathermy unit (Magnatherm SSP). (Courtesy of International Medical electronics. Ltd., Kansas City, MO.)

took on and has retained the same configuration of electronics and physical dimensions. Later devices, using the same energy parameters, applied solid-state electronics to the engineering of their PEMF and PRF equipment that reduced the weight and bulk of their equipment. Currently, miniaturized equipment is used for wound healing for patient populations including plastic surgery.[3] (See Figs. 24.7 and 24.8 for examples.)

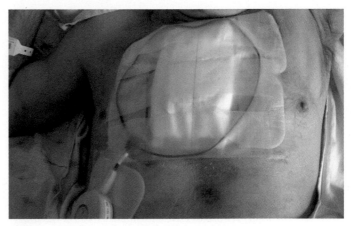

FIGURE 24.8 Ivivi SofPulse® device. (Courtesy of Dr. B. Strauch, Ivivi Health Sciences, San Francisco, CA.)

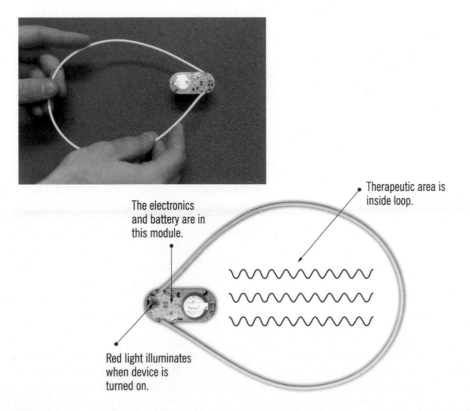

The electronics and battery are in this module.

Therapeutic area is inside loop.

Red light illuminates when device is turned on.

FIGURE 24.7 RecoveryRx™ (Courtesy of Dr. B. Strauch, Ivivi Health Sciences, San Francisco, CA.)

ownership, the MRT SofPulse® (Electropharmacology now disbanded) is no longer on the market, having been replaced by a new SofPulse®, sold by Ivivi Health Sciences (San Francisco, CA) with pulse durations from 2 to 5 µs and repetition rates from 1 to 5 pps. This new device requires less than 20 W input power and induces a magnetic field one-tenth the strength of the other two PRFS units.

Regulatory Approval

Regulatory approval in the United States falls into two categories. The Food and Drug Administration (FDA) regulates safe and effective marketing of medical devices. The Center for Medicare and Medicaid Services (CMS) regulates reimbursement for medical interventions including wound healing. Both categories regulate use of EMF devices.

Food and Drug Administration

Both PSWD and PRF are classified as diathermy by the FDA but in two separate classes: thermal and nonthermal. The first PRF device that was approved by the FDA for medical use and appeared on the market was the Diapulse. The FDA allowed the Diapulse Corporation to market the device as a short-wave diathermy class III device meaning it was nonthermal. Diathermy class III devices that are currently being marketed are described in the equipment section later PSWD and PRF send EMF signals to the tissues, but they are not considered synonymous therapies.

The CSWD and PSWD generators are classified as Class II shortwave diathermy devices, used for therapeutic deep heating for purposes of treatment of pain, muscle spasms, and joint contractures. PRF generators are classified as Class III shortwave diathermy for all other uses (except treatment of malignancy), intended to treat medical conditions by means other than deep heating as nonthermal units, and are sold to control pain and edema.[84]

Center for Medicare and Medicaid Services

The CMS now considers PEMF and PRF as reimbursable covered service for wound healing of Medicare beneficiaries when the patient meets specific criteria.[85] In the materials we have just reviewed, you learned that PEMF and PRF induce electrical current in the body; therefore, the coverage policy explanation, since 2004, states that PEMF and PRF are essentially equivalent therapy to electrical stimulation, but by a different application method.[86] The coverage policy can be accessed at www.hhs.cms.gov by searching for electrical stimulation coverage policy.

State licensing agencies regulate what is physical therapy. PSWD is considered a separate treatment and, thus, Medicare guidelines state that the use of diathermy should always be by or under the supervision of a licensed physical therapist or physician.

Clinical Practice Treatment Guidelines

Early published treatment guidelines for pressure ulcers did not distinguish PRFS-induced current from capacitive electrotherapy as an adjunctive treatment.[87–89] However, in 2009, the NPUAP and EPUAP Prevention and Treatment Guidelines for Pressure Ulcers made a distinction. Direct contact electrical stimulation is included as an A level recommended modality; however, due to the limited evidence, level 1 evidence, PRF, and PEMF are only designated as having a level B recommendation.[55]

EXHIBIT	24.5	
FDA Indications		
PSWD		**PRF**
Improved blood flow		Relief of pain and edema
Improved oxygenation		Increased blood flow
Increased metabolic rate		
Inflammatory conditions Relief of pain and edema		

Exhibit 24.4 lists FDA contraindications, and Exhibit 24.5 lists FDA indications.

Devices

In this subsection, you will learn about the specific technology of different devices on the market at this time including PSWD, Diapulse.

Pulsed Short-Wave Diathermy

A PSWD generator uses a coil mounted within a case (called a *head*) as the radiating element. This coil is driven by a crystal-controlled amplifier contained within the main chassis of the unit. The output of this head is an EMF with a radio frequency of 27.12 MHz. The head is mounted on a movable, adjustable arm. Depending on the unit design, the head may be rectangular or round. Some devices allow the frequency to be delivered continuously or pulsed. The range of heating and nonthermal effects will depend on the pulse rate and duration. A PSWD device that can be operated at a broad range of pulse rates and pulse durations will have the most potential clinical applications. Heating effects are the principal action of the device at high pulse rates of long duration, and nonthermal effects are achieved at low pulse rates and over short durations. At the nonthermal settings, the PSWD may have effects equivalent to those of the PRFS devices, which are limited to this range. PSWD devices are on the market, including the Magnatherm (International Medical Electronics, Kansas City, MO), the Curapulse (Enraf Nonius, Delft, The Netherlands, and Henley International, Sugarland, TX), and Megapulse (Electro-Medical Supplies, Ltd, UK, and PTI Corporation, Topeka, KS). They are considered equivalent; however, there are differences in available pulse rates, pulse duration, and average outputs.

The Curapulse method of creating the electric and magnetic fields uses a different technology than do the other devices described. Each field is delivered in isolation by means of the condenser electrodes and a monode head, and transformation to an EMF occurs within the body tissue. Curapulse is available with either one or two electrodes that can be operated with different protocols (see Fig. 24.9). For example, the pulse rate and the duration of treatment must remain constant for both heads, but the other parameters can be set separately for each. Two models are available: (1) Model 670 allows for variation of pulse duration from 65 to 400 µs, adjustable in seven steps, and an adjustment of frequency from 26 to 400 Hz, adjustable in 10 steps, that can be used for both thermal and nonthermal effects; (2) Model 970 has a fixed pulse duration of 400 µs and a

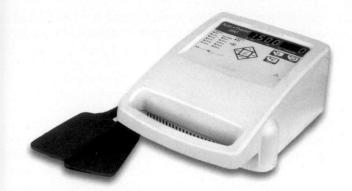

FIGURE 24.9 Autotherm 390 pulsed and continuous shortwave diathermy. (Courtesy of Mettler Electronics, Anaheim CA The Netherlands and Sugarland, TX.)

frequency of 15 to 200 pps, and is considered a thermal device. Maximum outputs are also different. Table 24.6 shows the available parameters for these different models.

The Megapulse pulse-width settings range from 25 to 400 µs. Three pulse modes are offered with the device on/off cycles consisting of one-third on time and two-thirds off time; two-thirds on time and one-third off time; and continuous. The pulse duration and frequency can be changed during those three modes. When longer on time and shorter off time are selected, there will be more thermal effects. Shorter on and longer off time will be less thermal, and the effects will be stimulation of the cells, rather than heating. It can be used like a PSWD or PRF device. The wide range of settings may be confusing to new users, but they enhance the choice and variety of applications and conditions that can be treated. The Magnatherm SSP unit is designed so that each of the two round inductive treatment heads can be set at the same or different settings to deliver controlled dosages for individualized treatment effects. Each is controlled and monitored from its own panel. There is a full range of pulse rates from which to choose. The unit is designed to be used on a cart for mobility, or to be lifted off the cart and

RESEARCH WISDOM

Pattern of Treatment Effect

The pattern of treatment effect for PSWD and PRF stimulators is in the form of the shape and size of the applicator head.

packed in its own carrying case for portability. However, the 25-pound weight would be a real workout for a therapist carrying it from car to house several times a day. A wheeled attachment would facilitate this application.

Pulsed Radio Frequency Stimulators

PRF generators, like PSWD generators, consist of a radiating treatment head or applicator coil and an electronic console with the power generator. The output of this head is an EMF with a radio frequency of 27.12 MHz that is the same for all three devices described here. Other parameters vary.

PRF

Diapulse

The Diapulse has a pulse length of 65 µs and an interpulse interval that can be varied from 12.4 to 1.6 milliseconds by altering the pulse frequency. This allows ample time for heat to be.[90] Electromagnetic effects at the cellular level are the actions to expect from these devices, not heating.[8] The Diapulse has a stronger magnetic field and a weaker electrical field, and both are emitted simultaneously.[91] The frequency can be set in six steps (80, 120, 200, 300, 400, 500 pps) in conjunction with six intensity settings. Peak power output is 38 W delivered to the tissues.

Provant Wound Closure System

The Provant Wound Closure System product is designed with a treatment coil enclosed in a pad and a lead attaching it to the power generator. The signal is a pulsed square wave with a pulse

TABLE 24.6	**Typical Equipment Parameters**			
Device	Operating Frequency (MHz)	Pulse Pulse Generated Rates (pps)	Widths (µs)	Power (W)
Magnatherm	27.12	700–7,000	95 Fixed	0.2%–100% (1,000 peak)
Megapulse	27.12	50–800	20–400	150 Peak, 5–40 average
Nonthermal mode < 200	<200			
Thermal mode > 200	>100			
Curapulse				
Model 970	27.12	15–200	400 Fixed	1,000 Peak, 80 average
Model 670	27.12	26–400	65–400	200 Peak, 32 average
Diapulse	27.12	80–600	65 Fixed	293–975 Peak, 1.5–38 average
SofPulse®	27.12			
Model Roma 1–5	2–5 ms	1–10 W		
Model Torino 2	3 ms	2 W		

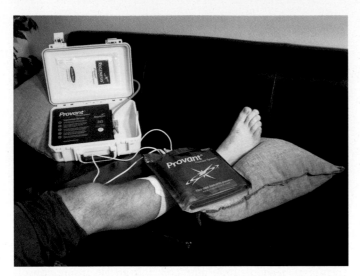

FIGURE 24.10 Provant device. (Regenesis Biomedical Scottsdale, AZ.)

duration of 42 μs and frequency of 1 KHz. Output strength delivered to the tissues is 187 V/m at 5 cm (Fig. 24.10).

Ivivi Health Sciences' Roma and Torino Models

The Ivivi Health Sciences' Roma model is a clinical model with three outputs for application to three wound areas. The treatment coil comes in different size diameters for treatment of different size wound or multiple wounds in a given area. The EMF field is projected equally in all directions around the coil and has the ability to reach and treat a large volume of tissue. For example, an 8-inch coil loop will treat the whole head. Since there is no sensation when using PRF, it is difficult to know that the active coil is transmitting the energy. To compensate for this the manufacturer has designed two failsafe alarm systems that are built into the unit. One alarm sends a flashing light error message letting the operator know that the output is not intact. The second alarm is a beeping sound to call attention to a problem. Based on the basic science research reported elsewhere in this chapter, the manufacturer has adjusted the energy delivery to provide longer duration signal (1 milliseconds) and reduced output from 300 to 10 W. The Torino model is a disposable single patient design that consists of a coil loop and a small generator (see Fig. 24.8).

The current state of knowledge of the mechanism of PRF's bioeffects has recently allowed the peak input power to the applicator to be reduced from 300 to less than 10 W. This leads to more efficacious and speedier therapeutic outcomes.[35] Like all PRF units in this class, the radio frequency used remains at 27.12 Hz, but with this low power output there is negligible radio frequency interference on monitoring and life-sustaining electronic equipment. The low power requirement of modern PRF devices has allowed the development of portable, battery-operated units which can be sent home with the patient. To achieve all of this, the PRF signal now typically has a burst duration of 3 milliseconds, versus 65 μs, which repeats at 5 bursts per second, as opposed to 600 per second, and a peak amplitude of 0.05 G, versus 2 G. So far, the only company to use this new technology is Ivivi, in their two SofPulse® models: the Roma clinical model and Torino portable and single-subject use model. Another innovation of this product line is the use of a

radiating coil loop instead of a drum housing the radiating coil. Loops come in varying sizes to assure adequate dosimetry for wounds of different sizes.

RecoveryRx™ (Bioelectronics Corp, Frederick, MD) came on the market after FDA approval in March 2004 and is a fourth-generation product. It weighs only a few ounces and radiates less total power but over a 24-hour period yet delivers 2.5 to 3 times the energy of the large second-generation devices described earlier. It is housed in a flexible plastic that contours to the body and comes in different sizes. The design of the antenna/coil is efficient and was designed to create an enveloping radiation field with potential for better penetration. The lifespan of this device is approximately 30 days and has an on/off switch to conserve the power source.[3] It was designed for the plastic surgery market but has potential for the larger wound market but needs testing in that population.

Manufacturers are marketing these devices for home use by patients and caregivers under a medical prescription and the supervision of a licensed healthcare practitioner. All are FDA-approved devices for pain, edema, and circulation but NOT for wound healing.

PATIENT TREATMENT

Next you will learn about procedures of patient treatment used for circulatory benefits and for wound healing with PSWD and PRF. The literature interchanges the terms PRF and PEMF even though we know that they may not be equivalent. Therefore, the information presented will be those used in the studies as presented. As research continues about use of EMF for wound healing, both new devices and protocols should be expected. Here we are giving guidance based on current practice.

Protocols

Protocols are established to achieve a predictable outcome. Consider using along with your clinical judgment.

PSWD

PSWD is a thermal agent that has predictable effects on tissue temperature and blood flow.[40,41] Normal resting body temperature is between 36.3°C and 37.5°C. PSWD at thermal levels has the ability to raise deep tissue temperature to 45°C. Vigorous heating is defined as raising tissue temperature to between 40°C and 45°C.[40] This is estimated to be the maximum safe upper limit to raise tissue temperature and corresponds to the pain threshold of the skin. Maintaining a tissue temperature of 45°C for a sufficiently long period will result in irreversible tissue damage. Three factors influence the maximum tissue temperature reached: the square of the intensity, the tissue impedance, and the length of time the tissue is heated. Also, tissue perfusion determines how quickly the blood flow will dissipate the heat.[8] The observable effect of heating is hyperemia due to increased blood flow. This is a mild inflammatory response, initiating the biologic cascade associated with the process of inflammation (see Chapter 2). Vasodilation occurs along with increased capillary hydrostatic pressure and vessel permeability. This promotes movement of fluid from the vessels into the interstitial spaces. Symptoms associated with this process are *edema*, *pain*, and *warmth*. Raising the tissue temperature within a 5- to 15-minute period will raise the tissue temperature to the maximum range.[40,41] The resulting vasodilation will produce a marked increase in blood flow that will then dissipate the heat and decrease the temperature by several degrees. A total exposure period of 20 to 30 minutes is described in the literature as the required time for the optimal therapeutic benefits of heating to occur. Studies show that this can be achieved with inductive coupling using PSWD or PRF over the area of the inguinal ligament and lower abdomen while avoiding excessive heating of the superficial tissues and subcutaneous fat.[1] Tissue heating below 40°C temperature is considered mild.[18]

PRF

PRF protocols used in the reported studies have a single set of parameters, regardless of whether perfusion, reduction of edema or pain, or tissue healing was the outcome. It is not currently known, however, what may be the optimal parameters of dosage that affect different levels of tissues at different stages of repair. This determination requires further research. In the current situation, the experimental protocols have validity and reliability, and can be used safely. At this time, it is recommended that you consult with the manufacturer for information about protocols.

Expected Outcomes

Change in temperature measures the change in tissue perfusion after the treatment. How the tissue responds functionally to the enhanced perfusion is the functional outcome (e.g., progression to the proliferative phase—red, neovascularized granulation tissue). The sequence of predictable biologic events occurs during the process of healing as the wound progresses from an initial phase of healing (inflammatory) to a later phase of healing (epithelialization or contraction). The steps of the progression are outcome measures for measuring and predicting wound healing. See Chapter 3 for possible wound outcomes and prognoses. The expected outcome for a chronic wound treated with a physical agent such as PSWD or PRF should progress from one phase to the next phase in a 2- to 4-week period. Research evidence can be used as a guide for the mean time for healing. For example, in two pressure ulcer studies using PRF (Diapulse),[61,64] closure was reported at a rate of 8.7% and 5.9% per week for stage III pressure ulcers. The healing time will be at the end of the range for patients with the factors that affect healing, such as older age, immobility, comorbidities, long duration of wound, large wound size, and the depth of tissue involvement. If reassessment does not confirm the expected outcomes, treatment must change. Change here can mean a change in protocol (e.g., mild heating changed to vigorous heating), an increase in the length of treatment time, a change in frequency from three times per week to daily, or a change in dressing or topical agent. Any or all of the above are ways to consider changing the treatment to affect the wound status and reach a predictable outcome. Below are expected outcomes for the protocols for both PSWD and PRF.

Wound Healing Phase Diagnosis: Acute or Chronic Inflammation

Expected Outcome Protocol
- Hyperemia: change in skin color to red, blue, or purplish, depending on color of surrounding skin

- Temperature: increased tissue temperature, due to increased tissue perfusion
- Edema: resolution or prevention and restoration of tissue turgor
- Wound progression to the proliferative phase

Wound Healing Phase Diagnosis: Subacute Inflammation

Expected Outcome Protocol
- Skin color: change to that of surrounding skin
- Temperature: change to that of adjacent tissues or same area on corresponding opposite side of the body
- Edema free
- Necrosis free
- Wound progression to the proliferative phase

Protocols for PSWD

Kloth and Ziskin[5] devised a protocol for using PSWD, based on the definitions of Lehman and deLateur[40] of vigorous and mild heating, to write a protocol for the acute, subacute, and chronic inflammatory phases of healing. The power level of the PSWD unit is divided into four levels. The four levels range from quarter power, which has a sensory effect below sensation of heat, to full power, which is vigorous heating. Table 24.7 shows the PSWD dosages and effects, and the aspect of the inflammation phase of healing to be treated at that level. Table 24.8 shows the dosage, level, duration, frequency, and expected temperature changes in the tissues.

Change Moist Dressing during PSWD Treatment

According to the PSWD instruction manual, it is necessary to remove wound dressings before PSWD.[81] To avoid burns of wound tissue during treatment with PSWD, replace any moist wound dressing with a dry sterile gauze pad. Check the gauze pad during the treatment when there is much wound exudate observed during the setup. If the dressing is moist, remove and replace it with another dry gauze dressing.

There are anecdotal clinical reports that the use of PSWD over wound dressings does not have harmful effects. Also, clinical practice for wound management has changed since the PSWD instruction cautions were first issued in 1981. Further evaluation of the effects of PSWD on wound fluids and dressing adhesives is needed to update this position.

Setup for Treatment with Pulsed Short-Wave Diathermy

1. Explain the procedure to the patient and caregiver.
2. Inspect and remove all metal items, including jewelry, wristwatches, brassieres with metal fasteners, and clothing with zippers.
3. Remove hearing aids and external electronic devices.
4. Place the patient on a nonmetal surface.
5. Avoid contact with synthetic materials, including pillows.
6. Remove clothing from body area.
7. Position the patient for comfort in a position that can be maintained for 30 minutes.
8. Remove the wound dressing and absorb excess exudate; cover with dry gauze.

TABLE	24.7	**PSWD Power, Effects, and Application**		

Dose	Level	Effect	Phase of Healing
I (1/4 power)	Lowest	Below sensation of heat	Acute inflammation
II (1/2 power)	Low	Mild heat sensation	Subacute, resolving inflammation
III (3/4 power)	Medium	Moderate, comfortable heat sensation	Subacute, resolving inflammation
IV (full power)	Heavy	Vigorous heating, well tolerated; reduce to just below maximum tolerance	Chronic conditions

Reprinted from Kloth L, Ziskin M. Diathermy and pulsed radio frequency radiation. In: Michlovitz S, ed. *Thermal Agents in Rehabilitation*. 3rd ed. Philadelphia, PA: F.A. Davis Company Publishers©; 1996, with permission.

9. Cleanse the wound of debris and metallic and petrolatum-based products; blot dry.
10. Cover the wound and surrounding skin with a 1/2-inch thickness of toweling.
11. Cover the drum with a disposable surgical head cap or terry cloth towel for hygiene.
12. Place the drum 0.5 to 1 cm above the terry cloth.
13. Set the protocol and treatment duration. Start.

Patient Monitoring

- Never leave a patient who is confused or disoriented alone and unsupervised while receiving treatment.
- When using PSWD, remember that pain is a warning that excessive heating is occurring. Give the patient a call light and pay immediate attention to a call. Reduce power level. Increase air space, either by positioning the drum farther from the target tissue or by layering towels between the drum and the body area.
- Check skin before application for unguents that may have been applied (e.g., oil of wintergreen, Ben-Gay); clean thoroughly and dry.

Aftercare for Pulsed Short-Wave Diathermy

Because the dressing is always removed before this treatment, it is important that the wound be dressed with the appropriate dressing as soon as possible after conclusion of the treatment.

A dressing should be selected that will match the frequency of the PSWD treatment and other components of the wound healing. Rapid redressing of the wound safeguards against wound contamination and desiccation of the wound tissues sustains the warmth of the wound that has occurred from the increased profusion and promotes optimal cell mitosis.

Setup Treatment with Pulsed Radio Frequency

Diapulse

1. Explain the procedure to the patient and caregiver.
2. Position the patient for comfort, with the treatment site accessible, so that it can be maintained for 30 minutes.
3. Cover the drum with a disposable surgical head cap or terry cloth towel for hygiene.
4. Place the drum 0.5 to 1 cm above the terry cloth over the wound site.
5. Leave clothes, dressings, casts, bandages, splints in place unless there is strikethrough or it is time to change dressing.
6. Drum can lie on top of bandages, casts, splints, Unna boot.
7. Set the protocol and treatment duration. Start.

SofPulse® and RecoveryRx™

Treatment is delivered automatically for 30-minute treatments. Dose of treatment will be equal to all areas regardless of coil loop size. Coil loops of different diameters are available to best

TABLE	24.8	**PSWD Dosage, Duration, and Outcomes**	

Dose	Duration	Outcome[a]
I	15 min one or two times daily for 1–2 wk	Temperature ↑ 37.5°C–38.5°C
II	15 min daily for 1–2 wk	Temperature ↑ 38.5°C–40.0°C
III	15–30 min daily for 1–2 wk	Temperature ↑ 40.0°C–42.0°C
IV	15–30 min daily or two times per week for 1 week to 1 mo	Temperature ↑ 42.0°C–44.0°C

[a]Continue for 2 wk. If outcomes are achieved through the phases of healing, continue.
Reprinted from Kloth L, Ziskin M. Diathermy and pulsed radio frequency radiation. In: Michlovitz S, ed. *Thermal Agents in Rehabilitation*. 3rd ed. Philadelphia, PA: F.A. Davis© Company Publishers; 1996, with permission.

CLINICAL WISDOM

PSWD (Magnatherm) for Venous Disease

Patients with venous disease do not tolerate high heating and subsequent effects of vasodilation. Two phases are used. For the first phase of treatment, energy is adjusted to deliver a pulse rate of 1,600 pps for 15 minutes. This is followed by a second phase at 700 pps for a 15-minute period. Power levels are kept at power level 12 (Frankenberger L, *personal communication*, 1997).

meet the wound size. Large coils could be laid over near wounds for example, hip and coccyx for more efficient treatment.

Precautions

1. Do not bend the loop into a different shape. If it is configured into a "U," the signal polarity will cancel itself out. If twisted into a pretzel or squeezed like a sausage, the area of treatment will be restricted and the depth of penetration reduced.
2. The coil loop is designed for single patient use and can be cleaned and disinfected between uses and discarded at end of care.

Setup

1. Explain the procedure to the patient and caregiver.
2. Position the patient for comfort, with the treatment site accessible, so that it can be maintained for 30 minutes.
3. Leave clothes, dressings, casts, bandages, splints in place unless there is strikethrough or it is time to change dressing.
4. Match loop coil size to the wound area to be treated.
5. Position the loop, so it stays in the position and is not likely to be dislodged by gravity or patient movement.
6. Lay the loop coil flat over the wound area and tape in place as shown in Figure 24.8.
7. Coil loop can lie on top of clothing, bandages, casts, splints.
8. DO NOT bend or twist the loop as this will interfere with delivery of the signal from the coil (see precaution 1 above).
9. Error alarm messages are built into this unit and include a flashing light that will indicate the output is not intact and also there is a beeping signal to alert patient and caregiver of operational problems.
10. A home care model (Torino) is also available that is totally disposable after use.
11. Preset protocols and 30-minute timer, 1 to 10 W; Torino 2 pps, 3 milliseconds, 2 W; Torino is designed for clinical

CLINICAL WISDOM

Tissue Perfusion

When tissue perfusion is the treatment effect, the wound will be warmed, and the cells will divide and proliferate faster in the warm environment. Therefore, dress the wound *immediately after* PSWD and before PRF.

or unattended home use. In either case, patient education should be provided.

Frequency for all the PRF devices described is once or twice daily or every 4 hours for pain management, 30 minutes per session.

Adjunctive or Multimodal Treatments

It has already been mentioned that PSWD and PRF can be used in conjunction with adjunctive treatments, such as compression bandages, casts, splints. It can also be used following whirlpool or pulsatile lavage with suction for cleansing or debridement. If dressings are to be removed, it may be preferable to treat with PSWD or PRF immediately after the other interventions to keep the wound temperature from declining. Another choice could be to treat the wound with ultraviolet light for bactericidal effects or to initiate a mild inflammatory process, then follow with either PSWD or PRF to enhance the circulation and cellular activation.

"Multimodal therapies" is a new term adopted to reflect the common practice of using such modalities either sequentially or concurrently to bring difficult wounds to closure.[92] In a case of a complex diabetic ulcer that was infected with necrotizing fasciitis, they chose to used advanced multimodal therapies of negative pressure therapy (see Chapter 29) and PRF to salvage the lower limb. Surgery was required to remove the necrotic tissue and this left a large draining open trans-metatarsal amputation and anterior compartment incision. Initially, the wound was treated with NPWT for 8 weeks, then a dermal graft was placed along with addition of PRF therapy (Provant) twice daily. After 24 weeks, the wound was ready for closure with a split-thickness skin graft.[92]

As reported in this case study by Frykberg et al., the combination of therapies could enhance results, since the mechanisms of action are different. Benefits of multiple treatments with different or multiple biophysical agents are reported in the literature and examples are noted in Chapters 23 and 26. This is an area that merits further research for best utilization management of services and best efficacy for the patient.

Another adjunctive treatment with well-established effects on circulation is exercise. Exercise following PSWD or PRF would use the muscle pump for exchange of nutrients and oxygen brought to the tissue by the PSWD or PRF treatment and removal of waste products, as well as to help dissipate the effects of heating and avoid burning. Exercise encourages movement of fluids from the venous system into the lymphatics and is a way to avoid stasis in the area of heating. For those patients who are unable to exercise actively, assisted or passive range of motion would encourage change in fluid dynamics in the affected area. Therapeutic positioning should also be considered as an adjunctive treatment because improper positioning may have blood flowing away from the target tissues or applying pressure to the area that is to be perfused (see Chapter 10).

Conclusions

In this chapter, the biophysical properties of EMF have been explained, preclinical biologic and animal studies and clinical cases and trials have been used to help you and understand and evaluate the scientific studies. Three EMF-related categories of devices—PSWD, PRF, and PEMF—were described and compared for their physical properties and for their therapeutic effects related to tissue repair and wound healing. PSWD and PRF are similar but not identical. They both are radio wave signals from the short-wave spectrum. PSWD has the ability to heat tissue; PRF does not. Both are able to increase perfusion and blood flow in normal adults. Only two studies by Santoro et al.[45] and Mayrovitz and Larsen[46] looked at the effect of PSWD and PRFS on blood flow changes in individuals with PVD. Cellular changes are reported for stimulation with PRFS but no studies were found that looked at such effects for PSWD, although that does not rule them out, and they should be investigated. Exhibits 24.1 and 24.6 list the characteristics and rationale for selecting PSWD and PRFS.

PSWD studies focus on thermotherapy changes to the circulatory system and the ANS, whereas the effects of PRF and PEMF are attributed to changes in the cellular activity of the tissues and mechanisms that control blood flow and edema that are not heat related. Both PSWD and PRF devices can increase blood flow, which increases oxygen transport essential to support the metabolic demands of the tissues and to control infection. All three modes of electromagnetic stimulation affect pain and edema during the inflammatory phase and PRF is considered to be anti-inflammatory. If the circulatory effects desired require deep heating such as to raise core body temperature, then PSWD would be a good choice. A protocol for PSWD that is based on the circulatory effect on acute, subacute, and chronic inflammation is provided. PRF has the ability to quench the escalation of free radicals and prevent ischemia reperfusion injury[10] (see Chapter 2). Best privative efficacy is reported when treatment begins soon after injury. The effects on the inflammatory and proliferative phases of healing are described. Enhanced circulation and oxygen are requirements of all the phases of healing, so continuation during all phases is appropriate. PRF is the preferred choice if the objective is to stimulate the body's bioelectric system at the cellular level, over a dressing, cast, or bandage; to increase peripheral microcirculation; to prevent or minimize edema; and to avoid and relieve pain. Treatment effects should be seen within hours for acute wounds in 3 to 7 days from the start of the protocol for chronic wounds.[62,64,65] Reported effects include increased wound exudate for the first 1 to 3 days. Progress through the phases of healing should continue throughout the episode of care.

PEMF stimulators have distinctly different parameters than the radio frequency stimulators. However, some are called PEMF when they have the characteristics of PRF and vise versa. Initially used for osteogenesis of nonunion fractures, PEMF has now been tested for soft tissue wound healing in venous ulcers with good outcomes in pilot studies. Although the results presented look promising, more new studies are needed. There remain many unknowns about mechanisms of action, and there is a need for improved study designs and reporting of the data with objective quantitative results. For example, the rate of healing has been identified as a predictor of healing outcome and the trigger for referral for adjunctive therapy.[93–97] The study data for many of the research projects testing these interventions did not provide quantitative information about the rate of healing of the control or the treatment groups, making it impossible to compare rate of healing between study intervention and controls and between other adjunctive therapy interventions. Except for two studies where the percentage of change could be derived from the data reported, the best available data are the percentage of patients that healed in a study and those that did not. One factor is evident from compiling the matrices of studies for different applications of PRF, namely that the Diapulse protocol, 400 pps, power level 4 over the epigastrium, and 600 pps peak power over the target tissue, has been followed consistently, with treatment efficacy reported for each application. Although many of the studies are reported as DBRCTs, it is also evident that the data reported are observational descriptive data, rather than quantitative. To review, the studies looked at seven components that you should consider when selecting this intervention.

1. PRF and PEMF stimulate cellular activity and cell permeability.
2. PRF and PEMF affect the body's bioelectric system.
3. PSWD and PRF affect edema formation but possibly through different processes.
4. PSWD, PRF, and PEMF prevent or modulate pain.
5. PSWD and PRF affect circulation, as measured by increased blood flow and tcPO2, but through different processes.
6. PRF promotes absorption of hematoma.
7. PSWD heats tissue; PRF does not.

EXHIBIT 24.6

Wound Classification and Characteristics

Wound Classification	PSWD/PRF
Level of tissue disruption	Superficial, partial thickness, full thickness, subcutaneous and deep tissues
Etiologies/diagnostic groups	Burns, neuropathic ulcers, pressure ulcers, surgical wounds, vascular ulcers
Wound phases	*Inflammatory phase:* necrosis, exudate, edema, pain *Proliferative phase:* Granulation, contraction, collagen synthesis, angiogenesis *Epithelialization phase:* epidermal migration *Remodeling:* collagen organization

Patients who were treated in the clinical studies had acute postsurgical wounds, including split-thickness skin grafts, or posttrauma, and chronic pressure ulcers, venous or arterial leg ulcers. The wounds were either partial- or full-thickness tissue disruption, extending into deeper tissues (e.g., stages II through IV pressure ulcers). None of the effects of treatment described are dependent on the medical diagnosis, the wound etiology, or the depth of the wound. However, wounds that are deep, large, or of long duration have been identified as slower to heal. Those wounds will probably heal faster with one of these adjunctive therapy interventions.

SELF-CARE TEACHING GUIDELINES

Both PSWD and PRF labels state that "federal law restricts the sale and use of this equipment to a licensed health practitioner."[53,80] However, the manufacturers and distributors of the PRF nonthermal devices report that patients are using them as home therapy units under physician prescription, after instruction by an appropriate provider, a caregiver, or patient. As explained, reduced power PRF devices like the Ivivi Torino™ and Recovery RX™ are safe, portable, battery operated, preprogramed, single patient specific, disposable, and have simple care requirements so they can be sent home with the patient. The Provant™ device is not battery operated but uses standard electrical current and can be used for self-administered home care with proper placement instruction. PSWD should not be used unsupervised and unattended in the home.

Chapter 23 outlines the requirements for selecting and teaching a candidate or caregiver biophysical agent home care. Instructions differ for PRF treatment that is administered over an in place dressing, leg wrap, or cast. Setup of the patient and the wound for treatment, write down all steps including those listed here. Review what is on paper, then do a demonstration and return demonstration to confirm understanding.

The ten steps of PRF instructions are as follows:

1. Place the coil or packet flat over the wound *over* the wound dressing and hold in place with dressing tape as shown in Figure 24.7.

2. If tape is used, apply a skin prep to the surrounding skin before attaching the tape for skin sparing. Depending on location of the wound, a gauze, not an elastic, wrap could be used for placement to hold the device in place, but take care NOT to bend the wire coil.

3. Place the coil or pack over the *wound area* that *is* inside of a cast or compression wrap and held in place with a wrap.

4. Inform the patient that the energy is primarily located inside of the circle of the coil and to NEVER bend or twist the coil as it will affect the energy delivery.

5. Tell the patient that they will not feel the energy just as they do not feel the energy from a radio but like a radio sound that passes through a wall the energy will pass into the body.

6. Instruct the patient/caregiver to turn the device ON twice daily at least 4 hours apart. It will automatically turn off after the 30-minute treatment session is completed.

7. If the coil or pack is not left in place as shown in Figure 24.8, then it should be wiped clean, laid flat, perhaps inside of a plastic-zippered storage bag, and stored in a safe place.

8. When the wound dressing is changed, the wound should be cleaned and examined and wound status documented.

9. Give a written list of expected signs and symptoms related to the treatment to the patient and the caregiver.

10. Provide written instruction about when and how to report any undesirable results and contact information about who to contact.

DOCUMENTATION

The functional outcome report (FOR) described in Chapter 1 is an accepted method to meet Medicare and third-party payer guidelines for documentation of the need for physical therapy intervention for wound healing. The two cases presented as examples of the use of PSWD and PRFS are documented by using the FOR method. A sample form and case are found in Chapter 1. Also, try to apply the method to wound cases in the clinic.[98] Data collected about treatment outcomes in a systematic manner can be of great value to report the success of the therapy and to predict outcomes.

Pictorial case study of a woman with surgical excision of breast tissue (see Fig. 24.11A–D)

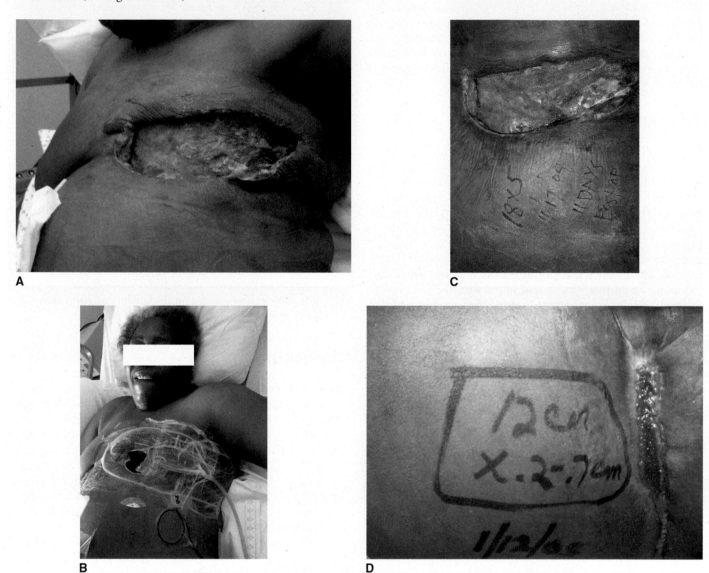

FIGURE 24.11 Case study Pictorial case study of a woman with surgical excision of breast tissue. Case study provided courtesy of Berish Strauch, MD, Department of Plastic and Reconstructive Surgery, Montefiore Medical Center, Albert Einstein college of Medicine of Yeshiva University. Bronx, NY). **A:** Postsurgical case of woman with surgical excision of breast tissue following radiation skin necrosis. Two prior flaps had been lost trying to close the defect. **B:** PRF with Ivivi Roma® (Courtesy of Dr. B. Strauch, Ivivi Health Sciences, San Francisco, CA) negative pressure devices in place. This combined treatment was provided for 1 week post-op, and then the negative pressure was discontinued. **C:** View of tissue 11 days post-op. Treatment now only PRF and dressings. **D:** View of epithelializing and contracting wound at 2 months post-op.

CASE STUDY

Pictorial case study of a patient with an incisional wound treated with pulsed radio frequency stimulation (PRFS) (see Fig. 24.12A,B).

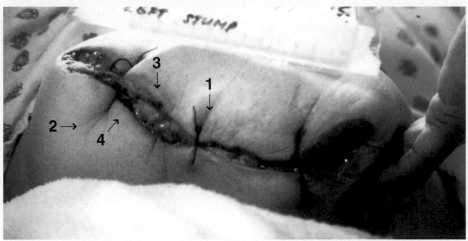

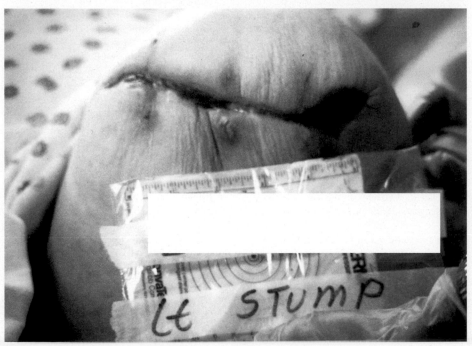

FIGURE 24.12 Case study of wound healing with PRFS. **A:** Patient with the incision from an above-the-knee amputation left open for delayed primary intention healing. Wound is in acute inflammatory phase. Start of treatment with PRFS began 8/3. Note: (1) Sutures placed (2) Edema (3) Erythema and tissue tension (4) Yellow, mucinous slough in incision line. **B:** Same incision wound as in Figure 24.12A, on 8/17 (14 days later). Note good outcomes: edema-free, necrosis-free, wound contraction, and granulation. The wound is in acute proliferative and epithelialization phases. (Copyright © C. Sussman.)

REVIEW QUESTIONS

1. Signal characteristics can differ in which way:
   A. Signal shape
   B. Pulse rate
   C. Depth and duration
   D. All of the above
2. Which statement regarding PSWD and PRF is true?
   A. Both PSWD and PRF are nonthermal
   B. PSWD heats the tissues and PRF is nonthermal
   C. PRF penetrates deeply while PSWD does not
   D. Both PSWD and PRF heat from the inside out
3. All the following are contraindications for PSWD and PRF, except
   A. Do not use over metal implants
   B. Do not treat over immature bone
   C. Do not use with patients with cardiac pacemakers
   D. Do not use over anesthetized areas

4. Expected treatment outcomes of PRF include all of the following, except
   A. Progression from one phase to the next in 2 to 4 weeks
   B. Healing times will be at the end range for patients who are older and immobile
   C. Comorbidities and wound duration will not affect healing times
   D. All are correct
5. Multimodal therapies is a new term reflecting the practice of
   A. Using at least three modalities to improve healing
   B. Treating a wound while the dressing is in place
   C. Using modalities sequentially or concurrently to improve healing
   D. Using a treatment modality with debridement

REFERENCES

1. Guy A, Lehmann J, Stonebridge J. Therapeutic applications of electromagnetic power. *Proc IEEE*. 1974;62:55–75.
2. Erdman W. Peripheral blood flow measurements during application of pulsed high frequency currents. *Orthopedics*. 1960;2:196–197.
3. Kinney BM. Pulsed electromagnetic field therapy in plastic surgery. *Aesthetic Surg* J. 2005;25:87–92.
4. Kellogg R. Magnetotherapy: potential clinical and therapeutic applications. In: Nelson R, Currier D, eds. *Clinical Electrotherapy*. Norwalk, CT: Appleton & Lange; 1991:390–391.
5. Kloth L, Ziskin M. Diathermy and pulsed radiofrequency radiation. In: Michlovitz SL, ed. *Thermal Agents in Rehabilitation*. Philadelphia, PA: FA Davis; 1996:213–254.
6. Pilla AA. Mechanisms and therapeutic applications of time-varying and static magnetic fields. In: Barnes F, Greenebaum B, eds. *Handbook of Biological Effects of Electromagnetic Fields*. 3rd ed. Boca Raton, FL: CRC Press; 2006.
7. Pilla AA. Weak time-varying and static magnetic fields: from mechanisms to therapeutic applications. In: Stavroulakis P, ed. *Biological Effects of Electromagnetic Fields*. Berlin: Springer Verlag; 2003:34–75.
8. Markov MS, Pilla A. Electromagnetic field stimulation of soft tissues: pulsed radio frequency treatment of postoperative pain and edema. *Wounds*. 1995;7(4):143–151.
9. Collins English Dictionary. Complete and Unabridged. Harper Collins Publishers. 1991,1994, 1998, 2000, 2003.
10. Gordon GA. Designed electromagnetic pulsed therapy: clinical applications. *J Cell. Physiol*. 2007;212:579–582.
11. Pienkowski D, Pollack SR, Brighton CT, et al. Comparison of asymmetrical and symmetrical pulse waveforms in electromagnetic stimulation. *J Orthop Res*. 1992;10(2):247–255.
12. Skerry TM, Pead MJ, Lanyon LE. Modulation of bone loss during disuse by pulsed electromagnetic fields. *J Ortho Res*. 1991;7:600–608.
13. Blumlein H, McDaniel J. Effect of the magnetic field component of the Kraus-Lechner method on the healing of experimental nonunion in dogs. In: Burny F, Herbst E, Hinsenkamp M, eds. *Electric Stimulation of Bone Growth and Repair*. New York, NY: Springer-Verlag; 1978:35–46.
14. Herber H. Cordey J, Perren SM. Influence of magnetic fields on growth and regeneration in organ culture. In: Burny F, Herbst E, Hinsenkamp M,
    eds. *Electric Stimulation of Bone Growth and Repair*. New York, NY: Springer-Verlag; 1978:35–40.
15. Mooney V. A randomized double-blind prospective study of efficacy of pulsed electromagnetic fields for interbody lumbar fusion. *Spine*. 1990;15:708–712.
16. Sharrard WJ. Double blind trials of pulsed electromagnetic fields of delayed union of tibial fractures. *J Bone Joint Surg*. 1990;72-B:347–355.
17. Skerry TM, Pead MJ, Lanyon LE. Modulation of bone loss during disuse by pulsed electromagnetic fields. *J Ortho Res*. 1991;9:600–608.
18. Rabkin J, Hunt TK. Local heat increases blood flow and oxygen tension in wounds. *Arch Surg*. 1987;122:221–225.
19. Seegers JC, Engelbrecht A, van Papendorp DH. Activation of signal-transduction mechanisms may underlie the therapeutic effects of an applied electric field. *Medical Hypotheses*. 2001;57(2):224–230.
20. Brighton CT, Wang W, Seldes R, et al. Signal transduction in electrically stimulated bone cells. *J Bone Joint Surg*. 2001;83A(10):1514–1523.
21. George FR, Lukas RJ, Moffett J, et al. In-vitro mechanisms of cell proliferation induction: a novel bioactive treatment for accelerating wound healing. *Wounds* 2002;14(3):107–115
22. Pilla A. A Synopsis of Published Peer Reviewed Studies, not dated, Ivivi Technologies, personal communication 2006.
23. Nindl G, Balcavage WX, Vesper DN, et al. Experiments showing that electromagnetic fields can be used to treat inflammatory diseases. *Bimed Sci Instrum*. 2000;36:7–13.
24. Canedo-Dorantes L, Garcia-Canto R, Barrera R, et al. Healing of chronic arterial and venous leg ulcers with systemic electromagnetic fields. *Arch Med Res*. 2002;33:281–289.
25. Bassett C. Low energy pulsing electromagnetic fields modify biomedical processes. *BioEssays*. 1987;6(1):36–40.
26. Aaron RK, Boyan BD, McKCiombor D, et al. Stimulation of growth factor synthesis by electric and electromagnetic fields. *Clin Orthop*. 2004;419:30–37.
27. Rohde C, Chiang A, et al. Effects of pulsed electromagnetic fields on interleukin-1β and postoperative pain: a double-blind, placebo-controlled, pilot study in breast reduction patients. *Plast Reconstr Surg*. 2010;125:1620–1629. www.PRSJournal.com.
28. Ionescu A, Ionescu D, et al. Study of efficiency of diapulse therapy on the dynamics of enzymes in burned wound. Presented at the Sixth International Congress on Burns; August 31, 1982; San Francisco, CA.

29. Barclay V, Collier R, Jones A. Treatment of various hand injuries by pulsed electromagnetic energy (Diapulse). *Physiotherapy*. 1983;69(6):186–188.

30. Pennington G, Daily D, Sumko M. Pulsed, non-thermal, high-frequency electromagnetic energy (Diapulse) in the treatment of grade I and grade II ankle sprains. *Mil Med*. 1993;158:101–104.

31. Sambasivan M. Pulsed electromagnetic field in management of head injuries. *Neurol India*. 1993;41(suppl):56–59.

32. Heden P, Pilla AA. Effects of pulsed electromagnetic fields on postoperative pain:a double-blind randomized pilot study in breast augmentation patients. *Anesth Plast Surg*. 2008;32:660–666.

33. Santiesteban J, Grant C. Post-surgical effect of pulsed shortwave therapy. *J Am Podiatr Med Assoc*. 1979;75:306–309.

34. Hill J, Lewis M, Mills P, et al. Pulsed short-wave diathermy effects on human fibroblast proliferation. *Arch Physical Med Rehabil*. 2002;83(6):832–836.

35. Strauch B, Patel M, Navarro JA, et al. Pulsed magnetic fields accelerate cutaneous wound healing in rats. *Plast Reconstr Surg*. 2007;120(2):425–430.

36. Park H-Y, Shon K, Phillips T. The effect of heat on inhibitory effects of chronic wound fluid on fibroblasts in vitro. *Wounds*. 1998;10(6):189–192.

37. Shields N, Gormley J, O'Hare N. Short-wave diathermy: current clinical and safety practices. *Physiother Res Int*. 2002;7(4):191–202.

38. Knighton D, Halliday B, Hunt TK. Oxygen as antibiotic: a comparison of inspired oxygen concentration and antibiotic administration on in vivo bacterial clearance. *Arch Surg*. 1986;121:191–195.

39. Jonsson K, Jensen J, Goodson WH III. Tissue oxygenation, anemia, and perfusion in relation to wound healing in surgical patients. *Ann Surg*. 1991;214(5):605–613.

40. Lehman JF, deLateur BJ. Therapeutic heat. In: Lehmann JF, ed. *Therapeutic Heat and Cold*. 4th ed. Baltimore, MD: Williams & Wilkins; 1990.

41. Draper DO, Knight K, et al. Temperature change in human muscle during and after pulsed short-wave diathermy. *J Orthop Sports Phys Ther*. 1999;29(1):13–22.

42. Brown G. Diathermy: a renewed interest in a proven therapy. *Phys Ther Today*. 1993 (spring):78–80.

43. Silverman D, Pendleton L. A comparison of the effects of continuous and pulsed short-wave diathermy on peripheral circulation. *Arch Phys Med Rehabil*. 1968;49:429–436.

44. Wessman HC, Kottke FJ. The effect of indirect heating on peripheral blood flow, pulse rate, blood pressure and temperature. *Arch Phys Med Rehabil*. 1967;48:567–576.

45. Santoro D, Ostranderl, Lee B, Cagir B. Inductive 27.12 MHz: diathermy in arterial peripheral vascular disease. 16th International IEEE/EMBS Conference; October 1994; Montreal, Canada.

46. Mayrovitz H, Larsen P. Effects of pulsed electromagnetic fields on skin microvascular blood perfusion. *Wounds*. 1992;4(5):197–202.

47. Mayrovitz H, Larsen P. A preliminary study to evaluate the effect of pulsed radio frequency field treatment on lower extremity peri-ulcer skin microcirculation of diabetic patients. *Wounds*. 1995;7(3):90–93.

48. Ankrom MA BR, Sprigle S, Langemo D, et al. National Pressure Ulcer Advisory Panel. Pressure-related deep tissue injury under intact skin and the current pressure ulcer staging systems. *Adv Skin Wound Care*. 2005;18(1):35–42.

49. National Pressure Ulcer Advisory Panel. *Deep Tissue Injury—White Paper*. Washington, DC: National Pressure Ulcer Advisory Panel; 2005.

50. Witkowski JA. Purple ulcers. *J ET Nurs*. 1993; 20:132.

51. Fenn JE. Effect of pulsed electromagnetic energy (Diapulse) on experimental hematomas. *Can Med Assoc J*. 1969;100:251.

52. Ginsberg AJ. Pearl Chain Phenomenon. Abstract. Presented at the 35th Annual Meeting of the American Congress of Physical Medicine and Rehabilitation; 1958;36:112–115.

53. Cameron BM. Experimental acceleration of wound healing. *Am J Orthop*. 1961;336–343.

54. Musaev AV, Guseinova SG, et al. The use of pulsed electromagnetic fields with complex modulation in the treatment of patients withdiabetic polyneuropathy. *Neurosci Behav Phys*. 2003;33(8):745–752.

55. National Pressure Ulcer Advisory Panel and European Pressure Ulcer Advisory Panel (EPUAP). *Pressure Ulcers Prevention and Treatment: Clinical Practice Guideline*, Washington, DC: National Pressure Ulcer Advisory Panel; 2009.

56. Dindar H, Renda N, Barlas M. The effects of electromagnetic field stimulation on corticosteroids-inhibited intestinal wound healing. *Tokai J Exp Clin Med*. 1993;18(1–2):49–55.

57. Patino O, Grana D, Bolgiani A. Pulsed electromagnetic fields in experimental cutanous wound healing in rats. *J Burn Care Rehabil*. 1996;17(6 Pt 1):528–531.

58. Scardino M, Swaim SF, Sartin, EA. Evaluation of treatment with a pulsed electromagnetic field on wound healing, clinicopathologic variables, and central nervous system activity of dogs. *Am J Vet Res*. 1998;59(9):1177–1181.

59. Lin Y, Nishimura R, Nozaki K. Effects of pulsing electromagnetic fields on the ligament healing in rabbits. *J Vet Med Sci*. 1992;54(5):1017–1022.

60. Lee E, Maffuli N, Li CK, et al. Pulsed magnetic and electromagnetic fields in experimental Achilles tendonitis in the rat: a prospective randomized study. *Arch Phys Med Rehabil*. 1997;78(4):399–404.

61. Itoh M, Montemayor J, Matsumoto E, et al. Accelerated wound healing of pressure ulcers by pulsed high peak power electromagnetic energy (Diapulse). *Decubitus*. 1991;4(1):24–34.

62. Wilson CM. Clinical Effects of Diapulse Technology in Treatment of Recalcitrant Pressure Ulcers. In *Clinical Symposium on Pressure Ulcer and Wound Management*. Orlando, FL: Silver Cross Hospital and *Decubitus*; 1992.

63. Patino O, Grana D, Bolgiani A. Effect of magnetic fields on skin wound healing. Experimental study. *Medicina (B Aires)*. 1996;56(1):41–44.

64. Salzberg A, Cooper-Vastola S, Perez F, et al. The effects of non-thermal pulsed electromagnetic energy (Diapulse) on wound healing of pressure ulcers in spinal cord-injured patients: a randomized, double-blind study. *Wounds*. 1995;7(1):11–16.

65. Seaborne D, Quirion-DeGirardi C, Rovsseau M, et al. The treatment of pressure sores using pulsed electromagnetic energy (PEME). *Physiother Can*. 1996;48(2):131–137.

66. Gupta A, Taly AB, et al. Efficacy of pulsed electromagnetic field therapy in healing of pressure ulcers: a randomized control trial. *Neurol India [cited 2011 Apr 28]* 2009;57:622–626. Available from: http://www.neurologyindia.com/text.asp?2009/57/5/622/57820.

67. Cameron BM. A three phase evaluation of pulsed high frequency radio short waves (Diapulse), 646 patients. *Am J Orthop*. 1964;6:72–78.

68. Goldin JH, Broadbent JD, et al. The effects of Diapulse on the healing of wounds: a double-blind randomised controlled trial in man. *Br J Plastic Surg*. 1981;34:267–270.

69. Kaplan EG, Weinstock R. Clinical evaluation of Diapulse as adjunctive therapy following foot surgery. *J Am Podiatr Assoc*. 1968;58(5):218.

70. Aronofsky DH. Reduction of dental postsurgical symptoms using non-thermal pulsed high peak power electromagnetic energy. *Oral Surg Oral Med Oral Pathol*. 1971;32(5):688–696.

71. Bentall R, Eckstein H. A trial involving the use of pulsed electromagnetic therapy on children undergoing orchidoplexy. *Hippokrates Verlag Stuttgart*. 1975;17(4):380–388.

72. Comorosan S, Paslaru L, Popovici Z. The stimulation of wound healing processes by pulsed electromagnetic energy. *Wounds*. 1992;4(1):31–32.

73. Ieran M, Zaffuto S. Effect of low frequency pulsing electromagnetic fields on skin ulcers of venous origin in humans: a double blind study. *J Orthop Rev*. 1990;8:276–282.

74. Duran V, Zamurovic A, Stojanovk S, et al. Therapy of venous ulcers using pulsating electromagnetic fields—personal results. *Med Pregl*. 1991;44(11–12):485–488.

75. Todd D, Heylings D, Allen G, et al. Treatment of chronic varicose ulcers with pulsed electromagnetic fields: a controlled pilot study. *Ir Med J.* 1991;84(2):54–55.

76. Stiller M, Pak G, Shupack J, et al. A portable pulsed electromagnetic field (PEMF) device to enhance healing of recalcitrant venous ulcers: a double-blind, placebo-controlled clinical trial. *Br J Dermatol.* 1992;127(2):147–154.

77. Kenkre J, Hobbs F, Carter Y, et al. A randomized controlled trial of electromagnetic therapy in the primary care management of venous leg ulceration. *Fam Pract.* 1996;13(3):236–240.

78. Frykberg RG, Driver VR, et al. The use of pulsed radio frequency energy therapy in treating lower extremity wounds: resuylts of a retrospective study of a wound registry. *Ostom Wound Manage.* 2011;57(3):22–29.

79. Larsen JA, Julia O. Pulsed radio frequency energy in the treatment of complex diabetic foot wounds: two cases. *J Wound Ostomy Continence Nurs.* 2008;35(5):523–527.

80. Electropharmacology. *MRT SofPulse User's Manual.* Pompano Beach, FL: Electropharmacology, Inc.; 1994.

81. Van Rijswijk L, Polansky M. Predictors of time to healing deep pressure ulcers. *Ostomy/Wound Manage.* 1994;40(8):40–42, 44, 46–48.

82. Martin CJ, McCallum HM, Strelley S, et al. Electromagnetic fields from therapeutic diathermy equipment: a review of hazards and precautions. *Physiotherapy.* 1991;77:3–7.

83. Ourllet-Hellstrom SR. Miscarriages among female physical therapists who report using radio- and microwave-frequency electromagnetic radiation. *Am J Epidemiol.* 1993;138:775–786.

84. CFR Ch. 1 (4–1–93 Edition). Device described in paragraph (BX1); see section 890.3, 48 FR 53047, Nov. 23, 1983, as amended in 52 FR 17742, May 11, 1987, Document No. A779269 (PSWD Instruction Manual).

85. Medicare Coverage Issues Manual (MCIM)—Medical Procedures, Section 35–98, 5 Medicare and Medicaid Guide (CCH). In: Health Care Financing Administration (HCFA). Baltimore, MD: Department of Health and Human Services; 1997:35–98.

86. National Coverage Decision for Electrical Stimulation (ES) and Electromagnetic Therapy for the Treatment of Wounds. Vol 270.1; 2004. Department of Health and Human Services, Center for Medicare and Medicaid Services.

87. Bergstrom N, Allman RM, Alvarez OM. Treatment of Pressure Ulcers. Clinical Practice Guideline. Rockville, MD: Agency for Health Care Research and Quality (AHRQ), formerly known as the Agency for Health Care Policy and Research (AHCPR), U.S. Department of Health and Human Services, Public Health Service; 1994.

88. Ovington LG. Dressings and adjunctive therapies: AHCPR guidelines revisited. *Ostomy/Wound Manage.* 1999;45(suppl 1A):94s–106s.

89. Dolynchuk K, Keast D, Campbell K. Best practices for the prevention and treatment of pressure ulcers. *Ostomy/Wound Manage.* 2000;46(11):38–52

90. Low JL. The nature and effects of pulsed electromagnetic radiations. *NZ J Physiother.* 1978;18–22.

91. Hayne CR. Pulsed high frequency energy—its place in physiotherapy. *Physiotherapy.* 1984;70:459.

92. Frykberg RG, Martin E, et al. A case history of multimodal therapy in healing a complicated diabetic foot wound: negative pressure dermal replacement and pulsed radio frequency energy therapies. *IntWound J.* 2011;8(2):132–139.

93. Bates-Jensen B. *A Quantitative Analysis of Wound Characteristics as Early Predictors of Healing in Pressure Sores.* Dissertation Abstracts International, Vol. 59, No. 11. Los Angeles, CA: University of California; 1999.

94. Margolis DJ, Gross EA, Wood CR, et al. Planimetric rate of healing in venous ulcers of the leg treated with pressure bandage and hydrocolloid dressing. *J Am Acad Dermatol.* 1993;28(3):418–421.

95. Robson MC, Hill DP, Woodske ME, et al. Wound healing trajectories as predictors of effectiveness of therapeutic agents. *Arch Surg.* 2000;135(7):773–777.

96. Van Rijswijk L. Full-thickness leg ulcers: Patient demographics and predictors of time to healing. Multi-center leg ulcer study group. *J Fam Pract.* 1993;36(6):625–632.

97. International Medical Electronics. *Megatherm (Model 1000) Shortwave Therapy Unit Instruction Manual.* Kansas City, MO: International Medical Electronics Ltd.; 1981.

98. Swanson G. Functional outcomes report: the next generation in physical therapy reporting. In: Stewart DL, Abeln SH, eds. *Documenting Functional Outcomes in Physical Therapy.* St. Louis, MO: Mosby-Year Book; 1993.

CHAPTER 25

Phototherapeutic Applications for Wound Management

Teresa Conner-Kerr, Karen W. Albaugh, and Autumn Bell

CHAPTER OBJECTIVES

At the completion of this chapter, the reader will be able to:

1. Define phototherapy and list the portions of the electromagnetic spectrum commonly used in the application of this therapeutic modality.
2. List the biologic effects of ultraviolet, visible, and infrared radiation.
3. Summarize the clinical evidence supporting the use of phototherapy in wound management.
4. List indications and contraindications to treatment of open wounds with phototherapy.
5. Describe the procedures for applying phototherapy to open wounds.

Phototherapy, also known as *light therapy*, is a form of radiant energy that has been used to promote healing for thousands of years.[1,2] Sunlight was recognized as having potential healing properties by many early cultures, among them the Egyptians, Romans, Greeks, Sumerians, Chinese, Indians, and Japanese.[3] While sunlight was used by many of these cultures, writings on its use all but disappeared with the advent of Christianity. It was not until the 18th century that an interest in sunlight as a possible medicinal therapy reemerged. In 1796, the German scientist Ebernaier proposed a relationship between the lack of sun exposure and the development of rickets.

Nearly a century later, Danish scientist Niels Finsen prepared a paper on the influence of light on skin.[1,2] Using his own forearm, he demonstrated the ability of sunlight to induce a delayed erythema on unprotected skin exposed to sunlight. During this same time, the bactericidal properties of light were first demonstrated. Between 1890 and 1909, ultraviolet (UV) light in particular was shown to kill many bacteria, including *Mycobacterium tuberculosis*, *Staphylococcus*, *Streptococcus*, *Bacillus*, and *Shigella dysenteriae*. As a result, UV radiation became a common treatment for tuberculosis of the skin. In fact, the Nobel Prize for Medicine and Science was awarded to Finsen in 1903 for his work on the treatment of tuberculosis-induced skin lesions with UV light.

Because of Finsen's early work, research began to focus on the use of UV light to control or prevent surgical wound infection.[1-3] This interest continues today with several groups investigating the utility of using UV light to prevent or control infection of orthopedic surgical wounds, acute wounds, and chronic wounds.[4-11] Similarly, interest in the potential health benefits of other wavelengths of light, as well as novel delivery systems such as lasers, has also evolved over the past 50 years.[12]

This chapter describes the science behind the various forms of phototherapy and its application in wound care. The first part of this chapter focuses on UV radiation and the latter half on lasers and diodes.

THE SCIENCE OF RADIANT ENERGY

Radiant energy is defined as energy in the form of electromagnetic waves.[13] Different forms of radiant energy are arranged into a spectrum—a distribution—called the *electromagnetic spectrum (EMS)* in order of their wavelength, frequency, or both. *Wavelengths* represent the distance between two adjacent peaks or troughs in an energy wave. Wavelengths of radiant energy extend from millions of meters (electrical power) to as short as a million-millionth (10^{-12}) of a meter (gamma and cosmic rays). *Frequency* refers to the number of times a wave travels past a specific point per second.

Penetration of light into skin is known to increase linearly as the wavelength of light increases. This fact is important clinically because longer wavelengths penetrate deeper into tissue than do their shorter counterparts. Light energy from the UV light and blue light portions of the visible light spectrum are absorbed mostly in the epidermis, while longer wavelengths of visible and infrared (IR) light penetrate into the dermis.[15] It is also important to distinguish between depth of penetration and depth of effect, as the biologic cascade of events set in motion by radiant energy treatment can extend beyond the treatment depth. The wavelength of radiant energy influences its depth of penetration.[14]

Term	Definition	Système International (SI unit)
Power	Rate at which work is performed	Watts
Power density (irradiance)	Power per unit area	Watts/cm^2
Energy (work)	Power (watts) × time (seconds)	Joules
Energy density (fluence)	Power density × time	Joules/cm^2
Dose	Reported as energy density	Joules/cm^2

FIGURE 25.1 Definition of radiant energy terms. (From Barham CD, Bounkeo JM, Brannon WM, et al. The efficacy of laser therapy in the treatment of wounds: a meta-analysis of the literature. Master's Thesis Graduate Program of Physical Therapy, North Georgia College and State University, Dahloneg, GA, 2003.)

In addition to wavelength, several other factors affect transmission of radiant energy.[14,15] These include

- Optical properties of tissues
- Angle of application of the light or radiant energy
- Intensity of the energy delivered

Optical properties of tissue are related to tissue pigmentation, composition (high levels of protein increase absorption), density, and architecture.[15] Less heavily pigmented skin or white skin is more sensitive to the effects of radiant energy because it has less melanin, which protects the nucleus of keratinocytes. Skin with greater melanin content, as well as dense tissues, may decrease light transmission, thereby preventing or limiting radiant energy from reaching deeper tissues. For example, UV light transmission is significantly lower for black versus white individuals. The effect of the angle of application and the intensity of power will be considered shortly.

Other terms used in phototherapy include power, power density, energy, and energy density (Fig. 25.1).[16] *Power* is the rate at which work is performed and is measured in watts. Power influences the duration of treatment, in an inverse relationship; that is, when power increases, treatment times generally decrease.

Power density describes the relationship of the power of the light source to the area irradiated or treated.[16] Thus, power density equals the average power divided by the area (in cm^2) irradiated. At a given power, if the area irradiated increases, then the power density decreases.

In phototherapy, *energy* is defined as power (in watts) multiplied by time (in seconds). *Energy density*, which is referred to as the *dose*, is the amount of energy per unit area and can be calculated by multiplying power density by time.[16]

Forms of Radiant Energy Used in Wound Care

Radiant energy is used by a number of health-care professionals for a variety of purposes. For example, therapeutic radiation involves the use of very short wavelength, high-energy radiant energy (x-rays and gamma rays) by medical physicists, oncologists, and surgeons in the management of tumors. We are not addressing these forms of radiant energy in this chapter, as our focus is on the radiant energy used in the management of open wounds.

The three forms of radiant energy used in the care of open wounds that are addressed in this chapter are all emitted from the central portion of the EMS. They are UV, visible, and IR energy.

Ultraviolet Energy

UV energy is a form of radiation that falls between x-rays and visible light on the EMS (Fig. 25.2). Although some people refer to it as UV *light*, this is a misnomer, as this portion of the EMS is largely invisible to the human eye. UV energy encompasses the wavelengths between 180 and 400 nm and has been separated into three distinct bands, UVA, UVB, and UVC,[17–19] based on their wavelength and associated biologic activities.

According to the International Commission on Illumination (CIE), UV wavelengths can be subdivided as follows: 400 to 315 nm (UVA), 315 to 280 nm (UVB), and 280 to 100 nm (UVC).[18] The World Health Organization (WHO) definition of the three UV bands differs somewhat as compared with the CIE. The WHO defines UVA as wavelengths 400 to 320 nm, UVB as wavelengths 320 to 280 nm, and UVC as wavelengths 280 to 200 nm. Recently, UVA has been subdivided into UVA1 and UVA2, since UVA2 rays are thought to have actions more

FIGURE 25.2 UV spectrum. (Courtesy of Teresa Conner-Kerr and John Kerr.)

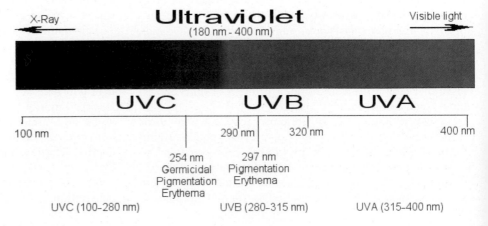

similar to those of UVB. UVA1 encompasses wavelengths from 340 to 400 nm while UVA2 encompasses wavelengths from 320 to 340 nm.[17]

- **UVA.** Long-wave UV radiation, or UVA, is referred to as *black light* or near UV radiation. It is closest to the visible light portion of the EMS. Just over 6% of summer sunlight is UVA.
- **UVB.** The middle band of UV radiation, or UVB, makes up only about 0.5% of summer sunlight. However, it's known as *sunburn radiation* because it is thought to mediate most of the harmful effects of sunlight on human skin, including photoaging and carcinogenesis.[20–24]
- **UVC.** Also called *shortwave UV*, UVC radiation is known for its germicidal effects. Almost all of these rays are prevented from reaching the earth by the ozone layer.

The wavelengths of visible light fall between 400 and 800 nm in length. When viewed together, we see the spectrum of visible light as *white light*. But we can separate white light into its different wavelengths, or colors, by reflecting it off a prism. A rainbow occurs when visible light is reflected off of raindrops, which act as a prism.

Infrared Energy

Whereas the wavelengths of UV energy are shorter than those of visible light, the wavelengths of IR energy are longer. They can be divided into two separate bands. Short (or near) IR wavelengths of light fall between 800 and 1,500 nm. Long (or far) IR wavelengths fall between 1,500 and 15,000 nm.

Physical Science of Phototherapy Radiant Energy Forms

A basic principle of radiant energy is that, as wavelength increases across the EMS, frequency decreases.[17] For example, gamma rays, which are produced by subatomic nuclear reactions, have wavelengths that can be smaller than an atom but are extremely high frequency. In contrast, the wavelengths used in wound care (UV through IR) are longer and have lower frequencies. As we noted earlier, in biologic tissues, longer wavelengths typically penetrate more deeply than do short ones. Therefore, longer wavelengths allow treatment of deeper structures.

Time to delivery of radiant energy is affected by the density of the tissue in which it travels.[14,15,17] Radiant energy travels in a straight line at high speed while in a vacuum. However, as the density of tissue increases (skin, muscle, bone), the speed of the radiant energy wave decreases. Delivery of radiant energy to a tissue is also reduced by the following mechanisms:

1. Reflection (decrease in energy to the medium as some waves are reflected away from the medium)
2. Absorption (energy captured by the medium with a decrease in waves traveling completely through the medium)
3. Refraction (bending and dividing wavelengths into component parts)
4. Penetration or transmission through the medium (decreased absorption by the medium with loss of energy from the medium)

Three physical laws govern the use of radiant energy in the treatment of biologic tissues.[17] The first, Grotthus-Draper law, states that the effect of a wavelength on a tissue is determined by the amount of energy that the tissue absorbs. Different wavelengths are known to produce different effects. The second law, the inverse square law, states that the intensity of the energy wave is inversely related to the square of the distance from the radiant source. The third law, the cosine law, states that energy absorption is at its greatest when energy waves strike a medium at right angles. All of these laws must be taken into consideration for the proper and optimal application of radiant energy.

PHOTOTHERAPY DELIVERY SYSTEMS

Modern approaches to phototherapy began with the use of UV light boxes and IR lamps in the early part of the 20th century.[1] By the late 1950s, new technologies had emerged that produced a uniform and coherent, monochromatic beam of light, the laser.[25–27] Early use of the laser focused on high-power units that operated at an intensity high enough to produce coagulation of body proteins due to thermal effects; hence, the term hot laser. In comparison, low-level or cold lasers, which do not produce significant elevation of tissue temperatures, were later adopted for applications in wound/tissue healing and pain control due to their photobiomodulation effects. Low-level lasers were first used in Europe, China, and Canada and have only recently gained acceptance in the United States for use in wound healing.

Recent developments in phototherapy involve the use of clusters of light-emitting diodes (LEDs), laser diodes (LDs), superluminescent (luminous) diodes (SLDs), or a mixture of these light sources (cluster probes).[26,27] Energy emitted from a laser differs from that emitted by an LED or SLD because it is a stimulated emission and not a spontaneous one. LDs, on the other hand, are true lasers.

Laser and Diodes

A laser is a device that emits a uniform and coherent beam of light.[26,27] Because the light that is produced is a single wavelength, it is monochromatic in nature. These single wavelengths of monochromatic light travel in parallel in a tightly focused beam. As a result, a pinpoint of light can be produced. Lasers are created by stimulating the release of photons from an atom in a high-energy state. These released photons produce the single wavelength of light described above. Hence, laser is an acronym for light amplification by stimulated emission of radiation.

A *diode* is an electronic device that has two points for receiving electric current, and then transmits the current in one direction. *Light-emitting diodes* (*LEDs*) transmit a form of energy in the visible or invisible range of the EMS. They are made from semiconductors and when a charge is applied to the material, electrons move from a conduction band to a lower energy orbital releasing photons of light. LEDs spontaneously release a narrow range of wavelengths with similar colors that are minimally divergent. Although the light produced by LEDs is polychromatic (multicolored), it is not directional or coherent.[21,28] Thus, it produces a wider beam of energy. The clinical importance of this is unknown, since beams from lasers are widened in tissues by refraction.

Two other diode devices are used therapeutically. *Laser diodes* (*LDs*) are true lasers that produce a directed and monochromatic beam of light. *Superluminescent diodes* (*SLDs*) are not lasers but LEDs. They produce a beam that is wider than that of an LD, but narrower than that of a conventional LED.

The above technologies may also be combined to produce *cluster probes* that take advantage of the unique properties of the different components. The advantage of combining these different technologies is that treatment times are reduced, larger tissue areas can be treated, and the biologic effects of different wavelengths may be accessed.

THERAPEUTIC EFFECTS OF ULTRAVIOLET ENERGY

UV energy has been used to treat a variety of skin conditions, including open wounds.[5,6,7,10,28–32] UV radiation is known to promote exfoliation of the outer skin layers, enhance healing through the induction of an erythematous response in the skin, and kill a variety of microorganisms.

The three bands of UV radiation differ in their ability to penetrate human skin (Fig. 25.2) and to produce certain biologic effects.[13,17,19] The UVA band constitutes the longest wavelengths of the UV energy spectrum, and these rays are known to penetrate human skin to the level of the upper dermis. In contrast, UVB rays penetrate only to the stratum basale, the lowermost level of the epidermis. The effects of high-level exposure to UVB radiation are listed in Exhibit 25.1. UVC rays (which have the least ability to penetrate human skin) reach only the upper layers of the epidermis. These rays are associated with germicidal properties (Figure 25.3).

Specific UV wavelengths have been associated with particular biologic responses (see Fig. 25.2). For example, the germicidal effects of UV radiation are associated with UV wavelengths from 250 to 270 nm,[13,17,19] while UV wavelengths of 254 and 297 nm have the greatest ability to induce an erythematous or reddening reaction in the skin. The tanning response, on the other hand, is predominantly associated with wavelengths of 254 and 299 nm.

UV-induced Skin Erythema

Skin reddening or erythema is a well-known effect of UV at certain exposure levels. UV radiation produces this reddening of the skin via stimulation of an inflammatory response that leads

EXHIBIT 25.1				

Immediate and Long-Term Effects of High-Level Exposure to UVB Radiation

Immediate
 Early (0–60 hours)
  Immediate hyperpigmentation
  Epidermal hyperplasia
  Inflammatory reactions
 Late (60–336 hours)
  Secondary hyperpigmentation
  Hyperplasia
  Fibrosis
 Long-standing (Chronic exposure)
  Elastosis
  Carcinoma

	UVC Treatment Times (seconds)				
	in vitro				*in vivo*
	3	5	15	30	30
Procaryotes *(bacteria)*					
MRSA		*			*
VRE		*			
Group A streptococcus		*			
Pseudomonas aeruginosa		*			
Mycobacterium abscesses		*			
Unicellular eucaryote *(yeast)*					
Candida albicans		*			
Multicellular procaryote *(fungi)*					
Aspergillus fumigatus			*		
Mixed cultures			*		
Pseudomonas aeruginosa					
Candida albicans					
Aspergillus fumigatus					

FIGURE 25.3 UV exposure times for 99.99% kill rate.

to increased vascularity of the dermis.[18,22,33] Erythema is most effectively produced by the 297 and 254 nm UV wavelengths.[13,17] These wavelengths encompass both the B and C bands of UV. Erythema that results from the longer wavelengths has a greater latency and lasts for a longer period of time than that produced by shorter wavelengths. However, the shorter wavelengths have a greater potency.

UV-induced erythema is associated with a latent period of 2 to 3 hours.[18] The exact mechanism that underlies this latent appearance of erythema is unknown, but several theories have been offered. The latent development of the erythemal response has been ascribed to the production of some diffusible biologic mediator from damaged epidermal cells.[18,33] It is thought that this mediator then diffuses to the dermis, where it enhances blood vessel permeability. The identity of this diffusible mediator is unknown. Several substances including histamine, bradykinin, and prostaglandins have been implicated in this role. In the past, prostaglandins were thought to be the most likely candidate for this role as a diffusible mediator. However, work by Hensby et al.[34] utilizing prostaglandin antagonists has been inconclusive, and the role that prostaglandins play in mediating erythema is unclear.

Studies by Brauchle et al.[35] have demonstrated a significant increase in vascular endothelial growth factor (VEGF) expression in cultured keratinocytes after irradiation with both sublethal and physiologic levels of UVB. Irradiation of quiescent keratinocytes leads to both an increase in mRNA levels as well as increased levels of VEGF. Since VEGF is known to enhance vascular permeability, it is thought that VEGF may be a potential target for the above-described diffusible mediator. However, the identity of this diffusible mediator(s) remains unknown. Congruent with the findings of Brauchle,[35] Holtz[36] has shown that UV-induced erythema is accompanied by an intercellular edema in the stratum spinosum of the epidermis and an accumulation of white cells in local blood vessels. The development of intercellular edema is also consistent with the separation of the upper and lower epidermal layers that occurs upon exposure to high-intensity UV radiation. These effects on the skin most likely underlie the ability of UV radiation to stimulate debridement. Debridement would result from this sloughing of the upper layers of the epidermis as well as recruitment of phagocytic white blood cells. Increased lysosomal activity and leakage of lysosomal enzymes that has been detected with UV exposure may also contribute to this debridement effect.

UV-induced Epidermal Hyperplasia

Work by Kaiser et al.[37] demonstrated that UVB stimulated epithelialization by enhancing IL-1 production. This work supports the current treatment approach of utilizing UV to enhance epithelialization, especially with indolent wounds that exhibit fibrotic edges. In these wounds, UV may stimulate or restart the epithelialization process.

When low-level UV radiation exposure occurs, it is thought that the above-described effect is confined to the upper third or one-half of the epidermis.[23] As a result, no long-lasting effects are thought to occur as the cells in these layers are differentiating in transit to becoming part of the outer dead layer of the skin. Therefore, this study supports the supposition that UV radiation stimulates repair processes and that these effects may be harnessed at a low enough level to prevent long-term damage. The wound clinician may find the induction of epidermal hyperplasia by UV radiation to be beneficial in promoting rapid epithelialization in acute and chronic wounds.

UV-induced Immunosuppression

High levels of UVB exposure have also been shown to affect Langerhans cells.[18,38,39] These cells inhabit the middle region of the epidermis and appear to have an immune function. They are part of the macrophage lineage and are derived from the bone marrow. High-level UVB exposure is known to produce Langerhans cell necrosis within 24 hours. This pattern of cellular necrosis is seen in both experimental rodent models and humans. The destruction of these cells is thought to account for the immunosuppressive ability of high levels of UVB. Interestingly, this immunosuppressive effect of high-level UVB exposure has been harnessed by researchers to enhance graft take in individuals with burn wounds.[40] However, since the Langerhans cells are derived from the bone marrow, no long-term effects are expected as a result of this local immunosuppression of the treated skin. Furthermore, the effects of short treatment times at low intensities with UVB or UVC are unknown. It is possible that the effects may be different from those seen with high-level UV radiation.

UV-mediated Bactericidal Effects

Research has shown that UV radiation from all three bands, A, B, and C, has the ability to kill numerous microorganisms. However, the effects of UVC are much greater than those associated with UVA or B. UVA and B when used for infection require much longer exposure times and often induce burning of the skin layers.

Because of continuing issues with surgical infections, there has been renewed interest in the potential role of UV light in preventing surgical wound infections. Taylor et al.[5,41] in the United Kingdom examined the effectiveness of UVC radiation on reducing bacterial numbers in individuals undergoing total joint arthroplasty. UVC energy was delivered by tubing placed overhead in a conventional plenum-ventilated surgical theatre. The UVC tubes were activated 10 minutes after the surgical procedure was initiated. Results of the study showed that UVC application was effective in significantly reducing bacterial levels in both the theatre air and surgical wounds. Bacterial levels in the surgical wounds fell 87% with UVC delivered at 100 μW/cm² (N = 18) and 92% with UVC delivered at 300 μW/cm² (N = 13).

In a similar study, Moggio et al.[6] also found that UV irradiation significantly lowered the average number of airborne bacteria detected over the surgical site. The rate of infection for 1,322 individuals who underwent hip arthroplasties was found to be only 0.15% with application of UVC. Similar findings were obtained by Berg et al.[7] when UVC application in operating rooms was compared with a sham blue light application. These authors concluded that the air quality was similar to that produced by ultraclean air ventilation systems. It is also interesting to note that both Berg et al.[7] and Taylor et al.[41] recorded no adverse effects of UVC exposure on operating room personnel.

A growing interest in the use of UV energy for treatment of established wound infections has also been seen in the past two decades. This renewed interest in UV light comes at a time when antimicrobial resistance is rampant among common wound pathogens and when the health-care community is increasingly under pressure to find the most cost-effective and time-efficient method of treatment for various health-care problems.

The effectiveness of UV radiation in killing microbes has been demonstrated by many researchers using in vitro testing. High and High[42] demonstrated that broad-spectrum UV radiation delivered by the Kromayer lamp (model 10), which produces wavelengths from all three UV bands, was effective in eliminating a wide range of wound pathogens in vitro. In contrast, Norback et al.[43] did not find a difference in colonization levels in rats with acute surgical wounds that were exposed to broad-spectrum UV radiation. Since the UV radiation source emitted a broad spectrum of UV A, B, and C wavelengths and the proportion of each type of wavelength is not described, it is difficult to determine if the wavelengths that are known to have the greatest germicidal activity (UVC at 250–270 nm) were present at adequate doses.

Using a halogen lamp that emits predominantly UVC, the authors have shown that a broad range of wound pathogens including those expressing antibiotic resistance can be effectively eliminated with short treatment times (Fig. 25.3).[44,45]

Using the V-254 lamp, which selectively emits UVC energy, we have been able to obtain a 99.99% kill rate for all tested common wound pathogens. Using an in vitro model with optimal growth characteristics for the microorganisms tested, we have shown that UVC irradiation is effective in eradicating both procaryotic organisms such as bacteria and eucaryotic organisms such as yeast or multicellular fungi at short exposure times. In fact, we have found that UVC is effective in killing multicellular eucaryotic wound pathogens at treatment times shorter than those currently advocated for procaryotic (bacterial) organisms. However, our data do indicate that multicellular eucaryotic organisms require 10 times the exposure time (30 seconds) for a 99.9% kill rate as compared with the most susceptible eucaryotic organism (3 seconds). Work conducted in our laboratory has also demonstrated that short UVC exposure times can produce a 99.99% kill rate for methicillin-resistant *Staphylococcus aureus*, both in vitro and in vivo.[8,9]

UV Preclinical Studies

The effects of UVA and UVB radiation on wound healing has been examined using a number of different animal models, including the rat, hairless guinea pig, rabbit, and pig.[46–50] Positive effects of UVB on wound healing were observed in both the rat[13] and rabbit[46] animal models but not in the hairless guinea pig[47–49] model. Irradiation of the acute surgical wound bed of rats with a UVA and UVB energy source resulted in a significantly increased rate of wound closure between the fourth and fifteenth days of treatment compared with untreated controls on the contralateral side of the animal.[43] Additionally, no decrement in wound tensile strength was found at either day 7 or 15 compared with the untreated controls. The results from this study also suggest that the effects of UVA and UVB are localized and not systemic, as healing of the contralateral wounds was not enhanced.

Similarly, El-Batouty et al.[46] found a modestly higher rate of tissue regeneration in acute full-thickness wounds to the pinna of rabbit ears using a hot quartz lamp (UVA and UVB). UV-treated wounds healed more rapidly than their untreated controls. Histopathologic analysis demonstrated significant increases in epithelialization rates and collagen deposition as compared with untreated controls.

In contrast, acute surgical wounds induced in hairless guinea pigs that had been pretreated with UVA or UVB radiation every other day for 16 weeks did not exhibit enhanced wound closure rates.[48,49] Additionally, wound tensile strength was found to be significantly less in both the UVA- and UVB-treated animals. Histopathologic analysis also demonstrated marked endothelial swelling and eosinophilic infiltration in the irradiated group. Similar findings for decreased wound tensile strength were found using hairless guinea pigs pretreated with pure UVA radiation prior to wounding. Due to the extraordinarily long duration of treatment (16 weeks in the first study and 21 weeks in the second study) and the use of a pretreatment UV paradigm rather than UV treatment postwounding, the relevance of these findings is not clear. Furthermore, additional work by the same investigators found that there were no significant differences in tensile strength of wounds made to UV-treated versus untreated skin by recovery day 90.[50]

At this point in time, examination of the effects of UVC on wound healing rates in both the pig and rodent model have shown no grossly detectable facilitation of wound closure. In the porcine model, no significant effect of UVC radiation on wound tensile strength was detected.[50] However, recent studies in our laboratory demonstrated that a 30-second UVC treatment once daily for 5 days in a rodent model resulted in a cleaner and smoother transition area between the periwound and the wound bed with no tissue curling.[11] This treatment paradigm also produced a change in wound morphology due to altered wound contraction. The induction of a change in wound contraction by UVC is consistent with the findings of Morykwas and Mark.[51] Using cultured fibroblasts, Morykwas and Mark[51] demonstrated increased secretion of fibronectin into the culture medium after UVC irradiation. Fibronectin is an extracellular matrix protein that appears to play a role in wound contraction.

UV Clinical Studies

Although there are significant experimental data to suggest a positive role for UV radiation in enhancing wound healing, relatively few clinical studies have been conducted. However, the majority of studies that have been conducted have found positive effects. Documented positive effects of UVA and UVB on wound healing can be found in the literature as far back as 1945.[29] Stein and Shorey[29] published an article detailing the increased rate of wound healing and reduction of wound infection in two soldiers, one with a traumatic wound and the other with a pressure wound. Both wounds had been resistant to healing prior to the institution of UV radiation. The traumatic wound healed within 10 days of the initiation of UV therapy, and the pressure wound healed in less than 2 months.

A randomized controlled trial examining the effects of both UVA and UVB energy on superficial pressure sores in the elderly has also demonstrated enhanced healing rates.[30] In this study, UV-treated ulcers closed in an average time of 6.25 weeks compared with an average of 10 weeks for control wounds. Additionally, a clinical study by Crous and Malherbe[28] also examined the effects of UVA and UVB on wound healing in individuals with venous insufficiency. UV radiation appeared to facilitate wound healing, but wound closure was not achieved with any of the wounds.

The effects of UVC on chronic wound healing have also been examined. A study by Nussbaum et al.[31] examined the effects of UVC combined with ultrasound on pressure ulcer healing. Their treatment parameters were similar to those used with the Crous and Malherbe[28] study. Combination of the UVC and ultrasound treatment was found to enhance healing over that of cold laser or moist wound healing. However, it is difficult to ascribe the enhanced healing effects observed in this study to a UVC-mediated effect, as the UVC treatment employed was delivered in combination with ultrasound. Therefore, it is not clear as to what effect either of the modalities had separately.

Taylor[32] also examined the effectiveness of UVC in treating 56 individuals with infections of the skin including the following lesions: tinea pedis, tinea capitis, sporotrichosis, and tinea corporis. The treatment times were between 2 and 5 minutes, with individuals receiving an average of 3.2 treatments over a period of 5 to 7 days. Fifty patients showed a good response to therapy, with most showing significant clearing of the infection within 1 week.

Recently, Thai et al.[10] found that UVC was effective in decreasing bacterial numbers in chronic wounds. *Pseudomonas aeruginosa*, *S. aureus*, and methicillin-resistant *S. aureus* numbers among other bacterial species were reduced with a single application of UVC for 180 seconds. Consistent with in vitro testing, UVC was shown to be most effective in reducing the level of *P. aeruginosa* in chronic wounds. However, the effects of UVC on MRSA were not as robust as the effects on other bacteria in the wounds with only a one-level reduction in numbers after the standard 180-second treatment time. The present data indicate that multiple treatments of 180 seconds may be required to completely eradicate common bacterial pathogens from chronic wounds.

UVC: Current Recommended Treatment Approaches
UVC Treatment

Based on work[8–10,44,45] by Conner-Kerr and Sullivan along with studies by Thai and Houghton, we propose the use of the algorithm found in Figure 25.4 to determine treatment times for infected wounds when using UVC radiation. This time-dose dependent approach is in place of the older system that utilized the production of varying degrees of skin erythema

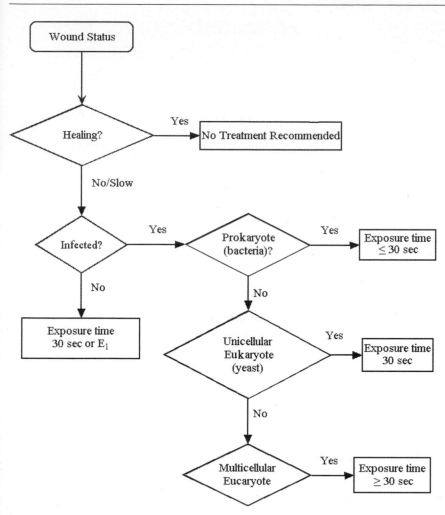

FIGURE 25.4 UVC treatment algorithm. (Courtesy of Teresa Conner-Kerr.)

to determine treatment times. Our algorithm is based on the theoretical principle of choosing UVC treatment times according to minimal lethal dose for the infecting organism. The author advocates this approach as it specifically addresses the susceptibility pattern of the infecting organism to UVC and not the response of the host to UVC. As a result, an adequate dose for killing or inactivation of a particular pathogen can be selected while preventing or minimizing any damage to host cells. Longer treatment times, especially those used with UVB, are known to produce deleterious effects.

PROCEDURE FOR ADMINISTERING UV THERAPY

Only clinicians trained in the application of physical agent modalities are authorized to administer UV therapy. To prevent overexposure to the wound bed and inappropriate exposure to other skin areas, UV treatment should not be administered by the individual receiving treatment, a family member, or other caregiver. Additionally, as with all physical agent modalities or procedures, it's important to reevaluate the necessity of using this modality frequently to ensure optimum treatment outcomes.

Equipment Selection

The primary decision when selecting a UV generator is whether a UVA/UVB or UVC energy source should be used for treatments. As discussed earlier, research appears to indicate that either source is germicidal; however, the peak germicidal wavelengths are in the UVC band from 250 to 270 nm. Thus, if infection control is the primary therapeutic goal, a UVC device should be used. Several different lamp types are available that selectively emit UVC radiation. These include the Birtcher cold quartz lamp and the "V-254" halogen lamp (Fig. 25.5). Cold quartz lamps emit better than 90% UVC at approximately 254 nm. This emission falls within the peak germicidal range for UV radiation. The V-254 halogen lamp has a similar emission

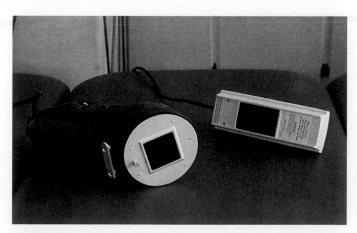

FIGURE 25.5 Laser types. (Courtesy Dr. Teresa Conner-Kerr.)

RESEARCH WISDOM

Select a UVC Lamp for Clinical Infections

The peak germicidal effects of UV radiation are seen with wavelengths of 250 to 270 nm. These wavelengths are found in the UVC band. Therefore, when treating fungal or bacterial skin or wound infections, use low-dose UVC radiation.

CLINICAL WISDOM

Cleanse Wound and Remove Necrotic Tissue Prior to UV Treatment

To maximize exposure of the wound bed to the UV rays, the wound should be cleansed with a gentle cleanser such as normal saline, and then debrided to remove as much necrotic tissue as possible.

Remove all dressings prior to treatment. Mackinnon and Cleek[53] had previously suggested that UV radiation could be used with transparent dressings. However, we were unable to detect any bacterial inactivation or killing when bacterial cultures covered with either Tegaderm™ or Bioclusive™ were irradiated with UVC for treatment times as long as 120 seconds.[45]

Remove Wound Dressings Prior to Treatment

All moist wound dressings should be removed prior to treatment of the wound bed with UV radiation so that the UV rays reach the wound tissue.

range. Either will provide a good germicidal effect; however, the halogen lamp is lighter and has a larger face plate that allows for more rapid treatment of larger wounds.

For wound healing, the decision as to which particular UV energy source to use is less clear. However, since the literature has linked chronic or prolonged exposure to high-dose UVB to carcinoma formation,[23,33] the author recommends the use of UVC or very low exposure to a UVA or B light source with the induction of a very minimal skin erythema (minimal erythemal dose [MED]) that appears in 4 to 6 hours but resolves within 24 hours (Fig. 25.6 for UVA-B dosing). A cost-effective approach would include the use of the UVC generator for both bioburden control and stimulating wound healing.

Preparation of Wound and Periwound Area

Protection is a primary consideration in preparing the wound bed for treatment with UV radiation. Most authorities recommend protecting the periwound and any nontreatment area with draping materials (Fig. 25.7). UV-resistant ointments such as petrolatum jelly may also be used to protect the periwound area that is immediately adjacent to the wound bed. On the other hand, it has been argued that protecting the adjacent periwound eliminates a potential source of epithelial cells and wound healing factors that would also be stimulated with the treatment.

Other considerations for preparation of the wound bed are removal of all dressing materials and cleansing of particulate matter in the wound bed. This can be accomplished by a variety of mechanisms, including pulsatile lavage with suction, low-frequency ultrasound sprays, or normal saline flush. At this point in time, there is one study that found added benefit to

decreasing microorganism numbers when coadministering jet lavage and UV radiation.[52] Cleansing of the wound bed is also important, as the depth of penetration for all UV wavelengths is only at best less than 100 to 200 μm.[18] Therefore, cleansing of particulate increases wound bed exposure.

Treatment Times

The authors recommend UVC treatment primarily for wounds with high levels of bioburden, particularly antibiotic-resistant bacteria. In the past, UV dose has been calculated according to a response called the *MED* response of each individual client.[17] However, the authors question the appropriateness of this system for determining UVC treatment times, especially for infection control. Findings in Conner-Kerr and Sullivan's laboratory[8,9] using both in vitro and in vivo testing along with those of Thai et al.[10] indicate that many wound pathogens, especially MRSA, can be eradicated with short treatment times. Therefore, the authors advocate the use of short exposure times

Dose	Skin Reaction	Time to Develop	Time to Resolution
SED	None noted		
E_1 (MED)	Subtle reddening	4–6 hrs	24 hrs
E_2	Similar to mild sunburn Skin exfoliation and pigmentation	4–6 hrs	3–4 days
E_3	Similar to severe sunburn Intense erythema Marked increase in exfoliation and pigmentation	2 hrs	Several days
E_4	Same as E_3 with significant tissue swelling and exudate	2 hrs	Several days

SED = suberythemal dose
E_1 (MED) = minimal erythemal dose
E_2 = second-degree erythemal dose
E_3 = third-degree erythemal dose
E_4 = fourth-degree erythemal dose

FIGURE 25.6 Erythemal dosages used in UVA-B treatments.

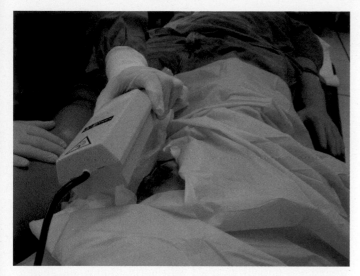

FIGURE 25.7 A Winston-Salem State University physical therapy graduate student has prepared a simulated wound on a human patient simulator for treatment with a UVC light. The wound is draped on all sides to protect periwound tissue. (Courtesy Dr. Teresa Conner-Kerr.)

(30–60 seconds but no more than 180 seconds) administered once daily for 1 week. Prior to the initiation or reinitiation of UVC treatment, the individual should be assessed for any clinical signs of infection, and the wound should be cultured to determine the level of bioburden present.

Treatment Distance

Place a UVC lamp so that there is a distance of 1 inch (or 2.54 cm) between the UVC energy source and the wound bed.[17,19] UVC lamps are available with built-in spacers. Alternatively, you can simply attach a spacer made of a 1-inch portion of a sterile swab or tongue depressor. Deliver the UVC energy perpendicular to the wound bed to maximize delivery according to the cosine law.

Step-by-Step Guide to UVC Application

1. Cleanse the face plate of the UVC lamp with an antimicrobial agent per manufacturer's guidelines.
2. As patient comfort permits, position for maximal exposure of the wound.
3. Remove all dressings.
4. Cleanse wound with normal saline.
5. Remove excess wound fluid and loose particulate matter.
6. Drape periwound area or coat with nontoxic UV-blocking ointment (avoid getting it in the wound bed).
7. Protect your own and the patient's eyes from UV radiation with UV-protective goggles or draping for the patient.
8. Place UVC lamp source 1 inch (or 2.5 cm) from wound.
9. Irradiate wound according to degree of bioburden present (30–180 seconds/day for 5 days; repeat if bioburden has not decreased as measured on culture and with clinical assessment for signs of wound infection).
10. Remove UV-blocking ointment and redress wound.

Step-by-Step Guide to UVA/UVB Application

1. Allow the UVA/UVB lamp adequate time to warm up according to manufacturer's guidelines.

CLINICAL WISDOM

Orient UV Lamp Parallel to Wound Bed

Observing the cosine law, orient the UV lamp parallel to the wound bed with UV rays delivered perpendicular to the wound to maximize energy delivery.

2. Determine MED dose with erythrometer over a nonpigmented area such as the inner arm, starting with 30 seconds of exposure (Fig. 25.6).
3. An MED dose is the exposure time that produces a subtle reddening or erythema that develops in 4 to 6 hours but resolves in 24 hours.
4. Follow steps 2 to 7 above for UVC application.
5. Place UVA/UVB source 30 inch from wound bed.
6. Irradiate wound according to individual skin response for an MED dose initially to stimulate epithelialization and increase vascularity.
7. Remove UV-blocking ointment and redress wound.

Indications and Contraindications

UV radiation appears to be indicated for the following:

1. Slow or nonhealing wounds
2. Necrotic wounds
3. Purulent or infected acute or chronic wounds

Commonly sited contraindications[17,19] to treatment include the following:

1. Diabetes
2. Pulmonary tuberculosis
3. Hyperthyroidism
4. Systemic lupus erythematosus
5. Cardiac, renal, and hepatic disease
6. Acute eczema or psoriasis
7. Herpes simplex
8. Cancerous growths

Also, do not apply UV over the eyes.
The following precautions should also be noted:

1. Generalized fever
2. Photosensitizing medications
3. Photosensitivity
4. Recent x-ray
5. Malignant wounds for palliative care

With any adverse reaction, such as severe pain, intense itching, or burning, UV therapy should be discontinued. Hydrogel moist wound dressings or other products that have been shown to decrease the pain associated with radiation or burn wounds may increase client comfort and speed healing.

Documentation

Document treatment times, duration, and angle of incidence along with the distance at which the UV energy source is placed from the wound bed. Client position during treatment and specific lamp model and serial number should also be documented, as should treatment outcomes.

CASE STUDY

Decontamination of a Wound Infected with MRSA Using UVC Radiation

Individual: M.G. Age: 79. Start of Care Date: 4/98

Medical History
M.G. was a 79-year-old nonambulatory female resident of a long-term care facility with a sacral wound. Her medical diagnoses included CHF with end-stage renal disease. She required mod-max assist of two therapists for all bed mobility. She had no prior history of pressure ulceration.

Reason for Referral
Client was referred to physical therapy due to impaired bed mobility and the presence of a nonhealing stage 3 sacral pressure ulcer.

Functional Diagnosis and Targeted Outcomes
Wound Examination

The wound was a stage 3 pressure ulcer located over the sacrum. Wound margins were indurated, and the periwound expressed moderate erythema. The periwound was also noted to be warmer than adjacent tissues. The wound bed was fully granulated and friable upon manual examination, and a distinctive odor of ammonia was detected upon initial examination. Semiquantitative swab cultures of this wound indicated that it contained high numbers of methicillin-resistant *S. aureus* (MRSA).

Functional Diagnosis

Impaired integumentary integrity secondary to full-thickness skin involvement and scar formation (from Guide to PT Practice, pattern 7D), chronic inflammation phase.

Targeted outcome: Wound decontamination for progression through stages of wound healing and resolution of chronic inflammation.

Need for Skilled Services: The Therapy Problem
The client had a nonhealing stage 3 pressure ulcer and exhibited clinical signs of wound infection. The wound required decontamination and appropriate moist wound therapy to stimulate the healing process.

Treatment Plan and Outcome
A single application of UVC was applied to the wound bed to determine if one application of UVC for 30 seconds was effective in immediately reducing the bacterial load (Fig. 25.3). The wound was initially cleansed with normal saline and then a semiquantitative swab culture was obtained using the 10-point culturing method. UVC was then applied to the wound bed with a V-254 halogen lamp with a calibrated output of 15 mW for 30 seconds. The periwound was completely covered with draping materials, and the UVC lamp was placed parallel to the wound bed at a distance of 2.5 cm. Immediately after the UVC treatment, a second semiquantitative swab culture was performed. Both cultures were immediately sent for processing in the clinical laboratory. The laboratory report derived from the swab culture taken immediately prior to the UVC treatment showed high numbers of MRSA present. Results from the swab culture taken immediately posttreatment of the wound bed for 30 seconds with UVC demonstrated very low growth. This case study demonstrates the utility and immediacy of UVC in decontaminating the surface of the wound bed. (Case study courtesy of Rhonda M. Jones, PT.)

LASERS AND LIGHT-EMITTING DIODES

Both low-level lasers and LEDs are capable of producing changes in cellular function. This effect is known as *photobiomodulation*.

Biologic and Therapeutic Effects of Lasers

Andre Mester was the first to demonstrate the effectiveness of low-power lasers (also called *cold or low-level lasers*) in facilitating healing of chronic wounds.[25,54] He purported to have achieved a 90% rate of healing in more than 1,000 patients. Low-level laser therapy has also increased rates of healing in surgical wounds, cutaneous fissures, and venous ulcerations.[12,25,55] Interestingly, studies of laser's effect on time to healing suggest that treatment of wounds around day 3 results in the greatest acceleration of wound healing. This finding is congruent with those from other studies that have demonstrated a cold-laser–induced acceleration in the inflammatory and proliferative phases of wound healing.

But how do these healing effects occur? It seems that cold or low-level lasers may modulate biologic processes in either a stimulatory or inhibitory manner. The changes appear to be prompted by interaction of low-level laser light with naturally occurring chromophores (light-absorbing pigments such as melanin, hemoglobin, and others) located in cells' mitochondria.[16,55] Specifically, absorption by the chromophores of low-level laser light from the visible and IR region of the EMS results in heightened cellular metabolism.[56]

Wavelengths of radiant energy between 600 and 1,200 nm are capable of penetrating the dermis and interacting with chromophores in human tissues.[16,55] Chromophores in cells that can absorb this low-level laser light include respiratory chain enzymes, melanin, hemoglobin, and myoglobin.[56] Longer wavelengths of light, which are produced by the gallium-arsenide laser (long IR waves), can interact with a wide variety of cellular chromophores. Visible and short IR waves, which are generated by the helium-neon laser, interact with a limited number of chromophores (melanin, hemoglobin, and myoglobin).

Biological effects of low-level laser that result from modulation of endogenous chromophores include

- Increased cellular proliferation and differentiation (muscle and fibroblast)[57–59]
- Increased mitochondrial production of ATP[59]
- Increased collagen synthesis[60,61]
- Increased activity of T and B lymphocytes including binding of pathogens[59,62,63]
- Increased macrophage activity[60,64]

EXHIBIT **25.2   Characteristics of Common Low-Level Lasers.**

Laser Type	Helium Neon	Gallium Arsenide	Gallium Aluminum Arsenide
Lasing medium	Gas	Semiconductor	Semiconductor
Wavelength	632.8 nm	904 nm	830 nm
Electromagnetic spectrum	Red portion of visible light	Infrared	Infrared
Depth of absorption	2–5 mm	1–2 cm	3–5 cm

The above biological phenomena are thought to partially explain the positive effect of low-level laser on wound healing.[12,25,55,65]

Biologic and Therapeutic Effects of LEDs

As noted earlier, photobiomodulation also occurs with LED therapy. For instance, cells exposed to IR LED lights have also been shown to grow 150% to 200% faster than untreated cells.[66] IR light produced by LEDs penetrates up to 5 cm and has been shown to stimulate a variety of cell types. Human muscle cells treated with an IR LED grew seven times faster than their untreated counterparts, and skin cells grew five times faster.

Procedure for Administering Laser Therapy

As with UV therapy, administration of low-level laser therapy should be performed only by a clinician skilled in the application of physical agent modalities. One of the greatest limitations in integrating laser therapy into clinical practice is the failure of many research studies to report parameters such as wavelength, delivery mode (pulsed vs. continuous), power density, exposure time, frequency, and total duration of the treatment.[67,68] Adding to the confusion is the scarcity of published studies comparing the effects of lasers and LEDs. They both appear to promote soft tissue healing; however, the therapeutic devices and research parameters should be clearly understood by the clinician using them and documented accordingly.

Equipment Selection

The primary characteristics that distinguish laser devices include a power range of 10^{-3} to 10^{-1} W and a wavelength between 300 and 10,600 nm.[69] A variety of media have been used to create lasers. These include gases such as helium and neon (632.8 nm), ruby (694 nm), and argon (488 nm). Newer laser technology employs semiconductor LDs, such as gallium arsenide (904 nm) and gallium aluminum arsenide (830 nm). We stated earlier that wavelength is the primary determinant of depth of penetration.[14,15] Helium-neon lasers have been shown to affect more superficial tissues, while gallium arsenide, which is longer in wavelength, appears to have an effect up to 5 cm of

CLINICAL WISDOM

A clear, transparent film should be placed over the wound to avoid contamination of the laser device.

depth (Exhibit 25.2). Whether a device is using continuous or pulsed mode also affects the average power output.[69]

Every device should have a description of the types of light sources incorporated in the unit, wavelength, power output, pulse rate, intensity, and total irradiation time. Energy density is reported in joules per square centimeter.[25] Note that all laser devices should bear an FDA warning label for class II or III devices. If the device is truly a laser in its construction, it will carry a warning label.

Any claim that a device produces temperature increases indicate that the device is not a low-power laser of the type that is currently approved for use by physical therapists in the rehabilitation setting. Low-power lasers do not produce a noticeable temperature increase in tissues.

Laser devices are classified according to their power and their biologic effects (Fig. 25.8). Physical therapists and other wound care clinicians trained in physical agent theory and practice use class 3B lasers.[25]

Preparation of Wound and Periwound

Prior to application of the laser, the wound and surrounding tissue should be cleansed thoroughly to remove loose slough and excess drainage. Presence of exudates diminishes laser penetration.

Treatment Times

The more powerful the laser (intensity), the less time is needed to treat the area. For example, a 1-mW laser would take 1,000 seconds to deliver 1 J of energy. A 10-mW laser would take 100 seconds to deliver the same energy. A 50-mW laser would take

Class I	< 0.5 mW	No hazards
Class 2	< 1 mW	Safe for momentary viewing
Class 3A	< 5 mW	
Class 3B	< 5 00 mW	Photobiomodulation
		No photothermal effect
		No harm to skin or clothing
		Potential damage to the eyes
		Used by wound care clinicians/rehab
Class 4	> 500 mW	Photothermal effects
		Harmful to skin, eyes, and clothing
		Use with extreme caution (medical use)

FIGURE 25.8 Power and biologic Effect of Laser Devices.

CLINICAL WISDOM

Studies have shown that larger doses or extended treatment times can be detrimental to healing.[71] Therefore, more is not necessarily better. Laser should be administered to the treatment area no more than once per day.

20 seconds.[70] Most devices offer a preset time of exposure in seconds to create a programmed activation cycle. Overall dosage is based on the output of the laser in mW, the time of exposure in seconds, and the beam surface area of the laser in square centimeters. Depending on the device, some manufacturers recommend a rotation of the laser at several intervals to ensure thorough treatment of the target area.

Treatment Distance

A common technique involves placing the head of the laser in direct contact with the transparent film covering the wound surface. The device is kept stationary for the prescribed treatment time. Sweeping motions are avoided to allow for maximal absorption of photons of light energy. Additionally, some clinicians advocate treatment with laser to the wound periphery.

Step-by-Step Guide to Laser Application

1. Cleanse the laser probe with 70% rubbing alcohol and a damp cloth or per manufacturer guidelines.
2. Position the patient comfortably, while permitting adequate exposure of the wound.
3. Remove all dressings.
4. Cleanse the wound with normal saline.
5. Remove excess wound fluid and loose debris.
6. Cover the wound with a clear semipermeable film that extends at least 1/2 inch beyond the wound margins. If the wound has significant depth, press plastic wrap into the cavity to cover all open areas.
7. Protect the clinician's and patient's eyes from laser radiation using laser protection goggles (Fig. 25.9).

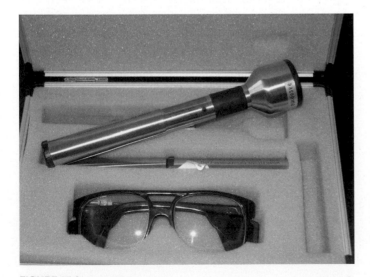

FIGURE 25.9 Protective eyewear.

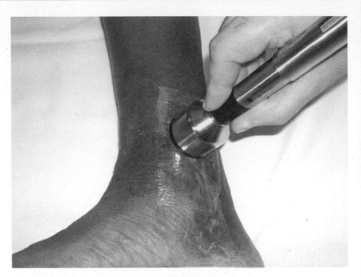

FIGURE 25.10 Low-level laser treatment of wound in medial malleolar region.

8. Place laser device in direct contact with the thin film dressing applied over the wound bed. Maintain direct contact throughout the treatment (Fig. 25.10).
9. Irradiate the area beneath the probe per manufacturer guidelines. If the wound is larger than the head of the device, move to the next untreated area and repeat the treatment until the entire wound surface is treated.
10. Remove the transparent film. Cleanse the wound with saline.
11. Redress with an appropriate wound dressing.
12. Cleanse the head of the laser with 70% rubbing alcohol and a damp cloth or per manufacturer guidelines.

Indications and Contraindications

Laser has not yet been approved by the FDA for use with wounds. Based on the available research related to wound healing, however, laser may be indicated for the following types of wounds[69,70,72]:

1. Acute or chronic wounds
2. Slow or nonhealing wounds
3. Infected or colonized wounds

CLINICAL WISDOM

Avoid direct exposure to the eyes due to possible retinal burns.

Self Care

Administration of low-level laser therapy should be performed by a skilled individual licensed in the application of physical agent modalities. To prevent overexposure or inappropriate exposure to other areas, laser should not be administered by the individual receiving treatment or by the caregiver. The clinician should monitor the necessity of this intervention on a regular basis to ensure optimal outcomes.

No adverse reactions have been reported in the literature. Contraindications and precautions for laser therapy include the following:

1. Do not use over cancerous growths.
2. Avoid direct exposure to the eyes, which could result in burn injury to the retina. Private treatment areas are recommended to avoid accidental eye exposure from reflected laser light.
3. As a general precaution, do not use during the first trimester of pregnancy.
4. Do not treat over the thyroid gland.

Documentation

Document location of the treatment, treatment parameters utilized, and response of the patient to the treatment. Wavelength, mode of treatment (pulsed vs. continuous), and energy density (dose) should also be documented, as well as frequency of application and total treatment sessions. Patient position during treatment and wound preparation will be helpful for subsequent treating clinicians. Documentation of treatment outcomes may include but is not limited to changes in wound size, pain, and bioburden.

CONCLUSION

Research evidence supports the use of UVC in managing wound bioburden. UVC provides an effective alternative to standard antibiotic therapies especially in the case of antibiotic-resistant wound pathogens. Evolving evidence also supports a role for UV energy, laser, and LED therapies in facilitating wound healing.

CASE STUDY

Promotion of Wound Closure with Helium-Neon Laser Treatment

Individual: S.P. Age: 67 Start of Care Date: 12/05

Medical History

S.P. was a 67-year-old ambulatory male who lives with his wife on a small family farm. He has a diabetic, neuropathic wound (Wagner Grade 2) on the distal plantar surface of his left great toe. His medical diagnoses included diabetes, HTN, and mild CHF. He has a past history of diabetic neuropathic ulcers over the left first metatarsal head.

Reason for Referral

The patient was referred to physical therapy because of impaired gait and balance with the presence of a nonhealing diabetic neuropathic ulcer.

Functional Diagnosis and Targeted Outcomes
Wound Examination

The wound was covered with a thick callus except for a 1.0-cm opening that revealed a dry, pink granulation bed. No exposed bone or significant odor was detected. Upon saucerization of the callus, a dry pink granulation bed with minimal necrosis and exudate was revealed.

Functional Diagnosis

Impaired integumentary integrity secondary to full-thickness skin involvement and scar formation (from Guide to PT Practice, pattern 7D), chronic inflammation phase; *Targeted outcome*: Wound stimulation for progression through stages of wound healing and resolution of chronic inflammation.

Need for Skilled Services: The Therapy Problem

The client had a Wagner stage 2 diabetic neuropathic ulcer that had failed to heal with traditional moist wound therapy and off-loading. The wound required debridement, cleansing, appropriate moist wound therapy, and laser treatment to stimulate the healing process. Off-loading continued with a diabetic walking boot.

Treatment Plan and Outcome

Helium-neon laser therapy was applied three times/week for 3 weeks until wound closure. Wound debridement was performed as needed along with wound cleansing prior to laser treatment. A transparent film dressing was placed over the wound and the wound was treated with the laser using a stroking method to produce a cross-hatch effect. A total treatment dose of 30 J/cm^2 was used at each treatment session. The wound closed with minimal scarring at the end of the third week.

REVIEW QUESTIONS

1. Which band of UV is used primarily to control wound bioburden?
   A. UVA
   B. UVB
   C. UVC
   D. UVD

2. Which of the following is an indication for UVC treatment?
   A. Slow-healing wounds
   B. Necrotic wounds
   C. Infected chronic wounds
   D. All

REVIEW QUESTIONS *(continued)*

3. Which of the following factors affect transmission of radiant energy?
   A. Optical properties of tissues
   B. Angle of light application
   C. Wavelength of light energy
   D. All
4. Which statement is correct?
   A. The effect of a wavelength on a tissue is determined by the amount of energy the tissue absorbs.
   B. Different wavelengths produce the same effects on tissue.
   C. The intensity of the energy wave is directly related to the distance from the radiant source.
   D. Energy absorption is least when energy waves strike at right angles.
5. Which is a precaution and not a contraindication to UV radiation?
   A. Diabetes
   B. Generalized fever
   C. Acute eczema
   D. Herpes simplex

REFERENCES

1. Licht S. History of ultraviolet light therapy. In: Licht S ed. *Therapeutic Electricity and Ultraviolet Radiation.* 2nd ed. New Haven, CT: Elizabeth Licht; 1967:191–212.
2. Licht S. History of ultraviolet therapy. In: Stillwell GK, ed. *Therapeutic Electricity and Ultraviolet Radiation.* 3rd ed. Baltimore, MA: Williams & Wilkins; 1983:228–261.
3. Hart D. Sterilization of the air in the operating room by special antibacterial radiant energy. *J Thorac Surg.* 1936;6:45.
4. Wu J, Barisoni D, Armato U. Prolongation of survival of alloskin grafts with no concurrent general suppression of the burned patient's immune system: a preliminary clinical investigation. *Burns.* 1996;22(5):353–358.
5. Taylor GJ, Chandler L. Ultraviolet light in the orthopaedic operating theatre. *Br J Theatre Nurs.* 1997;6(10):10–14.
6. Moggio M, Goldner JL, McCollum DE, et al. Wound infections in patients undergoing total hip arthroplasty. Ultraviolet light for the control of airborne bacteria. *Arch Surg.* 1979;114(7):815–823.
7. Berg M, Bergman BR, Hoborn J. Shortwave ultraviolet radiation in operating rooms. *J Bone Joint Surg.* 1989;71(3):483–485.
8. Conner-Kerr TA, Sullivan PK, Gaillard J, et al. The effects of ultraviolet radiation on antibiotic-resistant bacteria in vitro. *Ostomy/Wound Manage.* 1998;44(10):50–56.
9. Conner-Kerr TA, Sullivan PK, Keegan A, et al. UVC reduces antibiotic resistant bacterial numbers in living tissue. *Ostomy/Wound Manage.* 1999;45(4):84.
10. Thai TP, Keast DH, Campbell KE, et al. Effect of ultraviolet light C on bacterial colonization in chronic wounds. *Ostomy/Wound Manage.* 2005;51(10):32–45.
11. Sullivan PK, Conner-Kerr TA, Dixon S, et al. The effect of UVC irradiation on wound closure. *Presented at the 2000 Symposium on Advanced Wound Care & Medical Research Forum on Wound Repair,* April 2000, Dallas, TX.
12. Enwemeka C, Parker JC, Dowdy DS, et al. The efficacy of low power lasers in tissue repair and pain control: a meta-analysis study. *Photomed Laser Surg.* 2004;22:323–329.
13. Weisberg J. Electromagnetic spectrum. In: Hecox B, Mehreteab TA, Weisberg J, eds. *Physical Agents: A Comprehensive Text for Physical Therapists.* Norwalk, CT: Appleton & Lange; 1994:50.
14. Ackermann G, Hartmann M, Scherer K, et al. Correlations between light penetration into skin and the therapeutic outcome following laser therapy of port wine stains. *Lasers Med Sci.* 2002;17(2):70–78.
15. Grossweiner L. Tissue Optics Theories. In: Grossweiner L, ed. *The Science of Phototherapy.* Boca Raton, FL: CRC Press; 1994:87–100.
16. Barham CD, Bounkeo JM, Brannon WM, et al. The efficacy of laser therapy in the treatment of wounds: a meta-analysis of the literature. Master's Thesis Graduate Program of Physical Therapy, North Georgia College and State University, Dahloneg, GA, 2003.
17. Weisberg J. Ultraviolet irradiation. In: Hecox B, Mehreteab TA, Weisberg J, eds. *Physical Agents: A Comprehensive Text for Physical Therapists.* Norwalk, CT: Appleton & Lange; 1994:377–378.
18. Moseley H. Sources of ultraviolet radiation. In: Moseley H, ed. *Non-Ionising Radiation: Microwaves, Ultraviolet and Laser Radiation.* Philadelphia, PA: IOP Publishing Ltd; 1988:110.
19. Hayes KW. Ultraviolet radiation. In: Hayes KW, ed. *Manual for Physical Agents.* 5th ed. Norwalk, CT: Appleton & Lange; 1999:
20. Schwarz T, Urbanski A, Luger TA. Ultraviolet light and epidermal cell-derived cytokines. In: Luger TA, Schwarz T, eds. *Epidermal Growth Factors and Cytokines.* New York: Marcel Dekker, Inc.; 1994:303.
21. Scott BO. Clinical uses of ultraviolet radiation. In: Stillwell GK, ed. *Therapeutic Electricity and Ultraviolet Radiation.* 3rd ed. Baltimore, MA: Williams & Wilkins; 1983:228–261.
22. Stenback F. Health hazards from ultraviolet radiation. *Public Health Rev.* 1982;10:229.
23. Daniels F. Ultraviolet light and dermatology. In: Stillwell GK, ed. *Therapeutic Electricity and Ultraviolet Radiation.* 3rd ed. Baltimore, MA: Williams & Wilkins; 1983:263–303.
24. van der Leun JC. On the action spectrum of ultraviolet erythema. *Res Prog Org Biol Med Chem.* 1972;3:711–736.
25. Belanger AY. LASER. In: Belanger AY, ed. *Evidence-Based Guide to Therapeutic Physical Agents.* Philadelphia, PA: Lippincott Williams & Wilkins; 2003:191–221.
26. Cameron MH. A shining light. *Adv Dir Rehabil.* 2005;14(4):39–42.
27. Conner-Kerr T. Wound technology: The future is now. *ECPN.* 2005;104:34–39.
28. Crous L, Malherbe C. Laser and ultraviolet light irradiation in the treatment of chronic ulcers. *Physiotherapy.* 1988;44:73.
29. Stein I, Shorey MM. Ultraviolet radiation in the treatment of indolent, soft-tissue ulcerations. *Physiother Rev.* 1945;25(6):272–274.
30. Willis EE, Anderson TW, Beattie BL, et al. A randomized placebo controlled trial of ultraviolet light in the treatment of superficial pressure sores. *J Am Geriatr Soc.* 1983;31:131.
31. Nussbaum EL, Biemann, Mustard B. Comparison of ultrasound/ ultraviolet-C and laser for treatment of pressure ulcers in patients with spinal cord injury. *Phys Ther.* 1994;74(9):812–825.
32. Taylor R. Clinical study of ultraviolet in various skin conditions. *Phys Ther.* 1972;52(3):279–282.
33. Harm W. UV carcinogenesis. In: Harm W, ed. *Biological Effects of Ultraviolet Radiation.* New York: Cambridge University Press; 1980:191.
34. Hensby CN, Plummer NA, Black AK, et al. Time-course of arachidonic acid, prostaglandins E2 and F2 alpha production in human abdominal skin following irradiation with ultraviolet wavelengths (290–320 nm). *Adv Prostaglandin Thromboxane Res.* 1980;7:857–860.

35. Brauchle M, Funk JO, Kind P, et al. Ultraviolet B and H_2O_2 are potent inducers of vascular endothelial growth factor expression in cultured keratinocytes. *J Biol Chem*. 1996;271(36):21793–21797.

36. Holtz F. Pharmacology of ultraviolet radiation. *Br J Phys Med*. 1952;5:201.

37. Kaiser MR, Davis SC, Mertz PM. The effect of ultraviolet irradiation-in-duced inflammation on epidermal wound healing. *Wound Repair Regen*. 1995;3:311–315.

38. Fan J, Schoenfeld RJ, Hunter RA. A study of the epidermal clear cells with special reference to their relationship to the cells of Langerhans. *J Invest Dermatol*. 1959;32:445–450.

39. Bergstresser PR, Toews GB, Streilein JW. Natural and perturbed distribution of Langerhans cells: responses to ultraviolet light, heterotopic skin grafting and dinitrofluorobenzene sensitization. *J Invest Dermatol*. 1980;75:73–77.

40. Wu J, Barisoni D, Armato U. Prolongation of survival of alloskin grafts with no concurrent general suppression of the burned patient's immune system: a preliminary clinical investigation. *Burns*. 1996;22(5):353–358.

41. Taylor GJS, Bannister GC, Leeming JP. Wound disinfection with ultraviolet radiation. *J Hosp Infect*. 1995;30:85–93.

42. High AS, High JP. Treatment of infected skin wounds using ultra-violet radiation: An in vitro study. *Physiotherapy*. 1983;69(10):359–360.

43. Norback I, Kulmala R, Jarvinen M. Effect of ultraviolet therapy on rat skin wound healing. *J Surg Res*. 1990;48:68–71.

44. Sullivan PK, Conner-Kerr T. A comparative study of the effects of UVC irradiation on select procaryotic and eucaryotic wound pathogens. *Ostomy/Wound Manage*. 2000;46(10):44–50.

45. Sullivan PK, Conner-Kerr TA, Smith ST. The effects of UVC irradiation on Group A Streptococcus in vitro. *Ostomy/Wound Manage*. 1999;45(10):50–58.

46. El-Batouty MF, El-Gindy M, El-Shawaf I, et al. Comparative evaluation of the effects of ultrasonic and ultraviolet irradiation on tissue regeneration. *Scand J Rheumatol*. 1986;15:381–386.

47. Das SK, Brantley SK, Davidson SF. Wound tensile strength in the hairless guinea pig following irradiation with pure ultraviolet-A light. *Br J Plast Surg*. 1991;44(7):509–513.

48. Davidson SF, Brantley SK, Das SK. The effects of ultraviolet radiation on wound healing. *Br J Plast Surg*. 1991;44(3):210–214.

49. Davidson SF, Brantley SK, Das SK. The reversibility of UV-altered wound tensile strength in the hairless guinea pig following a 90-day recovery period. *Br J Plast Surg*. 1992;45(2):109–112.

50. Basford JR, Hallman HO, Sheffield CG, et al. Comparison of cold-quartz ultraviolet, low-energy laser, and occlusion in wound healing in a swine model. *Arch Phys Med Rehabil*. 1986;67:151.

51. Morykwas MJ, Mark MW. Effects of ultraviolet light on fibroblast fibronectin production and lattice contraction. *Wounds*. 1998;10(4):111–117.

52. Taylor GJ, Leeming JP, Bannister GC. Effects of antiseptics, ultraviolet light and lavage on airborne bacteria in a model wound. *J Bone Joint Surg Br*. 1993;75(5):724–730.

53. MacKinnon JL, Cleek PL. Therapeutic penetration of ultraviolet light through transparent dressing. *Phys Ther*. 1984;64:204.

54. Mester E, Spiry T, Szende B, et al. Effect of laser-rays on wound healing. *Am J Surg*. 1971;122(4):532–535.

55. Woodruff LD, Bounkeo JM, Brannon WM, et al. The efficacy of laser therapy in wound repair: a meta-analysis of the literature. *Photomed Laser Surg*. 2004;22(3):241–247.

56. Passarella S, Casamassima E, Molinari S, et al. Increase of proton electrochemical and ATP synthesis in rat liver mitochondria irradiated in vitro by HeNe. *FEBS Lett*. 1984;175:95–99.

57. Shefer G, Partridge TA, Heslop L, et al. Low energy laser irradiation promotes the survival and cell cycle entry of skeletal muscle satellite cells. *J Cell Sci*. 2002;115(Pt 7):1461–1469.

58. Abergel RP, Lyons RF, Castel JC, et al. Biostimulation of wound healing by lasers: experimental approaches in animal models and in fibroblast cultures. *J Dermatol Surg Oncol*. 1987;13(2):127–133.

59. Passarella S, Casamassima E, Quagliariello E, et al. Quantitative analysis of lymphocyte-salmonella interaction and effect of lymphocyte irradiation by helium-neon laser. *Biochem Biophys Res Commun*. 1985;130(2):546–552.

60. Rajaratnam S, Bolton P, Dyson M. Macrophage responsiveness to laser therapy with varying pulsing frequencies. *Laser Ther*. 1994;6:107–111.

61. Abergel RP, Lam TS, Meeker CA, et al. Biostimulation of procollagen production by low energy lasers in human skin fibroblast cultures. *Clin Res*. 1984;32:567A.

62. Kupin VI, Bykov VS, Ivanov AV, et al. Potentiating effects of laser radiation on some immunological traits. *Neoplasma* 1982;29:403–406.

63. Nussbaum EL, Lilge L, Mazzulli T. Effects of 630-, 660-, and 905-nm laser irradiation delivering radiant exposure of 1–50 J/cm^2 on three species of bacteria in vivo. *J Clin Laser Med Surg*. 2002;20(6):325–333.

64. Young S, Bolton P, Dyson M, et al. Macrophage responsiveness to light therapy. *Laser Surg Med*. 1989;9:497–505.

65. Mester E, Spiry T, Szende B, et al. Effect of laser rays on wound healing. *Am J Surg*. 1971;122:532–535.

66. Whelan HT, Smits RL, Buchman EV, et al. Effect of NASA light-emitting diode irradiation on wound healing. *J Clin Laser Med Surg*. 2001;19(6):305–314.

67. Reddy GK. Photobiological basis and clinical role of low-intensity lasers in biology and medicine. *J Clin Laser Med Surg*. 2004;22(2):141–150.

68. Calderhead RG. Watts a joule: on the importance of accurate and correct reporting of laser parameters in low-reactive-level laser therapy and photobioactivation research. *Laser Ther*. 1991;3(4):177–182.

69. Posten W, et al. Low-level laser therapy for wound healing: mechanism and efficacy. *Dermatol Surg*. 2005;31:334–340.

70. Schindl M, Kerschan K, Schindl A, et al. Induction of complete wound healing in recalcitrant ulcers by low-intensity laser irradiation depends on ulcer cause and size. *Photodermatol Photoimmunol Photomed*. 1999;15:18–21.

71. Mendez T, Pinheiro A, Pacheco M, et al. Dose and wavelength of laser light have influence on the repair of cutaneous wounds. *J Clin Laser Med Surg*. 2004;22(1):19–25.

72. DeSimone NA, Christiansen C, Dore D. Bactericidal effect of 0.95-mW helium-neon and 5-mW indium-gallium-aluminum-phosphate laser irradiation at exposure times of 30, 60, and 120 seconds on photosensitized *Staphylococcus aureus* and *Pseudomonas aeruginosa* in vitro. *Phys Ther*. 1999;79:8039–8846.

CHAPTER 26

Therapeutic and Diagnostic Ultrasound

Carrie Sussman and Mary Dyson

CHAPTER OBJECTIVES

At the completion of this chapter, the reader will be able to:

1. Discuss the terminology and properties of therapeutic and diagnostic ultrasound (US), explaining the significance of each.
2. Describe the equipment used to generate US, comparing and contrasting the essential features of the three classes of devices available.
3. Analyze the current evidence of the physical and physiologic effects of therapeutic US as they relate to wound healing.
4. Identify the therapeutic benefits of US in wound care.
5. Evaluate whether US treatment is appropriate based on the patient, the wound, and the evidence.
6. Explain recent advances in the use of high-resolution ultrasound (HRUS) to monitor the extent of soft tissue injury and repair.
7. Select the most appropriate therapeutic US device for the intended intervention and the most appropriate transmission medium to achieve the desired outcome.
8. Apply US treatment interventions, if appropriately trained to do so.

This chapter provides an introduction to the therapeutic and diagnostic use of ultrasound (US) in wound care. It provides you with the information you need about the physical properties and physiologic effects of ultrasound (US) that apply to wound healing. High-frequency and low-frequency applications are presented. In wound care, US can be used therapeutically to accelerate wound healing, debride tissue and diagnostically to assess the extent of soft tissue injuries and to monitor their repair in a quantitative manner. Each of these aspects will be presented and discussed.

Clinical studies in which US had been used for the healing of animals and humans are included. For therapeutic US, the therapist is provided with sufficient information to select the most appropriate method of US treatment for tissue repair in injuries of different etiologies and in different locations, as well as to clean and debride wounds. This chapter also describes recent advances in the use of high-resolution diagnostic US, which can be used to monitor the extent of soft tissue injury and its repair in a quantitative, objective manner.

As with other wound care intervention evidence of efficacy, there are no well-designed controlled clinical trials that have been conducted on the use of US in wound care. Thus, it is difficult to make definitive judgments about efficacy. However, several small, randomized trials have demonstrated the effectiveness of therapeutic US in the treatment of chronic leg ulcers, and the 2009 National Pressure Ulcer and European Pressure Ulcer Prevention and Treatment Guidelines said "consider low-frequency US (LFUS) as an adjunctive for debridement of necrotic soft tissue (not eschar) therapy (level of evidence C). Consider use of high-frequency US (HFUS) as an adjunct for the treatment of infected pressure ulcers (level of evidence C)."[1] A Cochrane Review reported in 2010 found that there is some weak evidence from what they called "poor-quality research" that ultrasound may increase the healing of venous leg ulcers.[2] However, the literature supporting US therapeutic efficacy for the treatment of pressure ulcers and human tissue repair in general is insufficient and inconclusive enough to not make a recommendation.[3] Further investigation with well-designed clinical trials is needed.

For now, the attention of the research community has shifted to the use of LFUS for wound debridement and bacteriacidal effects. HFUS for diagnostic purposes, specifically to determine the efficacy of wound-healing interventions and to diagnose the depth of tissue impairment, is another US application. These new applications of US show great promise, as we discuss later in this chapter.

TABLE 26.1	US Terminology
Term	**Definition**
Acoustic impedance	The acoustic impedance of a medium is the product of its density (p) and the velocity of US through it (c). The greater the difference in *acoustic impedance* (z) between the two materials forming the interface, the greater the amount of energy is reflected
AM	*AM* is defined as the movement of fluids along the acoustic boundaries (e.g., cell membranes) as a result of the mechanical pressure wave associated with the US beam.
Acoustic pressure	Beam of energy that advances as a pressure (acoustic) wave of energy.
Absorption	US beam is absorbed by tissues of different density depending on the frequency of the acoustic pressure wave
Attenuation	Loss of intensity and force of the acoustic pressure wave due to absorption
Beam	A stream of sound waves
Cavitation	Acoustic Cavitation involves the production and vibration of micron-sized gaseous bubbles within the coupling medium and fluids within the tissues by an US beam
Compression wave	The sound wave progression consists of compression and rarefaction of molecules of air
Continuous US	Continuous stream of sound energy, thermal and nonthermal effects; 100% duty cycle
Cycle	One cycle consists of one compression and one rarefaction
Duty cycle	Period sound beam is on and off per unit of time
Echogenic	Reflection of a sound wave. For example microbubbles have a high degree of echogenicity. When gas bubbles are caught in an ultrasonic frequency field, they compress, oscillate, and reflect a characteristic echo- this generates the strong and unique sonogram in contrast-enhanced US.
ERA	The area of transducer from which the radiating sound wave emanate. Always smaller than the size of the sound head
Far field (Fraunhofer zone)	The area at a given distance from the transducer head the sound wave diverges and where there is the most uniform distribution of the sound wave
Frequency	The number of compressions and rarefactions (or cycles) that occur per second (Hertz, Hz) based on the setting for the piezoelectric crystal to vibrate.
Half Value thickness	Depth of tissue at which the intensity of the US wave is ½ its initial intensity
High Frequency	A million or more cycles per second
Hyperechogenic	Higly reflective like reflection from the keratin layer of the epidermis or the interface between the epidermis and dermis are
Hypoechogenic	Fluid-containing spaces within the dermis and subcutaneous fat are hypoechogenic meaning that these spaces are hyporeflective and show up as black holes on the scans
Intensity	Power per unit area of the sound head expressed in Watts/centimeter squared (W/cm^2)
Intensity (Low)	The range is < 0.3 W/cm^2
Intensity (Medium)	The range is 0.3–1.2 W/cm^2
Intensity (High)	The range is >1.2–3.0 W/cm^2
Near Field (Fresnel zone)	Field generally within 10–30 cm of the sound head surface)
Period	The time it takes for one cycle to occur.
Piezoelectric crystal	Conversion of electrical energy into sound energy by use of a transducer, and visa versa
Phonophoresis/Sonophoresis	Transdermal drug delivery by driving the medication into the tissues with the US wave.
Pulsed US	The beam of US energy can be delivered in an interrupted stream by an on and off method called pulsing
Rarefaction	To make rare or thin as decreasing the density of air in a sound wave
Reflection	Reflection occurs at the interface between materials that differ in their acoustic properties, specifically in their acoustic impedance. Each reflection is termed an echo.
Stable Cavitation	*Stable cavitation* occurs when the bubbles in the field do not change much in size. The effect of stable cavitation can result in changes in diffusion of substances along across cell membranes

(continued)

TABLE 26.1	US Terminology (*continued*)
Term	**Definition**
Transducer	A device that converts one form of energy to another. Also a term for the sound head or applicator head.
US	Inaudible sound in the frequency above human hearing >20,000 cycles/s
Wavelength	The distance between beginning and end of a wave cycle

Mitragotri S, Kost J. Low-frequency sonophoresis: a review. *Adv Drug Deliv Rev.* 2004;56(5):589–601.

PROPERTIES AND TERMINOLOGY OF ULTRASOUND

Ultrasound is a type of sound generated when a mechanical vibration is transmitted at a frequency beyond the upper limit of human hearing.[4] Human hearing is from 16 to 20,000 cycles per second. Thus, US is sound that has a frequency greater than 20,000 cycles per second.[5] It causes the molecules of the media that can transmit it (e.g., biologic tissues) to oscillate or vibrate. Unlike electromagnetic waves of the electromagnetic spectrum (see Introduction to Part IV), such as visible light or electrical current, sound waves cannot travel through a vacuum. Sound requires a conductive medium to propagate the wave. Conductive media are discussed in the chapter's treatment section. When US is applied to the tissues, it is called **sonication.** The act is called sonation.

Like electrical stimulation (ES) and other biophysical agents, US has its own terminology and principles. Since they are important for the understanding of this technology, this chapter begins by introducing them. Table 26.1 provides a list of terms and definitions.

Instrumentation

Ultrasonic energy is produced when an electronic generator transforms AC line power to the US signal. The equipment used to produce therapeutic levels of US typically consists of a microcomputer-controlled high-frequency generator linked by a coaxial cable to an applicator (probe) or treatment head as shown in Figure 26.1. The treatment head contains a disc of a piezoelectric material, such as lead zirconate titanate, which acts as a transducer to change one form of energy into another. When an alternating voltage is applied across such a disc, the crystal expands and contracts at the same frequency as the oscillation, transducing and amplifying the electrical energy into a mechanical vibration/oscillation delivered through the applicator/handpiece, which is also called the transducer. The mechanical vibration frequency that causes the crystal to expand and contract is chosen either by the operator or by the manufacturer, creating a sound wave or beam of energy that advances as a pressure (acoustic) wave of energy. Transducers for kilohertz (kHz) devices are very narrow but transducers used with megahertz (MHz) are of varying widths, and the following information needs to be interpreted with those differences in mind. The terms kHz and MHz and acoustic pressure will be explained soon.

The region next to the applicator is termed the *near field*, or *Fresnel zone* (generally within 10 to 30 cm of the

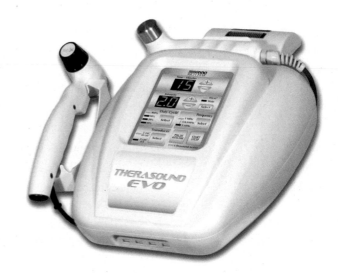

FIGURE 26.1 Therasound shows a typical US instrument panel. Note all the parameters which are described in this chapter section. (Used with permission from Richmar.)

sound head surface), and the energy distribution within it is extremely variable, meaning that the energy may vary from little or no intensity to very high peak intensities. Beyond this, the beam starts to diverge and the energy distribution within it becomes more regular. This region is termed the *far field*, or *Fraunhofer zone* (Fig. 26.2). The distance (d) from the transducer to the beginning of the far field is related to the radius (a) of the transducer and the wavelength (Δ) of the US: d = a²/Δ. Unless the body part to be treated is immersed in a water bath in which the transducer and target tissue can be separated by a distance sufficient for the target tissues to be in the far field, US therapy usually involves treatment of tissue in the nonuniform near field. The beam nonuniformity ratio (BNR) is a measure of this nonuniformity and is the ratio of the spatial peak intensity (I[SP]) to the spatial average intensity (I[SA]). These terms are defined in Table 26.1. For MHz transducers, BNR is listed on the equipment or in the equipment manual. Low BNRs have a more homogeneous beam pattern that give more predictable results and are safer than those with higher BNRs[6] (Fig. 26.2). Since the pressure wave intensity varies, across the surface of the applicator, as well as with the distance from it, the pressure changes experienced by the tissues being treated depend in part on their position relative to the size and shape of the transducer, on how it is mounted in the applicator, and on how it is delivered.

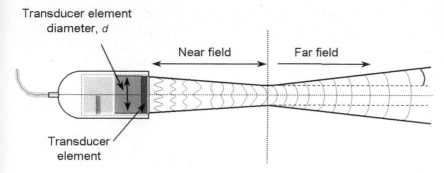

Transducer element
diameter, *d*

Near field   Far field

Transducer
element

FIGURE 26.2 Hour glass shaped US beam. Near field (zone) and far field (zone). The diameter of the beam is determined by both the frequency and the diameter of the element itself, also referred to as the aperture. The beam takes on a shape in the appearance of an hourglass. (Reprinted from Bushberg J. *The Essential Physics of Medical Imaging.* 2nd ed. Philadelphia, PA: Lippincott Williams & Wilkins; 2002:231, with permission.)

We list the properties to consider when selecting MHz US equipment in more detail later in this chapter. Similar sound systems are used for MHz and kilohertz (kHz) US, but the frequency of kHz vibration is much lower and the wavelength therefore longer.

Wavelength

The transducer produces a sound wave of specific wavelength. The *wavelength* is the shortest distance, measured parallel to the direction of wave propagation, between molecules that are at equivalent points of vibration in the repeated cycle of movement, which constitutes a wave (Fig. 26.3). The wavelength is related to the frequency (f) and *velocity* (c) of the wave by the equation: (= c/f). For example, the velocity of US in water, blood, interstitial fluid, and soft tissues is approximately 1,500 m/s.

An important principle in diagnostic US is that the shorter the wavelength, the greater the degree of resolution. Short wavelengths allow collagen fiber bundles and other components of intact and damaged soft connective tissues to be distinguished acoustically. Figure 26.4A,B shows use of diagnostic US to examine a wound as it is healing.

Frequency

The number of expansion and contraction cycles of the crystal per unit of time is usually expressed in terms of cycles per second or the frequency. This is the number of times per second that a molecule displaced by the US wave completes a cycle of movement (oscillation or vibration) and returns to its original position. The greater the number of oscillations or vibrations per unit of time, the more likely heating of tissues will

be produced as a byproduct. Frequencies are expressed in Hz, where 1 Hz = one cycle per second. The time taken to complete a cycle is termed a *period* (T). Devices with higher and lower frequencies are not inferior or superior in any general sense, but are simply appropriate for different treatment purposes. Many of the clinically relevant bioacoustic properties of US are related to its *frequency* (f) (Fig. 26.5). In the next section, we will consider high frequency (HFUS), MHz, followed by discussion of low frequency (LFUS), kHz.

High Frequency

HFUS is measured in Megahertz, or MHz, where 1 MHz = 1,000,000 cycles per second. It is also known as *short-wave US.* HFUS, typically between 0.5 and 3 MHz (i.e., between 0.5 and 3 million cycles per second), has been used for more than 40 years to stimulate healing, and for transdermal drug delivery. The higher the frequency, the shorter the wavelength and the shorter the wavelength, the greater the absorption. As mentioned, absorption, which is a major cause of attenuation (loss of intensity), is frequency dependent as are depth of penetration and quantity of energy delivered to a target tissue. At higher frequencies, more of the energy is absorbed by superficial structures than can penetrate into deeper structures. For example, the wavelength of a US beam at 3 MHz is shorter than at 1 MHz, and therefore absorption occurs more readily at the skin, reducing the half-value thickness by 3. In this example, the half-value thickness that the beam will penetrate would be 5/3 = 1.7 cm. Thus, US devices offering 3 MHz are widely used for wound healing when superficial. The higher the frequency, the more attenuation as the sound wave beam travels through tissue. For example, if 1 W per cm² of 1 MHz US (watt [W]

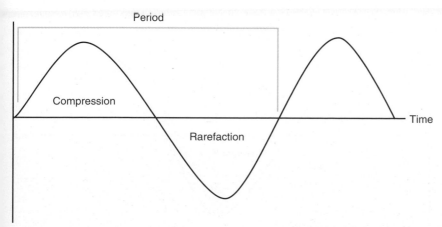

Period

Compression

Rarefaction

Time

FIGURE 26.3 Diagram of Period. Period is defined as the time it takes for one cycle to occur. One cycle consists of one compression and one rarefaction.

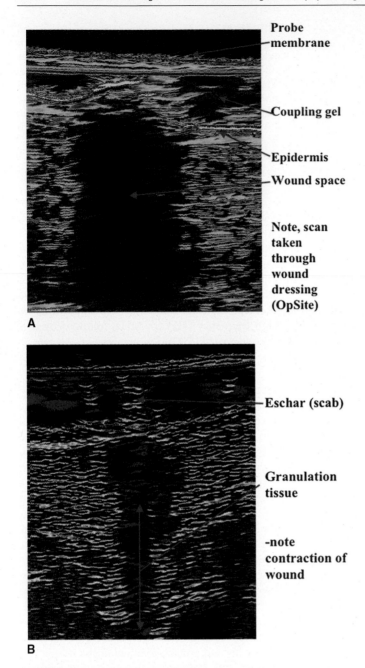

Probe
membrane

Coupling gel

Epidermis
Wound space

Note, scan
taken
through
wound
dressing
(OpSite)

A

Eschar (scab)

Granulation
tissue

-note
contraction of
wound

B

FIGURE 26.4 A. HRUS Scan of Punch Biopsy Wound day 3. (Copyright© P. Wilson, Longport, Inc.). **B.** HFUS Scan of Punch Biopsy Wound, day 14. (Copyright© P. Wilson, Longport, Inc.)

a unit of energy) is applied to the skin, at a depth of 5 cm, only 0.25 W per cm^2 of energy would be available. At lower frequencies, superficial tissue absorption is reduced and US energy penetrates more deeply. Thus, for decades, 1 MHz US was used for deep penetration into tissues such as injured muscle or bone or for treatment of deep wounds like stage IV pressure ulcers. Megahertz US is often used as direct contact application but may be noncontact when applied through water.

Diagnostic US uses the range of 20 to 50 MHz to image tissue. Current applications to wound healing include imaging tissue to identify its structures, and locating, diagnosing, and monitoring areas of tissue congestion and healing.

Low Frequency

LFUS is measured in kilohertz, typically between 20 and 50 kHz, and is also known as *long-wave US*. Kilohertz US, which has a long wave length, has less attenuation and absorption, and greater penetration of tissue. Attenuation and absorption are important elements that will be discussed in detail soon. Long-wave US, also called kHz, can penetrate skin, fat, and edematous tissues to reach a deeply located injury in, for example, a stage IV pressure ulcer that penetrates into muscle. Serena et al conducted experiments to assess noncontact 40 kHz LFUS penetration with the transducer head 0.5 to 1.5 cm from the wound bed. Experiments were conducted on full-thickness skin samples of Yorkshire pigs that were "wounded" by removal of superficial skin. The dye material used for this experiment, mixed with the saline solution in the canister used by the noncontact device, penetrated into the intact porcine skin 2.0 to 2.5 mm. In "wounded" samples, penetration was 3 to 3.5 mm. The penetration extended into the reticular dermis but not the underlying subcutaneous fat.[7] With kHz US, even bone and metal can be penetrated, with sufficient energy remaining to have an effect on deeper injured tissues. Devices exploiting kHz US are now used for wound care for bacteriacidal effects, debridement, and transdermal drug delivery. More about kHz US and applications will be presented in following chapter sections.

LFUS is used for both *contact* and *noncontact* delivery methods, which produce different outcomes.[8] Contact at low frequency appears to enhance fibrinolysis without visible destruction of adjacent granulation tissue and is transmitted at lower intensity. For example, LFUS at 25 kHz delivered at 0.25 to 0.75 W per cm^2 tends to produce stable bubbles associated

FIGURE 26.5 Diagram of Frequency. Frequency is defined as the number of cycles per second. (Used from Feigenbaum H. *Feigenbaum's Echocardiography.* 6th ed. Philadelphia, PA: Lippincott Williams & Wilkins; 2004, with permission.)

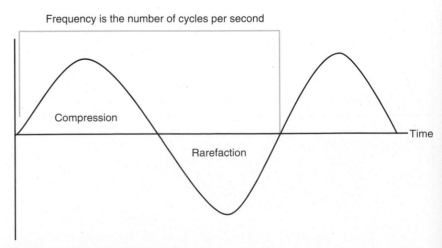

Frequency is the number of cycles per second

Compression

Rarefaction

Time

RESEARCH WISDOM

Analysis of an air sample following use of the noncontact US MIST Therapy System ™ (Celleration Corp, Eden Prairie, MN) showed no detectable production of aerosolized *Pseudomonas aeruginosa*. Protective clothing is therefore not required during treatment application.

with stable cavitation. Therefore, these devices are designed to be used for debridement of necrotic tissue and slough.[8]

When a noncontact application method is used and the transmission medium is a mist, the particles of the fluid are atomized or nebulized. The particles are projected with a high pressure wave that propels them through the air. When the pressure wave impacts tissue, cells there receive vibration that perturbates cell membranes and provides the mechanical stimulation that initiates intracellular signaling networks to produce chemical mediators as just discussed.[9] However, no clear evidence was located on a systematic review of the literature that the noncontact mist delivery method removes necrotic debris or necrotic tissue.[8] However, a retrospective review of 48 patients with 50 ulcers reported that the amount of healthy tissue in wound beds was 31% to 75% before noncontact LFUS mist delivered therapy and was 72% to 94% ($p = .02$) following.[10] A comparative randomized controlled trial would help to clarify this matter.

Frequency and Heat

Whenever US is absorbed, heat is produced. Kilohertz as well as MHz devices produce heat when used in the continuous mode. A medium intensity range of 1.0 to 2.0 W per cm² applied continuously for 5 to 10 minutes will elevate tissue temperatures to between 40°C and 45°C.[6] This is acceptable only in adequately vascularized tissues. Temperatures above this cause thermal *necrosis* and must be avoided. Thermal effects occur with both 1 and 3 MHz US when continuous wave US is applied, but at different tissue depths. As just discussed, at a frequency of 3 MHz, energy absorption occurs mainly in superficial tissues (1–2 cm beneath the surface). At a frequency of 1 MHz, less energy is absorbed by the superficial tissues, provided that there is adequate power output from the transducer. This frequency also penetrates into deeper tissues, with effective energy levels being available up to 5 cm below the surface. In contrast, therapeutic kHz US can be used in continuous mode without significant tissue heating and penetrates all the way through the body. Thermal effects are reduced by pulsing the wave, because this reduces the average intensity. Also, fluid is used in conjunction with the kHz US delivery not only for conduction but also to dissipate the heat produced during the application. For example, penetration of the acoustic wave was at least 1 mm below the surface on agar plate and the surface temperature of agar-plated sample decreased by 1.9°C with 60 mL solution application of MIST™.[11] While heating of tissue is mitigated, the tip of the applicator can become hot and should not directly touch the wound or be touched by the provider.

- If US increases the tissue temperature less than 1°C, this is not considered to be physiologically relevant; in such

circumstances, therapeutic effects are due primarily to non-thermal (not athermal) mechanisms. No addition of energy can be athermal.

- Because many wounds occur in ischemic tissues, care must be used when applying thermal US in the presence of arterial occlusive disease. In these areas, there is reduced ability to dissipate heat, and burns can result. US is contraindicated in the presence of arterial occlusion. However, nonthermal, pulsed US at low-intensity application has no reported adverse effects over areas of impaired circulation.

Continuous and Pulsed US Waves

The beam of US energy can be delivered in a continuous stream or it can be interrupted and delivered by an on and off method called pulsing. Continuous US is used where thermal effects are indicated. Pulsing the US wave changes the average intensity and reduces the thermal effects because the acoustic energy is only applied for a portion of the treatment time. A benefit of pulsing the beam during delivery is that it allows for heat dissipation to occur and thus thermal effects are minimized. If there is ischemia or occlusion, heat dissipation is reduced and this is a precaution when using US. For wound healing, the pulsed mode is employed for HFUS.

The period that the sound beam is on is called the *duty cycle*. For continuous US, the duty cycle is 100%. Pulsed beam duty cycle can be on for a percentage of time and off for the rest of the time (Fig. 26.6). A typical duty cycle is 20%. This signifies that the beam is streaming for 20% of the treatment time and off for 80% of the treatment time. Pulsing the US wave changes the average intensity and reduces the thermal effects because the acoustic energy is only applied for a portion of the treatment time.

Intensity

Intensity (I) is the amount of energy (in W) per unit area per unit time (W/cm²/× minutes) delivered by the transducer to the target. Treatment application parameters are based on intensity reported in W per cm². Therapeutic applications generally operate in an intensity range from 0.1 to 2.0 W per cm², with the safe upper limit having been established by the World Health Organization at 3.0 W per cm². Intensities over 3.0 W per cm² are used in surgical applications as ultrasonic scalpels and in tissue emulsification applications.

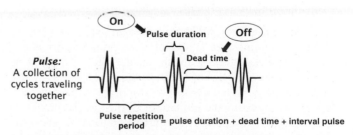

FIGURE 26.6 Duty Cycle. Comparison between pulse duration, duty cycle, and pulse repetition period. US energy is usually emitted from the transducer in a series of pulses, each one representing a collection of cycles. Each pulse has a duration and is separated from the next pulse by the interpulse interval (dead time).

FIGURE 26.7 Diagram indicating that amplitude and frequency are independent of each other. **A.** Two waves of identical frequency and different amplitudes.

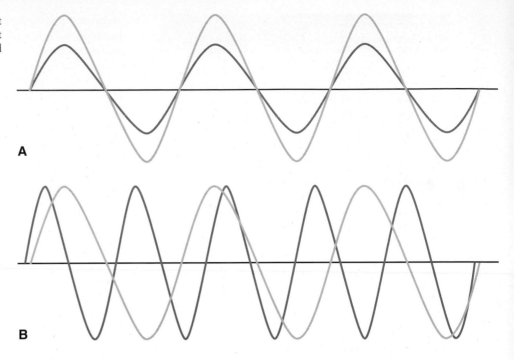

A

B

The movement of a device's piezoelectric crystal up and down is called its amplitude or intensity[12] (Fig. 26.7). Intensity is altered in different ways for different purposes including by choice of applicator, amplitude, power, treatment application methods, and intended use. The amplitude is adjusted by choosing the amount of power per unit area on the device instrument panel. By choosing a device with a low BNR, the amplitude will be more evenly delivered.[5]

The intensity can be averaged in space over the face of the applicator (termed *spatial average* [*SA*]) or in time (termed *temporal average* [*TA*]). *Spatial average temporal peak* (SATP) intensity is the SA peak intensity of the US during the time that the *pulse is on*. The type of intensity should be specified as either I(SATA), if continuous, or both I(SATA) and I(SAPA), if pulsed. This parameter is displayed on the instrument panel of US units. The SATP is often reported in research papers as is the *spatial average, temporal average* (SATA) intensity. Information provided about the SATA is useful in comparing US dosages reported in studies (Fig. 26.8).

Table 26.1 summarizes MHz US intensity terminology and gives examples.[5]

The following list is presented for additional guidance.

- Applicators used for MHz transmission typically have an effective radiating area (ERA) of a few square centimeters. Kilohertz devices have a much smaller ERA. The ERA is always less than the size of the transducer surface, so the size of the transducer is not a true indicator of the actual radiating surface. Recognizing the limitations of the ERA is significant because time and application must be adjusted to allow for this. For instance, one reason for moving the US transducer head in overlapping circles or bands is to make sure that the entire area of treatment receives adequate dosage of energy (see Fig. 26.9A,B).
- There is a direct relationship between amplitude and intensity, so that at low control settings there will be low amplitudes

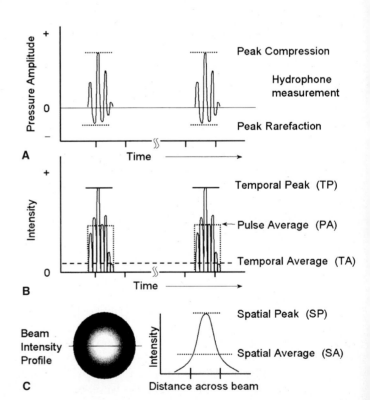

FIGURE 26.8 Intensities (Temporal and Spatial). **A.** Pressure amplitude variations are measured with a hydrophone and include peak compression and rarefaction variations with time. **B.** Temporal intensity variations of pulsed US vary widely, from temporal peak and TA values; pulse average intensity represents the average intensity measured over the pulse duration. **C.** Spatial intensity variations of pulsed US are described by the spatial peak value and the SA value, measured over the US. (Reprinted from Feigenbaum H. *Feigenbaum's Echocardiography*. 6th ed. Philadelphia, PA: Lippincott Williams & Wilkins; 2004, with permission.)

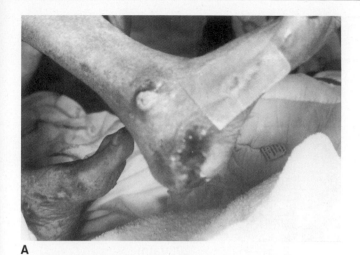

A

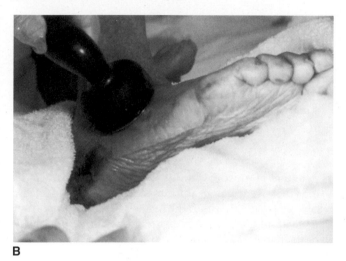

B

FIGURE 26.9 **A,B.** Application of MHz US through a hydroscan.

and low-intensity sonication. To achieve the desired intensity for a particular therapeutic application, the output control setting is critical.

- Variable power, the amount of energy per unit of time expressed in Watts (W) has a variable relationship with amplitude and intensity. At a low control setting, the device will have a low wattage reading if it is sonicating water, but if it is sonicating viscose tissue then at the same setting there will be a higher wattage reading because of the resistance of the tissues to the flow of the sound beam. The amplitude and intensity will be the same, but the power needed to drive the crystal to produce the same intensity and amplitude is greater.

Acoustic Pressure: Cavitation and Microstreaming

Acoustic cavitation is also known as the *acoustic pressure wave*. It has been suggested that stable *acoustic cavitation* and *acoustic microstreaming* (*AM*) are responsible for the cellular stimulatory effects of low-intensity US. These two physical properties of US, *acoustic cavitation* and *AM*, occur at a low SA intensity. These mechanisms act as a stimulus that reversibly modifies plasma membrane permeability and modulates cellular activity. In this section, you will learn about how they are achieved and their functions (Fig. 26.10).

Acoustic Cavitation

Acoustic cavitation involves the production and vibration of micron-sized gaseous bubbles within the coupling medium and fluids within the tissues. Sound travels in waves that transmit energy by alternate compression and rarefaction of the transmission material, in this case gaseous bubbles. Thus, the US beam affects small gaseous bubbles that move within the tissue fluids. As the bubbles collect and condense, they are compressed before moving on to the next area. The action of compression in one area causes a reduction of bubbles in the adjacent areas behind and in front of the wave. These are called the areas of *rarefaction*. This sequential movement of the bubbles along a path is the *acoustic pressure wave*. It is the movement and compression of the bubbles that can cause changes in the cellular activities of the tissues subjected to US. In cells treated in suspension, the suppression of cavitation also suppresses the stimulation of cellular activity. *Stable cavitation* occurs when the bubbles in the field do not change much in size. The effect of stable cavitation can result in changes in diffusion of substances along across cell membranes, thereby altering cell function and, therefore, this property is beneficial because of its ability to initiate cellular changes within the tissues. *Unstable* or *transient cavitation* refers to the collapse of these bubbles. Transient bubbles implode, causing local mechanical damage and free radical formation. This is potentially very hazardous. It occurs at high intensities, particularly when the sound head is not moved during treatment and standing waves, waves that do not move, develop. Unstable cavitation and standing wave formation are potentially damaging, but are easily avoided by using low intensities and keeping the applicator moving during treatment.

Acoustic Microstreaming

AM is defined as the movement of fluids along the acoustic boundaries (e.g., bubbles or cell membranes) as a result of the mechanical pressure wave associated with the US beam.[6] The ultrasonic stimulus is perceived by the cells and transduced by them; an amplified response then occurs of a type that varies according to the cell type involved. Cells close to

---

CLINICAL WISDOM

Clarification about Use of the Term Acoustic Pressure

Because the process of acoustic streaming creates a pressure wave, some studies in the literature refer to LFUS as "Acoustic Pressure Therapy." This came about when, for a period of time, "Acoustic Pressure" was a company attempt to use this as the generic term for noncontact LFUS MIST Therapy System™, (Celleration, Inc. Eden Prairie, MN). Studies reported under that title were supported by educational grants from this company that undeniably suggest a potential for bias when a manufacturer of a technology funds studies of that technology.[10,13–18] In another attempt at a generic term, the company has decided to change the term for the therapy to noncontact low-frequency ultrasound. Therefore, be aware of these caveats when you search for evidence about LFUS therapy for wounds and burns.

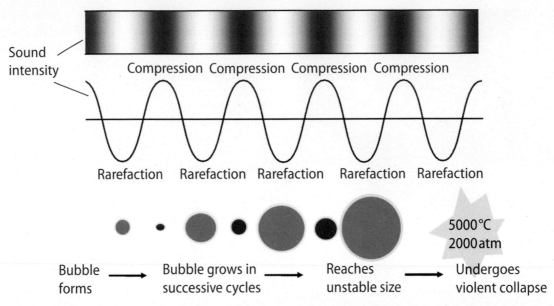

FIGURE 26.10 US Compression, Rarefaction, and Cavitation diagram. Like any sound wave US is transmitted via waves which alternately compress and stretch the molecular structure of the medium through which they pass. During each "stretching" phase (rarefaction), provided that the negative pressure is strong enough to overcome intermolecular binding forces, a fluid medium can be torn apart producing tiny cavities (microbubbles). (T.J. Mason, Educ. Chem., 2009, 46(5). Reproduced by permission of The Royal Society of Chemistry.)

stable bubbles are subject to bubble-associated microstreaming, which increases their plasma membrane permeability to calcium ions, temporarily acting as a stimulus to cell activity (e.g., cell migration, proliferation, synthesis of intracellular and extracellular materials) and the synthesis and release of growth factors by macrophages.[8,9] There is also increased endothelial nitric oxide (NO) synthesis and production of NO synthase, an enzymatic precursor of NO.[8] NO reduces vasoconstriction and allows increased blood flow to the tissues. More on blood flow effects is coming soon. More information about NO is found in Chapter 2.

Absorption and Attenuation

When US is transmitted through tissue, its intensity gradually decreases the deeper it travels as a result of absorption, scattering, and reflection. Absorption is a major cause of attenuation (loss of intensity). The amount of absorption varies with the composition of the tissues, as well as with the wavelength. During absorption, the mechanical energy of US is converted into heat. Tissues with the highest collagen content have highest absorption and are most likely to be heated.[5] Bone is more absorptive than highly proteinaceous tissues (e.g., dermis and muscle), protein is more absorptive than fat (e.g., adipose tissue), and fat is more absorptive than water-rich materials (e.g., plasma, edematous tissues). Attenuation refers to a reduction in the force of an US wave as the energy is absorbed into, scattered, or reflected by the tissues. Absorption, a primary cause of attenuation, is frequency dependent. Frequency discussion follows soon.

The thickness of tissue necessary for the intensity to be reduced by one half is termed the *half-value thickness*. The half-value thickness is the depth of tissue at which the intensity of the US is half its initial intensity. For instance, half-value of bone is

less than that of muscle, which is less than that of fat, which is less than that of edematous soft connective tissue.[5] The intensity available at any depth within the tissue is inversely proportional to the depth of penetration (i.e., the greater the depth, the less will be the remaining available intensity).

The acoustic impedance of a medium is the product of its density (p) and the velocity of US through it (c). The greater the difference in *acoustic impedance* (z) between the two materials forming the interface, the greater the amount of energy reflected. Reflection occurs at the interface between tissues. With MHz US, only a 0.2% reflection occurs at the interface between soft tissue and water, more than 50% between soft tissue and bone, and virtually complete reflection (99.9%) between soft tissue and air. Therefore, a transmission medium such as a gel or water is needed to conduct the sound energy into the body. Reflection reduces the amount of energy reaching the target tissues; if this falls below the stimulatory threshold (~0.1 W per cm² I [SATA]), US will be ineffective. Reflection concepts are discussed further under the section on high-resolution diagnostic US.

CLINICAL WISDOM

Move the Transducer Head

When there is reflection back into the soft tissues from bone, there is concentration of thermal energy at that interface. Thus, reflection at the interface between soft tissue and bone is a hazard that must be avoided by moving the transducer head continuously so as not to overheat one specific area.

PHYSIOLOGIC EFFECTS OF ULTRASOUND

Throughout this text, we have discussed the biological cascade of healing and how it is influenced by different endogenous and exogenous factors. This section begins by examining the effects of exogenously applied US on the four phases of wound healing. From the basic science research we learn that all phases of healing—inflammatory, proliferative, epithelialization, and remodeling—are impacted by this energy. Each phase is now examined for effects.

Inflammatory Phase

As you will recall, in normal wounding, the acute inflammatory state occurs following an initial clotting response that initiates a vascular response involving vasodilatation and invasion of the area by a large number of white blood cells that release the growth factors necessary to initiate repair. (See Chapter 2 regarding the physiology of wound healing.) These white blood cells include macrophages, polymorphonuclear leukocytes, and mast cells. The mast cells degranulate, releasing histamine hyaluronic acid and other proteoglycans that bind with the watery wound fluid to create a gel. Coagulated wound gel will later be replaced by a dense, binding scar. The inflammatory phase is a critical period of repair. US delivered during this time stimulates the release of growth factors from platelets, macrophages, and enhances degranulation of mast cells which, in turn, are chemotactic to the fibroblasts and endothelial cells that later form collagen-containing vascular granulation tissue. Early intervention with US accelerates the inflammatory phase, leading to more rapid entry into the proliferative phase of repair. It is not antiinflammatory and therefore should begin as soon as possible, during the acute inflammatory phase.[19–21] The influence of US on endothelial cells will be discussed soon under effects on circulation. Hart demonstrated that treatment with low-intensity nonthermal US in the early inflammatory phase influenced a positive outcome of scar collagen density and organization.[22] Later treatment is less effective.

Proliferative Phase

In the proliferative phase, US stimulates fibroblast migration and proliferation[19] reports that fibroblasts exposed to therapeutic levels of US in vivo were stimulated to synthesize more of the type of collagen that gives soft connective tissue its tensile

---

CLINICAL WISDOM

Use US to Restart the Inflammatory Phase

- Use US as soon as possible after injury to accelerate the inflammatory phase, leading to more rapid entry into the proliferative phase of repair.
- Use US to restart the inflammatory phase in chronic wounds. A single thermal treatment with US has been shown to induce the inflammatory phase in chronic diabetic foot ulcer and pressure wounds within 2 to 3 days. The protocol used involved 1 MHz, 0.5 W per cm^2 (SATP), 20% duty cycle, applied daily for 5 minutes to periwound area.[23]

---

strength. Endothelial cells, responsible for vascularization of the granulation tissue, are also affected by US at this stage to produce vascular endothelial growth factor and angiogenesis.[24] Under histologic examination, more angiogenesis is seen in granulation tissue that has been sonated at 0.75 MHz and 0.1 W per cm^2 than in untreated tissue.[19–21] There is a dose response outcome of treating human fibroblasts with 2:8 duty cycle of 1 MHz US at more than 1 W per cm^2. With the dose and intensities held constant, cells were treated for 30, 60, or 90 seconds. There was a control group (CG) of cells that received no sonation. Results showed that live cell counts diminished after a 30-second treatment and longer treatments of 60 and 90 seconds killed most of the fibroblasts after sonication.[25] Perhaps this report of fibroblast killing accounts for the insignificant effects on healing that are reported in clinical trials, reviewed here in a later section, where MHz US is used. In contrast, Emsen found that there was enhanced collagen formation and angiogenesis, functions of fibroblasts, after 5 minutes per day of LFUS at 0.1 W per cm^2 SATA.[26]

During the late phase of proliferation, the wound contracts. During this process, the wound is pulled together by the centripetal movement of the surrounding tissue. This results in less scar tissue formation. Fibroblasts transform into specialized contractile cells called *myofibroblasts*, which at this phase resemble smooth muscle cells. In some experiments, smooth muscle cells are reported to contract when treated with therapeutic levels of US. It has been postulated that myofibroblasts may be similarly affected. US, applied during the inflammatory and early proliferative phases, may accelerate wound contraction both by causing those cells to develop earlier and by increasing their efficiency. At this time, however, the mechanisms by which this occurs are not fully understood. Dyson states that no reports have been found of excessive pathologic contraction (contracture) following treatment with therapeutic US.[19,21] Intervention with low-intensity, nonthermal US within 72 hours following injury can therefore be used to promote wound contraction, which results in a reduction in size of the resulting scar.[22]

Epithelialization Phase

In the early hours after injury, epithelial cells begin migration and reproduction to restore the skin integrity and to protect the body from infection or admission of foreign substances. US stimulates the release of growth factors necessary for the regeneration of epithelial cells. US, therefore, appears to stimulate epithelialization and hasten it, by application to the periwound areas

Remodeling/Maturation Phase

Remodeling/maturation phase is affected by low-intensity US *only if* treatment is commenced in the inflammatory phase. If so, the effects are more rapid entry into the remodeling phase, increased wound tensile strength, increased capacity to absorb energy without mechanical damage, increased elasticity, and deposition of collagen fibers in a pattern closer to that of intact tissue. Several researchers have reported that application of thermal US during the remodeling phase mechanically affects collagen extensibility and organization as well as enzyme activity. Frieder et al.[27] reported improved collagen organization and Jackson et al.[28] reported improved tensile strength in the tendon repairs of US-treated animals. Emsen[26] reported that skin flaps treated with LFUS 5 to 10 minutes per day at 0.05 W per cm^2 SATA for 14 days had improved tensile strength compared to controls who were not sonicated.

Effects on Circulation

In this section, we will consider the effects of US on circulation from several aspects including

- **Blood flow**
- Shear stress
- Endothelial cell dysfunction
- Ischemic reperfusion damage (I/R)
- Thrombolysis/fibrinolysis

Blood Flow

Transcutaneous partial pressure of oxygen (tcPO$_2$) can be measured before and after treatment as a method of monitoring changes in blood flow (see Chapter 6). Byl and Hopf[29] found that, following pulsed low-intensity (0.5 W/cm^2) 1 MHz US, little increase in tissue temperature or oxygen transport occurred unless the individual was both well hydrated (three to four glasses of water), and receiving supplemental oxygen by nasal cannula. Well-hydrated subjects receiving supplemental oxygen had an increase in subcutaneous oxygen four times greater than that measured when breathing room air. Thermal application with HFUS, [(1.0 W/cm^2)(1 MHz)], produced vasodilatation and raised tissue oxygen levels and temperature significantly. Care must be taken to avoid excessive thermal effects whereby circulation is diminished and heat cannot be dissipated rapidly.[29]

In the body, blood flow provides constant vascular shear stress to vascular endothelial cells as it moves through the vessels. Shear stress depends on blood flow and also on blood and plasma viscosity, and membrane fluidity.[30] Vascular shear stress controls vascular tone, vessel wall remodeling, binding of circulating blood cells due to enhanced endothelial cell activation, production of NO and of autocrine, and paracrine vasoactive factors.[30] In some individuals, like diabetics, there are dysfunctional endothelial cell and US appears to have significant treatment potential for regulating this function that would benefit patients.

Ischemia reperfusion

(I/R) damage is characterized by low shear stress due to vasoconstriction of the microcirculatory vessels and excessive formation of reactive oxygen species (ROS). Reperfusion after ischemia in effect damages the endothelial cells by exposing them to abnormal shear stress and excessive formation of ROS biochemical events occurs in vascular endothelial cells[30] (see Chapter 2 for information about I/R).

Following low-intensity pulsed US (LIPUS), there is increased diameter of arterioles and terminal arterioles and increased capillary perfusion during post ischemic reperfusion. The LIPUS enhances the tolerance to post ischemic reperfusion including enhanced thrombolysis of clots due to the microbubbles of cavitation generated in the pressure wave that normalize the vascular shear stress.[30] Thrombolysis and US discussion is forthcoming.

Full-thickness skin flap survival is also dependent on adequate vasodilation and blood flow. Ischemic necrosis is a

> **CLINICAL WISDOM**

Increasing Circulation with HFUS

Ischemic tissues surrounding a chronic wound that have not responded to other types of wound treatments may benefit from periwound HFUS. If the wound bed is clean, expect increased serosanguineous exudate from the wound base to appear in 3 to 5 days. If the wound has necrotic tissue, expect to see lysis of the necrotic tissue, increased periwound erythema, and raised temperature due to the increased circulation associated with a change to the acute inflammatory phase. If this does not occur, repeat the single higher intensity treatment and follow with lower intensity treatments. Parameters of treatment are 1.0 to 1.4 W per cm^2 (SATP), 1 or 3 MHz, and continuous 5- to 10-minute duration, depending on the size of the area. Reduce intensity to 0.5 W per cm^2 (SATP), pulsed 20%, applied three to five times per week after one treatment.[31]

common adverse event following flap surgery that results in poor survival rate of acute skin flaps. Ischemia may be caused by vasospasm or I/R. In an animal study, there were three groups of rats where[26] Group I received pulsed US at .75 to 3.0 MHz at intensity 0.1 W per cm^2 SATA, 20% duty cycle; Group II received the same parameters except increased intensity of 0.18 W per cm^2; and Group III controls did not receive US. At the end of the study, there was statistically significant improved flap survival for the US-treated groups (p groups II and III = .001). Recommendation was to treat the flaps 5 minutes per day for 15 postoperative days to prevent ischemic changes in flaps. No adverse effects were reported. Clinical trials of patients are needed to confirm these results.

Thrombolysis (Fibrinolysis) and Deep Tissue Injury

Thrombosis, fibrin-rich clot, affects different aspects of the circulatory system including vessels of the brain (ischemic stroke) and veins (deep vein thrombosis [CVT]). Research has been concentrated on using low- and high-frequency US for thrombolysis of ischemic stroke alone and in conjunction with clot busting drugs and on treatment of DVT.[32-34] One mechanism of action is the mechanical forces resulting from collapsing microbubbles associated with stable cavitation which appear to be sufficient to break the fibrin bonds in thrombi, inducing fragmentation—hence the use of the term fibrinolysis. At higher frequencies, more power is needed to produce cavitation and more power can damage tissue. The intensity of the collapsing force is diminished at greater than 1 MHz, and not produced at greater than 2.5 MHz.[34,35] Pulsed mid-kHz exposure is more effective for thrombolysis than continuous exposure. It minimizes the probability of heating and improves absorption and the penetration of the sound wave into the tissues.[36,37]

There is a correlation of thrombus ablation with US and the elasticity of the arterial wall. A clot's low level of elasticity contributes to the fragmentation effect of the US, but the high elasticity of arterial walls resists damaging effects if HFUS

CASE STUDY

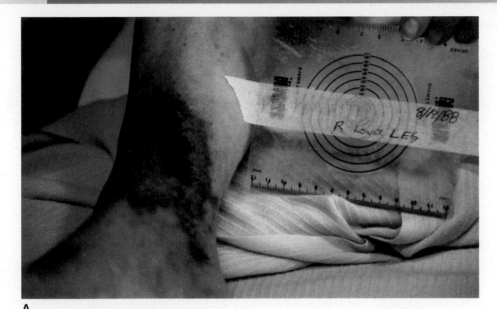

A

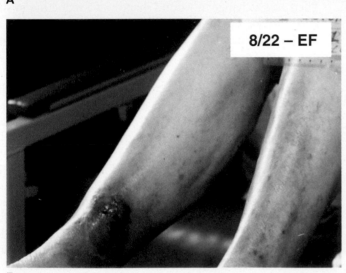

B

8/22 – EF

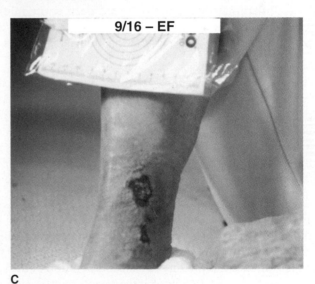

9/16 – EF

C

FIGURE 26.11 **A.** Wound is in acute inflammatory phase and shows subcutaneous hemorrhage (ecchymosis) associated with venous disease. (Copyright © C. Sussman.) **B.** Same wound as in (A), 4 days after two treatments with 1 MHz US. No other treatment provided including dressings and compression. Note absorption of the ecchymosis seen in earlier photo. There is partial-thickness skin loss. The wound is in acute inflammatory phase. (Copyright © C. Sussman.) **C.** Same wound as in (A) and (B), 4 weeks after start of US. Note wound contraction compared with that in (B). There are soft, irregular wound edges and new epitheliazation. The wound is in epithelialization phase. (Copyright © C. Sussman.)

Venous Ulcer Treated with US

Patient: E.F. Age: 82 years

Functional Outcome Report: Initial Assessment

Reason for Referral
The patient was referred to physical therapy for evaluation of ulceration of her left leg. The patient had a long history of Alzheimer disease and was noncompliant with all attempts to keep the wound dressed. Nurses in the nursing home where she lived were concerned about infection and healing of the ulcer and wanted a physical therapist's opinion.

Medical History
The patient had a cardiac pacemaker and venous insufficiency. As a consequence of neurologic system changes associated with Alzheimer disease, she was hyperactive and would not stay still for more than a couple of minutes at a time. Wound onset was 24 hours prior to referral.

Functional Diagnosis and Targeted Outcomes
Wound Examination

The wound is located above the left medial malleus. The surrounding skin is very friable, with extensive subcutaneous extravasation of blood (hemorrhaging) and epidermal necrosis; petechiae surround the open area. There is mild edema, which is reactive to touching. The wound tissue is pink, with partial-thickness loss of the skin surface area (Fig. 26.11A).

Functional Diagnosis

Impairment of the integumentary system; targeted outcome: wound closure; due date: 4 weeks.

Functional Diagnosis

Impairment of the venous system (venous insufficiency); targeted outcome: absorption of hematoma; due date: 2 weeks.

Functional Diagnosis

Acute inflammatory phase; suspected deep tissue injury, targeted outcome: thrombolysis of extravasated blood, tissue salvage, rapid wound contraction; due date: 4 weeks.

Psychosocial Examination

The patient had advanced Alzheimer dementia, thus she removed dressings and would not tolerate any topical medications, compression stockings, or staying off her feet. She walked all day long and was very accomplished at removing passive restraints in a flash. This was her second wound on her legs and nursing reported total noncompliance during the last episode of wounding due to mental status.

Functional Diagnosis

Impairment of mental functions. The functional loss causes her to be unaccepting of treatment interventions and yet she has undue susceptibility to venous ulceration of the legs and inability to heal without integumentary intervention. The patient has improvement potential and will heal after intervention, but she will continue to be at risk for venous ulceration.

Need for Skilled Services: The Therapy Problem

The patient has a history of recurrent ulceration above the left medial malleolus and impaired healing due to impairment of the venous system and impaired mental status. US is indicated during the first 72 hours after injury during acute inflammation. US would promote absorption of the hemorrhagic material and stimulate acceleration of the inflammatory phase, leading to rapid wound contraction.

Treatment Plan

Periwound US will be applied at 1 MHz, at 0.5 W per cm^2 (SATP), 20% pulsed for 5 minutes five times per week for 4 weeks. The nurses will attempt to do a wound dressing with a transparent film as tolerated.

Discharge Outcomes

Thrombolyis, absorption of hemorrhagic material within 3 days. Thrombolysis continued until all blood was absorbed. There was a change in wound shape and a reduction in size after 2 weeks. There was an 85% reduction in wound size at 4 weeks (see Fig. 26.11A–C for a pictorial review of the case).

Discussion

Behavioral information as well as medical history were important considerations in choosing the intervention. From all perspectives, US was the most practical choice for this patient because of the short duration of the nonpainful treatment (5 minutes), her short attention span, and intolerance of being handled. Electrotherapies were contraindicated due to her cardiac pacemaker. Because of her nonacceptance of any other treatment, it was also an opportunity to evaluate the effects of the HFUS. The absorption of the hemorrhagic material was unquestionable. The patient required constant engagement and diversionary activities by a physical therapy aide to tolerate the US by the physical therapist for even 5 minutes. By the end of 4 weeks, she refused to accept further treatment. Since the wound was closing, physical therapy was discontinued. On follow-up, it healed completely.

---

is used. This is a key factor in the safety of US thrombolysis.[35] Investigations of the effect of combining US with pharmacologic thrombolytic agents (e.g., tissue plasminogen activator or streptokinase) for enhanced thrombolysis report that there appears to be a synergistic effect on thrombus disruption that is not seen when US is used alone.[32–34,37,38] US has been described as increasing dispersal of the hemorrhagic material associated with bruising.[39] In patients with wounds like pressure ulcers, often the initial insult is a deep tissue injury with extraversion of blood, followed by coagulation, hematoma, and later by necrosis.[40] Initially, this looks like a hematoma or bruise or purple pressure ulcer (see Chapters 3 and 9). With the extensive use of anticoagulation and antiplatelet therapies, incidence rates of suspected deep tissue injury due to hematoma and thrombosis are likely to rise.

The onset of venous ulceration is often preceded by subcutaneous bleeding. Figure 26.11A–C shows a case example, at baseline 24 hours after onset of subcutaneous hemorrhage and the results of pulsed US, 1 MHz, at low-intensity treatment first 4 days post start of treatment and outcome over a 4-week course of care. Note the pronounced evidence of fibrinolysis following US treatment of the hemorrhagic area. These were closed wounds, initially. By the time the skin sloughed off, the area of involvement was significantly reduced, and the open ulcers went on to heal in a timely sequence, which is not common (see Case Study at end of chapter).

Intervention with US appears to have been efficacious in resolution of a rectus sheath hematoma.[41] A patient receiving oral anticoagulant therapy developed a large hematoma of the rectus sheath, confirmed with sonography and CT scan. The hematoma was stabilized with pharmacological treatment. Since MHz US has the ability to increase blood flow (as described above), the physical therapy team believed that early intervention with US would pose a risk of new bleeding during the acute phase of the hematoma. Therefore, US application was delayed until the hematoma showed a predominantly hypoechoic image (see Table 26.1) on sonogram due to pathologic change in tissue density, and coagulation parameters were within the correct range. This status was achieved 9 days after onset. Pulsed 1 MHz US at 1.5 to 2 W per cm² was subsequently applied around the hematoma 5 days a week for 4 weeks (20 sessions). By the end of one week pain was negligible, and by the end of 2 weeks the hematoma was reduced 50% in size. By the end of 4 weeks it was barely palpable, and a follow-up sonogram 2 weeks later showed that the hematoma had been resolved.

In all of these examples, the physical therapists used clinical reasoning based on their unique training and knowledge about the effect of US to safely and effectively treat the hematoma problems presented. The hypothesis that exogenous application of US to the adjacent skin can promote absorption and resolution of hematoma (deep tissue injury) or venous leakage needs further validation.

Figure 26.11A shows subcutaneous extravasation of blood secondary to venous insufficiency in the lower leg. Figure 26.11B shows the same area of the leg after 4 days and two treatments with MHz US.

Edema

Enhanced blood flow creates greater capillary pressure and fluid shift into the interstitial tissues, and the result is edema. Acoustic streaming may affect vascular permeability and help to control periwound edema. Edema-free outcomes are highly desirable because they accelerate and decrease the duration of the inflammatory process.[4,6,12,36,42]

CLINICAL WISDOM

HFUS for Skin Tears

Skin tears are a common problem for the elderly. They are often painful and surrounded with edema and ecchymosis. Application of nonthermal US with a conductive gel or lotion over a hydrogel transmission sheet or a transparent film dressing produces a reduction in pain and edema after one or two treatments, and dispersal and absorption of the ecchymosis within 6 to 10 sessions, depending on the size of the area involved. This method allows the dressing to remain in place between treatments, and will not disrupt the wound or cause skin damage. As healing progresses, expect the patient's mobility to increase. The protocol used involves 1 MHz, 0.5 W per cm² (SATP), 20% duty cycle, applied daily for 5 minutes to the periwound area.

INFECTION AND BACTERICIDAL EFFECTS

Bacterial infection is a common barrier to wound healing. Biophysical methods of bacterial reduction with interventions like US appear to be useful in the treatment of resistant organisms and biofilms. The bactericidal effects of US appear to occur on several levels: tissue level, cellular level, bacterial cell level, and chemical level. Effects at each of these levels are discussed in this section.

Tissue Level

On the tissue level, ultrasonic debridement has been shown to remove bacterial contamination.[7,43–45] In a retrospective study of heterogeneous patients with clinical signs of infected wounds there was significant improvement with treatment with LFUS ($p = .01$).[13] In another retrospective study of a heterogeneous group of patients, five infected wounds, 3/5 with methicillin-resistant *Staphylococcus aureus* (MRSA), were treated with systemic antibiotics and LFUS and all were infection free by the end of the course of care.[10] Healing is speeded by debriding the bioburden of necrotic tissue in leg ulcers with 25 kHz US.[46] Perhaps the effects were due to the reduction of bioburden through destruction of the bacteria and debridement of necrotic tissue by the LFUS treatment that turned these nonhealing wounds into healers.

Another retrospective study looked at using a combination regimen of LFUS and high voltage pulsed current (see Chapter 23) that reported faster closure of chronic leg ulcers than either alone. In two other studies, patients with postsurgical infected wounds including MRSA went on to heal or have significant reduction in wound volume after treatment with LFUS and negative pressure wound therapy.[14,15]

When two treatments are combined, teasing out the results of each is problematic. By looking at several studies here, there appears to be a trend developing that LFUS has a role in controlling bioburden and bacterial infection at the tissue level. These studies are small and of poor quality. Randomized controlled studies for single treatment interventions with LFUS as well as combining multiple interventions are needed.

Cellular Level

At the cellular level, US has been shown to modify plasma membrane permeability and transport properties.[7,47] For example, US enhances transport of systemic antibiotics like gentamicin through cell membranes.[48]

We have already discussed how US stimulates NO production and increases endothelial cell NO synthase activity.[49,50] NO kills pathogens when it reacts with peroxide oxygen ions, prevents replication of DNA viruses within cells, and serves as an immune regulator.[51]

Bacterial Cell Membranes and Biofilms

Killing effect is best when the frequency of the sound wave *decreases* and is reduced as the frequency increases.[48] Serena et al. conducted experiments to assess bacterial reduction in vitro and in vivo in an animal model after treatment with LFUS (40 kHz) mist. Bacteria quantified in the in vitro experiment were *P. aeruginosa*, *S. aureus*, MRSA, *Escherichia coli*, and *Enterococcus faecalis*, respectively.[7] They were then compared to sham treated samples. Treatment samples of dead bacteria were 33%, 40%, and 27% for *P. aeruginosa*, *E. Coli*, and *E. faecalis*, respectively. Using this treatment protocol, noncontact US at 40 kHz using mist delivery for 5 minutes had little or no effect on MRSA (1% increase live bacteria) and *S. aureus* (0% change). There were structural changes in *E. faecalis* indicating cell wall punctures or destruction. In a second experiment, this group examined effects of LFUS 40 kHz in pigs inoculated with *P. aeruginosa*, *Fusobacterium*, and Staphlococci into acute wounds. There was a comparison made with silver antimicrobial dressing and sham treatment. Each experimental wound was treated for 4 minutes per session with the applicator tip held 1 cm above the wound base every other day for 7 days. Between treatments wounds were treated with moistened Telfa gauze. Evaluation was made with punch biopsies. Histologically, there was no difference noted between the noncontact LFUS and sham treatment groups (TGs). Differences in overall bacteria counts in silver dressing group and LFUS group were minimal and due to small sample size not statistically analysed.[7]

Animal Clinical Studies

Animal studies allow investigation of different aspects of treatment effects. In this section, you will learn about some animal studies using US at different parameters exploiting its different properties to determine potential treatment benefits or adverse effects for patients with wounds. Properties that are discussed include the following.

Frequency

High Frequency—Low Intensity

a. **Heating**: High-frequency 5 MHz US was selected to determine whether there was a beneficial effects from US when applied daily for short periods to postsurgical incisional wounds.[52] Subjects were Fischer F344 male rats. The US frequency was chosen because less than 20% of the power would penetrate deeper than 1 cm below the surface of the skin, so that most of the US energy would be absorbed in the vicinity of the wound. The chosen intensity for a 5-minute exposure was 0.05 or 0.075 W per cm². Several experiments were performed at different thermal intensities (ranging from 0.05 to 0.15 W/cm²). Sonication was continuous. The extent of heat production by sonication and the effect on healing were the study variables.

Results:
1. Measurements at all intensities following 5 minutes of continuous sonication showed an increase in subcutaneous tissue temperatures that were progressively larger with higher intensities of sonication.[52]
2. At lower intensities (0.025 and 0.05 W/cm²), 10 minutes of sonication produced only a small additional elevation in subcutaneous tissue temperature, indicating that a plateau in temperature had been approached by 5 minutes.[52]
   b. **Effect on Proliferative Phase:** In the same study as above, treatment of the surgically induced incisional wounds began on the fourth postoperative day, when clips could be removed. The clips would have interfered

with the US beam, and, at that time, the wounds were entering the proliferative phase of healing. Expectation was that this was the optimal time to stimulate the fibroblasts to augment healing and improve the breaking strength of scars.

Results:
- The breaking strength of the sonicated wounds was equivalent but not greater than that of those treated by direct heating of the tissues.
- At the higher intensities (0.1 and 0.15 W/cm2), healing was impaired, and dermal burns occurred.[52]

In other studies, described below, treatment began within 24 hours of surgery; signs of healing were reported by the fourth postoperative day.

   c. **Histologic changes:** In another study of burn-induced wounds in rats, there was a CG and two groups of animals who were treated with pulsed (SATP 0.25 W/cm²) and continuous (0.3 W/cm²) US.[53]

Results: no stimulating effects were demonstrated in either US TG or against controls when evaluated by change in wound size and histologic examination. The investigators questioned the clinical benefit of treating burn wounds with US. There is no indication in the study report how soon after burn-induced wounding the US treatment commenced.

   d. **High frequency—High- and low-dose intensity:** There is a lack of consensus on the dosimetry for treatment with US. The purpose of this study was to learn more about dosage and wound healing. One property of healing is tensile or breaking strength of the healed wound. Thus, the tensile strength of wounds treated with different intensities, called *high-* and *low-dose US*, was tested by Byl et al.[54]

Method: Incisional wounds were made in the backs of miniature Yucatan pigs, and treatment was applied at different doses for different lengths of time. Forty-eight wounds were made, and the wounds were divided into three groups: 12 for control and 18 each for high-dose US and low-dose US. The groups were subdivided into two groups of 12 that received low dose or high dose for 5 days and two groups of six that received high dose or low dose for 10 days. All TGs received a frequency of 1 MHz for 5 minutes. The wounds were sonicated for approximately 1.25 minutes per cm of incisional length, beginning 24 hours after surgery. High-dose US was classified as 1.5 W per cm², continuous mode. Low-dose US was 0.5 W per cm², pulsed mode, 20% duty cycle. The wounds were covered with a moisture- and vapor-permeable adhesive dressing (Tegaderm, 3M Medical-Surgical Division, St. Paul, MN) that was left in place for up to 1 week. The dressing was found to permit transmission of US energy and could be left in place, avoiding disruption of the wound between treatment sessions.

Results:
1. Two variables were evaluated, the breaking strength of the incision, and the deposition of hydroxyproline, which is a measure of collagen deposition. The study found that the tensile strength for all TGs was significantly higher than that

of the controls, but there was no difference in hydroxyproline deposition.

2. A significant interaction was found between the number of days of treatment and the US dose. Hydroxyproline deposition was significantly higher and the breaking strength was higher for the low-dose group, compared with the high-dose group, after 10 days of treatment.

3. The study findings suggest that during the first week, either low- or high-dose US will enhance wound breaking strength but, to facilitate collagen deposition and wound strength, low-dose US should be used if treatment has to continue for 2 weeks or more.

4. A comparative study of the effect of US (0.1 W/cm² pulsed) MHz and ES (300 mA direct current, 30 min/d) on incisional wound healing in rats began within 2 hours of the surgical procedure.[55]

Results:

1. ES treatment allowed wounds to move to the proliferative phase earlier than in the US group, as indicated by the presence of more fibroblasts on the fourth day.

2. Although the density and arrangement of collagen was greater in the US group on the seventh day, the collagen was more regular in the ES group on the same day.

3. Breaking strength was higher in the US group than in the sham US group, but not as great as the ES group.

4. US affects the early phases of wound healing, but ES causes a beneficial effect on all phases.

5. US is more useful for the acute, uninfected, well-perfused wound, but ES is more useful for treatment of chronic or infected wounds, or wounds likely to be infected.[55] See Chapter 23 for more information about ES and wound healing.

REPORTED CLINICAL EFFECTS OF US

Reports in the literature attribute several clinical effects of US that pertain to the wound healing. In this section, we will review three of them including

1. Pain relief
2. Transdermal drug delivery
3. Wound debridement
4. Scar revision

Pain Relief

We know that pain prevention and/or relief is an essential part of wound healing. It has been theorized that the pain threshold can be raised with thermal application of therapeutic HFUS.[22] However, after careful systematic examination of the published reports, there is no conclusive evidence that pain is relieved by HFUS.[56]

There are reports in the literature that burns and wounds treated with LFUS have lower pain scores on visual analog scale (VAS). A retrospective chart review study of 14 burn patients found that pain resolved within 2 to 10 treatments of LFUS 40 kHz.[16] Another concurrent clinical study of six burn patients used the VAS to measure pain results. Patients reported no pain during the removal of fibrin, slough, and eschar and at end of study all patients reported no pain.[13] Haan and Lucich also did a retrospective chart review and found that the significance of the reduced pain levels was at $p < .0001$.[10] The delivery of LFUS mist method is also reported as not painful and therefore is well tolerated.[57]

Infection is often a contributing cause of pain. In a retrospective chart review, Gehling and Samies inclusion criteria excluded infection-related pain from their study.[58] Therefore, the 15 cases of nonhealing painful wounds examined had pain related to other causes (e.g., 10/15 were diabetics, 3/15 sickle cell). After 2 to 4 weeks of treatment with LFUS MIST, the mean pain scores decreased from 8.07 ± 1.91 to 1.67 ± 1.76 ($p < .0003$). All reported decreased pain from start of care and all reported using less narcotics for pain.

Transdermal Drug Delivery

High- and low-frequency US have been used successfully for many decades for enhanced transdermal drug delivery.[59] The current term used for this application of US is sonophoresis. The mechanism of action is enhanced diffusion through the structural layers of the stratum corneum. Pretreatment or co-treatment of skin with US of various frequencies almost completely eliminates the lag time typically associated with transdermal drug delivery, and is sustained after the US is turned off. Pretreatment of a short application of US enables permeation of the skin prior to the drug delivery, and the skin remains in this state of high permeability for several hours, so that drugs delivered by this method have sustained release. Current applications include sonophoresis of lidocaine, insulin, and macromolecular drugs.[59]

Wound Debridement

Surgeons have used ultrasonic dissection to surgically debride tissue for many years. Ultrasonic tools are now available for bedside and clinical debridement of contaminated soft tissue that may be used by nonphysicians. US is reported to be less traumatic to tissue than abrasive scrubbing, high-pressure jet irrigation, or sharp/surgical debridement.[36,43,44,60] US improves the outcome of bone debridement by maintaining the integrity of the directly involved bone trabecula, reducing contamination, preventing bacterial colonization, and decreasing possible infection.[43]

Technological advances have led to the development of several devices approved for wound debridement and cleansing by the Food and Drug Administration (FDA). These are the MIST Therapy System™ (Celleration, Eden Prairie, MN), Sonoca 18™ (Soring Inc. North Richland Hills, TX), and Sonic One™ (Misonix Inc. Farmingdale, NY) Qoustic Wound Therapy System™ (Arobella, Minnetonka, MN). See Table 26.2 for features of these different systems. These devices are pictured in Figures 26.12 to 26.15. All are LFUS, but the frequencies vary as do their delivery systems and their effects are not identical. MIST™ only functions as a noncontact system mist device and has been approved by the FDA for wound cleansing and debridement, and has an expanded indication for "promoting wound healing" since 2005.[4] Like other US devices, electrical energy in the MIST system is transmitted to a piezoelectric transducer where it is changed into mechanical energy. The transducer operates at 40 kHz. The transducer horn vibrates

TABLE 26.2 **Kilohertz Ultrasound Device Comparison**

Feature	Celleration MIST™ Therapy System 5.0	Arobella™	SÖRING/Sonoca™ 180	Misonix
Frequency	40 kHz	35 kHz	25 kHz	22.5 kHz
FDA 510k Clearance Indications	K032378/K050129 Indications for use: the MIST Therapy System produces a low energy US-generated mist used to promote wound healing through wound cleansing and maintenance debridement by the removal of yellow slough, fibrin, tissue exudates and bacteria.	Indications for use: uses ultrasonic energy combined with a 10 mm surgical curette for selective dissection and fragmentation of tissue, wound debridement with selective and excisional for acute and chronic wounds, burns, diseased and necrotic tissue using focused ultra sonic energy, and saline irrigation of the site for removal of debris, exudates, fragments, and other matter.	K012753 Indications for use: selective ultrasonic dissection and fragmentation of tissue at the operation site during multi medical discipline surgery including: general surgery, neuro, thoracic, urology, and gastrointestinal modalities http://www.fda.gov/cdrh/pdf/k012753.pdf	K050776 Indications for use: Fragmentation and aspiration of both soft and hard tissue in the following surgical specialties: neurosurgery, thoracic surgery, wound care, gastrointestinal surgery, urological surgery, general surgery, orthopedic surgery, plastic and reconstructive surgery, gynecology http://www.fda.gov/cdrh/pdf5/k050776.pdf
Surgical Procedure	No. Equivalent to stimulated autolytic debridement	NO. Equivalent to advanced sharp debridement	NO. Equivalent to advanced sharp debridement	NO. Equivalent to advanced sharp debridement
	Selective	Tissue emulsification	Tissue emulsification	Tissue emulsification
		Soft tissue sparing selectively removes non viable/necrotic tissue types with minimal damage to or removal of healthy/viable tissue types. May be more effective and accurate than sharp debridement. Can be used in an excisional manner.	Soft tissue sparing selectively removes non viable/necrotic tissue types with minimal damage to or removal of healthy/viable tissue types. May be more effective and accurate than sharp debridement.	Soft tissue sparing: selectively removes non viable/necrotic tissue types with minimal damage to or removal of healthy/viable tissue types. May be more effective and accurate than sharp debridement.
Clinician qualification	Physician, podiatrist, physical therapist, advanced practice nurse	Physician, podiatrist, physical therapist, advanced practice nurse, WOCN, WCC, CWS, PA, NP	Physician, podiatrist, physical therapist, advanced practice nurse	Physician, podiatrist, physical therapist, advanced practice nurse
	Licensing requirements for sharp debridement equivalency	Licensing requirements for sharp debridement equivalency	Licensing requirements for sharp debridement equivalency	Licensing requirements for sharp debridement equivalency
	Knowledge to appropriately use US	Training beyond needed for sharp debridement recommended	Training beyond needed for sharp debridement recommended	Training beyond needed for sharp debridement recommended
		Knowledge to appropriately use US	Knowledge to appropriately use US	Knowledge to appropriately use US
Intensity	Intensity (Therapeutic range) 0.1–0.5 W/cm^2	Adjustable treatment range: from 0.1 to 2.0 W/cm^2	Adjustable treatment range: from 0.1 to 2.0 W/cm^2	Adjustable Treatment range: from 0.1 to 2.0 W/cm^2

(continued)

TABLE 26.2	Kilohertz Ultrasound Device Comparison *(continued)*			

Feature	Celleration MIST™ Therapy System 5.0	Arobella™	SÖRING/Sonoca™ 180	Misonix
	Intensity(Maximum) 1.25 W/cm²	Less than 3 W/cm² Amplitude adjustment from 5–100. Can be combined with sharp skills.	Less than 3 W/cm²	Less than 3 W/cm².
	The intensity is preset not variable. The dose is calculated by size of wound and the device selects the treatment time based on wound size.		Amplitude adjustment from 20% to 100%.	Amplitude adjustment provided
	Intensities over 3.0 W/cm² are used in surgical applications as ultrasonic scalpels and in tissue emulsification applications		Higher intensity may be needed for thicker tissues e.g., necrotic tissues.	Higher intensity may be needed for thicker tissues e.g., necrotic tissues.
			Intensities over 3.0 W/cm² are used in surgical applications as ultrasonic scalpels and in tissue emulsification applications	Intensities over 3 W/cm² are used in surgical applications as ultrasonic scalpels and in tissue emulsification applications
Mode	Continuous	Continuous and pulsed	Continuous	Continuous and pulsed (50%–90% duty cycle choices)
Fluid dispensing	Disposable single use product specific sterile saline bottle.	No required disposable. Normal Saline and primary IV tubing set required.	Fluid dispensing	Fluid dispensing: Single use disposable required
			Preset and variable by practitioner	Increased amplitude allows the clinician to increase fluid output
			Suction equipment can be attached to control fluid	Suction equipment can be attached to control fluid
			Fluid selection by physician order	Fluid selection by physician order
Fluide delivery mode	Mist	1–3 drops of NSS per second. Decreased aroesolization.	Stream and mist	Clinician can use exact amount of fluid from a fine spray to a steady stream
Control mechanisms	Control button on hand held applicator	Foot panel or front panel control flexibility	Foot control pedal	Foot control pedal
Duration of treatment	3–5 min; wound size dependent.	Varies. Small wounds usually 3–5 min. Larger wounds 5–7 min.	Varies, usually 2–5 min patient tolerance, tissue quality, operator evaluation	Varies, patient tolerance, tissue quality, operator evaluation

(continued)

| TABLE 26.2 | Kilohertz Ultrasound Device Comparison *(continued)* | | | |

Feature	Celleration MIST™ Therapy System 5.0	Arobella™	SÖRING/Sonoca™ 180	Misonix
Wound bed contact	No. Treatment distance 0.5–1.5 cm. Note: at greater distance more US energy will be attenuated.	NO	Yes	Yes
Noncontact single Use Applicator	Yes	Yes	No	No
Selective Debridement	Yes, better for slough, softened necrotic tissue Use also for maintenance debridement	Yes, efficient	Yes, efficient	Yes, efficient
Pain with treatment	No	Occasionally a topical lidocaine.	Sometimes. Recommend use of lidocaine if needed	Sometimes. Sensitivity can be modulated with pulsed mode, recommend use of lidocaine if needed
Observation of Results	2–3 treatments slow effect	Immediate	Immediate	Immediate
Potential for thermal tissue destruction with misuse	No thermal effects	Yes, through frictional heat. Heat is dissipated in two ways: Use of a fluid and pulsed mode	Yes, through frictional heat. Heat dissipation with fluid	Yes, through frictional heat. Heat is dissipated in two ways: Use of a fluid and pulsed mode
Need to autoclave probe between patients	No, single use disposable applicator non contact	Yes	Yes	Yes, Probe life:~300–400 uses
Aerosolization Potential	No	No if operate correctly.	Yes	Yes
Infection control Requirements	No Aerosolization	Personal protection equipment recommended: masks, gloves, and gown being used. No need to have a separate room or drape the room.	Personal protection equipment recommended: masks, gloves, and gown being used	Personal protection equipment required: masks, gloves, and gown being used
	Disposable single use applicator		Private Room, drapes, Wipe down of surfaces pre and post procedure of unit	Private Room, drapes, PPE, Wipe down horizontal surfaces
	Germicidal wipes provided for disinfecting the transducer handle, cable, generator, and cradle			
	Figure 26.12	Figure 26.15	Figure 26.13	Fig. 26.14

Source: C Sussman, Sussman Physical Therapy, Inc.© Prepared from materials provided and evaluated by the companies listed.

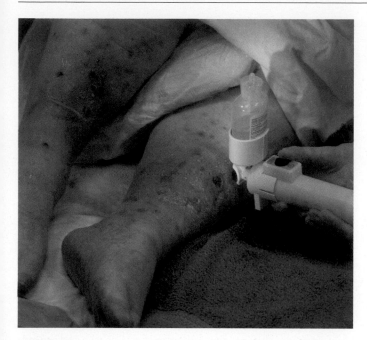

FIGURE 26.12 Celleration MIST therapy system 5.0. (Celleration, Eden Prairie, MN.)

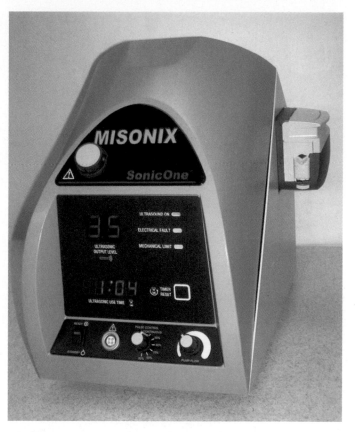

FIGURE 26.14 Misonix (Misonix Inc., Farmingdale, NY).

longitudinally. The maximum transducer intensity delivered to the tissues through the applicator tip is 1.25 W per cm². The therapeutic intensity range is 0.1 to 0.5 W per cm². The sound waves are transferred to the tissue in a mist.

The other devices offer a choice of fluid stream or mist applications (see Table 26.2). When in the contact mode, the instruments are coupled with the wound fluid if it is adequate, or with the addition of saline, and have tips that push the fluid forward. The various tips provided offer a distinct advantage when necrotic tissue is located in hard-to-reach places, such as tunnels and undermined areas. Clinically, the LFUS debriders have been

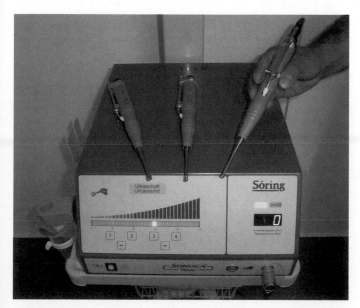

FIGURE 26.13 SÖRING/Sonoca 180 (Courtesy of Ferdinand Toro, National Sales Manager/Surgical Specialist, Soring Medical Technology. Doral, FL)

used and tested in tertiary wound care centers for several years. Clinical studies and reviews are being presented and published that indicate favorable results of the treatment.[8,10,13,36,44,46,61–63]

Benefits reported include

1. Selective removal of necrotic debris along with preservation of granulation tissue
2. Bactericidal effects—reduced infection
3. Cleansing of deep tunneling and undermining is facilitated
4. Deep tissue penetration of ultrasonic vibration and energy
5. Excellent wound bed preparation for grafting or flap closure
6. Improved flap survival rate
7. Reduced use of narcotics to control pain
8. Minimal blood loss despite anticoagulation therapy
9. Rapid removal of fibrin

This advanced technology is not likely to become part of the wound care toolbox overnight, as it is very costly and requires high level of knowledge and skill to use correctly. Clinical research is needed to determine the best treatment intervals, which wounds are candidates for treatment, and which will be most responsive to this treatment, and then compare the results with other debridement methods.[8,36,44]

It is not a benign intervention, even though negative effects are not well documented. In their multicenter study, Ennis et al.[4] reported on 12 adverse events that were possibly, probably, or definitely related to the use of the MIST Therapy System® device. These events included pain, erythema, blister, edema, ulcer enlargement, infection, additional ulcer development, and other unspecified. See the Case Study at end of this chapter about using LFUS for debridement of a leg ulcer.

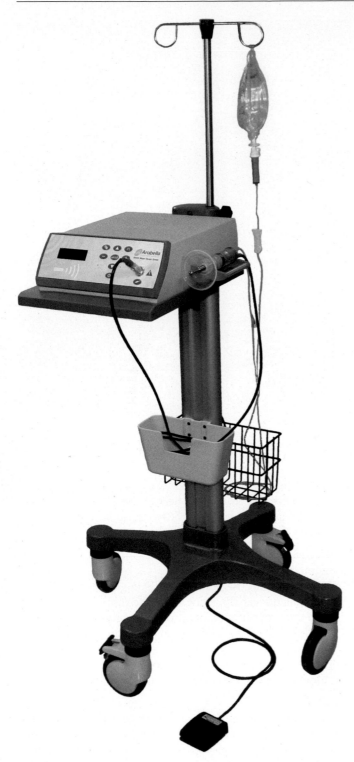

FIGURE 26.15 Arobella Qoustic Q Wound Therapy System (Arobella, Minnetonka, MN).

Scar Revision

Ward et al.[64] evaluated the therapeutic effects of US on the revision of scar contracture after burn injury, as well as the effect of standard burn physical therapy consisting of stretching. Elongation of collagen tissue following a combination of stretching and heat has been reported to be greater than stretching alone. Therefore, the study investigators wanted to

determine whether topical US would help patients with burns to progress to healed scar tissue. Joint range of motion and pain were the study variables chosen. The joints to be treated were randomized, and the patients and therapists were blinded to the TG. All treatments were performed every other day over a 2-week period with continuous US, 1 MHz, at 1 W per cm^2. Analysis of the data revealed no statistically significant differences in the two groups in either pain perception or joint range of motion. The lack of significance may be due to the fact that US has been demonstrated to be most effective during the inflammatory phase of healing, before scar formation is established, and to affect scar formation at that time by accelerating the healing response and the deposition and organization of the collagen. It is unlikely that US will be useful for healed scars.

CLINICAL EFFECTS SECTION SUMMARY

Studies on the efficacy of US suggest that it has the following important physiologic effects:

1. It affects all phases of wound recovery at the cellular level if applied during the inflammatory phase and speeds inflammation.
2. It accelerates the rate of progression through the phases of repair.
3. It affects different tissue types differently, according to the tissues' ability to absorb energy.
4. It appears that lower energy and lower frequency is more effective than HFUS and high energy for tissue, cellular, and bacteriacidal effects
5. It promotes thrombolysis/fibrinolysis of hemorrhagic material such as found in extravasation of blood into subcutaneous tissue. It increases circulation and tcPO$_2$ and is most effective if the patient is well hydrated and oxygenated.
6. It is useful for the debridement of necrotic tissue and reduction of biofilms.
7. It enables noninvasive, nontraumatic treatment of either deep or superficial tissue, depending on frequency.

Following is a summary of three mechanisms of action by which US interacts with biologic tissue.[64]

   a. Acoustic or microstreaming provides mechanical vibration that alters the tissue at the cellular or tissue levels.
   b. Acoustic cavitation is another property that has the ability to alter the cell membrane and noncellular structures. Cavitation occurs most easily and safely at lower frequencies. Cavitation appears to be responsible for bacteriacidal effects.
   c. Absorption of sonic energy produces increased tissue temperature, followed by increased blood flow with HFUS. Low frequency is nonthermal but increases blood flow by altering the microcirculation.

CLINICAL STUDIES OF WOUND HEALING

Clinical studies using US are reviewed next and are grouped as much as possible by wound etiology. Subsections include Pressure Ulcers, Venous Leg Ulcers, Diabetic Foot Ulcers, and Burns.

CASE STUDY

Debridement of Chronic Venous Ulcer

Venous Ulcer History

A 45-year-old female patient with a chronic venous insufficiency ulcer of the left lower leg of approximately 6 months duration was treated for approximately 4 months with compression therapy, Unna Boots, and various other dressings as guided by the University of Virginia Chronic Wound Clinic, with little success. (See Fig. 26.16A,B for before and after treatment photos.)

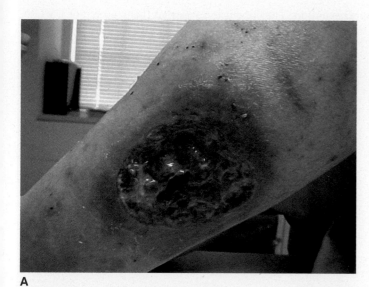

A

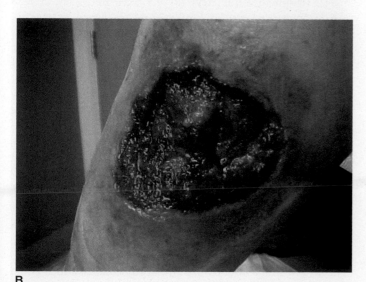

B

FIGURE 26.16 A. Venous Ulcer before debridement with Söring Sonoca 180. (Courtesy of Christine Newcomer, MSN, RN, WOCN, PhD Student University of Virginia, with permission.) **B.** Venous Ulcer after debridement with Söring Sonoca 180 (Courtesy of Christine Newcomer, MSN, RN, WOCN, PhD Student University of Virginia, with permission.)

Baseline Wound Assessment

Prior to LF ultrasonic therapy, there was a large wound (7.8 cm × 6.6 cm = 51.48 cm²) containing 80% well-adhered yellow slough, 15% pink moist tissue, and 5% dry black eschar in the center of the wound. The periwound skin was intact but was macerated at different points during therapy due to large amounts of exudate.

Plan of Wound Care

Skin Care

When her skin appeared macerated, skin protectant was used. This was effective for maintaining periwound skin throughout therapy.

Standard Wound Care

Unna Boot used for compression, and foam dressing over the wound to manage wound exudate between US sessions.

Biophysical Agent Care

A LFUS device (Sonoca 180) used once weekly for debridement.

Treatment Goals

Treatment goals were removal of necrotic debris and progression toward wound healing.

Outcomes

- After two US treatments, the wound bed had improved, as indicated by reduction in yellow slough from 80% to about 20% without eschar, and was starting to granulate and contract.
- After seven treatments, the wound showed 90% granulation tissue, and wound contraction without slough or eschar.
- After 7 treatments, the wound size had decreased to 4.8 cm × 3 5 cm = 16.8 cm². This was a 53% reduction in size in 8 weeks, demonstrating a positive healing trajectory.

This patient required local application of lidocaine jelly for pain management during the first three or four treatments. By the end of the treatments, she no longer required pain medication.

Results

The impression is that US debridement decreased the bioburden and restarted the healing process. Other patients treated at our clinic with the ultrasonic wound debridement therapy have not required any pain medications. The procedure used for this case study was supplied by Söring, Inc.

Acknowledgement

Thank you to Christine Newcomer, MSN, RN, WOCN, PhD candidate, University of Virginia, who supplied supporting information that is used in this section and kindly prepared the case study of her patient, who was treated with Sonoca 180. Wound debridement technology at University of Virginia. Thanks also to Catherine Ratliff, PhD, APRM-BC, CWOCN, for arranging and mentoring this collaboration.

Pressure Ulcers

1. A classic study was published in 1960, Paul et al.[65], reporting clinical observations of 23 patients with pressure ulcers, which suggested that ultrasonic therapy is effective in reducing tissue congestion, cleansing necrotic tissue, and promoting healing and the return of skin function to a near normal state, and that a "scientifically controlled study would be richly rewarding."[65]

2. In 1985, McDiarmid et al.[66] 25 years after the Paul study, undertook a double-blind randomized study to determine whether these nonthermal therapeutic effects could be used to treat/heal pressure ulcers.

Study groups: Patients with partial-thickness skin loss caused by pressure ulcers (stage II), but not extending beyond the dermis, were selected. Forty patients were entered into the study and randomized into a US treatment and a sham US TG.

Parameters of treatment: Parameters for the US treatment were 3 MHz, 0.8 W per cm² (SATP), pulse duration 2 milliseconds, duty cycle 20%, SATA intensity, 0.16 W per cm², effective radiating surface area 5.2 cm². Treatment duration was a minimum of 5 minutes for all pressure ulcers up to 3 cm². One additional minute was added for each 0.5 cm² area, for a maximum of 10 minutes. Frequency was three times per week.

Results: The sonated ulcers tended to heal more quickly, but the difference was not statistically significant.

1. When comparing clean ulcers with infected ulcers, the mean healing time for the clean ulcers was 30 versus 40 days for the infected ulcers.

2. Although US had little effect on the healing of clean pressure ulcers, there appeared to be a statistically significant effect of US on the healing of infected pressure ulcers, implying that the major factor influencing healing is whether the ulcer is clean or infected.

Discussion: McDiarmid et al.[66] speculated that, if the clean wound was already healing at an optimal biologic rate, the addition of a therapy such as US would not make a significant difference. On the other hand, slower healing infected ulcers may benefit from the effect of US stimulation of the large number of macrophages—the pivotal cell of the inflammatory phase and repair—present in infected wounds, with a resulting release of "wound factors" from those cells and other repair cells.[66] Based on recent information that is presented in the section about bacteriacidal effects of US, perhaps these wounds healed better because of the killing of bacteria by the perturbation and breakage of their cell walls from the US sonation.

3. Nussbaum et al.[67] conducted a comparison study of nursing care alone, nursing care with laser, and nursing care with an alternating protocol of US and ultraviolet C (UVC) on 20 spinal cord-injured patients with 22 pressure ulcers. Four of the initial subjects dropped out, leaving 16 subjects with 18 wounds to be considered for the analysis.

Plan of care:

1. Nursing care consisted of moist dressings and continuous pressure relief.

2. The laser regimen was provided three times per week.

3. The US/UVC regimen consisted of US treatment five times weekly, alternating the US and UVC daily, 5 days per week. If the ulcer had purulent drainage, the UVC was used three times per week; if not, US was used three times per week.

Methods: US protocol was frequency 3 MHz and intensity (SATA) of 0.2 W per cm² (1:4 pulse ratio) for 5 minutes per 5 cm² of wound area delivered to the periwound area.

Results:
- US/UVC treatment had a greater effect on wound healing than did the other treatment regimens.
- The mean treatment time to wound closure was 4.1 weeks.
- The trend was for ulcers to heal faster in sites where wound contraction was the primary mode of closure (e.g., over the coccyx).

Discussion: The conclusion was that this regimen of US/UVC may decrease the healing time for spinal cord-injured patients with pressure ulcers.[67] This was a small multimodal study that combined included several interventions, making it impossible to demonstrate the efficacy of each individually. Questions remain concerning whether the combination was essential, and what the effects of each treatment were.

4. Ter Riet et al.[68] studied pressure ulcer's response to HFUS treatment. Eighty-eight subjects were randomized into two groups: 45 for the TG and 43 for the CG. The trials lasted 12 weeks. Sixteen ulcers were stage IV, extending into muscle tissue, and 72 had less depth of tissue involvement.

Methods:
- Treatment was given directly to the wound surface (although how this was accomplished for the stage IV ulcers is not described) and to an extended radius 0.75 cm beyond the wound edge.
- The treatment parameters for US were frequency of 3.28 MHz, pulse duration of 2 milliseconds, SATA 0.1 W per cm², and BNR less than 4. The minimum treatment duration was 3 minutes, 45 seconds. Wounds with treatment areas larger than 5 cm² were treated longer. A wound with an area of 10 cm² was treated for 7 1/2 minutes.
- Local wound care included once or occasionally twice-daily cleansing or rinsing with sterile saline or chlorhexidine (0.1%) on gauze or in a syringe.
- Four wound characteristics (color of surrounding skin, necrotic tissue, granulation tissue, and deepest tissue involved) were each marked on a scale, with grading from 1 = bad to 10 = excellent. Two outcome variables were end points: surface area reduction (in cm²) and wound closure (yes or no).

Results: After 12 weeks, 40% of the ulcers (18/45) in the US group and 44% of the ulcers (19/43) in the sham US group were closed. The results showed a tendency for the US to be more effective in small wounds than in larger wounds, which could not be explained.[68]

Discussion: This multicenter clinical trial, published in 1996, did not support the hypothesis that US speeded up healing. However, examination of the methodology reveals that, although the US parameters were suitably controlled and described, there was a large variation in ulcer size and depth, patient health, and wound cleansing methods. The surface area of the pressure ulcers varied at the outset from less than 1 to more than 10 cm². Ulcer severity ranged from grade II to IV. The study sample had 16 patients with grade IV ulcers. Partial-thickness grade II ulcers heal faster than do full-thickness ulcers. To combine the two would bias the results. Furthermore, the patients were elderly (75–87 years); some were terminally ill and many incapacitated, those in the US-treated group being confined to bed from 14.4 to 24 hours per day, and those in the sham-irradiated CG from 14 to 20.5 hours per day. Chlorhexidine is a cytoxic agent to cells of repair, and using it for wound cleansing may have affected treatment results. Therefore, it is perhaps unreasonable to expect a significant improvement in healing to occur following US therapy (or possibly any other type of biophysical therapy). Ideally, the variability of both treatment parameters and patient characteristics in such studies should be minimized, and the physical condition of the patients should be such that healing is likely to occur. Only then can the efficacy of procedures designed to speed up healing rather than initiate it be adequately assessed.

5. Ennis reported on a study of five subjects with six pressure ulcers that was designed as a preliminary examination of the effects of LFUS (MIST®) 40 kHZ US on the size and appearance of pressure ulcers.

Plan of care: ulcers received a 5- to 10-minute treatment five to seven times weekly along with standard good wound care.
Results: The investigators found that after 4 weeks, ulcers receiving a 5- to 10-minute treatment five to seven times weekly along with standard good wound care were 73% of their original size.
Discussion: This is an interesting pilot study using LFUS for pressure ulcers. Now a large RCT is needed to support a recommendation.

Chronic Leg Ulcers

A. Dyson et al.[69] used MHz periwound US as a periwound treatment for a controlled trial among patients with chronic varicose ulcers.

Method: Two groups received either sonication or sham sonication three times per week for 4 weeks. Treatment parameters for the US treatment were 3 MHz, 1 W per cm² (SA, TP), pulse duration 2 milliseconds, delivered to the tissues every 10 milliseconds for up to 10 minutes. The treatment technique involved moving the head of the device over the skin immediately adjacent to the ulcer.
Results:
  a. At the end of 4 weeks, the experimental, sonicated group had statistically significant reduction in wound size compared with the CG (experimental group 66.4% ± 8.8%; CG 91.6% ± 8.9%).
  b. No adverse effects of treatment were found.
B. Weichenthal et al.[70] randomized into two groups of thirty-eight patients with chronic venous insufficiency who had leg ulcers.

Methods:
Standard Wound care: Both groups received standard wound care including compression bandaging, debridement, and antiseptics as needed.
Ultrasound Treatment: An experimental device that consisted of a water bath heated to 32°C to 34°C and a transducer that produced 30 kHz US at intensity of 100 mW per cm² was used for treatment given for 10 minutes to the area of the ulcer immersed in the water bath.
Results:
1. After 8 weeks of active and sham treatment, there was a statistically significant decrease in ulcer area of 41% for the US group compared to that of 11% for the controls.
2. Adverse effects included minor transient pain during the treatment, mild to moderate but not pain-related erythema after treatment persisting from 10 minutes to 2 hours.
3. Wound debridement effects were not observed.

C. Peschen et al.[71] treated 24 patients with chronic venous ulceration. All study and control patients were randomized and received either a conventional therapy of hydrocolloid dressings and compression or the conventional therapy plus US treatment.

Method: Application of 30 kHz US at an intensity (SATA) of 0.1 W per cm² via a water bath for 10 minutes three times weekly for 12 weeks.
Results: 1. At the end of a 12-week period, the experimental group showed an average decrease in ulcer area of 55.4%, compared with only 16.5% in the CG—a highly significant decrease ($p =.007$). The water bath method of delivering therapeutic US has found acceptance in Europe, but not in the United States.[71]

D. Meta-analysis of studies on the use of US therapy in the treatment of chronic leg ulcers was published in 1998.[72] While this meta-analysis is now dated and fails to include newer research, it is presented to illustrate what was known up to this point. Of the 14 studies found during a literature review, 6 were selected for inclusion. Of the six studies selected for inclusion, five used MHz US,[69,73-75] whereas the sixth used kHz US.[71] The frequency of US used was not evaluated as a treatment variable in the meta-analysis. The six studies are summarized in Table 26.3

Results:
1. The meta-analysis demonstrated that US therapy had a significant effect in decreasing ulcer surface area when compared with sham-irradiated controls.
2. It was suggested, on the basis of the meta-analysis, that US had its best effect when delivered in "low doses" around the edge of the ulcer, but it was noted that further studies would be required to confirm this possible effect and to evaluate a possible dose-response relationship. The authors did not specify what they meant by a low dose.
3. A statistically significant increase in the healing response, as demonstrated by a reduction in the surface area of the ulcers, was reported in four of the six studies.
4. The authors of this chapter reviewed the two studies used in the Johanson meta-anlysis that found no significant effect with the following findings.
  a. The study of Lundeberg et al.,[74] who used an unusual pulsing regimen (1:9), found no significant difference. The use of longer gaps between the pulses than were used in the other studies would reduce the TA intensity to 0.05 W per cm²; it is possible that such a low temporal intensity is below the level required to stimulate wound healing in chronic venous ulcers.

TABLE 26.3	Protocols and Results of Studies Used in Meta-analysis[76] of US Effects on chronic Leg Ulcers[76]					
Study Variable	Treatment	Roche and West[73]	Lundeberg et al.[74]	Callam et al.[75]	Dyson et al.[69]	Ericksson et al.[77]	Peschen et al.[71]
Ulcer etiology		Venous	Venous	Venous predominately (94/108)	Venous	Venous	Venous
Method of randomization		Random allocate	Permuted blocks	Permuted blocks	Alternately	Alternately	Alternately
Number of subjects	Control	13	15	41(15 dropouts)	12	13	12
	US	13	17	41(11 dropouts)	13	12	12
Area treated		Periwound	Wound surface	Periwound	Periwound	Wound surface	Wound surface and periwound
Frequency of treatment		3×/wk	3×/wk	1×/wk	3×/wk	2×/wk	3×/wk
Frequency of device		3 MHz	1 MHz	1 MHz	3 MHz	1 MHz	30 kHz
Intensity		1.0 W/cm²	0.5 W/cm²	0.5 W/cm²	1.0 W/cm²	1.0 W/cm²	100 mW/cm²
Pulsed or continuous/ duty cycle		1:4	1:9	Pulsed	1:5	Not stated	Continuous
Time		5–10 min	10 min	1 min/probe head area	5-10 min	Max 10 min	10 min
% Healing							
Results							
4 weeks	Control	↓ 28%	↓ 19	↓ 30%	↓ 7.4%	↓ 27	↓ 8
		SD 27.3	SD 9	SD 61.6	SD 8.9	SD 12	SD 20
			1 healed	5 healed		1 healed	
	US	↓ 35%	↓24	↓ 48	↓ 34%	↓ 35	↓ 27
		SD 21.9	SD 12	SD 49.8	SD 8.8	SD 14	SD 24
			2 healed	6 healed		2 healed	
8 weeks	Control	↓ 7%	↓ 47	↓ 60	Not reported after 4 wk	↓ 52	↓ 20
		SD 36.7	SD 10	SD 41.9		SD 13	SD 24
			3 healed	6 healed		4 healed	
	US	↓ 35.3	↓ 53	↓ 80	No. healed ulcers bit reported	↓ 68	↓ 40
		SD 30.1	SD 8	SD 24.6		SD 9	SD 23
		No. healed ulcers not reported	5 healed	14 healed		5 healed	No. healed ulcers not reported

Data from references listed in table.

b. The study of Eriksson et al.[77,78] failed to show statistically significant healing between controls and the US TG. Pulsed US was used, but pulsing ratio was not stated.

c. The sixth study reported by Peschen[71] was the only study where kHz US was used and can be considered as a pilot study to the studies that have followed using this frequency.

E. Johnson, in an attempt to reproduce the results of the Peschen and Weichenthal studies, performed a program evaluation of 15 chronic venous ulcers.[79]

Methods: Biophysical agent: LFUS, 30 kHz US, 100 mW per cm^2 in a water bath heated to 32°C to 34°C was used as the sound-conduction medium. Treatment was for 10 minutes, three times weekly over a 24-week period.

Results: All treated patients had reduction of wound size, exudate amount, and noticeable reduction in pain, with 50% achieving total healing. Clinical evaluation is an ideal way to test and evaluate research results.

F. Tan et al. sought to learn if Sonica 180™ was painless debridement. They studied 19 leg ulcers, 13 of which were venous ulcers and were included in this study. Patients served as their own controls.

Methods:
1. Standard wound care and compression.
2. Sonica 180, 25 kHz coupled with normal saline for 10 to 20 seconds per probe head area onto the ulcer surface repeated at 2- to 3-week intervals. Intensity not stated.
3. Total of five to seven treatments per patient, 5 to 20 minutes each.

Results:
1. Relief of pain and odor: eight patients no response; six patients greater than 50% (39%); seven patients healed 100% no pain.
2. Treatment is relatively painless.

G. Dolibog et al. evaluated the efficiency of using 1 MHz US for healing of venous leg ulcers in surgically treated patients ($N = 70$).

Method:
1. Standard wound care: elastic compression stockings, between 30 and 40 mm Hg at the ankle. Saline-soaked gauze dressings, oral medications micronized flavonoid fraction. Dressings changed daily.***
2. Biophysical agent: HFUS pulsed 1 MHz, 0.5 W per cm^2, duty cycle 1/5. In a water bath at 34°C. Transducer 10 cm^2; duration size dependent less than 5 cm^2 5 minutes plus one minute increase for each 1 cm^2 larger. For ulcers greater

than 20 cm^2, the wound was divided into two parts and each exposed for corresponding time. Frequency: once daily for 7 weeks.

Results: No statistically significant acceleration of healing (epithelialization) between groups. Progression of the treatment and CGs were parallel. Pus decreased statistically more in the US than other groups.

H. Watson used high frequency, 1 MHz, low dose US in a RCT ($N = 337$) for treatment of venous leg ulcers.

Methods
1. Standard wound care including compression.
2. 1.0 Hz pulsed US at 1:4 duty cycle and 0.5 W per cm^2 intensity was used for a range of 1 to 15 sessions. Average 11.

Results: No significant difference in time to heal between two groups.

Diabetic Foot Ulcers

A. In a multicenter trial, Ennis et al used the LFUS (MIST therapy system® 40 kHz) to study the effects of US on diabetic ulcer healing[4]. Patients in the study all had diabetic foot ulcers. Patients who met the study's inclusion criteria were randomized into two matched groups: 27 in the TG, 28 in the CG.

Methods:
1. Standard care was the same for both groups.
2. The duration of individual treatments was 4 minutes, delivered three times per week with LFUS (MIST® 40 kHz) therapy system.
3. The total treatment period was up to 12 weeks or closure.

Results:
1. Findings were that the LFUS group had a 40.7% closure (epithelialization) rate compared to a 14.3% rate for the controls.
2. Exudate diminished over time in the LFUS group, but not among the controls.
3. The use of LFUS did not significantly decrease the number of sharp/surgical debridement events in the TG.

Discussion:
B. Kavros et al.[63] used LFUS (MIST® therapy system 40 kHz) to conduct a RCT on patients with leg and foot ulcers who had critical ischemia (tcPO$_2$ levels between 20 and 40 mm Hg). A majority of subjects were diabetic.

Methods: Two groups were randomly selected for 12 weeks or until healed study period. TG received good standard wound care plus three times weekly treatment with LFUS MIST for 5 minutes regardless of wound size. The CG received only standard wound care of daily dressing changes and weekly debridement plus offloading and low stretch bandage compression as needed.

Results:
1. Target outcomes were to determine the percentage of patients whose wounds decreased greater than 50% in size from baseline: TG: 63% greater than 50%; CG 29% greater than 50% ($p < .001$). Failure to reach greater than 50% size decrease: TG 37%; CG 71%.

RESEARCH WISDOM

Knowing when to *stop* Treatment

If no improvement in wound healing was observed by five treatments with Sonica 180, no benefit can be expected with more treatment.[46]

CLINICAL WISDOM

MIST® Therapy System and Pulsed Lavage with Suction

If a wound is grossly infected and the tissue is sloughy or if the granulation tissue is poorly perfused, choose MIST® because, although there appears to be an angiogenic effect with both, the MIST® far exceeds the effect of the PLWS.[82]

2. TG had improvement in the dependent position measurement of tcPO$_2$.

Discussion: Using noncontact LFUS improved the rate of healing and closure in recalcitrant lower extremity ulcerations.

Clinical Studies Section Conclusions

Information about the effects of US on wound healing remains uncertain because of the limited number of clinical trials, the different parameters used for each study, the small sample sizes, and perhaps because the intervention was not appropriately applied. Nevertheless, findings are available to guide treatment decisions as listed here.

1. **Multiple interventions:** One study compared two interventions, US and UVC, with laser and there were good outcomes, but we cannot distinguish the effects of the US from the UVC.[67]

2. **No significant benefits for Pressure ulcers with HFUS:** Three RCT studies included subjects who had pressure ulcers treated with HFUS and none showed significant benefits.[66–68] LFUS appears to have promise in treatment of pressure ulcers but further evidence is needed to support.

3. **No significant benefits for chronic leg ulcers with HFUS.** Several studies included patients with chronic leg ulcers that suggest that HFUS is *not* the best choice for treatment of venous leg ulcers.[66–68,80,81] Yet, what appears evident is that LFUS is a fresh approach with the potential to accelerate the healing process possibly due to its effects on circulation and bacteriacidal effects and reduction of bioburden giving the host a chance to heal. RCT are needed to quantify results with LFUS.

4. **Diabetic patients with foot ulcers** appear to have potential benefit from treatment with LFUS, but the test group in the relevant study was so small that it is hard to generalize the results.

5. **Wound severity:** Pressure ulcer studies reported wound severity that ranged from partial thickness to full thickness, extending to tissue involvement at the level of muscle. The partial-thickness ulcers heal by re-epithelialization, deep ulcers by regeneration and contraction. Therefore, mixing results of these two groups cannot give a clear picture of the results of treatment.

6. **Bacteriacidal effects:** Bacteriacidal effects including increased microvascular enhancement are associated with both HFUS and LFUS. The results for infected pressure ulcers treated with HFUS were better than those for clean ulcers. However, the trend favors LFUS.

7. **Dosimetry:** More evaluation of the dosimetry parameters of US is still required. Nevertheless, after review of the studies presented, LFUS appears to have the edge over HFUS efficacy on all aspects of healing and infection. However, cases such as the examples described in the case studies at the end of this chapter where thrombolysis was the desired objective, the higher frequency may have greater impact.

HIGH-RESOLUTION DIAGNOSTIC ULTRASOUND

US is widely used as both a diagnostic and a therapeutic modality. It has an excellent safety record and can be used with confidence to image-sensitive structures such as a fetus, tumors, and granulation tissue. Originally developed to image macroscopic structures, high-resolution equipment that allows tissues to be viewed at the microscopic level is now available. This equipment uses higher frequencies of US than are available in lower resolution devices. High-frequency diagnostic US has utility in wound care to help clinicians better understand the pathogenesis of pressure ulcers and to detect soft tissue destruction and edema before visible clinical signs appear and plan appropriate care. It is a method to visually document the status of patients who test high risk for pressure ulcers (e.g., Braden score < 18 at the time of admission). In addition to better clinical management of patients, pressure ulcers that occur during a hospital or nursing home stay are considered to be avoidable and care is not compensated by government insurance plans (see Chapter 9). Therefore, for legal and regulatory reasons, such a piece of equipment should be considered as part of wound care clinic equipment.

Imaging

US imaging depends on the principle that different tissue components reflect and absorb US to varying degrees, depending on their acoustic properties, which, in turn, depend on their structure. For example, tissues rich in fat absorb less US than do tissues rich in protein. Reflection occurs at the interface between materials that differ in their acoustic properties, specifically in their acoustic impedance. Each reflection is termed an echo.

Piezoelectric materials not only transduce electrical signals into mechanical vibrations but also transduce mechanical vibrations into electrical signals. In US imaging, the reflected US, that is, each echo, is detected by the same transducer that produced it. The transducer listens for the echoes in the short intervals between the pulses of US emitted by the transducer. When a pulse of US travels through the tissues of the body, it meets many targets (interfaces and scatters) that generate echoes. The echoes return first from targets closest to the transducer, followed by echoes from targets further and further away from the transducer. The diagnostic US equipment determines the distance d of each target from the transducer by measuring the time t taken for the echo to return following the emission of the pulse (the go and return time), assuming a fixed value for the speed of sound c in human tissues (1,540 milliseconds). The echo returns to the transducer after a total go and return time of 2 d/c. The distance or depth of each target is calculated as $d = ct/2$.

A two-dimensional *B-mode image*, *B-scan* or *brightness scan*, typically consists of at least 100 adjacent pulse echo sequences (each termed a B-mode line) captured sequentially as the beam or pulse of US is moved across the tissues being scanned. A display spot on the viewing screen of the monitor moves from a point corresponding to the position of the transducer in a direction representing the path of the beam. Reflections, or echoes, increase the brightness of the spot. The stronger the reflection, the greater its amplitude, and the brighter the spot.

The reflections or echoes received at each beam position are displayed as spots on the display screen of the scanner, the brightness of each spot being related to the echo amplitude as a grayscale display. The grayscale can be replaced by different colors to assist in visual interpretation of the image, the colors representing differing levels of echogenicity from different tissue components. The distance down the screen at which each echo is displayed indicates d, the depth of the target producing the echo.

The tissue components, and hence the pattern and brightness of the reflections from them, vary with tissue type and are modified by injury and during repair. When high-resolution diagnostic US is used, the resultant image, which superficially resembles a histologic section, can be thought of as a noninvasive biopsy produced in a nontraumatic, painless manner, with no damage to the tissues that interact with the high-frequency/low-intensity US.

Visual Details

The detail that can be visualized ultrasonically is dependent on the resolution of the imaging equipment used, and this depends mainly on the wavelength of the US, which is determined by the frequency; the higher the frequency, the shorter the wavelength and, therefore, the greater the resolution. There is an inverse relationship between frequency and depth of penetration,

higher frequencies being less penetrative than lower frequencies (Teresa Conner-Kerr, *personal communication*, 2006). In one 1991 study, US at a frequency of 5 MHz (i.e., 5 million cycles of vibration per second) was described as providing "high resolution"[82] and was considered to be adequate to view, for example, the plantaris tendon, provided that this was at least 2 mm thick, when the aim was merely to demonstrate whether it was present and whether it was thick enough to be used as a graft.

More recently, improved instrumentation coupled with the use of higher frequencies and image analysis has resulted in the effective use of US to noninvasively visualize changes in tissue associated with the presence or development of injury and its repair. In 1993, O'Reilly and Massouh[83] published a pictorial essay in which they compared the ultrasonic appearance of normal and damaged Achilles tendons, using a real-time scanner equipped with a 7.5-MHz linear transducer and a 5-MHz sector transducer. They were able to detect and distinguish between tenosynovitis, acute and chronic tendinitis, peritendinitis, nodular tendinitis, and partial or complete tendon rupture on the basis of differences in echogenicity and measurements of tendon thickness, the changes detected ultrasonographically being confirmed invasively by fine-needle aspiration and histologic examination.

Higher frequencies, permitting greater resolution, can be used for more superficial structures, such as the components of skin, where less depth of penetration is required. In 1994, 20 MHz US was used by Karim et al.[84] to image skin from various parts of the body, and it was demonstrated that mathematical algorithms could be used to characterize and classify the dermal

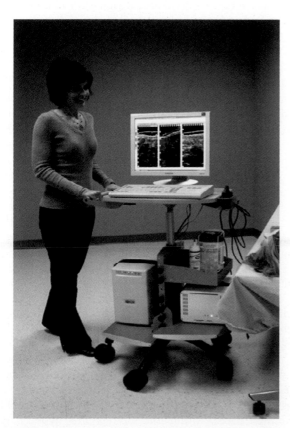

FIGURE 26.17 Photo of Longport Episcanner (Used with permission of Paul Wilson, Longport, Inc.)

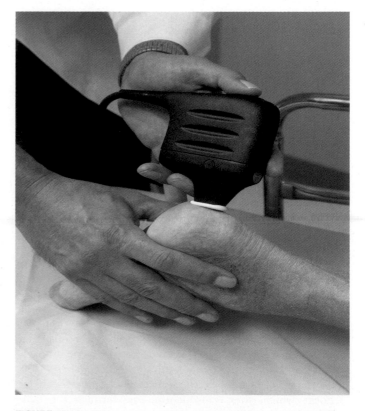

FIGURE 26.18 Taking a scan of heel with Episcan transducer/applicator. (Used with permission of Paul Wilson, Longport, Inc.)

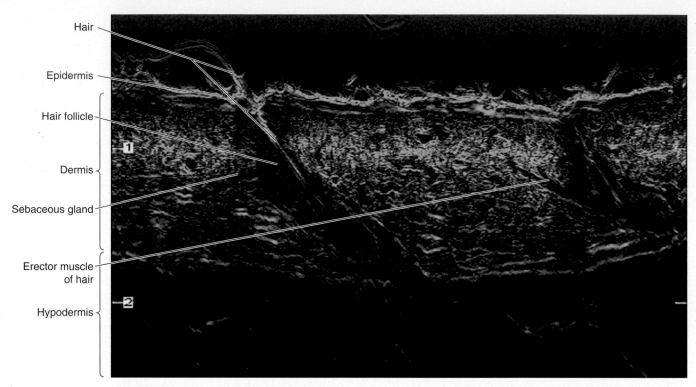

FIGURE 26.19 HRUS image of dermal structure captured at 50 MHz (Courtesy of Paul Wilson, Longport, Inc.)

monograms as to their site of origin. Two analytic techniques were investigated, fractal analysis and fast Fourier transform, the aim being to develop image analysis techniques sensitive enough to detect minute changes in the pattern of the ultrasonically produced images, and to avoid inter-observer differences in interpretation of these images (see Figure 26.17).

New High-Resolution Diagnostic Scanner

HRUS equipment with increased sensitivity is now available commercially. This equipment has evolved from prototypes developed at the United Medical and Dental Schools of Guy's and St. Thomas's Hospitals in London. Marketed by Longport Inc. (Silchester, UK) as the Episcanner, it is currently in use in the United States, Europe, and Australia to monitor changes in soft connective tissues associated with damage and repair. The equipment is portable and is fitted with a polyvinylidene difluoride piezoelectric polymer transducer incorporated into a handset filled with distilled water (Fig. 26.18). It emits a chain of single-cycle pulses at a frequency of between 10 and 50 MHz, although it is generally used at a center frequency of 20 MHz. This allows the production of images of the interfaces between acoustically different materials, with a resolution such that structures separated by approximately 65 micrometers (μm) in the direction of the US transmission can be distinguished. The transducer is moved within the probe by a stepper motor, producing pulses of US with a repetition frequency of 1 millisecond. The system has been designed to emit an ultrafast rise and fall time pulse of duration of less than 50 ns. These sharp pulses allow excellent detection of reflected signals (echoes), which, after transduction, pass through a preamp unit in the probe before passing to the main unit. As with other US imaging devices, including those operating at lower frequencies, time-gain compensation is used to control for the attenuation that occurs as the US is reflected back to the transducer. Digitization of the reflected signals produces data that can be stored and used for statistical analysis.[85,86] A digital scan converter stores information in the US scan format and displays it in the video format (see Fig. 26.19).

Practical Implications

High-resolution B-mode displays show the components of a slice of soft tissue, akin to a histological section, but without removal of these tissues for examination (Figs. 26.4A,B and 26.19). The same region of the body can be scanned repeatedly, showing, for example, the speed of tissue healing or the progression of the tissue damage.[78,87,88] Cross-sectional images of the skin produced by Longport's Episcanner have a very characteristic appearance. The hyperechogenic (highly reflective) keratinized layer of the epidermis can be distinguished from the less echogenic layers of living cells that collectively form the stratum malpighii. As shown with other high-resolution equipment, the interface between the epidermis and dermis can be identified as a hyperechogenic layer under the less echogenic layer.[31] The dermis shows variations in echogenicity; the pattern of echoes varying from a speckled appearance in the papillary zone of the dermis to a more linear appearance in its deeper reticular zone, where the collagen fiber bundles are thicker and more aligned. Hair follicles, blood vessels, tendon sheaths, tendons, ligaments, and adipose tissue can be identified, as can the interfaces between soft tissue and calcified tissue. Figure 26.19 shows images of dermal structures captured at 50 MHz. Fluid-containing spaces within the dermis are hypoechogenic, meaning that these spaces are hyporeflective and show up as black holes on the scan, as is subcutaneous fat, although this

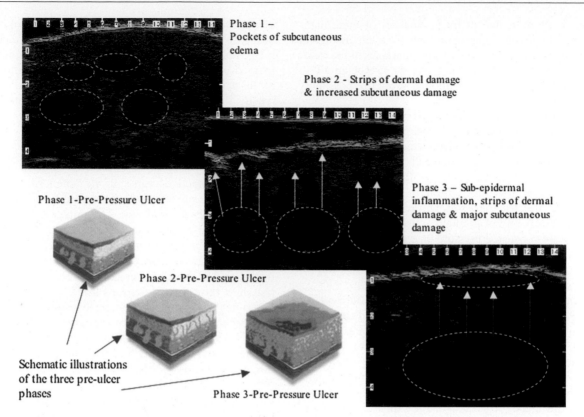

Phase 1 –
Pockets of subcutaneous
edema

Phase 2 - Strips of dermal damage
& increased subcutaneous damage

Phase 3 – Sub-epidermal
inflammation, strips of dermal
damage & major subcutaneous
damage

Phase 1-Pre-Pressure Ulcer

Phase 2-Pre-Pressure Ulcer

Schematic illustrations
of the three pre-ulcer
phases

Phase 3-Pre-Pressure Ulcer

FIGURE 26.20 Phases 1 to 3 Using the EPISCAN, pressure ulcers have been found to develop in the subcutaneous tissue over a hard prominence, typically a bone, and then spread out through the dermis to the epidermis, where at some point, an open wound often develops. Studies have shown that the early phases of pressure ulcer development shown below can be used to initiate earlier and mare targeted intervention, and that this can significantly and cost-effectively reduce the occurrence of open pressure ulcers. (Copyright P. Wilson.)

produces some thin linear echoes that may represent strands of collagenous fibrous connective tissue that support the fat. The scanner allows changes in soft tissue associated with the repair of injuries to be monitored (Fig. 26.4A,B) and subjected to fractal analysis, as did earlier, less informative and versatile instrumentation.[72,88,89]

More recently, high-resolution B-mode US has been used to detect the dermal changes associated with exposure to pressure[90,91] and as a means of quantifying the irritant response.[88,92] Deeper soft tissue injuries, such as developing pressure ulcers, can also be detected at pressure points close to the bone before they become visible at the surface of the skin. HRUS is very sensitive in detecting fluid changes within tissues. It has been reported that HRUS can detect the edema associated with developing pressure ulcers 48 to 72 hours before there are clinical signs.[91] This edema is first recognizable in the subcutaneous tissue near the bone (Fig. 26.20 Phase 1). It then extends superficially, first into the reticular layer of the dermis (Fig. 26.20 Phase 2), and then into the papillary layer of the dermis (Fig. 26.20 Phase 3). Early detection of deep tissue injury allows pressure relief measures to be implemented before the ulcer breaks through the skin, with considerable reduction of suffering. A 3-year cost analysis of the use of high-frequency (high-resolution) diagnostic US technology's use in managing soft tissue injuries in a nursing home showed costs were reduced when HRUS was used as an addition to the current pressure ulcer risk assessment and management tool.[93] The ability of the highly sensitive Episcanner to detect and

quantify muscle inflammation remains to be investigated. In 1990, Van Holsbeek and Introcaso[94] demonstrated echogenic differences between normal and inflamed muscle with less sensitive instrumentation.

Other uses of HRUS include monitoring changes in the thickness of the epidermis and underlying soft connective tissues, and in detecting lesions such as melanomas, potentially even those as small as 70 μm in thickness. As long ago as 1984, Shafir et al.[95] indicated that what were then considered to be high-resolution US scanners could measure the thickness of melanomas. Accurate measurement of a melanoma's thickness can provide useful prognostic information, because this dimension is directly related to metastatic potential.[96] Also of

CLINICAL WISDOM

Visualizing undermined and tunneled regions

Extent of undermined and tunneled areas are difficult to determine. Probing with an instrument like a cotton-tipped applicator shears the fragile interstitial fascia and has potential to increase the tunneled length and risk of infectious invasion. However, undermined/tunneled regions can be visualized in HRUS B-scans without tissue damage. This can be used to aide clinical decision making about plan of care.

importance is the potential of fractal analysis of these high-quality images to provide quantitative data for comparison and assessment of the effectiveness of various therapies in the treatment of injured tissues. Fractal analysis may also be an aid to the diagnosis of a variety of skin pathologies, but this possibility remains to be examined critically.

One area of concern is the inability of clinicians to detect stage I pressure ulcers accurately in people with darkly pigmented skin.[56,97–100] This is due to the reliance for assessment on the parameter of color change, specifically redness (unblanchable erythema), for all patients, rather than considering the hues of blue–purple that may appear in people with darkly pigmented skin. Because the assessment of color is affected by the quantity and quality of the light source used, its value as the only indicator of stage I pressure ulcers in persons of color is questionable. Therefore, inclusion of other characteristics, such as skin temperature, stiffness, and sensation has been proposed,[99] together with the use of HRUS B-scans.[98,100]

Although the specific characteristics of early pressure-related injury are yet to be defined, awareness of the need to educate clinicians in culturally sensitive assessment techniques is growing.[86] Use of the HRUS as described above greatly increases both the sensitivity and specificity of correctly identifying stage I pressure ulcers, particularly in darkly pigmented skin. Furthermore, dependence on less accurate measures to identify stage I pressure ulcers, regardless of the skin's pigmentation, could be eradicated by the use of this equipment. The implementation of appropriate preventative measures and treatment, such as the use of the physical modalities described in this section, could significantly decrease the incidence of pressure ulcers in those at risk, leading to improvement in the quality of life and savings in the cost of health care. The effectiveness of these measures can now be assessed easily, objectively, and without damage or discomfort to the patient.[88,91,93,100]

High-resolution diagnostic US or US biomicroscopy is of considerable clinical importance that will grow as more uses are demonstrated for it. Visual detection of clinical signs of dermal and subdermal edema and soft tissue damage can only infer that there is a problem.

Quintavalle et al. learned from studying 1,139 readable images of bony prominence from 119 long-term residents that are common sites of pressure ulcers (heels, sacrum, and ischial tuberosity), that 630 (55.3%) had HRUS patterns consistent with abnormal skin and soft tissue; 509 (44.7%) of the images were consistent with normal skin and soft tissue.[88] The high-resolution scanner can thus detect and document the changes

---

CLINICAL WISDOM

HRUS for Use in Telemedicine

The Longport Scanner is a portable device that can be used in many settings. The application of this technology and the resulting B scans, as seen in the color plates, take only a few seconds to produce, can be read immediately by a skilled clinician, transmitted for interpretation, or stored electronically, making them ideal for telemedicine applications.

---

in skin and soft tissues consistent with developing pressure ulcers, so that the clinician can see evidence of damage before it is visible on the surface. This can lead to earlier and more focused pressure ulcer prevention and treatment.[88] Adoption of this technology is progressing while more research of a high quality is currently being organized internationally.

EVALUATING CANDIDACY FOR THE INTERVENTION

With any interactive treatment, the benefit to the patient must outweigh any possible risk. Therefore, you must be able to assess both benefit and risk. The potential benefits of US in wound care have been described above. Now let us turn to risks.

There is a long list of contraindications in the literature, and the excellent safety record of US owes much to the constraints on treatment that these have engendered (Exhibit 26.1). However, not all of the contraindications listed here have been verified experimentally,[21] and it is possible that some patients who could have benefited from US treatment have been denied it.

To ensure safe use, you must also consider the basic precautions listed in Exhibit 26.2. The most fundamental precaution, of course, is to select the right candidate for treatment. A patient's medical history, the onset date, an injury's location and depth, and the size of the area to be treated should all guide you in deciding whether to use US. For example, review the medical history for information about the circulatory system. Look for information concerning arteriosclerotic vessels, ischemia, and occlusion from reports of vascular studies, or a noninvasive vascular examination (see Chapter 6). US is not recommended over deep vein thrombosis or thrombophlebitis because of the risk of dislodging thrombi. Likewise, hemophiliacs should not be treated with US because of the risk of disturbing clot formation (thrombolysis). This should also be considered a precaution at the least, if not a contraindication, for patients on anticoagulant medications. Also look for information about diabetes mellitus, as diabetic patients are likely to

---

EXHIBIT 26.1

Contraindications for US[21,101]

Do Not Use Us

Over the uterus during pregnancy
Over the gonads
Over malignancies and precancerous lesions
Over tissues previously treated with deep x-ray of irradiation
On patients with vascular abnormalities
    Deep vein thrombosis
    Emboli
    Severe atherosclerosis
Over the cardiac area in advanced heart disease
Over the stellate ganglion
For hemophiliacs not covered by factor replacement
Over the spinal cord after laminectomy

EXHIBIT	26.2

Precautions for Use of US[21]

Exercise Caution in Use of Us

In acute infections
Over subcutaneous bony prominences
Over epiphyseal plates
Over subcutaneous major nerves
Over the cranium
Over anesthetic areas

have vascular impairments. Over areas of poor use circulation ultrasound LFUS should be used.

A patient with loss of sensation—whether due to diabetes or any other cause—is not a candidate for HFUS but could be considered for LFUS.

In a patient with a history of spinal laminectomy, do not use US over the affected area, because of the as-yet undetermined but potentially harmful effects on the spinal cord. A history of malignant or precancerous lesions or tumors in the area to be treated would also be a contraindication, because US could stimulate cellular proliferation.[102] Injuries around the eye also should not be treated with US because the sensitive retina may be affected.

Refrain from treating over the uterus during pregnancy to ensure that an embryo or fetus is not exposed to the intensities used in therapeutic US, which are higher than those used diagnostically. Do not treat over the gonads. Metal implants, including foreign objects, which are often described in a medical history or directly by the patient, are another contraindication for HFUS but acceptable for LFUS.

Clearly, more investigation is warranted, so that the proper caveats can be used when determining patient candidacy. In all cases, conduct a thorough review before determining whether or not US therapy is indicated. If in doubt, do not sonate.

SELECTING EQUIPMENT FOR ULTRASOUND APPLICATIONS

Choice of devices for generation of therapeutic levels of US is based on the frequency and methods of delivery. Therefore, the criteria for section of the two classes of devices are separated into two subsections.

Selection of HFUS

The selection of therapeutic HFUS (MHz) equipment should be based on the following considerations:

1. Select a transducer with low BNR.
2. Select a transducer that is water immersible.
3. Select one transducer that is less than 2 cm² and another 5 cm². Avoid large transducers with small ERA.
4. Choose an ergonomically designed transducer that is comfortable to hold.

5. Select a unit with multiple frequencies for optimal treatment options, depending on desired depth of penetration.
6. Select a unit with a built-in feature that tests output performance every time the unit is powered up.

Maintenance Requirements for HFUS Equipment

The American Institute of Ultrasound in Medicine suggests that all US equipment should be kept in good working order and be evaluated and calibrated annually. Individual transducers should be scanned two or three times a year depending on the amount or use, by a skilled US technician to ensure proper calibration of intensity. Intensity can be averaged in space over the face of the applicator (termed SA) or in time (termed *TA*). When pulsed US is used, pulse average (PA) intensity (this is the TA, average amount of time that the energy is delivered), during the period of the pulse should be noted, as should the TA during the full pulse repetition cycle. The type of intensity should be specified as either I (SATA), if continuous, or both I (SATA) and I (SAPA), if pulsed. This will facilitate follow-up treatments by another clinician and allow identification of best treatment intensity to be used.

Selection of LFUS Devices

Choice of kHz equipment is much more limited than MHz because it is new technology and as of this writing, there are only a few products on the market that are approved by the FDA for medical use to treat wounds. Table 26.2 shows a comparison of four kHz products. These products are shown in Figures 26.12 to 26.15. Information about their parameters and utility is presented throughout this chapter. The main difference between devices is the frequency 25 to 40 kHz and whether they can be used for both mist and continuous stream or only mist delivery systems and are contact or noncontact. Frequency is not adjustable but intensity in W per cm² is.

PROCEDURES

Procedures for HFUS and LFUS are very different. Each type of application will be described separately in this section. The section begins with protocol considerations.

Protocol Considerations

After determining the patient's candidacy for US, you must then determine the appropriate treatment parameters. The following are considerations.

HFUS Considerations

A. The anatomic location of the wound is a very important consideration when using HFUS. For example, be aware of the location of major subcutaneous nerves, which absorb US energy very well and can become overheated.
B. When treating young people, take into account epiphyseal plates, the growth of which may not be complete. This varies with the bone and sex, and there are racial differences as well.
C. If the wound is located over a bony prominence, consider a method of sonication that will avoid increasing periosteal temperature. Choose one of the following: (1) select a high frequency (3 MHz), which is absorbed primarily in the more superficial tissues; (2) move the treatment head

continuously to avoid standing waves; (3) treat through water for a more uniform far field; (4) for deeper wounds, select a lower frequency (1 MHz); (5) use pulsed mode.

D. Consider the local circulation. If it is poor, always use pulsed US to avoid excessive heating, because it will take longer for heat to be dissipated from the area.

E. Assess the size of the area to be treated. Use this assessment to determine the duration of the treatment and the size of the applicator to select. Note that an applicator with a larger ERA will allow treatment of a large wound more rapidly than if an applicator with a smaller ERA is used. Small applicators, however, are very useful for being more selective in treating specific tissues. Select an appropriate intensity. If the wound is acute, make use of the nonthermal effects of US. The beam's intensity should be at the upper end of the low range (see Table 26.1). For chronic wounds, consider a single upper medium-intensity treatment and subsequent treatment at lower intensity.

F. Select the coupling medium based on whether the skin is intact or broken. Coupling media are described soon.

LFUS Considerations

1. Determine the nature of tissue to be debrided.
2. Noncontact LFUS is useful for autolytic and maintenance-type debridement (e.g., slough and fibrin).
3. Select direct contact LFUS, equivalent for advanced sharp debridement, it is not surgical debridement, for speedy selective removal of nonviable necrotic tissue.
4. High intensity may be needed to debride thick necrotic tissue (e.g., eschar).
5. Consider LFUS for treatment of infected wounds including biofilms.
6. Assess the size of the area to be treated. Use this assessment to determine the duration of the treatment. Time varies, usually 2 to 5 minutes.
7. Consider patient tolerance as well as size in determining the length of treatment time.
8. Premedicate with analgesic such as lidocaine before direct contact LFUS debridement.
9. Always use LFUS with a transmission fluid such as normal saline.
10. NEVER touch the tip of the transducer directly to tissue, because it will be hot and can cause burns.

Safety Precautions

To ensure the safe use of all frequencies of therapeutic US, the following basic precautions are recommended:

1. Use US only if adequately trained to do so.
2. Use US only to treat patients with conditions known to respond favorably to US therapy, unless it is being used experimentally with the understanding and approval of the patient, his or her medical advisors, and the local medical ethics committee or internal review board.
3. Use the lowest intensity that produces the required effect, because higher intensities may be damaging. Burns, for example, occur when the intensity is too high or the frequency is low, and when the treatment head is not moved continuously or is moved too slowly.

4. Move the applicator constantly throughout treatment to avoid the damaging effects of standing waves and, when treating in the nonuniform near field, of high intensity regions.
5. Make sure that there is adequate coupling media and that it is free of air bubbles.
6. Make sure that the equipment is calibrated regularly. A crystal may be broken, for instance, if the applicator head is dropped. Staff must report such incidents, so that the applicator head can be tested before reuse. A faulty piece of equipment can result in inadequate treatment for the patient, or can produce shear waves and standing waves that can cause burns or other harmful effects.[21]

Expected Outcomes

In acute wounds, US is most effective when treating in the acute inflammatory phase of healing. During this phase, expect an acceleration of the inflammatory phase and early progression to the proliferative and epithelialization phases of healing.

In chronic wounds, the first treatment outcome with MHz will be increased perfusion, observed as warmth, edema, and darkening of tissue color compared with adjacent skin color tones. In necrotic wounds, expect to see autolysis of the necrotic tissue; the outcome will be a clean wound bed. In two clinical trials, chronic wounds progressed to closure in a mean time of 4 to 6 weeks.[66,67] Closure times could be longer for patients with intrinsic and extrinsic factors that limit healing.

Predict the expected outcome at start of care, then reassessment should confirm the predicted outcomes. For more information on predicting outcomes see Chapter 4. If the wound does not change tissue characteristics, wound phase and/or reduce the size of surface area or overall size estimate within 2 to 4 weeks, the treatment regimen must change. There are several changes to US treatment to consider: enhance the inflammatory phase or restart it with the protocol for chronic wounds; change the frequency of the transducer; use a different size transducer for better ERA, or increase/decrease the treatment time; or recalculate the area if the wound has been debrided and become larger as a result. If using HVUS change to LFUS. With direct contact LFUS, debridement should be observable during the treatment sessions and with noncontact wound bed cleansing should be observable in one to two sessions. Pain should reduce within 2 to 10 treatments.

Wound Treatment Protocols

In this section, we are discussing some typical protocols for using the different US devices. It is not meant to propose that these are the only useful or tested protocols. As evidence accumulates, we can expect new protocols to be proposed and old protocols dropped or revised. Therefore, it is important to read journal articles, attend conference presentations, and keep abreast of changes. For example, the newest evidence regarding use of HFUS for leg ulcers says it is ineffective. Older evidence suggests the same for pressure ulcers. Why then are there protocols in this section applying HFUS? They are included because evidence exists that suggests they have utility for certain situations. Also, clinicians who use this text may not have access to LFUS devices but have a HFUS device available and need guidance for safe and best uses. On the other hand, recent evidence, as we have reviewed, is demonstrating that LFUS is a useful biophysical agent for wound debridement, wound healing, and the physiological processes involved. We begin by considering use of HFUS for acute wounds, then for chronic wounds of mixed etiologies. Later, protocols for LFUS will be presented.

Coupling Media

US requires a coupling medium that displaces air. All bubbles need to be smoothed out between the transducer head and the coupling interface. This is essential because as mentioned US is reflected from air/water or air/tissue interfaces. The ideal coupling medium would:

- have the same acoustic impedance as skin
- also act as a wound dressing (if using HFUS)
- be sterile, thixotropic, nonstaining, nonirritant, and chemically inert
- have slow absorption and evaporation rates
- be free from gas bubbles and other inclusions
- not break down when the US energy is transmitted through it
- be inexpensive and easily acquired

Wound care products are part of the treatment regimen also, and should be considered in the treatment planning. Will the dressing be part of the US treatment, as described above, or will the dressing be removed and replaced when the US treatment is given? Will the dressing be changed every other day? Can it be changed in conjunction with the US treatment to minimize disruption of the wound-healing environment? MDs, PTs, and RNS should collaborate about the application of topical agents, such as petrolatum or petrolatum-based products, which will interfere with US transmission. This will avoid conflicting treatment approaches and improve utilization management.

The ability of wound care dressings to transmit US affects the efficacy, efficiency, and cost of US treatment. A study of

wound care products identified four sheet hydrogels and four transparent film dressings with different transmission rates.[103] (see Exhibit 26.3). Intensities from 0.2 to 2.0 W per cm^2 were tested at a frequency of 3.3 MHz. US transmission gel was used on the skin and on top of the dressing to remove air. Plastic sheets that could have interfered with the sound energy transmission were removed from the tops and bottoms of the hydrogel sheets. Findings are listed in Exhibit 26.3 and should help guide the clinician in selecting the dressing that will optimize treatment effects with MHz US.

Suitable coupling media that displace air and that can be used along the wound perimeter include commercially available US-transmitting gel, and over-the-wound, sterile, transparent, US-transmitting wound dressings. Tegaderm was tested for transmission of US energy and found to transmit 40% of the acoustic energy.[54] Tests of the results of US stimulation on $tcPO_2$ measurements when energy was transmitted through Tegaderm showed no significant differences in the measurements, with or without the Tegaderm.[29] Tegaderm and similar transparent film dressings are useful for treating full-thickness wounds because the film will stretch down into the wound bed under the pressure of the transducer head. Make sure that the size of the film dressing is larger than the wound, so that the stress of the stretching does not pull the adhesive away from the skin. Using US transmission gel on the surface of the film makes gliding of the head easier.

Another method of coupling is use of underwater application. This method is useful for transmission of US, especially if the region to be treated is irregular and can be conveniently placed in the container. This includes the foot, ankle, hand, and elbow. In Europe, US at the kHz frequency is often delivered via a water bath, so that the wound can be cleaned and debrided by it. Kilohertz US applied in a water bath is reported to stimulate the healing of chronic venous ulcers[71] and facilitates the debridement of bacteria- and particulate-contaminated wounds.[64,104]

A metal whirlpool tank or basin should **not** be used to hold the water because the metal reflects sound energy and increases the intensity in the body area near the metal. A plastic or rubber basin or tub would be acceptable. Eliminate air bubbles by running the water and letting it stand for a few minutes before using it for US transmission. The applicator head and the body part must be submerged throughout the treatment, and the applicator should not touch the skin. Avoiding contact would be advantageous if the treatment area is painful. If possible, select a large container, such as a baby's plastic bathtub, where the target tissues can be placed at a significant distance from the applicator. At that distance, the target tissues will be in the far field, where the spatial intensity is more uniform. While there is no evidence of harm, it is suggested that you wear waterproof gloves that trap US reflecting air, so as to minimize your exposure to the US energy.

Manipulation of the Applicator

To avoid exposing tissue to regions of high intensity, move the MHz applicator throughout treatment. In the near field, where most treatments occur, the spatial peak intensity can be more than three times the SA. It is also essential to avoid excessive exposure to the peaks of pressure variation that

---

EXHIBIT 26.3

Wound Dressing MHz US Transmission Rates

Dressing Product US	Transmission Rate
Hydrogels	
Nu-Gel	77.2% (±4.6%)
ClearSite	72% (±2.2%)
Aquasorb Border	45.3% (±2.1%)
CarraDress	42.8% (±5.9%)
Film Dressings	
CarraSmart Film	60.5% (±4.4%)
J & J Bioclusive	53.2% (±2.4%)
Tegaderm	47.1% (±2.3%)
Opsite Flexigrid	31.5% (±4%)

Reprinted from Klucinec, B., et al. Effectiveness of wound care products in the transmission of acoustic energy. *Physical Therapy*. 2000;80(5):469–476, © with permission of the American Physical Therapy Association.

CLINICAL WISDOM

Application of the Transducer can Alter Results

Treat an area that is appropriate for the size of the transducer head. Traverse each area slowly with the face of the transducer interfacing with the tissue.

occur in *standing wave fields* produced by the interaction of incident and reflected waves of US. Standing waves can damage tissue components, endothelial cells in particular, and exposure to them must, therefore, be avoided. Move the applicator in short linear strokes a few centimeters long (3–4 cm/s) ensuring that they overlap, so that the entire region is treated. Alternatively, use small circular movements, also overlapping, so that the movement is essentially spiral. Treatment area should be two to three times the ERA of the transducer to produce therapeutic results with MHz US. Time needs to be selected that will apply a therapeutic dose of the energy to each area appropriately.

Setup for Treatment

- Explain the procedure to the patient and the caregiver.
- Place the patient in a comfortable position that can be maintained for up to 15 minutes
- Remove clothing from the area to be treated.
- Warm US gel by placing it in a warmer or between folds of a hot pack—always test a drop for temperature before applying to the patient.
- Remove the wound dressing, unless it is a dressing that is to be left in place. Check for bubbles under the dressing and

bleed them from the edges, if present by lifting the edge and squeezing out the air.
- Use either as a periwound treatment or direct application over a film, as described above.
- Treat deep wounds by a periwound application around the margins of the wound.
- Keep the sound head perpendicular to the surface in complete contact with the surface area throughout the treatment (Fig. 26.21).

Special Applications of HFUS
- #### Use US for Blisters

Treating blisters with US promotes absorption of the hemorrhagic material beneath the blister and healing of superficial and partial-thickness wounds. Absorption of hemorrhagic material may be due to enhanced macrophage activity via acoustic streaming and/or stable cavitation effecting thrombolysis. Use the protocol for acute inflammation and apply as a periwound application or in a water bath. Continue after the blister roof is removed as long as hemorrhagic material continues to be absorbed. Hemorrhagic material should shrink in size daily; when it is no longer shrinking, it has probably necrosed and will need to be debrided. Figure 26.22A–C illustrate a case in which US was the only treatment intervention, aside from a transparent film dressing, until it was determined that the focal area of necrosis needed debridement

- #### Sonication of Undermined/Tunneled Areas

One-MHz US is a very useful means to treat undermined/tunneled areas surrounding wounds. These areas can be "mapped" on the skin surface with a marker pen (see Chapter 4 for more information about measuring undermining and tunneled areas) to guide the treatment. Imagine the wound with a grid over the area, or use a plastic screen with cm markings and divide the wound into quarters at the 12:00, 3:00, 6:00, and 9:00 positions. Depending on the size of the applicator, sonicate at the rate of 1 minute per cm². For example, a 5 cm² applicator would be used to stimulate a 25 cm² wound area for 5 minutes.

Aftercare

If HFUS is used and the dressing is left intact, all that is required is to clean off excess US transmission gel/lotion. If a new dressing is to be applied, do so as soon as possible to avoid chilling of the wound tissues and slowing of epithelial migration and mitotic cell activity.

After use, handle the US applicator of both HFUS and LFUS devices carefully to avoid environmental contamination. Place the applicator in a rubber glove and transport it to a dirty sink area for cleansing with cold tap water and soap. Then disinfect per facility and manufacturer policies and procedures. It is useful to have two applicators, so that one can be used while the other is being disinfected, thus reducing down time.

HFUS and Acute Wounds

The onset, duration, and intensity of treatment vary for acute and chronic wounds.

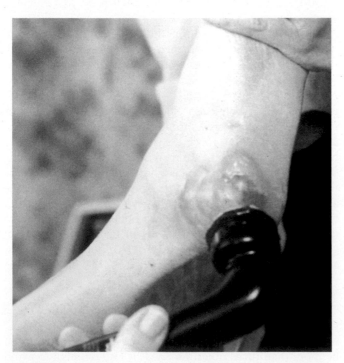

FIGURE 26.21 Periblister application of US gel.

CASE STUDY

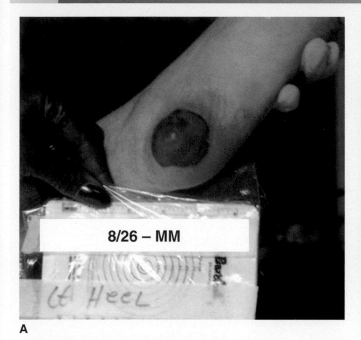

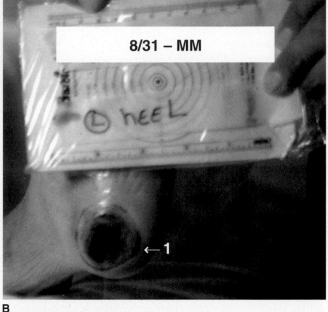

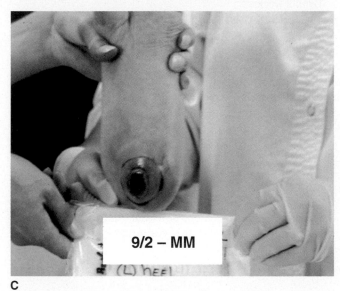

FIGURE 26.22 A. Wound Healing with US. Acute inflammatory phase. Blister with bloody fluid at day of identification. (Copyright © C. Sussman.) **B.** Same wound as in (A) without blister roof. The periwound skin was treated with daily US for 4 days prior. Note area of apparent necrosis and hematoma. There is an absence of inflammatory phase. (Copyright © C. Sussman.) **C.** Same wound as in (A) and (B) after two additional periwound US treatments. Note absorption of hematoma by reduced size of necrotic area and mild erythema surrounding the area of necrosis. The wound is acute inflammatory phase. (Copyright © C. Sussman.)

Blood Blister on the Heel Treated with US

Patient: M.M. Age: 83 years

Functional Outcome Report: Initial Assessment

Reason for Referral

The patient was referred to the physical therapist because the nursing staff had identified a blood blister on a heel.

Medical History

The patient had a below-the-knee amputation on the other leg due to peripheral vascular disease. The limb with the blister was thus at risk for amputation, and early intervention was

requested for limb salvage. Patient was alert/confused and nonambulatory. She could reposition but not consistently. She had a history of a cerebrovascular accident. The following medical problems are associated with this request for service.

Functional Diagnosis and Targeted Outcomes
Integumentary Examination

The surrounding skin on the heel was erythematous, edematous, and tender. There was a large blood-filled blister on the heel of the intact limb.

Wound Tissue Examination

The wound was covered with a bloody, fluid-filled blister. Bloody fluid suggests rupture of vessels beneath the blister.

It was an unstageable pressure ulcer with a suspicion of deep tissue injury.

Functional Diagnosis

Wound in acute inflammatory phase; targeted outcome: debridement of blister, conservation of healthy tissue under the blister; determine level and extent of tissue damage, due date: 2 weeks.

Associated Impairment

Suspicion of necrotic tissue beneath blister; targeted outcome: clean wound bed; due date: 4 weeks.

Functional Diagnosis

Impairment of integument, depth to be determined; targeted outcome: exhibits granulation tissue; due date: 6 weeks.

Vascular Examination

Visual examination showed an inflammatory response to wounding. Palpation indicated weak but palpable pulses. Because of the prior vascular history, the presence of peripheral vascular disease was assumed.

Functional Diagnosis

Vascular impairment; targeted outcome: enhanced perfusion; due date: 2 weeks.

Musculoskeletal Examination

The patient is nonambulatory, has limited mobility in bed, and needs verbal cues to reposition. Motor impairment from the stroke limits her mobility. Her Braden Risk Score is 15, indicating risk for pressure ulcers.

Functional Diagnosis

Undue susceptibility to pressure ulceration; targeted outcome: pressure elimination; due date: immediately.

Evaluation

The patient's loss of function in these systems is responsible for the undue susceptibility to skin breakdown on the legs and inability to heal without integumentary intervention. The patient has improvement potential, and the wound will heal with intervention to bring perfusion to tissues and relieve pressure.

Need for Skilled Services

The patient has a prior history of failed wound healing leading to amputation. Intervention that will enhance wound tissue perfusion to conserve tissues underneath the blister and stimulate healing will be required. Wound dressings will not address these issues. The blister needs to be debrided to assess tissue damage. Thrombolysis and absorption of hemorrhagic materials will conserve healthy tissues and result in a healed wound.

Treatment Plan

- Apply periwound nonthermal US to accelerate the inflammatory phase and promote absorption of hemorrhagic material (0.5 W/cm^2 [SATP] 1 MHz, 20% duty cycle pulsed for 5 minutes).
- Sharply debride the blister roof.
- Continue US until the extent of the wound depth is determined.

Outcomes

Periwound US and debridement were begun on August 26. On August 31, the blister was debrided, and a large hemorrhagic/necrotic area was seen under the tissues; inflammation in the surrounding tissues was subsiding. On September 2, there was a 50% reduction in the size of the hemorrhagic area and resolution of the inflammation in the surrounding tissues. Minimal reduction in the area of the hematoma in next 2 weeks indicated that the tissues had necrosed and debridement began. On October 8, the wound was progressing to the proliferative phase; there was a small area of necrosis. The US seemed to have had maximum benefit and treatment was changed to HVPC.

Discussion

Removal of the blister roof identified an area of focal necrosis or hematoma. The only other treatment intervention was transparent film dressing. The size of the hematoma was reduced 50% with seven US treatments. Inflammation was accelerated, and the wound progressed to the proliferative phase. At this point, treatment was changed to HVPC. Closure was achieved on November 2.

Onset

Begin as soon as possible, ideally within a few hours of injury, but always during the inflammatory phase of healing. As mentioned previously, treatment with MHz US during this phase has been shown to result in the liberation of stimulatory growth factors from platelets, mast cells, and macrophages, with the result that the inflammatory phase is accelerated, the proliferative and remodeling phases occur earlier, and the scar tissue becomes stronger. If treatment is delayed beyond the inflammatory phase, the strength of the scar tissue is not affected.[22]

Duration

Determine the duration of treatment on the surface area to be treated. The area is divided into zones, each 1.5 times the area of the ERA of the applicator, with 1 to 2 minutes being allowed for treating each zone. Some clinicians recommend 1 minute per cm^2. The maximum treatment time should be no longer than 15 minutes. If the wound is large, two sessions per day, one for each section of the wound, would be preferable. Three treatments per week have been found to be effective.

Intensity

In the interest of safety, the lowest possible intensity should be used. This is usually near the upper end of the low range (0.01–0.05). Note that, to obtain a significant increase in temperature, an I(SATA) of at least 0.5 W per cm^2 is required, but that primarily nonthermal effects can be achieved with lower SATA intensities, obtained by pulsing I(SATP) 0.5 W per cm^2 at, for example, 2 milliseconds on, 8 milliseconds off. Treatments should be pulsed if the local circulation is compromised and might be unable to dissipate heat efficiently.

Chronic Wounds

- *Onset.* Begin as soon as possible.
- *Duration.* Duration is the same as that for acute wounds.
- *Intensity.* Generally an I(SATA) at approximately the middle of the medium range is recommended (e.g., 0.5–1.0 W/cm² SA, TP). Pulsing should be used. Repair can be initiated by using *one* treatment at the upper end of the medium range (e.g., 1.2 W/cm²), after which lower intensities in the medium range are used, as described above. It has been suggested that the higher intensity may produce local trauma, followed by acute inflammation, which is necessary to initiate healing. Note that this hypothesis requires testing.

Frequency Selection

Equipment now on the market allows more flexibility in choosing US frequencies.

Consider the following when selecting a frequency for treatment:

- If the lesion is superficial, a higher frequency is appropriate because high-frequency US is absorbed superficially.
- Although it is not readily available in many clinics, kHz US is another frequency in use in select wound care centers. We examined the primary differences between kHz and MHz US earlier in this chapter. Points to remember are that kHz US is less attenuated, being less readily absorbed than MHz, and is readily transmitted through metal implants and bone; Nevertheless, sufficient absorption occurs to produce a stimulatory effect at the cellular and tissue levels.
- High frequencies (1 MHz or greater) are used if thermal changes are required in the tissues to increase blood flow, but evidence shows that LFUS changes the microcirculation mechanisms significantly.
- Lower frequencies (<1 MHz or kHz) are more appropriate if primarily nonthermal effects, such as stable cavitation and/or acoustic streaming, are required.

Low-Frequency Noncontact Ultrasound and Chronic Wounds

There is limited testing of protocols used with low-frequency noncontact US (**LFNCUS**) devices. Based on a review of case and retrospective studies reporting use of the Mist® Therapy System (Celleration, Eden Prairie, MN), protocols were listed as follows:[10,15,18]

Device: 40 kHz MIST

Time: wound size (10–180 cm²) dependent 3 to 20 minutes per session

Intensity: 0.1 to 0.8 W per cm².[63]

Frequency: two to three times per week

LFUS (25 kHz) Sonica 180 Policy and Procedure for Wound Debridement

The following clinical policy and application procedure for use of the Sonica 180 ultrasonic wound debridement system was developed by Mary M. Verhage, RN, BSN, CWOCN (Verhage, MM, *personal communication*, 2006.).

It has been used successfully in the wound clinic where she works and is provided here with the author's permission. However, the author notes that the use of this modality for wound treatment is in its infancy and the insights gained with repeated use are yet to be discovered.

Purpose

To provide a method of wound debridement that produces optimal removal of nonviable tissue and enhances wound healing by stimulating the viable cell through the use of guided US.

Policy

This policy provides guidelines for ultrasonic assisted wound therapy and debridement with the Söring Sonoca 180™ (Fig. 26.13).

1. LFUS assisted wound therapy (LFUSAW) is initiated by physician order and includes location to be treated and frequency of treatments (e.g., treatment of ulcer on right leg, PRN until necrotic tissue is removed).
2. Ultrasonic assisted wound therapy Söring Sonoca 180™ treatment is only to be administered by trained, licensed providers; MD, PA, APNP, PT, and trained RN.
3. Wounds are considered contaminated; therefore, LFUSAW treatments are considered clean, not sterile. The only time LFUSAW should be done using sterile technique is in the operating room when utilized prior to wound closure.
4. The Söring Sonoca 180™ user's manual is to be available for reference by the practitioner when the Sonoca is in use.

Equipment

1. Söring Sonoca 180 and probe attachment
2. Irrigation solution; 1,000 cc IV infusion bag of 0.9% NaCl, Ringer lactate, or other premixed solution as ordered. Primary and secondary IV tubing with drip chamber.
3. Personal protective equipment (PPE): gloves, fluid-resistant gown, face mask, eye protection, and shoe covers.
4. Equipment protection: disposable plastic covers
5. Disposable absorbent pads with impermeable layer
6. Suction equipment
7. Dressing change materials

Indications

- Locally infected wounds
- Wounds with impaired circulation
- Wounds with the need for debridement, irrigation, and topical treatment
- Pressure ulcers, diabetic foot ulcers, lower extremity diabetic ulcers, venous ulcers

Contraindications

- Untreated advancing cellulitis with signs of systemic response
- Wounds with metal components such as joint replacements, plates and screws, or implanted electronic devices within the treatment field
- Uncontrolled pain

Precautions

1. The thermal effects of US are multiplied if the sound waves are allowed to reflect back up to the probe tip, creating a standing wave.
2. Avoid putting the probe tip on intact skin without the fluid medium or it may create a burn.

3. The only irrigant that has been tested and approved for use with this device is 0.9% NaCl IV solution. Other potential choices, such as antibiotics, have not been tested and could potentially induce harm.

Key Points/Information

- Physician or other appropriately licenses health practitioner to assess patient and wound status to determine wound treatment and write or obtain orders.
- Establish expected outcome of treatment: for example, wound will be relieved of bioburden in X amount of time.
- Follow standard precautions for use of PPE for protection from dripping, splashing, and aerosolization of fluids.
- If patient is in contact isolation for a resistant organism, follow precautions infection control procedures per facility policy.
- Document predebridement wound condition; measure length, width, and depth; photograph.
- Premedicate with systemic analgesic or local anesthetic for example, lidocaine; use as directed prior to procedure, reassess pain frequently.
- Use one standard irrigant, sterile 0.9% NaCl IV solution.
- Use the angled horseshoe-shaped probe with a large flat surface for to lift or wedge under thick necrotic tissue or eschar to separate it from viable tissue.
- Use double ball tip probe to treat tunnels, cavities, and undermining.

Procedure

1. Obtain physician order as noted above.
2. Explain procedure to the patient.
3. Assess patient's comfort, current pain level, history of pain with debridement, and current analgesic regimen. Provide premedication for pain.
4. Obtain appropriate Sonoca Sonotrode attachment from sterile processing.
5. Set up the Sonoca machine as illustrated in user's manual, hang irrigation solution, and prime IV tubing. Attach probe to US cable and tubing to probe.
6. Position patient, the wound, and the operator for comfort and accessibility.
7. Protect patient and clothing with absorbent pads (chux).
8. Provide adequate lighting.
9. Wash hands and apply PPE gloves, mask, fluid-resistant gown, eye protection, and shoe covers. Apply equipment-protective covering.
10. Prime US wand with irrigant, set drip rate and use to wet surface of the wound before the start of treatment. DO NOT OPERATE SONOCA WITHOUT IRRIGATION FLUID. In order for US waves to be transmitted, the probe tip must be in contact with fluid or moist wound. Fluid is also needed to dissipate heat.
11. Turn unit on and set intensity to begin treatment. Activate US by depressing foot pedal.
    a. Start at low intensity and increase as patient tolerates. Power may be decreased to 20% or increased to 80% or 100% according to patient tolerance and tissue needs.
    b. Place probe in contact with wound bed/irrigant. Fluid placed on the wound bed will "bubble," but although heat is produced, do not confuse this bubbling with boiling. With probe in contact with fluid or wound

---

> **CLINICAL WISDOM**
>
> WARNING! To avoid burns, do not touch the metal tip of any of the low-frequency US debridement devices mentioned here.

bed, pass the probe tip with a slow continuous motion across the entire wound surface. DO NOT STOP IN ONE SPOT. Instead, sweep over and return for repeated treatment.

12. Continue the sweeping motion until treatment goals for the session are reached.
13. Treatment time: 20 seconds per cm^2 wound area
14. Limit the time of procedure to patient and clinician tolerance; discontinue if not tolerated because of pain, or when goals of treatment are achieved.
15. Turn off machine.
16. Gently wipe dry periwound tissue.
17. Assess patient condition and wound, measure and photograph as indicated.
18. Apply dressing or advanced therapy to wound as ordered.
19. Document procedure: location, treatment, dressing applied, intensity, duration, irrigation solution, patient tolerance, wound status after treatment.

Post Procedure

1. Remove equipment protection covering prior to moving it from area of use.
2. Wipe connector lines with facility-approved disinfectant.
3. Remove PPE and dispose of properly.
4. Have treatment room cleaned prior to next client use.
5. Remove Sonoca wand and probe tip.
6. Prepare for sterile processing of the tips used per user's manual/facility recommendations.

Figure 26.23A–C show a venous ulcer before, during, and after 5 minutes of debridement with Söring Sonoca 180.[62]

Adjunctive Treatments

Several attempts at using US with adjunctive treatments were discussed under the clinical studies section. However, we do not know enough about combining treatments to make a recommendation to do this or to offer protocols to follow.

SELF-CARE TEACHING GUIDELINES

US should *not* be taught to a patient or a caregiver as a home treatment. Although it appears very innocuous, US can result in tissue damage if performed by improperly trained and unsupervised individuals.

DOCUMENTATION

Documentation of US treatment outcomes is extremely valuable. The cases documented below are examples of the

A

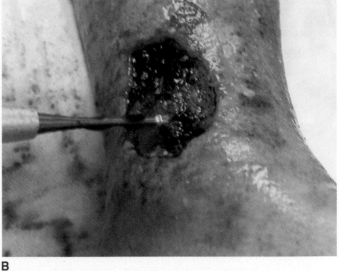

B

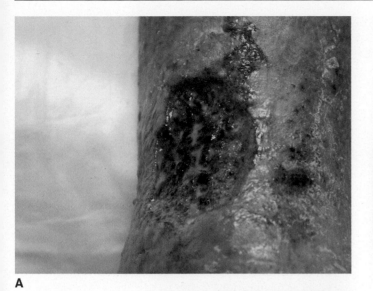

C

FIGURE 26.23 **A.** Venous Ulcer before treatment with Söring Sonoca 180. (Courtesy of Mary Verhage RN, BSN, CWOCN, with permission.) **B.** Venous Ulcer during treatment with Söring Sonoca 180 (Courtesy of Mary Verhage RN, BSN, CWOCN, with permission.) **C.** Venous Ulcer after treatment with Söring Sonoca 180 (Courtesy of Mary Verhage RN, BSN, CWOCN, with permission.)

value of recording on film those changes in wound healing that are produced by selected interventions. In both cases, US was the only intervention given. For example, it would be difficult to do a controlled, double-blind study of patients with new hematoma formation, as in the Case Study 26.1 (Figure 26.11). A single-subject design study would be one method of developing a body of knowledge about clinical outcomes. Another Case Study (Figure 26.22) was done to determine how US affects hematoma formation under a blister. Photography was done every 2 days to track the change in the hematoma. These are just two examples of many ways that you can present information about treatment interventions and advance clinical practice as part of the documentation process.

REVIEW QUESTIONS

1. Which statement is correct regarding low-frequency US?
   A. The wavelengths are shorter than high-frequency US.
   B. Depth of penetration is equal to low-frequency US.
   C. It can penetrate deeper than HFUS.
   D. It is only used for contact delivery methods.
2. Which frequency allows the penetration of energy into deeper tissues (up to 5 cm)?
   A. 1 MHz
   B. 3 MHz
   C. Therapeutic KHz
   D. All of the above
3. Early intervention with US:
   A. Reduces the inflammatory phase by being an antiinflammatory agent
   B. Stimulates the release of growth factors from platelets and macrophages

   C. Accelerates the inflammatory and postpones the proliferative phase
   D. Impairs degranulation of mast cells while influencing scar density
4. US can be useful for
   A. Thrombolysis and pain reduction in skin tears
   B. Controlling periwound edema and absorption of hematoma
   C. Removal of bacterial contamination and debridement of bioburden
   D. All of the above
5. Which is a precaution and not a contraindication to US?
   A. Over malignancies and precancerous lesions
   B. On patients with vascular abnormalities
   C. In acute infections
   D. Deep vein thrombosis

REFERENCES

1. National Pressure Ulcer Advisory Panel and European Pressure Ulcer Advisory Panel (EPUAP). *Pressure Ulcers Prevention and Treatment: Clinical Practice Guideline*, Washington, DC: National Pressure Ulcer Advisory Panel; 2009.
2. Cullum NA, Al-Kurdi D, et al. Therapeutic ultrasound for venous leg ulcers. *Cochrane Database Syst Rev*. 2010 Issue 6. Art. No.: CD001180. DOI: 10.1002/14651858.CD001180.pub3.
3. Reddy M, Gill SS, et al. Treatment of pressure ulcers a systematic review *JAMA*. 2008;300(22):2647–2662.
4. Ennis WJ, Formann P, Mozen N, et al. Ultrasound therapy for recalcitrant diabetic foot ulcers: results of a randomized, double-blind, controlled, multicenter study. *Ostomy Wound Manage*. 2005;51(8):24–39.
5. Cameron MH. Ultrasound. In: *Physical Agents in Rehabilitation*. Cameron MH, eds. Philadelphia, PA: WB Saunders; 1999:275–276.
6. Ziskin MC, Michlovitz SL. Therapeutic ultrasound. In: Michlovitz SL, ed. *Thermal Agents in Rehabilitation*. Philadelphia, PA: F.A. Davis; 1990.
7. Serena T, Lee SK, et al. The impact of noncontact, nonthermal, low-frequency ultrasound on bacterial counts in experimental and chronic wounds. *Ostom Wound Manage*. 2009;55(1):22–30.
8. Ramundo J, Gray M. Is ultrasonic mist therapy effective for debriding chronic wounds? *Wound Ostomy Continence Nurs*. 2008;35(6):579–583.
9. Lai J, Pittelkow MR. Physiological effects of ultrasound mist on fibroblasts. *Int J Dermatol*. 2007;46:587–593.
10. Haan J, Lucich S. A retrospective analysis of acoustic pressurewound therapy: effects on the healing progression of chronic wounds. *J Am Coll Certif Wound Spec*. 2009;1:28–34.
11. Sullivan PK, Conner-Kerr T. Effectiveness of non-contact mist ultrasound therapy (MUST). In: Removal of *Pseudomonas aeruginosa* in vitro. Presented at the Symposium for Advanced Wound Care and Medical Research Forum on Wound Repair, Las Vegas; 2001.
12. Misonex Inc. How Sonicators Work. Available at: www.misonix.com. Last accessed January 6, 2006.
13. Cole PS, Quisberg J, Melin MM. Adjuvant use of acoustic pressure wound therapy for treatmentof chronic wounds a retrospective analysis. *J Wound Ostomy Continence Nurs*. 2009;36(2):171–177.

14. Howell-Taylor M, Hall MG, et al. Negative pressure wopund therapy combined with acoustic pressure wouynd therapy for infected post surgery wounds: a case series. *Ostom Wound Manage*. 2008;54(9):49–52.
15. Liguori PA, Peters KL, et al. Combination of negative pressure wound therapy and acoustic pressure wound therapy for treatment of infected surgical wounds: a case series. *Ostom Wound Manage*. 2008;54(5):50–53.
16. Samies J, Gehling M. Acoustic pressure wound therapy for managemet of mixed partial and full-thickness burns in a rural wound center. *Ostom Wound Manage*. 2008;54(3):56–59.
17. Fleming, CP. Acoutsitc pressure wound therapy in the treatment of vasculopathy-associated digital ulcer: a case study. *Ostom Wound Manage*. 2008;54(4):62–65.
18. Lasko, J, Kochiik J, Serena T. Combining acoustic pressure wound therapy with electrical stimulation for treatment of chronic lower extremity ulcers: a case series. *Adv Skin Wound Care*. 2010;23(10):446–449.
19. Dyson M. Mechanisms involved in therapeutic ultrasound. *Physiother J Chartered Soc Physiother*. 1987;73(3):8.
20. Dyson M, Young SR. Acceleration of tissue repair by low intensity ultrasound applied during the inflammatory phase. Presented at the meeting of American Physical Therapy Association and Canadian Physical Therapy Association; Toronto; 1988.
21. Dyson M. Role of ultrasound in wound healing. In: McCulloch JM, Kloth LC, Feedar JA, eds. *Wound Healing: Alternatives in Management*. 2nd ed. Philadelphia, PA: FA Davis; 1995.
22. Hart J. The *Effect of Therapeutic Ultrasound on Dermal Repair with Emphasis on Fibroblasts Activity*. London: University of London; 1993.
23. Sussman C. Ultrasound for Wound Healing. In: *Monograph*. Houston, TX: The Chattanooga Group; 1993.
24. Young SR, L D, Dyson M, et al. The effects of therapeutic ultrasound on angiogenesis. *Ultrasound Med Biol*. 1990;16:261–269.
25. De Deyne PG, Kirsch-Volders. M. In vitro effects of therapeutic ultrasound on the nucleus of human fibroblasts. *Phys Ther*. 1995;75(7):629–634.
26. Emsen IM. The effect of ultrasound on flap survival: an experimental study in rats. *Burns*. 2007;33:369–371.

27. Frieder S, Weisberg J, Flemming B, et al. The therapeutic effects of ultrasound following partial rupture of Achilles tendons in male rats. *J Orthop Sports Phys Ther.* 1988;10:39–46.

28. Jackson BA, Schwane JA, Starcher BC. Effect of ultrasound therapy on the repair of Achilles tendon injuries in rats. *Med Sci Sports Exerc.* 1991;23:171–176.

29. Byl N, Hopf H. The use of oxygen in wound healing. In: McCulloch J, Kloth L, Feedar JA, eds. *Wound Healing: Alternatives in Management.* 2nd ed. Philadelphia, PA: FA Davis; 1996.

30. Bertuglia S. Mechanisms by which low-intensity ultrasound improve tolerance to ischemia-reperfusion injury. *Ultrasound Med Biol.* 2007;33(5):663–671.

31. Fornage BD, Deshayes JL. Ultrasound of normal skin. *J Clin Ultrasound.* 1986;14:619.

32. Daffertshofer M, Gass A, et al. Transcranial low-frequency ultrasound-mediated thrombolysis in brain ischemia: increased risk of hemorrhage with combined ultrasound and tissue plasminogen activator: results of a Phase II Clinical Trial. *Stroke.* 2005;36(7):1441–1446.

33. Tsivgoulis G, Eggers J, et al. Safety and efficacy of ultrasound-enhanced thrombolysis: a comprehensive review and meta-analysis of randomized and nonrandomized studies. *Stroke.* 2010;41(2):280–287.

34. Luo H, Nishioka T, et al. Transcutaneous ultrasound augments lysis of arterial thrombi in vivo. *Circulation.* 1996;94:775–778.

35. Hajri Z, Boukadoum M, Hamam H, et al. An investigation of the physical forces leading to thrombosis disruption by cavitation. *J Thromb Thrombolysis.* 2005;20(1):27–32.

36. Stanisic MM, Provo BJ, Larson DL, et al. Wound debridement with 25 kHz ultrasound. *Adv Skin Wound Care.* 2005;18(9):484–490.

37. Suchkova V, Carstensen EL, Francis CW. ultrasound enhancement of fibrinolysis at frequencies of 27–100 kHz. *Ultrasound Med Biol.* 2002;28(3):377–382.

38. Riggs PN, Francis CW, Bartos SR, et al. Ultrasound enhancement of rabbit femoral artery thrombolysis. *Cardiovasc Surg.* 1997;5(2):201–207.

39. McDiarmid T, Burns P. Clinical applications of therapeutic ultrasound. *Physiother J Chartered Soc Physiother.* 1987;73(4):14–21.

40. Parish CP. Decubitus ulcers: how to intervene effectively. *Drug Ther.* 1983.

41. Berna-Serna JD, Sanchez-Garre J, Madrigal M, et al. Ultrasound therapy in rectus sheath hematoma. *Phys Ther.* 2005;85(4):352–357.

42. Flemming K, Cullum N. Therapeutic ultrasound for venous leg ulcers (Review). *Cochrane Database Syst Rev.* 2000(4. Art.):No.: CD001180. DOI: 001110.001002/14651858.CD14001180.

43 West BR, Nichter LS, Halpern DE, et al. Ultrasound debridement of trabeculated bone: effective and atraumatic. *Plast Reconstr Surg.* 1994;93:561–566.

44. Breuing KH, Bayer L, Neuwalder J, et al. Early experience using low-frequency ultrtasound in chronic wounds. *Ann Plast Surg.* 2005;55(2):183–187.

45. Schoenbach SF, Song IC. Ultrasonic debridement: a new approach in the treatment of burn wounds. *Plast Reconstr Surg.* 1980;66:34.

46. Tan J, Abisi S, et al. A painless method of ultrasonically assisted debridement of chronic leg ulcers: a pilot study. *Eur J Vasc Endovasc Surg.* 2007;33:234E–238E.

47. Dinno MA, Young SR, Mortimer AJ, et al. The significance of membrane changes in the safe and effective use of therapeutic and diagnostic ultrasound. *Phys Med Biol.* 1989;34(11):1543–1552.

48. Qian Z, Sagers R, Pitt WG. Investigation of the mechanism of the bioacoustic effect. *J Biomed Mater Res.* 1999;44(2):198–205.

49. Atland OD, Daleck D, Suchkova VN, et al. Low-intensity ultrasound increases endothelial cell nitric oxide synthase activity and nitric oxide synthesis. *J Thromb Haemost.* 2004;2:637–643.

50. Reher P, Harris M, Whitemea M, et al. Ultrasound stimulates nitric oxide and protaglandin E2 production by human osteoblasts. *Bone.* 2002;31(1):236–241.

51. Witte M, Barbul A. General principles of wound healing. *Surg Clin North Am.* 1997;77(3):509–528.

52. Shamberger RC, Talbot TL, Tipton HW, et al. The effect of ultrasonic and thermal treatment on wounds. *Plast Reconstr Surg.* 1981;68(6):860–869.

53. Cambier DC, Vanderstraeten GG. Failure of therapuetic ultrasound in healing burn injuries. *Burns.* 1997;23(3):248–249.

54. Byl N, McKenze A, Wong T, et al. Incisional wound healing: a controlled study of low and high dose ultrasound. *Orthop Sports Phys Ther.* 1993;18:619–628.

55. Taskan I, Ozyazgan I, Tercan M, et al. A comparative study of the effect of ultrasound and electrostimulation on wound healing in rats. *Plast Reconstr Surg.* 1997;100(4):966–972.

56. Bennett M. Report of the task force on the implications for darkly pigmented intact skin in the prediction and prevention of pressure ulcers. *Adv Wound Care.* 1995;8:34–35.

57. Serena T. Wound closure and gradual involution of an infantile hemangioma using a noncontact, low frequency ultrasound therapy. *Ostom Wound Manage.* 2008;54(2):68–71.

58. Gehling M, Samies J. The effect of noncontact, low-intensity, low-frequency therapeutic ultrasound on lower extremity chronic wound pain: a retrospective chart review. *Ostom Wound Manage.* 2007;53(3):44–50.

59. Mitragotri S, Kost J. Low-frequency sonophoresis: a review. *Adv Drug Deliv Rev.* 2004;56(5):589–601.

60. Nicter LS, Williams J. Ultrasonic wound debridement. *J Hand Surg.* 1988;13A(1):142–146.

61. Niezgoda JA, Verhage MM, Walek D, et al. Clinical experience using ultrasonic assisted wound treatment. Presented at the Symposium for Advanced Wound Care, Las Vegas; 2003.

62. Verhage MM, Niezgoda JA, Nelson KM, et al. Ultrasonic-assisted wound tratment: a novel technique for wound debridement. Presented at the Symposium for Advanced Wound Care, Las Vegas; 2003.

63. Kavros SJ, Schenck EC. Use of noncontact low-frequency ultrasound in the treatment of chronic foot and leg ulcerations: a 51-patient analysis. *J am Podiatr Med Assoc.* 2007;97(2):95–101.

64. Ward RS, Hayes-Lundy C, Reddy R, et al. Evaluation of topical therapeutic ultrasound to improve response to physical therapy and lessen scar contracture after burn injury. *J Burn Care Rehabil.* 1994;15(1):74–79.

65. Paul BJ, Lafrattta CW, Dawson RA, et al. Use of ultrasound in the treatment of pressure sores in patients with spinal cord injury. *Arch Phys Med Rehabil.* 1960;41:438–440.

66. McDiarmid T, Burns P, Lewith GT, et al. Ultrasound and the treatment of pressure sores. *Physiotherapy.* 1985;71(2):66–70.

67. Nussbaum EL, Biemann I, Mustard B. Comparison of ultrasound/ultraviolet C and laser for treatment of pressure ulcers in patients with spinal cord injury. *Phys Ther.* 1994;74:812–825.

68. ter Riet G, Kessels AGH, Knipschild P. A randomized clinical trial of ultrasound in the treatment of pressure ulcers. *Phys Ther.* 1996;76:1301–1312.

69. Dyson M, Franks C, Suckling J. Stimulation of venous ulcers by ultrasound. *Ultrasonics.* 1976;14:232–236.

70. Weichenthal M, Mohr P, Stegman W, et al. Low-frequency ultrasound treatment of chronic venous ulcers. *Wound Repair Regen.* 1997;5:18–22.

71. Peschen M, Weichenthal M, Schopf E, et al. Low frequency ultrasound treatment of chronic venous leg ulcers in an outpatient therapy. *Acta Derm Venereol.* 1997;77(4):311–314.

72. Young SR, Lynch JA, Leipins PJ, et al. ultrasound imaging: a non-invasive method of wound assessment. In: Proceedings of the Second Conference on Advances in Wound Management. London: Macmillan Press; 1992.

73. Roche C, West J. A controlled trial investigating the effect of ultrasound on venous ulcers referred from general practitioners. *Physiotherapy.* 1984;70(12):475–477.

74. Lundberg T, Nordstrom F, Brodda-Jansen G, et al. Pulsed ultrasound does not improve healing of venous ulcers. *Scand J Rehabil Med.* 1990;22(4):195–197.

75. Callam MJ, Harper DR, Dale JJ, et al. A controlled trial of weekly ultrasound therapy in chronic leg ulceration. *Lancet.* 1987;2(8552):204–206.

76. Johannsen F, Gam AN, Karsmark T. Ultrasound therapy in chronic leg ulceration: a meta-analysis. *Wound Repair Regen.* 1998;6:121–126.

77. Eriksson S, Lundberg T, Malm M. A placebo controlled trial of ultrasound therapy in chronic leg ulceration. *Scand J Rehabil Med.* 1991;23(4):211–213.

78. Ebrecht M, Hextall J, Kirtley LG, et al. Perceived stress and cortisol levels predict speed of wound healing in healthy male adults. *Psychoneuroendocrinol.* 2004;29:798–809.

79. Johnson S. Low-frequency ultrasound to manage chronic venous leg ulcers. *Br J Nurs.* 2003;12(19 suppl):s14–s24.

80. Dolibog P, Franek A, et al. Efficiency of therapeutic ultrasound for healing venous leg ulcer in surgically-treated patients. *Wounds Compend Clin Res Pract.* 2008;20(12):334–340.

81. Watson JM, Kang'ombe AR, et al. "Use of weekly, low dose, high frequency ultrasound for hard to heal venous leg ulcers: the VenUS III randomised controlled trial. *BMJ.* 2011;342:1–9. d1092 doi:10.1136/bmj.d1092:

82. Simpson SL, Hertzog MS, Barja RH. The plantaris tendon graft: an ultrasound study. *J Hand Surg.* 1991;16:708–711.

83. O'Reilly MAR, Massouh H. Pictorial review: the sonographic diagnosis of pathology in the Achilles tendon. *Clin Radiol.* 1993;48:202–206.

84. Karim A, Young SR, Lynch JA, et al. A novel method of assessing skin ultrasound scans. *Wounds.* 1994;6:9–15.

85. Gonzalez RC, Wintz P. Digital image processing. In: Gonzalez RC, Winter P, eds. *Digital Image Fundamentals.* Reading, MA: Addison-Wesley; 1987.

86. Bamber JC, Tristam M. The physics of medical imaging. In: Webb S, ed. *Diagnostic Ultrasound.* Bristol, England: Adam Hilger; 1988.

87. Dyson M, Moodley S, Verjee L, et al. Wound healing assessment using 20 MHz ultrasound and photography. *Skin Res Technol.* 2003;9:116–121.

88. Quintavalle PR, Lyder CH, Mertz PJ, et al. Use of high resolution, high frequency diagnostic ultrasound to investigate the pathogenesis of pressure ulcer development. *Adv Skin Wound Care.* 2006;19(9):490–505.

89. Whiston RJ, Young SR, Lynch JA, et al. Application of high frequency ultrasound to the objective assessment of healing wounds. In: Proceedings of the Second Conference on Advances in Wound Management. London: Macmillan Press; 1992.

90. Miller M, Dyson M. *Principles of Wound Care.* London: Macmillan Magazines Ltd.; 1996.

91. Quintavalle PR. Getting a better view with high resolution ultrasound. *Podiatry Today.* 2002;15(10):30–36.

92. Liong JL. High frequency diagnostic ultrasound as an adjunct to irritant patch assessment. Thesis. London: University of London UMDS; 1996.

93. Mertz P. Cost analysis of utilizing high frequency ultrasound technology to manage soft tissue injuries. Thesis. Kennedy-Western University; 2004.

94. Van Holsbeek M, Introcaso JH. Sonography of muscle. In: *Musculoskeletal Ultrasound.* Chicago, IL: Mosby-Yearbook; 1990.

95. Shafir R, Itzchak Y, Heyman Z, et al. Preoperative ultrasonic measurements of the thickness of cutaneous malignant melanoma. *J Ultrasound Med.* 1984;3:205.

96. Breslow A. Thickness, cross-sectional areas and depth of invasion in the prognosis of cutaneous melanoma. *Ann Surg.* 1970;172:902.

97. Graves D. Stage I pressure ulcer in ebony complexion. *Decubitus.* 1990;3:4.

98. Lyder C. Examining the inclusion of ethnic minorities in pressure ulcer prediction studies. *JWOCN.* 1996;23:257–260.

99. Henderson C, Ayello C, Sussman C. Draft definition of stage I pressure ulcers: inclusion of person with darkly pigmented skin. *Adv Wound Care.* 1997;10:34–35.

100. Dyson M, Lyder C. Wound management with physical modalities. In: Morison M, ed. *The Prevention and Treatment of Pressure Ulcers.* Edinburgh: Mosby; 2001.

101. Sackett D. Rules of evidence and clinical recommendations on the use of antithrombotic agents. *Chest.* 1989;95(2):2s–4s.

102. Sicard-Rosenbaum L, Danoff JV, Guthrie JA, et al. Effects of energy-matched pulsed and continuous ultrasound on tumor growth in mice. *Phys Ther.* 1998;78:271–277.

103. Klucinec B, Scheidler M, Denegar C, et al. Effectiveness of wound care products in the transmission of acoustic energy. *Phys Ther.* 2000;80:469–476.

104. McDonald W, Nichter L. Debridement of bacterial and particulate contaminated wounds. *Ann Plast Surg.* 1994;33(2):142–147.

Carrie Sussman

CHAPTER OBJECTIVES

At the completion of this chapter, the reader will be able to:

1. Discuss the mechanisms of heat transfer and the regulation of body temperature.
2. Delineate the physiologic responses of the body to hydrotherapy.
3. Present evidence of the physiological effects of hydrotherapy for wound management.
4. Identify special patient populations and their candidacy for hydrotherapy.
5. Provide guidelines about the risks, benefits, and disadvantages of hydrotherapy.
6. Describe the methods of using hydrotherapy that provides the safest and most effective wound treatment.

Hydrotherapy is the immersion of the body in a water source for therapeutic effect.

Thermotherapy is an integral component of hydrotherapy and the safe and effective use of hydrotherapy depends on proper use of the thermal effects. The mechanisms of heat transfer and regulation, the physiologic responses of the body to hydrotherapy, the efficacy of hydrotherapy for wound management, and the safe and effective methods of application of hydrotherapy are discussed in detail in this chapter. The term hydrotherapy is used here rather than whirlpool because the effects described apply to water immersion in a tank or tub that is used everywhere. Whirlpool is primarily a mode of hydrotherapy used in the United States. Agitation, an important component of whirlpool, adds hydrodynamic features to the hydrotherapy system and will be discussed separately.

HISTORIC USE OF HYDROTHERAPY AND THERMOTHERAPY

The use of water and warmth—hydrotherapy and thermotherapy—for wound healing has been reported in the literature back in ancient times and is still used widely as a traditional therapy in many cultures. Therefore, it is essential to provide current information that aids clinicians everywhere. In current physical medicine wound care practice in the United States, whirlpool is often the hydrotherapy method selected for treating wounds.

Whirlpool hydrotherapy is a form of hydrotherapy in which the patient's body or body part is submerged in water in a tub or tank with underwater jets that keep the water in constant motion. It has been a standard treatment for chronic wounds

and burns for many years. Most of what we know about hydrotherapy is about the physiological effects of hydrotherapy on the circulatory, nervous, and neuroendocrine systems and the cells of repair.

Since circulation and tissue perfusion are key requirements for healing, how they are affected by hydrotherapy is the main focus of this chapter while the other physiological effects are included briefly. Little information is available about efficacy for wound healing because studies are small, have not been performed with current standards of rigor, and are older. However, that information is included because it provides some much needed evidence about the purported efficacy of hydrotherapy for wound healing. As we present in detail in this chapter, clinicians may select hydrotherapy to treat wounds because research suggests it has the following effects:

1. Thermal
   - To increase skin blood flow to transport oxygen and nutrients to the tissues and remove waste products
   - To improve vascular endothelial function
   - To improve vascular systemic hemodynamics
2. Neuronal
   - To facilitate neuronal mechanisms of analgesia for pain relief and increased mobility
   - To facilitate skin blood flow by changes in the neuroendocrine function of the renin-angiotensin system
3. Cellular
   - To stimulate cellular activities for regeneration
4. Mechanical débridement
   - To reduce wound contamination, bioburden, and infection by softening and removing debris and exudate

MECHANISMS OF HEAT TRANSFER AND THERMAL REGULATION

This section explores the physiology of heat transfer, which is the underlying mechanism for many of the therapeutic effects of hydrotherapy including hemodynamics and hypothalamic regulation of body temperature. *Hemodynamics* is the study of the physical aspects of blood circulation, including cardiac function and peripheral vascular physiology. The *hypothalamus* is a brain relay center with many regulatory functions including temperature.

Thermal Effects

Thermal effects of hydrotherapy that are involved in the safe and appropriate application of hydrotherapy are heat transfer, thermal regulation, hemodynamic effects, cellular effects, neuronal effects, and the temperature effects. Each of these topics is discussed here.

Moist Heat versus Dry

Another factor in increased cutaneous blood flow is skin moisture demonstrated by the evidence that during water immersion where skin moisture is increased there is greater increase in skin blood flow than with local dry heating.[1]

Heat Transfer

Heat is transferred from the water to the body by conduction and convection. *Conduction* is the exchange of thermal energy between two surfaces. According to the Second Law of Thermodynamics, heat can only flow down a temperature gradient. Heat will be transferred from the warmer to the cooler surface, for example, from warm water to the body.[1] Conduction also occurs between the ambient room air and the body so that the thermal energy (warm and cool) of the room is transferred to the skin and affects cutaneous blood flow.[2,3] In the cold ambient temperature of 16°C, blood flow is less for all age groups. At cooler room temperature (16°C) and thermally neutral ambient temperature (24°C), the response to the addition of local heat (30°C, 33°C, and 37°C), such as from water immersion, causes a significant increase of between 80% and 90% in skin blood flow and an increase in skin temperature as the heat is transferred to the venous blood. The blood flow, incurred by the addition of 37°C local heating at ambient air of 32°C, plateaus in older adults, with or without diabetes, raising skin temperature because the heat transfer is limited by an impaired vascular response increasing the risk of thermal burns.[3] More information about these special population responses to hydrotherapy is coming up shortly.

Convection is a transfer of heat that occurs when there is circulation of a current of air or fluid, such as when a fan blows cool air over the body surface, or when warm water flows over the skin.[1] Agitation increases the movement of the water over the body surface and promotes convection. Since heating occurs more rapidly by convection than by conduction when using the whirlpool, it is important to keep in mind that the moving water will speed heating. Together, conduction and convection bring heat from the warm water to the body core. Core heating is a consequence that has physiological benefits as well as risks. One risk is that heating may occur more rapidly than some patients can dissipate the heat.

So far the discussion has centered on direct contact heat transfer. Indirect heating refers to heating of an area away from the target area such as upper extremity immersion when the wound is located on the leg. It has been shown that indirect application of heat to a distant area also has the ability to increase blood flow and pulse rate systemically.[4]

PHYSIOLOGIC RESPONSES TO HYDROTHERAPY

Hydrotherapy can cause the following physiological responses in the body: changes in skin blood flow, alteration of systemic hemodynamics, and suppression of endocrine stimulation. Each response is described in this section.

Skin Blood Flow

Contact with local heat such as warm water induces vasodilation and increases local blood flow to the skin.[3–6] Physiologically, the local heating stimulates the skin thermo receptors that are involved in the continuous release of vasodilator nitric oxide (NO), which reduces impedance to blood flow.[3,7] It is known that infection rates of tissues are inversely proportional to blood flow, and oxygenation of tissues is totally dependent on perfusion.[2,8,9] NO is an agent for killing of pathogens and could be a contributing factor to this reduction in infection rates. NO is discussed in Chapter 2.

Local heating can increase peripheral perfusion an average of threefold and is the simplest and most effective way of enhancing blood flow and achieving an increased subcutaneous oxygen tension that is sustained even after the heat source is removed.[8,10] Tissues are totally dependent on blood flow to meet the metabolic demands of inflammation. Increased oxygen tension makes tissue more resistant to infection and supports the use of intermittent heating at normothermia.[10] Decreased tissue oxygen tension impairs the deposition of collagen and oxidative killing by the neutrophils.[11] Support for intermittent heating at normothermia has been demonstrated to increase subcutaneous oxygen tension and presumably reduce infection.[10] Three different temperatures (38°C, 42°C, and 46°C) were tested in healthy adults to determine effects of heating on local subcutaneous oxygen. Results of 100% increase in blood flow and 50% increase in subcutaneous oxygen were comparable for all three temperatures.[12]

Vascular Endothelial Function

In the *vascular endothelium*, which is the lining of the blood vessels, by a conversion process involving NO synthase, NO is formed. NO as we learned recently is an important vasodilator. It also is known to prevent atherosclerosis by maintaining vasodilation and inhibiting platelet aggregation, leukocyte adhesion, and proliferation of smooth muscle cells in the arterial wall. In addition to the benefits of increased blood flow already mentioned, repeated heat treatment induced vasodilation and increased blood flow provides shear stress to the vascular endothelium, which improves endothelial function by increasing NO synthase activity and reduces blood pressure. It has been suggested that there is a therapeutic role for thermotherapy such as hydrotherapy for patients with risk factors for atherosclerosis.[7] By extension, this should be beneficial for patients with low blood flow states who are at risk for or who have arterial ulcers.

Hemodynamics

Vasodilation

Hemodynamic changes begin when surface heating causes vasodilation of the peripheral compartment (extremities). Core body warming is accomplished by the shunting of blood from the arterioles to the venules and venous plexuses located in the hands, feet, and face. Then conduction and convection of warm moving water on the body warms venous blood and venous return towards the core. Hemodynamic changes that follow include (1) Initiation of the baroreflex regulation of vascular resistance and sympathetic nervous activity. As central blood volume increases, there is stimulation of the baroreceptors, which are stretch receptors located in the blood vessels and in the cardiopulmonary system, that respond by increasing the diameter and capacity of the major vessels and heart by vasodilation. (2) Systemic results from increased venous return include initial increase in systolic arterial blood pressure, followed by decrease as peripheral vasodilation occurs, increased cardiac filling and output, decreased heart rate and decreased systemic vascular resistance ($p < 0.05$).[13,14] (3) Both systemic and vascular resistance decreased significantly during immersion and significant change persists for 30 minutes afterward.[15] Respiration rate also decreases during immersion due to reduced peripheral vascular resistance.[15,16]

Neuroendocrine Effects

Another hemodynamic effect is neuroendocrine suppression of the *renin-angiotensin* system. The renin-angiotensin system has two key functions: (1) increase systemic vascular resistance by vasoconstriction and (2) increase in extracellular volume that contributes to water retention.[17] When central blood volume increases it is accompanied by suppression of the renin-angiotensin system and overall sympathetic nervous system which further contributes to the hemodynamic response by inhibition of vasoconstriction thus allowing vasodilation and systemic vascular resistance to decrease and blood flow to increase. These combined effects occur during 30 minutes of water immersion. After cessation of the treatment increased blood flow is quickly reversed.[13,18]

Hyperthermia

During hydrotherapy, the body's ability to transfer heat back to the environment, and therefore avoid hyperthermia, depends on the following factors:

1. The ability of the peripheral compartment vasculature to dilate
2. The function of the autonomic nervous system
3. Subcutaneous body fat
4. The area of body surface immersed
5. The temperature of the water and duration of application

Peripheral Compartment Vasculature

As just detailed, hydrotherapy adds heat to the body and the body must be able to distribute and disperse the heat quickly and efficiently to avoid hyperthermia. Vasodilation may be compromised due to age, artheriosclerosis, calcification of the vessels, or peripheral neuropathy so this becomes a risk that needs to be addressed when selecting this intervention. Very soon we will learn about specific issues pertaining to these special situations and how to manage treatment.

Subcutaneous Body Fat

Thick subcutaneous fat layers lessen and slow the transfer and conduction of heat to the body core, reduces the body's ability to dissipate heat and can cause skin temperature to rise to a dangerously high level. The thicker the fat layer the greater the impairment in heat transfer and the greater the skin temperature increase during the treatment.[19] This effect is most noticeable where treatment with rapid heating modalities such as hydrotherapy are used. Therefore, since obese persons are unable to dissipate heat well, the water temperature needs to be adjusted downward accordingly. It has been suggested that thermoneutral water temperature (35°C) would meet this criterion.[3]

Body Surface Area

Radiation transfers heat from the body surface to the atmosphere, but cannot take place from immersed body areas; therefore, heat dissipation is shifted to the exposed body areas that can sweat, and to the lungs. The greater the body surface area immersed, the less transpiration can take place on the skin surface, and the greater the risk of cutaneous hyperthermia and burns. Again water temperature is an important mitigating factor.

Thermal Regulation by Hypothalamus

The body's thermoregulatory system is centrally controlled by the hypothalamus to maintain a core temperature of about 37°C (98.6°F). Information from the skin surface, deep abdominals, thoracic tissue, spinal cord, and nonhypothalamic portions of the brain, as well as the temperature of the hypothalamus itself, each contribute roughly 20% of the information used by the hypothalamus for thermoregulatory control. Because of the effectiveness of the thermoregulatory defenses, body temperature rarely deviates more than a few tenths of a degree. The range of core temperature that does not trigger thermoregulatory responses is only 0.2°C and is called the *interthreshold range*.[20] Autonomic thermoregulatory defenses are not triggered unless the body temperature moves out of this interthreshold range.

Under normal conditions, the body maintains a temperature gradient between the core and periphery of 2°C to 4°C.[21] Because of the Second Law of Thermodynamics, heat can only flow *down* a temperature gradient, for example, from the peripheral compartment to the core. The gradient thus functions as a safety feature to maintain the normal temperature gradient between core and periphery, the purpose of which is to allow the dissipation of metabolic heat from the core to the periphery and subsequently to the environment. Core heating is achieved in two ways: by constraint of metabolic heat by greater body surface area immersion and by rapid heating that causes the reversal of the normal core to periphery temperature gradient.[22] Whirlpool hydrotherapy because of the conduction and convection effects of the moving water has the ability to make this reversal happen more quickly than conduction alone.

Both systemic and local tissue temperatures are of considerable importance in the control of body temperature. If the hypothalamus receives a signal from the skin that there is a rise in temperature, the response is sweating, which redistributes body heat from the core to the periphery and cooling results.

If the signal from the skin is cold, the response would be vasoconstriction, which conserves heat, and generates shivering. There is a linear relation near 20% between mean skin temperature and core temperatures at the vasoconstriction and shivering thresholds; however, there is individual variability.[23] The object is a redistribution of body heat from the core to the periphery.

All thermoregulatory responses are neuronally mediated. Thus, the administration of nerve blocks prevents the normal activation of thermoregulatory defenses, such as sweating, vasoconstriction, and shivering. Peripheral inhibition of thermoregulatory defenses is a major cause of hypothermia during regional anesthesia.[21]

Mild hypothermia impairs the oxidative killing by neutrophils and decreases cutaneous blood flow, which reduces tissue oxygen and contributes to decreased wound strength by reducing the deposition of collagen. Under the right thermal conditions, hydrotherapy can be used to treat mild core hypothermia and prevent impaired immune functions by vasoconstriction-induced hypoxia. Vasoconstriction-induced tissue hypoxia can decrease the strength of the healing wound because the process of collagen deposition and cross-linkages between strands of collagen is dependent on oxygen tension.[24] Nineteen percent of 104 control group postsurgical patients who experienced mild hypothermia during surgery developed postsurgical wound infection. Heating core body temperature to 37°C, normothermia, during surgery in an experimental study group of 96 patients was found to reduce significantly the incidence of postsurgical wound infection and to increase significantly collagen deposition near the wound.[24] Mild hypothermia also reduces platelet function and increases coagulation time.[25] These inhibitory effects were found to be completely reversible by rewarming the blood to 37°C.[4,8]

Circulatory Effects on Special Populations

After our discussions of hemodynamic changes during hydrotherapy in this chapter, it should now be apparent that "one size" hydrotherapy treatment should not be given to everyone. Special populations require mitigating measures to prevent unintended and undesirable consequences from occurring as well as to achieve maximum benefit from the therapy.

Six special populations whose responses to hydrotherapy differ from those of normal adults and require special consideration when planning a course of hydrotherapy intervention are discussed in this section. They include patients who are

- Elderly
- Diabetics
- Spinal cord injured
- Obese
- Patients with compensated heart failure
- Patients with venous insufficiency
- Patients with burns

CLINICAL WISDOM

Monitor Temperature

Use a thermometer to record tympanic membrane temperature during hydrotherapy treatment to monitor for changes in core body temperature.

All of these populations are likely to be treated for wounds as a secondary consequence of their primary disease. Therefore, it is necessary for you to be aware of potential issues when providing hydrotherapy treatment in order to deliver appropriate patient centered care.

Elderly

Elderly here is defined, based on the research evidence reviewed for this discussion, as greater than age 60. It is important to be aware of age-related changes in the cardiovascular system that affect cardiac and vascular performance before selecting hydrotherapy treatment. Aging slows and reduces blood flow to the skin for a number of reasons:

- Altered ability of vascular system to respond to thermal stimuli. Maximum blood flow increases seem to be capped in the elderly at higher room temperatures (32°C) related to impaired vascular responses.[3]
- Plateau of vasodilation with the addition of heat. The blood flow increase with addition of 37°C local heating to the skin at an ambient air of 32°C plateaus in older adults with or without diabetes raising skin temperature.[3]
- Reduction in red cell concentration and red cell velocity.[26]
- Impaired skin circulation due to damage of vascular endothelial cells with decreased production of NO and other vasodilators resulting in decreased ability to vasodilate and increase microcirculation of the skin adequately to dissipate heat.[3,27]
- Significantly reduced skin thickness and subcutaneous fat layers. Even if the body mass index is the same or greater than in younger people there is less subcutaneous fat.[26]
- Over age 80 there is very little effect of local heating on skin blood flow.[26]
- Impairment of the sympathetic nervous system causes decreased skin moisture (sweat) so that evaporative cooling of the skin is decreased and skin temperature rises.[3]
- Limited heat transfer from the surface to the deeper tissues due to reduced dermal epidermal adhesion (see Chapter 2).[27]

Therefore, room and water temperature need to be carefully selected so as to reduce heat stress to the skin and prevent thermal burns. Normothermal temperature of the air and water, soon to be discussed, would be one way of reducing heat stress.

Diabetics

What has just been presented about the responses of the elderly to hydrotherapy can also be applied to the diabetic population. Except that the diabetics may be younger in chronological age. Vasodilation is limited in this patient population who have calcified vessels as a secondary complication of the disease and an ankle-brachial index of greater than 1.0 (see Chapter 6 for vascular assessment). Both groups also experience a plateau in the skin blood flow response.[3] Therefore, in this group, the application of heat will at best have a muted response. By prewarming the body and treating in a warm environment, addition of more local heat may slightly increase vasodilation. More about environmental temperatures effects will be discussed on page 6. The condition of decreased blood flow response to local and global heating in both diabetics and the elderly is progressive.

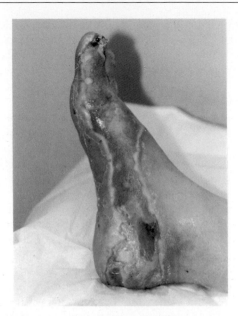

FIGURE 27.1 Burn resulting from putting neuropathic foot in hot water. (Copyright © Nancy Elftman.)

Peripheral neuropathy is usually identified in the lower extremities first and then progresses to the upper extremities. Application of heat to an extremity with impaired sensation likewise presents risk of burns because of lack of sympathetic nervous system input to mediate vasodilation required to dissipate and remove the heat and/or lack of sensory input to warn of overheating[28] Figure 27.1 shows the foot of a patient with diabetic neuropathy who suffered a burn when immersed in hot water. Diabetics and others with peripheral neuropathy also have peripheral inhibition of thermoregulatory defenses and are at risk for both mild core hypothermia and thermal injury from immersion.

Diabetics who often develop callus formation on the plantar surfaces of the feet should *not* be treated in hydrotherapy because calluses will be softened, and subsequent exposure to pressure from standing on the foot will result in skin breakdown. The break in the skin will become a portal for infection.

Spinal Cord Injured

Spinal cord–injured individuals just like diabetics also have peripheral inhibition of thermoregulatory defenses and are at risk for thermal injury and fluid shift similar to those with venous insufficiency. Therefore, attention should be paid to heat gain and changes in plasma volume.[28,29]

Obese

When using a rapid heating modality like whirlpool, heat transfer from the skin to the deeper tissues is significantly impaired by thicker subcutaneous fat layers because the subcutaneous fat acts as an insulator. Individuals with high body fat increase their deep tissue temperatures nearly **twice as slowly** as thin individuals. The greater the impairment the warmer the skin temperature increase during the treatment.[19] If the body fat exceeds 25% of the subjects weight 20 minutes of immersion is not long enough to change deep muscle temperature.[30] Depending on the water temperature and body fat, the length of immersion may need to be longer than 15 to 20 minutes and

at a normothermic temperature to raise body core temperature without causing overheating of the skin.[18] Normothermic temperature discussion follows on page 7.

Chronic Heart Failure

Warm water bathing has been generally considered inappropriate for patients with stable chronic heart failure (CHF). In CHF patients, peripheral vascular resistance is increased by sympathetic hypertonia to compensate for reduced cardiac output.[15] Since peripheral vasodilation occurs with addition of warmth, investigation of the comprehensive hemodynamic effects on this population has been undertaken in several studies and the findings suggest that this belief is wrong and that it is time to make this treatment option available to this population.[7,13,15,16] Hemodynamic responses, just described, including increased cardiac and stroke volume, decreased systemic vascular resistance and increased blood flow occur in this population but more slowly than in the normal population. The neuroendocrine system is also affected similarly.[13] This information is useful for two reasons: (1) in this patient population, vascular resistance is chronically high and cardiac output reduced and (2) hydrotherapy provides a nonpharmaceutical treatment option to reduce vascular resistance and to improve hemodynamics and blood flow to the tissues.[31] If the patient also has a wound, increased blood flow would have wound healing benefits as well.

Venous Insufficiency

Vasodilatation is a benefit for a patient with reduced perfusion, but it can be disastrous for a patient with venous insufficiency whose venous system has difficulty managing tissue fluids.[32] As learned throughout this text, vasodilation with increased blood flow is essential for wound healing. In earlier chapters on vascular and edema management it was explained that as the blood volume in the veins increases the fluid shifts from the vessels into the interstitial spaces and becomes edematous. If placed in a dependent position such as in the whirlpool tank the effect of the hydrostatic pressure of the blood exerted on the veins increases the pressure further and edema will increase. The fluid shift also occurs within a wound, which is usually in the gaiter area of the leg, with a loss of proteins, electrolytes, other nutrients, and growth factors found in wound fluid. If immersed in water, those fluids will pass out into the water. Fluid shifts can lead to dehydration and depletion of nutrients needed for healing.[33] Use of saline instead of tap water will prevent loss of fluids. Saline hydrotherapy solution can be made by adding salt to the water. But the amount of salt needed and the corrosive effects if the tank or turbine is metal may be barriers to this option. If fluid shift is of concern, another intervention for this patient population could better meet the goals of treatment.

Burns

Hydrotherapy is used to facilitate burn débridement. From the 1950s to mid 1980s, immersion hydrotherapy was a standard of care for burn débridement and then practice began to change from immersion to showering due to infection rates attributable to hydrotherapy services.[34] Still by the early 1990s over 80% of patients with burns received immersion hydrotherapy.[35] The chief concern is the transference of nosocomial infections between patients that have been traced to the hydrotherapy intervention

---

RESEARCH WISDOM

Hydrotherapy Implications for Venous Congestion

McCulloch and Boyd[32] reported that hydrotherapy treatment of a dependent leg resulted in increased hypotension and lower extremity vascular congestion, even in healthy individuals. The implications for the patient with a compromised venous system are very serious.

and the difficulty in decontaminating the agitators and aerators. Also iatrogenic care by caregivers who use inadequate hand washing and barriers is also implicated. Attempts to use disinfectants in the water is also unacceptable due to patient discomfort.[34] Change in burn management at a regional burn center occurred in 1999 and included no hydrotherapy. Evaluation of the results of change in care there over a 10-year period found that there was reduced mortality not all of which was attributable to the discontinuance of hydrotherapy.[36] Primary rationale for using hydrotherapy was wound débridement. Burn patients report severe pain with immersion hydrotherapy. Showering has been substituted because it is less painful and takes less time.[37] Also surgical excision which is faster and can be done under anesthesia has become a better débridement choice. For the burn population the goal of care is not enhanced circulatory effects. Further information about burn care is provided in Chapter 15.

Cellular Effects

Heat is infrared energy. Use of heat adds energy to the cells as well other body systems already described. Warmth stimulates cell mitosis and enhances leukocytic activity. Research on pigs has shown experimentally that the speed of production of new epidermal cells is enhanced if the temperature is maintained at 37°C. Similar results have been reported following in vitro testing of human skin cultures. Leukocyte activity may fall to zero when wound temperature is cooled, such as during a dressing change. This will impair the phagocytic activity of the leukocytes.[38] It has been observed that it takes 40 minutes for a freshly cleaned wound to return to normal temperature and 3 hours for mitotic cell division to resume.[39,40] However, at 33°C, the proliferative capacity of endothelial cells was potentiated.[41] Fibroblasts treated with heat at 38°C have increased cell division and metabolic activity[20] and this along with the mechanical stimulation of the fibroblasts during whirlpool stimulates granulation tissue formation.

Clotting factor activity is prolonged at temperatures below 35°C, resulting in decreased activation of the coagulation cascade (Chapter 2). More bleeding could be expected during débridement if a tepid hydrotherapy is used. Clotting function is restored with warming.[25] Chronic wound fluid is known to inhibit fibroblast activity. Heating of chronic wound fluid in a water bath showed that there was a temperature-dependent reduction in the inhibitory effect on fibroblasts. When the heated chronic wound fluid was added to fetal and adult fibroblasts, the fluid assisted in the growth of both fetal and adult fibroblasts.[42] Heating of wound fluid during hydrotherapy treatment may have a significant effect on restarting the growth of fibroblasts in chronic wounds.

Frequent changes in wound temperature may delay phagocytosis and wound healing. Therefore, the effect of temperature on cellular activity is an important consideration when choosing a treatment temperature for the whirlpool.

Neuronal Effects

Neural receptors for heat and cold are distributed all over the body. Signals from cold receptors travel along A-delta fibers and from warm receptors along C fibers. Neuronal mediation of thermoregulatory responses is the primary means of activation. Warm water has mild analgesic effects, reduces inflammation, is soothing, and relaxes muscle tension.[43–45] Patients experiencing severe pain or anxiety may find these effects soothing and analgesic. However, patients who are lethargic or semicomatose with already suppressed central nervous system function would be neurosuppressed to a point where they could become totally unresponsive. These patients should not be immersed in warm water. Analgesia from the warm water is often reported, but some wound patients, especially those with ischemic limbs or burns, find that the agitation stimulates pain receptors. Treatment at a very gentle agitation level directed away from the wound tissue can be used to soothe, rather than stimulate, the nerves. Patient tolerance should be evaluated and treatment modified as required.

Combining Hydrotherapy with Exercise

During hydrotherapy treatment, the patient should be encouraged to perform gentle exercise for muscle pump functions and strengthening. Both skin blood flow and sweating during exercise increase with a rise in water temperature and are notable at 35°C.[46] If exercise is to be performed during the wound treatment, consider the physiologic effects when choosing the water temperature and the extent of body area to be immersed. Heart rate and blood pressure can be expected to increase significantly during exercise in the water. CHF patients also have significant increase in cardiac output.[16] Joint range-of-motion extensibility is usually performed more easily and less painfully in warm water. The gentle stretching forces around the wound may stimulate tissue regeneration. Of course, stretching and exercise of a newly sutured wound should be avoided until the sutures are removed.

Physiologic Effects at Different Temperatures and Duration

In this section, we will discuss how different room, body and water temperatures and the duration of immersion effect physiology and how to use them to for the best clinical results.

Room temperature

If the patient is allowed to sit in a warm room (24°C–32°C) for 15 minutes before adding local heat (water immersion), the heat

CLINICAL WISDOM

Fluids

Provide patients with fluids during hydrotherapy to compensate for loss of fluids

of the room is transferred to the skin that is warmed, arterial dilation is initiated, blood flow increases, and heat is transferred across the skin layers and stored in the tissues below. It also appears that prewarming offers some protection from local heat damage to the skin. However, this benefit is blunted in the elderly whose skin is more sensitive to heating and burns.[27]

Water Temperature, Duration, Precautions
Water Temperature

Use the water temperature closest to the optimal that is consistent with the patient's medical status. We begin this section with definitions of water temperature ranges summarized as follows[47]:

- Nonthermal/tepid: 27°C to 33.5°C or 80°F to 92°F
- Neutral: 33.5°C to 35.5°C or 92°F to 96°F
- Normothermal: 37°C or 98.6°F
- Hot: 36.7°C to 40°C or 98°F to 104°F

Each temperature range exerts different degree of physiological effects on the body. To begin let us consider that the average skin temperature of the body is 34°C (93°F). The range of body indifference to temperature is 34°C to 38°C (93°F–100.4°F). At 27°C to 33.5°C (80°F–92°F), the temperature is tepid or nonthermal. At this temperature range, chilling with local vasoconstriction, decreased oxygen uptake, and tissue cooling that affects the cells of repair occurs.[5] Avoid mild core hypothermia at this thermal range by treating only a limited body area for a very short duration (e.g., 5 minutes) for cleansing or to soften dry tissue; keep the rest of the body and surrounding air temperature warm and slightly humid. Use a normothermic tap water rinse (35°C–37°C) immediately following the hydrotherapy to raise local wound temperatures. Temperatures of 36.5°C to 40°C (98°F–104°F) are typically used for therapeutic heating.[47] Above 37°C or 98°F is classified as hot. Higher temperature levels are *not* recommended because of physiologic stress. A tissue temperature rise of as much as 4°C at temperatures ranging from 37°C to 42°C has been measured after immersion for 20 minutes in a whirlpool.

If hydrotherapy is to be used, consider the neutral temperature choice for patients with venous insufficiency in whom wound débridement and cleansing is the objective and where vasodilation should be avoided since the added blood volume could overload incompetent veins. The warm rinse as described would reduce shock to local cells of repair.

Neutral warmth is 33.5°C to 35.5°C (92°F–96°F). The normothermic temperature range of 35.5°C to 37°C is best when treating the patient with peripheral vascular disease, sensory impairment, CHF, the elderly, diabetic, or obese.[13] At neutral warmth tissues will still be soaked, softened, and cleansed, and hemodynamics will be positively effected. The temperature range shown to optimize cellular functions and enzymatic and biochemical reactions is at normal body temperature, or normothermia, defined as 98.6°F or 37°C ± 1°C.[48]

Temperature Precautions

As reviewed, water temperature modifies circulatory responses. Use the following treatment modifications to modify the heating effects of hydrotherapy:

- Water temperature should not exceed local skin temperature (usually 34°C–35°C) in the presence of peripheral vascular disease and in the presence of cardiovascular and pulmonary disease.
- Water temperature of 32°C increases blood flow of 2.3 mL/dL of limb volume but will chill the wound and slow clotting and healing.[47,49]

Immersion Duration

Application of heat with hydrotherapy for 20 minutes at a hot temperature of 40°C produces an immediate increase in local blood flow[3] Also at this temperature and duration, mean cardiac output and oxygen consumption increase, but not significantly. Heart rate increases 1.3 to 1.5 times over the sitting or supine resting level, and mean blood pressure increases 1.1 times over the supine resting values. Core body temperature is increased when exposure to warm water ceases to increase local blood flow and the warm venous blood is carried to the core vessels.[15,50] In conjunction with the rise in core temperature, there is a rise in local skin temperature. As we learned if there is limited skin blood flow to dissipate the heat, burns may result. At this temperature, that can occur quickly before the rise in core temperature. Therefore the temperature and duration of the treatment needs to be adjusted to avoid this hazard and achieve desired outcomes. Normothermic temperature for longer duration can be better tolerated by the skin and still have desired physiological benefits.

The necessary duration of immersion for increased blood flow at 35°C, normothermia, is 30 minutes. In the elderly and those with diabetes, changes in blood flow are *not* noted until 15 minutes of immersion at normothermic temperature. So the customary 20-minute hydrotherapy immersion session is probably not long enough to promote the hemodynamic changes outlined in this chapter in these populations.

EVIDENCE OF THE EFFECT OF HYDROTHERAPY ON WOUND HEALING

Little direct evidence exists about the benefits of hydrotherapy on wound healing. What we have learned so far is evidence about the physiological effects of heat and water immersion on hemodynamics, neuronal activities, and cellular effects. In this section, evidence is presented from clinical studies reporting on the efficacy of whirlpool hydrotherapy for wound healing.

Clinical Practice Guidelines

Whirlpool, a form of hydrotherapy, has been a standard treatment for chronic wounds and burns for many years. In 1994, the Agency for Health Care Policy and Research, now known as the Agency for Health Care Research and Quality, panel

---

CLINICAL WISDOM

Avoid Chilling

When using lower temperatures, avoid chilling by maintaining warm room temperature and use only for single limbs, not the whole body. Reduce treatment duration from 20 to 5 or 10 minutes.

considered the evidence and, based on an absence of clinical trials, recommended a level "C" grade for this therapy based on expert opinion (refer to the book *Introduction for the AHCPR Evidence Grading System*[51]). The AHCPR recommendation was "to consider whirlpool hydrotherapy treatment for pressure ulcers that contain thick exudate, slough, or necrotic tissue and to discontinue hydrotherapy when the ulcer is clean."[51] Thus, many clinicians have moved away from use of the hydrotherapy because of a lack of evidence and cautions received from experts.

In 2009, the National Pressure Ulcer and European Pressure Ulcer Advisory Panels released new guidelines for treatment of pressure ulcers.[52] After an updated review of the evidence for these guidelines, whirlpool hydrotherapy was again found to have a level C strength of evidence for pressure ulcers but recommendations changed as follows: "consider a course of whirlpool as an adjunct for wound cleansing and facilitating healing and to reduce wound bioburden and infection"[52] According to the same source, no other method of débridement receives an evidence level greater than C. The guidelines go on to say that the débridement method selected should be the one most appropriate to the individual's "condition, the goals of care, ulcer status, type, quantity and location of necrotic tissue, the care setting and professional accessibility/capability."[52]

Published Clinical Studies

Review of the literature for other wound treatment interventions brought to light a number of studies in which hydrotherapy was used as either a cotreatment modality or the comparative standard wound care treatment. Since the AHCPR guidelines were published in 1994, one small randomized controlled clinical trial of clean, surgically débrided pressure ulcers treated with hydrotherapy has been published and with no negative findings reported and wounds healing.[53] Like most treatment intervention studies, the data from these studies often have gaps, such as treatment parameters used or the percentage of healing. The purpose of this review of the hydrotherapy clinical studies is to look at the reported data and the evidence that provides for choosing an intervention with whirlpool hydrotherapy. Table 27.1 summarizes the data derived from this literature review. The following text outlines the studies more extensively.

Randomized Clinical Trials

A randomized clinical trial was designed to test the effect of whirlpool hydrotherapy on surgically débrided, clean granulating, Stage III and IV pressure ulcers.[53] Group A was treated with moist wound dressings hydrotherapy ($N = 24$) at 96 to 97°F and the control group B with moist wound dressings ($N = 18$). One 20-minute session was given daily. The hydrotherapy group showed a significantly faster rate of wound healing, mean rate 0.39 cm/wk, in 58.33% of the whirlpool-treated ulcers, compared with a mean healing rate of 0.169 cm/wk for 27.78% of the nonhydrotherapy controls. Fewer wounds in the whirlpool hydrotherapy group (9 versus 11) deteriorated during the course of treatment. However, the investigators were concerned that there were so many deteriorating wounds in both groups that could not be explained.

Wood et al.[54] reported on results of a randomized controlled trial of 31 patients treated with whirlpool, saline wet-to-moist dressings, and compared the results with those of a group of 43 patients treated with low-intensity direct current.

The hydrotherapy and dressing group had 3% healing or had increased wound size while the low-voltage microamperage direct current group had 58% healing. Perhaps some of the poor results in the whirlpool/saline wet-to-moist dressing group were due to the dressings drying out, resulting in repeated trauma during dressing changes or other factors not described or considered.

Comparative Case Studies and Other Trials

Whirlpool hydrotherapy with povidone-iodine and low-energy infrared cold laser were combined treatments used for two patients in two case studies.[55] The patient in case study 1 had a 1.42 cm/wk or 7.12% per week (99.7% healing) reduction in size after 14 weeks of therapy. The patient in case study 2 had weekly reduction in size of 1.5 cm/wk or 5% per week (90% healing) in 18 weeks. A woman with septic autoamputation of a breast secondary to cancer was treated daily for 30 minutes with antimicrobial additives in the whirlpool for wound cleansing, nonselective débridement and the findings were that that tissue improvement took place within 2 weeks, that drainage ceased after 2 months, and that at 11 months the wound was closed and there was no evidence of the cancer. At a 2-year follow-up the wound remained closed.[56] Broad conclusions cannot be reached about use of these combined interventions. No negative effects were reported.

Another study is a small controlled comparative clinical trial ($N = 12$) of patients with pressure ulcers. The investigators followed daily 20-minute hydrotherapy with povidone-iodine intervention with 20-minute electrical stimulation (ES) in half the patients, and the control half of the study received only the 20-minute treatment of hydrotherapy with povidone-iodine.[57] Both groups received aftercare with saline wet-to-dry dressings. The hydrotherapy control group in this study had a 5.23% per week reduction in wound area and 28.37% per week reduction in depth.

Gault and Gatens[58] found that a hydrotherapy control group had a 14.7% per week rate of healing. They designated one ulcer on each of six patients as a control and assigned that ulcer to a hydrotherapy control group. Results for those ulcers were a 14.7% per week healing rate.[58] However, the electrotherapy that was administered to the other ulcer may have had some systemic effect that influenced the rate of healing in the control ulcer.

Akers and Gabrielson[59] compared three treatment regimens: (1) whirlpool, (2) whirlpool with electrical high-voltage pulsed current (HVPC) stimulation, and (3) HVPC alone in the healing of pressure ulcers of 14 spinal cord injured individuals. This controlled clinical trial reported that the hydrotherapy treatment was given once daily (QD), the HVPC was given twice daily (BID), and the hydrotherapy given QD plus HVPC BID. The treatment parameters and the rate or percentage of healing were not reported. Results reported that there was no statistical significance between the three groups. The best outcomes were achieved by the HVPC BID group, followed by the hydrotherapy QD group and the HVPC BID, and last, the hydrotherapy QD group. The study reported that numerous interval variations existed.

Thurman and Christian[60] reported a case study of a patient with diabetes who was scheduled for surgical amputation of a foot with an infected abscess. The ulcerated foot was treated with a mixture of interventions including hydrotherapy with hexachlorophene for 10 minutes daily, followed by treatment

TABLE **27.1**   **Clinical Studies Using Whirlpool**

Investigators and Type of Study	Disease States Treated	Whirlpool	Electrical Stimulation	Other Treatments	Effects on Healing
Akers and Gabrielson[59] (N = 14)	Pressure ulcers (full or partial denervation of spinal cord)	1. Once daily	2. HVPC BID	Not reported	ES only best
Controlled clinical trial-3 groups			3. WPL once and HVPC BID		ES with whirlpool second best
					Whirlpool only least
					No statistical significance between 3 groups. Lots of internal variation.
Burke et al.[53] (WPL N = 24 nonWPL N = 18) RCT	Pressure ulcers	Once daily, 20 min 96–98°F	N/A	Surgical débridement	WPL group[a]
				Saline wet-to-dry dressings	58.33% (14) mean 0.39 cm/wk reduction in size
					4.17% (1) no change
					37.5% (9) deterioration
					NonWPL group[a]
					27.78% (5) mean 0.169 cm/wk reduction in size
					11.11% (2) no change
					61.11% (11) deterioration
Carley and Wainapel[61] (WPL N = 4 LIDC N = 30)	Indolent ulcers below knee or sacral	4–5 ×/wk	LIDC	Wet-to-dry dressings	WP group
RCT			Direct, 2 h BID, 5 ×/wk	Dakin's or povidone-iodine, or hydrogel	45% healing (9%/wk)[a]
					LIDC group
					98.95% (19% wk)[*] healing in 5 wk
Gault and Gatens[58] (WPL N = 6 LIDC N = 6 subgroup)	Mixed	Once daily	LIDC		LIDC 30%/wk
Controlled trial			Direct, 2 h BID or TID		WP 14.7%/wk, 2/6 increased in size

(continued)

TABLE 27.1 **Clinical Studies Using Whirlpool (*continued*)**

Investigators and Type of Study	Disease States Treated	Whirlpool	Electrical Stimulation	Other Treatments	Effects on Healing
Gogia et al.[57] (*N* = 6)	Mixed	Once daily 20 min with povidone-iodine, 100°F	HVPC 20 min	Saline wet-to-dry dressings	WPL 20 d
Controlled trial			Direct, 5 ×/wk		27.19% reduction in area (9.51%/wk)
					56.76% reduction in depth (19.86%/wk)
					WPL and HVPC 20 d
					34.73% reduction area (12.15%/wk)
					30.30% reduction in depth (10.6%/wk)*
					Granulation, significant healing
Gogia, Hurt, and Zirn[55] (*N* = 2)		Whirlpool with povidone-iodine	N/A	Infrared cold laser	
Case Studies					
Haynes et al.[62] (WPL *N* = 15 PL *N* = 15)	Mixed	Whirlpool	N/A	Pulsed lavage varied	PL 12.2% healing/week
Controlled trial					WP 4.8% healing/week
Juve[43] (*N* = 63)	Major abdominal surgery	Whirlpool daily	N/A	Probably dressings (type unstated)	Pain reduction
Controlled trial		3 days postoperative			Reduced wound inflammation
					Positive signs of wound healing
Thurman and Christian[60] (*N* = 1)	Abscess, diabetes	Whirlpool with hexachlorophene detergent cleanser (pHisohex) 10 min	HVPC daily	Debridement	Decreased infection, exudate, and wound size 6 mo to closure
Case study				Hydrogen peroxide soaks	
				Antibiotic medication	

(continued)

Vetra and Whittaker[43]	Mixed	Whirlpool 40°C daily	Collagenase daily	80% closure
Uncontrolled clinical trial (N = 140)				Mean time 37.0 d (SD 27.5 d)
				7% good granulation and epithelialization
				3% healthy granulation
				10% reduction or cessation of drainage
Wood et al.[54] (WPL N = 31 PLIDC N = 43)	Pressure and venous ulcers	Whirlpool	Cleansing	Whirlpool and dressing group
		PLIDC		PLIDC
Randomized controlled trial			3×/wk	Saline wet-to-dry dressings	3% healed or increased in size
				PLIDC 58% healed
				Data for whirlpool only, ulcers not reported

[a]Percentage healing per week calculated study data to transform data for comparison.
WPL, whirlpool; HVPC, high-voltage pulsed current; LIDC, low-intensity direct current; PLIDC, pulsed low-intensity direct current; BID, twice daily; TID, three times daily.

Data from Petrofsky J, Laymon M. Heat transfer to deeptissue: the effect of body fat and heating modality. *J Med Eng Technol.* 2009;33(5):337–348; 46. Shimizu T, Kosaka M, Fujishima K. Human thermoregulatory responses during prolonged walking in water at 25, 30 and 35 degrees C. *Eur J Appl Physiol Occup Physiol.* 1998;78(6):473–478; Walsh M. Hydrotherapy: the use of water as a therapeutic agent. In: Michlovitz S, ed. *Thermal Agents in Rehabilitation.* Philadelphia, PA: FA Davis; third edition 1996:139–167; Kloth LC, et al. Effects of normothermic dressing on pressure ulcer healing. *Adv Wound Care.* 2000;13(2):69–74; Sussman C. The role of physical therapy in wound care. In: Krasner D, ed. *Chronic Wound Care: A Sourcebook for Health Care Professionals.* Wayne, PA: Health Management Publications; 1990:327–366; Petrofsky J, Bains G, Prowse M, et al. Does skin moisture influence the blood flow response to local heat? A re-evaluation of the Pennes model. *JMed Eng Technol.* 2009;33(7):532–537; Bergstrom N, Bennett MA, Carlson C, et al. *Treatment of Pressure Ulcers.* Clinical Practice Guideline No. 15. Rockville, MD: Agency for Health Care Research and Quality (AHRQ), formerly known as the Agency for Health Care Policy and Research (AHCPR), U.S. Public Health Service (PHS), U.S. Department of Health and Human Services (DHHS); AHRQ Publication No. 95–0652. December 1994:45–65; Burke DT, et al. Effects of hydrotherapy on pressure ulcer healing. *Am J Phys Med Rehabil.* 1998;77(5):394–398; Wood JM, Evans PE III, Schallreuter KU, et al. A multicenter study on the use of pulsed low intensity direct current for healing chronic Stage II and Stage III ulcers. *Arch Dermatol.* 1993;130(5):660–661; Gogia PP, Hurt BS, Zirn TT. Wound management with hydrotherapyand infrared cold laser. *Phys Ther.* 1988;68(8):1239–1242; Bohannon R. Hydrotherapy versus hydrotherapy and rinse for removal of bacteria from a venous stasis ulcer. *Phys Ther.* 1982;62:304–308.

with HVPC and other disinfecting agents and antimicrobials. Results were limb salvage, decreased infection, and exudate leading to wound closure in 4 months.

Carley and Wainapel's control group had a multitude of conventional dressing treatments, including mainly wet-to-dry dressings, gauze with Dakin's solution, or povidone-iodine.[61] Four were treated in the whirlpool. Results were not separated from the rest of the controls.

In another study, hydrotherapy efficacy was compared with pulsed lavage by measuring the rate of formation of granulation tissue in a variety of chronic wounds.[62] Although the rate of granulation tissue formation was greater at 12.2% per week, for the pulsed lavage group, the hydrotherapy group had a granulation rate of 4.8% per week. Hydrotherapy and collagenase were both used throughout the course of treatment for ulcers of mixed etiologies, and 80% reached closure in a median time of 37 days (SD 27.5 days).[63]

Major abdominal surgery is often followed by pain because of increased tension on muscles and tissues. Results of these events have been attributed to causing anxiety, stress, and altered tissue regeneration. Findings of a controlled clinical trial of postoperative patients ($N = 63$) who had major abdominal surgery and who received an intervention with hydrotherapy after surgery showed reduced pain behavior, fewer signs of wound inflammation, and positive signs of healing over a 3-day period following surgery.[43]

Vetra and Whittaker[63] found that patients with limited circulation and extensive necrotic tissue who most likely would have had to have limb amputation received benefit from the enhanced perfusion associated with heating in the whirlpool, combined with enzymatic débridement using collagenase.

Discussion about Clinical Studies

Review of the results of clinical studies suggest that there were extrinsic factors that may have influenced the results of the treatment interventions, such as use of cytotoxic agents like povidone iodine,[55,57,61] and hexachlorophene and hydrogen peroxide.[60] Two studies[53,54] reported conscientiously avoiding chemical and mechanical trauma to the wounds treated with whirlpool, yet both reported significant deterioration of the hydrotherapy groups that was not explained. Reports of healing at slower rates than comparative treatment are listed in Table 27.1. More studies need to be undertaken with good control standards in place. In the meantime, with all their flaws, what seems apparent from this review is that whirlpool hydrotherapy on a daily basis may be beneficial for wound cleansing, nonspecific débridement and healing for acute surgical as well as chronic wounds.

USE OF HYDROTHERAPY FOR WOUND CLEANSING AND DÉBRIDEMENT

Hydrotherapy is a method of both mechanical débridement and wound cleansing but should not be used or considered as bathing. It differs from other methods of wound cleansing, which uses a cleansing solution and a method of delivery that cleanses the wound. Use of mechanical and shearing force, such as turbulent water (agitation) that is a component of whirlpool, is an invasive procedure that scours and scrubs the necrotic tissue to loosen it from the healthy tissue but it is nonselective and

may damage healthy tissues. Trauma to granulation tissue and epithelial cells may occur if the wound is positioned too close to the high-pressure jets of the whirlpool.[64] Avoid trauma from shearing forces and turbulence by adjusting the level of aeration from the jet to minimal or by turning off the aerator if tissues are very fragile, such as new skin grafts.[47] Trauma from mechanical force prolongs inflammation and delays healing. Therefore, you must exercise care during delivery of the whirlpool treatment to minimize trauma to healthy granulation tissue as well as to surrounding soft tissues. Even trauma distant from the wound site can influence the occurrence of local wound infection.[65]

By performing a débridement procedure, the clinician minimizes the body's inflammatory response and removes a staging place for bacteria and fungi. Débridement methods, other than biophysical agents, are explored fully in Chapter 17.

Besides the physiological effects described in detail at the start of this chapter, physical effects of immersion in water are soaking, saturating, loosening, and softening of loosely adherent necrotic tissue, which aids phagocytosis and deodorization. Hydrotherapy has little or no effect on densely adherent fibrous tissue, and other methods of débridement should be considered. Hydrotherapy as a débridement intervention is often followed by other débridement methods; for example, sharp, enzymatic, biologic, autolytic, or surgical.

RISKS AND CANDIDACY FOR HYDROTHERAPY

Patients treated with hydrotherapy are at risk for a variety of associated risks, including exacerbation of systemic symptoms, tissue damage, and infection. Each of these risk factors should be considered when making the clinical decision about candidacy for hydrotherapy.

Cardiac, Vascular, and Pulmonary Systems

Until recently it has been considered a contraindication to immerse cardiopulmonary and peripheral vascular patients in warm water. As described under special populations, patients with cardiovascular problems including compensated congestive heart failure have improved hemodynamics and reduced vascular resistance when treated with warm water immersion. Therefore, it is now considered safe and good medical management to use warm water as a means of increasing blood flow for this population. Contraindication recommendation for patients with venous insufficiency remains unchanged for reasons just described. Medications that alter cardiac function such as beta blockers that reduce blood pressure and heart rate should be considered before selecting hydrotherapy because they will effect reaction to treatment.

Age related changes to the pulmonary system include diminished ventilation and gas exchange and this has been another factor for limiting use of hydrotherapy for this patient population. However, this is not supported by recent evidence. Patients with CHF have increased respiratory rates and improved pulmonary gas exchange because of decreased pulmonary arterial resistance.[15,16] Pulmonary risks, especially for the elderly and health-care providers that exist include inspiration of airborne respirable water vapor droplets resulting from the agitation of the water in the whirlpool which could result in a pneumonitis.[66] Thus, personal protective masks should be provided for patients during the agitation.

CLINICAL WISDOM

Use of a face mask by the patient as well as personnel would reduce risk of inhalation of respirable droplets during the hydrotherapy treatment.

In all patients, vital signs including blood pressure, heart rate, and respiration rates should be taken before, during, and after treatment. In addition, all patients should be monitored closely during the treatment for: dizziness, feeling faint, or changes in mental status.

Tissue Damage

Normally, the surface environment of the skin is unfavorable to most microflora because its pH is between 5 and 6.[67] Prolonged soaking supersaturates the wound tissue and surrounding skin, which may result in maceration, or the breaking down of the fibers of the skin, and a change in the pH that makes the skin more favorable to microbes.

Concern exists about tissue damage from the agitation force of the whirlpool jet on healthy tissue when it is used to provide nonselective mechanical wound débridement in a wound with granulation tissue.

Wound Infection

There is evidence that wounds treated with hydrotherapy are at risk for waterborne contamination and other complications. Reports in the literature demonstrate *Pseudomonas aeruginosa*–associated skin disease after immersion in public whirlpools.[35,68,69] Factors that influence host susceptibility include the anatomic and physiologic defenses of the skin, the skin surface microecology wherein the skin humidity is altered, and intrinsic factors such as disease and age. The skin's relative dryness may be a defense mechanism to resist infection which immersion in the hydrotherapy may negate. Increased skin tissue temperature has been associated with *P. aeruginosa* infections as well. Chronic antibiotic therapy changes the normal flora of the skin and can lead to colonization and superinfection with organisms such as *P. aeruginosa*.[68]

A variety of intrinsic factors, such as age and diabetes, also appear to increase this susceptibility to infection through the skin. Traumatic injuries such as burns, and immunosuppressive therapies also increase host susceptibility to skin infection with *P. aeruginosa*.[68] Hydration of the skin and increased skin tissue temperature have been associated with *P. aeruginosa* infections as well, and most likely negates many of the skin's normal defenses.

In experimental models, superhydration of the skin must be continuous for long periods of time before symptoms occur, and hydrotherapy usually offers considerably shorter exposure periods. However, repeated immersion and exposure to the hydrotherapy water may lead to colonization of *P. aeruginosa* despite drying of the skin surface between sessions. There is potential for the bacteria to be harbored in the invaginations of the skin appendages, where they release proteolytic enzymes and exotoxins that result in an inflammatory reaction of the surrounding tissues.[20]

Wound decontamination and infection control are cited as reasons to use hydrotherapy, but evidence of their efficacy is mixed. Two studies compared the effects of hydrotherapy treatment and hydrotherapy treatment followed by vigorous rinsing. Neiderhuber et al.[70] studied removal of bacterial load from the soles of the feet of 76 normal adults with intact skin. Factors considered in their investigation included water temperature, immersion time, agitation of the water versus soaking, spraying the part with clean water for 30 seconds, and agitation of the water during immersion, followed by spraying of the part with clean water for 30 seconds.[70] Findings showed that water temperature was not a significant factor in bacterial decontamination whereas duration of immersion was significant. There was a steady removal of bacterial load with longer duration treatment, 10 to 20 minutes being optimal. Agitation was best, compared with either soaking or spraying, in removal of skin surface bacteria, but the combination of immersion with agitation and spraying rinsed away 70% of the remaining contaminants, providing the best outcome.

Bohannon[71] studied a single subject with a venous ulcer and compared bacterial load following hydrotherapy with a low concentration of povidone iodine without and with rinsing for 30 to 90 seconds at the maximum pressure tolerated by the subject. More than four times as many bacteria were removed with rinsing added than without. Both studies support the use of hydrotherapy with rinse to reduce bacterial colonies present on skin and wound surface. Considerable documentation in the literature shows that when the bacterial content of an ulcer exceeds 10^5 organisms per gram of tissue, healing is impaired.[51] However, neither the Neiderhuber nor the Bohannon study identifies the organisms isolated, nor do they use the threshold standard of an infected wound as 10^5 organisms per gram of tissue measured by wound biopsy or culture.[72] Only one patient with a wound was evaluated. Another case mentioned above found relief of sepsis using antimicrobial agents in the whirlpool used to treat a breast cancer patient with a fumigating chest wound.[56]

Risk of infection for the patient with a burn or wound has been documented. Shankowsky et al.[35] surveyed 202 burn units in the United States and Canada, with 158 (75.7%) responding, and found that these facilities regularly use hydrotherapy as part of burn care. Hydrotherapy was implicated as a cause of nosocomial infection leading to sepsis with *P. aeruginosa* (52.9%), *Staphylococcus aureus* (25.5%), and *Candida albicans* (5.2%).[35] Cardany et al.[73] found that hydrotherapy did not reduce bacterial load on burned or normal skin, but the water contained heavy contamination with viable organisms that have the potential for contaminating clean wounds and for patient cross-contamination. A further documented complication is superhydration of the skin, which allows penetration of bacteria.[68,35] Water content of the skin may increase to 55% to 70% following a 20-minute immersion.[68] Intrinsic factors, such as immunosuppression, and diseases such as diabetes are known to increase susceptibility to infection. Hospitalized individuals, compared with healthy individuals, have a decreased resistance to infection and have the highest risk of secondary health effects.

Exposure to pathogens has been associated with many sources, including hydrotherapy tanks and associated equipment. Infectious organisms, particularly *P. aeruginosa*, have been identified in hydrotherapy equipment, despite rigorous efforts to disinfect properly and to monitor for cultures. For instance, Shankowsky et al.[35] reported a lethal outbreak of aminoglycoside-resistant *P. aeruginosa* in a newly constructed burn center in which stringent methods of disinfection were used and despite routine bacterial surveillance. Control of the outbreak was achieved when the hydrotherapy tanks were used for closed wounds during rehabilitation.[35] The following reports show how different clinical settings interpreted and responded to data collected from studies of infectious organisms in hydrotherapy tanks.

Over a 4-week period, cultures were taken in the morning before treatment and at the end of the day from whirlpools in two institutions in a university medical center commonly used by diabetic dysvascular patients. Special attention was directed toward recovery of *S. aureus*, *P. aeruginosa*, and *Escherichia coli* organisms. Results of the testing were that only 11 of 96 cultures (11.5%) were positive for these prospective pathogens. The opinion of the study authors was that immersion in these hydrotherapy tanks was not likely to expose patients with open wounds to potential iatrogenic contamination.[74]

Seventeen hydrotherapy baths in sixteen nursing homes were examined for presence of *P. aeruginosa*. Large numbers of these organisms were found in water samples taken from hydrotherapy baths after agitation, but only 1 patient out of 253 residents was known to have a *P. aeruginosa* wound infection. Results of these findings led the Health Commission to advise the local survey team that, although the prevalence of known *P. aeruginosa* infection was low, the hydrotherapy baths should continue to be used only by continent residents with intact skin to avoid an infection hazard to the residents.[75]

Although the reports in the literature provide considerable evidence of risk of wound contamination, hydrotherapy is used in 94.8% of the surveyed institutions. Despite the reported high incidence of infection, hydrotherapy immersion continues to be used in 118 burn units. Only 27 respondents to the survey have discontinued immersion in favor of showers. Patients who are mechanically ventilated and/or invasively monitored are regularly immersed at 47.6% of the responding burn units.[35] Local treatment appears to reduce risk of lethal sepsis. Alternative measures of controlling wound infection with hydrotherapy using irrigation with sterile solution applied by a syringe or pulsatile lavage with suction are described in Chapters 18 and 28. Risk of infection due to immersion in hydrotherapy is becoming more widely recognized, but has not yet significantly changed clinical practice.

SUMMARY

In the previous sections the physical principles and physiological effects and research evidence as well as risks of hydrotherapy intervention were reviewed. It was pointed out that it is critical for the PT to review the patient's medical history and do a systems review as guidelines for selection of an intervention with whirlpool.

Evaluation of study reports reviewed produced no evidence that hydrotherapy is harmful to granulation tissue. Good practice would be to take care that fragile granulation tissue or a new skin graft is protected from direct force of the whirlpool hydrotherapy jet and that the force of the aeration is modified to avoid any problems. The same is true for patients on anticoagulant therapy who are at risk for deep tissue injury and hematoma.[76]

Hydrotherapy will increase local blood flow for a sustained period of time after cessation of the treatment, increase subcutaneous oxygen, and stimulate the cells needed for healing. It is safe and effective to use, even after the wound is clean and free of exudate and necrotic debris.

Evidence of wound healing efficacy in treatment of patients with hydrotherapy is reported in two controlled clinical trials on pressure ulcers and surgical wounds,[43,53] as is evidence from studies in which it was the control treatment. Whirlpool hydrotherapy may be the most efficient way to treat multiple or extensive wounds. It can be used to heat a large body area or a limited body area and raise core body temperature; it is useful to relax tissue tension and provide relief for painful wounds. Although the evidence is still limited, additional study would be helpful to identify the best frequency of treatment and temperature that best speed healing.

CHOOSING AN INTERVENTION: CLINICAL REASONING

Historically, wounds of nearly every type had been treated with hydrotherapy. In recent time, the pendulum has swung away from using this intervention for the wound population. However, given the many evidence based benefits of hydrotherapy we have identified and examined here (e.g., circulation, cellular effects etc.), the use of hydrotherapy needs to be considered during the clinical reasoning process. Burns require special consideration and that is fully covered in Chapter 15. Appropriate patient centered use of hydrotherapy requires careful consideration of the potential benefits, disadvantages, precautions and contraindications for each patient. This section summarizes four ways for evaluating the choice of hydrotherapy.

- Benefits
- Disadvantages
- Precautions
- Contraindications

Benefits
- Mechanical débridement:
- Soaking and softening of eschar and other necrotic tissue
- Scrubbing and loosening of necrotic tissue
- Debriding by mechanical action of turbulence
- Deodorizing the wound through cleansing
- Soaking to remove dried dressings
- Removal of gelatinous exudate, debris and old topical agents
- Increased blood flow and tissue oxygen through enhancement of hemodynamics
- Enhanced immune system functions through NO production, increased oxygenation of tissue and removal of bacteria
- Ability to increase core body temperature
- Cellular effects:
- Stimulating cell mitosis
- Enhancing leukocytic activity
- Speeding epidermal cell production
- Bringing antibodies to wound area
- Neuronal effects of mild analgesia, comfort and pleasure

Disadvantages

- Superhydrating and macerating skin
- Changing of skin pH changes skin surface environment
- Potential risk of skin infection and wound infection
- Changing of mental status and possible dizziness
- Increasing edema with extremity in the dependent position
- Shifting fluids away from the body may lead to dehydration and nutrient depletion
- Potential traumatizing of the wound or surrounding tissues by mechanical forces
- Overheating (burns) of the tissues of insensate skin or ischemic tissue

Precautions

Whenever hydrotherapy is used, a variety of precautions are essential.

- For patients with venous disease, if cleansing is the intention, keep the water temperature tepid or neutral (33.5°C–35.5°C or 92°F–96°F). Minimize the time in the dependent position (e.g., treat for 5 minutes, not 20 minutes). Follow with a warm water rinse, then apply compression therapy.[77]
- If the wounded limb is edematous or has friable skin around the wound and should not be immersed, perfusion can be enhanced by reflexive vasodilatation through immersion of the opposite lower extremity or an upper extremity.
- Patients on anticoagulation therapy should use hydrotherapy with caution. A suggestion is to reduce the force jet or turn it off because the force of the jet has the potential to traumatize the tissue and cause internal bleeding.[76]
- Expect increasing heart and respiratory rates during the treatment and monitor for undesirable signs.
- Due to expected increased cardiac output, in patients with CHF, make sure that they are compensated and that temperature of water is in the normothermal range.
- Clean, granulating wounds are easily traumatized by the force of mild agitation. Direct the turbulence of the agitation away from the granulation tissue.
- Epithelializing wounds: Migrating epidermal cells may be damaged by even the least force. Do not use agitator jet.
- New skin grafts: Skin grafts will not tolerate high shearing forces and turbulence. Do not use agitator jet.
- New tissue flaps: New tissue flaps are very sensitive to shearing forces and vasoconstriction that can occur if the water or air temperature causes chilling. Shut off agitator jet, use normothermal temperature.
- Nonnecrotic diabetic ulcers: Callus often surrounds diabetic ulcers and will be softened and macerated. Macerated tissue will not tolerate pressure, and the wound will be enlarged. Moisture retention under the callus may become a source of infection. Therefore, do not immerse diabetic feet with callus.
- Impaired sensation. If the patient tests positive for impaired thermal.
- Sensation, lower water temperatures should be used as described.
- Patients with seizures or epilepsy patients should be treated at normothermic or nonthermal temperatures.
- Patients with multiple sclerosis should not be treated at temperatures about 31°C or 88°F due to potential increase in fatigue and weakness.[37]

Contraindications

Contraindications to use of hydrotherapy include the presence of any of the following:

- Moderate to severe extremity edema
- Lethargy
- Unresponsiveness
- Maceration
- Febrile conditions
- Compromised cardiovascular or pulmonary function
- Acute phlebitis
- Renal failure
- Dry gangrene (evaluate for ischemia) like those in Figure 27.2
- Incontinence of urine or feces (if tank and aerator will be contaminated)
- Limb contractures that prevent comfortable and safe positioning in the tank (e.g., fetal contracted posture)

Patients with dry gangrene should not have the tissues softened because the dry gangrene is nature's method of walling off the tissues and encapsulating the area. Softening of the tissue will reduce the barrier and allow infectious organisms to enter the body. Autoamputation of necrotic digits usually occurs anyway (see Chapter 12).

DELIVERY OF CARE

Delivery of care includes consideration of several factors that are discussed now including clinical skills required, equipment, and personal safety.

Clinical Skills Required

Hydrotherapy is not a benign procedure and, therefore, clinicians need to be adequately trained in the multifactorial nature of this clinical intervention. In some institutions, nurses are trained to provide hydrotherapy, in others it is the responsibility of physical medicine and delivered under the supervision of a physical therapist.

The survey of Thomson et al.[78] found that in most burn units (100 units polled), nurses perform hydrotherapy procedures, although there is no consensus on who does it. Shankowsky et al.[35] found that in most of the responding 118 burn units using immersion hydrotherapy, both débridement and rehabilitation/physical therapy treatments were included in a single hydrotherapy session (71.7%) and that hydrotherapy continued throughout the patient's length of stay. According to Medicare guidelines, hydrotherapy is considered a skilled physical therapy procedure when the patient's condition is complicated by disease processes, such as impaired circulation, areas of desensitization, open wounds (e.g., Stage III and IV pressure ulcers), or other complications that require the skills, knowledge, and judgment of a PT who is trained in hydrotherapy. Diagnosis or prognosis is not the sole factor in deciding whether the service is skilled or not.[79]

Recently, some Medicare contractors have issued specific guidelines for physical therapy skilled services for wound care. The guidelines state that interventions that will increase function using treatment modalities specific to physical therapy require the skills of a PT (e.g., treatment of an open wound or burn over a joint while undergoing functional mobility training in the whirlpool). Wound care alone does not require the skills

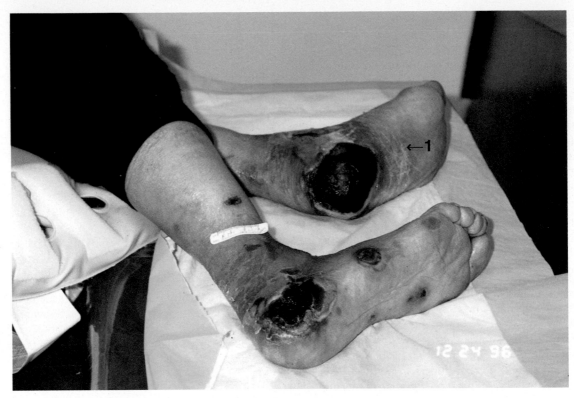

FIGURE 27.2 Dry gangrene.

of a PT.[80] Hydrotherapy has long been considered a physical therapy procedure for patients with burns and wounds because physical therapists receive education in the multifactorial nature of thermal agents for rehabilitation and are licensed in their use.

Equipment

Hydrotherapy tanks may be made of stainless steel, Plexiglas™, or tile (Fig. 27.3). They are used for immersion of either the full body or an extremity and are sized accordingly. Large hydrotherapy tanks are called *Hubbard tanks* and may be used for aquatic exercise as well as for wound healing. Select a tank sized for the wound or body area to be treated. If a patient has multiple wounds, the water should cover those areas that need soaking, cleansing, or debriding. The full-body tank or tub will allow the patient to extend the legs fully and may be more comfortable. If the patient is contracted, select a tank in which the patient can be comfortably positioned.

Hydrotherapy tanks have either an attached turbine or a built-in turbine, or the turbine might be suspended from the side of a bathtub. The whirlpool is created by a mixture of water and air to create controlled turbulence. The more the aeration, the greater will be the turbulence and pressure at the surface of the water.[47] The water-air mixture is adjustable, but the available

range varies from one piece of equipment to another. Force and direction of the agitation are also usually adjustable.

Hydraulic lift chairs and chaises or Hoyer lifts can be used to transfer a patient into the tank if the tank is too high or if the patient is nonambulatory. If the patient is seated on a chair for

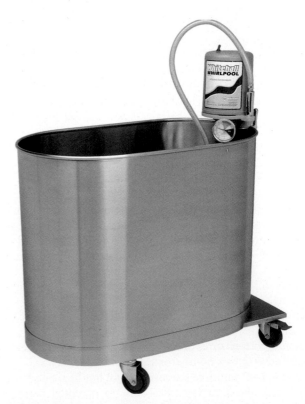

FIGURE 27.3 Whirlpool tank. (Courtesy of Whitehall Manufacturing/ Acorn Engineering, City of Industry, California.)

CLINICAL WISDOM

The physical therapist, nurse, and physician must collaborate on making a dressing selection that will provide the best wound environment and that is appropriate for frequency of whirlpool

CLINICAL WISDOM

Hydrotherapy Bathing

One situation that needs clarification is the common referral of patients with wounds for hydrotherapy treatment and the expectation that this will serve as the patient's bath. The hydrotherapy is not a bathing pool or shampoo basin. The water in the tank is dirty with wound exudate and debris. Soap, shampoo, and disinfectants have ingredients that are harmful to wounds and may irritate delicate skin during soaking. For personal hygiene, a shower is preferable because all substances are flushed away from the wound and the skin.

a leg hydrotherapy treatment be sure there is no pressure under the thigh.

Personnel Safety

Standard precautions should always be followed by hydrotherapy personnel. The hydrotherapy personnel are exposed to airborne water vapor. Inhalation or contact dermatitis of water droplets containing bacteria and antiseptic or disinfection products presents health risks. Isolation of the patient with an open wound during treatment in the hydrotherapy may be beneficial because of aerosolization of infectious organisms and production of respirable droplets from the agitation of the water.[66,81] Staff should use protective gear as barriers to infection including masks, gowns, caps, and goggles such as pictured in Chapter 28 (Fig. 28.5), Pulsed Lavage with Suction. Policies and procedures should be developed for each health-care facility to minimize staff exposure.[66]

PROCEDURES

Several procedural factors to be considered when providing hydrotherapy are now discussed including positioning, frequency and duration, monitoring of vital signs, and infection controls.

Positioning

Position in and the depth of water immersion influence the amount of hydrostatic pressure on the thorax. According to the studies of normal population and patients with CHF sitting in water up to the xyphoid process, nipple line or level of the depth of the right atrium is acceptable for a 30 minute session of immersion at water temperatures ranging from 33°C to 35°C but only for 10 minutes at 41°C.[13,15,16] Greater depth of immersion reduces the exposed skin and decreased ability for skin evaporation. Patient's exposed upper body should be covered with a blanket to prevent chilling.

Frequency and Duration

The care plan for the frequency and duration of hydrotherapy treatment should correspond to the goals of care and varies according to the patient's unique needs.

In the studies reviewed in Table 27.1, all whirlpool treatments were administered daily. Hemodynamic benefits are reported to occur when daily thermotherapy is provided.[7] In populations that we have discussed in this chapter where the

goal of treatment is improved hemodynamics, the duration of the treatment, as we have learned needs to be long enough to achieve those effects. In the case of elderly and diabetics that would most likely be 30 minutes at normothermia. (35°C–37°C). Higher temperature of 40°C produced hemodynamic changes in a 20 minutes session.

Once-daily or three-times-weekly hydrotherapy treatments minimize the frequency of dressing changes and exposure to infection, and maintain the wound temperature and the healing environment.

Monitoring Vital Signs

Monitor all patients' vital signs before, during, and after the hydrotherapy treatment. Record the patient's respiration and heart rate, and take blood pressure. Observe for change in mental status and any reports of lightheadedness. The latter is common with immersion of large body areas. The feeling of lightheadedness should go away after the patient sits for 5 to 10 minutes outside the hydrotherapy area. Also query the patient about the fifth vital sign, pain, both before and after treatment, and document the patient's report. Many individuals find warm water soothing.

Infection Control

Major controversies exist about the use of hydrotherapy and infection that are discussed in the following section. These included the pros and cons of using antiseptics in the hydrotherapy for treatment of infected wounds, comparison of clean tap water and saline on infection, the value of vigorous rinsing after hydrotherapy treatment to control infection, and treatment conferred transmission/cross-contamination from use of hydrotherapy equipment and associated care.

Use of Antiseptics

There is controversy about the use of antiseptic agents in hydrotherapy. Although using an antiseptic in the hydrotherapy tank is not generally encouraged, it is appropriate for certain wounds. These include necrotic, heavily exudating wounds, and wounds with antibiotic-resistant organisms such as *P. aeruginosa*. In these cases, wound decontamination is required. The rationale for using sodium hypochlorite solutions in hydrotherapy is to dissolve blood clots and that may be useful in solubilizing the clotted material that constitutes a considerable portion of necrotic tissue, but, as a consequence, delayed clotting may occur, and the wound exudate will become sanguineous.

When to use Antiseptics

Be sure that the intention for using the antiseptic is clear, monitor carefully, and stop when the desired outcome is met (e.g., the wound is exudate free or necrosis free). Use at low concentrations. Some commonly used antiseptics in the hydrotherapy are as follows:

- Povidone-iodine
- Sodium hypochlorite
- Chlorhexidine gluconate (Hibiclens)
- Chloramine-T (Chlorazene)

Cloramine-T

A hydrotherapy burn unit tested different concentrations of chloramine-T (Chlorazene) to determine its effect on gram-negative organisms.[82] Chloramine-T is an aqueous hypochlorite with a molecular structure that allows for slower release of free chlorine into the water, and this increases the bactericidal effects for a longer time.[83] Findings included negative cultures from patients and from the equipment after a 5-day treatment regimen using chloramine-T at a concentration of 200 parts per million (ppm). Patients' wounds, surrounding tissues, and staff reactions to the chloramine-T additive were carefully monitored, but no adverse side effects were found. Tank decontamination was achieved by running the turbine in the tank with the same solution after treatments. This reduced staff cleaning and disinfection time.

There has been heightened awareness of cytotoxicity to the cells of wound repair from antiseptics. Guinea pigs with an induced full-thickness wound were inoculated with *P. aeruginosa* to study the effects of chloramine-T on wound healing and wound decontamination.[84] One group of animals was immersed in tap water and the other set in water containing 300 ppm of chloramine-T solution at 36°C for 20 minutes. Results showed that, within 8 to 10 minutes of exposure to the chloramine-T solution, all microorganisms were killed. After immersion of the infected wounds in tap water on days 6 and 7 after wounding, there were a number of colony-forming units cultured from the water. There was no evidence of skin irritation in the chloramine-T group. Rates of wound healing of the full-thickness inoculated skin wounds were comparable in both the tap water and chloramine-T groups. After the 5 days, a wound culture, or clinical signs that show significant wound decontamination, the treatment should be changed to clear water, followed by vigorous rinse to rid the tissues of deposits of debris and bacteria. Longer use of the antiseptic agent may retard the healing process, due to the cytotoxic effects on the cells of repair.

In addition, antiseptics have limited effectiveness in reducing bacteria when high bacterial counts are measured, and they are inactivated by organic matter, such as pus and wound exudate.[35,40]

Also consider other methods of wound decontamination, such as photostimulation with ultraviolet light (described in Chapter 24) or ES (described in Chapter 23). Chapters 20 includes additional information on the use of antiseptics, their actions, indications, precautions, directions for use, packaging, and effects on wound healing. Chapter 18, Management of Infection also has useful strategies.

Use of Tap Water
Questions arise about the safety and efficacy of using plain tap water for wound cleansing and decontamination. A comparison study of 705 wounds looked at infection rates following wound cleansing with tap water and saline. It found that less infection occurred in wounds cleaned with tap water than

---

CLINICAL WISDOM

Chloramine-T could be put into the water at the manufacturer-recommended dilutions and agitated for 10 minutes *following* removal of the wound to disinfect the tank. Then the tank can be emptied, scrubbed with a disinfectant, and refilled with fresh water for the next treatment.[47]

with saline, and no bacteria were transferred to the wounds.[40] A comparison of normal saline and clean tap water wound irrigation used to remove bacteria from simple skin lacerations showed that both substances were comparable in reduction of bacterial counts.[85] Monitoring of local water supply for organisms has been useful in controlling nosocomial infection.[35]

Vigorous Rinsing
When a body or extremity is removed from the whirlpool, a layer of residue remains on the surfaces exposed to the water, just like the bathtub ring residue after a tub bath. This residue has many contaminants associated with it. A proven, safe method to reduce bacterial count is to follow hydrotherapy treatment with vigorous rinsing of the patient's skin and wound tissue with clean, warm water to remove the residue.[70,71] A shower may be the best method to cleanse a large body surface and is commonly used in burn centers

Transmission of Infection and Hydrotherapy Equipment
The Centers for Disease Control and Prevention and the American Physical Therapy Association (APTA) reviewed procedures for infection control in hydrotherapy and prepared a guide that is available through the APTA.[86] The procedures described here are adapted from the APTA guide. A copy of the guide would be valuable to all hydrotherapy departments.

Patients using whirlpools and other hydrotherapy tanks are often referred because of active infections. The infectious organisms and the organic debris are then deposited into the water. In warm water, steady temperature and agitation make it easy for bacterial pathogens to become harbored in the hydrotherapy equipment water pipes, drains, and other steel components associated with the device. These regions are difficult to clean and to disinfect or sterilize. In addition, the *Pseudomonas* bacteria has the ability to assume a sessile form, secreting a thick protective glycocalyx that colonizes the components described.[35] This increases the likelihood that highly contaminated water will contact the sites of open wounds, Foley catheters, and other percutaneous devices.

Besides the hydrotherapy tank and attached equipment, other equipment commonly used in the hydrotherapy department, such as Hoyer lifts, wheelchairs, and other transfer equipment, should be considered to be potential sources for colonization and transfer of infectious organisms.[86]

Culturing the Hydrotherapy and Related Equipment
Culturing of the hydrotherapy tank and associated equipment is a controversial topic in hydrotherapy. One rationale for culturing is to prevent infection. To contribute to the prevention of infection, the results must lead to specific actions.[85] One school of thought is that if the best methods of disinfection are already accepted procedures, routine culturing of hydrotherapy and associated equipment is not going to cause a change in procedure and, therefore, is superfluous. Conversely, there are reports that careful monitoring of equipment and the water supply to identify potential sources of bacteria is useful in preventing outbreaks.[35]

Aftercare
Immediately after termination of the treatment, it is ideal to wrap the patient in warm blankets for at least 30 minutes

to sustain the benefits of hemodynamic changes of the warm water.[4] It is also important to rinse the wound(s) with warm water,[71] manually debride the wound of any softened and loosened necrotic tissue, and then rinse again with warm tap water. After the final warm water rinse, protect the wound from cooling, contaminants, and desiccation. The best approach would be for the wound to be dressed immediately in the hydrotherapy area. If the setting does not allow for a complete dressing application while the patient is in hydrotherapy, place a protective moist dressing, such as warm, saline-soaked gauze in the wound and cover it with a secondary dry dressing. To maximize the circulatory benefits, keep the patient in a pre-warmed area (25°C–27°C) during a 30-minute post warming session.[4,13,15]

EXPECTED OUTCOMES

Hyperemia, the increased blood flow to the skin giving it a local bright red color in lightly pigmented skin and a reddish glow in dark skin accompanied by the increased warmth, is a desirable reaction to the application of heat and is called *reactive hyperemia*.

Prognosis for wounds treated by hydrotherapy is a change in tissue function in 2 to 4 weeks. Expect a wound treated for exudate and odor to be exudate and odor-free in 2 weeks. Wounds that are treated for débridement should be free of necrosis in 2 to 4 weeks, depending on volume of necrotic tissue present.

Wounds that have a wound-healing-phase diagnosis of chronic inflammatory phase or absence of inflammatory phase should progress toward a wound healing phase of *acute inflammatory phase* in 2 weeks and to a wound acute proliferative healing phase in 4 to 5 weeks. The signs and symptoms of acute inflammation would include hyperemia, increased skin temperature, and mild edema, followed by a decrease in temperature by the end of the inflammatory phase and a return of skin color to that of adjacent skin or comparable area on the opposite side of the body, progressing to a granulating, contracting wound in the proliferative phase, as seen in Figure 27.4.

The reported mean weekly healing rate from four studies in which hydrotherapy was used is 9.5% per week.[57,58,61,62,] Burke et al.[53] reported a 0.39 cm/wk reduction in size but did not state the size of wounds; they also reported a 37.5% wound deterioration in the hydrotherapy group, with an overall outcome of healing for the treatment group and a 28% improvement and 61% deterioration in the non hydrotherapy group.[53] Payer's data from 1989 showed that wounds treated with hydrotherapy were usually treated for 3 months, with the presumed outcome a clean wound.[87] Wounds treated with other physical agents and advanced therapies have average lengths of treatment that range from 7.5 to 10.5 weeks, with closure as the reported outcome (see Chapter 22). To be competitive, treatment with hydrotherapy must have comparable outcomes. If the wound is not progressing on the trajectory of healing, another intervention should be considered (Table 27.1)

Discontinue Treatment

Discontinue treatment when target outcomes are met, if the wound is not responding, or if other treatment options would better meet the needs of the wound and the patient. In most cases, once-daily treatment followed by application of moisture-retentive wound dressings or enzymes would be a good treatment protocol. Prompt wound dressing following the whirlpool/rinse treatment is needed so as not to cool the wound and stop cell mitosis.

SELF-CARE TEACHING GUIDELINES

After completing the diagnostic process, the PT may determine that hydrotherapy can be performed at home with a portable hydrotherapy unit attached to a bathtub. However, careful screening of the patient and caregiver must be made to have safe and effective treatment results.

Patients with grossly necrotic or purulent wounds are not candidates for home care until the necrosis and purulence are reduced to a level at which the patient and/or caregiver can manage them comfortably. Immunocompromised patients—including those who are diabetic, HIV-positive, or on chemotherapy or immune suppression drugs—should not use hydrotherapy at home. Patient's whose wound should not be placed into a tub can received benefits from indirect stimulation of systemic hemodynamic responses learned earlier. Best hemodynamic results can be expected if there is long-term adherence to the plan of care.[31]

Bathtub cleansing and disinfection of the portable hydrotherapy is extremely important to avoid infection and sepsis. If in doubt about the patient's or caregiver's ability to follow excellent disinfection procedures, do not recommend use of a portable whirlpool.

• Instruct the patient and/or caregiver in the correct water temperature, the duration of the immersion, how to rinse the wound after immersion, and the proper aftercare. Explain that it is critical to take the water temperature with a thermometer to prevent burns. Some people believe that the water must be as hot as tolerable to be beneficial. Emphasize to patients that this is not the case. Also cover proper cleaning and disinfection procedures for the tub and the portable agitator and thermometer.

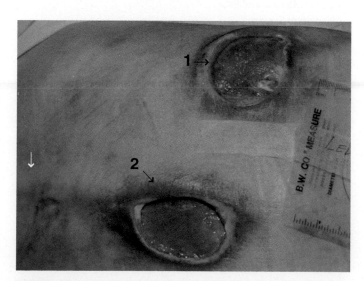

FIGURE 27.4 Wound healing phase: proliferative phase. Note: (*1*) Rolled epidermal ridge around granulation base (*2*) Brown hemosiderin staining (hemosiderosis). (Copyright © C. Sussman.)

CLINICAL WISDOM

Instruct patients and caregivers to turn the home hot water heater down to 120°F and to always use a thermometer to test the water temperature before immersion to avoid burn injury.

- Instruct patients with neuropathy that they should *never* do home foot soaks or hydrotherapy because of the high risk of self-inflicted injury.
- Lethargic patients should be limited to minimal soaking of a single limb in tepid water, primarily for the cleansing and softening of tissue.

- Instruct all patients and caregivers to monitor vital signs during the hydrotherapy treatment.
- Teach the side effects of the treatment and how to respond to symptoms such as lightheadedness, dizziness, or lethargy.
- Explain the desired effects of the treatment and any symptoms that are undesirable. If the patient is being seen through a home care agency, a demonstration and return demonstration in the home, including repetition of instructions, is essential to ensure the correct care delivery. If this is not possible, perhaps a mock setup can be simulated in the hospital or clinic.
- Accountability is essential and encourages compliance. Set up a regular reporting schedule. Give the patient a tracing of the wound, which the patient or caregiver can use to compare changes in size and shape. This will also help to reinforce compliance with the treatment regimen. Follow up by phone to assess changes in wound size or shape, and include periodic visits to monitor outcomes.

CASE STUDY

Patient with Eschar on Both Heels
Functional Outcome Report

Patient Name: G.W. Start of Care Date: 9/27

Medical History
An 84-year-old, alert, confused black female. Nonambulatory resident of long-term care facility. Sits up in wheelchair and attends activity program. Medical diagnosis of Alzheimer disease, and a prior history of cerebrovascular accident (CVA). No prior history of pressure ulceration.

Reason for Referral
1. Dry, leathery eschar on both heels not responding to treatment with occlusive dressings. Indicates loss of healing capacity.
2. Need to determine severity of pressure ulcers on the heels.
3. Severely limited mobility and activity levels.

Systems Review and Exam
Circulatory System
Circulatory perfusion adequate for healing indicated by palpable pulses, warm feet, no significant leg edema, and ankle/brachial index (ABI) of 0.8, but produces inadequate response to wounding due to motor and joint impairment of lower extremities (loss of muscle pump function for circulation).

Musculoskeletal System
Musculoskeletal impairments of the lower extremities due to weakness, joint pain, and stiffness with contractures (10 degrees) at the knees. Patient being positioned upright in wheelchair. Requires minimum assist to perform pivot transfer from bed to wheelchair. Weight bearing during transfer places stress on eschars. Unable to retain upright posture to ambulate and unable to reposition in wheelchair or bed for pressure relief. Braden risk assessment scores each for activity and for mobility 2/4.

Neuromuscular System
Loss of volitional movements due to impaired neuromotor system. Loss of cognitive awareness of position. Loss of protective sensation to reposition (sensory impairment).

Cardiopulmonary System
No clinical signs of cardiopulmonary impairment. Probable diminished ventilation due to inactive mobility status and age.

Integumentary System
Adjacent and surrounding skin has normal skin color tones and turgor, compared with adjacent areas. No pain responses in wounded tissues.

Wound Healing Tissue Assessment
Bilateral heels crusted with hard dry eschar; impairment of integumentary integrity. No thermal changes at the margins of the eschars compared with adjacent tissues. No edema or erythema (color changes) signifies impairment of inflammation response. Unable to see the tissue status under the eschar; unable to determine extent/severity of tissue loss. Size: 25 cm^2 area of eschar on each heel.

Psychosocial
Patient unable to understand directions to reposition or exercise independently. Will follow guided movements. Needs caregiver intervention for repositioning, exercise, and transfers.

Functional Impairments and Functional Diagnosis
Loss of function in above systems causes the following:

1. Wound severity diagnosis: unable to stage impaired integumentary integrity associated with eschar on both heels. Removal of eschar needed to determine extent of wound depth.
2. Wound healing phase diagnosis: absence of inflammatory phase and absence of proliferative phase. Needs restart of the inflammatory phase of healing after conversion to a clean wound that will progress through phases of healing.
3. Associated impairment of mobility and activity secondary to neuromuscular disability (Alzheimer disease and CVA).
4. Undue susceptibility to pressure ulceration on the feet due to motor and sensory impairment.
5. Low blood flow state but has adequate circulation to predict healing.

Short-Term Target Outcomes	Due Date
Wounds: Softening of eschar	3 days
Débridement of eschar	7 days
Shows evidence of inflammatory phase	14 days
Shows evidence of proliferative phase	28 days
Mobility: Nursing assistant will perform range-of-motion and guided exercise	3 days
Therapeutic positioning in bed and wheelchair willbe performed by nursing assistants all shifts	7 days
Transfers with Multi-Podus-type splint	5 days

Prognosis: A clean stable wound with potential for closure in 28 days. Undue susceptibility to pressure ulcers on the feet due to impaired mobility and cognition will continue after wounds are healed. Wound closure in 90 days both heels.

Plan of care with rationale for skilled services

1. Multiple débridement methods required to hasten progression to clean wound bed

Procedures:

- Score eschar—to allow penetration of moisture
- Hydrotherapy to soak and soften tissue, enhance circulation daily
- Sharp débridement—incremental as tissue softens and loosens PRN
- ES—enhance microcirculation and stimulate cells leading to progression through phases of healing daily
- Enzymatic débridement daily—to hasten solubilization of necrotic tissues
- Autolysis with transparent film—to maintain moist wound environment to soften eschar
2. Therapeutic positioning to reduce risk of pressure and shearing to feet during transfers, in wheelchair, and in bed
3. Instruction of nurses' aides in range-of-motion and guided exercises to stimulate delivery of circulation to the tissues
4. Therapeutic exercise performed while in the whirlpool
5. Fitting of Multi-Podus-type splint

Target Outcomes Achieved at First Reassessment 10/1

Wound status:

1. Eschar softened, partially debrided by day 4
2. Removal of outer eschar revealed two focal areas of necrosis covered by eschar
3. Wound has evidence of inflammatory phase: edema, increased warmth in surrounding tissues

Mobility:

1. Patient lying on pressure-relief support surface with pillows and pressure relief splint to relieve pressure
2. Patient sitting up in wheelchair with feet supported with pressure relief splint to relieve pressure during transfers
3. Range-of-motion and guided exercises by nurses' aide performed daily
4. Guided lower extremity exercise performed in the whirlpool

Reassessment 11/9

Wound status:

1. Eschar free, yellow slough
2. Wound depth greater than 0.2 cm
3. Two interconnecting wounds (medial and lateral sides of heel with viable tissue connecting)
4. Wound healing phase progressed to proliferation phase—presence of contraction and granulation tissue

Mobility:

1. Patient is participating in daily exercise and range-of-motion regimen
2. Therapeutic positioning is in place for all shifts

Functional impairments:

1. Integumentary impairment secondary to full-thickness pressure ulcer on the heels

Target outcome:

1. Clean proliferating and contracting wound—due date 21 days
2. Absence of epithelialization phase and sustained contraction

Target outcome:

Progress to epithelialization phase and sustained contraction—due date 21 days

Revised prognosis:

Wound will heal to closure in 60 days.

Revised Treatment Plan and Target Outcomes

Need for Continuation of Skilled Services

Patient failed to respond to routine dressing and conservative management, is now responding to the treatment program. Treatment is done as a collaborative effort between the PT and nurse. Change in treatment interventions required due to change in wound status. Patient has demonstrated potential for healing following interventions but will continue to be at risk for pressure ulceration.

Plan of Care (Intervention) with Rationale

- Discontinue hydrotherapy and sharp débridement tissue—neither needed to debride slough
- Continue ES for microcirculation and stimulation of healing
- Discontinue enzymatic débridement—not needed to debride slough
- Change dressing to hydrogel and secondary dressing—to débride slough, for moist wound healing environment compatible with ES treatment regimen

Target outcomes:

Clean wound bed 7 days

Proliferative phase:

Sustained contraction 14 days

Progress to epithelialization phase 21 days

Discharge outcome

Wounds on both heels healed in 90 days from start of care.

Functional Outcome Reporting System methodology used with permission of Swanson and Co., Long Beach, CA.

REVIEW QUESTIONS

1. Research has suggested that the use of hydrotherapy to treat wounds has all of the following effects except
   A. Improved vascular endothelial function
   B. Depressed vascular systemic hemodynamics
   C. Increased skin blood flow
   D. Increased removal of waste products

2. Which statement is most true regarding patients who are obese?
   A. Deep tissue temperatures increase twice as slowly as those for thin individuals.
   B. Heat transfer from the skin to deeper tissues is enhanced by subcutaneous fat
   C. If body fat exceeds 25%, length of immersion should be less than 15 minutes
   D. Deep tissue temperatures remain unchanged since body fat is an insulator

3. When exercise is performed during hydrotherapy wound treatment,
   A. Sweating will decrease with increases in water temperature
   B. Heart rate will decrease with increases in water temperature

C. Blood pressure will be unaffected by increases in water temperature
D. Gentle stretching forces may stimulate tissue regeneration

4. Benefits of mechanical débridement would include all of the following except
   A. Decrease of core body temperature
   B. Enhanced immune system functions
   C. Enhanced leukocyte activity
   D. Increased blood flow

5. Which statement is most true regarding convection?
   A. Agitation increases water movement, thus promoting convection.
   B. Heating occurs more slowly as compared to conduction.
   C. It will not bring heat to the body core.
   D. Heating will not occur faster than the patient can dissipate it.

REFERENCES

1. Petrofsky JS, Gunda S, Chinna R, et al. Impact of hydrotherapy on skin blood flow: how much is due to moisture and how much is due to heat? *Physiother Theory Pract*. 2010;26(2):107–112.
2. Pennes HH. Analysis of tisue and arterial blood temperatues in the resting human forearm. *J Appl Physiol*. 1998;85:5–34.
3. McLellan K, Petrofsky JS, Zimmerman G, et al. Multiple stressors and the response of vascular endothelial cells: the effect of aging and diabetes. *Diab Technol Ther*. 2009;11(2):73–77.
4. Wessman HC, Kottke FJ. The effect of indirect heating on peripheral blood flow, pulse rate, blood pressure and temperature. *Arch Phys Med Rehabil*. 1967;48:567–576.
5. Abramson D, et al. Changes in blood flow, oxygen uptake and tissue temperatures produced by the topical application of wet heat. *Arch Phys Med Rehabil*. 1961;42:305–317.
6. Taguchi A, Ratnaraj J, Kabon B, et al. Effects of a circulating-water garment and forced-air warming on ody heat content and core temperature. *Anesthesiology*. 2004;100(5):1058–1064.
7. Imamura M, Biro S, Kihara T, et al. Repeated thermal therapy improves impiared vascular endothelial function in patients with coronary risk factors. *J Am Coll Cardiol*. 2001;38(4):1083–1088.
8. Rabkin JM, Hunt TK. Local heat increases blood flow and oxygen tension in wounds. *Arch Surg*. 1987;122:221–225.
9. Hopf H. *The Role of Warming and Oxygen Tension in Wounds*. Symposium on thermoregulation in wound care. Oxford, England; 1999.
10. Ikeda T, et al. Local radiant heating increase subcutaneous oxygen tension. *Am J Surg*. 1998;175:33–37.
11. Plattner O, Akca O, Herbst F, et al. The influence of 2 surgical bandage systems on wound tissue oxygen tension. *Arch Surg*. 2000;135(7):818–822.
12. Ikeda T, et al. The effect of three different local temperatures on subcutaneous oxygen tension. *Anesthesiol Analg*. 1997;84(2S).
13. Gabrielsen A, Sørensen VB, Pump B, et al. Cardiovascular and neuroendocrine responses to water immersion in compensated heart failure. *J Physiol Heart Circ Physiol*. 2000;279:1931–1940.

14. Gabrielsen A, Pumpbie B, Christensen NJ, et al. Atrial distension, haemodilution, and acute control of renin release during water immersion in humans. *Acta Physiol Scand*. 2002;174:91–99.
15. Tei C, Horikiri Y, Park J-C, et al. Acute hemodynamic improvement by thermal vasodilation in congestive heart failure. *Circulation*. 1995;91:2582–2590.
16. Cider A, Svealy BG, Tang MS, et al. Immersion in warm water induces improvement in cardiac function in patients with chronic heart failure. *Eur J Heart Failure*. 2006;8:309–313.
17. Grimes K, Cohen M. Cardiovascular medications. In: Hillegass EA, Sadowsky HS, eds. *Essentials of Cardiopulmonary Physical Therapy*. 2nd ed. Philadelphia, PA: Saunders; 2001:556.
18. Petrofsky J, Gunda S, Raju C, et al. Impact of hydrotherapy on skin blood flow: How much is due to moisture and how much is due to heat? *Physiother Theory Pract*. 2010;26(2):107–112.
19. Petrofsky J, Bains G, Prowse M, et al. Dry heat, moist heat and body fat: are heating modalities really efective in people who are overweight? *J Med Eng Technol*. 2009;33(5):361–369.
20. Lopez M, et al. Rate and gender dependence of the sweating, vasoconstriction and shivering thresholds in humans. *Anesthesiology*. 1994;80(4):780–788.
21. Sessler DI. Mild perioperative hypothermia. *New Engl J Med*. 1997;336(24):1730–1736.
22. Wadhwa A, Komatsu R, Orhan-Sungur M, et al. New circulating-water devices warm more quickly than forced air in volunteers. *Anesth Analg*. 2007;105:1681–1687.
23. Lenhart R, et al. Relative contribution of skin and core temperatures to vasoconstriction and shivering thresholds during isoflurane anesthesia. *Anesthesiology*. 1999;91(2):422–429.
24. Kurz A, Sessler DI, Lenhart R. Perioperative normothermia to reduce the incidence of surgical-wound infection and shorten hospitalization. *New Engl J Med*. 1996;334(19):1209–1215.
25. Reed RL II, et al. Hypothermia and blood coagulation: dissociation between enzyme activity and clotting factor levels. *Circ Shock*. 1990;32(2):141–152.

26. Petrofsky JS, McLellan K, Prowse M, et al. The influence of ageing on the ability of the skin to dissipate heat. *Med Sci Monit.* 2009;15(6):CR261–CR268.

27. Petrofsky JS, Lohann III E, Suh HJ, et al. The effect of Aging on conductive heat exchange in the skin at two environmental temperatures. *Med Sci Monit.* 2006;12(10):CR400–CR408.

28. Hwang J, Himel H, Edlich R. Bilateral amputations following hydrotherapy tank burns in a paraplegic patient. *Burns.* 1995;21(1):70–71.

29. Gass EM, Gass GC, Pitetti K. Thermoregultory responses to exercise and war water immersion in physically trained men with tetraplegia. *Spinal Cord.* 2002;40:474–480.

30. Petrofsky J, Laymon M. Heat transfer to deeptissue: the effect of body fat and heating modality. *J Med Eng Technol.* 2009;33(5):337–348.

31. Michalsen A, Lüdtke R, Bühring M, et al. Thermal hydrotherapy improves quality of life and hemodynamic function in patients with chronic heart failure. *Am Heart J.* 2003;146(4):1–6.

32. McCulloch JM, Boyd VB. The effects of hydrotherapyand the dependent position on lower extremity volume. *J Orthop Sports Phys Ther.* 1992;16:169.

33. Guyton AC, ed. *Textbook of Medical Physiology,* 6th ed. Philadelphia, PA: WB Saunders; 1981.

34. Mayhall CG. Epidemiology of burn wound infections: then and now. *Clinical Infectious Diseases.* 2003;37:543–550.

35. Shankowsky HA, Callioux LS, Tredget EE. North American survey of hydrotherapy in modern burn care. *J Burn Care Rehabil.* 1994;15:143–146.

36. Gomez M, Cartotto R, Knighton J, et al. Improved survival following thermal injury in adult patients treated at a refional burn center. *J Burn Care Res.* 2008;29:130–137.

37. Cameron MH. Hydrotherapy. In: Cameron MH, ed. *Physical Agents in Rehabilitation.* Philadelphia, PA: WB Saunders; 1999:174–216.

38. Lock PM. The effect of temperature on mitosis at the edge of experimental wounds. In: Lundgren A, Soner AB, eds. *Symposia on Wound Healing: Plastic, Surgical and Dermatologic Aspects.* Sweden: Molndal; 1980:103–107.

39. Myers JA. Wound healing and the use of modern surgical dressing. *Pharm J.* 1982;229(6186):103–104.

40. Miller M, Dyson M. *Principles of Wound Care.* London: Macmillan Magazines Ltd.; 1996:29–36.

41. Yang Q, Berghe D. Effect of temperature on in vitro proliferative activity of human umbilical vein endothelial cells. *Experientia.* 1995;51(2):126–132.

42. Park H-Y, Shon K, Phillips T. The effect of heat on inhibitory effects of chronic wound fluid on fibroblasts in vitro. *Wounds.* 1998;10(6):189–192.

43. Juve MB. Hydrotherapytherapy on postoperative pain and surgical wound healing: an exploration. *Patient Educ Couns.* 1998;33(1):39–48.

44. Rush J, et al. The effects of hydrotherapybaths in labor: a randomized controlled trial. *Birth.* 1996;23(3):136–143.

45. Lenstrup C, et al. Warm tub bath during delivery. *Acta Obstet Gynecol Scand.* 1987;66(8):709–712.

46. Shimizu T, Kosaka M, Fujishima K. Human thermoregulatory responses during prolonged walking in water at 25, 30 and 35 degrees C. *Eur J Appl Physiol Occup Physiol.* 1998;78(6):473–478.

47. Walsh M. Hydrotherapy: the use of water as a therapeutic agent. In: Michlovitz S, ed. *Thermal Agents in Rehabilitation.* 3rd ed. Philadelphia, PA: FA Davis; 1996:139–167.

48. Kloth LC, et al. Effects of normothermic dressing on pressure ulcer healing. *Adv Wound Care.* 2000;13(2):69–74.

49. Sussman C. The role of physical therapy in wound care. In: Krasner D, ed. *Chronic Wound Care: A Sourcebook for Health Care Professionals.* Wayne, PA: Health Management Publications; 1990:327–366.

50. Petrofsky J, Bains G, Prowse M, et al. Does skin moisture influence the blood flow response to local heat? A re-evaluation of the Pennes model. *JMed Eng Technol.* 2009;33(7):532–537.

51. Bergstrom N, Bennett MA, Carlson C, et al. *Treatment of Pressure Ulcers.* Clinical Practice Guideline No. 15. Rockville, MD: Agency for Health Care Research and Quality (AHRQ), formerly known as the Agency for Health Care Policy and Research (AHCPR), U.S. Public Health Service (PHS), U.S. Department of Health and Human Services (DHHS); AHRQ Publication No. 95–0652. December 1994:45–65.

52. National Pressure Ulcer Advisory Panel, Panel EPUA. *Prevention and treatment of pressure ulcers: clinical practice guideline.* Washington, DC: National Pressure Ulcer Advisory Panel; 2009.

53. Burke DT, et al. Effects of hydrotherapy on pressure ulcer healing. *Am J Phys Med Rehabil.* 1998;77(5):394–398.

54. Wood JM, Evans PE III, Schallreuter KU, et al. A multicenter study on the use of pulsed low intensity direct current for healing chronic Stage II and Stage III ulcers. *Arch Dermatol.* 1993;130(5):660–661.

55. Gogia PP, Hurt BS, Zirn TT. Wound management with hydrotherapy- and infrared cold laser. *Phys Ther.* 1988;68(8):1239–1242.

56. Nash MS, Nash LH, Garcia RG, et al. Nonselective debridement and antimicrobial cleansing of a venting ductal breast carcinoma. *Arch Phys Med Rehabil.* 1999;80:118–121.

57. Gogia P, Marquez R, Minerbo G. Effects of high voltage galvanic stimulation on wound healing. *Ostomy/Wound Manage.* 1992;38(1):29–35.

58. Gault W, Gatens PF. Use of low intensity direct current in management of ischemic skin ulcers. *Phys Ther.* 1976;56(3):141:145.

59. Akers T, Gabrielson A. The effect of high voltage galvanic stimulation on the rate of healing of decubitus ulcers. *Biomed Sci Instrum J.* 1984;20:99–100.

60. Thurman B, Christian E. Response of a serious circulatory lesion to electrical stimulation. *Phys Ther.* 1971;51(10):137–140.

61. Carley PJ, Wainapel S. Electrotherapy of acceleration of wound healing: low intensity direct current. *Arch Phys Med Rehabil.* 1985;66:443–446.

62. Haynes L, et al. Comparison of Pulsavac and sterile hydrotherapy-regarding the promotion of tissue granulation (abstract). *Phys Ther.* 1994;74(suppl):S4.

63. Vetra H, Whittaker D. Hydrotherapy and topical collagenase for decubitus ulcers. *Geriatrics.* 1975;30:53–58.

64. Feedar JA, Kloth LC. Conservative management of chronic wounds. In: Kloth LC, McCulloch JM, Feedar JA, eds. *Wound Healing: Alternatives in Management.* Philadelphia, PA: FA Davis; 1990:135–172.

65. Conolly WB, et al. Influence of distant trauma on local wound infection. *Surg Gynecol Obstet.* 1969;128(4):713–717.

66. Baron R, Willeke K. Respirable droplets from whirlpools: measurement of size, distribution and estimation of disease potential. *Environ Res.* 1986;39:8–18.

67. Highsmith AK, Kaylor BM, Calhoun MT. Microbiology of therapeutic water. *Clin Manage.* 1991;11(1):34–37.

68. Solomon SL. Host factors in whirlpool-associated *Pseudomonas aeruginosa* skin disease. *Infect Control.* 1985;6:402–406.

69. Jacobson JA. Pool-associated *Pseudomonas aeruginosa* dermatitis and other bathing-associated infections. *Infect Control.* 1985;6:398–401.

70. Neiderhuber SS, Stribley RF, Koepke GH. Reduction of skin bacterial load with use of the therapeutic whirlpool. *Phys Ther.* 1975;5(5):482–486.

71. Bohannon R. Hydrotherapy versus hydrotherapy and rinse for removal of bacteria from a venous stasis ulcer. *Phys Ther.* 1982;62:304–308.

72. Swanson G. *Hydrotherapy Use in Standard Physical Therapist Practice Project.* Presented at class, University of Southern California, BKN 599. Los Angeles, CA; July 1997.

73. Cardany CR, Rodeheaver GT, Horowitz JH. Influence of hydrotherapy and antiseptic agents on burn wound bacterial contamination. *J Burn Care Rehabil.* 1985;6:230–232.

74. Stanwood W, Pinzur M. Risk of contamination of the wound in a hydrotherapeutic tank. *Foot Ankle Int.* 1998;19(3):173–176.

75. Hollyoak V, Boyd P, Freeman R. Hydrotherapybaths in nursing homes: use, maintenance and contamination with *Pseudomonas aeruginosa. Burn.* 1995;5(7):R102–R104.

76. Liefeldt L, Destanis P, Rupp K, et al. The hazards of whirlpooling. *Lancet,* 2003:361(9356):534.

77. McCulloch J. *Physical Modalities in Wound Management.* Preconference course. Presented at the Symposium on Advanced Wound Care; April 1995; San Diego, CA.

78. Thomson PD, Bowden ML, McDonald DK, et al. A survey of burn hydrotherapy in the United States. *J Burn Care Rehabil.* 1990;11(2):151–155.

79. Health Care Financing Administration. Coverage of Services, 3132.4. Woodlawn, MD: December 1987.

80. Blue Cross of North Carolina. Medicare Bulletin Number 98–9. December 1996, Part A Office, Durham, NC: 2–3.

81. Loehne HB, et al. *Aerosolization of Microorganisms During Pulsatile Lavage with Suction.* In Combined Sections Meeting, American Physical Therapy Association; 2000; New Orleans, LA: APTA.

82. Steve L, Goodhart P, Alexander J. Hydrotherapy burn treatment: Use of chloramine-T against resistant microorganisms. *Arch Phys Med Rehabil.* 1979;60:301–303.

83. Marquez RR. Wound debridement and hydrotherapy. In: Gogia P, ed. *Clinical Wound Management.* Thorofare, NJ: Slack; 1995: 122–126.

84. Henderson JD, Leming JT, Melon-Niksa DB. Chloramine-T solutions: Effect on wound healing in guinea pigs. *Arch Phys Med Rehabil.* 1989;70(8):628–631.

85. Moscati R, et al. Comparison of normal saline with tap water for wound irrigation. *Am J Emerg Med.* 1998;16(4):379–381.

86. American Physical Therapy Association. *Hydrotherapy/Therapeutic Pool Infection Control Guidelines.* Alexandria, VA: American Physical Therapy Association; 1995:8–11.

87. Swanson G. Use of cost data, provider experience, and clinical guidelines in the transition to managed care. *J Insurance Med.* 1991; 23(1):70–74.

CHAPTER 28

Pulsatile Lavage with Suction

Harriett Baugh Loehne

CHAPTER OBJECTIVES

At the completion of this chapter, the reader will be able to:

1. Identify four benefits of pulsatile lavage with suction for wound care.
2. Identify benefits for clinicians and facilities using pulsatile lavage with suction.
3. Discuss indications for treatment with pulsatile lavage with suction.
4. Discuss precautions for use of pulsatile lavage with suction.
5. Delineate outcome measures for pulsatile lavage with suction.
6. Follow national guidelines for infection control while providing pulsatile lavage with suction.
7. Explain the procedure for treatment with pulsatile lavage with suction.
8. Describe a device that provides jet lavage with and without suction.

Pulsatile lavage with suction (PLWS) is a method of wound care that provides cleansing and debridement with pulsed irrigation combined with suction. Battery-powered units are available, along with a selection of tips for cleansing and debridement of different wound configurations. The pulsed irrigant provides positive pressure, while suction provides negative pressure to remove the irrigant and debris to help reduce infection and to enhance granulation. This ultimately provides an improved foundation for wound healing.

Powered irrigation via the Water Pik™, a dental water jet, was first used by oral surgeons for soft tissue injuries in the Vietnam War.[1] Noting its efficacy, development of pulsed lavage with suction became a reality. Physicians have used these systems in the operating room since the early 1980s for irrigation in surgical procedures and to clean wounds of debris. Physical therapists (PT) have used the systems since the late 1980s for irrigation and debridement to enhance healing of soft tissue wounds, and subsequently nurses also are using PLWS.

In 1994, a study done by Haynes et al.[2] reported that the rate of granulation tissue formation was 12.2% per week for wounds treated with PLWS and 4.8% per week for those treated with WP. More physical therapists began to try and choose PLWS as an intervention for wound management.[3] Just as with whirlpool, there is limited research to support the use of PLWS for wound healing. A recent reference guide by the European and National Pressure Ulcer Advisory Panels gave PLWS and WP evidence ratings of "C."[4] There are numerous anecdotal reports and case studies that provide evidence of the following four therapeutic benefits of PLWS.[5–7]

BENEFITS OF PULSATILE LAVAGE WITH SUCTION

- It can be used at a gentle setting for wound cleansing.
- At a stronger setting, it provides irrigation and debridement.
- It reduces bacterial counts and infection.
- It promotes production of granulation tissue and reepithelialization. The negative pressure of the suction is thought to stimulate granulation of clean wounds.

In addition, patients themselves derive many benefits from PLWS therapy, as do clinicians and facilities. These benefits are discussed shortly.

Battery-powered, disposable PLWS devices modeled after operating and emergency room equipment are used for wound cleansing. These devices have been recommended to decrease treatment time, minimize cross-contamination, speed healing, and shorten length of hospital stays and for their versatility in enabling clinicians to personalize treatment to provide a best outcome for the patient and the wound.[8] Although research on the effects of PLWS on wound cleansing is scant, some studies have concluded that PLWS is a safe method of cleansing.[9,10] Research showed no evidence of bacteremia after lavage applications, regardless of pressure; however, until more research is done, low pressures should be used (between 4 and 15 pounds per square inch (psi), as discussed shortly).[11] However, if the impact pressure is too low, below 4 psi, the lavage will not cleanse effectively.

Mechanical Debridement

Irrigation is an effective mechanical debridement method to loosen and flush out debris from contaminated wounds. Fluid dynamics play an important role in expelling the loosened debris with a high-flowing irrigation stream. Different methods for irrigation of wounds include bulb syringe, Water Pik, shower spray, spray bottles, and pulsatile irrigation/lavage. Irrigation pressures vary with use of these different devices. Exhibit 28.1 includes the irrigation pressures obtained with these commonly used clinical devices.[12] Notice that the irrigation pressure of a spray bottle is 1.2 psi and of a bulb syringe is 2 psi. These pressures are not adequate to cleanse a wound.[12] Safe, effective irrigation pressures range from 4 to 15 psi.

Pulsed stimulation of the tissue also is thought to affect wound debridement.[13] The pulse phase rapidly compresses the tissue; then, during the interpulse phase, the tissue decompresses. This may be a mechanism for mechanically loosening debris. Because of the loosened and hydrated necrotic tissue, sharp debridement is easier following PLWS.

Management of Infection

Since we have learned that wound infection is a major concern in management of wounds and dead and dying tissue, debris, clotted blood, and foreign bodies are predisposing conditions to wound infection, rapid removal of these contaminants has been demonstrated to speed healing. A study in the literature reports that high-pressure pulsating irrigation in acute contaminated wounds decreases the presence of these contaminants and results in a lower incidence of wound infection.[14]

Irrigation pressures vary with the use of different devices. The incidence of wound infection is decreased as the amount of irrigation fluid increases.[15] Irrigation pressure of a bulb syringe is 2 psi, which is not adequate to reduce bacteria.[12] Stevenson et al.[6] reportedly calculated and tested combinations of syringe and needle sizes to determine wound irrigating pressure. The pressure produced by a 35-mL syringe and a 19-gauge needle was 8 psi, a pressure that has been found effective in removing bacteria and infection.[16] Irrigation at 13 psi has been attributed to reduction of inflammation in traumatic wounds. Irrigation pressures exceeding 15 psi may traumatize tissue and drive bacteria into the wound tissues.[17,18] The Water Pik™ ranges from 6 to more than 50 psi, which may cause trauma to a wound and drive bacteria into it.[17] Fortunately, the pulsatile lavage systems described later in this chapter allow the psi to be adjusted, but cannot be higher than 15 psi. The psi treatment setting chosen will depend on the amount of necrotic tissue/exudate, the location of the wound, and the patient's comfort. Pulse rate, as well as psi, has been demonstrated clinically to effect granulation formation and epithelialization of clean wounds.[5] From clinical experience, this author has learned that the higher the pulse rate, the more rapid the rate of granulation and epithelialization (as psi remains the same), though no clinical studies have been done. The pulse rate varies by brand of device.

Part of clinical decision making involves weighing the risk/benefit ratio. Sometimes multiple risks have to be considered when selecting a treatment intervention. For example, will the benefit of high-pressure cleansing of a highly contaminated wound outweigh the known risk of tissue trauma and have a better outcome than an inadequate response? PTs would not use high-pressure irrigation unless under the direct supervision of a physician. If patient assessment indicates that you should consider high-pressure irrigation, consultation with the physician is needed.

The author's clinical experience includes use of PLWS for both clean and infected wounds of many etiologies. Wounds that have benefited from this therapy are included in the list shown in Exhibit 28.2.

Pulsed jet lavage has been used for treatment of traumatic wounds in operating rooms and in the military for decades.[19] Delivery of vancomycin-, streptomycin-, and tetracycline-water solutions with pulsating jet lavage eliminated or reduced bacteria as early as the 2nd day, with earlier healing, less tissue loss, and reduced scarring. Infected diabetic foot lesions treated with pulsatile lavage and topical antibiotics had infection controlled, and the wounds were able to be closed surgically with grafts or flaps. Reduced inflammation has been reported following pulsed lavage treatment and was correlated to the extent of foreign material remaining in the tissues. Early cleansing with this therapy accelerated wound healing.[15]

Production of Granulation Tissue

Concurrent suction with pulsatile lavage appears to stimulate production of granulation tissue in "clean" wounds as a result of the negative pressure.[20] Negative pressure applies noncompressive mechanical forces to the tissues and dilates arterioles. Dilatation allows increased blood flow and transcutaneous oxygen delivery to the tissues.[21] Suction also removes debris, bacteria, and irrigant. In addition, the levels of pulsation and pressure have been demonstrated clinically to effect granulation formation and epithelialization of clean wounds.[5]

EXHIBIT 28.1

Irrigation Pressures Delivered by Various Devices

Device	Irrigation Impact Pressure (psi)
Spray bottle—Ultra Klenz	1.2
Bulb syringe	2.0
Piston irrigation syringe (60 mL) with catheter tip	4.2
Saline squeeze bottle (250 mL) with irrigation cap	4.5
Water Pik at lowest setting (1)	6.0
Irrijet DS syringe with tip	7.6
35-mL syringe with 19-gauge needle or angiocatheter	8.0
Water Pik at middle setting (3)	42
Water Pik at highest setting (5)	>50
Pressurized Cannister-Dey-Wash	>50

Reprinted from Bergstrom N, Bennett MA, Carlson CE, et al. Treatment of Pressure Ulcers, Clinical Practice Guideline No. 15, December, 1994; U.S. Department of Health and Human Services, Public Health Service, Agency for Health Care Policy and Research, AHCPR Publication No. 95–0652.

EXHIBIT	28.2

Examples of Indications for Pulsed Lavage

Type or Wound/Patient History	Rationale
Venous insufficiency ulcer	
A patient with a history of chronic leg wounds hit the pretibial area of his right lower extremity on a table leg 6 months ago. He has had open wounds on the lower extremity since then. The lower extremity is also edematous and there is periwound maceration. The patient is using a compression stocking.	If pulsed lavage with suction is used, the wounds can be treated with the lower extremity elevated to avoid increased edema. Treatment is site specific, so periwound maceration is not increased. Granulation and epithelialization can be stimulated, possibly by negative pressure of the suction.
Neuropathic ulcer	
A patient with diabetes and loss of protective sensation in both feet has an ulcer on the plantar surface of his left heel. He has a callus with a fragile area in the center at the head of the fifth metatarsal.	Instead of soaking the foot in a whirlpool, pulsed lavage with suction will offer site-specific treatment that will not compromise the callus and fragile area. In addition, the patient's lower extremity will not be in a dependent position, thereby avoiding edema, and the patient's skin will not be burned due to loss of sensation (a risk with whirlpool).
Pressure ulcer	
A paraplegic patient with bowel and bladder incontinence has a large sacral pressure ulcer.	An incontinent patient cannot be immersed in a whirlpool, but incontinence is not a contraindication to pulsed lavage with suction. Even if the patient were not incontinent, his wound would be difficult to treat in a whirlpool because he would have to lie on his sacrum, putting pressure on the wound site. In addition, he would have to be transported to physical therapy on a hard stretcher. This is not necessary with pulsed lavage because it is a bedside procedure.
Sternal wound	
Following coronary artery bypass graft surgery, a patient develops a wound infection and dehiscence. She is on a cardiac monitor and ventilator in the intensive care unit.	This patient's wound can be irrigated and debrided at the bedside using pulsed lavage with suction. Whirlpool immersion is not an option because of her medical equipment—cardiac electrodes cannot be placed in water.
Perineal wound	
A patient has Fournier gangrene with multiple deep, narrow tunnels; there is purulent drainage with a foul odor. The patient is septic with a temperature of 105°F.	Whirlpool is contraindicated for a febrile patient. Pulsed lavage with suction is the alternative, using a product with a flexible tip to allow irrigation and debridement of the tunnels and to decrease the bacterial count.
Partial-take split-thickness skin graft	
A patient with pyoderma gangrenosum has had a split-thickness skin graft on the right lower extremity. There has been only partial take, with eschar and necrotic slough at the failed site.	Because pulsed lavage with suction is site specific, it can be used to treat only the failed portion of the graft without compromising the remainder of the graft. Eschar will be hydrated enough to allow sharp debridement (escharotomy) following pulsed lavage.
Fasciotomies	
A patient with multiple fractures to his left lower extremity secondary to a motor vehicle accident is in skeletal traction. Medial and lateral fasciotomies have been performed, due to edema, and now there is periwound erythema and purulent drainage from tunnels and undermining.	Traction can be maintained and the wounds can be treated without disturbing the hardware if pulsed lavage with suction is used. The tracts can be irrigated using a device with a long, flexible tip.

Used with permission from *Adv Skin Wound Care* 2000;13(3):133–134, © Springhouse Corporation/ www.springnet.com.

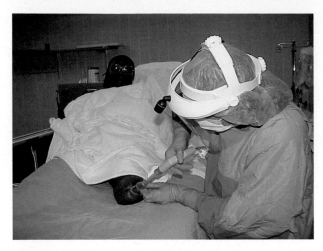

FIGURE 28.1 PLWS in a treatment room.

Patient Benefits

Patients derive many benefits from treatment by PLWS. Frequently, the patient can be treated by a nurse or PT at the bedside or by the PT in the PT department instead of by a physician in the operating room, with significant cost savings. Patient safety is improved, because PLWS requires no transfers such as would be needed getting into/out of the whirlpool, and comfort is increased because the therapy produces no changes in body temperature and the clinician has direct control over the pressure of the fluid on the wound.

A retrospective study by Ho et al.[22] in 2004 examined charts of 27 patients with pressure ulcers treated with PLWS over a 2-year period. The results indicated a favorable safety profile, with no moderate or severe bleeding, significant wound infection, or autonomic dysreflexia due to treatment. There was also no documented complaint of pain.

Patient benefits are summarized as follows:

- PLWS offers cost savings if operating room is not needed.
- It offers improved safety and comfort.
- Periwound maceration is avoided.
- It can be used for treatment of tracts, tunnels, and undermining (Fig. 28.1).
- It has contributed to the salvage of limbs.[5]
- Treatment is possible if whirlpool treatment is contraindicated.

Patients who would benefit from hydrotherapy but are contraindicated for whirlpool should be considered candidates for pulsatile lavage. This includes patients with the following conditions:

- Unresponsiveness
- Cardiopulmonary compromise
- Venous insufficiency
- Neuropathy/diabetes
- Fever
- Incontinence if body whirlpool is required

CLINICAL WISDOM

Irrigation and Debridement of Tracts and Tunnels

Pulsatile irrigation is an excellent choice for irrigation and debridement of tracts, tunnels, and/or undermining.

Treatment is possible in the following circumstances:

- Contractures—difficult body placement
- Ostomies
- Closed incisions with sutures intact
- IV placement
- Skeletal traction
- Casted extremities
- Obesity exceeding weight limit for stretcher/whirlpool
- Patient combative/restrained
- Patient in ICU, IMCU, burn unit, or isolation (negative pressure room)

Clinician Benefits

Clinicians are able to use time efficiently and effectively when performing PLWS. Because all supplies are disposable, a pulsatile lavage treatment can take only 15 to 30 minutes. This makes it possible to provide treatment to a greater number of patients.

The design of PLWS devices allows the user to control the intensity of the treatment, in psi, and to select the appropriate tip for specific effects. These features promote optimal results while safeguarding tissue. Some units allow greater control than others. Therefore, it is important to be aware of the features and the limitations of the available equipment.

Sharp debridement is significantly easier after PLWS treatment because it loosens and softens debris and hydrates necrotic tissue. Clinician benefits are summarized as follows:

- PLWS is time efficient.
- The clinician has the ability to control psi.
- There is no destruction of granulation tissue if 4 to 15 psi impact pressure is used.
- There is increased productivity.
- Ease of sharp debridement is increased after treatment.
- Treatment is convenient and cleanup is minimal.

Facility Benefits

In an acute care facility, PLWS contributes to a decreased length of stay because of the rapid rate of granulation and epithelialization. Thus, patients treated with PLWS can be discharged home with dressing changes sooner. Wounds treated with PLWS are ready for grafting/flap surgery more quickly. Physician and staff time is saved if the patient is treated with PLWS, either at the bedside or in the PT department, and does not have to be taken to the whirlpool tank or to the operating room for irrigation and debridement by the surgeon. Cross-contamination is virtually eliminated because all supplies are disposable. This is especially important with infection control issues for bloodborne pathogens (BBP) and the spread of methicillin-resistant *Staphylococcus aureus* (MRSA), vancomycin-resistant enterococci (VRE) and other multidrug-resistant organisms.

OUTCOME MEASURES

Clinical decision making involves evaluation of intervention choices to achieve a desired outcome. PLWS is a versatile treatment choice. As discussed earlier, it can be used for all wounds in which the expected functional outcome is a wound base free of infection, necrosis, inflammation, and exudate, and filled with good granulation, in preparation for closure by secondary intention or surgery.

Because there are no controlled clinical trials of this therapy, average length of time to achieve an expected outcome is undetermined. Clinical judgment of the author suggests that the clinician should

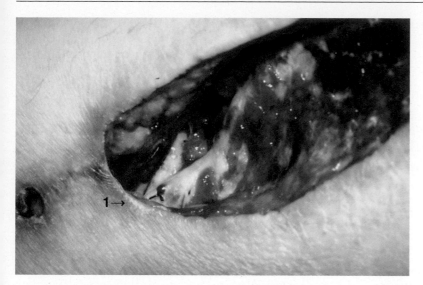

FIGURE 28.2 Exposed artery in infected bypass graft donor site in lower leg. (Copyright © H. Loehne.)

expect a decrease in necrotic tissue in 1 week and an increase in granulation/epithelialization in 1 week (see Figs. 28.3A and 28.3B). Following are some additional expected clinical outcomes:

- Odor and exudate free: 3 to 7 days
- Necrosis free: 2 weeks
- Progression from chronic inflammatory phase to acute inflammatory phase: 1 week
- Progression from acute inflammatory phase to proliferation phase: 2 weeks

A clinical outcome is one type of expected outcome. Another type of outcome to be considered is cost. The cost of an outcome includes many factors, such as labor, supplies, and length of stay. Since the average treatment time with pulsatile irrigation is 15 to 30 minutes, labor costs are reduced. Debridement with PLWS can be performed by a trained RN or PT at the bedside or in the PT department, so that surgeon and operating-room costs are avoided. Infection control costs are minimized because single-use, disposable components mean that cross-contamination is virtually eliminated. These are very important cost-management factors in facilities that must work continuously to control contamination with BBP, MRSA, and VRE.

Patient and caregiver satisfaction surveys monitor perceptions of how patients feel about the treatment they received and how it has affected function. Patients want to feel safe, secure, and comfortable during the treatment procedure, and confident that the therapy will help their wound to heal.

Treatment with pulsatile lavage can be given at the bedside, eliminating uncomfortable transfers and travel. Because of its portability and disposable components, it is an ideal modality for home treatment, often allowing for early discharge with Home Health providing continued treatment.

PRECAUTIONS AND CAUTIONS

The most important three words to remember when treating a patient with PLWS are ***know your anatomy!*** As with any method of debridement, it is imperative to have a strong anatomical background, enhanced by cadaver dissection, and to have an illustrated textbook in close proximity. Just as important is awareness of the possibility of anomalies. If you are unsure of the specific anatomy of exposed and nearby structures, consult the patient's surgeon. This is especially true when irrigating tracts and undermining.

There are no known absolute contraindications to treatment with PLWS. As with any wound care treatment, however,

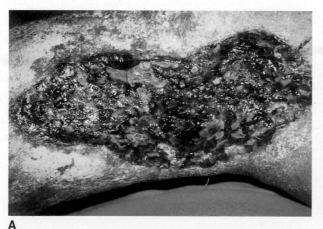

A

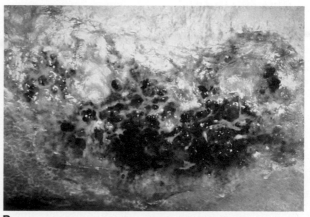

B

FIGURE 28.3 **A.** Pyoderma gangrenosum uylcer on medial lower leg of 8 year duration same ulcer shown. **B.** After treatment with pulsatile lavage with suction. Note new epitheliaization and granulation tissue after one week of treatment. (Copyright © H. Loehne.)

certain precautions should be observed. These precautions apply to treatment of the following:

- Insensate patients
- Those taking anticoagulant medication
- Those with wounds with tracts, tunnels, and/or undermining

Only experienced therapists should treat wounds that require extra attention to the entire procedure (Fig. 28.2). These include the following:

- Wounds near major vessels (e.g., in the groin or axilla)
- Wounds near a cavity lining (e.g., pericardium or peritoneum)
- Bypass graft sites, anastomoses
- Exposed vessel, nerve, tendon, bone
- Grafts, flaps
- Facial wounds

Certain wounds should be assessed carefully before being treated in a facility or home where a physician and emergency medical aid are not immediately available. Careful decision making is needed before treating wounds near major vessels, cavity linings, and bypass graft sites outside of an acute care hospital or hospital outpatient setting.

Stop treatment immediately if the patient complains of increased pain or is unable to tolerate treatment because of pain. A premedication order may be needed from the patient's physician. With an arterial bleeder, treatment must be stopped immediately and the physician called immediately. Hold firm pressure with gauze over bleeding. Use a hemostatic agent if available. Any bleeding not stopped with pressure held without pause for 10 minutes requires a physician consultation and/or an order to use silver nitrate to stop the bleeding. Also notify the physician if an abscess other than the one being treated is opened or a bone/joint disarticulation occurs. Cautions are summarized as follows:

- Stop treatment when the following occurs:
  1. Patient complains of increased pain.
  2. Patient is unable to tolerate treatment because of pain.
- Stop and call physician in any of the following circumstances:
  1. Patient has an arterial bleeder; notify physician *immediately*.
  2. Bleeding has not stopped after 10 minutes of pressure.
  3. Abscess is opened.
  4. Joint is disarticulated.

PROCEDURE FOR PLWS

PLWS can be performed along with negative pressure wound therapy (NPWT), the topic of the next chapter. Typically, NPWT uses a pump, attached by tubing to a foam dressing placed in the wound, to create a vacuum to remove fluid. The negative pressure on the wound helps to reduce edema,

---

CLINICAL WISDOM

Prevent Disruption of Clot Following Pressure to Stop Bleeding

After applying pressure over gauze packing until bleeding has stopped, leave the bottom layer of gauze in place to avoid disruption of the clot and restarting of the bleeding. Cover with the prescribed dressing.

---

increase blood supply, and decrease bacterial colonization. The procedure increases tension among the surrounding cells, which encourages cell growth and division, drawing the edges of the wound to the center and assisting wound closure. The technique also provides a moist wound environment to promote more effective cellular activity, and helps to prevent contamination of the wound site from outside bacteria.

There frequently is confusion among patients and clinical personnel due to the similarity in the names *VAC*, originally called *Decubivac* and *Dvac* (an NPWT product discussed in Chapter 29) and *Pulsavac (a PLWS product)*. These are two entirely different interventions for wound management, though, indeed, they complement each other. The combination of NPWT and pulsed lavage has healed wounds four times faster than nontreated wounds, producing extraordinary cost savings.

Frequency and Duration

Patients are usually treated once a day. If the wound has more than 50% necrotic/nonviable tissue with purulent drainage/foul odor, and especially if sepsis is present, treatment twice a day is reasonable. Treatment two or three times a week is recommended if there is a full granulation base, no odor, and no purulent drainage. If the wound is being treated with NPWT, then use PLWS with each NPWT change, usually two or three times a week. Discontinue PLWS when the wound is closed, there is no increase in granulation/epithelialization in 1 week, or there is no decrease in necrotic tissue in 1 week (Exhibit 28.3).

Procedure Setup

Most patients ideally are treated on a high-low stretcher, bed, or treatment table adjusted to a height that facilitates the therapist's proper body mechanics. Treatment may be delivered in a private treatment room in the physical therapy department or elsewhere or at the bedside in the patient's private room. Place a fluid-proof or fluid-resistant pad under the body part with the wound, and clean towels around the wound and covering adjacent body parts, IV sites, and other portals of entry. Set up an aseptic field, with treatment and dressing supplies in easy reach. A strong light source is important during pulsatile lavage and debridement.

Outpatients with lower extremity wounds can be treated while seated in a wheelchair with an elevating footrest, with towels padding the footrest. The therapist sits on a low footstool in front of the patient and in easy reach of the aseptic field setup of treatment and dressing supplies. Place a basin under the foot to catch any overflow of irrigant.

Recruit the assistance of an aide. Although an aide's duties will vary according to the patient needs and the system used, help with the following tasks can save you time and spare you from having to change gloves during treatment: connecting the tubing to the suction source, warming and spiking the bags of fluid, emptying and replacing the filled suction canisters and new fluid bags, and assisting with patient positioning. After the

---

CLINICAL WISDOM

NPWT and PLWS

NPWT and PLWS used in conjunction with each other provide an optimal intervention for management.

EXHIBIT 28.3

Frequency and Duration of Treatment

Frequency	Daily	Twice Daily	Three Times/Week	Discontinue
Most wounds	X			
>50% necrotic		X		
Purulent drainage		X		
Sepsis		X		
Full granulation base			X	
VAC being used			X	
Duration				
No increased granulation for 1 week				X
No decreased necrotic tissue for 1 week				X
Wound closed				X

treatment is completed, the aide also can dispose of the personal protective equipment (PPE), old dressings, and disposables while you complete the documentation.

Infection Control

Infection control procedures include standard precautions, use of PPE, and use of disposables.[23]

Standard Precautions

Protocols should adhere to each facility's policy, which can be more, but not less, stringent than Occupational Safety and Health Administration (OSHA) guidelines.[24] The importance of hand hygiene, including hand washing at the sink or use of an alcohol-based hand sanitizer, before and after the use of gloves, cannot be overemphasized.[25]

In 2003, there was an outbreak of multidrug-resistant bacteria in a hospital in the United States that was traced to patients being treated with PLWS. Some of the patients died.[26] The spread of the bacteria was apparently due to environmental contamination attributed to PLWS being utilized without proper PPE and other infection control techniques. As a result of their investigations, the CDC and FDA made the following recommendations for infection control guidelines for treatment with PLWS (Exhibit 28.4):[27,28]

Aerosolization of microorganisms occurs during treatment, as evidenced in a study by Loehne et al.[29] Therefore, the patient should be treated in a private room with walls and doors that shut, not privacy curtains or open areas. On admission to the facility, if wound management with PLWS at bedside is anticipated, the patient should be assigned a private room as a medical necessity. This should be included in the facility's policies and procedures.

When the patient is treated at the bedside, all visitors should leave the room during treatment. If treated at home, family members/visitors should leave the room during treatment. All IV sites and other portals of entry on the patient, as well as wounds not being treated, should be covered with a clean towel. Consider using a surgical mask for the patient during treatment.

All exposed linen used to control splash should be placed in a clear plastic biohazard bag after treatment for transport to the laundry. Disinfect the stretcher/wheelchair after each treatment if it is used to transport and treat the patient. Do not use a mattress or cushion with tears in the protective covering. With treatment of extremity wounds, use basins to contain the irrigant overflow. Disinfect the basin after each use. Clean the dressing cart with an approved disinfectant solution after each use. Reusable face shields should be cleaned with a disinfectant that has been approved as effective against HIV, hepatitis B, and tuberculosis. Dispose of all disposables in the appropriate waste stream per OSHA guidelines.

EXHIBIT 28.4

Summary of Infection Control Guidelines for Treatment with PLWS

1. Treat patient in private room, appropriately ventilated, with walls and doors that close
2. Cover any exposed supplies or patient's personal items
3. Cover any exposed tubes, ports, etc., and any wounds not being treated
4. Consider masking the patient
5. No family or visitors in room during treatment
6. Observe standard precautions, including hand hygiene
7. Staff must wear appropriate PPE
8. Dispose of disposables in appropriate waste stream
9. Discard suction canister or liner as appropriate, after each treatment
10. Do not reuse single-use-only items
11. After treatment, thoroughly disinfect all environmental surfaces touched

Thoroughly clean and disinfect all horizontal surfaces that can be touched by hand (e.g., bed rails, pumps) after treatment. There should be no supplies in open shelves or cabinets; do not open drawers during treatment. Cover any exposed supplies or personal articles with a clean towel. Do not reuse single-use-only items.

Personal Protective Equipment

Secondary to aerosolization and splashing, all staff present during treatment must wear PPE (Fig. 28.5). This includes the following items:[30]

- Surgical masks
- Hair covers (with ears covered)
- Face shields
- Fluid-proof (not fluid-resistant) gowns
- Fluid-resistant shoe covers (at the therapist's discretion for the aide)
- Nonsterile/sterile gloves with extra long cuffs to cover cuffs of gown

Disposables and Other Supplies

All disposables except two discussed below are marked for **single use only**. The FDA and OSHA mandate compliance. In fact, if used more than one time, Medicare and other payers consider the occurrence investigational and not reimbursable. Legal liability is possible.

Equipment manufacturers Davol and Stryker each offer suction diverter tips that allow the same handpiece to be used multiple times with the *same* patient, with a new tip at different treatment sessions (Fig. 28.5). This design diverts the suction mechanism from the interior of the product. Otherwise, units cannot be cleaned without damaging the product or being assured that all contaminants and/or disinfection material

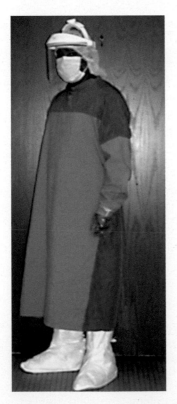

FIGURE 28.4 Personal protective equipment for hydrotherapy treatment.

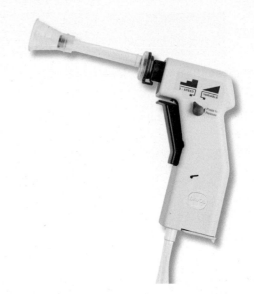

FIGURE 28.5 Simpulse VariCare System. (Courtesy of Davol, Inc, Cranston, Rhode Island.)

is removed. Store the handpieces used with suction diverter tips properly between treatments on the same patient. Plug the irrigation port, cap the IV tubing spike, and place everything in a storage bag labeled with the patient's name, medical record number, and date. The facility sets the maximum time to be used before disposal of the handpiece, usually 1 week or five treatments. Remember that with continued usage, the battery strength will be diminished and, therefore, so will the psi.

Although the Davol and Stryker products have FDA approval, this author has reservations about the ability to disinfect their external components, such that they can be stored and reused without concern for contamination. Disinfection and storage also require time, products, and space; more importantly, sterile procedure is precluded except for the first usage. The Davol VariCare now has a protective sleeve to cover the handpiece during treatment, which increases protection from contamination. The sleeve and a storage bag are provided with each tip package.

Latex Content

All battery products used are latex free. Therefore, latex-sensitive and latex-allergic patients may be treated with PLWS.[31]

Equipment Needed

Power Unit

All PLWS products are powered by batteries, and the products are completely disposable. See Exhibit 28.5 which lists

EXHIBIT 28.5			
Products Available and Power Source			
Power Source	**Davol**	**Stryker**	**Zimmer**
Batteries—unit disposable	VariCare	SurgiLav Plus	Pulsavac Plus LP
		InterPulse	

CLINICAL WISDOM

Single Use Only

Use of PLWS products only one time with disposal after use ensures no cross-contamination between patient treatments.

current products. The batteries in the Davol product can be removed easily without contamination and can be recycled. The batteries in the Stryker and Zimmer products cannot be easily removed from the battery case and should be discarded. Stryker offers also a rechargeable battery option. A rechargeable power pack, charger station, and rechargeable handpieces are available.

Tips

Sterile debridement tips include a small splash shield for soft tissue debridement and general irrigation, and long, flexible tips for undermining, tracts, and tunnels (Exhibit 28.6). Multiple other tips are available, depending on the manufacturer; however, most of these are utilized by physicians in the operating room. PLWS requires only the small splash shield and the long, narrow, flexible tips, although new tips are in product development (Figure 28.6).

If using the Zimmer Pulsavac Plus LP small splash shield, retract the hard shield covering the soft shield as it is not used during treatment. The small, pliable splash shield on all products placed in total contact with the tissue is recommended to obtain adequate suction for negative pressure, unless in undermining or tunnels. The flexible tips have measurement markings in centimeters to allow for safe and accurate measurement of extensive undermining, tracts, and tunnels. Insert and retract the flexible tips continuously during treatment to irrigate and débride the entire area of the wound. The same tip can be used for treating multiple wounds on the same patient in the same

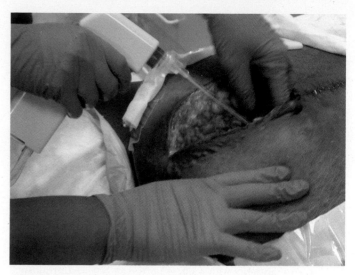

FIGURE 28.6 Simpulse being used with the long tunnel tip.

treatment session, if the least necrotic wounds are treated first. Figure 28.7 shows a handpiece with optional irrigation tips. All products have hand controls and tubing for spiking the saline bag Figure 28.8.

Irrigation Fluid

Normal saline (0.9% sodium chloride) is the preferred irrigation fluid. Water is not recommended because it is not physiologic. Antibiotics can be added with a physician's order. Do not use antiseptic agents or skin cleansers (povidone-iodine, iodophor, sodium hypochlorite, hydrogen peroxide, and acetic acid) because they can be cytotoxic to normal and/or wound tissue.[17]

Warm saline bags to 39°C to 41°C with a fluid warmer or in hot tap water. The number of bags used depends on the number and size of the wounds, the amount of necrotic tissue and exudate, and the patient's tolerance of the procedure.

EXHIBIT   28.6

Most Often Used Tips for Soft Tissue Wound Care

Tip	Davol	Stryker SurgiLav	Stryker InterPulse	Zimmer
Fan spray with splash shield	Yes	Yes	Yes	Yes
Retractable splash shield	Yes	No	No	No
Fan spray without splash shield	No	No	No	Yes
Shower with splash shield	No	Yes	No	Yes
Shower without splash shield	No	No	No	Yes
Open tract	Yes	No	No	No
Narrow open tract	Yes	No	No	No
Flexible, narrow open tract with suction	Yes	No	Yes	Yes
Flexible, narrow open tract without suction	No	No	Yes	No
Suction diverter tips	Yes	Yes		No

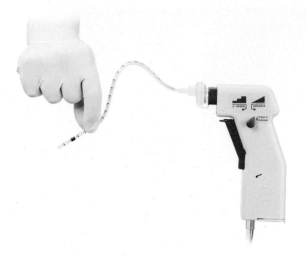

FIGURE 28.7 SurgiLav with a tip. (Courtesy of Stryker Instruments. Kalamazoo, MI.)

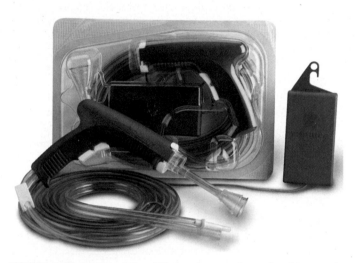

FIGURE 28.8 Pulsavac Plus LP, hand controls, and tubing pack. (Courtesy of Zimmer, Inc.)

CLINICAL WISDOM

Importance of Impact Pressure

It is very important to control and to know the impact pressure at all times during the treatment.

Suction

Either a wall suction or portable pump is necessary for this modality. Equipment includes canisters, a regulator, and connecting tubing, which is required if the suction source is too far away from the wound with the tubing provided.

The suction removes debris, bacteria, and the irrigant and provides negative pressure to increase the rate of granulation tissue.[12] Parameters are usually 60 to 100 mm Hg of continuous suction. Decrease the pressure if there is bleeding, if the wound is near a vessel or cavity, or if the patient complains of pain.

Pressure

As noted earlier, pressure is measured in psi. If the pressure is too high, bacteria and foreign matter can be forced into viable tissue, and granulation and epithelial tissues can be damaged. The Agency for Health Care Research and Quality recommends a treatment range of 4 to 15 psi.[12]

Initiation of treatment is usually 4 to 6 psi, with a typical range of 8 to 12 psi. A setting of 4 to 6 psi is advised for tracts, tunnels, and undermining, where you would be unable to visualize the wound base and nearby structures. Avoid pressures greater than 15 psi unless the physician is present and has issued a specific written order (Exhibit 28.7).

During treatment, increase psi in the presence of tough eschar and excessive necrotic tissue. Decrease if the patient complains of pain, if bleeding occurs, or if the tip is near a major or exposed vessel, nerve, tendon, or cavity lining. Exhibit 28.8 provides the pressure range and control available on various pressure products.

EXHIBIT 28.7

Pressure Used

Pulsatile Lavage with Suction

psi	4–6 psi	4 psi	8–12 psi	15 psi	16+ psi
Initiation	X				
Tracts/undermining	X				
Minimum effective		X			
Typical range			X		
Maximum—PT				X	
With physician present					X

EXHIBIT 28.8

Pressure Range and Control Available (On/Off Control on All Handpieces)

Product	psi Range	Adjust at Source	Vary at Hand Control
Davol	Small splash shield:	No	Dial controls—variable and three settings: low, medium, high settings: low, medium, high
VariCare	• Low: 3.8		
	• Medium: 9.6		
	• High: 11.2		
	• Variable: 0–11.3		
	Flexible: 2–6		
Stryker	Shower: 8–14	No	Switch with two settings
SurgiLav Plus	Fan: 2–4		
	Concentrated spray: 4–6		
Interpulse	Fan: 4–6	No	Trigger with variable control
	Coaxial fan: 4–8		
	Soft tissue: 10–12		
	Flexible with suction: 6–9		
	Flexible no suction: 12–14		
Zimmer	Fan: 6.3–12.6	No	Trigger control
Pulsavac Plus LP	Shower: 3.2–5.8		
	Flexible: 8.6–12.2		

JET LAVAGE

Jet lavage is a relatively painless wound cleansing and debridement system that does not provide pulsed lavage and is without a power source. Instead, it uses compressed oxygen with a small amount of saline (1.5 mL/min) solution to administer a gentle jet stream. The products currently on the market, which were developed in Israel in the 1990s and patented in the United States in 2001, include Jetox™-ND without suction and Jetox™-HDC with suction (manufactured by DeRoyal).

The recommended saline solution is 0.9% sodium chloride. The microdrops are between 5 and 100 μm and are accelerated up to 200 m/s. The air generated through the oxygen source has a desensitizing effect, making jet lavage beneficial for those patients whose wounds are hypersensitive.

Portable and disposable, this latex-free device can be used in the clinic, at the bedside, or in the home, requiring only an oxygen source. Proper PPE is required for treatment with jet lavage, as with all lavage therapies. The shield should be placed against the treatment area to maintain optimum treatment distance. psi is listed in Exhibit 28.9. Continue treatment with Jetox-ND until loose debris and exudate are sufficiently removed. There are at present no published studies addressing the efficacy of Jetox-ND treatment.

CONCLUSION

PLWS is an optimal strategy for irrigation and debridement for all wounds. With control of impact psi; site-specific treatment; the ability to treat tunnels, tracts, and undermining; enhancement of sharp debridement; avoidance of cross-contamination; and an increased rate of granulation and epithelialization, PLWS offers a valuable intervention for wound management. Treatment with PLWS, resulting in decreased length of stay and avoidance of facility-acquired infections with increased rate of wound closure, contributes to cost-effective wound management.[2]

EXHIBIT 28.9

psi with Jetox-ND, Determined by Oxygen Setting

L/min	psi
9	4
11	6
13	9
15	12

This case study uses the clinical decision-making process described in Chapter 1 to document the need for skilled intervention using PLWS. The methodology of the functional outcome report is provided.

Gunshot Wound Treated with Pulsatile Lavage with Suction

Patient ID: W.S. **Age:** 29 **Onset:** January 2

INITIAL ASSESSMENT

Reason for Referral

The patient was referred for a blasted shoulder wound with buckshot, necrotic tissue, tunnels, and undermining in the wound.

Medical History and Systems Review

The patient, previously fully functionally independent with no prior medical history, suffered a self-inflicted gunshot wound to the left shoulder. On the day of the injury and admission to the hospital, January 2, he had surgical exploration of the blasted shoulder wound. The humeral head was resected; fragments were resected from the laterally pulverized clavicle. There was no injury to the brachial plexus or axillary vasculature. The left upper extremity was placed in traction with pins. He had subsequent surgical incisions and drainage of the wound in the operating room on January 3, 4, 5, and 6, with closure of the shoulder capsule on January 6 (see Fig. 28.1).

Evaluation

The patient was admitted to the burn unit after the initial surgery because of the severity of the wounds and the complicated dressing changes required. The presence of necrotic tissue, purulent exudate, buckshot, and numerous tunnels and undermining were indications for treatment with pulsatile lavage with concurrent suction.

EXAMINATION—JANUARY 13

Joint Integrity

The left humeral head has been resected. The left upper extremity is in skeletal traction with pins, with shoulder abducted to 90 degrees. The lateral clavicle is pulverized.

Circulation

There is no injury to the axillary vasculature; there is edema in the left upper extremity.

Sensation

There is no injury to the brachial plexus.

Mobility

The patient is restricted to the supine position.

Integumentary

The left shoulder has a through-and-through wound, with the shotgun entrance wound on the anterior and the exit wound on the posterior.

Size

- Anterior border—118.75-cm surface open area
- Posterior border—50.0-cm surface open area
- Medial depth—2.0 cm
- Lateral depth—1.75 cm
- Tunneling and undermining cannot be measured because of proximity of vessels

Tissue Assessment The wound has red granulation with scattered areas of yellow and brown necrotic tissue; there is buckshot present. The periwound tissue is erythematous and edematous.

Wound Healing Phase The wound is in acute inflammatory phase.

FUNCTIONAL DIAGNOSIS

- Soft tissue injury

1. Absence of proliferative phase
2. Absence of epithelialization phase
3. Undue susceptibility to infection caused by debris in wound

- Functional loss of mobility associated with shoulder injury leading to inability to perform self-care and undue susceptibility to pressure ulcers

Need for Skilled Services

PLWS by PT is indicated in an attempt to avoid another surgical incision and drainage and to prepare the wound for a subsequent skin graft. Increased mobility will be allowed with an accelerated healing process. Therapeutic positioning is necessary to avoid pressure ulcers.

Targeted Outcomes

- The wound bed will be clean, including tunnels and undermining.
- The wound will progress through the phases of healing from inflammatory to epithelialization.
- The patient will be properly positioned to remove pressure.

Treatment Plan

- Irrigate and mechanically débride the wound with the Pulsavac System, including tunnels and undermining. Remove the buckshot. Treat with 1 L of normal saline, 4 to 12 psi, 80 mm Hg suction.
- Perform sharp debridement of necrotic tissue with forceps and scissors. On January 19, the pins are removed and

traction is discontinued by the physician. The patient is transferred from the burn unit.

- Maintain moist wound bed and obliterate dead space with dressing changes of wet to damp Dakin solution–soaked gauze; cover with a five 9-inch gauze pad and secure with dry gauze and paper tape. Tunnels and undermining will be loosely packed.
- Perform therapeutic positioning.

Prognosis

There will be no necrotic tissue and no debris. The wound will have a red granulation base and be ready for skin grafting by the physician.

Target Date 2 weeks.

Frequency Once a day, 6 days per week.

REEXAMINATION BY PHYSICAL THERAPY ON JANUARY 20

Size

- Anterior wound—68.25-cm surface open area
- Posterior wound—28.75-cm surface open area
- Medial depth—1.5 cm
- Lateral depth—1.0 cm

Tissue Assessment The wound has no necrotic tissue. There is a full red granulation base and increased epithelialization. There is no periwound erythema. Tunneling and undermining are present only in the proximal portion of the anterior wound.

Wound Healing Phase Proliferative phase.

Intervention

Physical Therapy Six treatments of PLWS, followed by sharp debridement as needed.

Physical Therapy and Nursing Dressing changes.

Physicians On January 19, the pins are removed and traction is discontinued. The patient is transferred from the burn unit to a regular room.

Revised Prognosis

Closure of the wound by secondary intention.

DISCHARGE OUTCOME

The patient's wounds not only required no further surgical incisions and drainage, but also had a significant increase in granulation and epithelialization with no necrotic tissue present. Anterior and posterior wounds had a decreased surface open area of 42%. Medial depth decreased 25% and lateral depth decreased 43% within 7 days. The physicians decided to allow the wound to close by secondary intention rather than a skin graft. The patient was discharged home on January 21, to continue dressing changes by his mother. Future surgical procedures were anticipated to replace the shoulder joint. He was lost to follow-up.

REVIEW QUESTIONS

1. PLWS can be utilized to
   A. irrigate and debride
   B. reduce bacterial counts and infection
   C. increase inflammation with some damage to healthy tissues
   D. produce granulation tissue but reduced reepithelialization
   E. a and b
   F. a and d
2. Irrigation pressures should be at least
   A. 1.2 psi
   B. 2 psi
   C. 3 psi
   D. 4 psi
3. All of the following are effective in removing bacteria from a wound except
   A. 19-gauge needle
   B. bulb syringe
   C. PLWS
   D. 35-mL syringe
4. Negative pressure and suction
   A. applies noncompression mechanical forces to the tissues
   B. dilates arterioles
   C. removes debris and bacteria
   D. all of the above
5. Clinical outcomes could include all of the following except
   A. decreased wound size
   B. patient satisfaction
   C. efficiency of treatment
   D. cost
6. Contraindications to PLWS include
   A. insensate patients
   B. wounds with tract, tunnels, and/or undermining
   C. anticoagulant medication
   D. none of the above

REFERENCES

1. Keblish DJ, DeMaio M. Early pulsatile lavage for the decontamination of combat wounds: historical review and point proposal. *Mil Med.* 1998;163:844–846.

2. Haynes LJ, Handley C, Brown MH, et al. *Comparison of Pulsavac and Sterile Whirlpool Regarding the Promotion of Tissue Granulation.* Lubbock, TX: University Medical Center and Methodist Hospital; 1994.

3. Kloth LC. Roles of physical therapists in wound management, part III: select biophysical technologies and management of patients with diabetic foot ulceration. *J Am Coll Certif Wound Specialists.* 2009;1:81.

4. European Pressure Ulcer Advisory Panel and National Pressure Ulcer Advisory Panel. *Treatment of Pressure Ulcers: Quick Reference Guide.* Washington, DC: National Pressure Ulcer Advisory Panel; 2009.

5. Loehne HB. Enhanced wound care using pulsavac system: case studies. *Acute Care Perspect.* 1995;9:13–15.

6. Morgan D, Hoelscher J. Pulsed lavage: promoting comfort and healing in home care. *Ostomy Wound Manage* 2000;46:44–49.

7. Mustoe T. Understanding chronic wounds: a unifying hypothesis on their pathogenesis and implications for therapy. *Am J Surg.* 2004;187:65S–70S.

8. Rodeheaver GT. Pressure ulcer debridement and cleansing: a review of current literature. *Ostomy Wound Manage.* 1999;45(Suppl):80S–85S.

9. Niederhuber SS, Stribley RF, Koepke GH. Reduction of skin bacterial load with use of the therapeutic whirlpool. *Phys Ther.* 1975;55:482–486.

10. Bohannon R. Whirlpool versus whirlpool and rinse for removal of bacteria from a venous stasis ulcer. *Phys Ther.* 1982;62:304–308.

11. Luedtke-Hoffmann KA, Schafer DS. Pulsed lavage in wound cleansing. *Phys Ther.* 2000;80:292–300.

12. U.S. Department of Health and Human Services. Treatment of pressure ulcers. *AHCPR Clin Pract Guideline.* 1994;15:50–53.

13. Streed SA, Loehne HB. Outcomes research—preventing infections to improve wound care outcomes: an epidemiological approach. *Wounds.* 2007;19.

14. Saxe A, Goldstein E, Dixon S, et al. Pulsatile lavage in the management of postoperative wound infections. *Am Surg.* 1980;46:391–397.

15. Bierbaum B. *High Pressure, Pulsatile Lavage in Wound Management: A Literature Review.* Cranston, RI: Davol, Inc.; 1986.

16. Stevenson TR, Thacker JG, Rodeheaver GT, et al. Cleansing the traumatic wound by high pressure syringe irrigation. *JACEP.* 1976;5(1):17–21.

17. Bhaskar SN, Cutright DT, Gross A. Effect of water lavage on infected wounds in the rat. *J Periodont.* 1969;40:671.

18. Wheeler CB, Rodeheaver GT, Thacker JG, et al. Side effects of high pressure irrigation. *Surg Gynecol Obstet.* 1976;143:775–778.

19. Bhaskar SN, Cutright DE, Hunsuck EE, et al. Pulsating water jet devices in debridement of combat wounds. *Mil Med.* 1971;136:274–276.

20. Morykwas MJ, Argenta LC. Use of negative pressure to increase the rate of granulation tissue formation in chronic open wounds. Presented at the annual meeting of the Federation of American Societies of Experimental Biology; March 28–April 1, 1993; New Orleans, LA.

21. Argenta LC, Morykwas M, Rouchard R. The use of negative pressure to promote healing of pressure ulcers and chronic wounds. Presented at the joint meeting of the Wound Healing Society and the European Tissue Repair Society; August 22–25, 1993; Amsterdam, The Netherlands.

22. Ho CH, Bogie KM, Banks PG, et al. Pulsatile lavage for pressure ulcer management: safety profile. Poster presentation at SAWC. April 2005.

23. Fuller J. Help prevent deadly infections when using pulsed lavage. *LPN2009.* 2007;3:9.

24. Occupational Safety and Health Administration. Bloodborne pathogen standard. *Fed Regist.* 1991;56(235):64175–64182.

25. Maragakis L. Multidrug-Resistant (MDR) Acinetobacter. Johns Hopkins Web site: http://hopkins-heic.org/infectious_diseases/acinetobacter.html 07/03/2005

26. Preventing Lethal Patient Infections from Pulsatile Lavage Treatment. *FDA Patient Safety News.* www/fda/gov/psn. *#36*; February 2005.

27. Maragakis LL, Cosgrove SE, Song X, et al. An outbreak of multidrug-resistant *Acinetobacter baumannii* associated with pulsatile lavage wound treatment. *JAMA.* 2004;292:3006–3011.

28. Fuller J. Cover up and clean up to prevent deadly infections. *Nursing 2005.* 2005;35:31.

29. Loehne HB, Streed SA, Gaither B, et al. Aerosolization of microorganisms during pulsatile lavage with suction. *Ostomy Wound Manage.* Abstract. 2002;48:75.

30. Goodman CC, Boissonnault WG. *Pathology: Implications for the Physical Therapist.* 2nd ed. Philadelphia, PA: WB Saunders; 2003.

31. U.S. Food and Drug Administration. Allergic reactions to latex-containing medical devices. *FDA Med Bull.* 1991.

CHAPTER 29

Management of the Wound Environment with Negative Pressure Wound Therapy

Allen Gabriel and Subhas Gupta

CHAPTER OBJECTIVES

At the completion of this chapter, the reader will be able to:

1. Identify the science behind negative pressure wound therapy (NPWT).
2. Describe applications of NPWT based on the peer-reviewed literature.
3. Explain indications and contraindications for the use of NPWT therapy.

While advances in medical technology during the past 20 years have increased life expectancies, growth in the aging population has contributed to rising disease burdens within the health-care system. Management of acute and chronic wounds of diverse etiologies remains a major challenge to society because of its magnitude, complexity, and cost. Over 2.8 million patients with chronic wounds are treated at an annual cost of billions of dollars in the United States.[1] Chronic, nonhealing wounds pose a continual challenge in medicine due to variable management strategies and inconsistent response to treatment.[2] Chronic wounds may be associated with pressure, trauma, venous insufficiency, diabetes, vascular disease, or prolonged immobilization. Treatment is variable and costly, demanding lengthy hospital stays or specialized home care requiring skilled nursing and costly supplies. Faster healing of chronic wounds typically results in decreased hospitalization and earlier return of function.

During the past decade, technological advances have resulted in an explosion of new products for managing acute and chronic wounds. Countless advanced wound treatments have been introduced to enhance wound healing, all supported by widely varying levels of scientific evidence. One adjunctive technology that has seen tremendous growth, both in usage and related publications, is negative pressure wound therapy (NPWT). The first commercialized NPWT device, called Vacuum-Assisted Closure (V.A.C.®, KCI Licensing Inc, San Antonio, TX), was cleared in 1995 by the U.S. Food and Drug Administration. Since then, NPWT has played an increasingly important role in wound management strategies within multiple surgical and nonsurgical specialties. In addition, over the last 5 years, we have seen an increase in the number of NPWT devices introduced to the market place (see Table 29.1).

Negative pressure wound therapy, also termed *vacuum-assisted closure, wound V.A.C., vacuum sealing,* and *topical negative pressure*, is the process of applying negative pressure to the wound site via foam or gauze dressing, tubing, and vacuum device. A polyurethane reticulated open-cell foam (ROCF) as shown in Figure 29.1A or polyvinyl alcohol foam dressing as shown in Figure 29.1B or gauze is placed into the wound cavity. An airtight thin film drape is sealed over the foam/gauze, and a tubing pad is applied over a hole cut into the drape. Controlled negative pressure, typically 125 mm Hg below ambient pressure, is applied and distributed through the porous foam over the entire wound surface. Excessive fluid and debris are drained into the canister. Removal of these infectious fluids has been shown to decrease interstitial edema, increase capillary blood flow, and promote granulation tissue formation by facilitating cell migration and proliferation.[3] The technique provides both adequate wound drainage and a moist environment necessary for wound healing, thus combining the benefits of open and closed wound healing systems.

HISTORY OF NPWT

Negative pressure has been employed for thousands of years in China as an adjunct to acupuncture techniques. A technique called *cupping*, whereby a heated glass sphere is applied to the skin, is a method of applying a pressure to a specific acupuncture site. It was not until the 17th century when the first report of sustained vacuum was made by Galileo's Italian assistant, Evangelista Torricelli.[4] This was then followed by both the Frenchman, Blaise Pascal, and the Dutchman, Christian Huygens, who created the syringe and vacuum pump, respectively.[4]

The application of negative pressure to an open wound was first described by several Russian authors in the 1970s[5] and 1980s;[5-8] however, critical evaluation of these studies by English-speaking clinicians was limited due to the paucity of

TABLE 29.1	Negative Pressure Wound Therapy Devices Marketed in the United States
Manufacturer	**Trade or Brand Names of Negative Pressure Wound Therapy Devices**
Boehringer Wound Systems, LLC	Engenex® Advanced NPWT System (Boehringer Laboratory Suction Pump System) ConvaTec (Skillman, NJ) markets and distributes the Engenex®
Innovative Therapies Inc.	SVEDMAN™ and SVED™ Wound Treatment Systems
KCI, USA Inc. (Kinetic Concepts, Inc.)	InfoV.A.C.® Therapy Unit (stationary unit) V.A.C.® ATS™ (stationary unit) V.A.C.® Freedom™ (portable unit) ActiV.A.C.® Therapy Unit (portable unit) V.A.C.® Instill System (delivery of topical solutions) ABThera™ Open Abdomen NPWT System Prevena™ Incision Management System
Medela, Inc.	Invia Liberty Wound Therapy (portable) Invia Vario 18 c/i Wound Therapy (stationary, mobile with battery)
MediTop BV/The Medical & Woundcare Company	Exsudex® wound drainage pump
Premco Medical Systems, Inc.	Prodigy™ NPWT System (PMS-800 and PMS-800V)
Prospera Technologies LLC	PRO-I™ (stationary and portable) PRO-II™ (portable) PRO-III™(stationary and portable)
Smith & Nephew, Inc.	V1STA Negative Pressure Wound Therapy (portable unit) EZCARE Negative Pressure Wound Therapy (stationary unit) RENASYS™ EZ Negative Pressure Wound Therapy
Talley Group Ltd.	Venturi™ Negative Pressure Wound Therapy (portable or stationary)

ECRI Institute, July 29, 2009 (https://www.ecri.org/Documents/Press%20Releases/Negative_Pressure_Wound_Therapy_Devices.pdf)

English abstracts. In 1993, Fleishman et al.[9] of Germany were the first group to report on vacuum sealing, which is similar to what is now known as NPWT in the United States. Subsequent studies have described successful vacuum sealing outcomes in open wounds with up to 14 months of follow-up.[10–12] All of the original Russian and German studies were performed using wall suction devices or surgical vacuum bottles. Downfalls of these systems included a lack of safety controls in fluid management and pressure delivery, as well as lack of portability.[13]

In 1997, Argenta and Morykwas[14,15] described in two seminal studies the effects of the first controlled negative pressure device, the V.A.C.®, in combination with a polyurethane ROCF interface. The clinical study reported that 296 of 300 acute, subacute, and chronic wounds responded favorably to subatmospheric pressure, showing an increase in granulation tissue formation.[14] The scientific study performed in porcine models documented significantly increased blood flow, granulation tissue formation, bacterial clearance, and random-pattern flap survival rates in NPWT/ROCF-treated wounds, compared to controls.[15] Fleishman et al described an advanced method of vacuum sealing in 1998, which included intermittent topical instillation of antiseptics and antibiotics to infected wounds.[16] This technology was introduced in the United States in 2003 and is known as NPWT Instillation (e.g., V.A.C.® Instill™).[17]

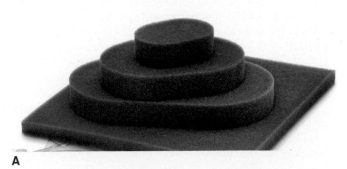

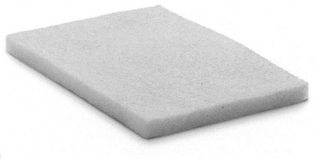

A   **B**

FIGURE 29.1 Types of foam for use with NPWT. **A.** Polyurethane ROCF. **B.** Polyvinyl alcohol foam.

PATHOPHYSIOLOGY

Wound healing is a complex and dynamic process that includes an immediate sequence of cell migration leading to repair and closure. This begins with removal of debris, control of infection, clearance of inflammation, angiogenesis, deposition of granulation tissue, contraction, remodeling of the connective tissue matrix, and maturation.[13,18] As growth factors, cytokines, proteases, and cellular and extracellular elements all play important roles in different stages of the healing process, alterations in one or more of these components could account for the impaired healing observed in chronic or compromised wounds. Levels of various matrix metalloproteinase (MMPs-1 [collagenase], 2 [gelatinase A], and 9 [gelatinase B]) and serine proteases are markedly increased in fluids from chronic wounds,[19] whereas they are decreased in wounds undergoing deposition of granulation tissue.[20] Other proteases, such as neutrophil elastase, have also been observed to be significantly higher in chronic wounds.[21] Elevated levels of serine proteases degrade fibronectin, an essential protein involved in the remodeling of the extracellular matrix (ECM).[19,22]

The main pathophysiology of necrotic tissue formation is the result of inadequate local blood supply. The necrotic tissue contains dead cells and debris that are a consequence of the fragmentation of dying cells. On the other hand, some wounds contain a yellow fibrinous tissue that mostly consists of fibrin and pertinacious material. This is frequently referred to as 'slough'. In compromised wounds, due to underlying pathogenic abnormalities and the altered biochemical and cellular environment, necrotic tissue and slough tend to continually accumulate.[23] Accumulation of necrotic tissue or slough in a wound promotes bacterial colonization and prevents complete repair of the wound. This halts wound progress to the next stage, and the wound remains in the inflammatory stage indefinitely, since the continued presence of bacteria in a wound leads to production of proinflammatory mediators such as IL-1, TNF-α, prostaglandin E2, and thromboxane.[24] Although inflammation is part of normal wound healing, healing may be prolonged if inflammation is excessive.[25]

Not all bacteria in a wound have deleterious effects, and therefore, they can be divided into three distinct categories; contamination, colonization, and infection. Both contamination (presence of nonreplicating organisms) and colonization (replicating organisms without tissue necrosis) do not produce a host response, whereas a severe infection produces a host response that has deleterious effects to wound healing. It is also important to be cognizant of age as a factor in wound healing since the biochemical and cytokine milieu that is present as age increases is similarly present in chronic wounds. In animal models, a delayed inflammatory response has been observed after acute wounding in middle-aged and aged compared to young mice.[26,27] Additionally, cellular and molecular characteristics of aged skin can impede the healing process. There is an up-regulation of MMP-2 in normal aged skin, and MMP-2 and MMP-9 in acute wounds in aged skin in comparison with young adults.[26,27] These factors may combine to predispose the remodeled wound in aged populations to recurrent breakdown.

Wound healing involves a complex series of events that begins at the moment of injury and continues for months to years. After wounding, edema and interstitial fluid create an oxygen-poor environment due to the collapse of the microcirculation. The thin-walled capillaries collapse, due to the increase in interstitial fluid and pressure exerted on the vessels. This causes the collapse and backup of the microcirculation, leading to localized thrombosis and a poor wound healing environment.

With the advent of NPWT, improved healing has been shown in animal and clinical studies.[14,15,28] The physiological and molecular biological mechanisms by which NPWT accelerates wound healing are still somewhat unknown; however, it is generally agreed that multiple mechanisms play a role.[3,29] Proposed mechanisms of action include reduction in localized edema, increased blood flow, removal of inhibitory agents, promotion of granulation tissue formation, a moist wound healing environment, enhancement of epithelial migration, and wound contraction.[30] For the purpose of this discussion, authors have divided scientific evidence into five categories: (1) blood flow; (2) granulation tissue formation; (3) bacterial clearance; (4) flap survival; and (5) cytokine milieu.

Blood Flow

All tissues need oxygen and nutrients for metabolism and cell turnover. Any impediment to localized blood flow has deleterious effects to wound healing. In order to understand the mechanisms involved in improving blood flow, a brief review of physiology is needed.

The movement of fluid and accompanying solutes between compartments (mostly water, electrolytes, and smaller molecular weight solutes) is governed by physical factors such as hydrostatic and oncotic forces. These forces are normally balanced in such a manner that the fluid volume remains relatively constant between the compartments. When the fluid volume within the interstitial compartment increases, this compartment will increase in size, leading to tissue swelling (i.e., edema). In most capillary systems of the body, there is a net filtration of fluid from the intravascular to the extravascular compartment. In other words, capillary fluid filtration exceeds reabsorption. This would cause fluid to accumulate within the interstitium if it were not for the lymphatic system that removes excess fluid from the interstitium and returns it to the intravascular compartment.

Circumstances, however, can arise where net capillary filtration exceeds the capacity of the lymphatics to remove the fluid (i.e., net filtration > lymph flow). When this occurs, the interstitium will swell with fluid, thereby become edematous. Some of the precipitating factors of edema that can be related to wound healing include (1) decreased plasma oncotic pressure (as occurs with hypoproteinemia), (2) increased capillary permeability caused by proinflammatory mediators (e.g., histamine, bradykinin) or by damage to the structural integrity of capillaries so that they become more "leaky" (as occurs in tissue trauma, burns, and severe inflammation), and (3) lymphatic obstruction.

NPWT has been shown to alter wound edge microvascular blood flow in several controlled studies.[15,31] In the first series of experiments, the role of NPWT on blood flow was evaluated in the back wounds of anesthetized swine.[15] Results indicated that flow increased with increasing levels of negative pressure, peaking at 125 mm Hg. While an increase in blood flow equivalent to four times the baseline value occurred with negative pressure values of 125 mm Hg, blood flow was decreased with higher levels and completely inhibited by negative pressures of 400 mm

TABLE 29.2	Guidelines for NPWT Intermittent Versus Continuous Mode

Continuous Mode	Intermittent Mode
Flaps	Minimally exudating
Difficult dressing application	Stalled progress
Highly exudating	
Meshed grafts	
Painful wounds	
Tunnels or undermining	
Unstable structures	

Hg and above.[15] A negative pressure value of 125 mm Hg was therefore selected for use in subsequent studies. In a more recent study, investigators determined that −80 mm Hg has similar blood flow effects as the clinical standard, −125 mm Hg, which suggests pressures may be lowered to accommodate wound type and tissue composition without compromise in blood flow.[32]

The same study also evaluated the effect of an intermittent negative pressure mode with 5 minutes on and 2 minutes off, on the local blood flow. Results showed this intermittent mode maintained local blood flow at four times the baseline blood flow after 2 minutes in the off mode. Thus, the intermittent mode is considered to be the optimal mode for certain wound characteristics (see Table 29.2).The proposed mechanism for improved blood flow involves removing the interstitial fluid from the tissues immediately surrounding the wound, decompressing the microcirculation, and restoring blood flow.

In a different study evaluating NPWT effects on blood flow in wounds of white rabbits, investigators found that NPWT promoted a significant increase in capillary blood flow velocity and capillary blood volume.[33] It was also shown that NPWT stimulated endothelial proliferation and angiogenesis, narrowed endothelial spaces, and restored the integrity of the capillary basement membrane.[33] This study confirms the hypothesis of edema reduction with use of NPWT, as seen with restoration of the basement membranes, leading to less leaky capillaries. This is also directly related to the change in the cytokine milieu that we see with use of NPWT, which will be discussed in detail later in this chapter.

Granulation Tissue Formation

Granulation tissue is a mix of small vessels and connective tissue in the wound base. The base forms a nutrient-rich matrix that can support the migration of epidermal cells across the wound bed. A well-granulated wound provides an optimal bed for epidermal migration and for a skin graft as the newly formed capillaries support the inhibition or diffusion of exudates through the host bed. The rate of granulation tissue production with NPWT was originally determined using a swine model, and measured by the reduction in wound volume over time.[15] Compared with control wounds dressed with saline-soaked gauze, significantly increased rates of granulation tissue formation occurred with both continuous (mean 63.3%, ± standard deviation [SD] 26.1%) and intermittent (5 minutes

on and 2 minutes off) (mean 103%, SD 35.3%) application of negative pressure at 125 mm Hg.[15]

A more recent study demonstrated that NPWT's micromechanical force at 125 mm Hg caused cell stretch at in vitro strain levels shown to promote cellular proliferation.[34] It has been suggested that cells, while undergoing an optimal degree of strain, can be induced to respond to growth factors and proliferate.[35–38] However, soluble growth factors and attachment to ECM proteins, although essential, are not sufficient to stimulate cell proliferation.[37] Cell cycle progression requires a sufficient physical framework to respond to chemical stimuli. If the normal matrix is altered such that it cannot form the scaffold on which cells normally stretch and build up isometric tension, Saxena et al.[34] suggested the mechanical strain generated by NPT/ROCF may overcome this loss of tissue integrity and substitute for the missing structural basis necessary for cell proliferation.

The effect of mechanical suction on wound healing is not surprising. In 1911, mechanical forces on wounds were thought to result in angiogenesis and tissue growth.[39] The extensive use of tissue expanders and the Ilizarov bone distraction technique in the last 20 years demonstrates how tissue moves and grows in response to the application of mechanical force, with viscoelastic flow, increased mitotic rate, and angiogenesis.[40,41] Vacuum-assisted closure moves distensible soft tissue by an effect similar to tissue expansion. At the same time, it stimulates more rapid wound healing with increased rates of granulation tissue formation.

The observation that intermittent or cycled treatment appears more effective than continuous therapy is interesting although the reasons for this are not fully understood. Philbeck et al.[42] suggested that intermittent cycling results in rhythmic perfusion of the tissue, which is maintained because the process of capillary autoregulation is not activated. They also suggested that as cells that are undergoing mitosis must go through a cycle of rest, cellular component production, and division, constant stimulation may cause the cells to "ignore" the stimulus and thus become ineffective. Intermittent stimulation allows the cells time to rest and prepare for the next cycle. For this reason, it is suggested that intermittent negative pressure should be used clinically, although some authors recommend a 48-hour period of continuous vacuum, which can be applied to exert a rapid initial cleansing effect, prior to initiating an intermittent cycle.[43] Tables 29.2 and 29.3 display the types of wounds best suited for intermittent versus continuous negative pressure, and suggested pressure settings for each wound type.

Bacterial Clearance

The definition of clinical infection is equivalent to greater than 10^5 organisms per gram of tissue. It has been postulated that the microorganisms consume the nutrients and oxygen that would otherwise be directed toward tissue repair. In addition, they release enzymes that break down protein, which is a crucial part of wound regeneration. Recently, Schmidtchen et al.[44] showed that elastase-producing bacterial isolates significantly degraded plasma proteins, extracellular products of human skin and fibroblasts, and inhibited fibroblast growth. These effects, in conjunction with the finding that proteinase production was detected in wound fluid ex vivo, suggest that bacterial proteinases play a pathogenic role in chronic wounds. Reducing the bacterial load of a wound improves its healing capacity

| TABLE 29.3 | **Recommended Guidelines for Treating Wound Types** |

Wound Type	Cycle	Subsequent Cycle	Target Pressure (Black Foam)	Target Pressure (Versa Foam)	Dressing Change Interval
Acute - Traumatic	Continuous first 48 h	Intermittent (5 min. ON/2 min OFF) for rest of therapy	125 mm Hg	125–175 mm Hg; Titrate up for more drainage	Every 48 h (every 12 h with infection)
Pressure Ulcers	Continuous first 48 h	Intermittent (5 min. ON/2 min OFF) for rest of therapy	125 mm Hg	125–175 mm Hg; Titrate up for more drainage	Every 48 h (every 12 h with infection)
Surgical Wound Dehiscence	Continuous first 48 h	Intermittent (5 min. ON/2 min OFF) for rest of therapy	125 mm Hg	125–175 mm Hg; Titrate up for more drainage	Every 48 h (every 12 h with infection)
Meshed Grafts & Bioengineered Tissues	Continuous for duration of therapy		75–125 mm Hg	125 mm Hg; Titrate up for more drainage	Remove dressing after 3–5 d (drainage should taper prior to removal)
Chronic Ulcers	Continuous first 48 h	Intermittent (5 min. ON/2 min OFF) for rest of therapy	50–125 mm Hg	125- 175 mm Hg; Titrate up for more drainage	Every 48 h (every 12 h with infection)
Flaps	Continuous for duration of therapy		125–150 mm Hg	125–175 mm Hg; Titrate up for more drainage	Fresh = every 72 h Complicated = every 48 h (every 12 h with infection)

The V.A.C.®—V.A.C.® Therapy™ Clinical Guidelines, January 2003 KCI USA, Inc.

because the body can then concentrate on healing rather than on fighting invasion of microorganisms.

In the original swine study, Morykwas et al.[15] deliberately infected wounds (*Staphylococcus aureus* and *Staphylococcus epidermidis*) and measured the number of colony-forming units per gram of tissue over time in wet-to-moist gauze-treated wounds versus NPWT-treated wounds. No antibiotics were used to treat the infection. NPWT-treated wounds showed a significant decrease in the number of bacterial colony-forming units from 10^7 organisms per gram of tissue to 10^4 by the fifth day of treatment.[15]

Since the original study, however, the effect of NPWT on bioburden has been debated in the literature. While various studies have reported decreased infection rates with NPWT,[45–47] other comparative studies have shown similar infection rates between NPWT- and moist wound care–treated wounds.[48,49] Mouës et al[50] found that the total quantitative bacterial load remained stable during NPWT. While nonfermentative gram-negative bacilli showed a significant decrease during NPWT, *S. aureus* showed a significant increase.[50] In comparative studies with similarly sustained bioburden levels in NPWT versus moist wound care groups, however, wounds in the NPWT groups healed faster on average.[48–50] This wound healing progress, despite quantitative bacterial load, may be due in part to negative pressure's role in reducing dead space, removing infectious byproducts known to contribute to wound breakdown, and improving local blood flow.

Flap Survival

In the seminal swine study, wounds pretreated and post-treated with NPWT demonstrated a 72.2% flap survival rate, a significant increase of 21% in random pattern flap survival

rate, compared to controls.[15] Other studies have reported successful rescue of jeopardized flaps (clinically observed venous congestion) with the use of NPWT as well.[51] One small series reported good outcomes in 11 of 14 free vastus lateralis muscle flaps with concurrent use of NPWT in lower extremity limb reconstruction.[52]

In a scientific study, the posterior compartment of rabbit hind limbs was crushed for 4 hours with 15-kg weights. Following removal, fasciotomies were made and NPWT was applied to the wounds of four rabbits. Serum samples for myoglobin in control animals showed a rapidly rising level versus the NPWT-treated group, which remained at baseline.[53] The proposed mechanism for these observed results is removal of excess interstitial fluid and increased local blood flow.

Cytokine milieu

Acute wounds typically heal by a complex and interdependent sequence of events that are divided into the different wound healing phases. Within these phases, cytokines and chemokines guide the normal healing progression and are fundamental components of the cellular and biochemical events that occur during wound healing.[54] Cytokines mediate cellular function by binding cell membrane receptors. They stimulate a variety of cellular activities via endocrine, paracrine, autocrine, or intracrine pathways.[55] Cytokines peak at different time points, and critical factors and their change in concentration over time in the wound are yet to be reliably determined.[55]

Recent research has been focused on the biochemical components of chronic wounds. There is growing support for the concept that a chronic wound is "stuck" in the inflammatory phase of healing.[56] Evidence suggests that mitogenic cellular activity decreases in chronic wound fluid, whereas acute wound fluid promotes DNA synthesis.[57,58] Research also has been directed in evaluating the cytokines found in wound fluid. Harris et al.[57] showed that higher levels of cytokines were found in nonhealing ulcers, and, interestingly, cytokine levels decreased when a chronic wound began to heal. However, it is important to differentiate between cytokines in the different wound healing stages.

Stechmiller et al.[59] showed a significant and sustained decrease in TNF-α, a potent proinflammatory cytokine active in the early inflammatory phase of wound healing, from day 0 to day 1 in wound fluid of NPWT-treated pressure ulcers. TNF-α has been shown to be in high concentrations in nonhealing wound fluid.[60,61] Studies have suggested that levels of TNF-α may be reduced with the application of negative pressure,[59,62] but larger, controlled studies are needed to substantiate this claim.

Chronic wounds have also shown higher levels of MMP than acute wounds.[21,63–65] This is supported by a study that shows higher levels of MMP degrade proteins and the exogenous growth factors needed for wound healing.[63] Shi et al.[66] evaluated the changes of MMP 1, 2, and 13 in granulating wounds after the treatment of NPWT in humans. Results demonstrated that NPWT may promote healing of chronic wounds by depressing the expressions of MMP-1, 2, 13 mRNA and protein synthesis, resulting in a decrease of the degradation of collagen and gelatin.[66] On the other hand, Tang et al.[67] explored the influence of NPWT on expression of Bcl-2 and NGF during wound healing in Sprague-Dawley rats. They concluded that application of NPWT during wound healing increases the expression of the apoptotic modulation related protein Bcl-2 and affects the expression of NGF/NGFmRNA, which may promote the wound healing process.[67] Basic science research continues to evolve regarding the mechanisms of action of NPWT in chronic and acute wound healing.

INDICATIONS FOR THERAPY

NPWT is intended to create an environment that promotes wound healing via secondary or tertiary intention by preparing the wound bed for closure, reducing edema, promoting granulation tissue formation and perfusion, and removing exudate and infectious material. NPWT is indicated for patients with chronic, acute, traumatic, subacute, and dehisced wounds, partial-thickness burns, ulcers (diabetic, pressure, or venous insufficiency), muscle flaps and split-thickness meshed skin grafts. FDA-cleared indications for NPWT are listed in Table 29.4.

Hundreds of publications have described effective use of NPWT in the treatment of a variety of wound etiologies including extensive degloving injuries, infected sternotomy wounds, acute open abdomen, infected complex deep spinal wounds with exposed instrumentation, gastroschisis, giant omphalocele, dehisced incisions, and various other soft tissue injuries or defects prior to surgical closure, grafting, or reconstructive surgery. Numerous controlled and uncontrolled studies have also been published, describing the use of NPWT in a variety of nonhealing chronic wounds, such as pressure, venous stasis, and diabetic ulcers.

In increasing numbers of geriatric and polymorbid patients, NPWT is used as an alternative treatment modality to more complex reconstructive operations. In patients who are not candidates to undergo prolonged anesthesia, NPWT is used as

TABLE 29.4	General Indication for NPWT
Pressure ulcers	
Diabetic ulcers	
Venous stasis ulcers	
Dehisced surgical wounds	
Chronic wounds	
Acute wounds	
Traumatic wounds	
Partial-thickness burns	
Grafts	
Flaps	

a temporizing bridge between debridement and final closure in complicated wounds. With adequate protection and precaution, NPWT can be applied over any type of tissue or material, including dermis, fat, fascia, muscle, mucosa, tendon, blood vessel, bone, synthetic graft, synthetic mesh, hardware, and synthetic skin substitute.[68] The authors have also successfully used NPWT conservatively on select wounds complicated by fistulae, as an off-label application.

CONTRAINDICATIONS AND PRECAUTIONS

NPWT is contraindicated for patients with nondebrided necrotic tissue or eschar, untreated or nondebrided osteomyelitis, unresected malignancy in the wound, and nonenteric and unexplored fistulae. Adequate, localized blood supply to the wound bed is required. The NPWT dressing must not be placed directly in contact with exposed blood vessels, organs, or nerves. Therapy can be initiated over vessels, organs, and nerves if they are completely covered with natural tissues, a thick layer of compatible bioengineered tissue, or several layers of a fine-meshed, nonadherent synthetic material that form a complete barrier.

NPWT should not be used in the presence of uncontrolled hemorrhage, blood dyscrasia, or coagulopathy and should be used with extreme caution in the presence of dysrhythmias.[68] Extreme caution should be exercised in cases of vascular anastomosis protected only by a nontissue barrier. Sharp edges or bone fragments must be eliminated from wound areas or covered to prevent them from puncturing blood vessels or organs before initiating NPWT. Patients at increased risk of potentially fatal bleeding must be closely monitored during NPWT.[69]

A published clinical review of infected wound treatment advises that NPWT should not be used in cases of gross infection, when the patient is persistently septic or the wound remains infected or becomes reinfected following a course of antibiotic therapy.[70] Patients who cannot tolerate the therapy are contraindicated. In all cases, the treating physician/surgeon or wound care specialist must have adequate experience or knowledge of the technique to safely apply and remove the dressing in association with the treatment course, irrigate and debride the wound, and ensure that there is no excessive or uncontrolled bleeding before NPWT is initiated. A multifactorial approach in evaluating the candidacy of a patient must take place.

APPLICATION OF THERAPY

Several combinations of devices and dressings are available to deliver NPWT (Table 29.1). Wound type, amount of exudate, and level of patient mobility required are important considerations when choosing an NPWT delivery system. Some systems are portable and some are stationary. Dressings are available in different sizes and materials (see Figs. 29.1A,B), with or without a protective visceral layer. Foam use guidelines are listed in Table 29.5. Guidelines for application of NPWT are largely similar across all wound types, with some exceptions (see Table 29.5). A foam or gauze dressing is placed into the wound cavity. An airtight thin film drape is sealed over the foam/gauze and a 3- to 5-cm border of intact periwound skin. Tubing is applied over a hole cut into the drape and connected to a canister within a vacuum device. Controlled negative pressure, typically 125 mm Hg below ambient pressure, is applied and distributed over the entire wound surface. The digital readout on the pump guides the user through different options, such as pressure settings and problem solving.

Obtaining a lasting seal can be particularly difficult near the anus or vagina or where the surrounding skin is moist. Leaks can sometimes be overcome by the use of a hydrocolloid dressing, which is first applied around the wound and used as a base for the adhesive membrane.[14] Practical techniques for successful dressing application on sacral pressure ulcers close to the anus and for multiple large ulcers on the lower extremities have been previously discussed.[71]

Despite the relatively simple concept of NPWT, unfamiliar equipment can be intimidating and confusing for health-care providers. Therefore, the authors recommend that institutions develop a technique for applying NPWT. Users should be educated on the equipment, application, removal, and monitoring of the therapy in order to achieve optimal outcomes.

WOUND-SPECIFIC APPLICATIONS OF NPWT

A number of NPWT systems have been developed for specific wound types, including the acute open abdomen; clean, closed incisions; and wounds requiring instillation of topical solutions. A brief discussion of these wound types and NPWT application is listed below.

Acute Open Abdomen

The open abdomen is an increasingly common strategy for the management of abdominal emergencies in trauma and general surgery. The use of an abbreviated laparotomy can reduce mortality associated with conditions such as abdominal compartment syndrome; however, the resulting open abdomen is a complex clinical problem. NPWT is an increasingly used method of temporary abdominal closure in patients with acute open abdomen following severe trauma, secondary peritonitis, necrotizing pancreatitis, acute postoperative intestinal failure, aortic surgery, abdominal compartment syndrome, and abdominal sepsis.

NPWT as a dynamic closure device allows access for multiple abdominal reexplorations, controls peritoneal fluid and third space loss, minimizes increases in intra-abdominal pressure, reduces dressing change frequency and wound exposure, and protects intra-abdominal contents.[72] Authors have reported relevant advantages of this technique to include prevention of abdominal compartment syndrome, simplified nursing of patients, and reduced time to abdominal closure.[73] Three prospective studies provide level III evidence that NPWT allows delayed primary fascial closure in the majority of laparotomy wounds up to 21 days after occurrence, but not where duration of NPWT was less than 9 days.[74]

Use of sequential fascial closure techniques, in tandem with NPWT dressings, to avoid fascial retraction, have also been

TABLE 29.5 Recommended Guidelines for Foam Use			
Indications	Polyurethane (Black Foam)	Versa Foam (White Foam)	Either
Deep, acute wounds with moderate granulation tissue present	X		
Deep pressure ulcers	X		
Flaps	X		
Exquisitely painful wounds		X	
Superficial wounds		X	
Tunneling/sinus tracks/undermining		X	
Deep trauma wounds			
Wounds that require controlled growth of granulation tissue			X
Diabetic ulcers			X
Dry wounds			X
Post graft placement (including Bioengineered tissues)			X
Shallow chronic ulcers			X

The V.A.C.®—V.A.C.® Therapy™ Clinical Guidelines, January 2003 KCI USA, Inc.

described.[75,76] The vast majority of case series report limited morbidity with this temporary closure technique in severely compromised patients. Prospective studies have reported occurrence of fistulae in a minority of NPWT-treated laparostomy wounds complicated by multiorgan failure or sepsis, but they could not be attributed to NPWT itself.

Clean, Closed Incisions

Disruption in optimal incision healing can lead to postoperative wound infection, dehiscence, seromas, hematomas, and additional surgeries. These surgical procedure incision types include sternotomies, caesarean sections, open hysterectomies, hip and knee arthroplasties, traumatic wounds such as pilon and tibia fractures, and lower extremity bypasses. Traditionally, surgical incisions have been closed by primary intention using sutures, staples, tissue adhesives, paper tape, or a combination of these methods. These closure methods, however, are not sufficient for some incisions, which reopen as a result of excessive edema or other factors, including patient comorbidities and location of incision.

Closure technologies also have drawbacks. Sutures and staples are tensioning devices, which concentrate the spreading force to small points along the incision and can result in tissue ischemia or necrosis at the tension points.[77] A disadvantage of tissue adhesive over incisions is that the adhesive may interfere with healing since it can act as a barrier to epithelialization.[78] A disadvantage to the use of paper tape is that it is not effective in moist or bleeding wounds, as moisture may wash away the adhesive or compromise the integrity of the paper itself.[79]

Many adjunctive therapies have, therefore, been used to aid treatment of clean closed surgical incisions, including gauze dressings and advanced therapies such as hydrocolloids, growth factors, cultured skin, low-energy ultrasound, and NPWT. The NPWT system protects the incision from external contamination, helps hold the closed incision edges together, reduces edema, removes exudates, and may allow for improved fluid flow beneath the incision.[80] Publications have documented successful outcomes with NPWT over clean closed incisions in high-risk patients with sternal wounds[81] and orthopedic fractures,[82,83] and in morbidly obese patients with acetabular fractures.[84] Stannard and colleagues'[83] data showed that postincision use of NPWT resulted in a 50.0% lower incidence of infection and 51.1% lower dehiscence rate, compared to traditional postoperative dressings.

Instillation of Antiseptics or Other Solutions with NPWT

NPWT-instillation was introduced to the US acute care market in 2003 as an evolutionary addition to standard NPWT. It combines standard NPWT with timed, intermittent delivery of an instilled topical solution. This technology is indicated for patients who would benefit from vacuum-assisted drainage and controlled delivery of topical wound treatment solutions and suspensions over the wound bed. It is intended for use with aqueous solutions in a physiologic pH range defined as 6.0 to 7.4. Alcohol- or hydrogen peroxide–based solutions are contraindicated because of their potential negative effect on

the foam dressing. Appropriate solutions for instillation with NPWT include antimicrobial irrigation or analgesic solutions.

Fleischmann[16] is generally credited for pioneering the NPWT-instillation technique in orthopedic medicine. He and his colleagues reported only one instance of recurrent infection (3 to 14 months of follow-up) out of a group of 27 patients with acute infections of bone and soft tissues, chronic osteomyelitis, or chronic wounds treated with vacuum sealing and instillation.[16]

NPWT-instillation setup differs from the standard NPWT devices in that it has an additional set of ingress tubing that allows gravity feed of solutions into the dressing. An intravenous pole that accommodates standard intravenous fluid bags is attached to the device. A mechanical clamp opens and closes the intravenous tubing per set instillation and hold times. Negative pressure resumes at the end of the hold time to remove the remaining instilled topical solution and wound exudate, as well as collapse the foam.

In the first published US case series exploring the use of NPWT-instillation, Wolvos[17] concluded that culture-directed antibiotic wound irrigation appeared to effectively decrease the bacterial burden of infected wounds, changing the apearance of some wounds from infected to clean, and converting wound culture data from positive cultures to no growth or normal flora.[17]

In a subsequent series, NPWT-instillation demonstrated a significant reduction in the mean time to infection clearance, wound closure, and hospital discharge compared to traditional advanced wound care methods.[85] Patient tolerance and compliance with the therapy are enhanced with the decreased time to closure and quicker hospital discharge. The improved outcomes also affect indirect costs such as loss of work days, recovery time, and mortality. In a pilot study, Lehner and Bernd[86] reported hip and knee prosthesis salvage in three patients with early periprosthetic infection treated with antiseptic irrigation and NPWT. Guidelines for use as well as novel application techniques of NPWT-instillation have been published.[87] Additional studies with larger patient samples are needed to further substantiate the results of this novel wound treatment therapy.

NPWT AND SILVER

Ionic silver has long been recognized as an effective antimicrobial against a broad spectrum of pathogens and is considered to be biocompatible with mammalian tissue.[88,89] The resurgence of interest in silver products for wound care stems from the increase in the level of bacterial resistance to traditional antibiotics. For example, rates of methicillin-resistant *S. aureus* increased steadily from about 30% in 1989 to approximately 40% in 1997 among ICU patients.[90] Unlike traditional antibiotics, ionic silver has multiple mechanisms of action, such as inhibiting cellular respiration, denaturing nucleic acids, and altering cellular membrane permeability.[91,92] Appropriately high concentrations of silver coupled with its various mechanisms of action make it difficult for microorganisms to develop resistance to silver because they would have to undergo several mutations in order to develop defense mechanisms against silver's multipronged attack. Silver also has low mammalian cell toxicity, and is now known to have potent anti-inflammatory properties when delivered at the appropriate concentrations.[93]

NPWT dressings are available with and without a micro-bonded metallic silver interface layer. Silver-coated NPWT dressings are recommended in cases of infected wounds or wounds at high risk for infection. One advantage of silver-coated foam dressings in a negative pressure environment is its conformity to the contours of the wound, reducing the areas of noncontact where bacteria may proliferate.[94] Although numerous studies have been published regarding the effectiveness of silver in wound care, publications specifically related to NPWT use with silver dressings are limited to a few case studies. One case study describes complete reepithelialization over a 40% failed graft of a third degree burn after 9 days with NPWT and silver foam.[95] In combination with antibiotics, the need for regrafting was prevented. In another case, NPWT and the silver foam dressings were successfully used to achieve complete closure in a necrotizing fasciitis wound of a newborn with acute myeloid leukemia.[96]

NPWT AND SKIN GRAFTS

Contoured wounds requiring skin grafts are often located in complex anatomic regions or are in unusual positions, which make conventional skin graft stabilization techniques cumbersome and ineffective. Use of NPWT in conjunction with split-thickness skin grafts is well documented in the treatment of burns and degloving injuries, and particularly over body sites with irregular or deep contours.[97–101]

In 1998, Blackburn et al.[102] first described the use of NPWT as a bolster for split-thickness skin grafts. They concluded that its use was efficacious, with increased graft take due to total immobilization of the graft, thereby limiting shear forces, eliminating fluid collection underneath the graft, bridging of the graft, and decreasing bacterial contamination.[102] NPWT has also been used successfully as a bolster in single-stage skin grafting over full-thickness loss of the scalp following a burn injury or excision of an extensive carcinoma.[103] Effective use of NPWT over split-thickness skin grafts has been reinforced in vulvo-vaginal and lower extremity reconstruction studies as well.[104,105]

Molnar et al.[106] showed that adjunctive NPWT improved the take rate and time to vascularization of Integra (Ethicon, Inc., Somerville, NJ), compared with previous published results, even in complicated wounds. In this series, bone was exposed in 62.5% of cases, joint in 50%, tendon in 37.5%, and bowel in 25%. The estimated Integra take rate was 96%. Authors concluded that this technique may be a practical alternative to flap closure.[106] Similarly, successful use of NPWT to facilitate incorporation of small intestinal submucosa (SIS, Cook Surgical, Bloomington, Ind.) has also been documented in neonates.[107]

PEDIATRICS

NPWT has been used in patients of all ages.[108] Mooney et al.[109] (2000) concluded in the first published pediatric series that adjunctive use of NPWT in pediatric patients with complex soft tissue wounds led to a decrease in complex microvascular surgeries. Later, Arca et al.[110] showed that NPWT was safe in premature neonates weighing less than 1,500 g.

A growing number of larger series have been subsequently published regarding successful use of NPWT in children with abdominal compartment syndrome, enterocutaneous fistulae, and a wide variety of tissue defects.[111–113]

COST-EFFECTIVENESS OF NPWT

Research and case studies have demonstrated that the use of NPWT may decrease hospital stays, nursing time, amputation rates, complex surgical closures, and office or home visits.[48,114–116] However, budget constraints require that advantages of advanced wound care technologies be weighed with their comparatively higher daily cost. When developing a wound healing strategy that includes advanced technology as part of the overall treatment plan, cost decisions should be based on overall cost and not individual product cost. Cost studies have shown that NPWT has higher material costs than modern or saline gauze dressings, but costs appear to be compensated by a lower number of dressing changes and shorter duration in the hospital.[117,118] Overall, costs were similar between NPWT and other modern wound care dressings and gauze dressings in two studies, the advantages of NPWT being patient comfort and a more satisfied nursing staff.[117, 119]

In a study that evaluated cost-effectiveness of NPWT versus advanced wound care in patients with complex wounds in a long-term acute care (LTAC) facility, the cost per cubic centimeter wound reduction was $11.90/cm^3 in the NPWT group versus $30.92/cm^3 in the moist wound healing group, based on cost of procedures performed, wound care products and devices used, and costs associated with treatment.[120] Postsurgical LTAC patients treated with NPWT had a more accelerated rate of wound closure, compared to the control.[120] A Swedish study determined that for patients who underwent coronary artery bypass grafting surgery followed by deep sternal wound infection, NPWT treatment was cost-effective, compared to gauze dressings, and had a low mortality rate.[121]

A study examining resource utilization and costs of NPWT in treating diabetic patients with postamputation wounds showed no difference between NPWT and standard moist wound therapy groups in hospital stay.[122] However, fewer surgical procedures and dressing changes were required in the NPWT group. The average direct cost per patient treated for 8 weeks or longer (independent of clinical outcome) was $27,270 and $36,096 in the NPWT and moist wound care groups, respectively. The average total cost to achieve healing was $25,954 for patients treated with NPWT ($N = 43$) compared with $38,806 for the moist wound care group ($N = 33$).[122]

Evidence also suggests that earlier initiation of NPWT may help reduce overall costs, particularly with traumatic wounds. One study has shown that patients with complex trauma wounds who received NPWT within 2 days of their hospital admission, versus day 3 or later, demonstrated significant reductions in length of stay, treatment days, and ICU stay, which resulted in significantly reduced patient treatment costs.[123]

Costs for NPWT equipment rental and dressing supplies will vary among institutions and geographic locations. Caregivers are advised to stay abreast of federal, state, and managed care contracts regarding NPWT reimbursement regulations and revisions.

Three photo case studies show how NPWT is used for different wound etiologies and for different outcomes. Figure 29.2 presents a photo case study of NPWT used on an ankle wound post debridement. In this case, NPWT was used until the wound fully healed. As can be seen in the photos, the wound was healed in a 15-day time period.

Figure 29.3 presents a series showing NPWT used on a patient with an infected right knee wound with hardware from prior knee replacement visible. In this case, the NPWT was used to help manage the infection and to prepare the wound for surgical closure. The final case series presented in Figure 29.4 shows NPWT used for a brief time period to prepare the wound for closure with a split-thickness skin graft.

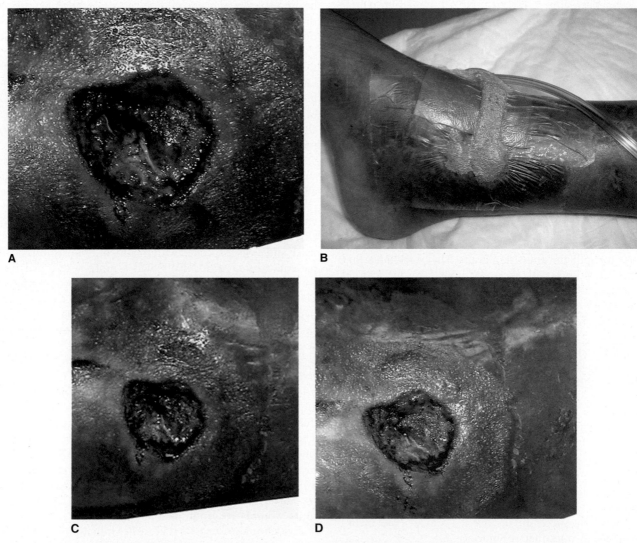

FIGURE 29.2 A. Wound at admission, postdebridement. **B.** Day 1 of V.A.C.® GranuFoam® Silver™ Dressing. **C.** Day 3 of V.A.C.® GranuFoam® Silver™ Dressing. **D.** Day 5 of V.A.C.® GranuFoam® Silver™ Dressing.

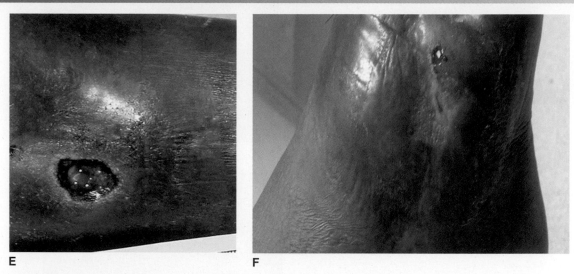

FIGURE 29.2 *(Continued)* **E.** Day 9 of V.A.C.® GranuFoam® Silver™ Dressing. **F.** Day 15: The patient is discharged with a closed wound.

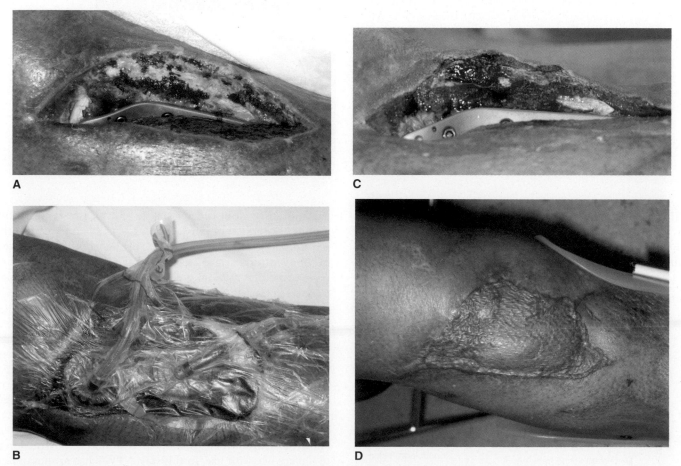

FIGURE 29.3 A 65-year-old male with infected open right knee joint with exposed hardware **A.** Infection present for 3 months following an open reduction with internal fixation procedure. NPWT instillation was initiated. **B.** With normal saline irrigation, and followed on day 3 with silver nitrate irrigation. By day 5, the wound culture returned negative, and the knee was closed via local flap on day 10. **C.** Illustrates the granulating knee the day it was closed, and **D.** shows the knee closed and viable at 6-month follow-up.

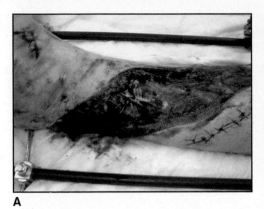

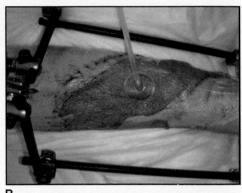

A

B

FIGURE 29.4 **A.** A 14-year-old male with open tibial fracture and bone exposure. **B.** Managed with VAC therapy and GranuFoam silver foam. **C.** The wound progressed over a 5-day period and was successfully closed with adjacent tissue transfer and STSG.

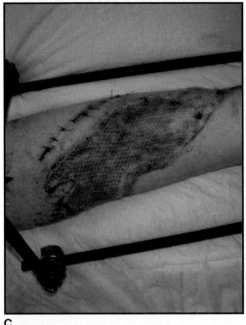

C

SUMMARY

Closure of any wound is evaluated with a reconstructive mindset that includes the following goals: (1) close wound, (2) prevent infection, (3) provide stable and robust coverage,

Reconstructive Ladder
Elevator

N
P
W
T

➢ Healing by secondary intention
➢ Direct tissue closure
  ✓ primary
  ✓ delayed
➢ Local tissue transfers
➢ Distant tissue transfers
➢ Free tissue transfer

High tech healing

• Tissue engineering
• Tissue expansion
• HBO
• Cytokine Therapy
• Xeno/Allograft skin
• **Negative Pressure**

FIGURE 29.5 Revised reconstructive ladder.

(4) minimize donor defect, and (5) maximize function. Taking those factors into account, plastic surgeons use the *reconstructive ladder* to proceed through the various levels of intervention used to close wounds. The *ladder* consists of basic principles of wound closure along with more complex closures such as using local, distant, and free flaps. As such, the *reconstructive ladder* is similar to an elevator as presented in the literature.[124] At some point along that elevator, clinicians must be able to make "stops" to implement adjunctive high-tech tools, including NPWT, at any level of treatment or intervention on the reconstructive elevator (see Fig. 29.5).

Deciding which tools to use and how to adapt the elevator to each patient is far more important to understand. The patient's overall condition, in terms of critical care issues, nutrition, and immunosuppression is a key determining factor, as is the class and type of wound. The main goal in wound reconstruction is to replace like with like. In this way, NPWT has revolutionized wound care, serving both as a temporizing bridge to closure while other factors are maximized (i.e., nutrition) and as a final therapeutic technology.

REVIEW QUESTIONS

1. A 19-year-old female presents with a 5 × 4 cm forearm wound. The wound has a good base of granulation tissue and is progressing well. Granulation tissue mainly consists of
   A. fibrinous tissue
   B. mix of small vessels and connective tissue
   C. MMPs
   D. Collagenase

2. The original scientific studies involving negative pressure wound therapy were performed in
   A. adult patient population
   B. pediatric patient population
   C. swine
   D. rabbits

3. The effect of the mechanical suction force of the vacuum device on wound healing was first noted in
   A. 1995
   B. 1911

   C. 1993
   D. 1984

4. Ilizarov bone distraction technique demonstrates
   A. how tissue moves and grows in response to the application of mechanical force
   B. an increase in angiogenesis
   C. an increase in mitotic figures
   D. all of the above

5. The proposed mechanism in negative pressure therapy for improved blood flow involves:
   A. Removal of interstitial fluid around the wound
   B. Decompressing the microcirculation
   C. A and B
   D. None of the above

REFERENCES

1. Gupta S, Baharestani M, Baranoski S. et al. Guidelines for managing pressure ulcers with negative pressure wound therapy. *Adv Skin Wound Care.* 2004;17(suppl 2):1.
2. Brown KM, Harper FV, Aston WJ, et al. Vacuum-assisted closure in the treatment of a 9-year-old child with severe and multiple dog bite injuries of the thorax. *Ann Thorac Surg.* 2001;72:1409.
3. Banwell PE, Musgrave M. Topical negative pressure therapy: mechanisms and indications. *Int Wound J.* 2008;5(4):511–529.
4. A Short History of Vacuum Terminology and Technology. http://www.mcallister.com/vacuum.html. McAllister Technical Services. Updated April 2010. Accessed September 3, 2010.
5. Zhivotaev VM. Vacuum therapy of postoperative infected wounds of the urinary bladder. *Klin Khir.* 1970;5:36.
6. Davydov Iu A, Larichev AB, Men'kov KG. Bacteriologic and cytologic evaluation of vacuum therapy of suppurative wounds. *Vestn Khir Im I Grek.* 1988;141:48.
7. Davydov IA, Larichev AB, Smirnov AP, et al. Vacuum therapy of acute suppurative diseases of soft tissues and suppurative wounds. *Vestn Khir Im I I Grek.* 1988;141:43.
8. Davydov IA, Larichev AB, Kozlov AG. Pathogenetic mechanisms of the effect of vacuum therapy on the course of the wound process. *Khirurgiia (Mosk).* 1990;66:42.
9. Fleischmann W, Strecker W, Bombelli M, et al. Vacuum sealing as treatment of soft tissue damage in open fractures. *Unfallchirurg.* 1993;96:488.
10. Fleischmann W, Becker U, Bischoff M, et al. Vacuum sealing: indication, technique and results. *Eur Orthop Surg Trauma.* 1995;5:37.
11. Fleischmann W, Russ M, Marquardt C. Closure of defect wounds by combined vacuum sealing with instrumental skin expansion. *Unfallchirurg.* 1996;99:970.
12. Fleischmann W, Lang E, Kinzl L. Vacuum assisted wound closure after dermatofasciotomy of the lower extremity. *Unfallchirurg.* 1996;99:283.
13. Banwell P, Withey S, Holten I. The use of negative pressure to promote healing. *Br J Plast Surg.* 51:79:1998.
14. Argenta LC, Morykwas MJ. Vacuum-assisted closure: a new method for wound control and treatment: clinical experience. *Ann Plast Surg.* 1997;38:563.

15. Morykwas MJ, Argenta LC, Shelton-Brown EI, et al. Vacuum-assisted closure: a new method for wound control and treatment: animal studies and basic foundation. *Ann Plast Surg.* 1997;38:553.
16. Fleischmann W, Russ M, Westhauser A, et al. Vacuum sealing as carrier system for controlled local drug administration in wound infection. *Unfallchirurg.* 1998;101:649.
17. Wolvos T. Wound instillation with negative pressure wound therapy. *Ostomy Wound Manage.* 2005;51:21.
18. Banwell P. Topical negative pressure therapy in wound care. *J Wound Care.* 1999;8:79.
19. Yager DR, Zhang LY, Liang HX, et al. Wound fluids from human pressure ulcers contain elevated matrix metalloproteinase levels and activity compared to surgical wound fluids. *J Invest Dermatol.* 1996;107:743.
20. Cook H, Davies KJ, Harding KG, et al. Defective extracellular matrix reorganization by chronic wound fibroblasts is associated with alterations in TIMP-1, TIMP-2, and MMP-2 activity. *J Invest Dermatol.* 2000;115:225.
21. Grinnell F, Zhu M, Parks WC. Collagenase-1 complexes with alpha2-macroglobulin in the acute and chronic wound environments. *J Invest Dermatol.* 1998;110:771.
22. Wlaschek M, Peus D, Achterberg V, et al. Protease inhibitors protect growth factor activity in chronic wounds. *Br J Dermatol.* 1997;137:646.
23. Falabella AF, Carson P, Eaglstein WH, et al. The safety and efficacy of a proteolytic ointment in the treatment of chronic ulcers of the lower extremity. *J Am Acad Dermatol.* 1998;39:737.
24. Ladwig GP, Robson MC, Liu R, et al. Ratios of activated matrix metalloproteinase-9 to tissue inhibitor of matrix metalloproteinase-1 in wound fluids are inversely correlated with healing of pressure ulcers. *Wound Repair Regen.* 2002;10:26, 2002.
25. Davey ME, O'Toole GA. Microbial biofilms: from ecology to molecular genetics. *Microbiol Mol Biol Rev.* 2000;64:847.
26. Ashcroft GS, Horan MA, Herrick SE, et al. Age-related differences in the temporal and spatial regulation of matrix metalloproteinases (MMPs) in normal skin and acute cutaneous wounds of healthy humans. *Cell Tissue Res.* 1997;290:581.
27. Ashcroft GS, Herrick SE, Tarnuzzer RW, et al. Human ageing impairs injury-induced in vivo expression of tissue inhibitor of matrix metalloproteinases (TIMP)-1 and -2 proteins and mRNA. *J Pathol.* 1997;183:169.

28. Argenta PA, Rahaman J, Gretz HF III, et al. Vacuum-assisted closure in the treatment of complex gynecologic wound failures. *Obstet Gynecol.* 2002;99: 497.

29. Morykwas MJ, Simpson J, Punger K, et al. Vacuum-assisted closure: state of basic research and physiologic foundation. *Plast Reconstr Surg.* 2006;117(7 suppl):121S–126S.

30. Lambert KV, Hayes P, McCarthy M. Vacuum assisted closure: a review of development and current applications. *Eur J Vasc Endovasc Surg.* 2005;29:219.

31. Wackenfors A, Sjögren J, Gustafsson R, et al. Effects of vacuum-assisted closure therapy on inguinal wound edge microvascular blood flow. *Wound Repair Regen.* 2004;12(6):600–606.

32. Borgquist O, Ingemansson R, Malmsjö M. Wound edge microvascular blood flow during negative-pressure wound therapy: examining the effects of pressures from −10 to −175 mm Hg. *Plast Reconstr Surg.* 2010;125(2):502–509.

33. Chen SZ, Li J, Li XY, et al. Effects of vacuum-assisted closure on wound microcirculation: an experimental study. *Asian J Surg.* 2005;28:211, 2005.

34. Saxena V, Hwang CW, Huang S, et al. Vacuum-assisted closure: microdeformations of wounds and cell proliferation. *Plast Reconstr Surg.* 2004;114:1086.

35. Chen CS, Mrksich M, Huang S, et al. Geometric control of cell life and death. *Science.* 1997;276:1425.

36. Ingber DE. Fibronectin controls capillary endothelial cell growth by modulating cell shape. *Proc Natl Acad Sci U S A.* 1990;87:3579.

37. Huang S, Ingber DE. The structural and mechanical complexity of cell-growth control. *Nat Cell Biol.* 1999;1:E131.

38. Ingber DE, Prusty D, Sun Z, et al. Cell shape, cytoskeletal mechanics, and cell cycle control in angiogenesis. *J. Biomech.* 1995;28:1471.

39. Thoma R. Ueber die Histomechanik des Gefasssystems und die Pathogenese der Angioskleroose. *Virchows Arch F Pathol Anat.* 1911;204:120–126.

40. Olenius M, Dalsgaard CJ, Wickman M. Mitotic activity in expanded human skin. *Plast Reconstr Surg.* 1993;91:213.

41. Urschel JD, Scott PG, Williams HT. The effect of mechanical stress on soft and hard tissue repair; a review. *Br J Plast Surg.* 1988;41:182. Sternal wound infection following cardiac surgery. *J Wound Care.* 2000;9:229.

42. Philbeck TE Jr, Whittington KT, Millsap MH, et al. The clinical and cost effectiveness of externally applied negative pressure wound therapy in the treatment of wounds in home healthcare Medicare patients. *Ostomy Wound Manage.* 1999;45:41.

43. Tang AT, Okri SK, Haw MP. Vacuum-assisted closure to treat deep sternal wound infection following cardiac surgery. *J Wound Care.* 2000;9:229.

44. Schmidtchen A, Holst E, Tapper H, et al. Elastase-producing Pseudomonas aeruginosa degrade plasma proteins and extracellular products of human skin and fibroblasts, and inhibit fibroblast growth. *Microb Pathog.* 2003;34:47.

45. Dedmond BT, Kortesis B, Punger K, et al. The use of negative-pressure wound therapy (NPWT) in the temporary treatment of soft-tissue injuries associated with high-energy open tibial shaft fractures. *J Orthop Trauma.* 2007;21:11–17.

46. Li JQ, Chen SZ, Li WZ, et al. Therapeutic effect of vacuum-assisted closure technology on infected explosion wound of pig. *Zhonghua Shao Shang Za Zhi.* 2008;24:13–17. Chinese.

47. Petzina R, Hoffmann J, Navasardyan A, et al. Negative pressure wound therapy for post-sternotomy mediastinitis reduces mortality rate and sternal re-infection rate compared to conventional treatment. *Eur J Cardiothorac Surg.* 2010;110–113.

48. Armstrong, DG, Lavery LA. Negative pressure wound therapy after partial diabetic foot amputation: a multicentre, randomised controlled trial. *Lancet.* 2005;366:1704–1710.

49. Blume PA, Walters J, Payne W, et al. Comparison of negative pressure wound therapy utilizing vacuum-assisted closure to advanced moist wound therapy in the treatment of diabetic foot ulcers: a multicenter randomized controlled trial. *Diabetes Care.* 2008;31:631–636.

50. Mouës CM, Vos MC, van den Bemd GL, et al. Bacterial load in relation to vacuum-assisted closure wound therapy: a prospective randomized trial. *Wound Repair Regen.* 2004;12:11–17.

51. Stannard JP, Singanamala N, Volgas DA. Fix and flap in the era of vacuum suction devices: what do we know in terms of evidence based medicine? *Injury.* 2010;41(8):780–786.

52. Nelson JA, Kim EM, Serletti JM, et al. A novel technique for lower extremity limb salvage: the vastus lateralis muscle flap with concurrent use of the vacuum-assisted closure device. *J Reconstr Microsurg.* 2010;26(7):427–431.

53. Morykwas MJ, Howell H, Bleyer AJ, et al. The effect of externally applied sub-atmospheric pressure on serum myoglobin levels following a prolonged crush/ischemia injury. *Trauma.* 2002; 53:537.

54. Robson MC, Steed DL, Franz MG. Wound healing: biologic features and approaches to maximize healing trajectories. *Curr Probl Surg.* 2001;38:72–140.

55. Schultz G. Molecular regulation of wound healing. In: Bryant R, Nix D. *Acute and Chronic Wounds: Current Management Concepts.* 3rd ed. St Louis, MO: Mosby; 2007:82–96.

56. Ayello EA, Cuddigan JE. Debridement: controlling the necrotic/cellular burden. *Adv Skin Wound Care.* 2004;17:66.

57. Harris IR, Yee KC, Walters CE, et al. Cytokine and protease levels in healing and non-healing chronic venous leg ulcers. *Exp Dermatol.* 1995;4:342.

58. Katz MH, Alvarez AF, Kirsner RS, et al. Human wound fluid from acute wounds stimulates fibroblast and endothelial cell growth. *J Am Acad Dermatol.* 1991;25:1054.

59. Stechmiller JK, Kilpadi DV, Childress B, et al. Effect of vacuum-assisted closure therapy on the expression of cytokines and proteases in wound fluid of adults with pressure ulcers. *Wound Repair Regen.* 2006;14(3):371–374.

60. Labler L, Rancan M, Mica L, et al. Vacuum-assisted closure therapy increases local interleukin-8 and vascular endothelial growth factor levels in traumatic wounds. *J Trauma.* 2009;66(3):749–757.

61. Hawksworth JS, Stojadinovic A, Gage FA, et al. Inflammatory biomarkers in combat wound healing. *Annal Surg.* 2009;250(3):1–6.

62. Wang JH, Li ZQ, Chen J, et al. Sequential management of residual wounds in burn patients. *Zhonghua Shao Shang Za Zhi.* 2007;23(1):16–19. Chinese.

63. Watelet JB, Claeys C, Van Cauwenberge P, et al. Predictive and monitoring value of matrix metalloproteinase-9 for healing quality after sinus surgery. *Wound Repair Regen.* 2004;12:412.

64. Bullen EC, Longaker MT, Updike DL, et al. Tissue inhibitor of metalloproteinases-1 is decreased and activated gelatinases are increased in chronic wounds. *J Invest Dermatol.* 1995;104:236.

65. Wysocki AB, Staiano-Coico L, Grinnell F. Wound fluid from chronic leg ulcers contains elevated levels of metalloproteinases MMP-2 and MMP-9. *J Invest Dermatol.* 1993;101:64.

66. Shi B, Chen SZ, Zhang P, et al. Effects of vacuum-assisted closure (VAC) on the expressions of MMP-1, 2, 13 in human granulation wound. *Zhonghua Zheng Xing Wai Ke Za Zhi.* 2003;19:279.

67. Tang SY, Chen SZ, Hu ZH, et al. Influence of vacuum-assisted closure technique on expression of Bcl-2 and NGF/NGFmRNA during wound healing. *Zhonghua Zheng Xing Wai Ke Za Zhi.* 2004; 20:139.

68. Venturi ML, Attinger CE, Mesbahi AN, et al. Mechanisms and clinical applications of the vacuum-assisted closure (VAC) Device: a review. *Am J Clin Dermatol.* 2005;6:185.

69. V.A.C. therapy clinical guidelines. San Antonio, TX: Kinetic Concepts Incorporated; 2010:1–22.

70. Gabriel A, Shores J, Bernstein B, et al. A clinical review of infected wound treatment with Vacuum Assisted Closure (V.A.C.) Therapy: Experience and case series. *Int Wound J.* 2009;6(suppl 2):1–25.

71. Greer SE, Duthie E, Cartolano B, et al. Techniques for applying sub-atmospheric pressure dressing to wounds in difficult regions of anatomy. *J Wound Ostomy Continence Nurs.* 1999;26:250.

72. Kaplan M, Banwell P, Orgill DP, et al. Guidelines for the management of the open abdomen. *Wounds.* 2005;17:S1–S24

73. Sermoneta D, Di Mugno M, Spada PL, et al. Intra-abdominal vacuum-assisted closure (VAC) after necrosectomy for acute necrotising pancreatitis: preliminary experience. *Int Wound J.* 2010.

74. Stevens P. Vacuum-assisted closure of laparostomy wounds: a critical review of the literature. *Int Wound J.* 2009;6(4):259–66.

75. Cothren CC, Moore EE, Johnson JL, et al. One hundred percent fascial approximation with sequential abdominal closure of the open abdomen. *Am J Surg.* 2006;192:238–242

76. Koss W, Ho HC, Yu M, et al. Preventing loss of domain: a management strategy for closure of the "open abdomen" during the initial hospitalization. *J Surg Educ.* 2009;66(2):89–95.

77. Easterlin B, Bromberg W, Linscott J. A novel technique of vacuum assisted wound closure that functions as a delayed primary closure. *Wounds.* 2007;19(12):331–333.

78. Toriumi DM, O'Grady K, Desai D, et al. Use of octyl-2-cyanoacrylate for skin closure in facial plastic surgery. *Plast Reconstr Surg.* 1998;102(6):2209–2219.

79. Shamiyeh A, Schrenk P, Stelzer T, et al. Prospective randomized blind controlled trial comparing sutures, tape, and octylcyanoacrylate tissue adhesive for skin closure after phlebectomy. *Dermatol Surg.* 2001;27(10):877–880.

80. Kinetic Concepts I. 510(k) Summary: prevena incision management system. San Antonio, TX: Kinetic Concepts, Inc.; 2010 Jun 11. Report No.: K100821.

81. Atkins BZ, Wooten MK, Kistler J, et al. Does negative pressure wound therapy have a role in preventing poststernotomy wound complications? *Surg Innov.* 2009;16(2):140–146.

82. Gomoll AH, Lin A, Harris MB. Incisional vacuum-assisted closure therapy. *J Orthop Trauma.* 2006;20(10):705–709.

83. Stannard JP, Robinson JT, Anderson ER, et al. Negative pressure wound therapy to treat hematomas and surgical incisions following high-energy trauma. *J Trauma.* 2006;60(6):1301–1306.

84. Reddix RN Jr, Tyler HK, Kulp B, et al. Incisional Vacuum-Assisted Wound Closure in morbidly obese patients undergoing acetabular fracture surgery. *Am J Orthop.* 2009;38(9):32–35.

85. Gabriel A, Heinrich C, Shores JT, et al. Negative pressure wound therapy with instillation: a pilot study describing a new method for treating infected wounds. *Int Wound J.* 2008;5(3):399–413.

86. Lehner B, Bernd L. V.A.C.-instill therapy in periprosthetic infection of hip and knee arthroplasty. *Zentralbl Chir.* 2006;131(suppl 1):S160–S164. German

87. Jerome D. Advances in negative pressure wound therapy: the VAC instill. *J Wound Ostomy Continence Nurs.* 2007;34(2):191–194.

88. Vanscheidt W, Lazareth I, Routkovsky-Norval C. Safety evaluation of a new ionic silver dressing in the management of chronic ulcers. *Wounds.* 2003;15:371.

89. Demling RH, DiSanti L. The role of silver technology in wound healing: effects of silver on wound management. *Wounds.* 2001;13:15.

90. Fridkin SK, Gaynes RP. Antimicrobial resistance in intensive care units. *Clin Chest Med.* 1999;20:303.

91. Ovington LG. The truth about silver. *Ostomy Wound Manage.* 2004;50:1S.

92. Driver VR. Silver dressings in clinical practice. *Ostomy Wound Manage.* 2004;50:11S.

93. Wright JB, Hansen DL, Burrell RE. The comparative efficacy of two antimicrobial barrier dressings: in vitro examination of two controlled release of silver dressings. *Wounds.* 1998;10:179.

94. Jones S, Bowler PG, Walker M. Antimircrobial activity of silver-containing dressings is influenced by dressing conformability with a wound surface. *Wounds.* 2005;17:263.

95. Poulakidas S, Kowal-Vern A. Facilitating residual wound closure after partial graft loss with vacuum assisted closure therapy. *J Burn Care Res.* 2008;29(4):663–665.

96. Negosanti L, Aceti A, Bianchi T, et al. Adapting a Vacuum Assisted Closure dressing to challenging wounds: negative pressure treatment for perineal necrotizing fasciitis with rectal prolapse in a newborn affected by acute myeloid leukaemia. *Eur J Dermatol.* 2010;20(4):501–503.

97. Meara JG, Guo L, Smith JD, et al. Vacuum-assisted closure in the treatment of degloving injuries. *Ann Plast Surg.* 1999;42:589.

98. Josty IC, Ramaswamy R, Laing JH. Vaccum assisted closure: an alternative strategy in the management of degloving injuries of the foot. *Br J Plast Surg.* 2001;54:363.

99. Bovill E, Banwell PE, Teot L, et al. Topical negative pressure wound therapy: a review of its role and guidelines for its use in the management of acute wounds. *Int Wound J.* 2008;5(4):511–529.

100. Landau AG, Hudson DA, Adams K, et al. Full-thickness skin grafts: maximizing graft take using negative pressure dressings to prepare the graft bed. *Ann Plast Surg.* 2008;60(6):661–666.

101. Roka J, Karle B, Andel H, et al. Use of V.A.C. Therapy in the surgical treatment of severe burns: the Viennese concept. *Handchir Mikrochir Plast Chir.* 2007;39(5):322–327. German.

102. Blackburn JH 2nd, Boemi L, Hall WW, et al. Negative-pressure dressings as a bolster for skin grafts. *Ann Plast Surg.* 1998;40:453.

103. Molnar JA, DeFranzo AJ, Marks MW. Single-stage approach to skin grafting the exposed skull. *Plast Reconstr Surg.* 2000;105:174, 2000.

104. Carson SN, Overall K, Lee-Jahshan S, et al. Vacuum-assisted closure used for healing chronic wounds and skin grafts in the lower extremities. *Ostomy Wound Manage.* 2004;50:52.

105. Dainty LA, Bosco JJ, McBroom JW, et al. Novel techniques to improve split-thickness skin graft viability during vulvo-vaginal reconstruction. *Gynecol Oncol.* 2005;97:949.

106. Molnar JA, DeFranzo AJ, Hadaegh A, et al. Acceleration of Integra incorporation in complex tissue defects with subatmospheric pressure. *Plast Reconstr Surg.* 2004;113:1339.

107. Gabriel A, Gollin G. Management of complicated gastroschisis with porcine small intestinal submucosa and negative pressure wound therapy. *J Pediatr Surg.* 2006;41(11):1836–1840.

108. Baharestani M, Amjad I, Bookout K, et al. Therapy in the management of paediatric wounds: clinical review and experience. *Int Wound J.* 2009;6(suppl 1):1–26.

109. Mooney JF 3rd, Argenta LC, Marks MW, et al. Treatment of soft tissue defects in pediatric patients using the V.A.C. system. *Clin Orthop Relat Res.* 2000;26.

110. Arca MJ, Somers KK, Derks TE, et al. Use of vacuum-assisted closure system in the management of complex wounds in the neonate. *Pediatr Surg Int.* 2005.

111. Caniano DA, Ruth B, Teich S. Wound management with vacuum-assisted closure: experience in 51 pediatric patients. *J Pediatr Surg.* 2005;40:128.

112. Gabriel A, Heinrich C, Shores J, et al. Outcomes of vacuum-assisted closure for the treatment of wounds in a paediatric population: case series of 58 patients. *J Plast Reconstr Aesthet Surg.* 2009;62(11):1428–1436.

113. McCord SS, Naik-Mathuria BJ, Murphy KM, et al. Negative pressure therapy is effective to manage a variety of wounds in infants and children. *Wound Repair Regen.* 2007;15(3):296–301.

114. Frykberg RG, Williams DV. Negative-pressure wound therapy and diabetic foot amputations: a retrospective study of payer claims data. *J Am Podiatr Med Assoc.* 2007;97(5):351–359.

115. Horch RE, Nord D, Augustin M, et al. Economic aspects of surgical wound therapies. *Chirurg.* 2008;79(6):518–525. [Article in German].

116. Parrett BM, Matros E, Pribaz JJ, et al. Lower extremity trauma: trends in the management of soft-tissue reconstruction of open tibia-fibula fractures. *Plast Reconstr Surg.* 2006;117(4):1315–1322.

117. Mouës CM, van den Bemd GJ, Meerding WJ, et al. An economic evaluation of the use of TNP on full-thickness wounds. *J Wound Care.* 2005;14(5):224–227.

118. Sadat U, Chang G, Noorani A, et al. Efficacy of TNP on lower limb wounds: a meta-analysis. *J Wound Care.* 2008;17(1):45–48.

119. Braakenburg A, Obdeijn MC, Feitz R, et al. The clinical efficacy and cost effectiveness of the vacuum-assisted closure technique in the management of acute and chronic wounds: a randomized controlled trial. *Plast Reconstr Surg.* 2006;118(2):390–397; discussion 398–400.

120. de Leon JM, Barnes S, Nagel M, et al. Cost-effectiveness of negative pressure wound therapy for postsurgical patients in long-term acute care. *Adv Skin Wound Care.* 2009;22(3):122–127.

121. Mokhtari A, Sjögren J, Nilsson J, et al. The cost of vacuum-assisted closure therapy in treatment of deep sternal wound infection. *Scand Cardiovasc J.* 2008;42(1):85–89.

122. Apelqvist J, Armstrong DG, Lavery LA, et al. Resource utilization and economic costs of care based on a randomized trial of vacuum-assisted closure therapy in the treatment of diabetic foot wounds. *Am J Surg.* 2008;195(6):782–788.

123. Kaplan M, Daly D, Stemkowski S. Early intervention of negative pressure wound therapy using Vacuum-Assisted Closure in trauma patients: impact on hospital length of stay and cost. *Adv Skin Wound Care.* 2009;22(3):128–132.

124. Bennett N, Choudhary S. Why climb a ladder when you can take the elevator? *Plast Reconstr Surg.* 2000;105:2266.

Hyperbaric Oxygen Therapy: Management of the Hypoxic Wound

Jeffrey A. Niezgoda

CHAPTER OBJECTIVES

At the completion of this chapter, the reader will be able to:

1. State the definition of hyperbaric oxygen therapy (HBOT).
2. Describe the basic physiology and the potential side effects, risks, and contraindications of hyperbaric therapy.
3. Explain the mechanisms of action of HBOT in the management of hypoxic wounds.
4. List several of the approved indications for use of HBOT.
5. Identify the required criteria for utilization of HBOT in the patient with a diabetic foot ulcer.

This chapter provides the reader with an overview of hyperbaric oxygen therapy (HBOT). The basic mechanisms, physiology, chamber environment, and potential risks of hyperbaric oxygen will be discussed. The indications and approved uses of hyperbaric oxygen will be presented accompanied by a brief review of the supporting literature. While many factors are cited as contributing to wound chronicity, impaired tissue perfusion ultimately resulting in poor tissue oxygenation and tissue hypoxia is often top on the list. Wound care providers must appreciate the importance of oxygen in wound healing and know when and how to use adjunctive technology to meet the oxygen demands of the hypoxic wound. Therefore, the synopsis of HBOT provided in this chapter will also include an introduction to the use of this technology in the management of the hypoxic wound.

HBOT is defined as treatment during which a patient inhales 100% oxygen inside a pressure vessel capable of the delivery of pressures exceeding 1.4 atmospheres absolute (ATA). HBOT can be administered either in a multiplace chamber (see Fig. 30.1), capable of treating multiple patients, or in a smaller single-patient monoplace chamber (see Fig. 30.2). While multiplace chambers traditionally tend to be quite large and expensive in design, construction, and operation, technological advances over the past 15 to 20 years have led to an increase in the number of monoplace chambers in use in the world today. Multiplace chambers are pressured with air, and oxygen is administered to the patients via mask or hood tent (see Fig. 30.3). Multiplace chambers allow for hands-on care of the patient during the hyperbaric treatment by a physician, nurse, or trained inside attendant. In a monoplace chamber, a single patient is placed in an environment of pure oxygen under the desired treatment pressure. Monoplace care is typically reserved for those patients with more minor conditions, while the multiplace setting best serves complex and critically ill patients in addition to the more common ambulatory patients and outpatients. For routine conditions, HBOT is typically administered between 2.0 and 2.5 ATA, with 90 minutes of oxygen breathing, interrupted briefly by an "air break" (5–10 minutes of air breathing). Hyperbaric therapy has been used worldwide for more than 50 years in the treatment of many chronic nonhealing wounds and ulcers.[1] The safety record of HBOT in this country is excellent, and the technology has become a vital part of the growth of comprehensive wound care programs across the nation.[2,3]

THE HISTORY OF HYPERBARIC OXYGEN

The first nondiving use of HBO was for cardiac surgery by the Dutch surgeon Ite Boerema in 1956. Before the heart-lung machine was available, Boerema was able to extend circulatory arrest time for several minutes by compressing both the patient and the surgical team in the hyperbaric chamber. While under pressure, the patient breathed 100% O_2 in order to "drench" the tissues with oxygen, as Boerema termed it. Soon the investigators in Amsterdam also discovered its dramatic effect in treating gas gangrene. Other surgeons began building chambers in England and the United States. Smith and Sharp in Glasgow were the first to treat carbon monoxide poisoning in 1960.[1] As the use of the heart-lung machine in the late 1960s became commonplace, the need for hyperbaric surgery became vanishingly small, and surgeons who had been the principle researchers began to leave the field and many large and expensive surgical chambers closed.[4]

In 1976, there were less than 50 clinical chambers operating in the United States. To provide insurers with guidance regarding appropriate clinical utilization of HBOT, the Undersea Medical Society (now known as the Undersea and Hyperbaric

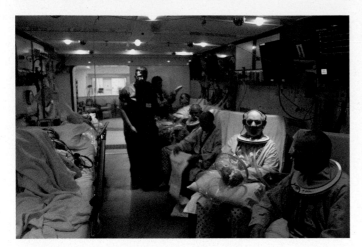

FIGURE 30.1 Multiplace hyperbaric chamber.

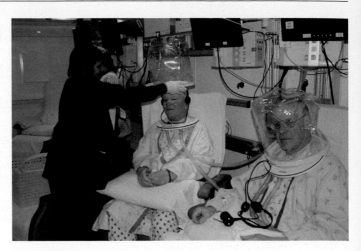

FIGURE 30.3 Patients breathing 100% oxygen via hood tent inside a multiplace hyperbaric chamber.

Medical Society) established the Committee on Hyperbaric Oxygen. The committee surveyed the field and published a short list of disorders treated with HBOT that had a scientific basis and had been clinically demonstrated to have merit. These were deemed reimbursable as Blue Cross/Blue Shield adopted it as their source document.[5] With a scientific basis and payment for services established, the number of chamber facilities began to grow. In the early 1980s, there were approximately 100 chambers in operation. Today, the number of clinical chambers is estimated to exceed 1,000. Typically, new hyperbaric facilities are established as an integral component of wound care clinics, and few are listed purely as hyperbaric facilities.

HYPERBARIC OXYGEN PHYSIOLOGY

Oxygen is the third most common element, and it comprises approximately 21% of the air we breathe. The majority of oxygen exists in a bi-atomic form as O_2 molecules, which fortunately is the form that can be best utilized by living organisms. The remaining composition of air consists of about

79% nitrogen, and less than 1% inert gases such as argon, carbon dioxide, neon, helium, and hydrogen. Air enters the alveoli, diffuses into the pneumonocytes and then into the blood stream. Given an atmospheric pressure of about 760 mm Hg at sea level, the partial pressure of oxygen (pO_2) in the air is around 150 mm Hg, but losses due to vapor pressure and pulmonary diffusion gradients further decrease the partial pressure of oxygen actually reaching the bloodstream.[6]

Once in the blood, oxygen is preferentially bound to the hemoglobin molecules on the red blood cells, and at sea level the average person has essentially 100% saturation of the hemoglobin molecules. However, the plasma can also carry dissolved oxygen, and in fact this system provides a great reserve in oxygen-carrying capacity. Under normal atmospheric pressure, the average person has about 0.3 volume percent of dissolved oxygen in his or her plasma. Thus when breathing air at sea level, an uncompromised patient will have an arterial pO_2 of approximately 100 mm Hg with the majority of this oxygen carried bound to hemoglobin and only a small percent of oxygen transported as dissolved in the plasma. In this setting, the normal diffusion radius for an oxygen molecule is 64 μm at the end arteriole and about 36 μm from the venous system where the pO_2 might be as low as 34 mm Hg (see Fig. 30.4).

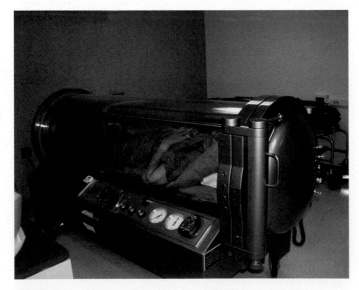

FIGURE 30.2 Monoplace hyperbaric chamber.

Normobaric Conditions

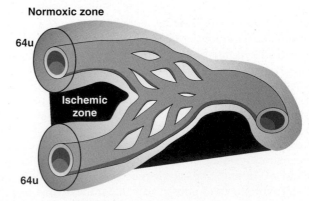

FIGURE 30.4 Oxygen diffusion normobaric air. (Courtesy Bob Bartlett MD.)

Oxygenated blood flows to distal tissues, and under normal physiologic conditions, the oxygen is offloaded to provide the energy substrates to fuel tissue metabolism. Oxygen delivery can be negatively impacted by conditions that inhibit uncoupling of oxyhemoglobin (such as tissue acidosis) or in conditions that prevent adequate tissue perfusion (i.e., peripheral arterial disease [PAD], edema, and conditions causing vessel sludging or trauma). In regard to wound healing, normal tissue oxygenation is critical to collagen synthesis, epithelialization, angiogenesis, and bacterial killing.[7–10]

The oxygen-carrying capacity of the plasma is immense, and this reserve capacity is exactly the target of the supraphysiologic oxygen levels provided by HBOT.[6,11] A patient breathing 100% oxygen at 3 ATA will have an enormous increase in the amount of oxygen physically dissolved in the plasma (6.9 volume percent) compared to the volume of oxygen dissolved at 1 ATA (0.3 volume percent). The brain only uses 6.1 volumes percent per pass, so the brain is fully oxygenated from oxygen dissolved in the plasma. In fact, plasma pO_2 values well in excess of 1,500 to 1,800 mm Hg are routinely achieved in hyperbaric patients. In this setting the hemoglobin never desaturates, and thus hemoglobin plays a minimal role in the transport of oxygen. Tissue oxygen partial pressures can reach 250 to 300 mm Hg, far above the normal 30 to 40 mm Hg when breathing air at one atmosphere. This 18- to 20-fold rise in dissolved oxygen establishes a tremendous gradient between the plasma and the peripheral tissues. It is this steep oxygen gradient that stimulates and initiates neoangiogenesis.

In addition to the supraphysiologic oxygen gradient, there is a significant increase in oxygen diffusion distance from the tissue capillary beds (247 μm) (see Fig. 30.5).[12] Given that the intercapillary distance in living tissue is less than 247 μm, it should be apparent that the fourfold increase in the oxygen diffusion radius provided by HBOT is an effective countermeasure against any tissue hypoxia that may be present. In addition, the supraphysiologic oxygen levels seen in hyperbaric patients can also reduce tissue edema through a compensatory vasoconstriction effect caused by an autoregulatory mechanism inherent to the vasculature. Thus, hyperbaric oxygen has a multifactorial mode of action: increased oxygen levels in the plasma available to diffuse farther into hypoxic tissues, while reducing tissue edema through compensatory vasoconstriction.[1]

Hyperbaric Conditions

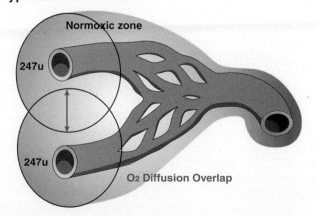

FIGURE 30.5 Oxygen diffusion hyperbaric oxygen. (Courtesy Bob Bartlett MD.)

Cellular Effects of HBOT

It is well documented that HBOT can induce angiogenesis and neovascularization in hypoxic tissues. Lee et al demonstrated that hyperbaric oxygen induces expression of Vascular Endothelial Growth Factor (VEGF) in human umbilical vein endothelial cells, through both transcription and translation within the cells.[13] They also showed that pure oxygen given at normobaric pressures (1 ATA) had no similar effect and therefore concluded that the benefits of pure oxygen seem to be unrealized unless the pressure at which it is given is significantly increased. Sheikh et al. showed that VEGF levels in hypoxic wounds rose by approximately 40% within 5 days of starting HBOT, but then dropped to control levels within 3 days of stopping the treatment.[14] They concluded that the angiogenic effect of HBOT was due to an increase in VEGF levels induced by hyperbaric oxygen, and that hypoxia was not necessarily the only requirement for wound VEGF production. Ahmad and Shiekh also demonstrated via laser Doppler imaging that in addition to an increase in angiogenesis, there was a 20% increase in wound bed perfusion following 10 days of HBOT.[15] Marx et al. showed that normobaric oxygen had no angiogenic properties above those associated with normal revascularization in rabbit mandibles irradiated with 60 Gy of gamma radiation.[16] They observed that hyperbaric oxygen demonstrated an eight- to ninefold increase in vascular density over both normobaric oxygen and air-breathing controls. Therefore the angiogenic benefits of HBOT in hypoxic, hypovascular tissue seem to be quite significant. Interim analysis of the Radiation Research Registry conducted by The American College of Hyperbaric Medicine found that the collective clinical outcomes of over 2,000 patients treated with HBOT due to the late effects of radiation tissue damage support this observation.[17]

Molecular oxygen is universally considered to be simply a consumable substrate to support our metabolism. At the time Boerema conducted his initial surgical experiments, this was considered to be its only property or function. But as research has delved deeper into the mechanisms of why HBOT produces the results seen clinically, oxygen was found to have other properties. Under increased pressure, it becomes a pharmacologic agent having the properties of a drug, but in excess can also be toxic to the body.

In only a limited number of circumstances is a great surfeit of oxygen necessary or even desirable. But in treating some disorders, we make use of the drug-like attributes of HBO alluded to above. For example, HBO acts as a potent vasoconstrictive agent that can reduce intracranial pressure by one-half. However, it does not cause vasoconstriction in postischemic muscle, sustaining blood flow to damaged tissues. It preserves adenosine triphosphate in cell membranes and dramatically reduces edema, allowing cells to control their own osmolarity. It prevents reperfusion injury in posthypoxic tissue.[18–20]

HBOT has been demonstrated to have a positive impact on limiting the deleterious effects of reperfusion injury. It blocks guanylate cyclase, the trigger molecule for beta-2-integrin that forms the leukocyte adhesion molecule. Thus, following ischemia or sepsis, leukocytes do not stick to the capillary walls to block circulation when the patient is treated early with HBOT. Every leukocyte in the body is rendered "nonsticky" for about 8 hours following a single HBO exposure. It also blocks the action of the intracellular adhesion molecule (the ICAM mechanism)

Oxygen Response Curves (90 min tx)

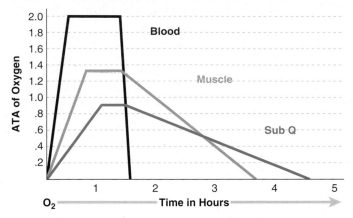

FIGURE 30.6 Hyperbaric oxygen response curves. (Courtesy Bob Bartlett, MD.)

that causes any leukocytes that become adherent to the capillary wall to bore through to the tissues surrounding the vessel, releasing the superoxide anion, proteinases, and elastase that liquefy tissue following crush injury and other forms of ischemia.[20,21]

Many nonhealing wounds do not heal because they are chronically infected or hypoxic. Because oxygen levels below 40 mm Hg do not allow leukocytes to kill bacteria, raising the tissue levels much higher than normal improves white cell bactericidal function. At oxygen partial pressures of 150 mm Hg, white cell killing ability is doubled or tripled beyond that found in even normally oxygenated leukocytes.[22]

It is important to note that oxygen levels remain high for a prolonged period following HBOT. After a 90-minute treatment at 2.0 ATA, the arterial levels fall to normal within a couple of minutes of cessation of treatment, but oxygen levels in muscle tissue remain significantly elevated for up to 3 hours and in subcutaneous tissues for 4 hours from the start of treatment (see Fig. 30.6). This phenomenon allows the use of bid or tid HBOT sessions to enhance tissue oxygenation for extended periods of time, rather than only when the patient is actually in the chamber.

For all the above reasons, wound healing centers have eagerly adopted HBO as its mechanisms have been clarified and clinical outcomes substantiated by research validation.

HYPERBARIC OXYGEN THERAPY INDICATIONS

The Centers for Medicare and Medicaid Services (CMS) has evaluated the use of HBOT in this country and has issued a National Coverage Determination (NCD) to define its policy regarding the reimbursement for hyperbaric services. While they are not obligated to follow the CMS guidelines, most insurance providers in this country do indeed follow the NCD when considering reimbursement for these services. A list of both approved diagnoses as well as other conditions (e.g., stroke, cerebral palsy) that are not considered to be reimbursable conditions can be found on the CMS website.[23] There are free-standing hyperbaric centers that offer treatment to patients with a noncovered diagnosis, typically on a cash basis. Indeed, there have been both published and anecdotal reports that HBOT may be efficacious in the treatment of certain conditions. Definitive randomized trials are clearly needed to investigate these claims.

Of the diagnoses listed as covered by CMS, some of the more common conditions treated with HBOT include

- Diabetic foot ulcer (DFU)
- Chronic refractory osteomyelitis
- Failing surgical flaps and grafts
- Osteoradionecrosis
- Soft tissue radionecrosis

Less common indications for HBOT include necrotizing soft tissue infections, decompression sickness (DCS) and carbon monoxide (CO) poisoning. HBOT is the treatment of choice for DCS and CO poisoning, and the timely treatment of both of these conditions can prevent many of the long-term neurologic sequelae often seen in patients not receiving hyperbaric oxygen.[2,24]

Hyperbaric Oxygen Therapy Treatment Protocols

While it is beyond the scope of this chapter to discuss the nuances of the treatment plans for each of these conditions, some generalizations can be made. For most patients, HBOT is administered on a daily basis. Although more serious conditions such as necrotizing soft tissue infections, DCS, and CO poisoning often require the use of HBOT on a more frequent basis, twice or three times daily (bid or tid), most chronic conditions can be treated using daily treatments. The patient is placed within the hyperbaric chamber for 90 to 120 minutes for a total of 20 to 35 treatments. Oftentimes, the use of HBOT is, in conjunction with both medical and surgical treatment modalities, aimed at correction of the underlying cause(s) of the nonhealing wound. As standard of care, HBOT should always be used as part of a multidisciplinary treatment plan with ongoing wound care on a regular basis and not simply as stand-alone therapy. While there certainly may be exceptions to this rule (DCS and CO poisoning), this important point should not be forgotten. Thus, if you are considering the use of HBOT for one of your patients, it would probably be best to also consider a general evaluation by a wound specialist who will look for other causes of the nonhealing wound.

HYPERBARIC OXYGEN THERAPY CONTRAINDICATIONS

As with any drug, there is a proper therapeutic range and overdoses are toxic. HBOT is never given at pressures greater than 3.0 ATA as higher pressures will evoke generalized seizures (Paul Bert effect). For this reason, clinical protocols limit the maximum exposure time at 3.0 ATA to 90 minutes. In the clinical practice of treating wounds, longest protocol typically used is 2 hours at 2.0 ATA.

Likewise, there may be significant contraindications in some patients. An absolute contraindication to HBOT, particularly in the monoplace chamber, is untreated pneumothorax. The danger is that this could develop into an expanding tension pneumothorax during treatment. Significant expansion of extrapleural air during decompression could severely compromise the patient's respirations and even block blood return to the heart. This problem can be circumvented in patients with a pneumothorax by inserting a chest tube on the affected side prior to treatment.

Other contraindications are the concomitant administration of doxorubicin (Adriamycin) and bleomycin with HBOT. Both are cancer chemotherapeutic drugs, and doxorubicin in animals has caused 70% mortality when combined with HBOT, presumably due to cardiac toxicity. Bleomycin is known to cause "bleomycin lung" and it is made fulminant by the addition of oxygen. It has been reported that therapeutic levels of one-atmosphere oxygen given years after bleomycin therapy was complete could re-evoke bleomycin lung. However, recent reports show that patients with a previous history of bleomycin therapy have been treated successfully with HBOT. It is probably safe to use HBOT if the bleomycin was discontinued more than 6 months previous to treatment. Nevertheless, pulmonary function should be closely monitored in these patients.[3,25]

HYPERBARIC OXYGEN THERAPY RISKS AND SIDE EFFECTS

While the use of HBOT is widely considered to be quite safe, there are certain conditions that might make a patient an unsuitable candidate for the hyperbaric chamber. Ear squeeze or failure to equalize the middle ear during compression is the most frequent side effect of HBO therapy. Equalizing the pressure in the middle ear during compression is a learned technique but may be made difficult by excess mucus from allergies or upper respiratory infections. Thus, a relative contraindication to HBOT includes an upper respiratory infection that could make ear equalization difficult or impossible. Oral decongestants and nasal sprays can be helpful to manage this condition. Serous otitis or fluid retention in the ear secondary to oxygen breathing may rarely occur and can also be managed with decongestants. The policy of utilizing gentle and slow compression and decompression rates will minimize the risks of barotrauma for both pulmonary and tympanic membrane injury. As patients are very carefully pressurized during their initial treatment, ruptured eardrums should not occur because pressurization is halted when the patient indicates distress.

Sinus squeeze is much less common, and the only remedy is to use decongestants. If the problem persists, the services of an ENT specialist should be enlisted. Frontal sinus squeeze is the most painful, and a patient who experiences it must not be forced to continue except in an absolute emergency as the pain can be unbearably severe.

Pulmonary oxygen toxicity does not occur with any of the treatment protocols in use clinically. Oxygen is toxic to the lung if administered for more that 6 continuous hours at 2.0 ATA. There is a drop in vital capacity as surfactant production ceases and patchy atelectasis becomes evident on x-ray. Repeated and prolonged exposure to pure oxygen at higher pressures is thought to cause an increased amount of oxygen free radical production, with subsequent tissue injury manifesting as a fibrotic response. Acutely, the appearance of pulmonary edema, increasing alveolar oxygen gradients, and pulmonary hemorrhage eventually results in interstitial fibrosis and Type 2 pneumonocyte production. If exposure continues, microhemorrhages appear, and eventually, the result is irreversible fibrosis. Needless to say, this is rarely seen clinically as the longest continuous exposure is only for 2 hours at 2.0 ATA. Even with repetitive exposures on the same day, the lung recovers well between treatments. Even 5-minute "air breaks" or air breathing periods every 20 minutes will double the time required before toxicity appears.[3,25]

Cerebral or CNS oxygen toxicity can occur at pressures greater than 2.0 ATA. A common wound treatment protocol is 2.4 ATA for 90 minutes, divided into three 30-minute periods separated by a 5-minute air break. Every hyperbaric clinician will eventually encounter a patient who has a lower than normal seizure threshold and manifest CNS toxicity as a generalized seizure. Febrile patients or those with a known seizure disorder may be at increased risk of CNS oxygen toxicity. This is probably mediated by an inhibition of the GABA pathways, with concomitant loss of GABA-mediated inhibitory neurochemical activity. Oxygen seizures are benign and management simply consists of lowering the FiO_2. This is done by removing the mask or hood in the multiplace chamber. In the monoplace chamber, the patient is decompressed after the tonic phase of the seizure is completed, usually in short bursts to avoid breath holding and air trapping that could cause a gas embolism.[3,25]

Pneumothorax occurring in the chamber is a potential risk, but fortunately, it is extremely rare. By definition, treatment in a hyperbaric chamber occurs at pressures in excess of 1.4 atmospheres; thus, the possibility exists that excess pressure can accumulate in inadequately ventilated portions of the lung, predisposing those areas to rupture under pressure. Therefore, any patients with a history of an air-trapping condition such as asthma, emphysema, or COPD must have a thorough evaluation with low threshold for pulmonology medicine consultation. Pneumothorax occurring in the monoplace chamber poses a particular problem because there is no way to insert a chest tube prior to decompression. If it occurs, a thoracentesis tray is obtained and the patient is rapidly decompressed to the surface where the physician quickly inserts a chest tube to relieve the intrathoracic pressure. In the multiplace chamber, a chest tube is inserted prior to decompression and this obviates the problem.[3,25]

Visual changes in the form of lens refraction can be a side effect of HBOT. Distant vision or myopia worsens in many patients after 20 to 30 treatments, particularly if they are over the age of 40. On the other hand, presbyopia is improved, and some patients say they can read again without reading glasses. These changes are usually temporary and revert to the pretreatment state within 6 weeks of the cessation of HBOT. Patients with early cataracts may not completely regain their pretreatment status, however, and may require a new prescription for glasses.

In the past, there was concern that a history of optic neuritis (with the possibility of HBOT causing blindness), a history of thoracic surgery (fear of air trapping), and pregnancy (retinitis of the newborn and premature closure of the patent ductus) were contraindications to HBOT. None of the above has been proven to be a serious threat in practice. Glaucoma is not a contraindication to HBOT as the eye consists of solids, gels, and liquids that are incompressible and do not deform. Only gas-containing spaces in the body or in hardware accompanying the patient can cause problems secondary to pressure changes. Confinement anxiety may occasionally occur. It is best managed by reassurance and sedatives.[3,25] Finally, diabetic patients require close monitoring of blood sugar levels especially prior to each hyperbaric treatment as they are at increased risk for hypoglycemia while they are receiving HBOT. While the exact mechanism for hypoglycemia is unclear, it is postulated that causes may include increased endogenous insulin production by pancreatic beta cells or enhancement of insulin receptors due to hyperbaric oxygen stimulation.

Safety Considerations

Considerable attention to safety is paramount for hyperbaric operations due to the risk of fire. While pure oxygen is not flammable, it vigorously supports combustion, and therefore, this concern is valid. However this risk can be managed very effectively through the use of environmental controls. Strict contraband monitoring and precautions against potential sources of combustion are vigorously enforced. Patients should not wear lipstick or alcohol-based perfumes or hairspray. Volatile flammable liquids such as alcohol should not be allowed in the chamber as static electricity has ignited liquids in pure oxygen in laboratory tests. It is essential that patients never be treated in their street clothes as there have been serious, fatal chamber fires where patients have brought ignition sources into the chamber in their pockets. Hospital cotton clothing is routinely worn to minimize this concern and decrease the risk of static discharge. In the monoplace chamber, as additional precaution, patients are also grounded via a wrist strap and grounding wire. The multiplace chamber patient is compressed in air (rather than 100% oxygen) and breathes 100% oxygen via a mask; thus, the issue of static discharge is not as pronounced as with the monoplace environment. Nonetheless, every effort is made to insure that all potential sources of combustion are eliminated from the hyperbaric chamber environment.

The many "foreign objects" or items of hardware that are attached to or accompany patients in the chamber have often caused worry. Internal cardiac pacemakers and internally implanted defibrillators are typically safe at therapeutic pressures. Most manufacturers will provide clearance guidelines for device usage with the hyperbaric environment. External metal fixators for fractures as well as fiberglass casts are safe. The removal of electronic hearing aids and watches is advised. Petrolatum or Vaseline® gauze dressings have been safely used for over 40 years, even in the monoplace chamber, as there is no ignition source. They are simply covered with a cloth covering during treatment.

Given all of the aforementioned safety precautions, patients treated with HBOT in the United States routinely complete 40 to 60 hyperbaric treatments without any untoward side effects during the course of their treatment.[3,25]

HYPERBARIC OXYGEN THERAPY FOR THE HYPOXIC WOUND

Wounds that have failed to progress through the normal stages of wound healing in an orderly fashion to produce anatomic tissue integrity and restored functional capability are considered to be chronic, nonhealing wounds, especially if they have persisted longer than 4 to 6 weeks.[26] The four stages of normal wound healing and their durations include hemostasis (0–3 hours), inflammatory (0–3 days), proliferative (3–21 days), and maturation (21 days–1.5 years). Although the process may go awry anywhere along the pathway, chronic wounds are generally considered to be stagnant within either the inflammatory or the proliferative stages of the normal healing cascade. Therefore the treatment of these nonhealing wounds and ulcers generally involves exploration, discovery, and correction of the factors that prevent normal healing from proceeding in an orderly fashion. Although poor tissue perfusion and resultant tissue hypoxia (tissue oxygen tensions <30 mmHg) is a common cause of wound healing compromise, other factors can also pose a significant impediment to normal wound healing. These include infection, tissue edema, tissue trauma, unrelieved pressure, or underlying medical conditions which unfortunately too often remain undiagnosed (such as diabetes,

collagen vascular disease, renal insufficiency, protein energy malnutrition) and can challenge the restoration of normal healing. Any or all of these conditions can arrest wound healing and in fact can occur simultaneously. Thus, recognition and correction of the underlying conditions responsible for the delay in wound healing are not always straightforward.

Generally speaking, living tissue needs oxygen and nutrients to thrive and in the case of wound healing, to regenerate. In normal wound healing, both hypoxia and normal amounts of oxygen are necessary for progression of the phases of the healing. Hypoxia stimulates macrophages to release mitogens, which in turn stimulate fibroblast replication and the release of angiogenic factors.[10] Oxygen is also essential for collagen synthesis by fibroblasts. Intermittent tissue hyperoxygenation allows for periods of hypoxia. During the hypoxic periods, angiogenic factors are released, initiating neoangiogenesis and propagation of the healing cascade. New capillaries, however, cannot advance unless they are surrounded by a supportive collagen matrix. The role of oxygen in wound healing has become increasingly more apparent. The maturation of collagen, development of new endothelium, and obliteration of dead space by healthy granulation tissue are all oxygen-dependent processes. With the development of a healthy collagen matrix, capillary buds invade rapidly and new capillary arcades are formed in the advancing vascular system. Referred to as granulation tissue formation, granulation obliterates dead space, allowing wound healing to proceed.[27–29]

Although white cells can phagocytize bacteria at relatively low oxygen tensions, they are unable to kill bacteria via normal oxidative mechanisms unless they are in an environment of at least 30 mm Hg partial pressure of oxygen. In patients with ischemic wounds, such as DFUs, oxygen tensions in peripheral soft tissue and bone are often much lower than 30 mm Hg. Under these circumstances, infections quickly become fulminant. Edema, frequently associated with infection, potentiates the tissue ischemia and creates a vicious circle of ischemia, more edema, and increasing tissue injury.[22]

It is clear that in the setting of tissue hypoxia (<30 mm Hg), healing will be impaired. Likewise, correction of tissue ischemia and improved oxygen delivery has been clearly shown to improve wound healing. In patients with large vessel stenosis, this is accomplished by vascular bypass or by endovascular intervention. However, in those areas where smaller vessels are damaged such as in radiation injury or diabetes, improved oxygen carrying capacity, increased oxygen diffusion, and correction of localized ischemia at a cellular level may allow neovascularization and healing to occur in tissues that were previously unresponsive. While the obvious solution to this problem seems to be the restoration of normal blood flow, in reality it is often much more complicated than this, as the patient's underlying medical condition(s) often prevents the complete reversal of the hypoxic process. In these cases, it is often advantageous to consider the use of supplemental oxygen to augment the normal healing process. In fact, this is one of the main reasons to use hyperbaric oxygen in the treatment of such patients.

The Classic Hypoxic Wound: Diabetic Foot Ulcer

HBOT is appropriate and indicated for the management of several classifications of compromised wound types. The majority of these wounds have similar pathergy in that they all manifest wound healing compromise due to varying degrees of tissue hypoxia. It is well established that local-tissue hypoxia and infection are two of the primary defects underlying compromised healing in the DFU. HBOT specifically treats both of these underlying factors. Thus a short discussion of the utilization of hyperbaric oxygen as an adjunct in the management of the DFU will be presented as an example of the benefit of HBOT in the generic "hypoxic wound." The use of HBOT in the care of the patient with a DFU is based on a rational physiologic basis, favorable in vitro studies, and animal research that has elucidated mechanisms of action in aerobic and anaerobic infections and wound healing.[30–33] These effects are corroborated by extensive clinical experience.[34–36]

HBOT provides a significant increase in tissue oxygenation in the hypoperfused, infected wound. Elevation in oxygen tension in the hypoxic wound induces powerful positive changes in the wound repair process. HBOT promotes wound healing by directly enhancing fibroblast replication, collagen synthesis, and the process of neovascularization in ischemic tissue.[27–29] By providing molecular oxygen at the cellular level, it also significantly increases leukocyte bactericidal activity. The increase in tissue oxygenation, which leads to the increased formation of oxygen radicals within the leukocyte, is bactericidal or bacteriostatic to anaerobic organisms, and it may be as effective as specific antibiotic therapy, providing an added effect.

The Centers for Medicare & Medicaid Services (CMS) recently approved the use of HBOT for the management of the DFU.[23] Strict criteria have been established. The patient must have diabetes (Type I or Type II) and a lower extremity wound (Wagner grade III or higher) due to diabetic disease. The wound must have failed standard wound care as demonstrated by no measurable signs of healing for 30 days (decrease in volume or size, decrease in exudate, or decrease in necrotic tissue). Standard therapy must include assessment of vascular status, optimization of nutrition/glucose control, debridement, moist dressings, off-loading, and treatment of infection. Once these criteria have been satisfied and HBOT initiated, the wound must be reevaluated every 30 days during HBOT course. Continued HBOT will not be covered if there are no measurable signs of healing during the 30-day period.

CLINICAL EVIDENCE SUPPORTING USE OF HYPERBARIC OXYGEN THERAPY

Although there is an extensive literature describing the surgical management of the diabetic foot, it is difficult to adequately compare different approaches to therapy. The principal obstacles to interpretation of most studies are the influence of the bias introduced by "clinical judgment" and the lack of objective documentation of the severity of complicating local and systemic factors. Recently, a protocol for the management of diabetic foot wounds has been tested in a prospective, randomized fashion.[37]

Several decades ago, a retrospective report of 70 patients with nonhealing wounds treated with adjuvant HBOT suggested beneficial effects for this modality. This report included diabetic patients with soft tissue infection, underlying osteomyelitis, failed skin grafts, and nonhealing amputation sites. In this series, 60% of the patients healed or showed significant improvement despite the presence of ischemia, infection, or neuropathic changes.[38]

In a prospective controlled study, Baroni et al. studied the effect of HBOT on the management of grade III and IV diabetic foot lesions.[39] The groups were matched for lesion size, subfascial involvement, and duration and severity of diabetes. All patients were hospitalized, underwent daily debridement, and were maintained under strict metabolic control. The study (HBO) group consisted of 18 patients, of whom 16 healed and two underwent amputation. In the control group ($N = 10$), 1 patient healed, five showed no change, and four underwent amputations ($p = 0.001$). A retrospective review in the same center revealed an amputation rate of 40%, between 1979 and 1981. Once HBO therapy became available, the amputation rate dropped dramatically to 11%. Baroni concluded that HBOT was effective in the treatment of grade III and IV diabetic foot lesions as evidenced by a higher healing rate and a dramatic decrease in amputation rate.

In a large clinical series of 168 patients with grade III and IV diabetic foot lesions, Davis reported a 70% success rate with a combined management protocol consisting of daily debridement, specific antibiotic therapy, aggressive wound care, metabolic control, and daily HBOT for 30 to 60 days.[40] Most treatment failures were seen in older patients with significant occlusive vascular disease and absent pedal pulses. Oriani and colleagues reported on the effect of HBO for the treatment of grade IV diabetic foot lesions.[41] In this series, the HBO group consisted of 62 patients while the matched control group had 18. There was no significant difference in age, severity or duration of diabetes, or its complications. All patients were hospitalized, underwent daily debridement, maintained strict metabolic control and received specific antibiotic therapy. In the HBO group, 96% of the patients healed, while 4% underwent amputation. In the control group, 66% achieved primary healing, and 33% required amputation ($p < 0.001$).

Wattel et al. evaluated the role of transcutaneous oximetry in predicting outcome in a prospective series of 59 consecutive patients with diabetic foot lesions treated with HBO therapy.[42] In this study, the patients received an average of 29 ± 19 treatment sessions at 2.5 ATA, 100% O_2 for 90 minutes, twice daily. The benefit of HBO therapy was shown in this study with a healing rate of 87% and an amputation rate of 13%. More importantly, the outcome was predicted by $TcPO_2$ measurements in the hyperbaric chamber. The healed group attained a chamber $TcPO_2$ of 786 ± 258 mm Hg as compared to 323 ± 214 mm Hg for the amputation group ($p < 0.005$). In this study, a minimum value of 450 mm Hg was shown to correlate with a successful outcome. In another large retrospective series of patients with diabetic foot lesions, Stone et al. showed that the HBO-treated group ($N = 87$) had a higher limb salvage rate (73% versus 53%) than the nontreated group ($N = 382$).[43]

In a prospective, randomized study, Faglia et al. evaluated the effectiveness of HBOT in decreasing major lower extremity amputations in diabetic patients with Wagner's grade II, III, and IV lesions.[37] All patients were evaluated and treated following a comprehensive protocol including aggressive surgical debridement, culture-specific antibiotics, appropriate revascularization, strict diabetic metabolic control, daily wound care,

RESEARCH WISDOM

HBOT and the Diabetic Foot

Multiple studies strongly suggest that HBO therapy should be an integral part of the treatment regimen of the diabetic foot to minimize lower extremity amputations and that $TcPO_2$ measurements may be of significant value in predicting outcome.

and prevention of mechanical stress. The HBO group consisted of 35 patients with the following Wagner's classification lesions: grade IV ($N = 22$), grade III ($N = 9$), and grade II ($N = 4$). The control group consisted of 33 patients with grade IV ($N = 20$), grade III ($N = 8$), and grade II ($N = 5$). The transcutaneous oxygen measurements on the dorsum of the foot for the HBO group were 23.25 ± 10.6 mm Hg, as compared to 21.29 ± 10.7 mm Hg in the control group. There were no significant differences in the clinical characteristics of the groups, including presence of infection, sensory motor neuropathy, or severity of peripheral vascular disease. The treated group underwent an average of 38 ± 8 sessions at 2.5 ATA on 100% O_2 for 90 minutes. The average chamber $TcPO_2$ value was 493 ± 152 mm Hg.

In this trial, a significant difference in major amputation rates was observed between the two groups. The HBO group underwent 3 major amputations (8.6%, 1 AKA, 2 BKA) with 11(33.3%, 4 AKA, 7BKA) major amputations in the control group ($p = .016$). Furthermore, the foot $TcPO_2$ values were significantly higher in the HBO-treated group (37 ± 16.1 mm Hg) than in the control group (26 ± 13.5 mm Hg) at the time of discharge ($p = .0002$). The results of this trial clearly document and define the effectiveness of HBO therapy, in addition to a comprehensive protocol, in decreasing major amputations in the diabetic with a compromised foot. Moreover, the transcutaneous oximetry data provide objective documentation of improved tissue oxygenation post-HBO treatment (see Fig. 30.7).

More recently, a well-designed randomized, single-center, double-blinded, placebo-controlled clinical trial reported by Londahl et al. showed that adjunctive treatment with HBOT facilitates healing in patients with DFUs.[44] Ninety-four patients with Wagner grade II, III, or IV ulcers, which had been present for 3 months, were studied in an ambulatory setting. Study treatment was given as an adjunct to regular treatment at the multidisciplinary diabetes foot clinic, which included treatment of infection, revascularization, debridement, off-loading, and metabolic control according to high international standards. All patients were assessed by a vascular surgeon at the time of inclusion, and only patients with adequate distal perfusion or nonreconstructible peripheral vascular disease were included in the study. Patients having an acute foot infection were included when the acute phase was resolved. Oral or local antibiotic treatment did not exclude patients from study.

Treatments were given in a multiplace hyperbaric chamber (2.5 ATA) for 85 minutes daily (session duration 95 minutes), 5 days a week for 8 weeks (40 treatment sessions). Both groups were treated in a pressurized chamber, with the study group breathing 100% oxygen while the control group received air in a blinded fashion. The outcomes for the group receiving HBOT were compared with those of the group receiving treatment

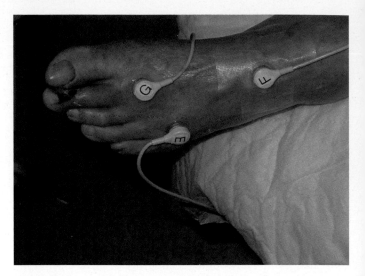

FIGURE 30.7 Transcutaneous oximetry examination of a DFU.

with hyperbaric air. In the intention-to-treat analysis, complete healing of the index ulcer was achieved in 37 patients at 1 year of follow-up: 25/48 (52%) in the HBOT group and 12/42 (29%) in the placebo group ($p = 0.03$). In a subanalysis of those patients completing 35 HBOT sessions, healing of the index ulcer occurred in 23/38 (61%) in the HBOT group and 10/37 (27%) in the placebo group ($p = 0.009$). The frequency of adverse events was low. The results obtained in this landmark randomized, double-blinded, placebo-controlled trial clearly demonstrates the effectiveness of HBOT complementary to a comprehensive protocol in the management of the patient with a hypoxic DFU.

PATIENT SELECTION

As previously mentioned, not all patients are good candidates for HBOT. Besides the contraindications mentioned above, not all patients will respond to HBOT, for various reasons. Therefore, in order to predict whether or not a patient might receive benefit from this treatment modality, especially in the case of a non-healing lower extremity wound or ulceration, transcutaneous oximetry is often a very useful tool. Transcutaneous Oxygen Mapping (TCOM) is the technique where a specialized instrument is used to simultaneously measure transcutaneous oxygen pressures in several areas of the skin. It is painless, is inexpensive, and can usually be performed quite easily at the bedside.

The concept of measuring the oxygen delivery to the cutaneous tissue is fairly straightforward. After a small area of the skin is thoroughly cleaned of any loose debris, a specialized electrode is placed on the skin to warm it to a specified temperature. This warming action induces vasodilation in small vessels within the skin, and the oxygen content is then measured by the same electrode. Tissue oxygen levels of 35 to 40 mm Hg and higher, obtained in room air at normobaric pressures are generally considered to be normal; and thus wound healing in these areas is not likely to be compromised due to hypoxia. However, values of 30 mm Hg or less indicate impaired wound healing, with impaired immune function and fibroblast proliferation rates being the two most significant impediments to the normal healing process in these patients. It is also important to note that abnormally low transcutaneous oxygen values can

CLINICAL WISDOM

Assessment of Tissue Hypoxia

Transcutaneous oximetry is a simple, reliable noninvasive diagnostic technique that provides an objective assessment of local tissue perfusion and oxygenation. It can be used for serial assessment of the soft tissue envelope surrounding the problem wound. Uses of transcutaneous oximetry in the evaluation of the diabetic ulcer include the assessment of healing potential, selection of amputation level, and patient selection for HBO therapy.

CLINICAL WISDOM

Tissue Criteria for HBOT

HBOT will not accelerate tissue repair in wounds with normal oxygen tensions and will only do so effectively in diabetic ulcers in which oxygen tension can be elevated to therapeutic levels. It is essential in clinical practice to demonstrate and evaluate critical tissue ischemia before considering the use of HBOT.

be caused by several disease processes, and once an abnormal value has been documented, further diagnostic workup is indicated to more fully define the exact cause for the tissue hypoxia.

For example, while patients having either PAD or diabetes may have abnormally low transcutaneous oximetry values, the mechanism behind each is vastly different. In the case of the patient with PAD, it is often macrovascular disease that accounts for the diminished distal blood flow; thus, these patients will likely benefit from a vascular workup with referral to the vascular specialist. In contrast is the patient with diabetes, which tends to more dramatically affect the microvasculature. However, as there could certainly be components of both microvascular and macrovascular disease in each of these patients, both deserve further evaluation prior to considering HBOT.

Besides indicating that a basic problem with tissue hypoxia exists, the TCOM study also helps to predict the potential success of HBOT. When normobaric oximetry values are less than 35 to 40 mm Hg, a 100% normobaric oxygen challenge is given via a nonrebreathing face mask. If the abnormally low TCOM values rise to 100 mm Hg or more, the patient will likely benefit from HBOT. However, this fact does not excuse the patient from a vascular workup, as many patients have multifactorial components to tissue hypoxia. Thus, the absence of reconstructible arterial disease is a CMS prerequisite for the use of HBOT.[45–47]

TOPICAL OXYGEN

A chapter devoted to HBOT would not be complete without a brief discussion of topical oxygen. Topical oxygen therapy is the application of oxygen to the surface of a wound. This

is generally accomplished by placing the affected limb in an enclosed acrylic or plastic box and filling it with oxygen (see Fig. 30.8). This should not be confused with systemic HBOT, in which the patients breathe 100% oxygen while they are inside of a monoplace or multiplace chamber under greater-than-normal atmospheric pressure. Topical oxygen is frequently (and inappropriately) called "topical hyperbaric oxygen." Use of this term simply adds confusion and is a misapplication of the word hyperbaric. Hyperbaric oxygen as defined by the American College of Hyperbaric Medicine is the inhalation of 100% oxygen while the entire patient is enclosed within a chamber at pressures of at least 1.4 ATA or greater. Advocates claim that topical oxygen dissolves in tissue fluids, is bacteriostatic, and stimulates angiogenesis and wound healing.[48] Clinical trials comparing topical oxygen and hyperbaric oxygen have been undertaken in centers in the United States. However, there are only two quantitative studies involving topical oxygen which have been reported in the literature, one controlled and the other using electron microscopy to assess results. Both show an impediment to healing.[49,50]

SUMMARY

HBOT is an advanced technology that can have a significant positive and powerful effect in the management of patients with compromised wound healing, especially when the primary deficit is tissue hypoxia. When patients are carefully selected and appropriately managed with HBOT as part of a comprehensive wound care strategy, wound healing enhancement can be realized and limb loss avoided.

CLINICAL WISDOM

Vascular Evaluation and Intervention is Critical to Outcomes

Even before HBOT is considered, in the absence of infection, it is vital that the patient receive a complete vascular workup and that all possibilities for endovascular or surgical correction of the ischemia be exhausted. Patients with evidence of critical ischemia and DFUs should be aggressively revascularized, unless a contraindication exists.

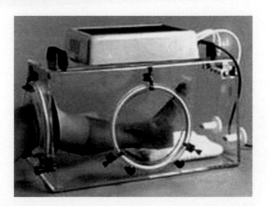

FIGURE 30.8 Topical oxygen device does not provide HBOT.

Case Study—Necrotizing Fasciitis

A 28-year-old female delivered a healthy infant via cesarean section on June 15, 2007. Her postoperative course was complicated by the onset of partial incisional dehiscence and drainage 12 days post-op. Several days later, she presented to the hospital with severe abdominal pain, erythema and subcutaneous crepitation in the periwound region, and fever. She was admitted and surgical evaluated. Necrotizing fasciitis was confirmed intraoperatively. Hyperbaric consultation followed, and the patient was started on HBOT within 12 hours of admission (see Fig. 30.9A).

The patient received broad spectrum antibiotics and aggressive wound care efforts that included negative pressure wound therapy. HBOT was continued at 2.4 ATA with bid sessions for the first 72 hours followed by daily treatments (see Fig. 30.9B).

The patient showed complete resolution of tissue ischemia, with no evidence of infection, and a well-granulated wound base. She underwent wound closure on hospital day 16 and was discharged 4 days later without recurrent problems. She received a total of 22 HBOTx's (see Fig. 30.9C).

Case Key Points

- HBOT is adjunctive therapy for the management of necrotizing fasciitis and compliments an aggressive surgical approach.
- HBOT can augment the effectiveness of antibiotic therapy in patients with necrotizing soft tissue infections.
- Aggressive wound care efforts with negative pressure therapy can be synergistically enhanced by HBOT.
- Early utilization of HBOT in patients with necrotizing fasciitis can decrease the number of surgical debridements and shorted hospitalizations.
- HBOT positively affects angiogenesis, collagen synthesis, and leucocyte function in patients with hypoxic wounds.

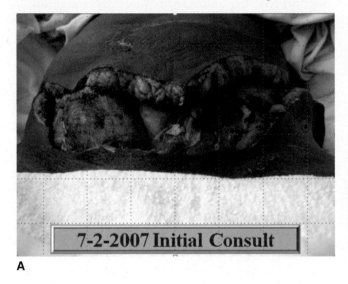

A

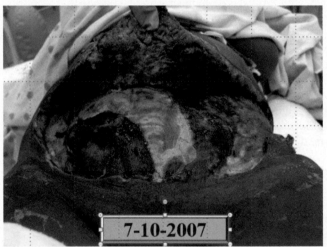

B

FIGURE 30.9 **A.** Necrotizing fasciitis initial consult. **B.** Same patient as in (**A**) after treatment with antibiotics, NPWT and HBOT. **C.** Same patient as in (**A**) and (**B**) after successful surgery for wound closure.

C

Case Study—Infected Diabetic Foot Ulcer

This 48-year-old male with a long history of insulin-dependent diabetes and plantar foot ulceration presented to the Emergency Department with fever, malaise, and septic left foot. The patient reported a rapid onset of foot swelling, erythema, and drainage over the prior 48 hours. The patient was admitted to the hospital with referral to the Center for Comprehensive Wound Care and Hyperbaric Oxygen Therapy. HBOT was initiated within 4 hours of admission (see Fig. 30.10A).

The patient underwent surgical exploration and debridement. A deep plantar abscess was found with necrotic muscle and fascia. The patient was managed with broad-spectrum antibiotics and negative pressure wound therapy in addition to continued HBOT. HBOT was administered at 2.4 ATA with twice daily sessions for the first 3 days (see Fig. 30.10B).

After approximately 2 weeks of therapy, all evidence of infection and tissue ischemia had resolved and the wound showed robust granulation. The patient was taken back to the OR for his second surgical procedure, placement of an

AlloDerm matrix to cover exposed tendons and bone and to decrease the tissue deficit and (see Fig. 30.10C)

The patient was discharged after a total of 19 days' hospitalization for continued outpatient care. HBOT was continued as an outpatient, and the patient received a total of 28 sessions. The patient was monitored closely and showed complete healing by secondary intent. Once healed, the patient was fitted for custom diabetic shoes with orthotic inserts. He was advised to perform daily foot monitoring and moisturization and continue with routine podiatric foot care (see Fig. 30.10D).

Case Key Points

- Diabetic patients are at high risk for foot ulceration, which can lead to partial foot or more proximal amputation.
- The risk of developing complicated skin, soft tissue, or bone infection once a DFU is present is significant.
- HBOT is appropriate as an adjunctive therapy in the management of a patient with a DFU (wagner stage III-V).
- HBOT positively affects angiogenesis, collagen synthesis, and leukocyte function in patients with hypoxic wounds.

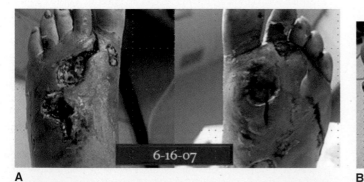

A

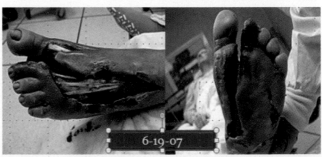

B

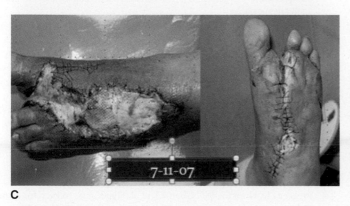

C

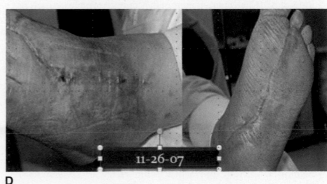

D

FIGURE 30.10 A. Patient with infected DFU on initial presentation. **B.** Same patient as in (**A**) during surgery with debridement of deep plantar abscess. **C.** Same patient as in (**A**) and (**B**) following treatment with HBOT; patient status post application of AlloDerm matrix to cover exposed tendon and bone. (**D**) Same patient as in (**A–C**) with complete wound closure.

REVIEW QUESTIONS

1. Insulin dependent diabetic patients receiving HBOT require close monitoring as they are at increased risk for
   A. hyperglycemia
   B. hypoglycemia
   C. oxygen toxicity
   D. hypertensive Crisis

2. HBOT is indicated for patients with the following classification of DFU.
   A. Wagner III or greater
   B. Strauss II-III
   C. Castillo 3 or greater
   D. Apache IV

3. Hyperbaric oxygen therapy is NOT an approved indication for HBOT by the American College of Hyperbaric Medicine:
   A. Wager III and IV Diabetic Foot Ulcers
   B. Necrotizing Fasciitis

   C. Learning Disorders
   D. Failing Grafts and Flaps

4. The reasons for using HBO in treating gas gangrene include all of the following EXCEPT
   A. inhibits production of alpha toxin
   B. enhances the line of demarcation between healthy and dead tissue
   C. eliminates the need for surgical debridement
   D. improves tissue oxygenation

5. All of the following are relative contraindications to hyperbaric oxygen treatments except
   A. Untreated pneumothorax.
   B. Administration of doxorubicin with HBOT.
   C. Osteoradionecrosis.
   D. Administration of bleomycin with HBOT.

REFERENCES

1. Hammarlund C. The physiologic effects of hyperbaric oxygenation. In: Kindwall EP, Whelan HT, eds. *Hyperbaric Medicine Practice*. Flagstaff, AZ: Best; 2004:37–68.

2. Weaver LK, Valentine KJ, Hopkins RO. Carbon monoxide poisoning: risk factors for cognitive sequelae and the role of hyperbaric oxygen. *Am J Res Crit Care Med*. 2007;176:491–497.

3. Kindwall EP, Niezgoda JA, eds. *Hyperbaric Medicine Procedures: The Kindwall HBO Handbook*. Milwaukee, WI: Aurora Heath Care; 2006.

4. Kindwall EP. The history of hyperbaric medicine. In: Kindwall EP, Whelan HT, eds. *Hyperbaric Medicine Practice*. Flagstaff, AZ: Best; 2004:1–20.

5. Kindwall EP (Chairman). Report of the committee on hyperbaric oxygenation. Bethesda, MD: Undersea medical Society; 1977.

6. Guyton AC. Textbook of medical physiology. Chapter 40. *Physical Principles of Gaseous Exchange*. Philadelphia, PA: Saunders; 1981:491–500.

7. Davis JC, Hunt TK. *Problem Wounds: The Role of Oxygen*. New York: Elsevier Science Publishing CO.; Inc.; 1988.

8. Niinikoski J. Oxygen and wound healing. *Clin Plast Surg*. 1977;4(3):361–374.

9. Niinikoski J, Rajamaki A, Kulonene E. Healing of open wounds: effects of oxygen, disturbed blood supply and hyperemia by infrared irradiation. *Acta Chir Scand*. 1971;137(5):399–401.

10. Knighton DR, Hunt TK, Scheuenstuhl H, et al. Oxygen tension regulates the expression of angiogenesis factor by macrophages. *Science*. 1983;221:1283–1285.

11. Guyton AC. Textbook of medical physiology. Chapter 41. *Transport of Oxygen and Carbon Dioxide in the Blood and Body Tissues*. Philadelphia, PA: Saunders; 1981:504–514.

12. Krough A. The number and distribution of capillaries in muscle with calculations of the oxygen pressure head necessary for supplying the tissue. *J Physiol*. 1919;52:409–415.

13. Lee CC, Chen SC, Tsai SC, et al. Hyperbaric oxygen induces VEGF expression through ERK, JNK and c-Jun/AP-1 activation in human umbilical vein endothelial cells. *J Biomed Sci*. 2006;13(1):143–156.

14. Sheikh AY, Gibson JJ, Rollins MD, et al. Effect of hyperoxia on vascular endothelial growth factor levels in a wound model. *Arch Surg*. 2000;135(11):1293–1297.

15. Ahmad Y, Sheikh MD, Mark D, et al. Hyperoxia improves microvascular perfusion in a murine wound model. *Wound Repair Regen*. 2005;13(3):303–308.

16. Marx RE, Ehler WJ, Tayapongsak P, et al. Relationship of oxygen dose to angiogenesis induction in irradiated tissue. *Am J Surg*. 1990;160:519–524.

17. https://www.achm.org/index.php/Registry/General/Registry-Home.html

18. Min L, Yizhang C, Meiping D, et al. Involvement of the mitochondrial ATP-sensitive potassium channel in the neuroprotective effect of hyperbaric oxygenation after cerebral ischemia. *Brain Res Bull*. 2006;69(2):109–116.

19. Buras JA, Stahl GL, Svoboda KKH, et al. Hyperbaric oxygen downregulates ICAM-1 expression induced by hypoxia and hypoglycemia: the role of NOS. *Am J Physiol Cell Physiol*. 2000;278:C292–C302.

20. Nylander G, Nordström H, Franzén L, et al. Effects of hyperbaric oxygen treatment in post-ischemic muscle. A quantitative morphological study. *Scand J Plast Reconstr Surg Hand Surg*. 1988;22(1):31–39.

21. Buras J. Basic mechanisms of hyperbaric oxygen in the treatment of ischemia-reperfusion injury. *Int Anesthesiol Clin*. 2000;38(1):91–109.

22. Hopf HW, Hunt TK, West JM, et al. Wound tissue oxygen tension predicts the risk of wound infection in surgical patients. *Arch Surg*. 1997;132:997–1004.

23. http://www.cms.hhs.gov/

24. Weaver LK, Hopkins RO, Chan KJ, et al. Hyperbaric oxygen for acute carbon monoxide poisoning. *N Engl J Med*. 2002;347:1057–1067.

25. Kindwall EP, Whelan HT, eds. *Hyperbaric Medicine Practice*. Flagstaff, AZ: Best; 2004.

26. Lawrence WT. Clinical management of non healing wounds. In: Cohen IK, Diegelmann RF, Lindblad WJ, eds. *Wound Healing. Biochemical and Clinical Aspects*. Philadelphia, PA: Saunders; 1992:541–561.

27. Stillman RM. Effects of hypoxia and hyperoxia on progression of intimal healing. *Arch Surg*. 1983;118(6):732–737.

28. Hunt TK, Hopf H, Hussian Z. Physiology of wound healing. *Adv Skin Wound Care*. 2000;13(2 suppl):6–11.

29. Knighton DR, Silver IA, Hunt TK. Regulation of wound healing angiogenesis-effect of oxygen gradients and inspired oxygen concentration. *Surgery* 1981;2:262–270.

30. Bassett BE, Bennett PB. Introduction to the physical and physiological bases of hyperbaric therapy. Davis JC, Hunt TK, eds. Bethesda, MD: Undersea Medical Society, Inc.; 1977:11–24.

31. LaVan FB, Hunt TK. Oxygen and wound healing. *Clin Plastic Surg.* 1990;17(3):463–472.

32. Mader JT, ed. *Hyperbaric Oxygen Therapy: A Committee Report.* The Undersea and Hyperbaric Medical Society Bethesda, MD: 1989;37–44.

33. Rabkin JM, Hunt TK. Infection and oxygen. In: Davis J, Hunt TK, eds. *Problem Wounds: The Role of Oxygen.* New York: Elsevier; 1988;1–16.

34. Davis JC. Enhancement of healing. In: Camporesi E, Barker AC, eds. *Hyperbaric Oxygen Therapy: A Critical Review.* Bethesda, MD: Undersea and Hyperbaric Medical Society, Inc.; 1991:127–140.

35. Davis JC, Buckley CJ, Barr PO. Compromised soft tissue wounds: correction of wound hypoxia. In: Davis JC, Hunt TK, eds. *Problem Wounds: The Role of Oxygen.* New York: Elsevier; 1988:143–152.

36. Perrins DJ, Davis JC. Enhancement of healing in soft tissue wounds. In: Davis JC, Hunt TK, eds. *Hyperbaric Oxygen Therapy.* Bethesda, MD: Undersea Medical Society, Inc.; 1977:229–248.

37. Faglia E. Adjunctive systemic hyperbaric oxygen therapy in treatment of severe prevalently ischemic diabetic foot ulcer. *Diabetes Care* 1996;19(12):1338–1343.

38. Matos LA. Preliminary report of the use of hyperbarics as adjunctive therapy in diabetics with chronic non-healing wounds. *HBO Rev.* 1983;4(2):88–89.

39. Baroni G, Porro T, Faglia E. Hyperbaric oxygen in diabetic gangrene treatment. *Diabetes Care.* 1987;10(1):81–86.

40. Davis JC. The use of adjuvant hyperbaric oxygen in treatment of the diabetic foot. *Clin Pediatr Med Surg.* 1987;4(2):429–437.

41. Oriani G, Meazza D, Favales F. Hyperbaric oxygen therapy in diabetic gangrene. *J Hyperb Med.* 1990;5(3):171–175.

42. Wattel FE, Mathieu DM, Fossati P, et al. Hyperbaric oxygen in the treatment of diabetic foot lesions. *J Hyperbaric Med.* 1991;6: 263–268.

43. Stone JA, Scott R, Brill LR, et al. The role of hyperbaric oxygen in the treatment of diabetic foot wounds. *Diabetes.* 1995;44(suppl 1): 71A.

44. Londahl M, Nilsson A, Katzman P, et al. Hyperbaric oxygen therapy facilitates healing of chronic foot ulcers in patients with diabetes. *Diabetes Care.* 2010;33:998–1003.

45. Sheffield PJ, Workman WT. Transcutaneous tissue oxygen monitoring in patients undergoing hyperbaric oxygen therapy. In: Huch R, Huch A, eds. *Continuous Transcutaneous Blood Gas Monitoring.* New York, NY: Marcel Dekker; 1983:655–60.

46. Fife CE, Buyukecakir C, Otto G, et al. The predictive value of transcutaneous oxygen tension measurement in diabetic lower extremity ulcers treated with hyperbaric oxygen therapy: a retrospective analysis of 1144 patients. *Wound Rep Regen.* 2002;10:198–207.

47. Ballard JL, Eke CC, Bunt TJ, et al. A prospective evaluation of transcutaneous oxygen measurements in the management of diabetic foot problems. *J Vasc Surg.* 1995;22:485–92.

48. Heng MCY. Topical hyperbaric therapy for problem skin wounds. *J Dermatol Surg Oncol.* 1993;19:784–793.

49. Heng, MCY, Kloss, SG. Endothelial cell toxicity in leg ulcers treated with topical hyperbaric oxygen. *Am J Dermatopath.* 1986;8(5): 403–410.

50. Leslie, CA, Sapico FL, Ginunas, VJ, et al. Randomized control trial of topical hyperbaric oxygen for treatment of diabetic foot ulcers. *Diabetes Care* 1988;11:111–115.

INDEX

CCS0811